Cox's SURGICAL TREATMENT of ATRIAL FIBRILLATION and *Other Cardiac Arrhythmias*

Cox's SURGICAL TREATMENT of ATRIAL FIBRILLATION

and Other Cardiac Arrhythmias

JAMES L. COX, MD
Professor of Surgery
Division of Cardiac Surgery
Feinberg School of Medicine
Surgical Director, Center for Heart Rhythm Disorders
Director, Comprehensive Atrial Fibrillation Program
Bluhm Cardiovascular Institute
Northwestern University
Chicago, Illinois

PATRICK M. McCARTHY, MD
Heller-Sacks Professor of Surgery
Division of Cardiac Surgery
Feinberg School of Medicine
Vice President, Northwestern Medical Group
Executive Director, Bluhm Cardiovascular Institute
Northwestern University
Chicago, Illinois

S. CHRIS MALAISRIE, MD
Professor of Surgery
Division of Cardiac Surgery
Feinberg School of Medicine
Bluhm Cardiovascular Institute
Northwestern University
Chicago, Illinois

ELSEVIER

Elsevier
1600 John F. Kennedy Blvd.
Suite 1600
Philadelphia, PA 19103-2899

COX'S SURGICAL TREATMENT OF ATRIAL FIBRILLATION AND OTHER CARDIAC ARRHYTHMIAS

ISBN: 978-0-443-28554-7

Content Strategist: Jessica McCool
Content Development Specialist: Lisa M. Barnes
Publishing Services Manager: Deepthi Unni
Project Manager: Prasanna Kalyanaraman
Design Direction: Patrick Ferguson

Printed in India

Last digit is the print number: 9 8 7 6 5 4 3 2 1

I would like to dedicate this book to my mentors:
John P. Boineau, MD
Will C. Sealy, MD
David C. Sabiston, Jr., MD

James L. Cox

I would like to dedicate this book to the three people with the most influence over my early career:
Norman E. Shumway, MD
Hartzell V. Schaff, MD
James L. Cox, MD

Patrick M. McCarthy

I would like to dedicate this book to:
Joseph S. Coselli, MD
D. Craig Miller, MD
Patrick M. McCarthy, MD

S. Chris Malaisrie

CONTRIBUTORS

Niv Ad, MD
Adjunct Professor of Surgery
Department of Cardiac Surgery
Johns Hopkins University
Baltimore, Maryland
Adjunct Professor of Surgery
Department of Cardiac Surgery
University of Vienna
Vienna, Austria

Vinay Badhwar, MD
Professor of Surgery
Chairman, Department of Cardiovascular and Thoracic Surgery
West Virginia University School of Medicine
Morgantown, West Virginia

Emilie Belley-Cote, MD
Associate Professor of Medicine
McMaster University
Hamilton, Ontario, Canada

Stefano Benussi, MD, PhD
Associate Professor of Cardiac Surgery
Chief, Division of Cardiac Surgery
Director, Cardio-thoracic Department
Spedali Civili Brescia University Hospital Piazzale Spedali Civili
Lombardy, Italy

Gianluigi Bisleri, MD, FRCSC
Associate Professor of Surgery
Department of Surgery
University of Toronto
Toronto, Ontario Canada
Director, Minimally Invasive Cardiac Surgery
Department of Surgery
St. Michael's Hospital

Steven F. Bolling, MD
Professor of Cardiac Surgery
Department of Cardiac Surgery
University of Michigan
Ann Arbor, Michigan

Stefano Branzoli, MD
Cardiac Surgery Unit
Santa Chiara Hospital
Trento, Italy

Etem Caliskan, MD
Deutsches Herzzentrum der Charité
Department of Cardiothoracic and Vascular Surgery
Charité – Universitätsmedizin Berlin
Corporate member of Freie Universität Berlin and Humboldt-Universität
Berlin, Germany

Michael Carrel
President and CEO
AtriCure, Inc.
Mason, Ohio

Manuel Castella, MD, PhD
Professor of Surgery
Chief, Department of Cardiovascular Surgery
University of Barcelona
Barcelona, Spain

W. Randolph Chitwood, Jr., MD
Emeritus Professor of Cardiothoracic Surgery
Department of Cardiovascular Sciences
Brody School of Medicine
East Carolina University
Greenville, North Carolina

Stephen F. Chiu, MD
Assistant Professor of Surgery
Division of Cardiac Surgery
Feinberg School of Medicine
Bluhm Cardiovascular Institute
Northwestern University
Chicago, Illinois

Andrei Churyla, MD
Medical Director of Cardiac Surgery
Department of Surgery
Northwestern Medicine Palos Hospital
Palos Heights, Illinois

James L. Cox, MD
Professor of Surgery
Division of Cardiac Surgery
Feinberg School of Medicine
Surgical Director, Center for Heart Rhythm Disorders
Director, Comprehensive Atrial Fibrillation Program
Bluhm Cardiovascular Institute
Northwestern University
Chicago, Illinois

Ralph J. Damiano, Jr., MD
Evarts Graham Professor of Surgery
Chief, Division of Cardiothoracic Surgery
Washington University School of Medicine
Barnes-Jewish Hospital
St. Louis, Missouri

Giuseppe D'Ancona, MD, PhD
Internal Intensive Care Unit
Department of Cardiology
Berlin Heart Rhythm Center
Vivantes Clinic Am Urban
Berlin, Germany

Gansevoort H. Dunnington, MD
Director of Cardiothoracic Surgery
St. Helena Hospital
St. Helena, California

James Edgerton, MD
Adjunct Professor of Surgery
Department of Surgery
Washington University School of Medicine
St. Louis, Missouri

Maximilian Y. Emmert, MD
Department of Cardiothoracic and Vascular Surgery
Deutsches Herzzentrum der Charite
Charité-Universitätsmedizin Berlin
Corporate Member of Freie Universität Berlin and Humboldt-Universität zu Berlin
Berlin, Germany
Institute for Regenerative Medicine
University of Zurich
Schlieren, Switzerland

Marek P. Ehrlich, MD
Cardiothoracic Surgeon
Department of Cardiac Surgery
Medical University of Vienna
Vienna, Austria

Whitney W. Fu, MD
General Surgery Resident
Department of Cardiac Surgery
University of Michigan School of Medicine
Ann Arbor, Michigan

Sydney L. Gaynor, MD
Medical Director
AtriCure, Inc.
Mason, Ohio

Marc W. Gerdisch, MD
Adjunct Associate Professor of Surgery
Loyola University Medical Center
Chicago, Illinois
Chief, Department of Cardiothoracic Surgery
Franciscan Health Indianapolis
Indianapolis, Indiana

Marc Gillinov, MD
Professor and Chair
Department of Thoracic and Cardiovascular Surgery
Judith Dion Pyle Chair in Heart Valve Research
Cleveland Clinic
Cleveland, Ohio

Douglas R. Johnston, MD
Professor of Surgery
Chief, Division of Cardiac Surgery
Feinberg School of Medicine
Northwestern University
Chicago, Illinois

Armin Kiankhooy, MD
Associate Professor of Surgery
Department of Cardiac Surgery
Cedars-Sinai Medical Center
Los Angeles, California

Olga N. Kislitsina, MD, PhD
Associate Professor of Medicine
Division of Cardiology
Feinberg School of Medicine
Associate Director, Center for Heart Failure Research
Bluhm Cardiovascular Institute
Northwestern University
Chicago, Illinois

Jane Kruse, BSN
Research and Publication Coordinator
Division of Cardiac Surgery
Feinberg School of Medicine
Bluhm Cardiovascular Institute
Northwestern University
Chicago, Illinois

Taras Lysyy, MD
Senior Surgery Fellow
Division of Cardiothoracic Surgery
Washington University School of Medicine
St. Louis, Missouri

Kevin J. Makati, MD
Assistant Professor
Department of Cardiology
University of South Florida
Director, Department of Electrophysiology
BayCare Health System
Tampa, Florida

S. Chris Malaisrie, MD
Professor of Surgery
Division of Cardiac Surgery
Feinberg School of Medicine
Bluhm Cardiovascular Institute
Northwestern University
Chicago, Illinois

Patrick M. McCarthy, MD
Heller-Sacks Professor of Surgery
Division of Cardiac Surgery
Feinberg School of Medicine
Vice President, Northwestern Medical Group
Executive Director, Bluhm Cardiovascular Institute
Northwestern University
Chicago, Illinois

Christopher K. Mehta, MD
Assistant Professor of Surgery
Division of Cardiac Surgery
Feinberg School of Medicine
Bluhm Cardiovascular Institute
Chicago, Illinois

Mark La Meir, MD, PhD
Professor of Surgery
Department of Cardiac Surgery
UZ Brussels
Brussels, Belgium

Emilio Osorio-Jaramillo, MD
Cardiothoracic Surgeon
Department of Cardiac Surgery
Medical University of Vienna
Vienna, Austria

Amiran Sh Revishvili, MD, PhD
Professor of Cardiac Surgery
Chairman, Department of Cardiac Surgery
Vishnevsky Institute of Surgery
Moscow, Russian Federation

Harold G. Roberts, Jr., MD
Associate Professor of Surgery
Division of Cardiothoracic Surgery
Washington University School of Medicine
St. Louis, Missouri

Fabrizio Rosati, MD
Adjunct Professor of Cardiac Surgery
University of Brescia
Brescia, Italy

Sacha P. Salzberg, MD
Cardiac Surgeon
Surgical Electrophysiologist
Department of Cardiac Surgery
Swiss Ablation Clinic
Zurich, Switzerland

Richard B. Schuessler, PhD
Professor of Surgery and Biomedical Engineering
Director Emeritus, Cardiothoracic Surgery Research Laboratory
Division of Cardiothoracic Surgery
Washington University School of Medicine
St. Louis, Missouri

Douglas Seith, BA
Chief Operating Officer
AtriCure, Inc.
Mason, Ohio

Andrew J. Sherman, MD
Chief, Department of Cardiac, Vascular, and Thoracic Surgery
St. Joseph's Hospital
Co-chair, Adult Cardiac Surgery/Structural Heart
BayCare Health System
Tampa, Florida

Edward G. Soltesz, MD
Cardiovascular Surgeon
Cleveland Clinic Foundation
Cleveland, Ohio

Piotr Suwalski, MD, PhD
Director of Institute and Head of Department
Department of Cardiac Surgery and Transplantology
National Medical Institute of the Ministry of Interior and Administration
Centre of Postgraduate Medical Education
Warsaw, Poland

Bart P. van Putte, MD, PhD
Cardiothoracic Surgeon
Department of Cardiothoracic Surgery
St. Antonius Hospital
Nieuwegein, Netherlands
Principal Investigator
Department of Cardiothoracic Surgery
University Medical Center, Amsterdam, Netherlands

Stephen D. Waterford, MD
Northwell Health
New Hyde Park, New York

Richard Whitlock, MD, PhD
Professor of Surgery
Department of Surgery
McMaster University
Hamilton, Ontario, Canada

DISCLOSURES

Niv Ad, MD
AtriCure: consultant and PI of ICE-ABLATE IDE Trial
VGS: advisory board
Cardiosight: board of directors
Helios Cardio: advisory board
Pulse Biosciences: consultant (options)
GBI: advisory board

Vinay Badhwar, MD
No disclosures

Emilie Belley-Cote
Supported by career awards from the Department of Medicine at McMaster University and the Population Health Research Institute
Received grants from Abbott Laboratories, Bayer, BMS-Pfizer
Received consulting fees from Trimedic Therapeutics and Abbott Laboratories

Stefano Benussi, MD, PhD
No disclosures

Gianluigi Bisleri, MD, FRCSC
No disclosures

Steven F. Bolling, MD
No disclosures

Stefano Branzoli, MD
No disclosures

Etem Caliskan, MD
No disclosures

Michael Carrel
No disclosures

Manuel Castella, MD, PhD
AtriCure: Consultant
Medtronic: Consultant

W. Randolph Chitwood, Jr., MD
Scanlan: Consultant

Stephen F. Chiu, MD
No disclosures

Andrei Churyla, MD
No disclosures

James L. Cox, MD
Adagio Medical: Co-Founder, Board of Directors
Atricure: Consultant
Lucid Diagnostics: Board of Directors

Ralph J. Damiano, Jr., MD
Edwards Lifesciences, Medtronic, AtriCure: consultant, speaking honoraria
AtriCure, Pulse Biosciences: research grants

Giuseppe D'Ancona, MD, PhD
No disclosures

Gansevoort H. Dunnington, MD
AtriCure: proctor, speaker, research grant, consultant
Pulse Biosciences: consultant, stock options, salary

James Edgarton, MD
No disclosures

Marek P. Ehrlich, MD
No disclosures

Maximilian Y. Emmert, MD
No disclosures

Whitney W. Fu, MD
No disclosures

Sydney L. Gaynor, BSc. (Hon), MB BS, FRCS (Ed.)
AtriCure: medical director

Marc W. Gerdisch, MD, FACS, FACC, FHRS
Consultant: Atricure, Arthrex, Artivion, CorVivo, Edwards, Abbott
Advisory board: Dasi

Marc Gillinov, MD
No disclosures

Douglas R. Johnston, MD, FACS
No disclosures

Armin Kiankhooy, MD
AtriCure: unpaid consultant; paid consultant until September 30, 2025

Olga N. Kislitsina, MD, PhD
No disclosures

Jane Kruse, BSN
No disclosures

Taras Lysyy, MD, MCh
No disclosures

Kevin J. Makati, MD, FACC, FHRS
Boston Scientific, AtriCure. Siemens Healthineers. Phillips. Cordis. Medtronic: consultant, speaker, research grant

S. Chris Malaisrie, MD
Consultant: Atricure, Artivion, Edwards, Medtronic, Terumo Aortic

Patrick M. McCarthy, MD
Abbott: principal investigator, REPAIR MR Trial (unfunded)
Edwards Lifesciences: royalties; honorarium for lectures
AtriCure: honorarium for lectures
Arthrex: advisory board
Genesee: royalties

Christopher K. Mehta, MD
W.L. Gore & Associates: consultant
Terumo Aortic: consultant

Mark La Meir, MD, PhD
No disclosures

Emilio Osorio-Jaramillo, MD
Co-founder: Aortic Technologies
Consultant: Biotronik, Terumo Aortic AATS James L. Cox Fellowship in Atrial Fibrillation Surgery

Amiran Sh. Revishvili, MD
No disclosures

Harold G. Roberts, Jr., MD
No disclosures

Fabrizio Rosati, MD
No disclosures

Sacha P. Salzberg, MD
No disclosures

Richard B. Schuessler, PhD
No disclosures

Douglas Seith, BA
No disclosures

Andrew J. Sherman, MD
AtriCure: teacher and consultant

Edward Soltesz, MD MPH
Abbott: honoraria (speaking and training)
Abiomed: honoraria (speaking and training), national Co-PI IMPACT Trial
Dilon: honoraria (speaking)
Atricure: honoraria (speaking and training)

Piotr Suwalski, MD, PhD
No disclosures

Bart P. van Putte, MD, PhD
AtriCure: consultant
Pulse Biosciences: consultant

Stephen D. Waterford, MD
No disclosures

Richard Whitlock, MD, PhD, FRCSC
No disclosures

FOREWORD

I was fortunate to join the faculty at Northwestern University Feinberg School of Medicine when this book was in its earlier stages. Taking on a leadership role at a new institution is never without its challenges; however, I was the beneficiary of the combined wisdom and experience of two senior surgical leaders in Drs. Patrick McCarthy and James Cox, both of whom have been instrumental in our subsequent success, and both editors of this very unique volume. At the time I joined, I related to Dr. Cox that my first exposure to the surgical treatment of patients with atrial fibrillation (AF) was as a cardiothoracic fellow at Cleveland Clinic, scrubbing in on a concomitant procedure with mitral valve repair. This involved two surgeons, one performing the repair and another the cryo lesions. In response to my question about the rationale for placement of the lesions, the senior surgeon replied, "The only one who understands this operation is Jim Cox." Although that was an overstatement even in 2005, the explosion of, and clinical dissemination of Dr. Cox's work in the intervening two decades is a remarkable story. I've also come to appreciate much more deeply how the collaboration between McCarthy and Cox and their ability to standardize a procedure many surgeons find daunting have transformative potential for the care of patients.

As a general surgical resident at the Massachusetts General Hospital, I developed a simplistic understanding of AF as an entity to be managed, often poorly, in the middle of the night with metoprolol and digoxin and perhaps to be avoided with judicious fluid management. That the science of AF surgery was already rapidly developing and patients were free of AF years after initial human operations was entirely unknown to me. For a cardiothoracic trainee 20 years ago, "cut-and-sew Maze" was a relatively exotic procedure performed by few surgeons, and concomitant ablation was applied variably and seemingly without scientific rationale. That surgery for AF would become an important and standardized part of my practice was at the time inconceivable.

Although I understood Cox as being intimately associated with the Cox-Maze procedure, it was hearing Dr. Cox speak at a Society of Thoracic Surgeons meeting that raised the curtain on what a unique achievement the procedure itself was, and what a unique individual was necessary for its development. I was first introduced to him personally by Dr. Bruce Lytle, who was fond of saying, "You can tell about 2 minutes into a conversation when someone is truly serious about the technical practice of cardiac surgery." Dr. Cox clearly exceeded that bar. What I did not know during that first conversation was that the combination of technical and scientific mastery that led to the creation of an entirely new procedure was the result of an early career that embodies the concept of "range."

As 81st president of the American Association for Thoracic Surgery, director of the American Board of Thoracic Surgery, and member of the Surgical Study Section of the National Institutes of Health, Dr. Cox's national and international influence on multiple generations of surgeons is well known. What may not be as well known is that before he redefined the science and practice of arrhythmia therapy. Dr. Cox was a three-sport athlete on a scholarship at the University of Mississippi and was subsequently drafted by the Los Angeles Dodgers in 1963. Luckily for our profession, he pivoted from baseball to medicine, attending the University of Tennessee School of Medicine, where he was recognized as the outstanding student in his graduating class. There is something to be said for being in the right place at the right time. The small group of investigators doing meaningful work on the pathogenesis of arrhythmias at the time included Horan and Flowers at the University of Tennessee. Thus, an opportunity arose for a future giant in the field to make an early foray into the research that would define his career. Lucky accidents of geography continued while he was a surgical resident at Duke, where he was surrounded by a confluence of innovation in cardiac surgical technique under David Sabiston and arrhythmia research in collaboration with John Boineau. While a surgical resident at Duke, Dr. Cox was called to military service in 1970. He rose to the rank of major in the US Army Medical Corps before returning to Duke to complete training in cardiothoracic surgery.

Dr. Cox went on to become the first Evarts A. Graham Professor of Surgery and led the Division of Cardiothoracic Surgery at Washington University School of Medicine in St. Louis for many years, training a generation of leaders in the field. It was during his time at Washington University that he began the herculean task of translating scientific understanding of the pathology of AF first into animal models and from there into an operation performed on patients with no other therapeutic option. Unlike some other eponymous operations in surgical history, the Cox-Maze procedure was not invented in the operating room in response to an anatomic challenge but arose from systematic research into a physiologic one, applying the surgeon's knowledge of the anatomy as endgame. I have never read a better illustration of the inventor's art than taking a marking pen to animal atrium as Dr. Cox describes in Chapter 1. Although it is the *depth* of understanding of a single subject that leads to mastery, it is the *range* of interest and experience that allows for successful implementation and the flexibility to adapt as necessary. That Dr. Cox not only was able to produce the science behind the procedure that bears his name but also had the courage to transition rapidly to a first-in-human procedure and then refine the technique aggressively in response to new technology is a story that represents the very best of our specialty.

In my first meeting with Dr. Cox, having taken over as chief of cardiac surgery at Northwestern, he in typical fashion left me with several leadership pearls in a few short minutes and kindly offered to be a source of advice "should I find it useful from time to time." Since then, I have been fortunate to be able to rely on him as a colleague, mentor, and friend. Those who know him only as the "Father of Cardiac Arrhythmia Surgery" will have missed a great wit and a fount of wisdom on all subjects, not least the trials of surgical leadership. Dr. Cox exemplifies the epitome of both range and depth. He continues to inspire those of us lucky enough to follow in his footsteps.

In the following pages, readers will be reminded of the scale of the burden of AF in cardiac disease, the relative ineffectiveness of pharmacotherapy and much current intervention, and the remarkable success of even the earliest forms of the Maze procedure in achieving what had not before been possible—a durable return to sinus rhythm, often without supplementary pharmacology. Readers will also, I hope, understand that there are few fields in surgery that have been shaped so profoundly by one individual. This book is a monument to dedication, scientific rigor, and creativity across a career spanning more than six decades. It is important to note that Drs. Cox, McCarthy, and Malaisrie represent three surgical generations of the dissemination of procedural technique. If there is a central message in this work, it is that interventional for AF should not be an occasional effort, but rather thoughtfully and widely applied based on an avalanche of sound science. It is an honor to have the opportunity to introduce this work. I hope you will find it, as I do, both the very practical work a textbook should be and an inspiration to push the boundaries of what we can achieve as physicians and surgeons.

Douglas R. Johnston, MD

PREFACE

As the number of people with atrial fibrillation (AF) has grown exponentially around the world, so, too, has the collaboration of the best clinicians, scientists, and medical device experts committed to healing patients. This integrated ecosystem has transformed AF treatment globally and unlocked solutions for millions of patients who might otherwise have continued to suffer the burden of this unresolved disease.

For decades, we have been honored to partner with Dr. James Cox as he provided the genesis and led the evolution of the interventional treatment of AF and then dispersed his knowledge around the globe. This book highlights his passionate pursuit of the treatment of patients with AF and the accelerated pace of advancement he has generated since performing the first Cox-Maze procedure in 1987. Dr. Cox is an influential and preeminent researcher and a cardiothoracic surgeon whose knowledge of and expertise in the treatment of patients with AF are unrivaled. The breakthroughs documented within these pages represent a life's work that has benefited millions of people in immeasurable ways.

Like our surgical colleagues, we believe deeply that patients are the focus of how and why we do what we do. More than a decade ago, when our company was young, we devoted ourselves solely to the surgical treatment of patients with AF; therefore, we recognized the importance of partnering with Dr. Cox to advance the education, innovation, and clinical science that profoundly impact patients who have this burdensome condition. We knew then, as we do today, that his passion for solutions and prodigious scientific acumen were key to our mission to defeat AF.

Initially, our collaboration focused on building a world-class education and training platform to help physicians treat their patients with AF more safely and effectively. Dr. Cox led the development of a series of educational courses with the help and participation of a foundational group of other esteemed surgical educators. This dynamic partnership continues to fuel the exchange of ideas, research, and resources, and it multiplies the number of physicians trained in the optimal interventional treatment of patients with AF. Along the way, our engineers and clinical education staff have been continuously and actively engaged with clinical surgeons in transforming new ideas into real-world solutions.

We have also worked to strategize and support scientific discovery through groundbreaking clinical trials led by renowned surgeons, many of whom have benefited from Dr. Cox's mentorship in this field. These trials have led to changes in societal guidelines worldwide and have significantly impacted the treatment of patients with AF. We also continue to work with Dr. Cox and other surgical leaders on the development of new surgical devices that will hopefully be even safer and more effective. The development of such surgical tools and clinical trials evolves from ideas to reality only when all partners convene in support of a common goal, and we believe that this scientist–industry collaboration has only just begun.

The knowledge and experience described in this book by world-renowned arrhythmia surgeons highlight the challenges and triumphs encountered when navigating all sectors and aspects of patient care. The insights that are provided shed light on the importance of fostering open lines of communication, building trust, and nurturing a shared vision among all stakeholders. This collaboration is essential for maintaining the fertile ground necessary to provide meaningful research, innovation, and solutions and is proof of the incredible possibilities that are revealed when we work together for a healthier world.

Finally, this book serves as a testament to the profound impact Dr. James Cox has had on the lives of patients. It is a call to action and urges all involved parties to embrace the spirit of collaboration and recognize the immense potential that lies in treating patients with this progressive and relentless disease. It is our sincere hope that Dr. Cox's enlightening exploration of the wide-ranging universe of AF and related heart conditions will spark conversation, foster new collaboration, and inspire the next generation of innovators to push the boundaries of what is possible in AF treatment. By doing so, we can continue to be united in our commitment to transforming and improving lives.

Michael Carrel
Douglas Seith

EDITOR'S PREFACE

Atrial fibrillation (AF) is the most common arrhythmia of the heart, occurring in approximately 1% of the general population and in more than 10% of the population older than the age of 65 years. AF is usually symptomatic, is associated with a fivefold increase in life-threatening or fatal strokes, is a major component of health care costs, and is predicted to double in incidence by the year 2050. Despite these foreboding statistics, until the last two decades of the 20th century, AF was approached by most physicians as if it were an innocuous problem. Thus, we chose near the beginning of this book (Chapter 2) to provide a description of the epidemiology of AF so that physicians and the lay public will better appreciate the fact that AF is a serious problem. Previously, patients with AF were treated within acceptable contemporary standards of the time by physicians who possessed only a superficial understanding of the arrhythmia itself, and the only options for treatment were relatively ineffective drugs. However, the introduction of surgery for AF in 1987 and catheter ablation for AF in 1998 increased the requirements for therapeutic competence on the part of health care providers. Despite this fact, patients with AF, even today, are treated far more commonly by primary care physicians and other noncardiologists than by electrophysiologists and arrhythmia surgeons who are specialists in arrhythmias.

There are essentially two ways to treat patients who have cardiac arrhythmias: (1) pharmacologically (i.e., with drugs) and (2) nonpharmacologically (i.e, with scars). Drug therapy is directed at altering the basic electrophysiologic characteristics of cardiac tissue such as the refractory period, velocity of conduction, synchronicity of depolarizaton, uniformity of repolarization, and so on. However, interventional therapy, whether it is surgery or catheter ablation, is focused on creating sites of conduction block with scars that either *isolate* the arrhythmia or its triggers from the rest of the heart or actually *ablate* the arrhythmia itself by interrupting or destroying its underlying mechanisms.

From 1914, when reentry was first described, until 1968, conduction blocks created by scars were used only to *study* arrhythmias. The first time a scar was used to *treat* an arrhythmia was May 2, 1968, when Dr. Will C. Sealy of Duke University divided an accessory atrioventricular connection responsible for the Wolff-Parkinson-White (WPW) syndrome in a fisherman from the Outer Banks of North Carolina. The success of Sealy's first surgical arrhythmia procedure eventually led to the development of other surgical procedures to treat patients with both ischemic and nonischemic ventricular tachycardia (VT), automatic atrial tachycardias, atrioventricular node reentry tachycardia (AVNRT), atrial flutter, and, finally, AF.

After more than two decades of performing surgery for various types of cardiac arrhythmias, a new category of nonsurgeon physicians (i.e., interventional electrophysiologists) successfully converted most of the earlier surgical procedures to catheter-based radiofrequency (RF) procedures, thus precluding the need for surgery. The chart that follows demonstrates a rough approximation of the lag times between the first surgical procedure for a specific arrhythmia and the ability to treat patients with that arrhythmia reliably by catheter ablation.

Arrhythmia	Surgical Treatment	Catheter Treatment	Lag Time (years)
WPW syndrome	1968	Early 1990s	~20
Ischemic VT	1978	Mid-1990s	~15
Nonischemic VT	1979	Mid-1990s	~15
Atrial tachycardias	1980	Early 1990s	~10
AVNRT	1982	Early 1990s	~10
Atrial Flutter	1986	Mid-1990s	~10
Atrial Fibrillation	1987	Late 1990s	~10

Despite lag times of 10 to 20 years after successful surgical therapy, the eventual success of RF catheter ablation for essentially all clinical arrhthmias except the persistent forms of AF ranks among the most impressive accomplishments in the history of heart disease therapy and represents a vast improvement over previous surgical therapy. It is still remarkable to us as surgeons that interventional electrophysiologists have been able to attain essentially the same success rates with the tip of a catheter that we once accomplished only by submitting patients to open-heart surgery.

After many years of developing surgical procedures for the treatment of patients with other types of supraventricular and ventricular arrhythmias, we decided in 1980 to focus on the one remaining arrhythmia for which there was no interventional therapy available except elective His bundle ablation and insertion of a permanent ventricular pacemaker. It was apparent that if we were to design an ablative treatment for patients with AF as effective as the procedures for those with WPW syndrome, AVNRT, and other arrhythmias, we would need to have a better understanding of the underlying pathophysiology of AF. This required the creation of new clinically relevant animal models of AF, the construction of multi-electrode arrays, and the design of computerized mapping programs that would allow us to marry the three-dimensional (3D) electrophysiologic events responsible for AF to 3D atrial anatomy. It was helpful that we already had a source of patients in whom AF could be mapped. These were patients who were being referred to us in large numbers for surgical correction of WPW syndrome. Approximately 30% of those patients also had AF, and we were granted institutaional review board approval by Barnes Hospital in St. Louis to map their cases of AF in the operating room at the time of their WPW surgery. Intensive study and interpretation of both experimental and human electrophysiological maps of AF, especially by Drs. John Boineau and Richard Schuessler, eventually provided the electrophysiologic insight that allowed the Maze procedure to be conceived. However, the Maze procedure was based solely on the mechanism by which AF is *maintained*, because at that time neither we nor anyone else knew about the atrial triggers that some 10 to 12 years were shown to *induce* AF.

The first Maze procedure was performed on September 25, 1987, at Barnes Hospital/Washington University in St. Louis, Missouri, and by 1990 we had performed a total of only seven Maze procedures. Clinical progression was purposely slow because we waited 6 months after each of the first seven procedures to be sure that each one had been successful. The Maze procedure was initially, and has remained, highly successful for treating patients with all forms of AF, though its original technique proved to be too invasive surgically to be used as routine therapy.

Although a few attempts at recreating the Maze procedure by RF catheter ablation were attempted in the early 1990s, the experience proved to be futile. Successful catheter ablation for AF awaited the discovery of pulmonary vein "triggers" and their catheter-based isolation, first described by Michel Haissaguerre in 1998. For the first time we learned how individual episodes of paroxysmal AF are usually *induced*, thereby enhancing our understanding of the basic electrophysiology of AF.

Unfortunately, many readers misinterpreted Haissaguerre's seminal article to suggest that the pulmonary vein triggers were the sole problem causing AF, thinking that the triggers were responsible not only for the *initiation* of AF but also for its *maintenance*. This misconception led to a number of misguided interventional catheter and surgical approaches to the more complex types of AF over the ensuing 20 years, some of which are still being practiced by both arrhythmia surgeons and interventional electrophysiologists. This is one reason that despite the relative success of catheter ablation for paroxysmal AF, the impact of catheter ablation on the societal problem of AF is less than it should be. Catheter ablation for AF has now been available for more than 25 years, has been applied in millions of patients, and has received billions of investment dollars from industry and government, yet it is used in fewer than 4% of all patients with AF and has a combined overall 5-year success rate for all patients with AF of around 25% for single catheter ablation and 60% to 70% for multiple catheter ablations.

Although these results seem dismal at first glance, the fact is that catheter ablation precludes the necessity for more invasive surgical intervention or resorting to simply leaving half of the patients in AF permanently. Catheter ablation is currently the treatment of choice for paroxysmal AF, and new catheter-based tools are being developed that are specifically designed to create reliable transmural linear lesions in the atria for the treatment of long-standing persistent AF. Coupled with the sophisticated mapping systems now available, these tools are likely to yield future results for the catheter ablation of AF comparable to those for all other cardiac arrhythmias.

Until recently, even so-called minimally invasive surgery remained too invasive to be considered a first-line therapy for patients with AF. However, the introduction of thoracoscopic surgical techniques in the past several years has resulted in the increasing practice of performing "hybrid procedures" in which the thoracoscopic surgeon and the interventional electrophysiologist combine their techniques to treat persistent and long-standing persistent (i.e., nonparoxysmal) AF. At least in the near future, this appears to be the most promising approach to these complex problems.

This book has been written to provide a single source of essential information that we hope will be useful to practitioners in the field of AF interventional therapy, especially surgical ablation. Our objective is to focus on the information critical to a sound clinical practice in the interventional treatment of AF and, hopefully, for the development of better interventional therapies in the future.

SUMMARY AND SPECIAL ACKNOWLEDGMENTS

Describing history, much like describing beauty, is subject to the vagaries inherent in the eye of the beholder, and the first chapter of this book is definitely a personal version of the history of cardiac arrhythmia surgery as I witnessed and participated in it. There are numerous individuals not mentioned in this account, and without them much of this history would not have happened. Chief among them is Dr. Demetrios Lappas, the brilliant professor and chief of Cardiac Anesthesiology at Washington University and Barnes Hospital during my tenure there. Without Lappas, the clinical results we attained with the Maze procedure would have remained only a pipe dream. He was my closest clinical associate and supporter during those exciting and sometimes trying days, and above all, he made it possible for me to perform this new, rather complex operation safely.

In addition to the original group of Duke surgical electrophysiology research fellows, Mark Williams, Ross Ungerleider, Gary Lofland, Peter Smith, Bill Holman, Bruce Ferguson, Jim Douglas, and Ralph Damiano, significant contributions were also made to the field of cardiac arrhythmia surgery by surgical research fellows Jim Levett, Patricia Penkoske, Harry D'Agostino, Constance Stone, Todd Shuman, and Jim Tweddell. Especially important were the contributions made by Robert "Jake" Jaquiss, who was instrumental in the modification and conversion of the original versions of the Maze procedure into its final version as the Maze-III procedure. Major contributions were also made by the many surgeons from abroad who spent periods varying from a few months to as long as 4 years in our research laboratories at Duke or in St. Louis. They include Drs. Masatoshi Ikeshita (Japan), Phillipe Gersbach (Switzerland), Jorge Martinell (Spain), Riccardo Sinatra (Italy), Tetusu Asano (Japan), Atsushi Harada (Japan), Byung-Chul Chang (South Korea), Yoko Yagi (Japan), Shigeo Sato (Japan), Yasuhiro Matsunaga (Japan), Shigeo Yamauchi (Japan), Tomohide Kawamoto (Japan), Takashi Nitta (Japan), Masataka Mitsuno (Japan), Fumitaka Isobe (Japan), Ki-Bong Kim (South Korea), Vladimir Goriatchev (Russia), David Johnson (Australia), and Monica Robotin-Johnson (Australia).

In addition to these research fellows, several surgeons also contributed significantly as clinical arrhythmia surgery fellows. They include Tom Canavan (Albany, New York), Eva Berglin (Goteborg, Sweden), David Haydock (Auckland, New Zealand), Hans Fieguth (Hannover, Germany), John Goldblatt (Victoria, Australia), and Stefano Benussi (Milan, Italy). Especially important contributions were made, and continue to be made, by Niv Ad (Tel Aviv, Israel), who developed the post-operative protocol for patients underoing Maze procedures and made significant contributions to the conversion of the Maze procedure into a minimally invasive operation that could be applied in a larger group of patients with AF.

Whatever success I enjoyed personally in this field was the direct result of having grown up in the laboratories of Drs. Leo Horan, Nancy Flowers, and John Boineau; having been supported by the untiring efforts of laboratory director George Quick and computer scientist Barry Branham; having learned surgery under the tutelage of Drs. David C. Sabiston, Jr. and Will C. Sealy; having the late, and dearly missed, surgical assistant Steve Fitzpatrick, RN, at my side in the operating room for virtually every Maze procedure I ever performed; having a supremely talented and irreplaceable scrub nurse Maria Marafiotti, RN, as a constant source of support for nearly two decades; having a loyal and tireless clinical nurse specialist Terry Palazzo to watch over the inpatients and follow up on the outpatients; and having been surrounded throughout my career by a multitude of brilliant residents and fellows who constantly challenged any and all assumptions and who added their own insights, intellect, and hard work to the development of this field of surgery.

One final important acknowledgment. The first time I ever gave a talk publicly on the Maze procedure was at the Cleveland Clinic in 1989. The head of cardiac surgery there at the time, Dr. Floyd ("Fred") Loop, became immediately enamoured with the procedure and thereafter was the biggest supporter of the Maze procedure during that early period of heavy criticism, especially from clinical electrophysiologists. As a result, I performed several Maze procedures at the Cleveland Clinic over the next few years. During that time, a young surgeon who had just finished his training at the Mayo Clinic and Stanford, Dr. Patrick McCarthy, joined the faculty at the Cleveland Clinic, and Dr. Loop assigned him to learn all that he could about the Maze procedure. Of all the numerous cardiac surgeons who visited St. Louis during those early years to learn how to perform the Maze procedure, Pat McCarthy approached the task far more diligently than any of them. He arranged for my administrative assistant to call him the day before I had a Maze procedure scheduled so that he could fly into St. Louis the night before for the case. During the time that we were gaining experience and learning the problems with the Maze-I procedure, struggling technically with the Maze-II procedure, and introducing the Maze-III procedure, Dr. McCarthy returned to St. Louis for nearly every case, peering over my shoulder and talking into his dictaphone (which was mildly distracting). For the next few years, Dr. McCarthy and I were the only two surgeons in the world who were able to accumulate a "personal series" of Maze patients. As a result, we had almost weekly phone calls and frequently exchanged visits between St. Louis and Cleveland to perform surgery together. Ten years later, we partnered as the two primary consultants for

St Jude Medical when they were introducing the high-intensity focused ultrasound device for the surgical treatment of patients with AF. As fate would have it, 15 years after that, Dr. McCarthy enticed me out of retirement to join his faculty at Northwestern University in Chicago, and he has now been my boss since January 1, 2017. I am pleased and honored that both Pat McCarthy and our brilliant surgical colleague, Dr. Chris Malaisrie, agreed to join me as co-editors of this book. Both Pat McCarthy and Chris Malaisrie are master heart surgeons, and they surgically ablate concomitant AF in 98% of all mitral valve patients and in roughly 75% of all cardiac surgery patients who have associated AF. I sometimes go over to the operating theater at Northwestern to watch Chris perform a difficult thoracic aortic case or to peer over Pat's shoulder to watch a Maze/double-valve procedure. I trust that they appreciate the fact that I never bring a dictaphone.

James L. Cox, MD

ACKNOWLEDGMENT

The authors would like to acknowledge the enormous contribution of Jane Kruse, BSN, the Coordinator of Cardiac Surgery Research at Northwestern University, to the completion of this book. Without her indispensable and untiring dedication, this project could not possibly have been completed.

We would also like to acknowledge the cooperation and support of the editors and publishers at Elsevier, particularly Lisa Barnes, who served as our primary point of contact for all matters related to the creation and publication of this book.

We would also like to thank the invited national and international authors for their expert and invaluable contributions to the content of this book.

CONTENTS

VIDEO CONTENTS

Chapter 1: A History of Cardiac Arrhythmia Surgery

Video 1.1 Postoperative Dynamic Magnetic Resonance Imaging Scan After a Maze Procedure, Circa 1985.

Chapter 5: Clinical Electrophysiology of Atrial Flutter and Atrial Fibrillation Pertinent to Interventional Therapy

Video 5.1 First Three-Dimensional Mapping of the Atria, Circa 1986

Chapter 9: Arrhythmia Surgery Prior to Atrial Fibrillation Surgery

Video 9.1 Wolff-Parkinson-White Surgery for a Left Free-Wall Accessory Pathway, Circa 1983.

Video 9.2 Surgery for Ischemic Ventricular Tachycardia, Circa 1985.

Chapter 12: Development and Evolution of the Maze Procedure for Atrial Fibrillation

Video 12.1 The First Maze Procedure, September 25, 1987.

Video 12.2 Cut-and-Sew Maze-III Procedure for Atrial Fibrillation, 1992.

Chapter 16: Robotic Cox CryoMaze-III Procedure

Video 16.1 Robotic Cox CryoMaze-III Procedure.

Chapter 17: The Cox Maze-IV Procedure for Atrial Fibrillation

Video 17.1 Cox Maze IV Procedure from Atricure.

Chapter 35: Thoracoscopic Non-Maze Hybrid Procedure for Stand-Alone Atrial Fibrillation

Video 35.1 Highlights of Key Technical Steps of Thoracoscopic Non-Maze Hybrid Ablation Procedure for Stand-Alone Atrial Fibrillation. Key steps include (1) left pulmonary vein (PV) mobilization with the lighted tip dissector and isolation with a radiofrequency clamp, (2) roof and floor ablation with simultaneous unidirectional devices, (3) left atrial appendage exclusion with an AtriClip, (4) oblique and transverse sinus mobilization, (5) right PV mobilization and ablation, and (6) completion of the left atrial "box" with right-sided roof and floor ablation.

1

A History of Cardiac Arrhythmia Surgery

James L. Cox

CHAPTER OUTLINE

PERSPECTIVE

Any attempt to describe the historical development of a specific era or discipline in the medical field is ultimately a personal view of that history. This chapter is no different. Having been present at the very beginning of cardiac arrhythmia surgery on May 2, 1968, and having spent 60 years (1964–2024) of focused interest and active participation in the evolution of surgery for cardiac arrhythmias, this chapter describes my own personal journey and is not meant to be the definitive history of cardiac arrhythmia surgery. Many of the great electrophysiologists (EPs) and surgeons who contributed to the basic knowledge that allowed us and others to devise surgical procedures to cure almost all clinical arrhythmias are not mentioned. If they were given their full due, it would take a book, not a book chapter, to describe the complete history of cardiac arrhythmia surgery. Hence, this chapter is presented as "A History," not "The History."

THE ORIGINS OF CARDIAC ARRHYTHMIA SURGERY

In 1930, the renowned Boston cardiologist Paul Dudley White visited the equally renowned London physician John Parkinson so they could update one another on the latest developments in the world of medicine. As was customary in those days, White brought along one of his young residents, Louis Wolff, to assist him on the long trans-Atlantic journey (Fig. 1.1). White was anxious to show Parkinson a few electrocardiograms (ECGs) he had recorded from several healthy young people in Boston who had recurrent bouts of sudden unexplained tachycardia. White had noted that when these patients were in normal sinus rhythm (i.e., between episodes of tachycardia), their ECGs showed a short P-R interval, an early deflection off the baseline immediately preceding the QRS complex (later termed the "delta wave"), and a wide QRS complex. The tachycardia, however, was characterized by a regular, narrow-complex rate of 240 beats/min with no delta wave.

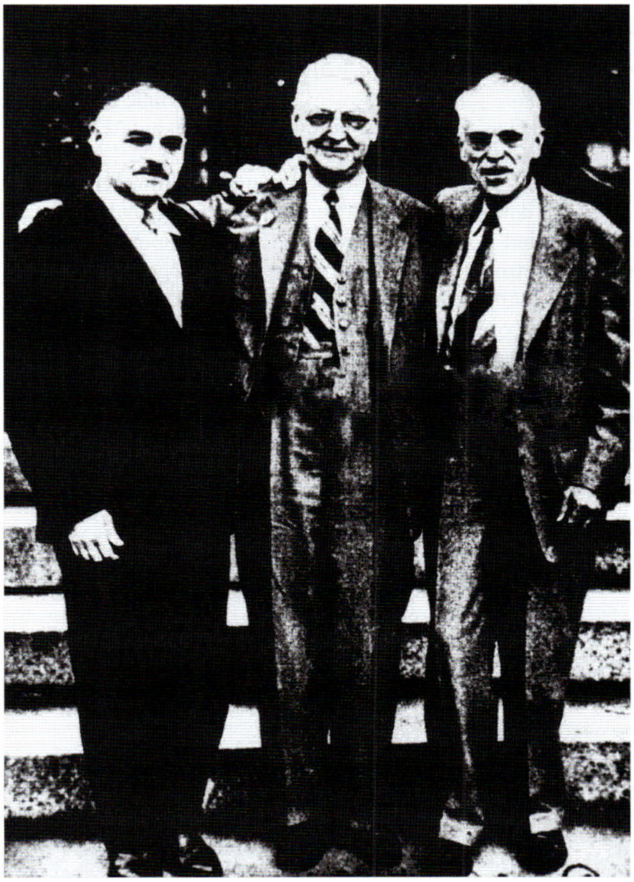

Fig. 1.1 The only known photograph of (from left to right) Drs. Louis Wolff, John Parkinson, and Paul Dudley White. Date unknown.

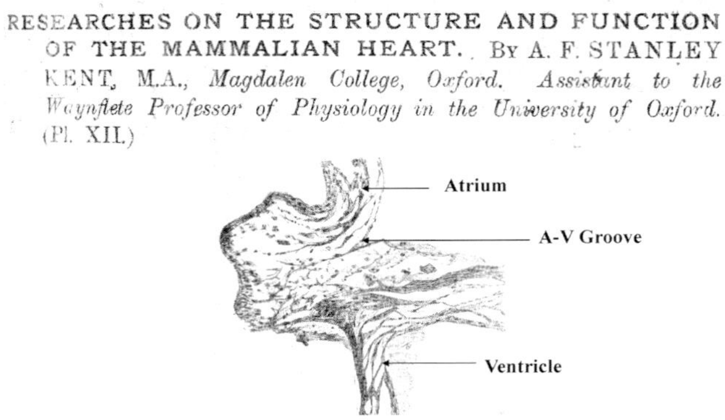

Fig. 1.2 Photomicrograph from Stanley Kent's 1893 article showing an accessory atrioventricular connection (aka, "Kent bundle," "accessory pathway"). The entire connection from atrium to ventricle is not seen because its full length was not in the exact plane of this histologic section.

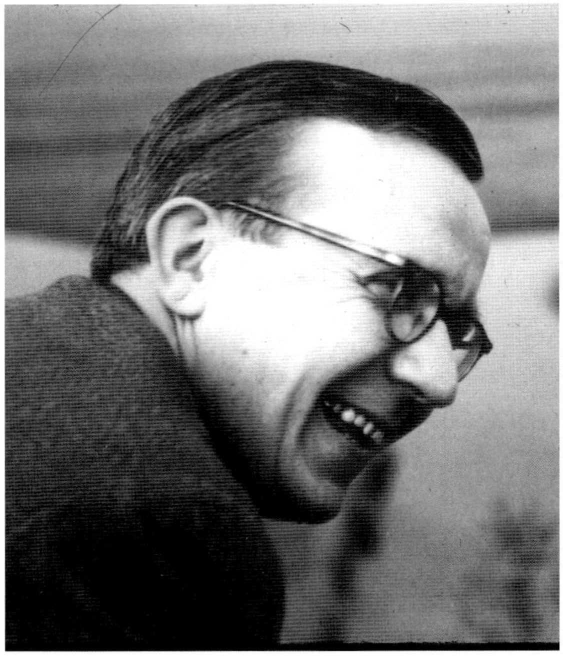

Fig. 1.3 Photo of Professor Durrer taken by John Boineau during his year studying with Durrer in 1963 to 1964 as the professor was leaning out an open window of a Dutch windmill near Amsterdam.

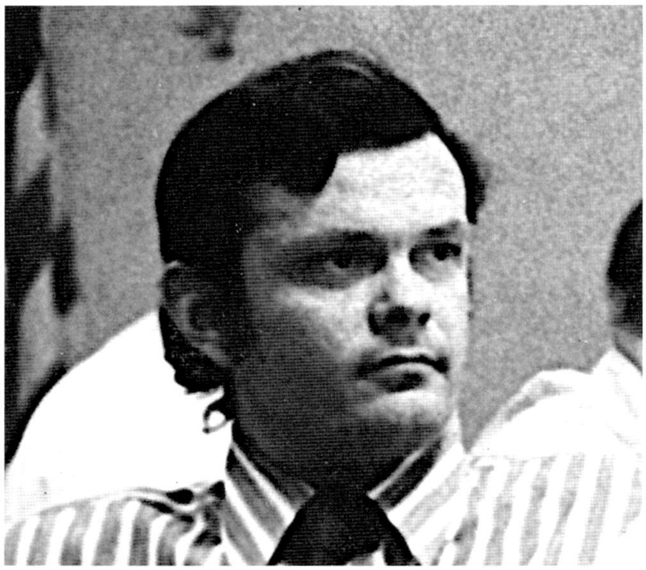

Fig. 1.4 Photo of a young John Boineau (c. 1964) at the time he returned to Duke University after spending a year with Durrer in the Netherlands.

Upon arrival in London, and much to White's surprise, Parkinson promptly produced several similar ECGs recorded from his own patients who had similar clinical histories of sudden tachycardia. Louis Wolff, being the most junior physician in attendance, was assigned the task of researching the literature and writing a paper on their observations,[1] which led to the designation of the condition known thereafter as the Wolff-Parkinson-White (WPW) syndrome. Even though Stanley Kent had described abnormal anatomic connections between the atria and the ventricles in mammalian hearts in 1893[2] (Fig. 1.2), Drs. Wolff, Parkinson, and White did not know that these "Kent bundles" were actually responsible for their newly identified syndrome. Indeed, it took more than three decades for this association to be documented, but it eventually led to a new field of medicine . . . clinical electrophysiology. However, before this could happen, electrophysiologic mapping techniques and a new method of controlling the onset and termination of arrhythmias had to be developed.

For some reason, a disproportionate number of the seminal observations and developments related to the electrical activity of the heart have emanated from the Netherlands. Thus, it is not surprising that although electrophysiological mapping was first reported at the beginning of the 20th century,[3,4] the technique was not fully developed until mid-century by A.M. Scher in Seattle, who used intramural needle electrodes in the ventricle[5] and most particularly by a Dutch physician, Dirk Durrer (Fig. 1.3), who developed a method for recording local electrograms directly from the surface of the heart.[6] Durrer realized that by comparing the timing of a "roving" handheld epicardial electrode with a fixed electrode, he could reconstruct the timing sequence of the electrical activation of the heart or at least of its epicardial surface. This became known as "activation time mapping" (see Chapter 6). Durrer's protégé, Hein J.J. Wellens, who was also from the Netherlands, subsequently developed a pacing technique called "programmed electrical stimulation" that provided a means of inducing and terminating most clinical arrhythmias.[7] Activation mapping and programmed electrical stimulation became the foundation of all subsequent clinical electrophysiology, cardiac arrhythmia surgery, and the catheter ablation of arrhythmias.

In 1963, John Boineau (Fig. 1.4), a young assistant professor of pediatric cardiology at Duke University, spent a year studying with Durrer in Amsterdam. Boineau returned to Duke in the summer of 1964 to work with Dr. Madison Spach, the revered chief of pediatric cardiology at Duke, on various arrhythmia problems in children and young adults, the most important of which was WPW syndrome. Ironically, Andrew Wallace, a colleague in cardiology (and Boineau's undergraduate classmate at Duke), had also just returned to Duke from the National Institutes of Health, where interest was also increasing in this newly emerging clinical electrophysiology field. Wallace asked Dr. Will Sealy, a renowned professor of thoracic surgery at Duke, for some space in his research laboratory where he could study the WPW syndrome, and Sealy graciously provided the necessary space. Thus, in 1964 Boineau and Wallace independently and simultaneously established two of the earliest, most productive, and most competitive electrophysiology laboratories in the world that were located less than 100 yards from one another on the Duke University campus.

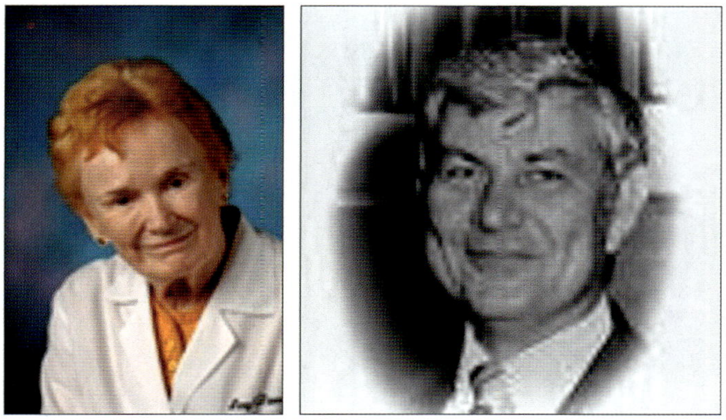

Fig. 1.5 (From left to right) Drs. Nancy Flowers and Leo Horan, who had one of the few experimental electrophysiological laboratories in the world in the early 1960s at the University of Tennessee School of Medicine in Memphis. They believed that ischemic ventricular tachycardia secondary to myocardial infarction (MI) most likely arose from myocardium located between the dead tissue in the center and normal tissue outside of the infarct. However, such an "ischemic zone" surrounding an MI had never been documented histologically. To identify it, in 1964 they provided the author, a freshman medical student, with an assistant and a small laboratory that harbored a grocer's standard meat slicer, a cryotome, a tank of liquid nitrogen, and a copy of Pearce's *Textbook of Histochemistry*. They also provided financial support and a lot of encouragement.

Several other individuals in the United States were active in this young field of clinical electrophysiology by that time, most notably Brian Hoffman and Paul Cranefield at Columbia-Presbyterian in New York City, E. Neil Moore at the University of Pennsylvania in Philadelphia, and Dan Brody, Leo Horan, and Nancy Flowers at the University of Tennessee in Memphis. I was privileged to begin my own career in the electrophysiology laboratory of Horan and Flowers (Fig. 1.5) in Memphis in that seminal year of 1964 as Boineau and Wallace were returning to Duke. In November 1966, I presented a paper at the American Heart Association (AHA) in New York City that was the first to delineate and characterize the "ischemic border zone" surrounding acute myocardial infarction (MI) and to suggest this zone as being the source of ischemic ventricular tachyarrhythmias.[8] During that meeting, Nancy Flowers introduced me to John Boineau, a person who would have a powerful influence on me for the remainder of his life.

In 1967, the long-standing controversy regarding the anatomic–electrophysiologic basis of the WPW syndrome was seemingly solved when Boineau and Moore provided the most convincing evidence to date that Kent bundles were indeed responsible for the abnormal electrical activation in the WPW syndrome. They first performed detailed mapping of a dog with the WPW syndrome and then asked Duke's renowned cardiac pathologist Don Hackel to cross-section the atrioventricular (AV) groove serially in the general region of earliest ventricular activation. Hackel documented the presence of an anatomic accessory pathway (Kent bundle) that spanned the AV groove between the atrium and the ventricle at the precise anatomic site of ventricular preexcitation (Fig. 1.6). Although this laboratory observation was made in 1967, it was not published until 1970.[9] Nevertheless, it immediately convinced the EPs at Duke that accessory AV connections (aka, accessory pathways, or Kent bundles) were responsible for the WPW syndrome and suggested that the problem might be curable by surgical division.

In 1967, Howard Burchell of the Mayo Clinic successfully blocked conduction across an accessory pathway in a patient undergoing surgery for closure of an atrial septal defect by Dwight Magoon (Fig. 1.7).

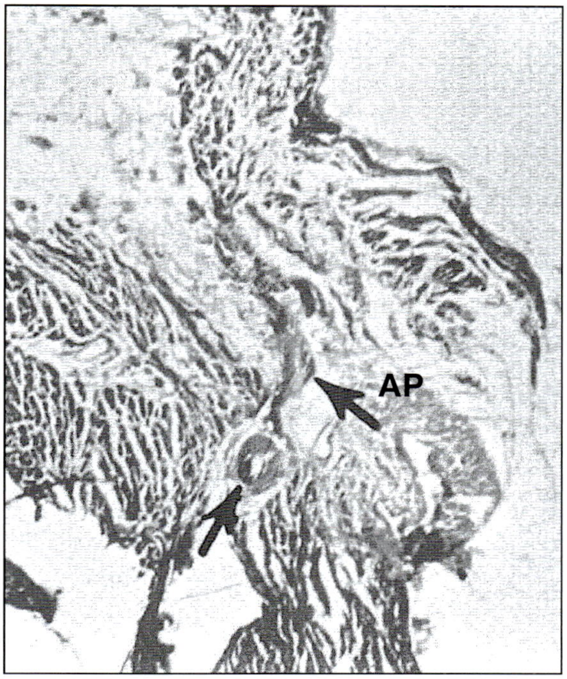

Fig. 1.6 The accessory pathway (AP) in a dog that was identified by John Boineau and Neil Moore in 1967 documenting that the Wolff-Parkinson-White syndrome was caused by these abnormal connections between the atrium and ventricle. (Reproduced from Boineau JP, Moore EN. Evidence for propagation of activation across an accessory atrioventricular connection in types A and B pre-excitation. *Circulation.* 1970:41(3):375–397.)

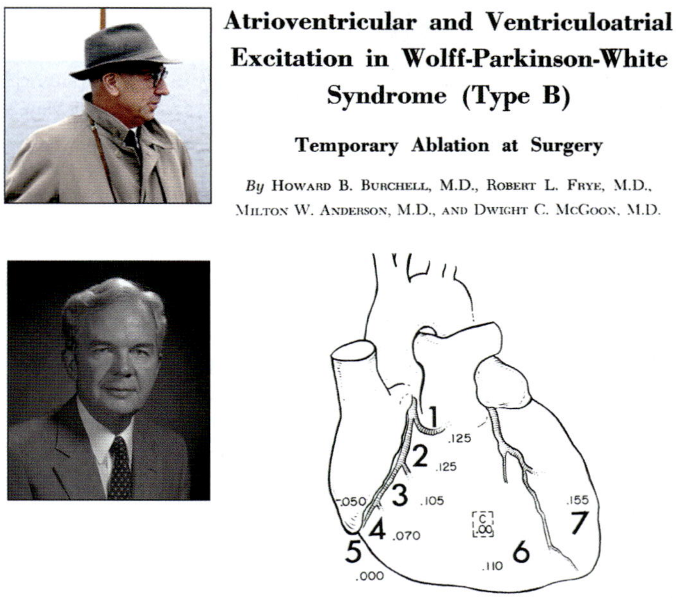

Fig. 1.7 Drs. Howard Burchell (top) and Dwight Magoon (bottom) of the Mayo Clinic were the first to temporarily block conduction across an accessory pathway in a patient with the Wolff-Parkinson-White syndrome in early 1968. The site of earliest ventricular and atrial preexcitation is on the right free-wall at the curvature of the right ventricle. See text for further description. (Reproduced from Burchell HB, Frye RL, Anderson MW, et al. Atrial-ventricular and ventricular-atrial excitation in Wolff-Parkinson-White syndrome (type B): temporary ablation at surgery. *Circulation.* 1976:36:663.)

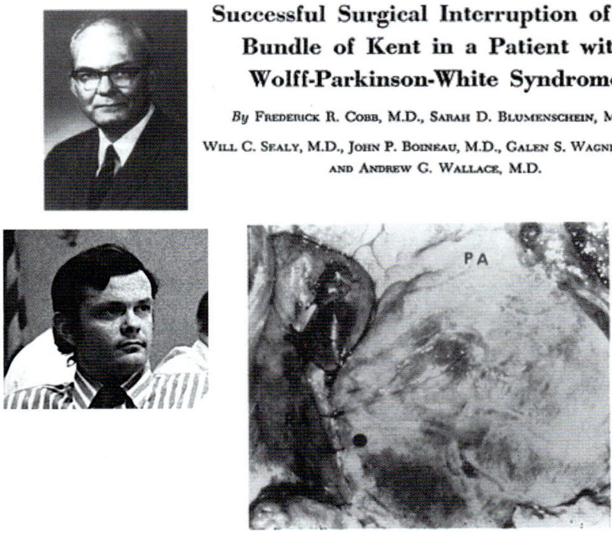

Fig. 1.8 John P. Boineau (bottom) and Will C. Sealy (top) of Duke University were the first to permanently block conduction across an accessory pathway on May 2, 1968. This successful operation initiated the era of surgery for cardiac arrhythmias. The right atrioventricular groove was dissected from the epicardial approach for approximately 1 cm on either side of the mapped location of the accessory pathway *(black dot)*. See text for further discussion.

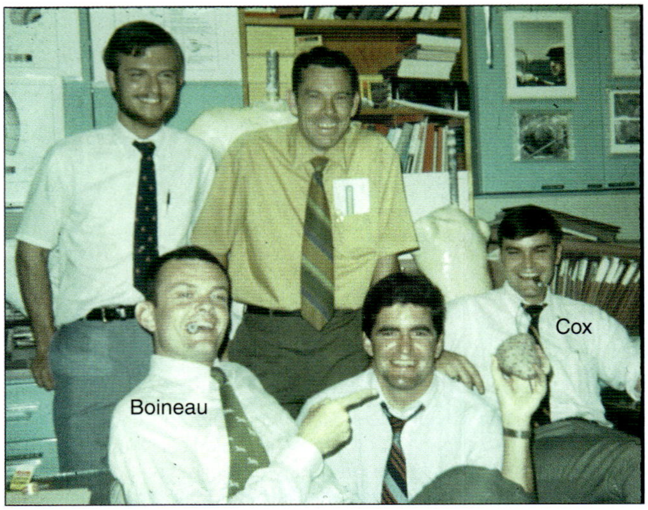

Fig. 1.9 John Boineau's electrophysiology laboratory crew at Duke University in 1969. Boineau and the author are identified. The man in the yellow shirt is Jack Kasell, who built all of the electrical stimulators, electrodes, and mapping devices used in the laboratory to study arrhythmias. The man kneeling in the center is Dr. Tom Daniel, who was also a Duke surgical resident several years senior to me in the program. Dr. Sabiston called us into his office one day and asked Tom if we wanted to be an "arrhythmia surgeon" in the future. Tom said he wasn't exactly sure what that meant, so he answered "no." Dr. Sabiston then asked me the same question and I answered "yes" even though the meaning of the designation "arrhythmia surgeon" was not clear to me either. Tom later became a highly respected professor of thoracic surgery at the University of Virginia.

The site of the accessory pathway in the AV groove of the right free wall was first identified by intraoperative mapping, and the AV groove was then injected with lidocaine at that site. The abnormal conduction across the accessory pathway abruptly stopped and did not return until several hours after surgery when the effects of the drug had abated.

Documentation of the anatomic-physiologic relationship between accessory AV connections and the WPW syndrome by Boineau and Moore,[9] coupled with the clinical experiment of Burchell and McGoon,[10] emboldened the involved parties at Duke University to attempt a surgical approach in a patient with the WPW syndrome. As a result, on May 2, 1968, with Drs. John Boineau performing the preliminary intraoperative mapping procedure, Dr. Will Sealy performed the first operation ever devised specifically for the treatment of a cardiac arrhythmia.[11] He divided the accessory pathway responsible for the WPW syndrome in a fisherman from the outer banks of North Carolina (Fig. 1.8). The fisherman lived for another 32 years and never again experienced a single episode of tachycardia.

Despite the success of this famous landmark surgical procedure, the second patient, on whom I was the third surgical assistant as a surgical intern at Duke, was not so fortunate. Her accessory pathway was located in an area that was later designated as the "anterior septal space," but at the time of her surgery the septum had not yet been recognized as a potential site of accessory pathways. Long hours of intraoperative mapping and surgical dissection resulted in her perioperative death, and a gloom settled over the entire concept of subjecting patients to such a risky surgical procedure to cure an elusive problem that was not life threatening.

THE MATURING OF CARDIAC ARRHYTHMIA SURGERY

I went to Duke in 1967 not because of my interest in electrophysiology but as a surgical intern interested in being trained as a cardiothoracic surgeon by David C. Sabiston, Jr. Nevertheless, having already spent 3 years during medical school in the electrophysiology research laboratory of Horan and Flowers in Memphis, I became involved rather early in my surgical residency with the electrophysiology pioneers at Duke who were quietly creating this new specialty of clinical electrophysiology. During my second year of surgical training, John Boineau came up to me in the surgical intensive care unit one day and asked if I was the same person who had worked with Horan and Flowers whom he had met at the AHA meeting in New York 2 years earlier. When I answered yes, he asked if I would consider working in his research laboratory, and thus began our lifelong association.

Boineau's laboratory (Fig. 1.9) was primarily focused on further elucidating the genesis of ischemic ventricular arrhythmias in the "ischemic border zone" surrounding acute myocardial infarctions,[12,13] the subject of my previous research with Horan and Flowers.[14,15] Also during that year, we continued to try to explain the vagaries and persistent mysteries of the WPW syndrome. Even though Boineau and Moore had already demonstrated the anatomic basis of the syndrome in its simplest form and Sealy had cured a patient with surgery based on that knowledge, the syndrome was still poorly understood. In fact, many authorities persisted in their belief that the WPW syndrome was caused by a phenomenon called "longitudinal dissociation in the His bundle." Thus, in the summer of 1969, the elucidation of the basis of the WPW syndrome with all its ramifications remained a challenge.

This problem was substantially clarified by two fortuitous events that occurred that year. First, Neil Moore, a PhD, DVM, and EP from the University of Pennsylvania, brought a huge black dog with a ventricular septal defect and the WPW syndrome down to Duke in the back of his station wagon one day so that he and Boineau could map its electrical abnormality. That study revealed for the first time that accessory pathways could occur in the *septum*, which was unknown at the time. It was an observation that many years later would be recognized by John Gallagher as the source of the problem that had occurred with Sealy's second patient who had died during surgery. In retrospect, she

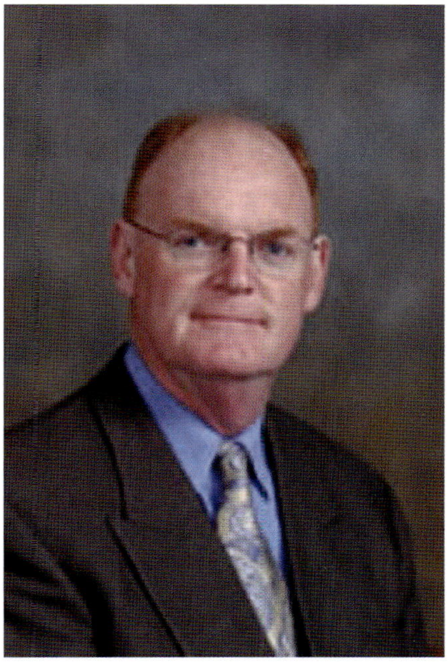

Fig. 1.10 John Gallagher, chief of clinical electrophysiology at Duke University from 1970 to 1983. It was primarily through his efforts, brilliance, and devotion that cardiac arrhythmia surgery eventually developed into an identifiable subspecialty of clinical medicine.

had an unrecognized anterior septal pathway that could simply not be reached surgically from the epicardial surface of the heart.

A few weeks later, Boineau received a call from Bowman-Gray Medical School at Wake Forest University in Winston-Salem, North Carolina, about one of the rhesus monkeys in their arteriosclerosis colony that had the pattern of the WPW syndrome on its ECG. The next day, Boineau and I drove to Winston-Salem, some 80 miles away, and transported the monkey back to his laboratory in Durham in the back seat of the car. We mapped the monkey extensively that very evening and Boineau finally deduced that the monkey had not one, but *two* accessory pathways. This finding, along with that from Neil Moore's dog, provided most of the final pieces of the puzzle of the WPW syndrome in humans.

In 1970, John Gallagher became the head of Duke's newly formed "Clinical Electrophysiology Service" (Fig. 1.10) as I was beginning a 2-year tour of active military duty in the US Army. Dr. Sealy was still working on developing surgical techniques for the different types of the WPW Syndrome. Unfortunately for me, Boineau left Duke for the University of Southern California during the 2 years that I was away from Duke on active duty in the Army. During the subsequent decade of the 1970s, while I was completing my residency in cardiothoracic surgery at Duke, Sealy and Gallagher continued to clarify the anatomic–electrophysiologic basis of WPW syndrome and its surgical treatment.

SURGERY FOR ALL CARDIAC ARRHYTHMIAS EXCEPT ATRIAL FIBRILLATION (NON–ATRIAL FIBRILLATION ARRHYTHMIAS)

Because of the enormous strides that were made in clinical electrophysiology from Durrer's first activation time mapping in 1957, through the seminal experimental observations of the 1960s, to the ability to cure the WPW syndrome surgically on a routine basis in the 1970s, the stage was set to develop surgical procedures that would cure all other clinical cardiac arrhythmias. The interest in surgery for cardiac arrhythmias shifted in the late 1970s from the WPW syndrome to ischemic ventricular tachycardia (VT) primarily because of the efforts in Paris of Dr. Gerard Guiraudon (surgeon) and Guy Fontaine (EP) (Fig. 1.11). Guiraudon visited Duke in 1976, and Drs. Sealy, John Gallagher, Guiraudon, and I had a memorable dinner one evening when we spent several hours cutting napkins into multiple patterns trying to create a way to treat ischemic VT. Shortly thereafter, Guiraudon and I performed an "encircling endocardial ventriculotomy" together in Paris for ischemic VT (Fig. 1.12). Almost simultaneously and totally independently, Drs. Alden Harken (surgeon) and Mark Josephson (EP) at the University of Pennsylvania (Fig. 1.13) performed a "subendocardial resection," which quickly became the procedure of choice for the surgical treatment of ischemic VT.

Also in 1978, I joined the surgical faculty at Duke, and during the next 5 years, I was privileged to have eight surgical research fellows from the Duke surgical residency program in my research laboratory for 2 to 3 years each (Fig. 1.14). In addition, many surgeons from other US institutions and from abroad joined us as surgical research fellows

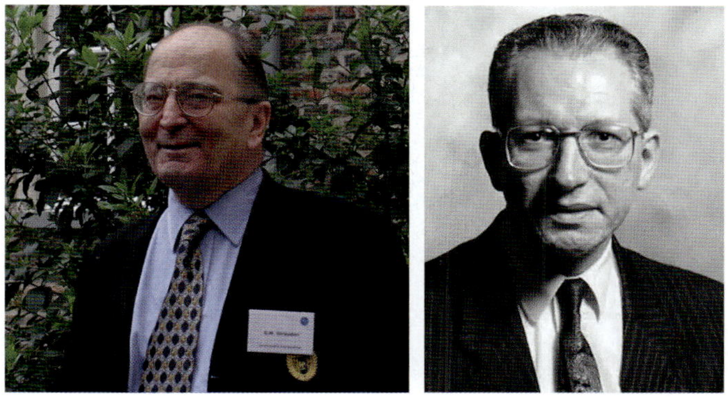

Fig. 1.11 Drs. Gerard Guiraudon (left) and Guy Fontaine (right) of Pitié Salpêtrière Hospital of the Sorbonne in Paris, two of the earliest pioneers in the surgical treatment of ischemic ventricular tachycardia (VT), who developed the encircling endocardial ventriculotomy. The procedure was soon abandoned because of the unacceptable operative mortality rate, but nevertheless, it contributed significantly to the understanding of ischemic VT and its surgical treatment. Fontaine was also the first to describe arrhythmogenic right ventricular dysplasia, a frequent cause of non-ischemic VT.

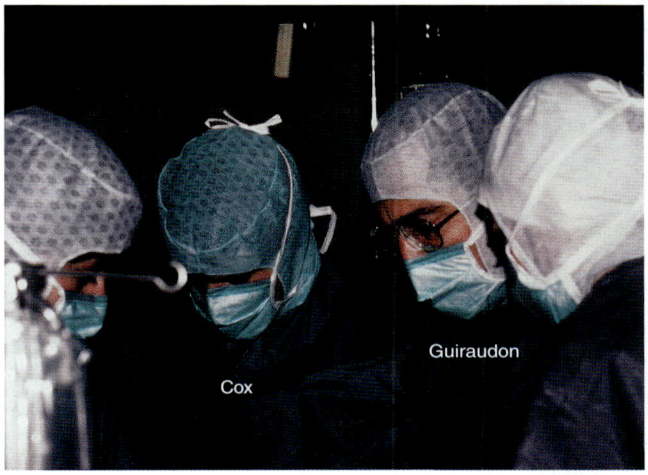

Fig. 1.12 Guiraudon and the author performing one of the earliest encircling endocardial ventriculotomies together in Paris on November 22, 1978. Both John Gallagher and Guy Fontaine were in the operating room with us and Gallagher took this photo during the operation. Photo by John J. Gallagher, MD.

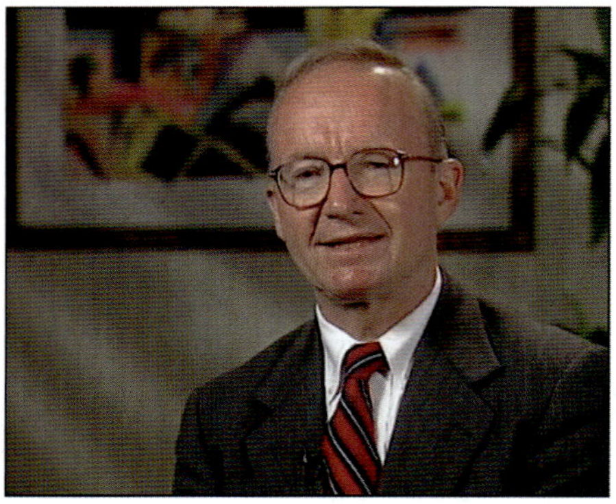
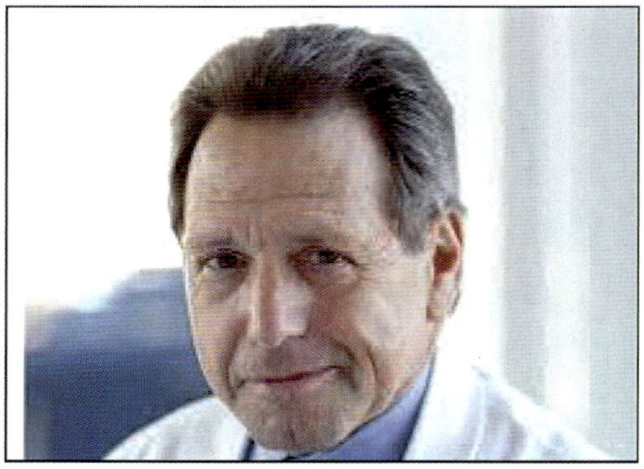

Fig. 1.13 Drs. Alden Harken (left) and Mark Josephson (right) of the University of Pennsylvania in Philadelphia were also two of the earliest pioneers in the surgical treatment of ischemic ventricular tachycardia. Completely independent of Guiraudon and Fontaine and nearly simultaneously, they developed the subendocardial resection procedure for ischemic ventricular tachycardia that became the standard of the industry during the late 1970s and early 1980s.

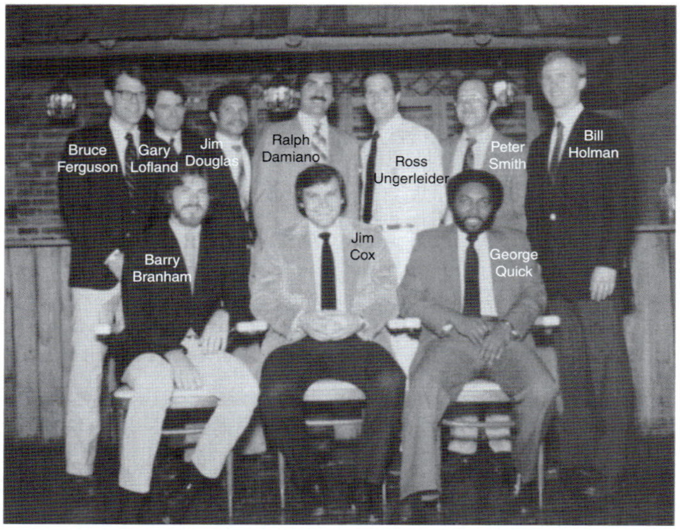

Fig. 1.14 Members of the Surgical Electrophysiology Laboratory at Duke University between 1978 and 1983.

for varying periods during that time (see Preface). These brilliant young investigators contributed to a veritable explosion of productivity in the field of cardiac arrhythmia surgery. In that 5-year period of time successful surgical procedures were developed for essentially all of the clinical arrhythmias except atrial fibrillation (AF). Indeed, by 1982, the armamentarium of cardiac surgeons included specifically designed and clinically successful surgical procedures for the following non-AF clinical arrhythmias:

1. Revised surgery for the WPW syndrome (Cox)[16,17]
2. Endocardial ablation procedures for ischemic VT
   - Encircling endocardial ventriculotomy (Giraudon)[18]
   - Subendocardial resection (Harken)[19]
   - Endocardial resection and cryoablation (Cox)[20–23]
3. Surgical isolation procedures for non-ischemic right ventricular tachycardias[24,25]
   - Idiopathic right VT (Cox)
   - Arrhythmogenic right ventricular dysplasia (Cox)
4. Left atrial isolation procedure for automatic left atrial tachycardia (Cox)[26]
5. Discrete cryosurgery procedure for AV node reentry tachycardia (Cox)[27–31]
6. Right atrial isolation for automatic right atrial tachycardias (Cox)[32,33]

INITIAL INABILITY TO ABLATE ATRIAL FIBRILLATION SURGICALLY

The lessons learned from surgery for the WPW syndrome and other non-AF arrhythmias provided a solid foundation for the development of successful surgery for AF. The first indication that we might be able to alter some of the detrimental effects of AF by surgery came with the development of the left atrial isolation procedure (see Chapter 9). Surgical isolation of the left atrium (LA) confined AF to the LA and allowed the remainder of the heart to remain in sinus rhythm. However, the left atrial isolation procedure was developed specifically for the treatment of patients with automatic LA tachycardias, so we never considered it to be a viable method for treating AF because left-sided AV synchrony was not restored and the problem of systemic thromboembolism remained.

The first step toward developing a way to ablate AF surgically was to create a realistic experimental model of AF. At the time, experimental models of AF had little or no relevance to the clinical arrhythmia. We decided to create mitral insufficiency in dogs by cutting the chordae tendineae of the mitral valve, but we needed to do it without opening the pericardium to avoid pericardial inflammation and adhesions that might irritate the atria and mislead us regarding the electrophysiology of "naturally occurring" AF. In addition, we knew that we must avoid placing any lesions in the atrium that could leave atrial scars that might cause areas of abnormal conduction block, thereby disrupting the spontaneous electrical patterns during AF. I assigned the task of developing a more clinically applicable animal model of AF to a young Duke surgical resident, Peter Smith, who began a 3-year tenure in our research laboratory in the summer of 1980. Years later, Dr. Smith would serve as the chief of cardiac surgery at Duke for more than 2 decades. His solution was elegant simplicity and is described in Chapter 5, Figure 5.2.

Just as we were beginning to use this animal model at Duke in 1983, I moved to Washington University in St. Louis. In 1984, John Boineau joined us in St. Louis and brought Richard (Rick) Schuessler, a brilliant biomedical engineer who had worked with Boineau for several years at the Medical College of Georgia (Fig. 1.15). By that time, we had finally begun using our animal model of AF routinely, but we still lacked a multipoint mapping system that would allow us to study AF in detail. As a result, we tried numerous surgical procedures by trial and error in an attempt to disrupt AF in the animal model; these procedures are described in Chapter 11, Figure 11.8. By 1985, Boineau and Schuessler had developed a system to map AF experimentally, but we were still limited to trial-and error surgical procedures because the electrophysiology of AF remained unclear. By 1986 these procedures culminated in the

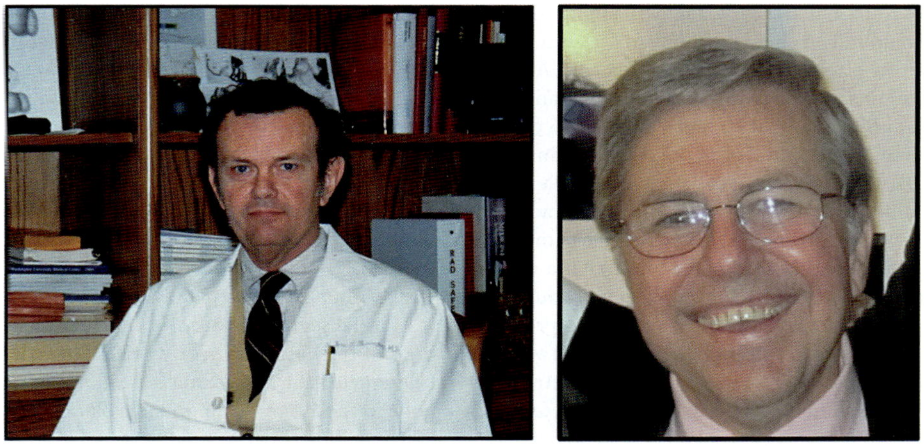

Fig. 1.15 Drs. John P. Boineau (left) and Richard (Rick) Schuessler (right), who directed the Cardiothoracic Surgery Research Laboratories at Washington University in St. Louis between 1984 and 2021. They led the development of the experimental, three-dimensional, multipoint computerized mapping systems that ultimately resulted in the concept of the Maze procedure for the treatment of patients with atrial fibrillation.

so-called "atrial transsection procedure" (see Chapter 11, Figure 11.10), which proved to be 100% successful in ablating AF in our animal model.

That summer, I received a call from an airline pilot in Cypress, Captain George Dheere. He was 37 years old and was in line to become the chief pilot for Cypress Airways. Unfortunately, Captain Dheere had recently experienced a transient ischemic attack (TIA) during which he lost use of his left arm and one side of his face. The TIA lasted for 4 hours and then spontaneously resolved. He was evaluated and found to have AF for which he was immediately anticoagulated and grounded from flying.

Captain Dheere had read a rather obscure book chapter that I had written in the early 1980s on the surgical treatment of AF in which I described eliminating AF in selected patients with WPW syndrome by surgical ablation of the WPW rather than by directly attacking the AF itself. The chapter was published in a book of the proceedings of The Midnight Sun Symposium on Atrial Fibrillation held in Kiruna, Sweden, in June 1981.[34] Probably because of its somewhat misleading title, Captain Dheere misunderstood the gist of the chapter and was insistent that he wanted to have surgery for his AF because he had already failed all medical therapy, including amiodarone. The problem was that he did not have the WPW syndrome or any other "arrhythmia trigger" causing his AF that we could actually treat surgically. I told him we had nothing to offer him specifically for the treatment of his AF, but he flew to St. Louis from Cypress 2 days later anyway. After a few days in St. Louis, he finally accepted the fact that although we were working on some possibilities, it was premature to try anything clinically at that point, so he returned to Cypress quite disgruntled.

After calling various members of our team for progress reports on a weekly basis for the next few months, Captain Dheere returned to St. Louis uninvited, insisting that we had to do something to stop his AF, or he simply was not going to leave. After several days of deliberation with Boineau, Schuessler, and our clinical electrophysiology colleagues Michael Cain and Bruce Lindsay (Fig. 1.16), we secured permission from the investigational review board (IRB) at Barnes Hospital for a "one-time" atrial transection procedure. As mentioned, the procedure was based on what we knew about the electrophysiology of AF at that time and that it had proven to be quite successful in our animal model. Thus, I rather reluctantly performed the atrial transection procedure for AF on Captain Dheere in September 1986. This was the first procedure ever developed specifically to *ablate* AF rather than to *isolate* its detrimental effects. Captain Dheere remained in sinus rhythm on no antiarrhythmic medication for 5 months when AF recurred during a flu-like episode complicated by pericarditis.

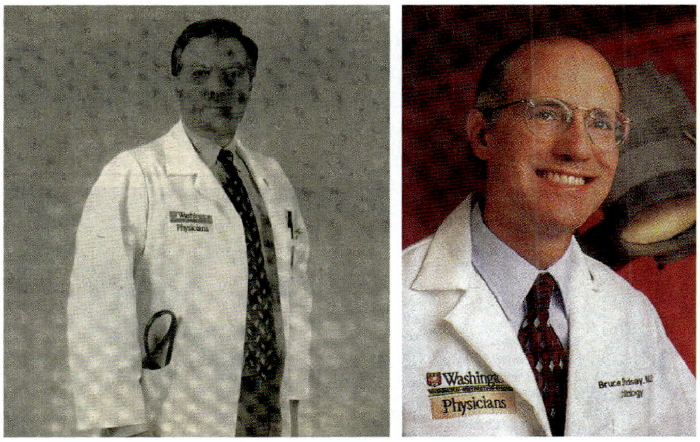

Fig. 1.16 Drs. Michael E. Cain (left) and Bruce D. Lindsay (right), the clinical electrophysiologists at Washington University in St. Louis who provided the clinical expertise that played a large role in the success of the Maze procedure for atrial fibrillation. They also did all of the postoperative follow-up and testing of the patients who underwent the Maze procedures.

CONCEPTION AND DEVELOPMENT OF THE MAZE PROCEDURE FOR ATRIAL FIBRILLATION

During the following months, Boineau and Schuessler continued to map AF in our experimental animal model using an array of more than 250 bipolar atrial electrodes and the computer programs developed by Barry Branham. Concurrently, we continued to map AF in patients undergoing surgery for WPW syndrome with the support of Michael Cain, Bruce Lindsay, and Peter Corr. Although the data were still incomplete, it became clear that when an episode of AF had been established, it was characterized by the simultaneous presence of multiple (at least two) large macro-reentrant circuits in the atria. Much to our disappointment, the maps also showed that the macro-reentrant circuits frequently changed anatomic locations, often remaining in one location for only 200 ms, making it impossible to ablate AF by "chasing" the individual reentrant circuits that were sustaining the AF episodes. This meant that unlike surgery for all other cardiac arrhythmias, *electrical mapping could not be used to guide the placement of atrial lesions for the treatment of patients with AF.* Even if we had enjoyed access to real-time atrial maps, which did not exist at the time, we realized that the constantly changing characteristics of sustained AF would still preclude the ability to use even those maps of the future to guide the placement of lesions to ablate the AF.

The macro-reentrant circuits that we mapped in both dogs and patients were physically relatively large, that is, more than 5 to 6 cm in diameter in the LA and even larger than that in the right atrium (RA; see Chapter 4, Figure 4.15). Therefore, atrial incisions placed no more than 5 to 6 cm apart should theoretically prevent the development of macro-reentrant circuits *anywhere* in the atria. It was clear that if macro-reentrant circuits could not develop in the atria, then the atria could not fibrillate. One way of preventing atrial macro-reentry would be to "bread-loaf" the heart with lesions placed close enough to prevent the development of the large macro-reentrant circuits, but that would destroy the very purpose of the atria by rendering them electrically inactive postoperatively. The dilemma was how to place enough lesions in the atria to preclude the development of atrial macro-reentry (fibrillation) and leave behind an atrium that could still be activated by the sinus node and that could still function effectively.

To take the next step, it seemed to me that we needed to assimilate all of this information into a workable concept by illustrating the relationship between atrial anatomy and the electrophysiology of AF in a more simplistic manner. Therefore, I created a series of cartoonish diagrams to include both anatomy and electrophysiology (Fig. 1.17) to better visualize the possibilities of some type of surgical ablation procedure for AF, which is described in detail in Chapter 5. While focusing on one of these simplistic anatomic–electrophysiologic cartoons for several long minutes one Saturday afternoon in early 1987, it suddenly occurred to me that if atrial lesions were placed in the pattern of a maze, they should still prevent atrial macro-reentry as effectively as "bread-loafing" but it would leave the atria capable of being activated by a sinus impulse afterwards.

Although this looked simple enough on a two-dimensional cartoon drawing of the atria, it was clear that I needed to transfer the maze concept to a three-dimensional (3D) atrium if it were to be of any value. Unfortunately in those days, we did not have the immediate and ubiquitous ability to construct 3D images of the atria as we do today. However, I remembered that John Boineau had several canine hearts stored in formaldehyde in our research laboratory, so I went to our laboratory and dissected several complete atrial blocks (RA, atrial septum, and LA) completely away from the remaining portions of the heart and great vessels. After drying the atria thoroughly, I designated the approximate location of the anatomic sinoatrial (SA) node in the RA by placing a large black dot at its usual site with a large felt-tipped marking pen. I then partially "enclosed" this SA node site on three sides by drawing black lines on the RA to simulate the locations of potential incisions (i.e., permanent lines of conduction block). By leaving one side of the three-sided "enclosure" around the SA node open, any subsequent sinus-generated impulse would have to exit the region of the SA node in only one direction (i.e., through the open side of the "enclosure"). I then placed subsequent black lines sequentially throughout both atria to "guide" the propagation of a postoperative sinus-generated wavefront to all of the atrial myocardium except the isolated pulmonary veins and the excised atrial appendages. After the pattern was completed, I confirmed visually that the impulse could not circle back on itself, thereby creating one large macro-reentrant

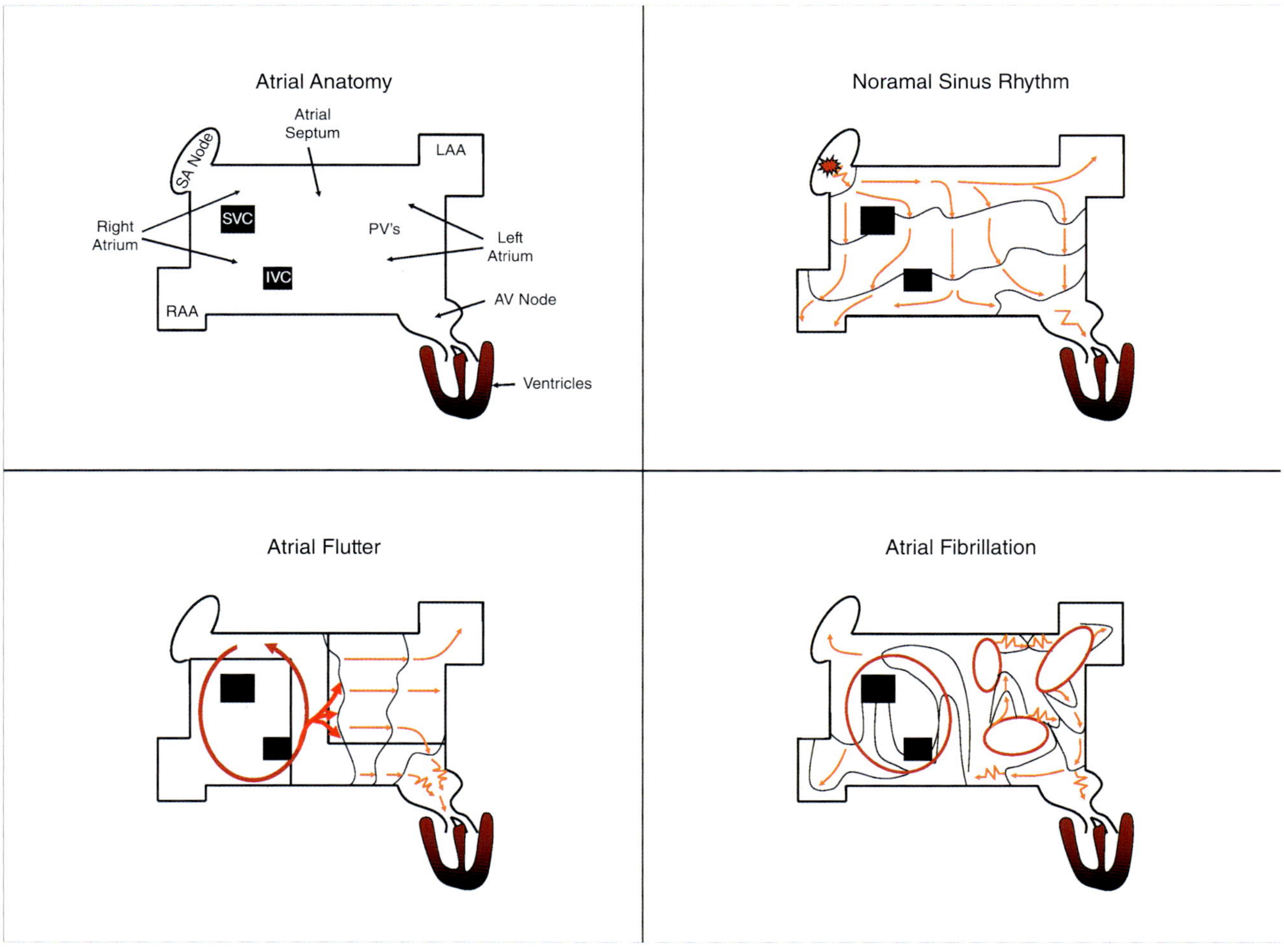

Fig. 1.17 Simple anatomic–electrophysiologic diagrams used in the conceptional development of the Maze procedure. See text and Chapter 5 for further discussion.

circuit. Obviously, care was also taken to avoid creating any lesions that might prevent the sinus-generated wavefront from reaching the AV Node so that normal AV synchrony could be preserved. Thus, there was one contiguous "true route" of conduction between the entrance (SA node) and exit (AV node) sites of the atria and multiple "blind alleys" off this main conduction route that allowed activation of all of the atrial myocardium, thereby preserving atrial contractility. One entrance, one exit, one true route between the two, with multiple blind alleys along the way . . . the pattern and principle of a maze.

The atrial block with its black marker lines was then used as a guide for the creation of the same maze pattern of incisions in a freshly excised canine heart. After closing the incisions with running sutures, the heart was fixed in formaldehyde and used thereafter as a visual guide for the performance of this new "Maze procedure" in live animals (Fig. 1.18). A number of these procedures were performed in normal animals to establish the optimal sequence of lesion placement and the general conduct of this new, rather complex surgical procedure. The Maze procedure was subsequently performed in our animal models and was 100% successful in ablating AF. Long-term experimental studies proved that it was safe and that the atria still functioned after the procedure (Fig. 1.19 and Video 1.1).

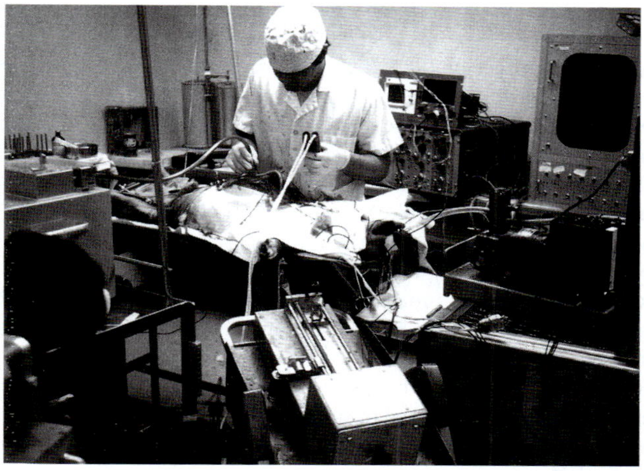

Fig. 1.18 The author performing the first experimental Maze procedure in the Cardiothoracic Surgery Research Laboratory at Washington University in early 1987. Photo taken by research fellow Byung-Chul Chang, who later became the chief of cardiac surgery at Yonsei University in Seoul, Korea.

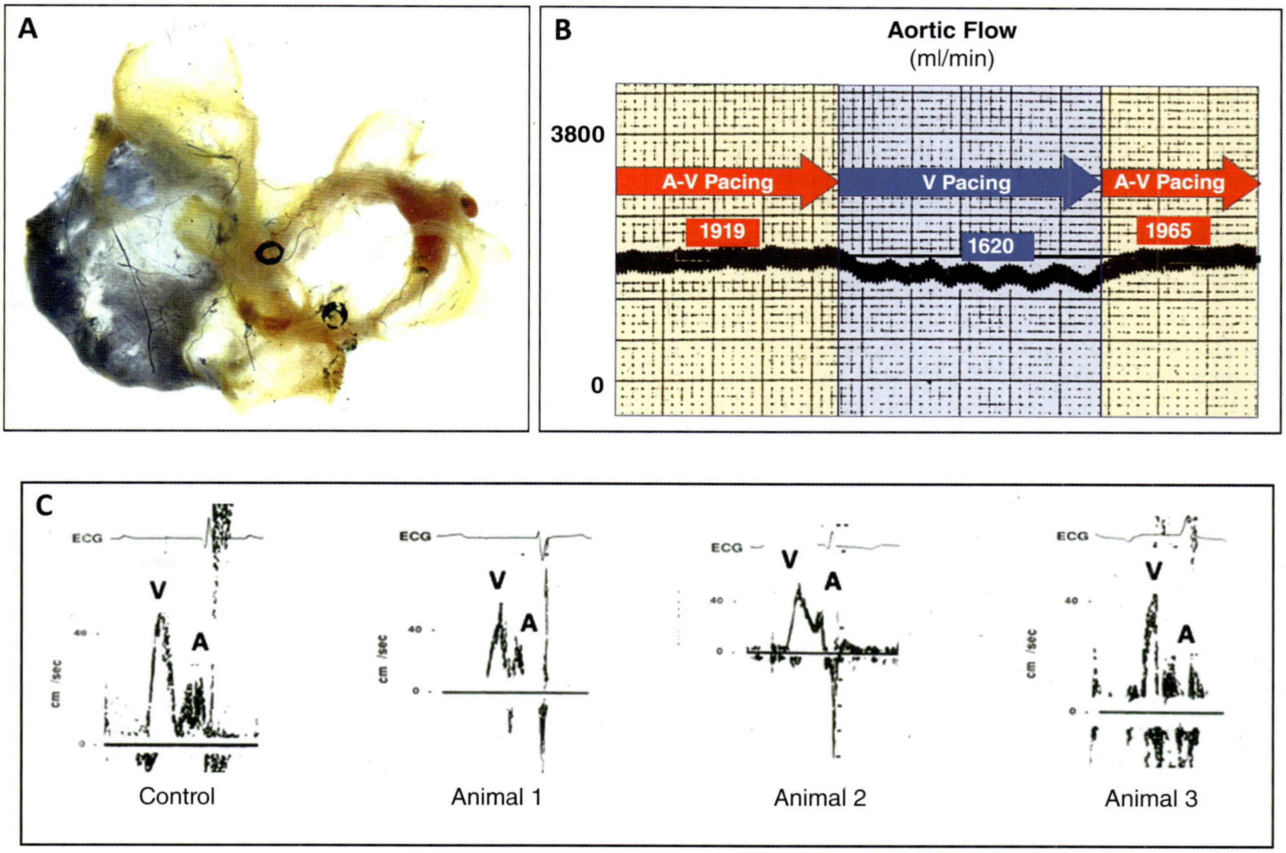

Fig. 1.19 Extensive evaluation of the safety and results of the Maze procedure was done for months before it was first applied clinically. This shows some examples of the type of experimental evaluations that were performed. (A) To be certain that the Maze procedure did not devascularize the atria, the right coronary artery was injected with blue dye and the left coronary artery with red dye following each experimental Maze in dogs. This photo documents that the Maze procedure did not cause atrial ischemia. Histologic studies confirmed this finding as well. (B) Postoperative function of the atria after an experimental Maze procedure. During A-V sequential pacing (when atrial contraction is present), the cardiac output (aortic flow measured with an electromagnetic flow meter) was higher than when the atria were not contributing during V-pacing only. The only way this can happen is if the atria are functioning. (C) Postoperative cardiac echocardiography of the mitral valve showing the presence of an "a-wave" in every animal. This indicated that the left atrium was still functioning after an experimental Maze procedure.

THE FIRST MAZE PROCEDURE

In the late summer of 1987, a cardiologist from Alton, Illinois, near St. Louis called about his cousin who had severe atrial flutter and AF. He had failed all medical therapy including amiodarone. After a long, detailed workup and several intense discussions, the Barnes Hospital IRB again approved a "one-time" trial of the Maze procedure, so we performed the first clinical Maze procedure on September 25, 1987. The patient remained in sinus rhythm until the seventh postoperative day when, much to my dismay, he developed postoperative AF. We instituted digoxin and procainamide (remember, this was 1987!), and the AF quickly converted to sinus rhythm. One month after hospital discharge, the patient presented with a severe case of procainamide-induced lupus syndrome, so the procainamide was discontinued. During the next month, he remained in sinus rhythm, and his lupus syndrome disappeared. Digoxin was then discontinued, and he remained in sinus rhythm at his 3-month postoperative evaluation. At his 3-month return outpatient visit, the eminent AF expert Prof. Maurits Allessie, a colleague of Prof. Hein Wellens at the University of Limburg in Maastricht, the Netherlands, happened to be visiting our institution, and I asked him to examine the patient with Bruce Lindsay and me. Professor Allessie was quite surprised to learn that the patient had undergone an operation for AF 3 months before, and he was even more surprised that the patient was now in normal sinus rhythm and on no antiarrhythmic drugs or anticoagulants. The patient had no further episodes of atrial flutter or AF, was not anticoagulated, and took no antiarrhythmic drugs. Six months after the Maze procedure, he underwent a complete endocardial electrophysiology study by Lindsay, including a full programmed electrical stimulation protocol and burst-pacing protocol with and without intravenous isoproterenol, but neither atrial flutter nor AF could be induced.

Interestingly, the first patient to receive a Maze procedure remained arrhythmia free for 19 years, 11 months, and 1 week on no antiarrhythmia drugs and no anticoagulation. On the 20th anniversary of the first Maze procedure, September 25, 2007, Rick Schuessler called to remind me of the Maze procedure's important anniversary and to tell me that the first patient to receive a Maze procedure had experienced a recurrence of his AF for the first time only 3 weeks earlier. Fortunately, this recurrence was controlled with routine antiarrhythmic drugs, but it would have been more satisfying for both of us had the patient chosen to wait for at least another 3 weeks to have his recurrence!

Having maintained weekly telephone contact with my office and directly with the first Maze patient himself during late 1987, Captain Dheere knew exactly what was unfolding in St. Louis. Thus, after a few months, he insisted on having his previous atrial transection procedure "converted" to a Maze procedure. Thus, 5 months after the first Maze procedure, we performed the "conversion" from an atrial transection procedure to a Maze procedure on Captain Dheere in February 1988. This conversion resulted in a pattern of combined atrial lesions that was very similar to the pattern that we would later call the "Maze-III" procedure.

Unfortunately, on the eighth postoperative day, Captain Dheere developed intractable atrial flutter, which we dubbed "atypical left atrial flutter" at that time but is now called "peri-mitral flutter." To our knowledge, this was the first ever occurrence of peri-mitral flutter since it is an iatrogenic arrhythmia resulting from successful isolation of the pulmonary veins and posterior walll of the LA (box lesion). Captain Dheere remained in peri-mitral flutter, which was even more symptomatic than his AF had been, until September 7, 1988. We interpreted the presence and persistence of Captain Dheere's atypical left atrial flutter to mean that the cryolesion that had been placed on the coronary sinus at the time of his second surgery had failed. This was before the availability of radiofrequency catheter ablation, so we used catheter fulguration and chose to interrupt the circuit at a narrow site of conduction just beneath the atrial septal lesion.

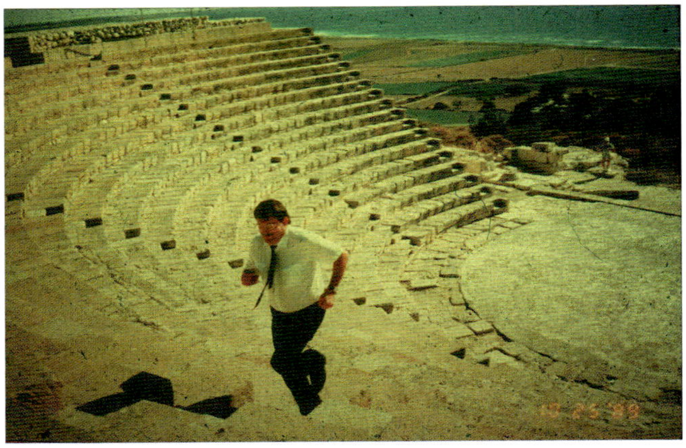

Fig. 1.20 Photo of Captain George Dheere taken by the author on October 25, 1989, which was 1 year and 8 months after his conversion from an atrial transection procedure to a Maze procedure, the second Maze procedure ever performed. We were initially standing on the floor of the Kourion Ancient Amphitheater near Limassol on the southern coast of Cyprus when he suddenly challenged me to a "race" to the top of the steps. I refused the race but climbed the stairs so I could take this photo of him as he ran up the steps.

Captain Dheere remained free of all atrial arrhythmias afterward on no antiarrhythmic drugs or anticoagulation. In addition, he ultimately was reinstated as a commercial airline pilot with his beloved Cypress Airways (Fig. 1.20). One of my saddest days occurred in the summer of 2003 when I was called by one of Captain Dheere's daughters in Cyprus and told that he had died suddenly of a heart attack. I have often said that without the courage and persistence of Captain Dheere, the development of the Maze procedure would have been delayed by at least 10 years and perhaps would never have occurred at all.

Because of the early recurrences and late successes in our first two patients, we waited approximately 6 months before performing the third Maze procedure. When the third patient had recovered from surgery and again proved to be a success, the fourth was done 6 months later, and so on. By early 1990, we had performed a total of 7 Maze procedures, each done under a separate "one-time" IRB approval. We submitted our work to the *Journal of Thoracic and Cardiovascular Surgery* in the form of four individual but "packaged" papers. The four papers were sent to 11 different reviewers, who returned a total of 44 reviews! After collating and answering these reviews, the editor, Dr. John Kirklin, requested a personal meeting with me to review our concepts, experimental studies, and clinical experience. He made several invaluable suggestions that were heeded and in 1991, the Maze procedure was introduced into the surgical literature.[35–39]

The evolution of the surgical treatment of AF from the original Maze procedure (Maze-I) to the present time is described in detail in subsequent chapters of this book.

REFERENCES

1. Wolff L, Parkinson J, White PD. Bundle branch block with short PR interval in healthy young people prone to paroxysmal tachycardia. *Am. Heart J.* 1930;5:685.
2. Kent AFS. Researches on structure and function of mammalian heart. *J. Physiol.* 1893;14:233.

3. Rothberger CJ, Winterberg H. Studien uber die bestimmung des ausgangspunktes ventrikularer extrasystolen mit hilfe des elektrokardiogramms. *Pflugers Arch Physiol.* 1913;154:571–598.
4. Lewis T, Rothschild MA. The excitatory process in the dog's heart. II. The ventricles. *London Philos Trans R Soc.* 1915;206:181.
5. Scher AM, Young AC, Malmgren AL, Paton RR. Spread of electrical activity through the wall of the ventricle. *Circ. Res.* 1953;6:539.
6. Durrer D, Roos JP. Epicardial excitation of the ventricles in a patient with Wolff-Parkinson-White syndrome (type B). *Circulation.* 1967;35:15.
7. Brugada P, Wellens HJJ. *Preface to Cardiac Arrhythmias: Where to Go From Here?.* Futura Publishing Company; 1987 (Eds.).
8. Cox JL, McLaughlin VW, Flowers NC, Horan LG. Changes in cellular dehydrogenase enzymes in acute myocardial infarction. *Circulation.* 1966;34:III–80.
9. Boineau JP, Moore EN. Evidence for propagation of activation across an accessory atrioventricular connection in types A and B pre-excitation. *Circulation.* 1970;41(3):375–397.
10. Burchell HB, Frye RL, Anderson MW, et al. Atrial-ventricular and ventricular-atrial excitation inWolff-Parkinson-White syndrome (type B): temporary ablation at surgery. *Circulation.* 1967;36:663.
11. Cobb FR, Blumenschein SD, Sealy WC, Boineau JP, Wagner GS, Wallace AG. Successful surgical interruption of the bundle of Kent in a patient with Wolff-Parkinson-White syndrome. *Circulation.* 1968;38:1018.
12. Boineau JP, Cox JL. Slow ventricular activation in acute myocardial infarction—a source of re-entrant premature ventricular contractions. *Circulation.* 1973;48:702–713.
13. Cox JL, Daniel TM, Boineau JP. The electrophysiologic time-course of acute myocardial ischemia and the effects of early coronary artery reperfusion. *Circulation.* 1973;48:971–983.
14. Cox JL, McLaughlin VW, Flowers NC, Horan LG. The ischemic zone surrounding acute myocardial infarction. Its morphology as detected by dehydrogenase staining. *Am Heart J.* 1968;76:650.
15. Citation Classic™Cox JL, McLaughlin VW, Flowers NC, Horan LG. The ischemic zone surrounding acute myocardial infarction. Its morphology as detected by dehydrogenase staining. *Am Heart J.* 1968;76:6509. *Curr Contents,* 12(16), 1984.
16. Edited by Gallagher JJ, Sealy WC, Cox JL, et al. Results of surgery for pre-excitation caused by accessory atrioventricular pathways in 267 consecutive cases. In: Josephson ME, Wellens HJJ, eds. *Tachycardias: Mechanisms, Diagnosis, and Treatment.* Lea & Febiger; 1984:259–269.
17. Cox JL, Gallagher JJ, Cain ME. Experience with 118 consecutive patients undergoing surgery for the WolffParkinsonWhite syndrome. *J Thorac Cardiovasc Surg.* 1985;90:490–501.
18. Guiraudon G, Fontaine G, Frank R, Escande G, Etievent P, Cabrol C. Encircling endocardial ventriculotomy: a new surgical treatment for life-threatening ventricular tachycardias resistant to medical treatment following myocardial infarction. *Ann Thor Surg.* 1978;26(5):438–444.
19. Miller JM, Kienzie MG, Harken AH. Josephson ME: Subendocardial resection for ventricular tachycardia: predictors of surgical success. *Circulation.* 1984;70(4):624–631.
20. Gallagher JJ, Cox JL. Status of surgery for ventricular arrhythmias. *Circulation.* 1979;60:1440.
21. Cox JL, Gallagher JJ, Ungerleider RM. Encircling endocardial ventriculotomy (EEV) for refractory ischemic ventricular tachycardia: IV: clinical indications, surgical technique, mechanism of action, and results. *J Thorac Cardiovasc Surg.* 1982;83:865–872.
22. Boineau JP, Cox JL. Rationale for a direct surgical approach to control ventricular arrhythmias: relation of specific intraoperative techniques to mechanism and location of arrhythmic circuit. *Am J Cardiol.* 1983;198:119–129.
23. Cox JL. Treatment of ventricular arrhythmias: surgery. In: Steinbach K, ed. *Proceedings of the VIIth World Symposium on Cardiac Pacing.* Steinkopff Verlag Darmstadt; 1983:909–919.
24. Cox JL, Bardy GH, Damiano RJ, et al. Right ventricular isolation procedures for n on-ischemic ventricular tachycardia. *J Thorac Cardiovasc Surg.* 1985;90:212.
25. Cox JL. Surgical treatment of ischemic and non-ischemic ventricular tachyarrhythmias. In: Cohn LH, ed. Futura Publ. Co.; 1985. *Modern Technics in Surgery.* 118.
26. Williams JM, Ungerleider RM, Lofland GK, Cox JL. Left atrial isolation: new technique for the treatment of supraventricular arrhythmias. *J Thorac Cardiovasc Surg.* 1980;80:373.
27. Holman WL, Ikeshita M, Lease JG, Smith PK, Ferguson Jr TB, Cox JL. Elective prolongation of atrioventricular conduction by multiple discrete cryolesions: a new technique for the treatment of paroxysmal supraventricular tachycardia. *J Thorac Cardiovasc Surg.* 1982;84:554.
28. Holman WL, Ikeshita M, Lease JG, Ferguson Jr TB, Lofland GK, Cox JL. Alteration of antegrade atrioventricular conduction by cryoablation of peri-atrioventricular nodal tissue. implications for the surgical treatment of AV node reentry tachycardia. *J Thorac Cardiovasc Surg.* 1984;88:67–75.
29. Holman WL, Ikeshita M, Lease JG, Smith PK, Lofland GK, Cox JL. Cryosurgical modification of retrograde atrioventricular conduction: implications for the surgical treatment of A-V node reentry tachycardia. *J Thorac Cardiovasc Surg.* 1986;91:826–834.
30. Cox JL, Holman WL, Cain ME. Cryosurgical treatment of atrioventricular node reentry tachycardia. *Circulation.* 1987;76:1329–1336.
31. Cox JL. Surgery for cardiac arrhythmias. Current Problems in CardiologyVIII. Yearbook Medical Publishers; 1983.
32. Harada A, D'Agostino Jr HJ, Boineau JP, Cox JL. Right atrial isolation: a new surgical treatment for supraventricular tachycardia. I. Surgical technique and electrophysiologic effects. *J Thorac Cardiovasc Surg.* 1988;95:643–650.
33. Harada A, D'Agostino Jr HJ, Boineau JP, Cox JL. Right atrial isolation: a new surgical treatment for supraventricular tachycardia. II: hemodynamic effects. *J Thorac Cardiovasc Surg.* 1988;95:651–657.
34. Cox JL, Williams JM, Smith PK, Sabiston Jr DC. Surgical management of atrial fibrillation. In: Kulbertus HE, Olsson SB, Schlepper M, eds. *Atrial Fibrillation.* AB Hassle Publ. Co.; 1982:321–335.
35. Cox JL, Schuessler RB, Boineau JP. The surgical treatment of atrial fibrillation: I. Summary of the current concepts of the mechanisms of atrial flutter and atrial fibrillation. *J Thorac Cardiovasc Surg.* 1991;101:402–405.
36. Cox JL, Canavan TE, Schuessler RB, et al. The surgical treatment of atrial fibrillation: II. Intraoperative electrophysiologic mapping and description of the electrophysiologic basis of atrial flutter and atrial fibrillation. *J Thorac Cardiovasc Surg.* 1991;101:406–426.
37. Cox JL, Schuessler RB, D'Agostino Jr HJ, et al. The surgical treatment of atrial fibrillation: III. Development of a definitive surgical procedure. *J Thorac Cardiovasc Surg.* 1991;101:569–583.
38. Cox JL. The surgical treatment of atrial fibrillation: IV. Surgical technique. *J Thorac Cardiovasc Surg.* 1991;101:584–592.
39. Cox JL. The first Maze procedure. *J Thorac Cardiovasc Surg.* 2011;141(5):1093–1097.

2

Epidemiology and Economics of Atrial Fibrillation

James L. Cox, S. Chris Malaisrie

CHAPTER OUTLINE

PREVALENCE AND INCIDENCE OF ATRIAL FIBRILLATION

Determination of the prevalence of atrial fibrillation (AF) in a given population depends on cohort selection and the methods used for the identification and validation of AF. The US Census Bureau states that in 2010, the population of the United States was 309 million people,[1] and 5.2 million of them were estimated to have AF.[2] This suggests a prevalence of AF in the general population of 1.7%. By 2020, the population of the United States had increased to 329.5 million.[1] At a prevalence of 1.7%, this would suggest that in 2020, approximately 5.6 million people in the United States had AF. In 2020, the global population was 7.8 billion people,[3] and 50 million were estimated to have AF (Fig. 2.1).[4] This suggests a prevalence of AF in the world's population of 0.6%. These ranges of data are consistent with historical estimates and provide a basis for the general "rule of thumb" that at least 1% of any general population can be expected to have AF.

In 2010, the incidence of newly diagnosed AF was estimated to be 1.2 million per year in the United States.[2] The lifetime risks of AF are 1 in 3 among Whites, 1 in 5 among Blacks, and 1 in 7 among Asians.[5,6] Asian males had a higher lifetime risk of AF than Asian females (16.9% versus 14.6%, respectively),[6] but a European study showed that differences in AF incidence observed by sex may be explained by a sex-specific distribution of risk factors.[7] The incidence of AF has remained

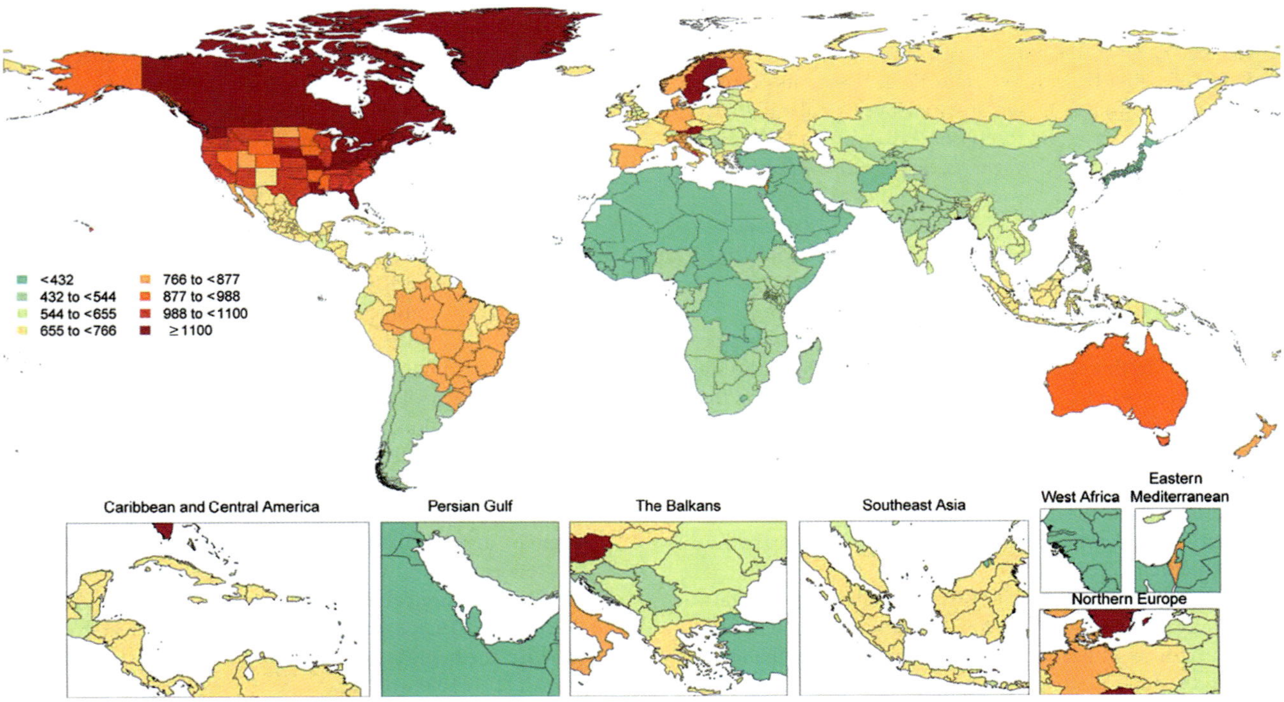

Fig. 2.1 Age-standardized global prevalence of AF and atrial flutter per 100,000 distributed by country. (Source: Institute for Health Metrics and Evaluation. Used with permission. All rights reserved).

relatively stable over time, contributing to a tripling of AF prevalence over the past 50 years.[8] Projections for the next 50 years indicate that AF prevalence will double in the United States by 2050, with nearly 16 million US citizens having AF (Fig. 2.2).[9,10] It is also predicted that by 2060, nearly 18 million people in the European Union will have AF (Fig. 2.3).[11,12]

The onset of AF can be accompanied by the sensation of palpitations, diaphoresis, shortness of breath, dyspnea on exertion, fatigue, malaise, worsening heart failure, or exacerbation of angina pectoris. Although these symptoms range from being only troublesome in some patients to being debilitating in others, AF can also be asymptomatic, leaving patients completely unaware that they have AF even over a period of years. In cardiac surgery patients, the cause of AF is usually left-heart disease, including mitral valve, aortic valve, and/or coronary artery disease, as well as systemic hypertension and/or left ventricular (LV) failure. However, in asymptomatic patients without

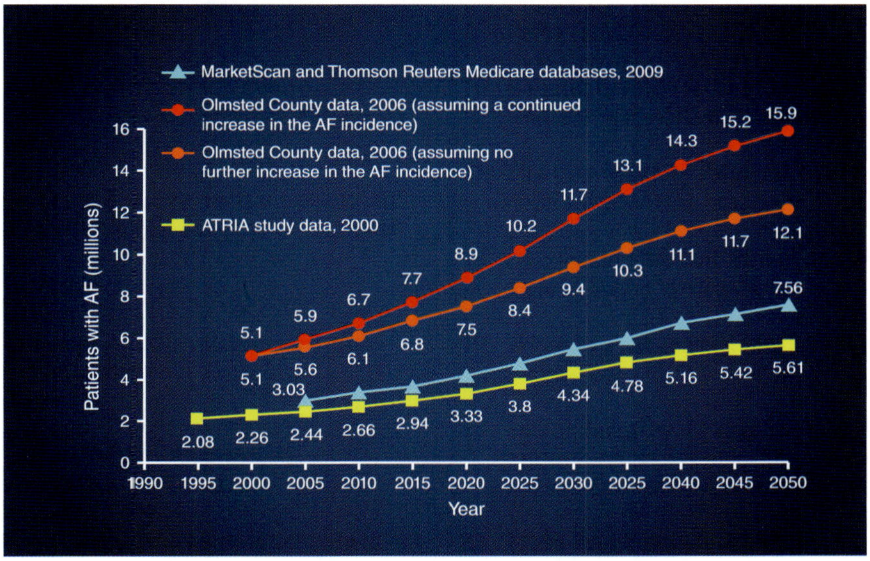

Fig. 2.2 Projected number of people in the United States with atrial fibrillation (AF). It will reach nearly 16 million by 2050. (Reproduced from Go AS, Hylek EM, Phillips KA, et al. Prevalence of diagnosed atrial fibrillation in adults: national implications for rhythm management and stroke prevention: the Anticoagulation and Risk Factors in Atrial Fibrillation (ATRIA) study. *J Am Med Assoc.* 2001;285(18):2370–2375 and Miyasaka Y, Barnes ME, Gersh BJ, et al. Secular trends in incidence of atrial fibrillation in Olmsted County, Minnesota, 1980 to 2000, and implications on the projections for future prevalence. *Circulation.* 2006;114(2):119–125.)

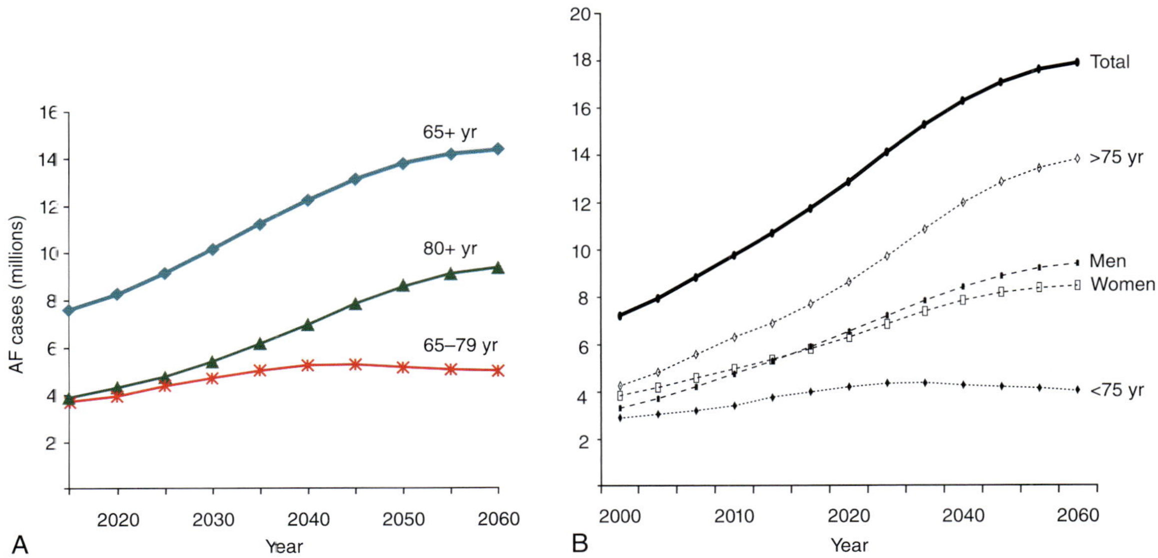

Fig. 2.3 Projected number of people in the European Union with atrial fibrillation (AF). It will reach nearly 18 million by 2060. (A) The Di Carlo and coworkers[12] prediction for patients in three different age groups. (B) The Krijthe and coworkers[11] prediction for patients younger and older than 75 years of age and for men and women. (Modified from Krijthe BP, Kunst A, Benjamin EJ, et al. Projections on the number of individuals with atrial fibrillation in the European Union, from 2000 to 2060. *Eur Heart J.* 2013;34(35):2746–2751 and Di Carlo A, Bellino L, Domenico C, et al. Prevalence of atrial fibrillation in the Italian elderly population and projections from 2020 to 2060 for Italy and the European Union: the FAI project. *Europace.* 2019;21(10):1468–1475.)

structural heart disease, both the presence of AF and its cause are often unknown ("cryptogenic AF"). AF is the most common arrhythmia encountered in clinical medicine. It is also the most common arrhythmia encountered by cardiac surgeons because many patients who require surgery also have AF (see Chapter 23), and roughly 35% of all patients undergoing cardiac surgery develop postoperative AF (see Chapter 47).

IMPACT OF ATRIAL FIBRILLATION ON SURVIVAL

AF is second only to ventricular fibrillation in its lethality. Piccini and colleagues[13] examined rates and risk factors for clinical events after new-onset AF in 230,940 hospitalized Medicare patients. AF increased the incidence of death, heart failure, myocardial infarction, stroke, and gastrointestinal bleeding, with the cumulative risk of death approaching 50% at 5 years (Fig. 2.4).[13] By tabulating the available statistics from the National Cancer Institute[14] with Piccini and colleagues' study of more than 230,000 Medicare patients, it is possible to compare the 5-year survival rate after new-onset AF with the 25 most common cancers in the United States. Such a comparison shows that AF places number 11 on the list (Fig. 2.5). Most hospitalized Medicare-age men would likely prefer a diagnosis of AF rather than melanoma, but their 5-year survival rate is better with melanoma than with new-onset AF. Likewise, most hospitalized Medicare-age women would probably prefer to be

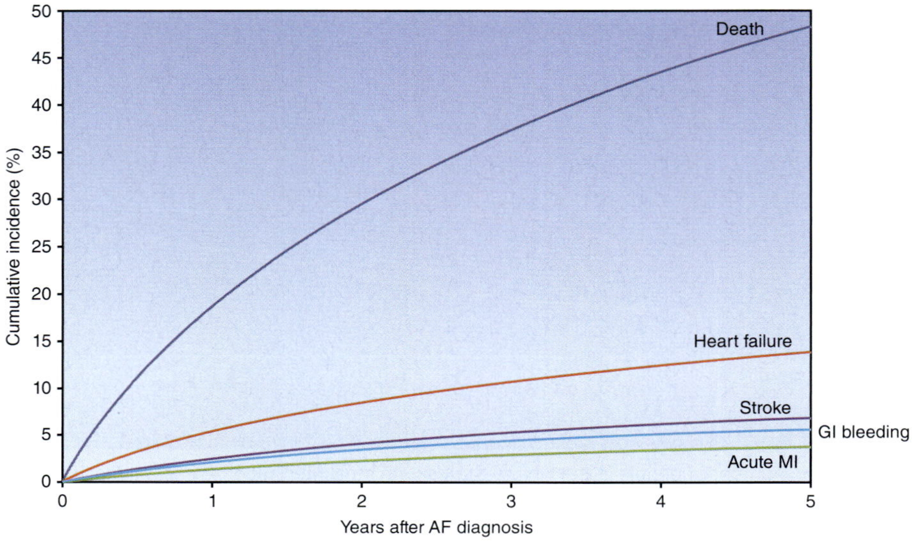

Fig. 2.4 Cumulative incidence of events in the 5 years after diagnosis of in-hospital atrial fibrillation (AF) in Medicare patients. *GI*, Gastrointestinal; *MI*, myocardial infarction. (Reproduced from Piccini JP, Hammill BG, Sinner MF, et al. Clinical course of atrial fibrillation in older adults: the importance of cardiovascular events beyond stroke. *Eur Heart J.* 2014;35(4):250–256.)

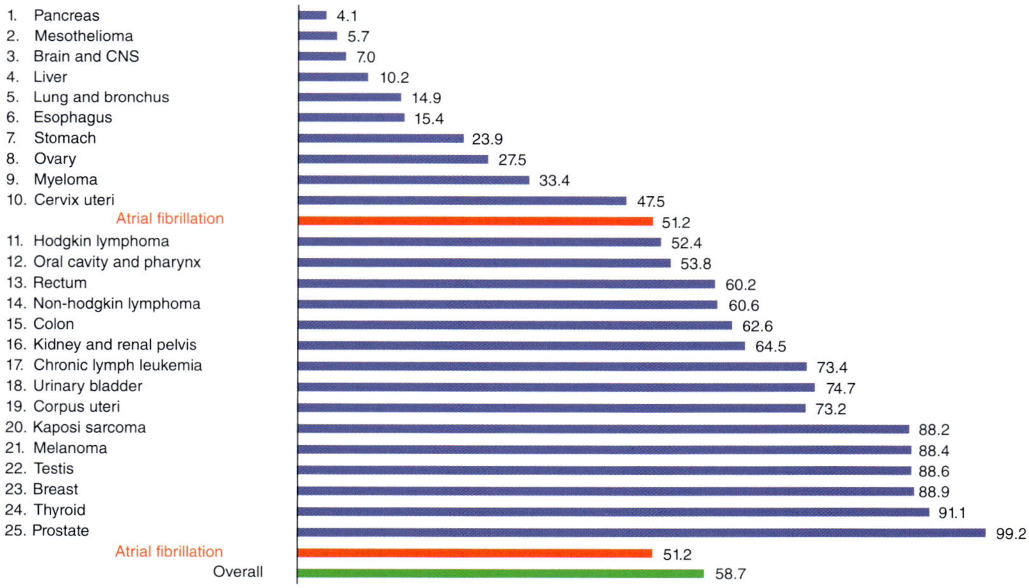

Fig. 2.5 Five-year survival rates for the top 25 cancers in the United States compared with the 5-year survival rate for new-onset atrial fibrillation in Medicare patients. *CNS*, Central nervous system. (Adapted from Piccini JP, Hammill BG, Sinner MF, et al. Clinical course of atrial fibrillation in older adults: the importance of cardiovascular events beyond stroke. *Eur Heart J.* 2014;35(4):250–256 and National Cancer Institute. 2013. https://seer.cancer.gov/statfacts/html/common.html).

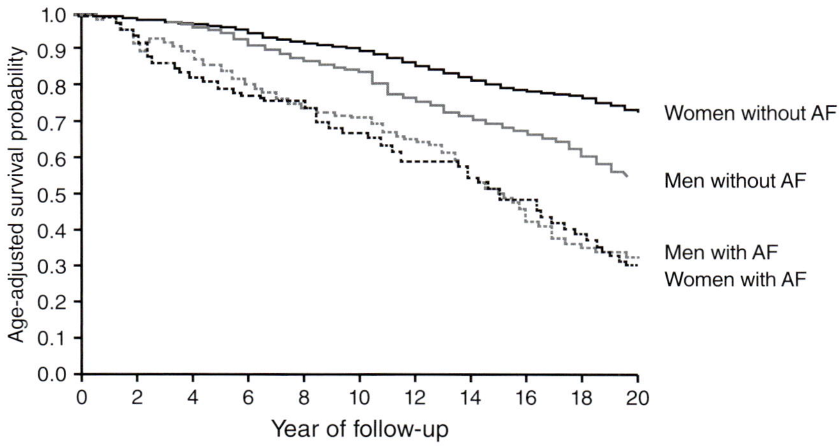

Fig. 2.6 Atrial fibrillation (AF) decreases the survival rate in women far greater than it does in men. Without AF, women have a higher life expectancy. However, the survival rate is the same in men and women who AF. (Reproduced from Stewart S, Hart MA, Hole DJ, McMurray JJV. A population-based study of the long-term risks associated with atrial fibrillation: 20-year follow-up of the Renfrew/Paisley study. *Am J Med.* 2002;113:359–364.)

told that they have new-onset AF than that they have breast cancer, but their likelihood of being alive in 5 years is substantially better if they have newly diagnosed breast cancer than if they have newly diagnosed AF.

AF has a significantly worse impact on survival in women than in men. In the Renfrew/Paisley Study from Scotland, 7052 men and 8354 women (age 45–64 years) with and without AF were followed for 20 years.[15] In patients without AF, the survival rate in women was roughly 20% higher than in men (Fig. 2.6). AF caused a survival decrease of 25% in men and a 45% decrease in women. The worse impact of AF in women resulted in their having essentially the same 20-year survival rate as men, indicating that AF in women is far more lethal than it is in men.

IMPACT OF ATRIAL FIBRILLATION ON STROKE

The 1991 Framingham Study of 5070 patients followed for 34 years documented that patients with AF were five times more likely to have a stroke than patients without AF.[16] Approximately 90% of all strokes are ischemic, and the other 10% are hemorrhagic (Fig. 2.7).[17] Hemorrhagic strokes are more lethal than ischemic strokes.[18] Patients with AF can have ischemic strokes because of systemic thromboembolism

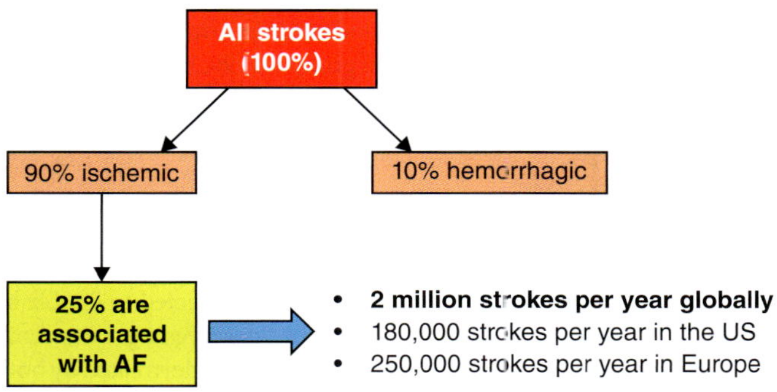

Fig. 2.7 Approximately 90% of all strokes are ischemic, and 10% are hemorrhagic. Atrial fibrillation (AF) is associated with approximately 25% of all ischemic strokes. This means that AF is associated with roughly 2 million strokes per year globally, 180,000 per year in the United States, and 250,000 per year in Europe.

or hemorrhagic strokes caused by overanticoagulation. Approximately 25% of thromboembolic strokes are associated with AF.[19] Globally, the number of ischemic strokes was 7.86 million in 2020,[20] so the number of ischemic strokes caused by AF globally was approximately 2 million. Of the 800,000 annual strokes in the United States, 90% are ischemic, and 180,000 are associated with AF.[21] Europeans have approximately 1.12 million strokes per year, 90% of which are ischemic, meaning that approximately 250,000 strokes occur annually in association with AF.[22] The cause of ischemic strokes associated with AF is systemic thromboembolism, usually originating from the left atrial appendage (LAA; see Section V). The ability to treat patients with AF successfully and to close the LAA by catheter and surgical techniques raises the possibility that the frequency of stroke in patients with AF might be decreased in the future.

ATRIAL FIBRILLATION AND HEART FAILURE

New-onset AF in hospitalized Medicare patients results in the development of heart failure in approximately 13% of patients within 5 years (see Fig. 2.4). However, not only can AF cause heart failure, but heart failure can also cause AF. A recent Mayo Clinic review of this relationship stated, "Atrial fibrillation (AF) is the most common arrhythmia among patients with heart failure (HF), and HF is the most common cause of death for patients presenting with clinical AF."[23] There are two major types of clinical heart failure: heart failure with *reduced* ejection fraction (HFrEF) and heart failure with *preserved* ejection fraction (HFpEF).

Sustained AF with a rapid ventricular response can cause HFrEF because of tachycardia-induced ventricular cardiomyopathy. Elimination of AF in these patients by catheter or surgical ablation commonly results in a return of the left ventricular ejection fraction (LVEF) toward normal and amelioration of the heart failure.[24] However, most patients with HFrEF develop secondary AF because of a chronically low LVEF, and the elimination of AF may have little salutary effect on the heart failure. Thus, in patients who present with simultaneous AF and HFrEF, it is often challenging to determine if the AF has caused tachycardia-induced HF or if a primary LV cardiomyopathy has caused the AF. The relationship between AF and HF in this clinical situation is a bit like the conundrum of "Which came first, the chicken or the egg?" The distinction is critical because it determines whether or not AF ablation will be beneficial to the patient.

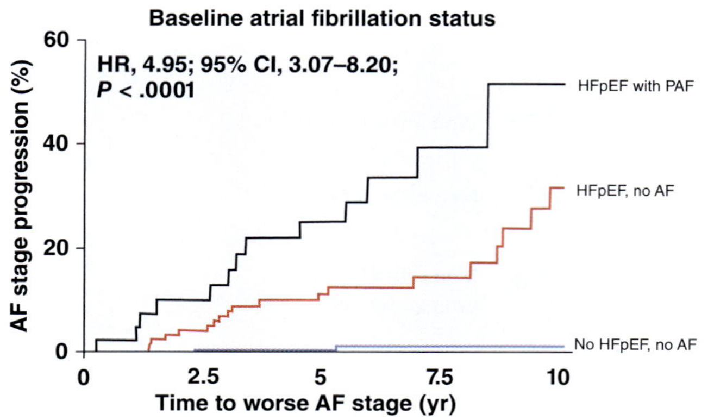

Fig. 2.8 The highest risk of progression of atrial fibrillation (AF) stage is seen in paroxysmal AF heart failure with preserved ejection fraction (HFpEF) with lower risk for HFpEF in patients in sinus rhythm. In contrast, control participants with normal exercise hemodynamics at baseline have almost no AF at follow-up. *HR,* Hazard ratio; *LV,* left ventricular; *PAF,* paroxysmal atrial fibrillation. (Modified from permission from Reddy YNV, Obokata M, Verbrugge FH, Lin G, Borlaug BA. Atrial dysfunction in patients with heart failure with preserved ejection fraction and atrial fibrillation. *J Am Coll Cardiol.* 2020;76:1051–1064.)

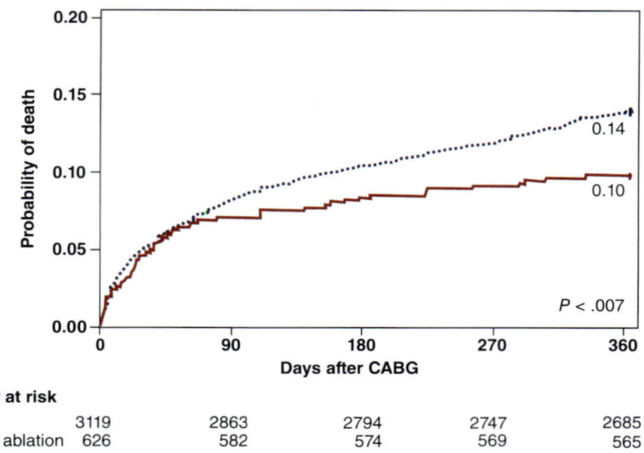

Fig. 2.9 Unadjusted mortality curves for Medicare beneficiaries who had coronary artery bypass grafting (CABG) and did (*solid line; n* = 626) or did not (*dashed line; n* = 3119) undergo concomitant surgical atrial fibrillation ablation. Curves derived using product-limit (Kaplan-Meier) survival analysis. Mortality rates are compared with the log-rank test. (Reproduced from Rankin JS, Lerner DJ, Braid-Forbes MJ, Ferguson MA, Badhwar V. One-year mortality and costs associated with surgical ablation for atrial fibrillation concomitant to coronary artery bypass grafting. *Eur J Cardiothorac Surg.* 2017;52(3):471–477.)

The pathogenesis of AF in patients with HFpEF is distinctly different from that in patients with HFrEF. AF in patients with HFpEF is thought to be caused by systemic inflammation resulting in abnormal myocardial remodeling and functional reserve.[25] This results in LV diastolic dysfunction while leaving LV systolic function intact. The left atrium often enlarges in response to this abnormal LV physiology, leading to AF. Development of secondary AF in HFpEF patients can have a profoundly negative effect on the severity of clinical heart failure, and the risk of progression of paroxysmal AF to persistent AF is dramatic (Fig. 2.8).[26] Drug-refractory AF in patients with HFpEF may require catheter ablation, but if surgery for AF is required in these patients, one should be careful about occluding the LAA if the LV diastolic dysfunction is severe (see Chapter 40).

ECONOMICS OF ATRIAL FIBRILLATION

In 2011, Wolowacz et al.[27] reported that AF increased health care costs by $2000 to $14,200 per patient in the United States.[27] Two years later, a systematic review concluded that "Unless action is taken to improve detection of AF and reduce its consequences, a considerable increase in the social and economic burden associated with AF-related stroke is likely."[28] A 2022 comparison of 79,621 patients with AF and a similar number without AF showed that the incremental health care cost of AF in the United States had increased to approximately $25,000 per patient.[29] If an AF patient has an ischemic stroke, the costs increase to approximately $37,000 per patient, and ischemic strokes are twice as costly in patients older than the age of 75 years.[30] Total health care spending on atrial flutter or AF currently ranks number 33 among 154 health conditions in the United States at a cost of $28.4 billion per year.[31]

ECONOMICS OF ATRIAL FIBRILLATION INTERVENTION

Catheter ablation for patients with AF increases health care expenditures because it requires specialized catheters, mapping systems, cardiac imaging, and routine hospitalization expenditures. In the first peer-reviewed analysis of its kind, Winkle et al.[32] reported in 2013 that the costs of catheter ablation equipment alone ranged from $6637 to $22,284 per patient depending on the preferred type of catheter, energy source, and navigation system.[32] Imaging procedures performed before, during, and after catheter ablation add an additional 6% (mean, $39,000) to the overall procedural costs.[33] The 2022 Catheter Ablation vs Anti-arrhythmic Drug Therapy for Atrial Fibrillation Trial (CABANA) randomized trial showed that the average 5-year cost for catheter ablation was $19,245 higher than for drug therapy, but the cost-effectiveness ratio of catheter ablation was $57,893 better per quality-adjusted life-years.[34] The conclusion was that catheter ablation was "economically attractive" compared with drug therapy.

Surgical ablation is rarely performed for stand-alone AF, and there are no direct comparisons between the cost-effectiveness of surgery versus catheter ablation for the treatment of patients with AF. However, 28% of Medicare patients undergoing cardiac surgery have preoperative AF, and many undergo concomitant AF surgical ablation at the time of their primary cardiac surgical procedures (see Chapter 23).[35]

In 2017, Rankin et al.[36] published a cost analysis of 3745 Medicare patients with AF undergoing coronary artery bypass grafting (CABG) as their primary procedure.[36] There was no difference in the operative mortality rate or perioperative morbidity rate in patients having concomitant AF surgical ablation and those who had no AF ablation. However, concomitant AF surgical ablation increased the hospital costs by $2225 (11%) per patient during the index CABG hospitalization. The 1-year survival rate of the AF-ablation group was 90.3% compared with 86.1% in the nonablated group (P = .007) (Fig. 2.9), and the overall cost per patient was only 6% higher in the AF-ablated group.

SUMMARY

AF should be recognized as a growing epidemic that creates heavy financial burdens on society, and its prevalence is expected to double by midcentury. It is as lethal as most cancers and deserves a greater sense of urgency because patients with AF are currently undertreated by both physicians and surgeons. Despite the demonstration that catheter ablation is superior to drug therapy for the treatment of patients with AF, only some 4% of all patients with AF in the United States are treated interventionally. Likewise, less than 1 in 4 patients with preoperative AF undergoing cardiac surgery receive concomitant surgical ablation of their AF despite irrefutable evidence that treated patients have far better outcomes. The continued treatment of AF primarily as a nuisance rather than as a serious and expanding lethal epidemic can only lead to undesirable results for society in the future.

REFERENCES

1. United States Census Bureau. 2023. https://www.census.gov/quickfacts/fact/table/US/POP010210#POP010210.
2. Colilla S, Crow A, Petkun W, Singer DE, Simon T, Liu X. Estimates of current and future incidence and prevalence of atrial fibrillation in the U.S. adult population. *Am J Cardiol.* 2013;112(8):1142–1147.
3. World Population (2010–2020). 2023. www.globaldata.com.
4. Tsao CW, Aday AW, Almarzoog Z, et al. Heart disease and stroke statistics-2023 update: a report from the American Heart Association. *Circulation.* 2023;147(8):e93–e621.
5. Mou L, Norby FL, Chen LY, et al. Lifetime risk of atrial fibrillation by race and socioeconomic status: ARIC study (Atherosclerosis Risk in Communities). *Circ Arrhythm Electrophysiol.* 2018;11(7):e006350.
6. Chao T-F, Liu C-J Tuan T-C, et al. Lifetime risks, projected numbers, and adverse outcomes in asian patients with atrial fibrillation: a report from the Taiwan nationwide AF cohort study. *Chest.* 2018;153(2):453–466.
7. Magnussen C, Niiranen TJ, Ojeda FM, et al. Sex differences and similarities in atrial fibrillation epidemiology, risk factors, and mortality in community cohorts: results from the BiomarCaRE Consortium (Biomarker for Cardiovascular Risk Assessment in Europe). *Circulation.* 2017;136(17):1588–1597.
8. Schnabel RB, Yin X, Gona P, et al. 50 Year trends in atrial fibrillation prevalence, incidence, risk factors, and mortality in the Framingham heart study: a cohort study. *Lancet.* 2015;386:154–162.
9. Go AS, Hylek EM, Phillips KA, et al. Prevalence of diagnosed atrial fibrillation in adults: national implications for rhythm management and stroke prevention: the anticoagulation and risk factors in atrial fibrillation (ATRIA) study. *J Am Med Assoc.* 2001;285(18):2370–2375.
10. Miyasaka Y, Barnes ME, Gersh BJ, et al. Secular trends in incidence of atrial fibrillation in Olmsted County, Minnesota, 1980 to 2000, and implications on the projections for future prevalence. *Circulation.* 2006;114(2):119–125.
11. Krijthe BP, Kunst A, Benjamin EJ, et al. Projections on the number of individuals with atrial fibrillation in the European Union, from 2000 to 2060. *Eur Heart J.* 2013;34(35):2746–2751.
12. Di Carlo A, Bellino L, Domenico C, et al. Prevalence of atrial fibrillation in the Italian elderly population and projections from 2020 to 2060 for Italy and the European Union: the FAI project. *Europace.* 2019;21(10):1468–1475.
13. Piccini J P, Hammill BG, Sinner MF, et al. Clinical course of atrial fibrillation in older adults: the importance of cardiovascular events beyond stroke. *Eur Heart J.* 2014;35(4):250–256.
14. National Cancer Institute. 2013. https://www.cdc.gov/stroke/data-research/facts-stats/.
15. Stewart S, Hart MA, Hole DJ, McMurray JJV. A population-based study of the long-term risks associated with atrial fibrillation: 20-year follow-up of the Renfrew/Paisley study. *Am J Med.* 2002;113:359–364.
16. Wolf PA, Abbott RD, Kannel WB. Atrial fibrillation as an independent risk factor for stroke: the Framingham study. *Stroke.* 1991;8:983–988.
17. Virani SS, Alonso A, Benjamin EJ, et al. Heart disease and stroke statistics-2020 update: a report from the American Heart Association. *Circulation.* 2020;141:e139–e596.
18. Balami JS, Buchan AM. Complications of intracerebral haemorrhage. *Lancet Neurol.* 2012;11:101–118.
19. Marini C, De Santis F, Sacco S, et al. Contribution of atrial fibrillation to incidence and outcome of ischemic stroke: results from a population-based study. *Stroke.* 2005;36:1115–1119.
20. Pu L, Wang L, Zhang R, Zhao T, Jiang Y, Han L. Projected global trends in ischemic stroke incidence, deaths and disability-adjusted life years from 2020 to 2030. *Stroke.* 2023;54:1330–1339.
21. Centers for Disease Control and Prevention. https://www.cdc.gov/stroke/data-research/facts-stats/.
22. Wafa HA, Wolfe CDA, Emmett E, Roth GA, Johnson CO, Wang Y. Burden of stroke in Europe: thirty-year projections of incidence, prevalence, deaths and disability-adjusted life years. *Stroke.* 2020;51:2418–2427.
23. Reddy YNV, Borlaug BA, Gersh BJ. Management of atrial fibrillation across the spectrum of heart failure with preserved and reduced ejection fraction. *Circulation.* 2022;146(4):339–357.
24. Marrouche NF, Brachmann J, Andresen D, et al. Catheter ablation for atrial fibrillation with heart failure. *N Engl J Med.* 2018;378:417–427.
25. Schiattarella GG, Altamirano F, Tong D, et al. Nitrosative stress drives heart failure with preserved ejection fraction. *Nature.* 2019;568:351–356.
26. Reddy YNV, Obokata M, Verbrugge FH, Lin G, Borlaug BA. Atrial dysfunction in patients with heart failure with preserved ejection fraction and atrial fibrillation. *J Am Coll Cardiol.* 2020;76:1051–1064.
27. Wolowacz SE, Samuel M, Brennan VK, Jasso-Mosqueda JG, Van Gelder IC. The cost of illness of atrial fibrillation: a systematic review of the recent literature. *Europace.* 2011;13(10):1375–1385.
28. Andrew NE, Thrift AG, Cadilhac DA. The prevalence, impact and economic implications of atrial fibrillation in stroke: what progress has been made? *Neuroepidemiology.* 2013;40(4):227–239.
29. Abhishek D, Iglesias M, Khanna R, Beaulieu T. Healthcare utilization and costs associated with a diagnosis of incident atrial fibrillation. *Heart Rhythm.* 2022;3(5):577–586.
30. Li X, Tse VC, Au-Doung LW, Wong ICK, Chan EW. The impact of ischaemic stroke on atrial fibrillation-related healthcare cost: a systematic review. *Europace.* 2017;19(6):937–947.
31. Dieleman JL, Cao J, Chapin A, et al. US health care spending by payer and health condition, 1996-2016. *J Am Med Assoc.* 2020;323(9):863–884.
32. Winkle RA, Mead RH, Engel G, Kong MH, Patrawala RA. Physician-controlled costs: the choice of equipment used for atrial fibrillation ablation. *J Interv Card Electrophysiol.* 2013;36(2):157–165.
33. Pokorney SD, Hammill BG, Quails LG, Steinberg BA, Curtis LH, Piccini JP. Cost analysis of periprocedural imaging in patients undergoing catheter ablation for atrial fibrillation. *Am J Cardiol.* 2014;114(2):266–271.
34. Chew DS, Li Y, Cowper PA, et al. Cost-effectiveness of catheter ablation versus antiarrhythmic drug therapy in atrial fibrillation: The CABANA randomized clinical trial. *Circulation.* 2022;146(7):535–547.
35. McCarthy PM, Davidson CJ, Kruse J, et al. Prevalence of atrial fibrillation before cardiac surgery and factors associated with concomitant ablation. *J Thorac Cardiovasc Surg.* 2020;159(6):2245–2253.
36. Rankin JS, Lerner DJ, Braid-Forbes MJ, Ferguson MA, Badhwar V. One-year mortality and costs associated with surgical ablation for atrial fibrillation concomitant to coronary artery bypass grafting. *Eur J Cardiothorac Surg.* 2017;52(3):471–477.

3

Cardiac Anatomy Pertinent to Atrial Fibrillation Surgery

James L. Cox, Olga N. Kislitsina

CHAPTER OUTLINE

Most cardiac surgeons do not learn the anatomy that is pertinent to arrhythmia surgery even though cardiac surgical training programs are traditionally steeped in the teaching of anatomy. Indeed, the first surgical procedure designed specifically to treat a clinical cardiac arrhythmia (Wolff-Parkinson-White [WPW] syndrome) demanded that the surgeon perform extensive dissection within the atrioventricular (AV) groove, an anatomic space that cardiac surgeons had traditionally avoided. In addition, the incomplete understanding of cardiac anatomy that is characteristic of many nonsurgical physicians has been considered relatively unimportant in the past, even to interventional electrophysiologists. However, with the recent advances in cardiac imaging and the development of new medical devices and catheter delivery systems to treat patients with atrial fibrillation (AF), both arrhythmia surgeons and interventional electrophysiologists have been forced to learn the cardiac anatomy that is pertinent to cardiac arrhythmias.

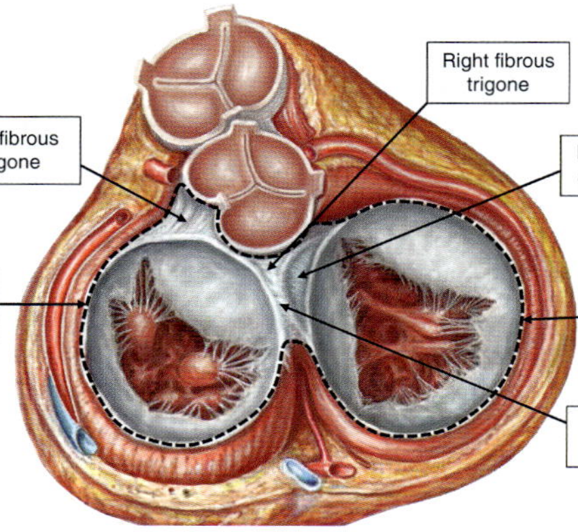

Fig. 3.1 Fibrous skeleton of the heart *(dashed line)*. The components of the fibrous skeleton include the mitral valve annulus, tricuspid valve annulus, central fibrous body, and right and left fibrous trigones.

FIBROUS SKELETON OF THE HEART

For any muscle to perform work, it is necessary for the muscle to have a solid support against which to contract. For example, if a skeletal muscle such as the biceps were excised, placed on a table, and stimulated with an electrical current, it would contract. Because it would have no solid attachments, however, its contraction would not result in any work. This is why skeletal muscles are attached to the bony skeleton. The ability to perform work is no different for cardiac muscle; that is, it must have a relatively solid support against which to contract, or it cannot perform any work. Although the skeletal muscles have the bony skeleton for support, the heart's support is made of cartilage rather than bone and is called the *fibrous skeleton of the heart* (Fig. 3.1). The fibrous skeleton of the heart consists primarily of the mitral valve annulus but also includes the tricuspid valve annulus. Where the mitral and tricuspid annuli become contiguous, the fibrous skeleton is slightly thicker and is called the *central fibrous body*.

The anterior portion of the central fibrous body adjacent to the aortic valve has been designated the *right fibrous trigone*. Some authors in the past have erroneously used the terms *central fibrous body* and *right fibrous trigone* interchangeably, but the latter is actually only the anterior portion of the central fibrous body where the anterior leaflet of the mitral annulus is contiguous with the aortic valve. Where these two valves converge laterally, the fibrous skeleton thickens and is called the *left fibrous trigone*.

The mitral annulus is slightly "bowed" between the right and left fibrous trigones, and in many patients it is somewhat thicker than its free-wall component. The cusps of the aortic valve are thickened at their attachments to the aorta, and together they form a scalloped ridge of tissue inside the aortic root that is commonly referred to as the *aortic valve annulus*. However, histologically, there is no evidence of fibrous tissue in the aortic root comparable to that seen in the mitral or tricuspid valve annuli, so technically there is no true "aortic valve annulus."

ATRIAL SEPTUM

To understand the anatomy of the atrial septum, it is necessary to have a clear three-dimensional (3D) concept of the center of the heart where the fibrous skeleton, both ventricles, and both atria intersect. This 3D picture begins with the understanding that the plane of the tricuspid valve annulus is not in the same plane as the mitral valve annulus because the tricuspid valve is slightly closer to the apex of the

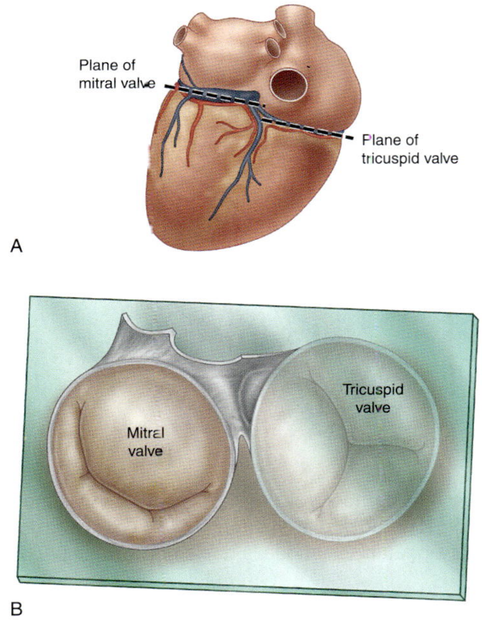

Fig. 3.2 The mitral valve annulus and tricuspid valve annulus are not in the same plane. The tricuspid valve is located in a more apical position than the mitral valve. (A) Posterior view of the heart with designation of the levels of the mitral and tricuspid valves showing that the tricuspid valve is more apically located than is the mitral valve. (B) If one placed a pane of glass across the heart at the level of the tricuspid valve annulus, everything else in this plane of the heart would be above the pane of glass, and the tricuspid valve would be below it.

heart than the mitral annulus (Fig. 3.2). This slightly more apical plane of the tricuspid valve relative to the mitral valve results in the membranous portion of the ventricular septum extending above the level of the tricuspid annulus medially to become the membranous portion of the atrial septum (Fig. 3.3). Thus, if one were to pass a probe through the membranous portion of the atrial septum from the right atrial side, the tip of the probe would pass below the level of the mitral valve annulus into the left ventricular cavity. This is why infections in this area can result in right atrial-to-left ventricular fistulas. This difference in the horizontal planes of the mitral and tricuspid valves also contributes to the coronary sinus emptying into the right atrium (RA) well above the level of the tricuspid valve annulus (Fig. 3.4).

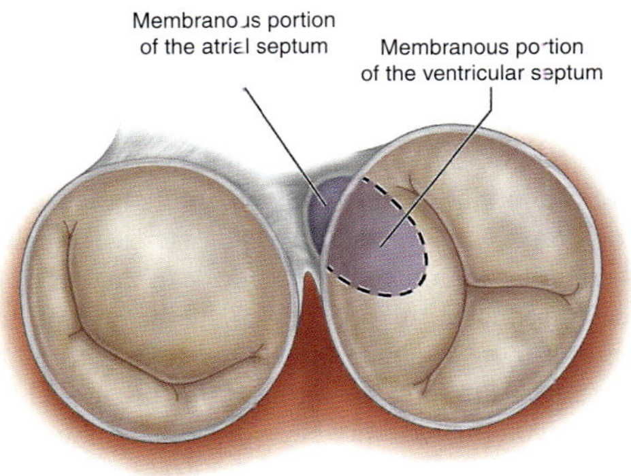

Fig. 3.3 The disparity in the planes of the mitral and tricuspid valves results in the superior tip of the membranous ventricular septum extending slightly above the level of the tricuspid annulus to become the membranous portion of the atrial septum. This membrane actually separates the right atrium from the left ventricle.

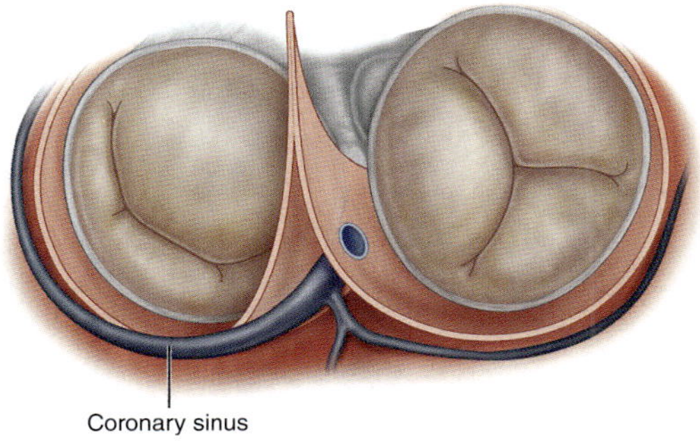

Fig. 3.4 The disparity in the planes of the mitral and tricuspid valves also contributes to the coronary sinus emptying into the right atrium well above the level of the tricuspid valve annulus.

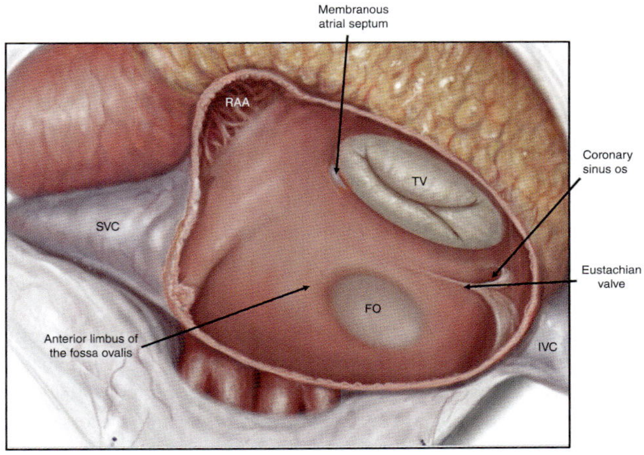

Fig. 3.5 Surgeon's view of the internal right atrium. *IVC,* Inferior vena cava; *FO, Fossa Ovalis*; *RAA,* right atrial appendage; *RV,* right ventricle; *SVC,* superior vena cava.

The most prominent anatomic feature of the atrial septum is the fossa ovalis, which is bordered superiorly by a thick bundle of muscle called the *anterior limbus of the fossa ovalis* (Fig. 3.5). Posterior to the fossa ovalis, the two medial free walls of the right and left atria may be adjacent and adherent, but there is a potential space between them (Fig. 3.6). This is the potential plane

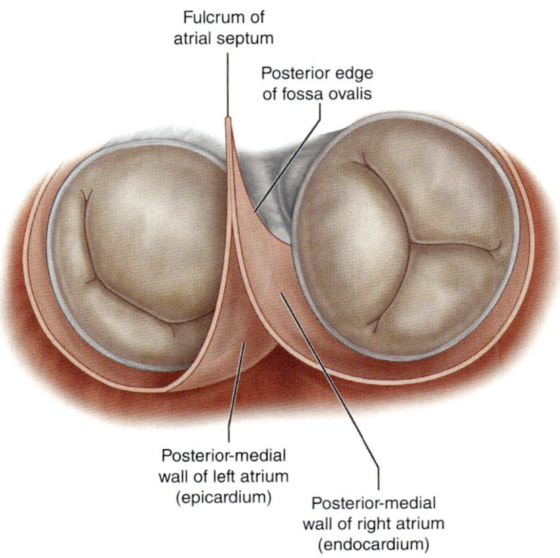

Fig. 3.6 Three-dimensional diagram of the relationship between the medial walls of the right and left atria to form the atrial septum.

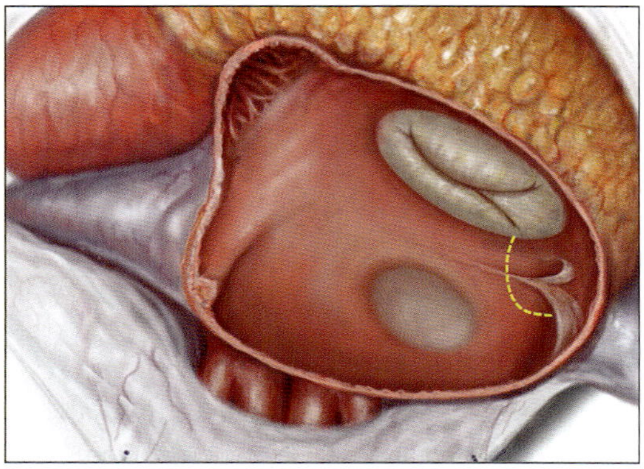

Fig. 3.7 The cavo-tricuspid isthmus (CTI) is the area of the right atrium (RA) between the IVC orifice and the tricuspid annulus in the RA. Classic right atrial flutter uses the CTI in virtually all patients, and a lesion *(yellow dashed line)* placed across the CTI cures most classic atrial flutter. This lesion must be placed from inside the RA because it cannot be exposed from the epicardial side without extensive surgical dissection. The successful catheter-based treatment of atrial flutter has resulted in this lesion being called the "flutter line." However, the CTI can support other right atrial reentrant circuits that can contribute to atrial fibrillation (AF). Therefore, under certain circumstances, a CTI lesion can improve the results of ablation procedures for AF as well as for atrial flutter.

called *Waterston's groove* that surgeons develop in preparation for performing mitral valve surgery or before encircling the pulmonary veins. The anatomic fusion between the two atrial walls anteriorly forms the posterior boundary of the fossa ovalis. Dissection in Waterston's groove is safe until the fossa ovalis is reached. As most cardiac surgeons know from experience, further dissection in this plane will result in the inadvertent entrance into both atria.

The isthmus of the right atrial wall between the IVC orifice and the tricuspid annulus is called the *cavotricuspid isthmus* (CTI) (Fig. 3.7). Classic atrial flutter can be caused by one of three different macro-reentrant circuits, and all three of them use the CTI.[1] Therefore placing a lesion across this CTI ("flutter line") is highly successful for the treatment of classic atrial flutter.[2]

SPECIALIZED CONDUCTION SYSTEM

Sinoatrial Node

The anatomic sinus node is commonly located near the junction of the superior vena cava (SVC) and RA in the superior lateral portion of the right atrial free wall (Fig. 3.8). The specialized cells in the sinus node are capable of generating an electrical impulse spontaneously however often one is needed to maintain an optimal heart rate. The generation of these impulses results from a natural phenomenon called *spontaneous phase 4 depolarization*, which is discussed in Chapter 4.

For decades it was assumed that all sinus rhythm beats originated from this anatomic sinus node, which is a definitive anatomic structure that can be identified histologically. However, electrophysiological studies performed over the past several years documented that sinus impulses can originate from disparate regions of the RA depending on the heart rate. This electrically active region has been called the *atrial pacemaker complex* (Fig. 3.9), and sinus rhythm beats normally originate from one of three different regions within this pacemaker complex.[3]

During sinus rhythm at normal heart rates of 60 to 100 beats/min, the sinus impulses originate from within or near the anatomic sinus node in the midportion of the atrial pacemaker complex. However, during sinus tachycardia, regardless of whether it is neurally or humorally mediated, the sinus impulses consistently originate from a small area located in the upper right atrial free wall immediately anterior to the

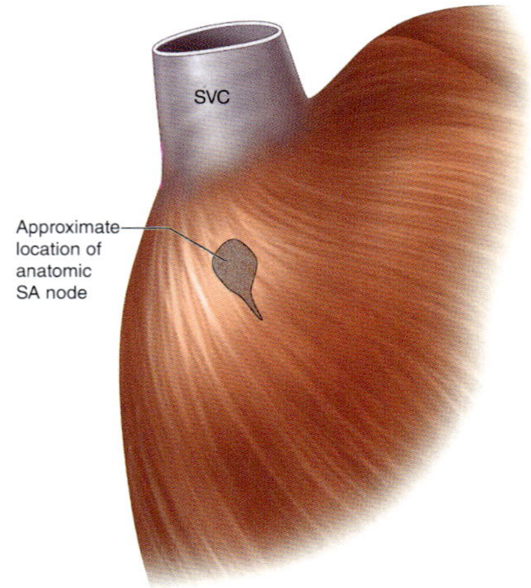

Fig. 3.8 The muscle fibers of the right atrial free-wall are arranged diagonally as highlighted in this illustration. The most common location of the anatomic sinoatrial (SA) node is depicted. *SVC,* Superior vena cava.

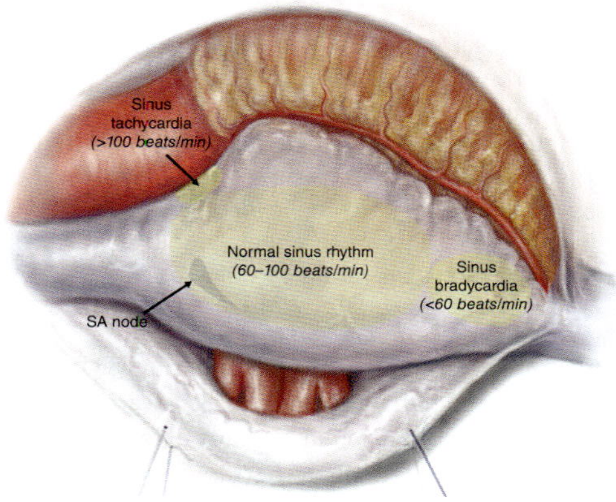

Fig. 3.9 The atrial pacemaker complex consists of three areas in the right atrium (RA). The lateral right atrial free wall includes the anatomic sinoatrial (SA) node and generates normal sinus rhythm beats at a rate of 60 to 100 beats/min. The small area at the junction of the superior vena cava and anterior RA is called the *sinus tachycardia site* and generates sinus impulses at a rate greater than 100 beats/min. The *sinus bradycardia site* is in the lower RA near the inferior vena cava and coronary sinus and it generates sinus impulses at a rate below 60 beats/min. (Reproduced from Cox JL, Ad N, Churyla A, et al. The maze procedure and postoperative pacemakers. *Ann Thorac Surg.* 2018;106(5):1561–1569.)

junction of the SVC and RA. The importance of this so-called *sinus tachycardia site* is that if it is damaged during surgery, patients will be unable to generate an appropriate chronotropic response to exercise postoperatively. Injury of this particular portion of the atrial pacemaker complex most commonly occurs as a result of an atrial incision or ablative lesion being placed immediately anterior to the orifice of the SVC. As will be discussed later, this was one of the major problems with the pattern of lesions in the original Maze-I procedure, which had two incisions directly across the sinus tachycardia site, because at the time, the atrial pacemaker complex had not been described in humans.

During sinus bradycardia, the sinus impulses usually originate from the lower portion of the atrial pacemaker complex. Thus, if one administers propranolol to decrease the heart rate, the resultant sinus rhythm beats will originate near the inferior vena cava on the lateral right atrial free wall. The same is true when the normal sinus rhythm rate slows naturally during sleep.

One of the frequently quoted myths in electrophysiology and cardiac surgery is that injury of the sinoatrial (SA) node artery causes sinus node dysfunction. The legendary cardiologist and cardiac pathologist Thomas James once told the author the following:

> *"The SA node artery, which has few if any branches to the anatomic AV node, reminds me of those interstate highways that pass through small towns and have no exit-ramps. I have never seen any evidence that the so-called "SA node artery" has anything to do with SA node function"*[4] (Fig. 3.10).

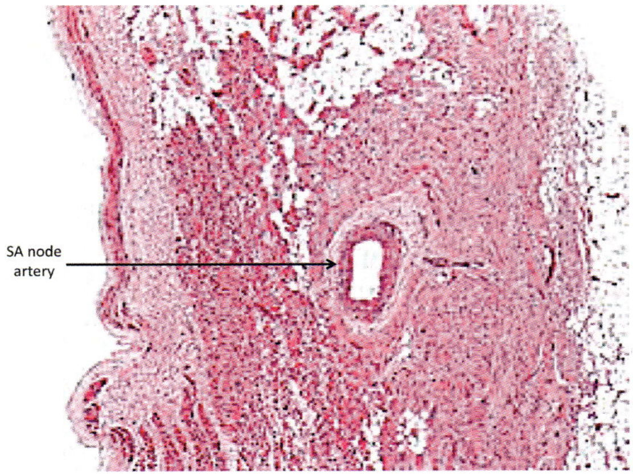

Fig. 3.10 The sinoatrial (SA) node artery typically passes through the anatomic SA node but does not normally provide identifiable branches specifically to the nodal tissue. Many authorities believe that ligation of the SA node artery does not lead to SA node dysfunction because it is not an "end artery."

James' observation is supported by the fact that neither the presence nor the severity of coronary artery disease in the right coronary artery system correlates with SA node dysfunction.[5] Furthermore, a meta-analysis of 66 studies of the anatomy of the so-called SA node artery in 21,455 human hearts documented that it most commonly originates as a single branch from the right coronary artery and takes a retrocaval course to reach the SA node in 47% of patients, but its location is highly variable (Fig. 3.11).[6]

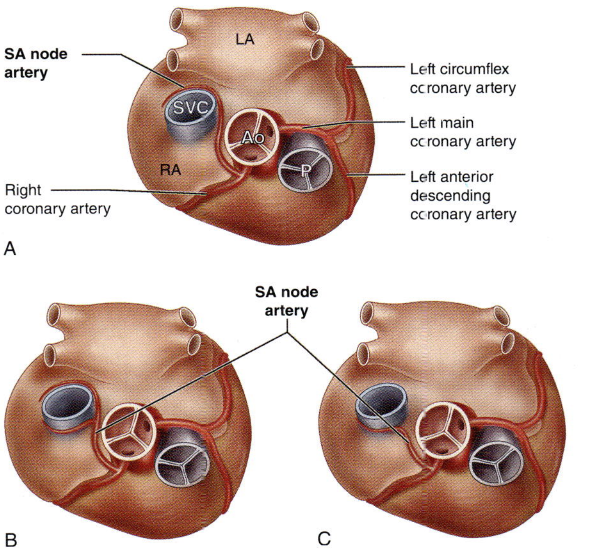

Fig. 3.11 The various courses of the sinoatrial nodal artery as seen from a superior view. (A) Retrocaval course. (B) Pericaval course. (C) Precaval course. *Ao*, Aorta; *LA*, left atrium; *P*, pulmonary trunk; *RA*, right atrium; *SVC*, superior vena cava.

These observations argue that the SA node artery, like the AV node artery (see later discussion), is not an "end artery," so its occlusion should not cause sinus node dysfunction unless there is associated coronary artery disease elsewhere. Supporting this concept is the fact that all four iterations of the Maze procedure include a lesion in the RA that extends posterior to the anatomic SA node and up into the SVC. That lesion has been performed thousands of times, including as a surgical incision in the original cut-and-sew technique, two different types of cryogens (nitrous oxide, argon gas), and bipolar radiofrequency clamps. It is inconceivable that the SA node artery has not been interrupted in a significant number of these patients because of the variability of its anatomy. Yet postoperative SA node dysfunction after a properly performed Maze procedure is less than 5%, and most postoperative pacemakers are required because of "unmasking" a sick sinus syndrome.[7] Furthermore, our original Maze procedure series is one of the few in which the *preoperative* function of the SA node was actually assessed by electrophysiologic studies, including sinus node recovery time. Ninety-five patients with paroxysmal AF had normal SA node function preoperatively, and not one of them developed SA node dysfunction after a Maze-I, Maze-II, or Maze-III procedure.[8] Although surgical injury or interruption of the SA node artery is highly unlikely to cause SA node dysfunction, it seems prudent to avoid its transsection if possible.

Internodal Conduction Pathways

When the sinus node impulse exits the atrial pacemaker complex, it travels to adjacent areas of the RA, atrial septum, left atrium (LA), and AV node via four main conduction routes (Fig. 3.12). The three primary conduction routes from the SA node to the AV node are the anterior, middle, and posterior internodal tracts. Unlike the specialized conduction system in the ventricles, these primary conduction routes in the atrium are not made up of specialized conduction tissue; rather, they consist of normal atrial myocytes. The reason that electrical conduction occurs preferentially along these four routes is that they are thicker than other areas of the atria, and their dominant fiber orientation is parallel to the direction of propagation. The impact of fiber orientation on the velocity of impulse propagation is a basic electrophysiologic characteristic of

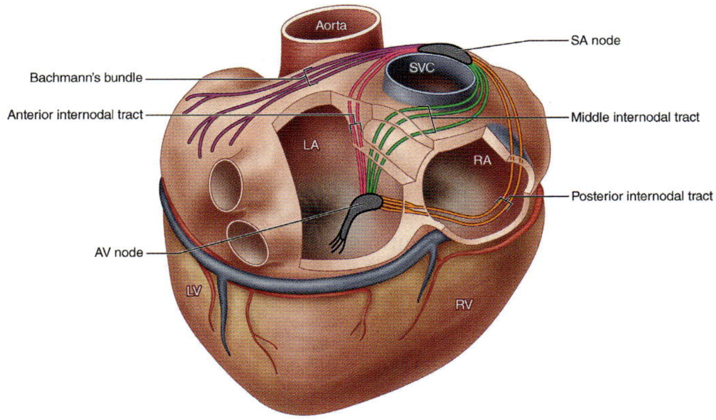

Fig. 3.12 Preferential pathways of conduction in the atria. There are three preferential internodal pathways between the sinoatrial (SA) node and atrioventricular (AV) node: the anterior, middle, and posterior internodal tracts. There is one preferential conduction pathway between the right atrium (RA) and left atrium (LA), Bachmann's bundle, which is located in the superior portion of both atria. See text for further discussion. *LV*, Left ventricle; *RV*, right ventricle; *SVC*, superior vena cava.

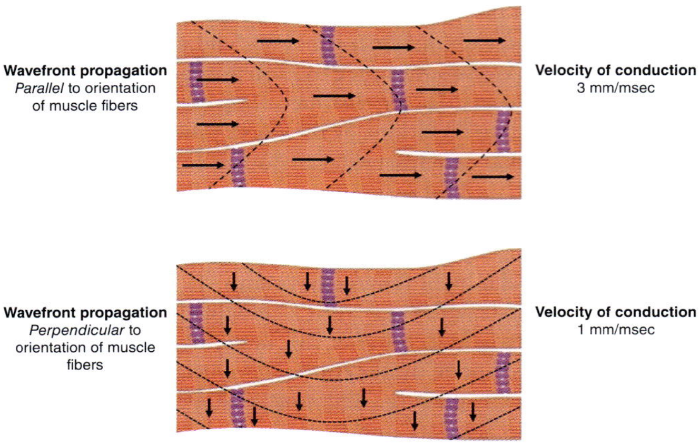

Fig. 3.13 Anisotropy of conduction. The velocity of wavefront propagation through myocardium depends on the orientation of the muscle fibers in relation to the direction of wavefront propagation. Wavefront propagation is faster (3 mm/ms) if the orientation of muscle fibers is parallel to the direction of electrical propagation. Wavefront propagation is slower (1 mm/ms) if the orientation of muscle fibers is perpendicular to the direction of electrical propagation.

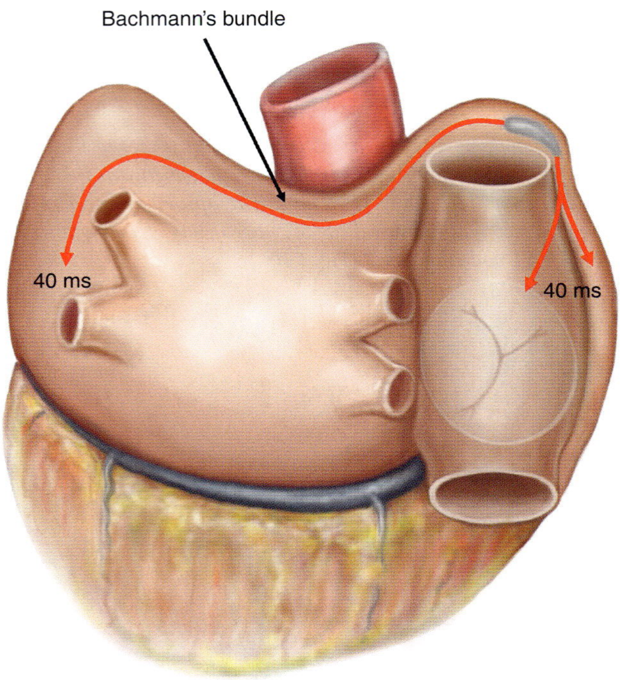

Fig. 3.14 Wavefront propagation is extremely fast from the right atrium to the left atrium across Bachmann's bundle because its muscle fibers are parallel to the direction of impulse propagation. This allows the upper right and left atria to be activated almost simultaneously.

myocardial cells called the *anisotropy of conduction* (Fig. 3.13). The fact that the atrial muscle is thicker in the preferential internodal pathways also promotes the accumulation of a greater electromotive force (EMF) as the impulse propagates from one myocyte to another. The greater EMF also results in more rapid electrical conduction through these thick muscle bundles than across the thinner areas of the atria. Thus, there are two reasons that impulses propagate along these preferential pathways even though they do not harbor any specialized conduction tissue: parallel fiber orientation and increased muscle thickness.

Interatrial Conduction Pathway (Bachmann's Bundle)

Bachmann's bundle is a finger-size muscle bundle that serves as the preferential interatrial conduction route. It extends from the top of the RA to the top of the LA at the base of the left atrial appendage and can be identified during surgery by retracting the ascending aorta off the top of the LA. The primary orientation of muscle fibers in Bachmann's bundle is parallel to the direction of an SA node impulse from the RA to the LA. Bachmann's bundle is critical to optimal atrial transport function because it allows the sinus impulse originating near the top of the RA to arrive at the top of the LA within 40 ms (Fig. 3.14). The virtually instantaneous arrival of the sinus impulse in the top of the LA results in both atria being activated almost simultaneously in a superior to inferior direction, and atrial mechanical contraction follows the same sequence. Contraction of both atria from top to bottom likely provides optimal atrial augmentation of the delivery of atrial blood into the respective ventricles during ventricular diastole.

If Bachmann's bundle is surgically interrupted, it can take as long as 150 ms for an SA node impulse to fully activate the LA (Fig. 3.15). Because this is the same length of time it normally takes the SA node impulse to activate the ventricles, the LA is activated at the same time as the LV, which means that the LA is contracting against a closed mitral valve. Thus the interatrial conduction delay caused by an interruption of conduction across Bachmann's bundle can eliminate all left atrial transport function despite the persistence of normal RA and right ventricle (RV) synchrony.

This was one of the problems with the pattern of lesions in the Maze-I procedure.[9] It is also a potential problem with the "Dallas Lesion Set," the "Five Box Maze," and any other procedure in which a lesion is placed

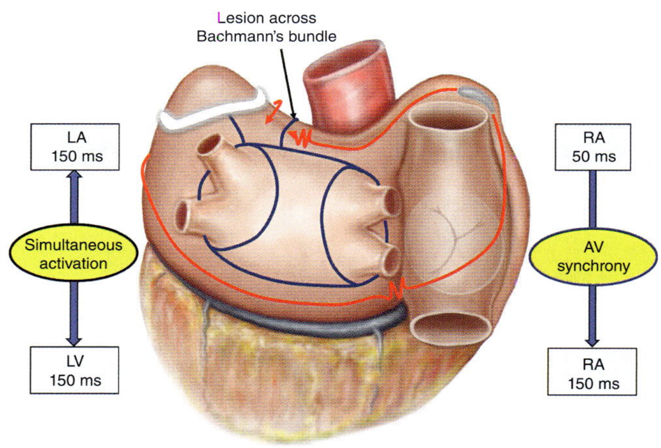

Fig. 3.15 If conduction is blocked across Bachmann's bundle, it can take as long as 150 ms after right atrial activation for complete left atrial activation to occur. This interatrial conduction delay does not affect right atrial–right ventricular synchrony, but the delay in left atrial activation can result in the left atrium (LA) and left ventricle (LV) to contract simultaneously. This problem can occur in all patients subjected to an "anterior trigone lesion" from the upper pulmonary veins to the mitral annulus anteriorly. It was one of the problems with the Maze-I procedure because the LA was exposed through an anterior left atrial septotomy that blocked conduction across Bachmann's bundle. It is also the reason that performing a Maze procedure through an anterior approach is not recommended. Although the efficacy of the procedure performed through an anterior approach is unaffected, little or no information has been published on the potential adverse effects that the anterior approach can have on subsequent left atrial function. *RA,* Right atrium; *RV,* right ventricle.

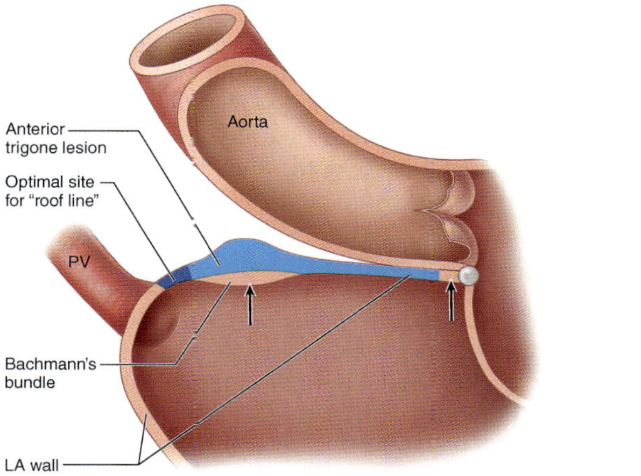

Fig. 3.16 The thickness of Bachmann's bundle can prevent anterior lesions between the upper pulmonary veins and the anterior mitral annulus from being transmural. n addition, it is very difficult to extend such a lesion all the way down to the true annulus of the mitral valve. Thus, there are two places where these anterior lines are vulnerable to failure, the subendocardium of Bachmann's bundle and at the mitral annulus *(small arrows)*. *LA,* Left atrium; *PV, Pulmonary vein.*

from the upper pulmonary veins anteriorly to the mitral annulus or left fibrous trigone. A separate anatomic problem with this lesion is that it is virtually impossible to create a completely contiguous, uniformly transmural lesion in this area with unipolar epicardial energy sources, including unipolar radiofrequency and cryothermia. Bachmann's bundle is commonly too thick even in normal atria to allow transmurality, and in addition, it is virtually impossible to reach the true mitral annulus anteriorly with an epicardial energy source (Fig. 3.16).

Atrioventricular Node

The AV node is a compact group of highly specialized cells located in the lower portion of the atrial septum that serves as a filter for electrical impulses traveling from the atrium to the ventricle (Fig. 3.17). The AV node resides in the plane of the mitral valve annulus as it tapers into the proximal portion of the His bundle. The AV node is located anterior to the os of the coronary sinus at the apex of an anatomic triangle called

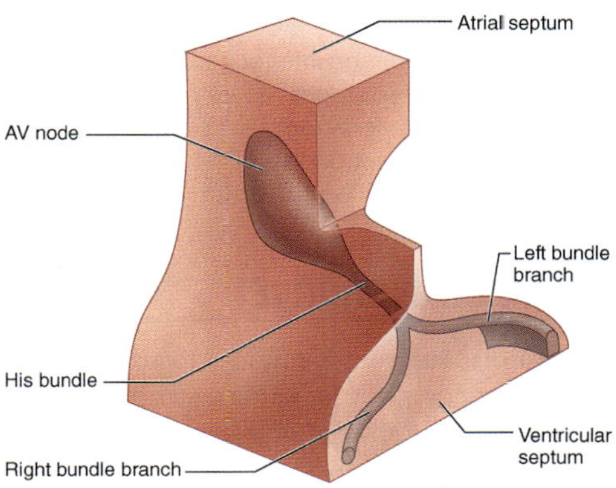

Fig. 3.17 The atrioventricular (AV) node and His bundle are located entirely within the atrial septum. The His bundle lies immediately inferior to the membranous portion of the interatrial septum, penetrates the upper ventricular septum, and then divides into the right and left bundle branches. It is anatomically impossible to damage this AV node–His bundle complex with a Maze procedure that has no septal lesion, such as the Maze-IV procedure.

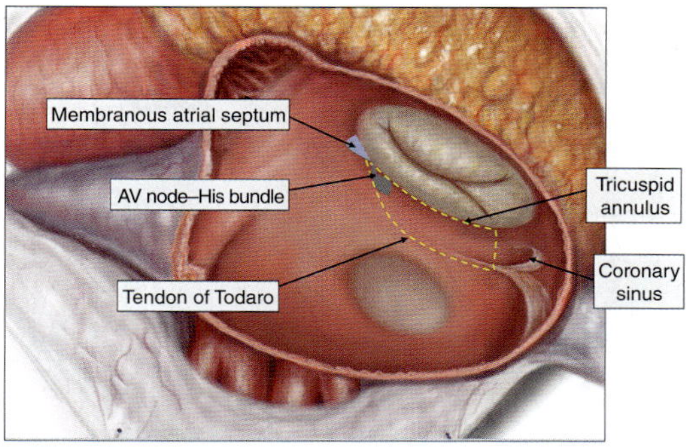

Fig. 3.18 Surgeon's view of the triangle of Koch in the right atrial septum that is bounded by the tendon of Todaro superiorly, the tricuspid annulus inferiorly, the os of the coronary sinus laterally, and the membranous atrial septum medially. The triangle harbors the atrioventricular (AV) node and the proximal portion of the His bundle. It is anatomically impossible to injure the AV node–His bundle complex surgically without entering the triangle of Koch.

the *triangle of Koch* (Fig. 3.18). This triangle is bordered superiorly by the tendon of Todaro that extends from the top of the os of the coronary sinus to the posterior extent of the membranous interatrial septum. Its location can be identified by placing posterior traction in the coronary sinus os, which stretches the tendon into prominence. The other borders of the triangle of Koch are the tricuspid valve annulus and a line drawn straight to the annulus from the top of the os of the coronary sinus. The triangle of Koch and the tendon of Todaro are critical landmarks for arrhythmia surgeons because a surgical lesion that does not extend into the triangle of Koch cannot possibly injure the AV node, and the tendon is a definitive barrier to prevent inadvertent entry into this triangle.

The AV nodal artery most commonly originates from the right coronary artery (Fig. 3.19) at a site that requires it to penetrate

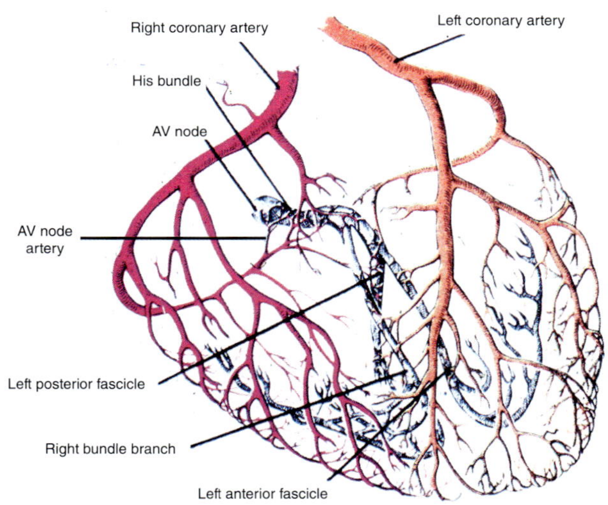

Fig. 3.19 Blood supply of the specialized conduction system. The atrioventricular (AV) node artery usually originates from the terminal branches of the right coronary artery. It was purposely divided in 115 patients with Wolff-Parkinson-White syndrome because of a posterior-septal accessory pathway. No patients developed postoperative heart block, confirming that the AV node artery is not an end artery, and its inadvertent occlusion during catheter or surgical ablation of atrial fibrillation will not result in heart block. (Reproduced from Cox JL, Churyla A, Kislitsina ON, Malaisrie SC, McCarthy PM. Cardiac anatomy pertinent to the catheter and surgical treatment of atrial fibrillation. *J Cardiovasc Electrophysiol.* 2020;31(8):2118–2127.)

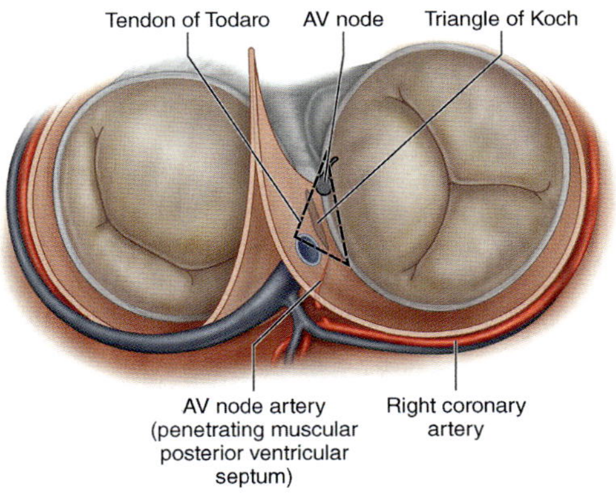

Fig. 3.20 The atrioventricular (AV) node artery typically penetrates the posterior ventricular septum to exit from the floor of the posterior septal space before entering the atrial septum to reach the AV node.

the muscular posterior ventricular septum before emerging from the floor of the posterior septal space on its way to the AV node in the anterior atrial septum (Fig. 3.20). Thus, when dissecting in the posterior septal space between its muscular floor and the overlying fat pad, one almost always encounters the AV node artery emerging from the top of the posterior ventricular septum. Posterior septal accessory pathways responsible for the WPW syndrome commonly accompany the AV nodal artery, and to interrupt them surgically, it is usually necessary to divide the AV node artery as well. The author has surgically divided the AV node artery more than 100 times purposely as a part of the dissection of the posterior septal space to divide accessory AV connections in patients with WPW syndrome without creating a single case of heart block.[8] Clearly, the AV nodal artery is not an "end artery," so it can be divided with impunity.

His Bundle and Bundle Branches

The AV node narrows distally to become the His bundle which passes beneath the border of the membranous septum before entering the muscular mass of the top of the ventricular septum where it divides into the right bundle branch (RBB) and the left bundle branch (LBB). The RBB is a narrow, round bundle of specialized conduction fibers that course down the right side of the ventricular septum just beneath the endocardial surface. It traverses the moderator band near the right ventricular apex to reach the right ventricular free-wall and then divides into Purkinje fibers. The LBB is a broad flat bundle of specialized conduction fibers located at the top of the left side of the ventricular septum (see Fig. 3.17). After it penetrates the ventricular septal musculature to reach the endocardial surface of the left ventricle, it quickly branches into anterior and posterior fascicles.

The specialized conduction fibers that make up the His bundle, both bundle branches, and the Purkinje fibers are distinct from the contracting myocytes of the ventricles. Conduction velocity through contracting ventricular myocardium is approximately 1 mm/ms, but in the specialized conduction tissue, the conduction velocity is approximately 3 mm/ms. The rapidity of conduction through these specialized tissues allows the electrical impulse exiting the AV node to reach the free walls of both ventricles within approximately 50 to 60 ms, resulting in near-simultaneous activation of the endocardium of both ventricles with subsequent activation of the ventricular myocardium of both ventricles from the endocardium to the epicardium. This near-simultaneous activation of the two ventricles results in a narrow QRS complex on the standard electrocardiogram, and it also results in stabilization of the ventricular septum during ventricular systole. If either bundle branch is blocked, the QRS complex becomes wider, and the pumping efficiency of the heart is hampered because of the dyssynchrony of contraction between the two ventricles.

LEFT ATRIAL ISTHMUS

The left atrial isthmus is the posterior-inferior wall of the LA between the inferior pulmonary veins and the posterior mitral valve annulus (Fig. 3.21). After successful isolation of the pulmonary veins and posterior left atrial wall, the left atrial isthmus can become a part of a large reentrant circuit responsible for "peri-mitral atrial flutter," which is described in Chapter 48.

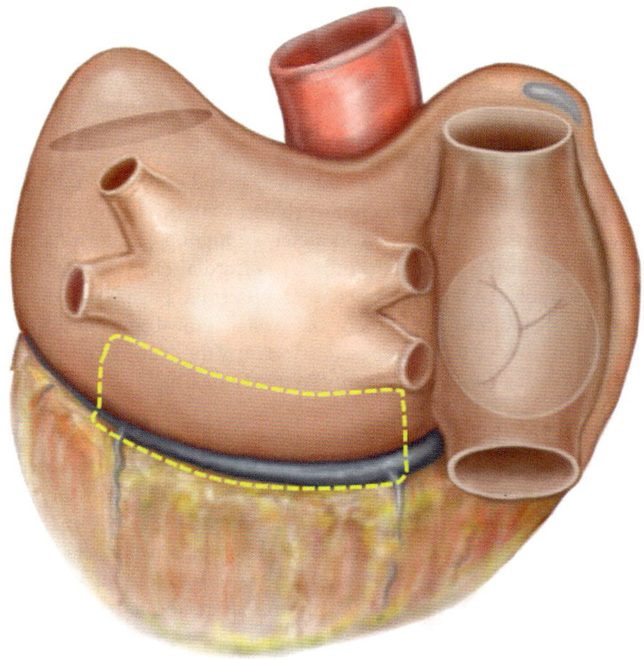

Fig. 3.21 The left atrial isthmus is the portion of the posterior inferior left atrial wall located between the inferior pulmonary veins and the posterior mitral valve annulus (encompassed in the *yellow dashed lines*). It serves as one part of the macro-reentrant circuit responsible for perimitral flutter, the most common mode of failure after surgery or catheter ablation for atrial fibrillation (see Chapter 48).

ATRIOVENTRICULAR GROOVE

Although most cardiac surgeons are trained to avoid the AV groove, it is an important anatomic space for cardiac arrhythmia surgeons. The anatomy, hazards, and methods of safe surgical entry and closure of the AV groove were learned from WPW surgery in which the surgical dissection to divide accessory AV connections was performed entirely within the AV groove.

In the left heart, the LA and LV walls join the mitral annulus without actually contacting one another at the level of the annulus (Fig. 3.22, *left panel*).[9] However, in the right heart, the free walls of the RA and RV "fold over" one another so that the true tricuspid valve annulus is buried between them and not in actual contact with the AV groove fat

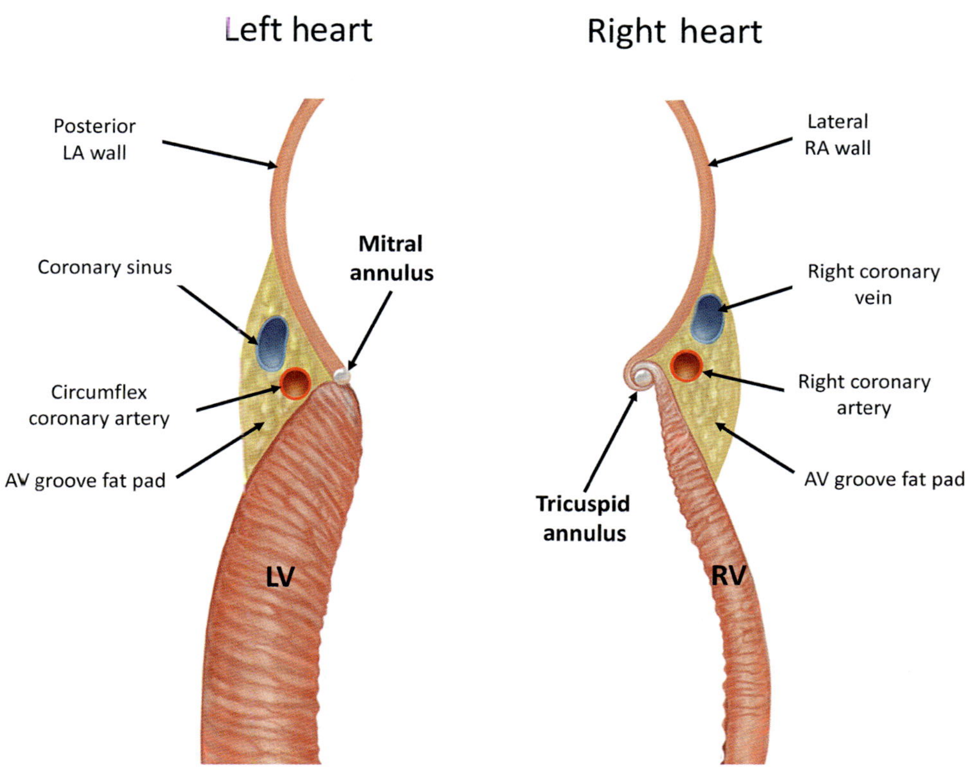

Fig. 3 22 *Left panel,* The left atrium (LA) and left ventricle (LV) join the mitral annulus from opposite directions, and therefore they normally are not in contact in the region of the atrioventricular (AV) groove. *Right panel,* In marked contrast, there is a "folding over" of the right atrium (RA) and right ventricle (RV) free wall at the level of the tricuspid annulus, which is the main reason that any RA lesion that terminates at the tricuspid annulus should have a cryolesion placed at its terminal end. (Reproduced from Cox JL, Churyla A, Kislitsina ON, Malaisrie SC, McCarthy PM. Cardiac anatomy pertinent to the catheter and surgical treatment of atrial fibrillation. *J Cardiovasc Electrophysiol.* 2020;31(8):2118–2127.)

pad (Fig. 3.22, *right panel*). This anatomic peculiarity is important in AF surgery if one wishes to extend a line of conduction block in the RA all the way down to the tricuspid valve annulus. This is the reason that a cryolesion should always be placed at the end of any RA or septal lesion that extends to the tricuspid valve.

The AV groove is covered by the same layer of epicardium that covers the surface of the atria and ventricles. The ventricular epicardium reflects off the ventricular surface to cover the space created by the curving of the atria and ventricles toward the mitral and tricuspid valve annuli and then reflects back onto the atria to become the atrial epicardial surface at the superior edge of the AV groove. The underlying space in the AV groove contains only fat and blood vessels. Whereas the vessels in the left AV groove are the coronary sinus and the circumflex coronary artery, the right AV groove contains the right coronary artery and vein. This view of the left AV groove graphically illustrates why it is virtually impossible to create a "mitral line" all the way to the mitral annulus from outside the heart or to create a circumferential coronary sinus cryolesion from inside the heart.

REFERENCES

1. Santucci PA, Varma N, Cytron J, et al. Electroanatomic mapping of postpacing intervals clarifies complete active circuit and variants in atrial flutter. *Heart Rhythm.* 2009;6(11):1586–1595.
2. Fischer B, Jais P, Shah D, et al. Radiofrequency catheter ablation of common atrial flutter in 200 patients. *J Cardiovasc Electrophysiol.* 1996;7(12):1225–1233.
3. Boineau JP, Schuessler RB, Canavan TE, Corr PB, Cain ME, Cox JL. The human atrial pacemaker complex. *J Electrocardiol (Suppl).* 1989;22:189–197.
4. Thomas James MD. *Personal communication with author JLC.* 1981.
5. Engel TR, Meister SG, Feitosa GS, Fischer HA, Frankl WS. Appraisal of sinus node artery disease. *Circulation.* 1975;52(2):286–291.
6. Vikse J, Henry BM, Roy J, et al. Anatomical variations in the sinoatrial nodal artery: a meta-analysis and clinical considerations. *PLoS One.* 2016;11(2):e0148331.
7. Ad N, Holmes SD, Ali Rabia, Pritchard G, Lamont D. A single center's experience with pacemaker implantation after the Cox maze procedure for atrial fibrillation. *J Thor Cardiovasc Surg.* 2017;154(1):139–146.
8. Cox JL, Ad N, Churyla A, et al. The maze procedure and postoperative pacemakers. *Ann Thorac Surg.* 2018;106(5):1561–1569.
9. Cox JL, Churyla A, Kislitsina ON, Malaisrie SC, McCarthy PM. Cardiac anatomy pertinent to the catheter and surgical treatment of atrial fibrillation. *J Cardiovasc Electrophysiol.* 2020;31(8):2118–2127.

4

Electrophysiologic Concepts Basic to the Understanding of How to Treat Atrial Fibrillation by Surgical or Catheter Intervention

James L. Cox, Richard B. Schuessler

CHAPTER OUTLINE

Clinical arrhythmias occur on the basis of one the following electrophysiologic mechanisms:

1. Automaticity
2. Reentry
   A. Micro-reentry
   B. Macro-reentry
      - Small-diameter macro-reentrant circuits (rotors)
      - Large-diameter macro-reentrant circuits

Although all reentry is abnormal, automaticity is essential for certain critical components of normal cardiac activation. For example, the sinoatrial (SA) node functions by virtue of the fact that its cells are capable of spontaneously generating an electrical impulse on the basis of normal automaticity. However, the transmembrane action potentials of pacemaker cells and normal myocytes are different, which explains why the pacemaker cells generate spontaneous electrical impulses and normal myocytes do not.

NORMAL AUTOMATICITY

Normal Contractile Myocytes

When normal myocardial cells are at rest, there is an electrical differential across the cellular membrane of approximately 90 millivolts that is traditionally expressed as −90 mV because the outside of the cell membrane is negatively charged relative to the inside of the cell. This resting membrane potential (RMP) is maintained primarily by the potassium channel IK1, which is an inward potassium current that keeps the RMP from becoming too negative (Fig. 4.1). It is time independent, which means that it reacts instantaneously to changes in the RMP so that above the RMP, the IK1 channel becomes an outward potassium current. In phase 0 when the fast inward sodium current is activated, IK1 decreases to zero. When the RMP reaches its peak voltage, an inward current calcium channel is activated that is responsible for the plateau of phase 2. At the same time, the outward current potassium channel starts to bring down the voltage toward the RMP. As the voltage decreases, IK1, the sodium–potassium (Na^+/K^+) pump and the sodium-calcium (Na^+/Ca^{2+}) exchanger are activated and reestablish the RMP to normal resting levels.

Anything that causes the RMP to increase to the threshold level of approximately −60 mV results in sudden depolarization of that individual myocyte (i.e., it results in an instantaneous reversal of the charge on the outside of the cell from negative to positive). When the

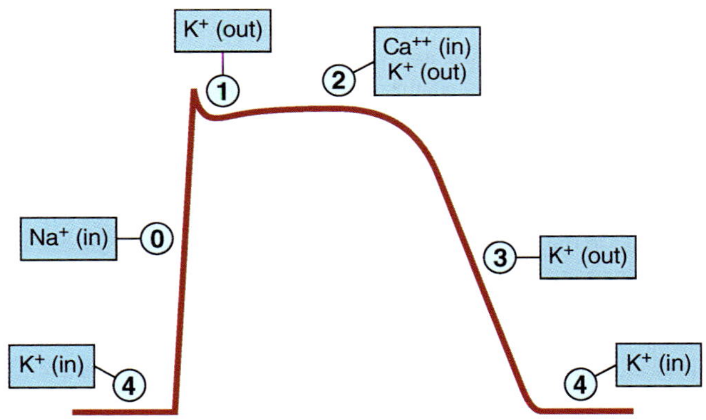

Fig. 4.1 Normal transmembrane action potential in nonpacemaker myocytes. *Ca^{++}*, Calcium; *(in)*, flow from outside the cell to inside the cell; *K^+*, potassium; *Na^+*, sodium; *(out)*, flow from inside the cell to outside the cell. See text for further discussion.

transmembrane potential again drops below the threshold potential of −60 mV, the cell is capable of being depolarized again. Sudden cellular depolarization of a myocyte can be caused by a variety of external stimuli such as a change in autonomic neural input or a mechanical external stimulus such as trauma or pacing.

Pacemaker Cells

The cellular electrophysiology of pacemaker cells differs from that of normal contractile myocytes by possessing the characteristic of *spontaneous phase 4 depolarization* (Fig. 4.2). This critical trait of pacemaker cells is possible for several reasons:

1. Pacemaker cells do not have an IK1 channel, which is one of the reasons that spontaneous phase 4 depolarization can occur.
2. In pacemaker cells, nonspecific cation channels produce an inward current that further contribute to spontaneous phase 4 depolarization.
3. In pacemaker cells, the action potential is produced by the calcium current, but they do not have the fast sodium current seen in nonpacemaker myocytes.

Factors that decrease the heart rate, including drugs such as beta-blockers, do so by *decreasing the slope* of phase 4 depolarization of pacemaker cells, thereby lengthening the time between heartbeats (Fig. 4.3). Humoral agents, neural stimuli, and drugs such as isoproterenol that increase the heart rate do so by *increasing the slope* of the phase 4 depolarization, thereby shortening the time between heartbeats.

Depolarization of a single cell causes immediate depolarization of adjacent myocardial cells, and the resultant electrical "wavefront" propagates away from this site in all directions. If multiple electrodes are arrayed around this region of the heart, the site where the original cell first depolarized appears to be a single spot or "focus" on an activation time map. Thus during normal sinus rhythm, the sinus impulse appears to originate from a single site.

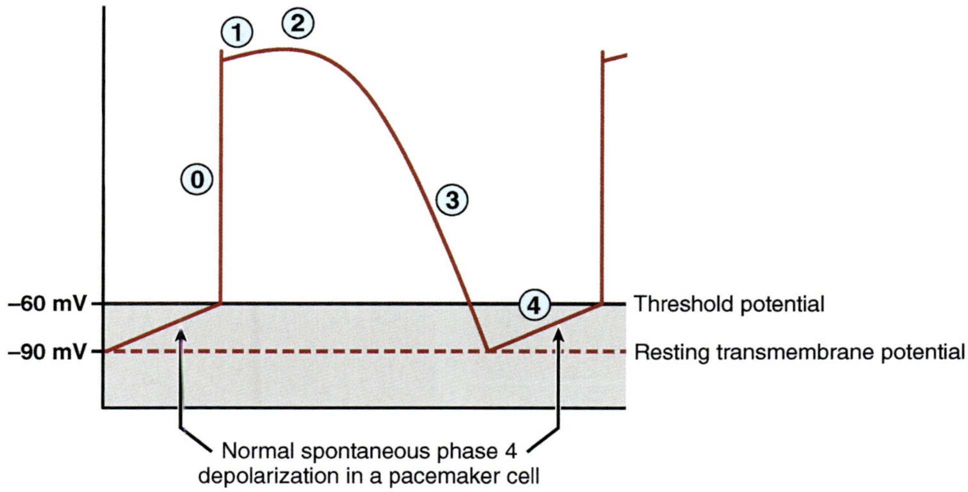

Fig. 4.2 Normal action potential of a pacemaker myocyte emphasizing normal phase 4 depolarization. See text for further discussion.

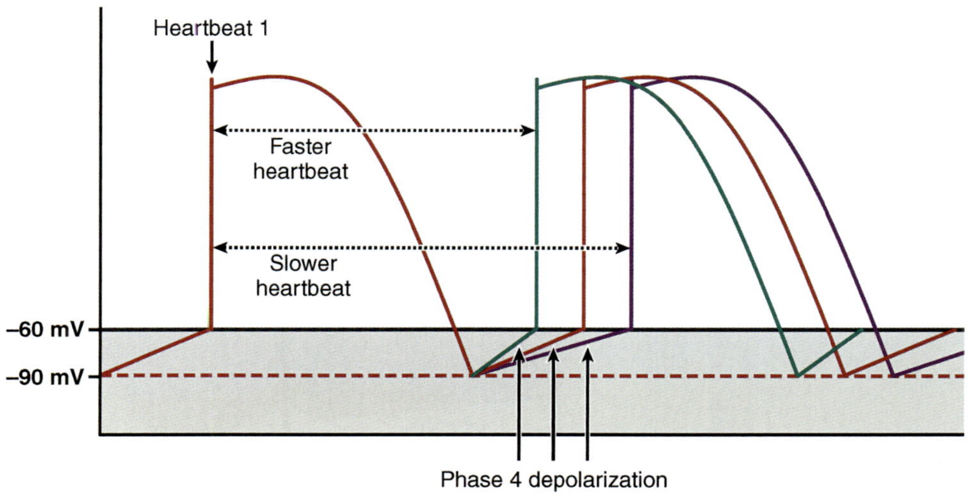

Fig. 4.3 Most stimulants and antiarrhythmic medications, as well as neurological events, change the heart rate by altering the slope of phase 4 depolarization. See text for further discussion.

NORMAL WAVEFRONT PROPAGATION AND COMPLEX FRAGMENTED ATRIAL ELECTROGRAMS

Cardiac myocytes are coupled by intercalated disks that are traversed by gap junctions between adjacent myocytes (Fig. 4.4). Gap junctions are tiny "pores" between cells that allow current to flow between a depolarized cell and one that is in the phase 4 resting state. As the current from the depolarized cell passes through the gap junction, it increases the voltage of the resting cell enough to trigger the inward sodium channel (INa) to cause its depolarization and thus propagate the electrical wavefront.

Electrical activity propagates across the atrial myocardium in "waves" characterized by a leading edge of depolarization where billions of individual cells are undergoing simultaneous depolarization (Fig. 4.5). When these cells are depolarized, they cannot be further depolarized for a certain period of time, the so-called effective refractory period (ERP). Allessie and coworkers[1] have referred to the distance between the leading edge and trailing edge of a wavefront as the "wavelength" of propagating electrical activity. Their formula for calculating the wavelength of a given propagating wavefront is as follows:

$$\text{Wavelength (mm)} = \text{Conduction velocity (mm/ms)} \times \text{ERP (ms)}$$

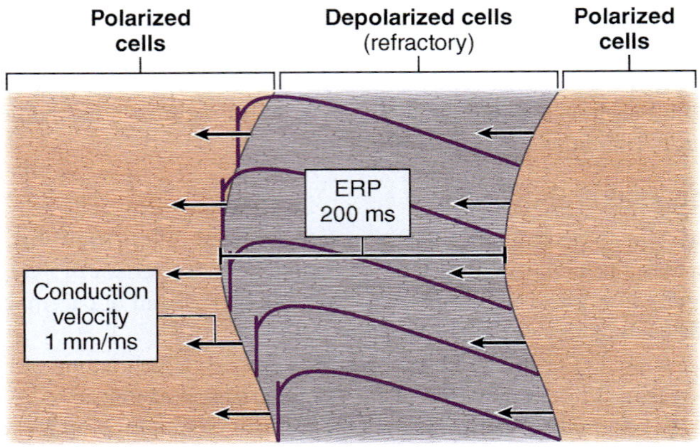

Fig. 4.5 Diagrammatic illustration of an electrical wavefront propagating across atrial myocardium from right to left. The leading edge of the wavefront is where the cells are simultaneously depolarizing ("phase 0" of the action potentials) and the trailing edge is where they are repolarizing. The distance between the two is the effective refractory period of the atrial tissue at this site. *ERP,* Effective refractory period.

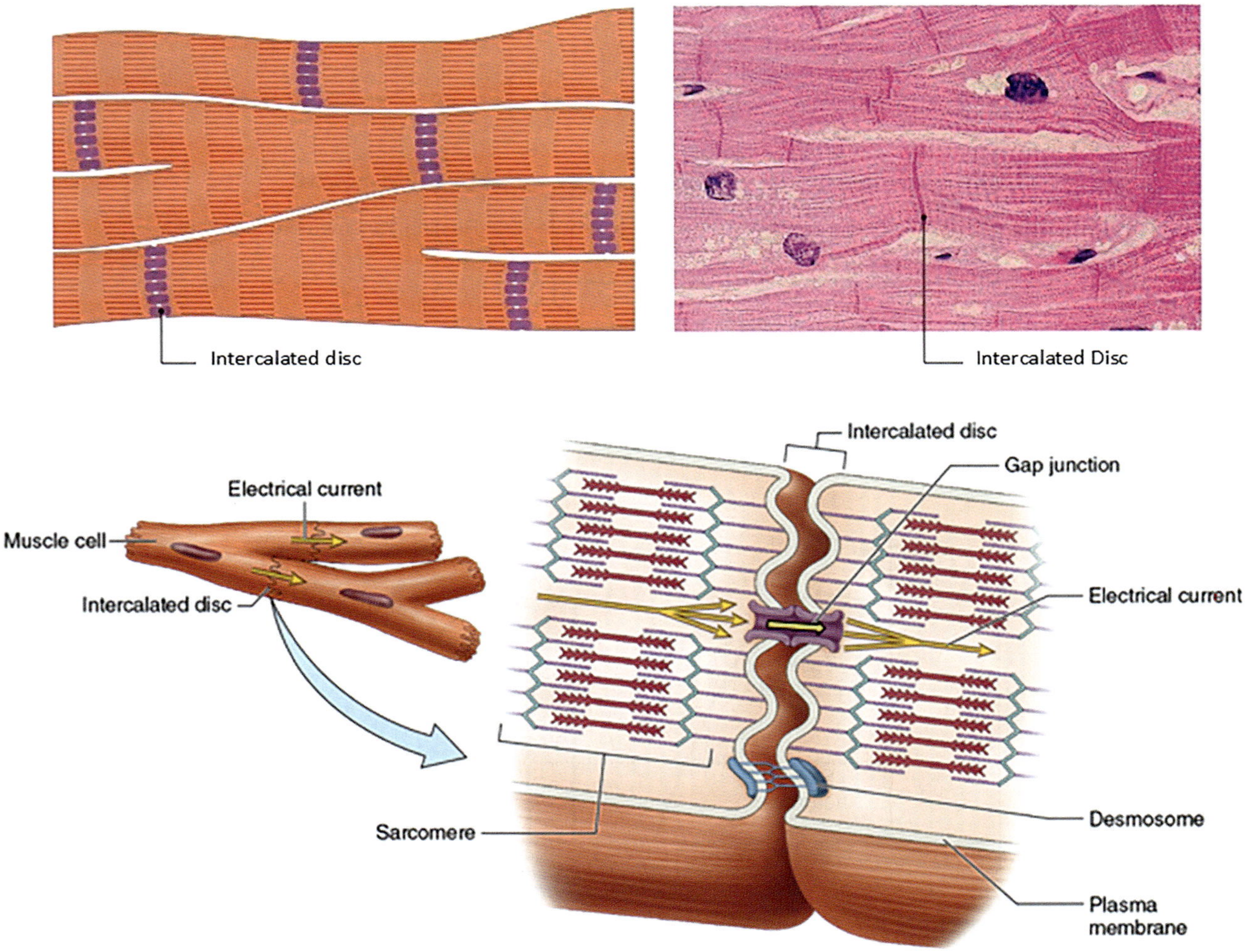

Fig. 4.4 *Left upper panel,* Diagrammatic illustration of myofibrils showing that the individual myocytes are connected by intercalated disks. *Right upper panel,* Photomicrograph of myofibrils showing the intercalated disks. *Lower panels*: Diagrammatic illustration of the details of adjacent myofibrils showing how gap junctions span the connecting intercalated disk between the myofibrils and conducts electrical current from one to the other.

For example, if a particular site in the atrium has a conduction velocity of 1 mm/ms and an ERP of 200 mm as in Fig. 4.5, a potential reentrant circuit in this area would require a path length of 200 mm or 20 cm.

$$1\,\text{mm/ms (CV)} \times 200\,\text{mm (ERP)} = 200\,\text{mm (wavelength)}$$

The wavelength of a propagating impulse is critical because it determines how large an area of the atrium is necessary for reentry to occur (i.e., it determines the smallest that a reentrant circuit can be in this region of the atrium). In the example given, it means that a potential reentrant pathway of *at least* 200 mm (20 cm) is needed to sustain a reentrant circuit. Although such reentrant circuits are traditionally illustrated as perfect circles (see later) for clarity's sake, in reality they can be very circuitous and even out of plane. However, they can only form and sustain themselves in contiguous areas of the atrium that are large enough to allow a wavefront with a given wavelength to circle back and reenter the same area where it began. This concept is fundamentally different from Moe's hypothesis of "multiple wandering wavelets" as the basis of atrial fibrillation (AF; see Chapter 5).

Abnormal Repolarization

Under abnormal conditions such as ischemia, scarring, or inflammation, the earliest measurable electrophysiologic abnormality is frequently an aggravation in the disparity between the repolarization times of individual cells or individual clusters of cells within a small region of the heart. The electrophysiological terms used to describe this pathological condition, which is highly arrhythmogenic in all cardiac tissues, have been changed many times over the years, and the lack of a single descriptive term has led to much confusion. These terms, which all refer to the same electrophysiologic abnormality, include *nonuniform recovery, dispersion of refractoriness, inhomogeneity of repolarization,* and *inhomogeneity of recovery*. In this situation, the trailing edge of repolarization of a wavefront is much more ragged and less well defined. Abnormal repolarization is one of the fundamental essentials for the genesis and perpetuation of arrhythmias.

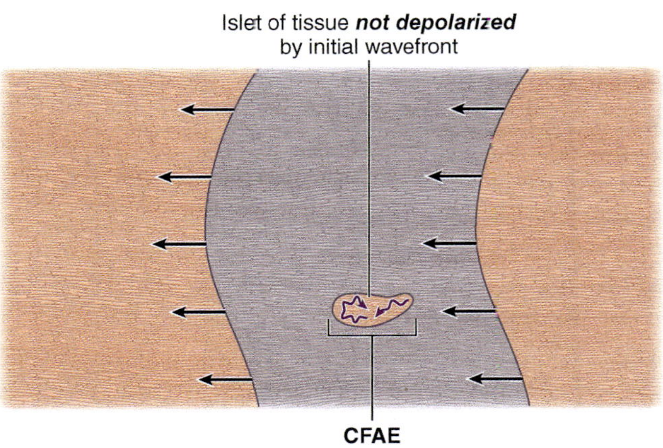

Fig. 4.6 An example of "desynchronized activation" caused by slow conduction in a small islet of atrial tissue. Such an islet of inhomogeneous scar, fat, or ischemia contains atrial myocytes that were not depolarized by the initial wavefront. The tissue around this nondepolarized islet is refractory so that any electrical activity in this area of slow conduction is effectively "trapped" throughout the refractory period of the wavefront. Local electrograms during that time show continuous fractionated electrical electrograms or (CFAEs).

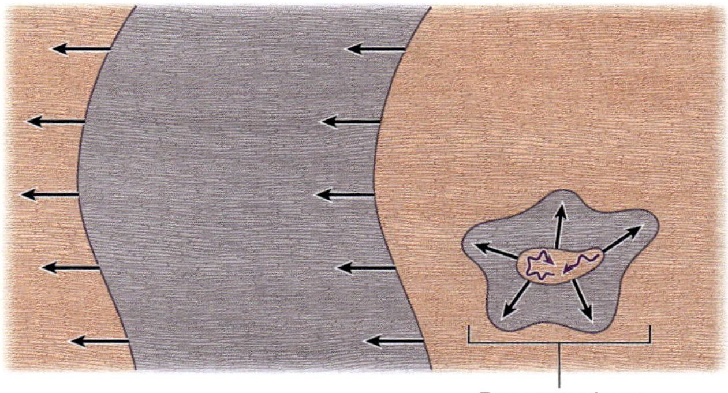

Fig. 4.7 After the original electrical wave passes through and the surrounding atrial myocardium becomes repolarized, the "trapped" electrical activity in the abnormal isolated islet escapes, causing a premature atrial beat. Such continuous fractionated electrical electrogram (CFAE) spots are likely the basis of some extrapulmonary vein atrial triggers that induce atrial fibrillation (AF). However, CFAE spots are not capable of sustaining AF.

Abnormal Depolarization and Complex Fragmented Atrial Electrogram Sites

Arrhythmogenic tissue can also be characterized by *desynchronized activation*, a term that describes the nonsimultaneous *depolarization* of individual cells or clusters of cells in the same region of the heart. In this case, the *leading* edge of a wavefront may become more ragged and actually leave behind islets of tissue where the electrical activity is delayed so long that the surrounding cells have time to repolarize before the depolarization of all the cells in the isolated islet has been completed (Fig. 4.6). Electrical conduction within such an isolated islet is characterized by slow local conduction and micro-reentry that is confined to that islet because the surrounding tissue is refractory. On local electrograms, this appears as complex fragmented atrial electrograms (CFAEs). The primary wave continues to propagate, and as the trailing repolarization edge clears the area, the confined electrical activity quickly escapes and causes a premature atrial beat (Fig. 4.7). These so-called CFAE spots at various local sites within the atrium have been proposed as drivers that are capable of sustaining AF that should be ablated.[2] However, the systematic ablation of hundreds of these CFAE spots per patient has had no discernible benefit when done in conjunction with catheter ablation of AF.[3]

Although it is clear that these CFAE spots do not act as "drivers" that *sustain* AF, it is possible that they might act as "triggers" that *induce* AF. We demonstrated many years ago that such isolated focal sites of abnormal conduction and micro-reentry located in the ischemic border zone surrounding myocardial infarctions (Fig. 4.8) lead to continuous fractionated electrical activity and were responsible for the development of premature ventricular beats that could trigger ventricular tachycardia (Fig. 4.9).[4,5] Thus although it is possible that CFAE sites might occasionally act as extrapulmonary vein triggers that induce AF, there is nothing to suggest that they are involved in sustaining AF. In addition, recording CFAE is critically dependent on the recording technique. CFAE can result from the recording electrodes "seeing" multiple wavefronts in the nearby regions, and if the area is being recorded in a bipolar mode, both electrodes can be recording potentials individually. The farther the bipolar electrodes are apart, the more likely that double potential and multiple deflections will be recorded. During AF these events occur all over the atria and necessarily in the most critical areas of interest. For these reasons, it is likely that most CFAE sites represent false positive targets for ablation coming from areas of slow conduction or block that have nothing to do with the induction, and certainly not the maintenance, of AF. Thus it is no surprise that their ablation has little efficacy in the treatment of patients with AF.

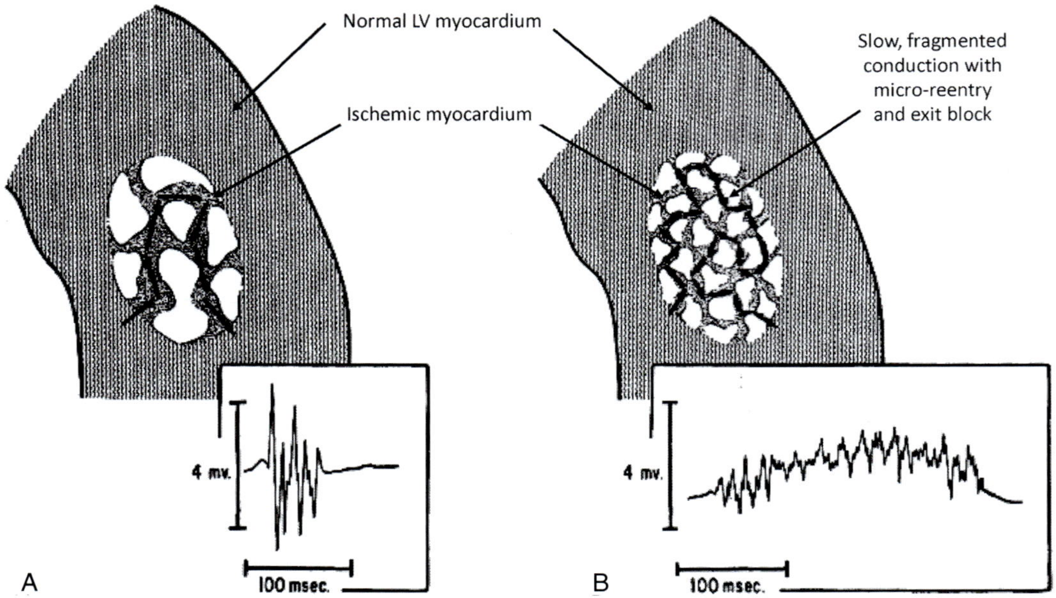

Fig. 4.8 Mechanism of complex desynchronization and slow propagation in an area of myocardial ischemia. In this schematic, the *white areas* represent severely depressed (unexcitable) myocardium. The *stippled areas* represent less severely depressed, nonhomogeneously excitable myocardium. The *area of wavy lines* represents normally excited myocardium in the absolute refractory period. (A) The more coarsely distributed nonhomogeneity results in fewer spikes of larger amplitude and a shorter duration of the activity than in B. (B) The more finely distributed nonhomogeneity of depressed excitability results in more complex and effectively longer pathways. The greater degree of asynchronous excitation in B results in a larger number of spikes of smaller amplitude and a markedly prolonged duration of the circuitous activity confined to this region. The activity is confined by the absolute refractory state of the surrounding myocardium, which has previously been excited by the normally propagated wavefront through this region. In this example, there is interplay between the duration of persistent desynchronized activity and the duration of the recovery period of the surrounding myocardium, a factor which determines whether reentrant premature ventricular contractions are generated or not. *LV*, Left ventricular. (Reproduced from Boineau JP, Cox JL. Slow ventricular activation in acute myocardial infarction—a source of re-entrant premature ventricular contractions. *Circulation*. 1973;48:702-713.)

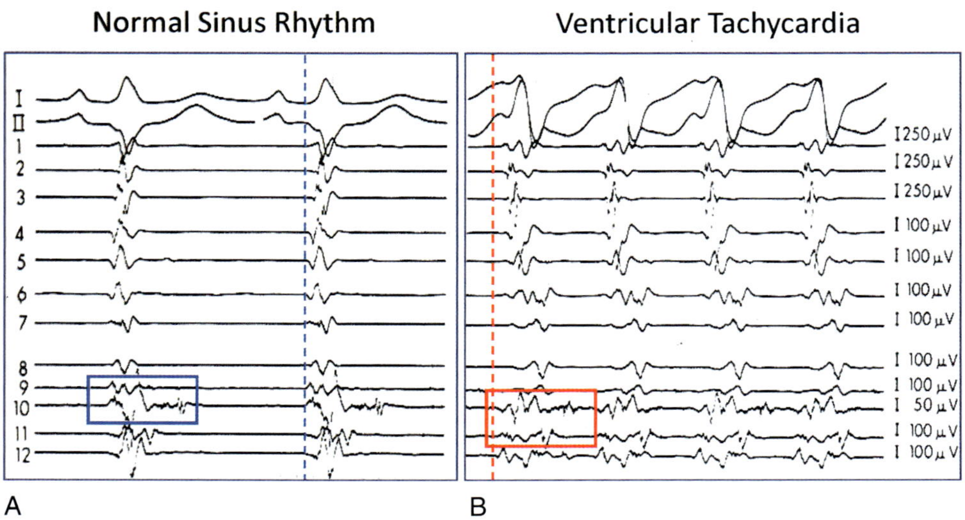

Fig. 4.9 (A) Continuous fractionated electrical activity (CFAE) recorded during normal sinus rhythm (NSR) in the ischemic border zone surrounding myocardial infarctions that were associated with the induction of ventricular tachycardia. The *blue box* shows local site of fractionated electrical activity. Note that the earliest normal activation during sinus rhythm is at electrodes 5 at 6 *(blue line)*, but the fractionated electrical activity begins simultaneously in electrodes 9, 10, and 11. (B) Local recordings from the same electrodes show that the site of origin of the ventricular tachycardia is at sites 10 and 11 *(red box)*, confirming the association between the local fractionated electrical activity and the development of ventricular tachycardia.

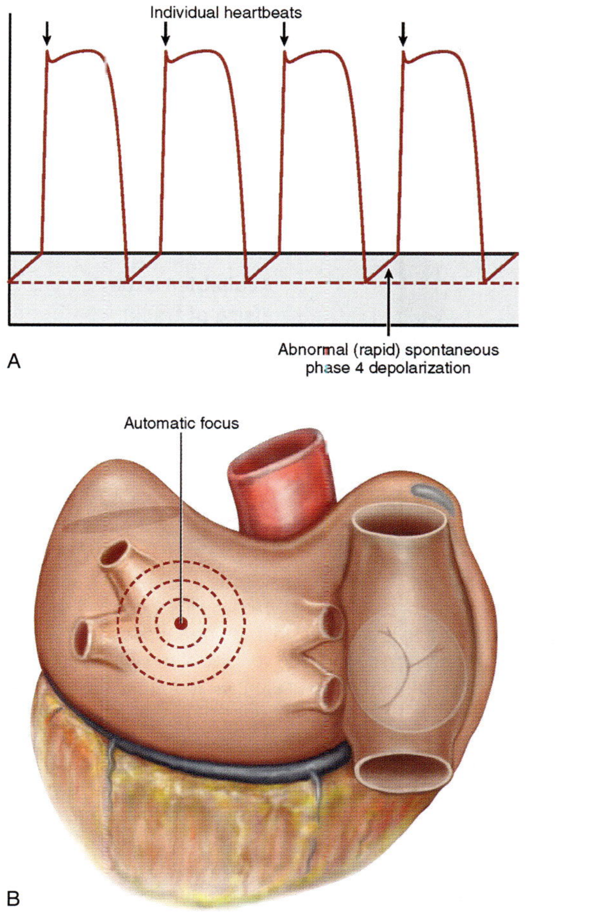

Fig. 4.10 (A) Automatic atrial tachycardias are caused by abnormally rapid spontaneous phase 4 depolarization in nonpacemaker myocytes. (B) When mapped, the site of this abnormal activity appears as a single pinpoint spot on the atrium with wavefronts propagating radially.

CLINICAL PRESENTATION OF AUTOMATIC ARRHYTHMIAS

Automatic Atrial Tachycardia

The most common clinical arrhythmias that occur on the basis of automaticity are the "automatic atrial tachycardias." These tachycardias are usually caused by abnormally rapid spontaneous phase 4 depolarization of one or more abnormal cells in a small localized site in the atrium (Fig. 4.10). *Automatic left atrial tachycardias* usually arise from a single site that can be located anywhere in the left atrium, and they typically remain fixed in one position (Fig. 4.11). They also occasionally occur as a result of congenital "cell rests" located near the left superior pulmonary vein orifice in the mirror-image position of the SA node in the right atrium.[6] Automatic left atrial tachycardia is typically quite regular. It is exceedingly rare for an automatic left atrial tachycardia to have multiple sites of origin. Thus if a left atrial focus can be mapped precisely, it is quite amenable to being ablated either by surgical or catheter-based techniques. If an automatic left atrial focus cannot be located precisely by mapping techniques, either the general region of the automatic focus (e.g., the pulmonary vein orifices) or the entire left atrium can be surgically isolated from the rest of the heart.[7]

Conversely, *automatic right atrial tachycardias* are most commonly multifocal in origin (i.e., there are several different automatic foci in the right atrium of a single patient). Because these arrhythmias are usually multifocal in origin, they are difficult to ablate by focal ablative techniques. If they are resistant to medical therapy and focal catheter ablation, they may require surgical isolation of the right atrium for control.[8]

Inappropriate Sinus Tachycardia and Postural Orthostatic Tachycardia Syndrome

Inappropriate sinus tachycardia (IST) is a diagnosis of exclusion defined by an unexplained sinus tachycardia with a resting heart rate of greater than 100 beats/min and an average 24-hour heart rate of greater than 90 beats/min. It can be associated with multiple different symptoms, including anxiety, dizziness, and syncope, and is often a debilitating arrhythmia in otherwise healthy people associated with a significant

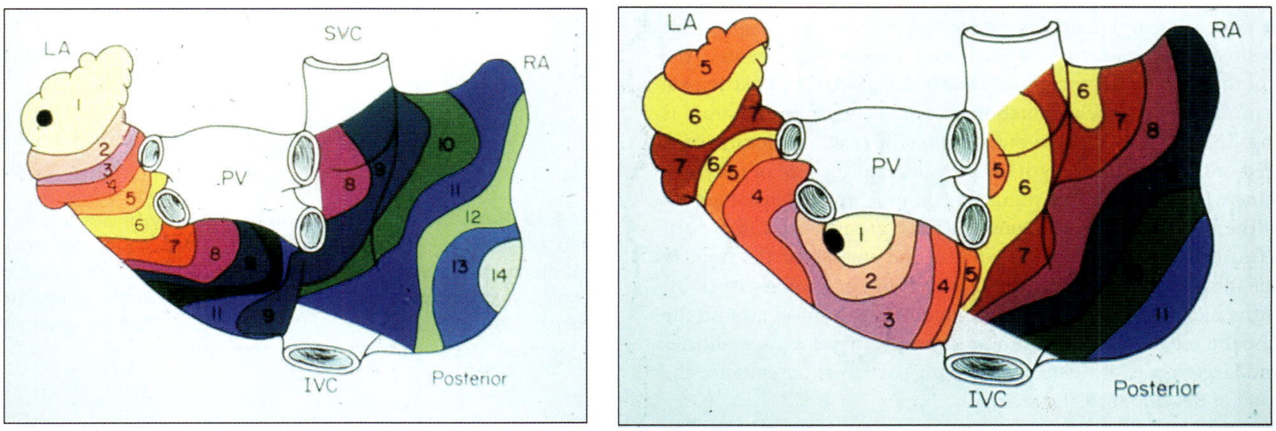

Fig. 4.11 Activation time maps recorded in the early 1980s from two different patients with automatic left atrial tachycardia. (A) The patient was a 14-year-old male who had a continuous, regular atrial tachycardia of 200 beats/min for 2 years before we successfully ablated his automatic focus *(black dot)* with a 2-cm diameter N_2O cryoprobe. (B) The patient was a young female in whom we ablated the site of origin *(black dot)* shown on the map but without success. We finally recognized that the apparent "site of origin" of the tachycardia could not be "bracketed" and that therefore the actual site of origin was most likely within one of the pulmonary veins (PVs) or in the posterior left atrial free wall between the right and left PVs. Therefore, we performed a surgical incision around the entire posterior wall of the left atrium (LA) encompassing all four PVs and the intervening posterior left atrial wall, today referred to as a "box lesion," which cured her tachycardia by confining the automatic focus to the isolated PV cuff. To our knowledge, this was the first PV isolation procedure of any type ever performed, and it was done out of necessity only. The sites of origin of automatic atrial tachycardias tend to be fixed in one position, and they usually discharge at a fixed, regular rate. *IVC,* Inferior vena cava; *RA,* right atrium; *SVC,* superior vena cava.

loss of quality of life.[9] Although the pathogenesis of IST is poorly understood, the central abnormality is autonomic dysfunction. Multiple drug and catheter-based therapies have been used to treat patients with IST with less than optimal results.

Postural orthostatic tachycardia syndrome (POTS) is a systemic illness on the spectrum of an autonomic dysfunction characterized by lightheadedness, palpitations, tremor, weakness, blurred vision, exercise intolerance, and fatigue that occur with standing. These symptoms are associated with an increase in heart rate of greater than 30 beats/min with standing and the absence of orthostatic hypotension. The sinus tachycardia that occurs is often greater than 120 beats/min.

The most successful treatment for patients with these abnormal tachycardias to date has been a hybrid thoracoscopic–catheter procedure developed by a group in Brussels led by Drs. La Meir and de Asmundis.[10]

FUNDAMENTALS OF REENTRY

Reentry was first described by GR Mines in 1914.[11] Understanding the pathophysiology of reentry is critical because it is the most common electrical abnormality responsible for clinical arrhythmias. Reentry can occur only when circumstances exist that allow a wavefront to propagate away from a particular local region and then return ("reenter") to that same local region. Reentry results from an interplay between three electrophysiologic factors:

1. *The conduction velocity of wavefront propagation*
   - The velocity of electrical conduction in normal myocardium is about 1 m/s, or 1 mm/ms. The slower the conduction velocity, the more likely reentry can be initiated and sustained.
2. *The effective refractory period of the involved tissue*
   - The shorter the effective refractory period and the more nonuniform the recovery, the more likely reentry can be initiated and sustained.
3. *The physical size (circumference) of the potential reentrant circuit*
   - The larger the area of atrium available to participate in the reentrant circuit, the more likely reentry can be initiated and sustained.

An analogy of the electrophysiology of atrial reentry can be made to that of a train traveling around a circular track. (Fig. 4.12). The fact that the train can travel in only one direction establishes the equivalent of a unidirectional conduction block, which is essential to reentry. The length of the track represents the area of tissue available to participate in a reentrant circuit. The conduction velocity is the speed the train is traveling. The ERP is the length of the train. The relationships between the speed of the train, the length of the train, and the size of the track determine whether or not the train can run indefinitely (sustained reentry). The result of those relationships must always result in at least some "free track" immediately in front of the engine for the train to continue moving. A slower train, a shorter train, or a longer track increases the likelihood that the train can continue to travel around the track indefinitely. Likewise, a slower conduction velocity, a shorter ERP, and larger areas of tissue available for participation enhance the likelihood of developing atrial reentry.

Thus for a reentrant circuit to develop, a unidirectional block in conduction must be present in the potential pathway, and there must always be a critical area of excitable tissue available in front of the propagating wave of activation. When a wavefront starts to propagate, if the head of the wavefront encounters the tail and that tissue is still refractory, it will block. However, if the head of the wavefront encounters tissue that is no longer refractory, it can reenter into the original site and establish a reentrant circuit. Thus for the reentrant circuit to sustain itself, it is essential that there to be a "gap" between the leading edge of the electrical wavefront (depolarization) and the trailing edge of the electrical wave (repolarization). This is called the "excitable gap"

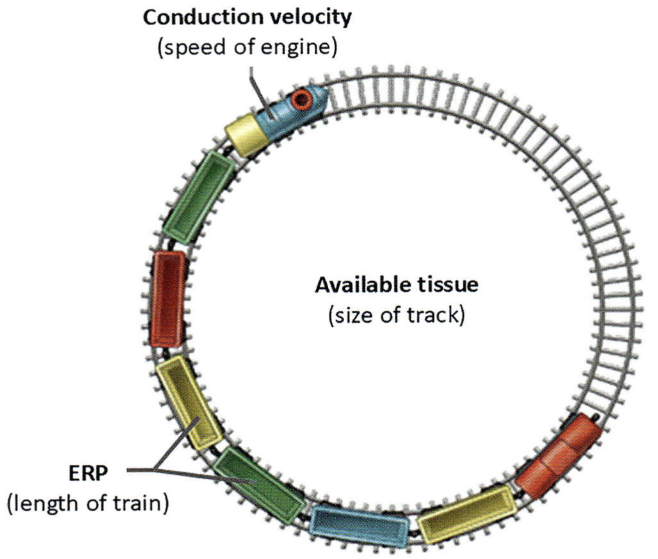

Fig. 4.12 Reentrant circuits are analogous to trains on a circular track. The train can go in only one direction, which is analogous to the unidirectional conduction block that is essential in all reentrant circuits. The speed of the train is analogous to the conduction velocity of the wavefront in a reentrant circuit. The length of the train is analogous to the duration of the effective refractory period (ERP) in the reentrant circuit that follows initial wave of depolarization. The size of the track is analogous to the area of atrium available to participate in the reentrant circuit. A slower conduction velocity, a shorter ERP, and a larger track enhance the stability of a reentrant circuit.

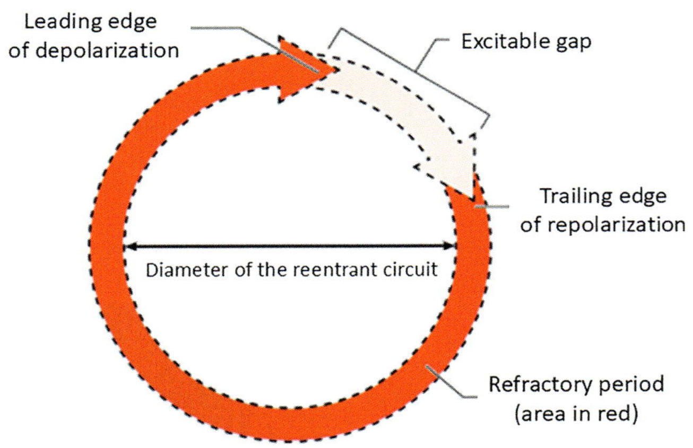

Fig. 4.13 Reentrant circuits involve an interplay between the area of tissue available to participate and support the circuit, the local velocity of electrical conduction, and the local tissue refractory period, all of which may vary from one part of the atrium to another. However, in all instances, an "excitable gap" within the circuit must be maintained for the reentrant circuit to become self-perpetuating.

(Fig. 4.13) because the tissue in this gap has recovered from the previous passage of the wavefront through the tissue and can therefore be depolarized again.

Assuming a stable conduction velocity, the duration of the local refractory period determines the *minimum* size that a macro-reentrant circuit can be in a given area of the atrium (Fig. 4.14).[12] Imagine the refractory period as an arrow with the point of the arrow at the leading edge of depolarization and the tail of the arrow at the trailing edge of repolarization. Now bend the arrow so that its point almost, but not quite, touches its feathers. (This maintains the equivalent of the "excitable gap.") This is the smallest that a macro-reentrant circuit can be in

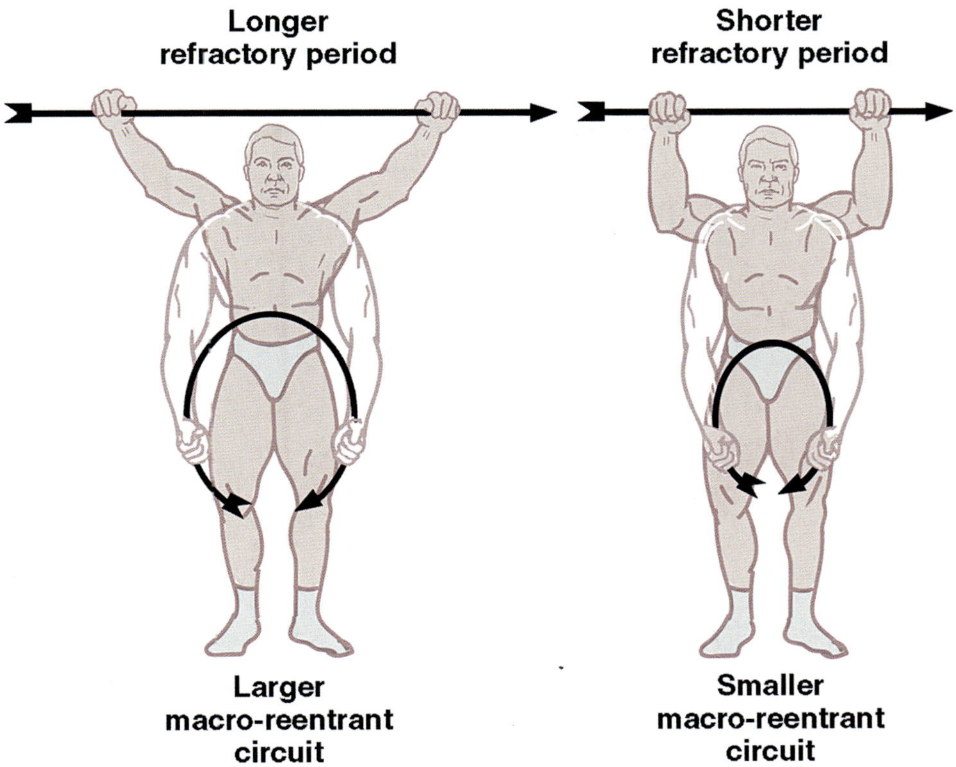

Fig. 4.14 The physical size of the macro-reentrant circuits that sustain atrial fibrillation varies from one area to another. Assuming a stable conduction velocity, the *minimum* size that a macro-reentrant circuit can be in a given area depends on the refractory period of the atrial tissue in that area. See text for further discussion. (Reproduced by permission)[10]

an area of the atrium with that particular refractory period. If the arrow were bent more, the gap between the point and the feathers would disappear, and reentry would be abolished. Thus the longer the refractory period, the bigger the reentrant circuit has to be to sustain macro-reentry. Smaller macro-reentrant circuits can occur in areas where the refractory periods are shorter. The refractory periods in the left atrium are shorter than those in the right atrium, so the macro-reentrant circuits in the left atrium are smaller than those in the right atrium (Fig. 4.15).

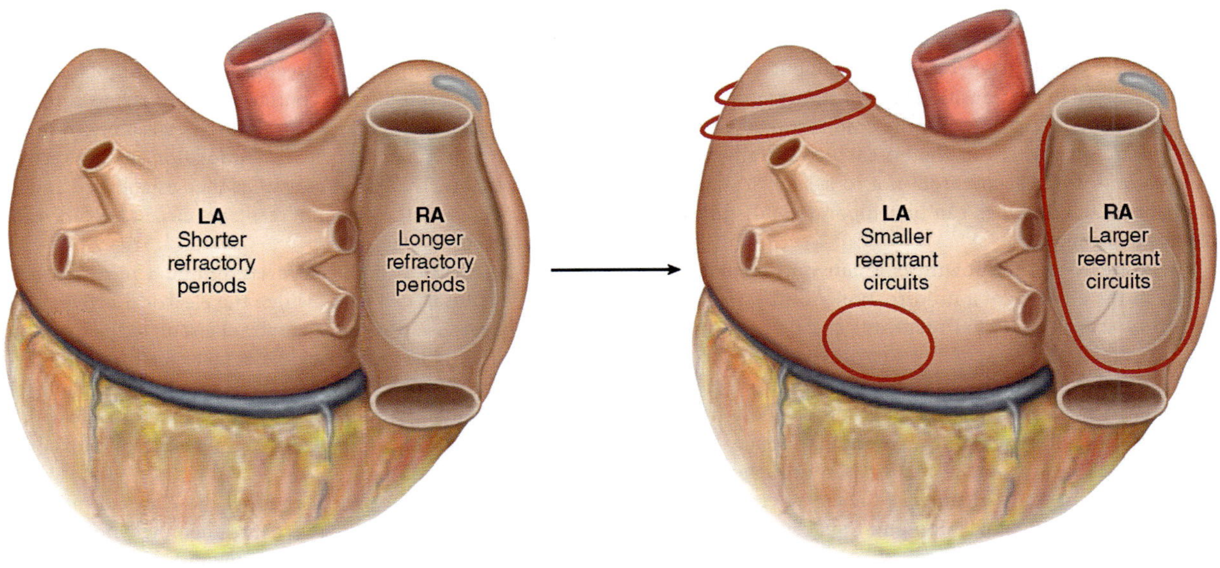

Fig. 4.15 The local refractory periods in the left atrium (LA) are shorter than the local refractory periods in the right atrium (RA). Therefore, macro-reentrant circuits can be smaller in the LA than they can be in the RA. In fact, the refractory periods in a normal RA are so long that the only macro-reentrant circuit that the normal RA can support is the large circuit responsible for classic atrial flutter.

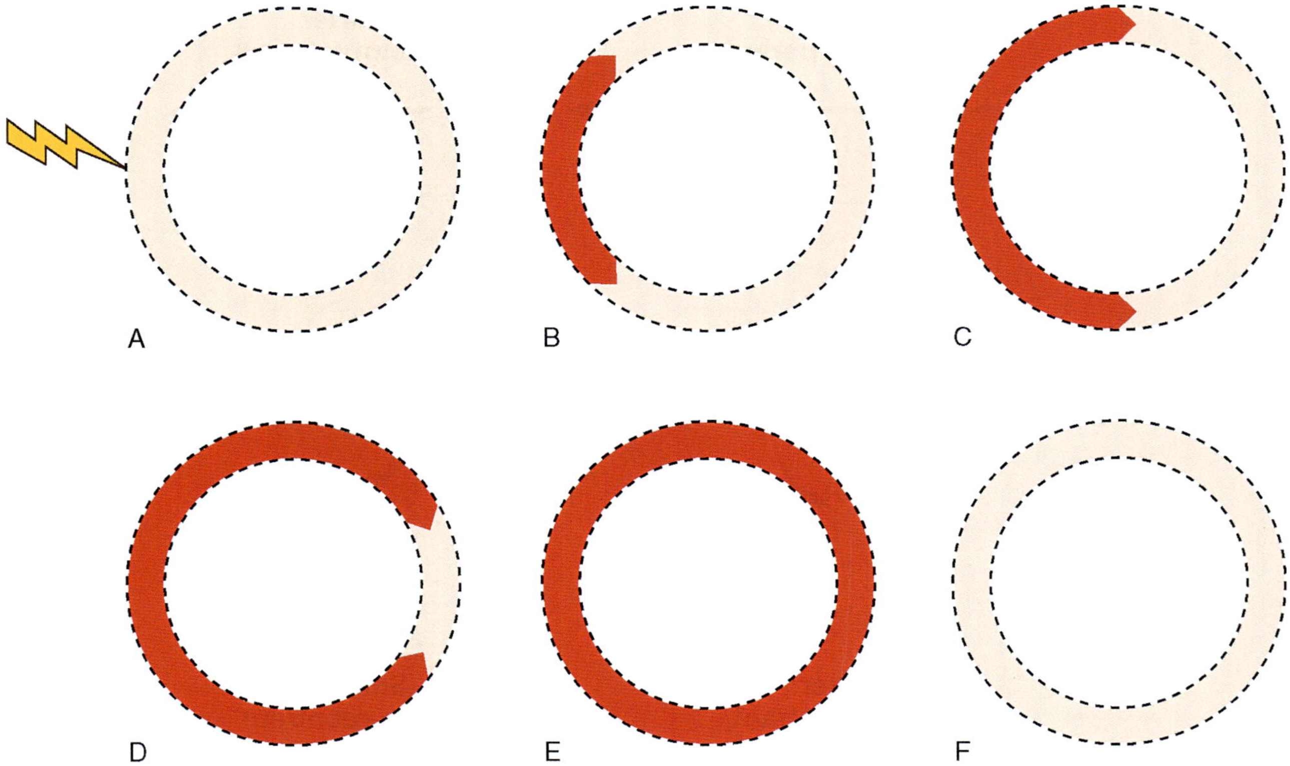

Fig. 4.16 Under normal circumstances, electrical stimulation of atrial tissue does not cause reentry to develop even though the area of the entire atrium is more than enough to sustain reentry. See text for further discussion.

This observation is critical to the proper understanding of the electrophysiology of AF and to understanding the optimal way to treat it interventionally.

Traditionally, it has been taught that there are two components necessary for reentry to develop: (1) a region of slow electrical conduction and (2) an area of unidirectional conduction block (i.e., a region of myocardium that will conduct an electrical impulse in one direction but not in the reverse direction). Because "slow conduction" is a relative term, the real culprit in the transition of a *potential* reentrant circuit into an *actual* reentrant circuit is usually the unidirectional block. This unidirectional block somewhere in the potential reentrant circuit is essential only to *initiate* the tachycardia not to sustain it. Therefore, a unidirectional conduction block can be temporary and still cause a reentrant circuit to form.

Virtually any area of either atrium is a *potential* reentrant circuit. However, in the absence of a unidirectional block, the electrical stimulation of such a potential reentrant circuit causes no abnormality, and in fact, the presence of the potential circuit is not even detectable (Fig. 4.16). In this example, the potential reentrant circuit is stimulated by an electrical impulse (the yellow lightning bolt), and the resulting electrical impulse (red) is propagated away from the stimulation site in both directions around the potential circuit. No reentry occurs, and ultimately, the entire circuit is completely depolarized in a normal fashion and then returns to its normal resting state.

The problem occurs when the potential reentrant circuit contains a region of unidirectional conduction block (Fig. 4.17). In this example, the same potential reentrant circuit is stimulated in the same manner as in the previous figure. The electrical impulse again propagates away from the stimulation site in both directions. However, as one part of the electrical impulse encounters the unidirectional block, its propagation stops. Meanwhile, the other limb of the impulse continues its propagation in the normal fashion around the circuit in a clockwise fashion (in this example). As the leading edge of this wavefront encounters the site of the unidirectional conduction block from the opposite direction, it simply continues to propagate across the region unimpeded because conduction in this area is blocked in only one direction. By this time, the original stimulation site has recovered and is again excitable. The "excitable gap" is then established and maintained as described, and the *potential* reentrant circuit becomes an *actual* reentrant circuit.

As the electrical impulse travels around a reentrant circuit, it encounters natural "exit sites" where the electrical activity in the circuit can propagate away from the reentrant circuit to the surrounding myocardium that is not a part of the actual reentrant circuit (Fig. 4.18). Because the electrical activity travels around this circuit quickly, the circuit continually stimulates the heart via the exit site with each cycle, thus becoming what amounts to a perpetual "generator" or "driver" for the clinical arrhythmia.

It is important to understand that these are not necessarily round or elliptical circuits, and they are most definitely not two dimensional. This is an anatomic reentry that can involve multiple layers of the atrial wall and multiple normal anatomic muscle bundles and areas of block such as vessel orifices and scar tissue.

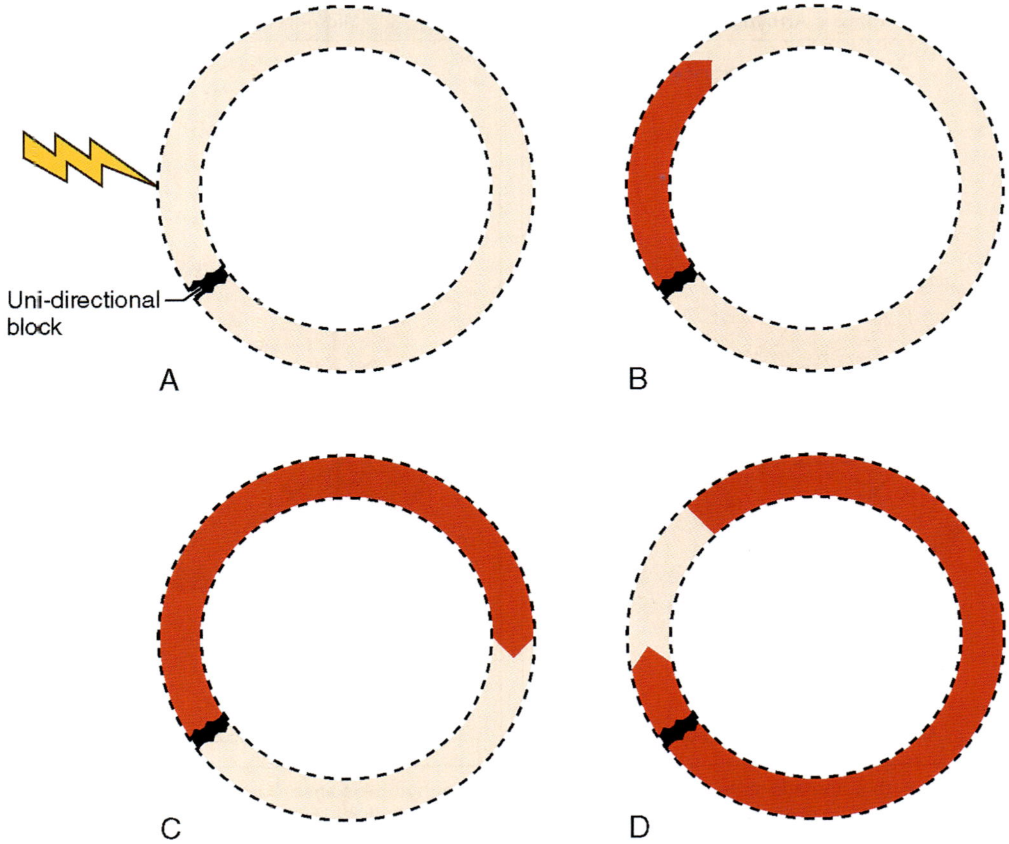

Fig. 4.17 (A) If an abnormal area of atrium can conduct electrical activity in only one direction, it is said to have a "unidirectional conduction block," which sets up one of the circumstances in which reentry can occur. (B) Electrical stimulation of such a potential reentrant circuit results in electrical wave propagation in only one direction. (C) Depending on the size of the area of the atrium available to participate, the local conduction velocity, and the local refractory period, the electrical wave can travel around the circuit as long as there is an excitable gap between the leading edge of the depolarization wavefront and refractory tissue. (D) This allows the leading edge of the wavefront to "reenter" back into its original area and become self-perpetuating). As the wavefront passes through the area of unidirectional block, its conduction velocity usually slows, which helps to maintain the excitable gap and stabilize the reentrant circuit.

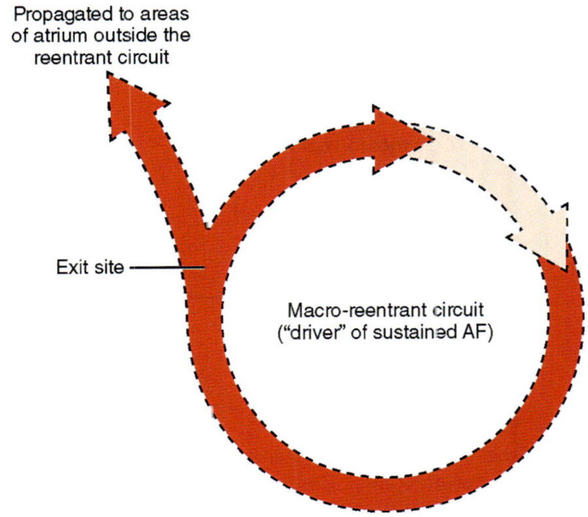

Fig. 4.18 Reentrant circuits typically have an "exit site" where the electrical activity in the circuit can exit and stimulate the rest of the atrium. This can happen with every cycle around the circuit. Because the reentrant circuit is self-perpetuating, it serves as a sustaining "driver" of atrial flutter or fibrillation until the reentrant circuit is broken. See text for further discussion. *AF,* Atrial fibrillation.

ELECTROPHYSIOLOGIC BASIS OF THE SURGICAL TREATMENT OF ATRIAL FIBRILLATION

An arrhythmia that is caused by a focal site of automaticity or micro-reentry (Fig. 4.19) is usually simple to ablate or isolate because the automatic or micro-reentrant focus involves only a few cells. However, it is essential in treating automatic or micro-reentrant arrhythmias by surgical or catheter intervention to identify their precise site of origin by electrophysiological mapping. In 2001, the Joint Expert Group from the Working Group of Arrhythmias of the European Society of Cardiology and the North American Society of Pacing and Electrophysiology (now called the Heart Rhythm Society) classified focal atrial tachycardias according to electrophysiologic mechanisms and anatomy.[13] The Joint Expert Group defined focal atrial tachycardia as "being characterized by atrial activation starting rhythmically at a small area (focus) from where it spreads centrifugally." This definition indicates that the arrhythmia arises from an area that is smaller than would be required for classical macro-reentry, which conventionally is considered to be a circuit larger than 2 cm in diameter. These focal sites of either automaticity or micro-reentry not only cause premature atrial beats and focal atrial tachycardias, but they can also serve as focal triggers that *induce* AF.

There has been disagreement for many years about the relative importance of small-diameter macro-reentrant circuits ("rotors") versus

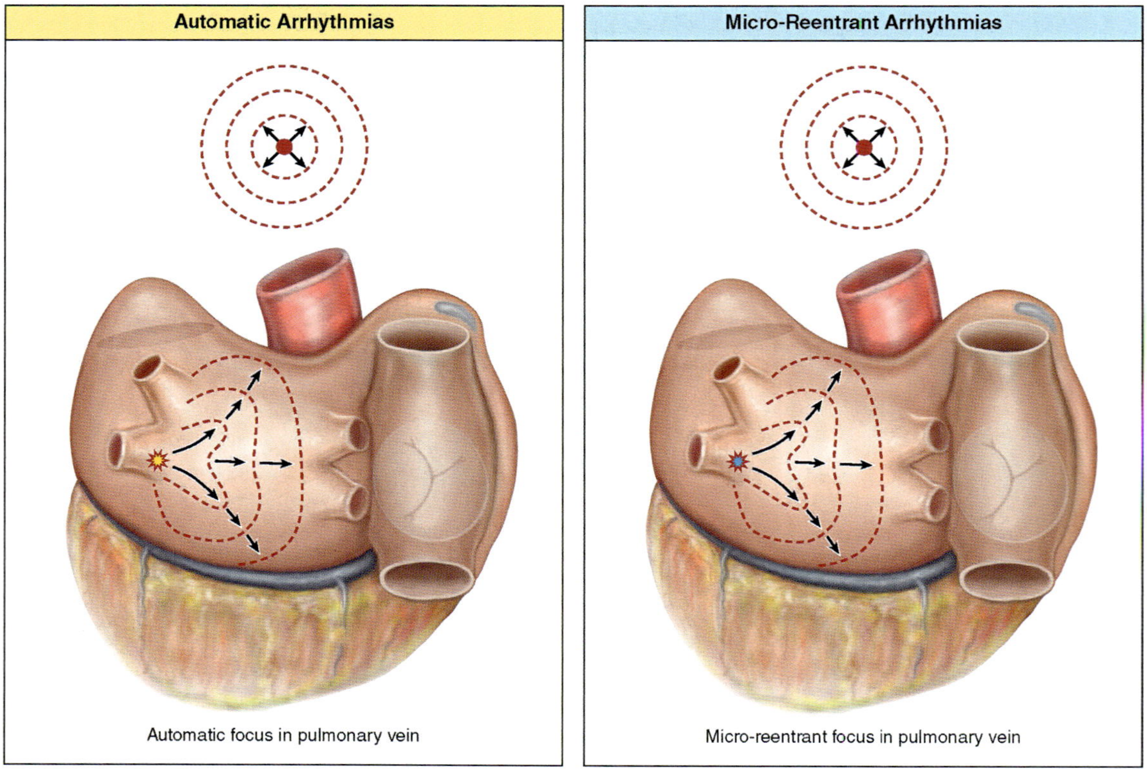

Fig. 4.19 Both automatic arrhythmias and micro-reentrant arrhythmias arise from a pinpoint focus, and the generated wavefront propagates radially from that focus as if a pebble had been dropped in a still pond *(upper panels)*. Automatic foci cannot be differentiated from micro-reentrant foci by simple electrophysiological mapping. For example, a global activation time map of an automatic focus *(left lower panel)* and a micro-reentrant focus *(right lower panel)* in the left inferior pulmonary vein look identical.

large-diameter macro-reentrant circuits in *sustaining* AF after it has been initiated by focal atrial triggers (Fig. 4.20). It is puzzling that the long-term success of the surgical Maze procedure[14] has not put to rest any doubt that after being established, AF is sustained primarily by *large* macro-reentrant circuits because otherwise, the procedure simply would not have worked. If, as some suggest, the drivers that sustain AF are small and focal, they would persist postoperatively between the linear lesions of the Maze procedure (Fig. 4.21). However, despite "surviving" the Maze procedure, these persistent small focal drivers would not be capable of driving AF postoperatively because there is not enough distance between the Maze lesions for the large macro-reentrant circuits of AF to form. Moreover, the persistence of these small focal drivers postoperatively would result in virtually all Maze procedures being followed by sustained episodes of *atrial tachycardia* because of the continuous firing of these microscopic "drivers." Certainly, this is *not* what happens after the Maze procedure. Again, this is an example of how we can deduce the mechanism of an arrhythmia by observing how it responds to the creation and precise placement of surgical scars. The *only* explanation for why critically placed linear lesions in the atria reproducibly ablate prolonged episodes of AF is that those episodes are sustained by the large macro-reentrant circuits themselves.

These lessons learned from our experience with the Maze procedure are why we have never wavered in our insistence that although the large atrial macro-reentrant circuits of AF are *induced* by triggers, they themselves subsequently become the self-perpetuating "drivers" that *sustain* the episodes in the majority of patients with persistent and long-standing persistent AF. It is true that at least some episodes of prolonged AF can be sustained by focal drivers or "rotors" that can be ablated locally to terminate the arrhythmia,[15] and that in other cases

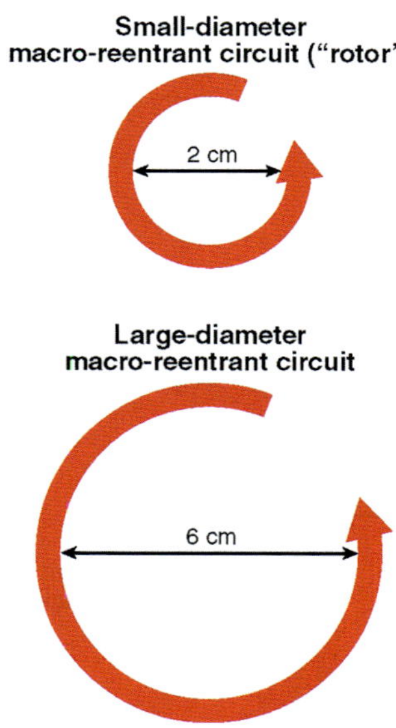

Fig. 4.20 Small-diameter macro-reentrant circuits or drivers *(upper panel)* are often called "rotors." They can have an active reentrant circuit with a diameter of only 2 cm in which case they are technically "focal," though they are distinguished from automatic and micro-reentrant foci by the fact that the impulses that they generate do not propagate away from the focus in a radial manner. Instead, they produce exactly the same pattern of spiral activation in the atrium as do larger macro-reentrant circuits *(lower panel)*. The larger reentrant circuits usually have a diameter of 5 to 6 cm or more.

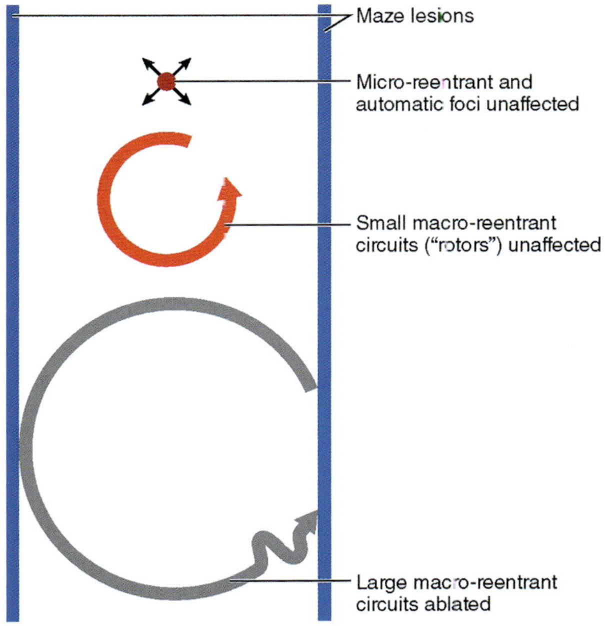

Fig. 4.21 If atrial fibrillation (AF) were sustained by focal triggers (automatic or micro-reentrant), the Maze procedure would be completely ineffective. Likewise, if AF were sustained primarily by small macro-reentrant drivers (rotors) that are only 2 cm in diameter, it is unlikely that the Maze procedure would be as effective as reported. Some authors suggest that the Maze procedure would ablate most AF even if, as they believe, it is sustained by these small rotors because the rotors move often and are extinguished when they run into one of the multiple lesions of the Maze procedure. The authors agree that these small rotors can occasionally drive AF but that AF is far more often driven by large macro-reentrant circuits, explaining the proven long-term success of the Maze procedure.

so-called pulmonary vein tachycardia[16] may rarely play a role in sustaining some episodes of AF for prolonged periods of time. However, as previously mentioned, such focal drivers are not active continuously for prolonged periods of time, and the instant they stop firing and the AF continues, some mechanism other than focal triggers is necessary to explain why the AF continues without the triggers. In our experience, focal drivers, including pulmonary vein tachycardia are *rarely* the drivers for prolonged episodes of AF and are *almost never* the drivers for the type of AF that is present continuously for years. Rather, in the majority of patients with continuous AF, the large atrial macro-reentrant circuits themselves become self-perpetuating "drivers," and it is essential to interrupt them to ablate nonparoxysmal AF effectively.

DECISION REGARDING *HOW* TO ABLATE THE MACRO-REENTRANT CIRCUITS THAT SUSTAIN ATRIAL FIBRILLATION

Electrophysiological maps are obviously the basis for our understanding of the mechanisms underlying the induction and maintenance of AF. However, despite the wealth of critical information that maps provide, real-time maps do not come with an interpretation. For example, a dynamic (video) map of a reentrant arrhythmia frequently shows electrical activity spinning around a central "hinge point" that may be fixed in one location or more commonly is constantly changing location. Electrophysiologists usually interpret the map to mean that the active part of the circuit is at its central hinge point and that the wavefront that is spinning around the hinge point is entirely passive (Fig. 4.22, *left panel*). An analogy would be holding one end of a rope and twirling it above one's head. Clearly, the active part of the rope's movement driving the twirling would be the hand (central), and the movement of the rope would be passive. However, the other way to

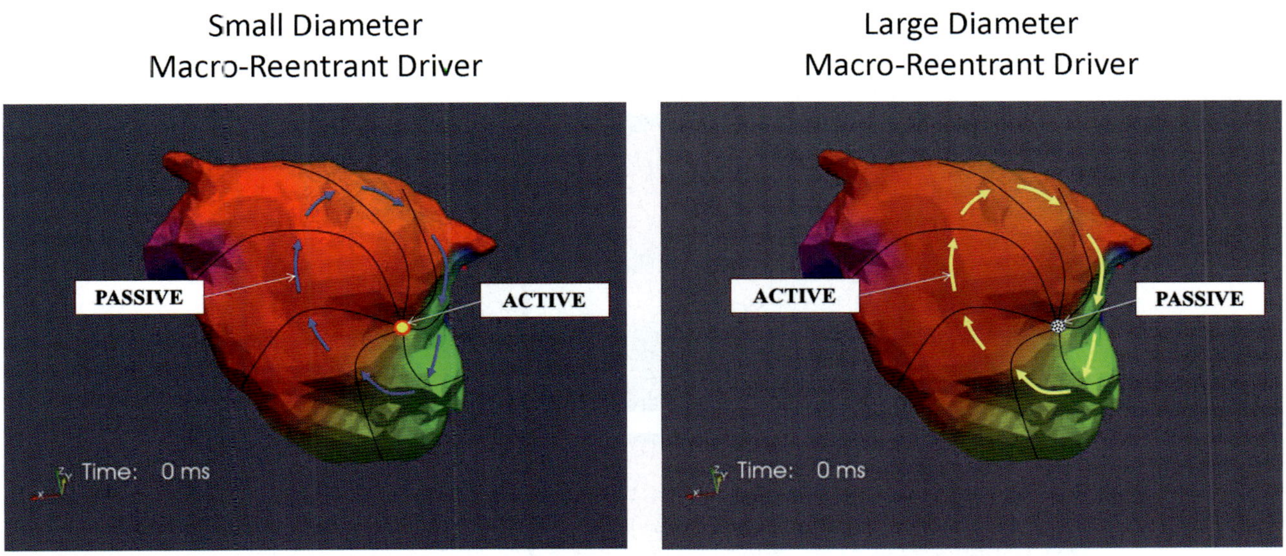

Fig. 4.22 The similar activations patterns caused by small-diameter macro-reentrant drivers and large-diameter macro-reentrant drivers makes it difficult, and sometimes impossible, to distinguish between the two. For example, some would interpret this map of a macro-reentrant driver during atrial fibrillation to be a small-diameter macro-reentrant driver ("rotor"), and the atrial activation is all passive *(left panel)*. Others would interpret this same map to show a large-diameter macro-reentrant driver rotating around a central area of functional conduction block *(right panel)* like atrial flutter, which is a large-diameter macro-reentrant driver in the right atrium that rotates around a central area of functional conduction block in the crista terminalis (See Fig. 5-4 in Chapter 5.)

interpret the same map is that the active part of the macro-reentrant circuit is in the wavefront that is spinning around and that the central hinge point is simply an area of functional conduction block created by the edge of the wavefront (Fig. 4.22, *right panel*). This would be analogous to having a rope attached to a pole and someone holding the other end of the rope while running in circles around the pole. In this analogy, the movement of the rope would be caused by the person running around the pole, and the pole itself would be passive.

Correct interpretation of the map is absolutely critical because it dictates the goal of the interventional procedure, whether it is by catheter or surgery (Fig. 4.23). For example, if the map shows that the active part of the reentrant circuit is its center and then one ablates that center, the arrhythmia will stop. However, if the active part of the reentrant circuit is actually the spinning wavefront itself and the central "hinge point" is only an area of functional block, ablation of the central area will fail to stop the arrhythmia (Fig. 4.24). In this case, the large reen-

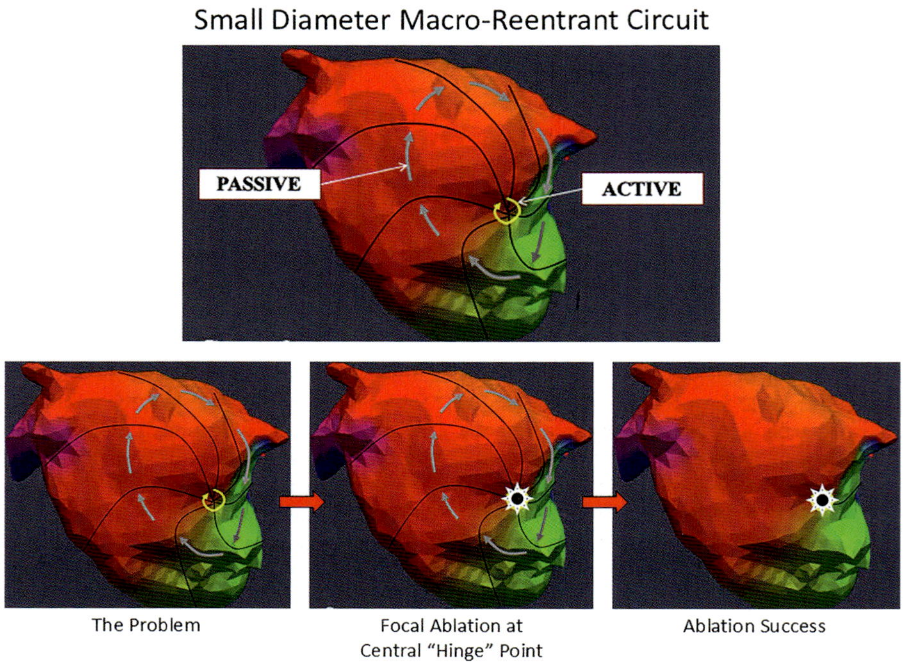

Fig. 4.23 Correct interpretation of this map during atrial fibrillation (AF) is essential to successful intervention. For example, if this activation pattern during AF is attributable to a small-diameter macro-reentrant driver *(upper panel)* and its central "hinge" area is ablated with a catheter *(lower panels),* the driver will be terminated successfully.

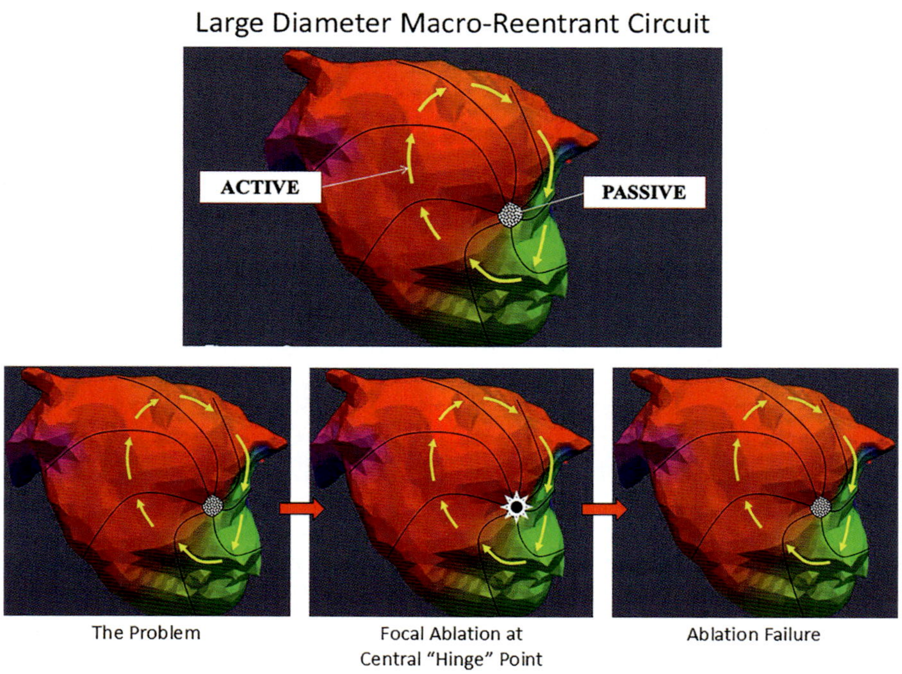

Fig. 4.24 However, if this activation pattern is attributable to a large-diameter macro-reentrant driver *(upper panel),* ablation of its central "hinge" area has no effect whatsoever on the driver, so the intervention for atrial fibrillation will fail *(lower panel).*

trant circuit itself will have to be blocked with a linear lesion, or the arrhythmia will persist. Misinterpretation of electrophysiologic maps and the constant motion of the apparent "hinge point" of large macro-reentrant circuits combine to make it virtually impossible to treat patients with sustained AF by focal ablation based on intraoperative mapping. This fact is the main reason that the results of catheter ablation for long-standing persistent AF have been so dismal.[17,18]

REFERENCES

1. Allessie MA, Dirchhof CJ, Konings KT. Unravelling the electrical mysteries of atrial fibrillation. *Eur Heart J*. 1996;17(Suppl C):2–9 Review.
2. Caldwell J, Redfearn D. Ablation of complex fractionated atrial electrograms in catheter ablation for AF; where have we been and where are we going? *Curr Cardiol Rev*. 2012;8(4):347–353.
3. Wong KCK, Faisey JR, Sopher M, et al. No benefit of complex fractionated atrial electrogram ablation in addition to circumferential pulmonary vein ablation and linear ablation. *Circ Arrhyth Electrophysiol*. 2015;8:1316–1324.
4. Cox JL, Daniel TM, Sabiston Jr DC, Boineau JP. De-synchronized activation in myocardial infarction—a reentry basis for ventricular arrhythmias. *Circulation*. 1969;40:III63.
5. Boineau JP, Cox JL. Slow ventricular activation in acute myocardial infarction—a source of reentrant premature ventricular contractions. *Circulation*. 1973;48:702–713.
6. Iwa T, Ichihashi T, Hashizume Y, Ishida K, Okada R. Successful surgical treatment of left atrial tachycardia. *Am Heart J*. 1985;109(1):160–162.
7. Williams JM, Ungerleider RM, Lofland GK, Cox JL. Left atrial isolation: new technique for the treatment of supraventricular arrhythmias. *J Thorac Cardiovasc Surg*. 1980;80:373.
8. Harada A, D'Agostino Jr HJ, Boineau JP, Cox JL. Right atrial isolation: a new surgical treatment for supraventricular tachycardia. I. Surgical technique and electrophysiologic effects. *J Thorac Cardiovasc Surg*. 1988;95:643–650.
9. Ahmed A, Pothineni NVK, Charate R, et al. Inappropriate sinus tachycardia: etiology, pathophysiology, and management: JACC review topic of the week. *J Am Coll Cardiol*. 2022;79(24):2450–2462.
10. de Asmundis C, Chierchia GB, Lakkireddy D, et al. Sinus node sparing novel hybrid approach for treatment of inappropriate sinus tachycardia/postural sinus tachycardia: multicenter experience. *J Interv Card Electrophysiol*. 2022;63(3):531–544.
11. Mines GR. On circulating excitations in heart muscle and their possible relation to tachycardia and fibrillation. *Trans Roy Soc Can*. 1914;8:43–52.
12. Cox JL, Boineau JP, Schuessler RB, Kater KM, Lappas DG. Five-year experience with the maze procedure for atrial fibrillation. *Ann Thorac Surg*. 1994;56:814–824.
13. Saoudi N, Coxio F, Waldo A, et al. Classification of atrial flutter and regular atrial tachycardia according to electrophysiologic mechanism and anatomic bases: a statement from a joint expert group from the Working Group of Arrhythmias of the European Society of Cardiology and the North American Society of pacing and electrophysiology. *J Cardiovasc Electrophysiol*. 2001;12(7):852–866.
14. Prasad SM, Maniar HS, Camillo CJ, et al. The Cox maze III procedure for atrial fibrillation: long-term efficacy in patients undergoing lone versus concomitant procedures. *J Thorac Cardiovasc Surg*. 2003;126(6):1822–1828.
15. Jais P, Haissaguerre M, Shah DC, et al. A focal source of atrial fibrillation treated by discrete radiofrequency ablation. *Circulation*. 1997;95(3):572–576.
16. O'Shea C, Lau DH, Kistler PM, Kalman JM, Sanders P. Pulmonary vein tachycardia: do we really need to isolate or freeze? *J Interv Card Electrophysiol*. 2020;59(2):299–301.
17. Tilz RR, Rillig A, Thum AM, et al. Catheter ablation of long-standing persistent atrial fibrillation: 5-year outcomes of the Hamburg sequential ablation strategy. *J Am Coll Card*. 2012;60(19):1921–1929.
18. Winkle RA, Mead RH, Engel G, et al. Very long term outcomes of atrial fibrillation ablation. *Heart Rhythm*. 2023;20:680–688.

5

Clinical Electrophysiology of Atrial Flutter and Atrial Fibrillation Pertinent to Interventional Therapy

James L. Cox, Richard B. Schuessler

CHAPTER OUTLINE

BACKGROUND

In 1912, Walter Garrey of Washington University in St. Louis published several of the basic concepts explaining why, 75 years later, the surgical Maze procedure was successful in ablating atrial fibrillation.[1] This is the frontispiece of that article:

THE NATURE OF FIBRILLARY CONTRACTION OF THE HEART. - ITS RELATION TO TISSUE MASS AND FORM

BY WALTER E. GARREY

[From the Physiological Laboratory of Washington University, St. Louis.]

The main features of this work were reported to the St. Louis Medical Science Club, November 12, 1912, and a synopsis appears in the Proceedings of the Society, Interstate medical journal, December, 1912, xix, p. 1081.

Garrey's seminal studies showed that although atrial fibrillation (AF) could be *induced* by rapid stimulation at a focal site, the fibrillation continued after the initiating stimulus (triggers) had stopped discharging electrical impulses. Therefore, some mechanism other than the triggering focus had to be *sustaining* the fibrillation. His studies also showed that when the focal triggering stimulus stopped, the maintenance of AF depended on the availability of a critical mass of myocardium to sustain the fibrillation. Interestingly, Garrey also demonstrated that "fibrillation was impossible in sufficiently narrow strips" and that if the strips of myocardium remained connected to each other by narrow bands of tissue, they would all contract synchronously in response to a regular stimulus.

Garrey's experiments were contemporaneous with those of GR Mines, who first described reentry as a mechanism for cardiac arrhythmias in an article published posthumously in 1914.[2] Sir Thomas Lewis subsequently used a string galvanometer to record electrical activity directly from the heart.[3] He mapped both normal sinus rhythm and atrial flutter and was the first to show fibrillatory conduction in a dog with atrial flutter and irregular left atrial electrograms. Lewis believed that AF was caused by a single right atrial reentrant circuit with fibrillatory conduction and partial atrioventricular (AV) block. Some 50 years later, Gordon Moe suggested that AF was characterized by multiple and random wandering waves of electrical activity that he called the "multiple wavelet hypothesis" (Fig. 5.1).[4] He

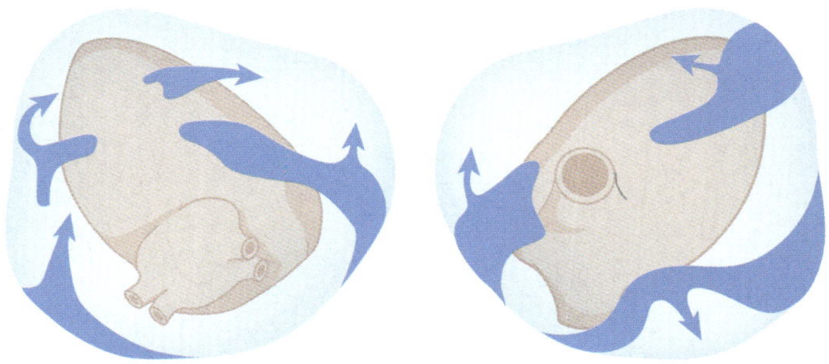

Fig. 5.1 Moe hypothesized that atrial fibrillation (AF) was caused by "multiple wavelets" propagating randomly throughout both atria, causing them to look like a "bag of worms." His "multiple wavelet theory" was debunked years ago. It is important to understand that this theory is fundamentally different from the concept that multiple macro-reentrant circuits serve as the drivers of AF. Even some recognized authorities in electrophysiology still do not understand the difference. (Reproduced from Moe GK. On the multiple wavelet hypothesis of atrial fibrillation. *Arch Int Pharmacodyn.* 1962;140:183–188.)

then developed a computer model of AF,[5] and his multiple wavelet hypothesis became widely accepted as the electrophysiologic basis of AF. Allessie then published some of the early multi-electrode maps of AF showing the presence of multiple wavelets that he described as a "circus movement" pattern of atrial activation,[6] thus seeming to confirm Moe's multiple wavelet hypothesis as the mechanism by which AF is sustained

When we began to use multipoint computerized mapping systems for the study of human AF some 20 years later, it quickly became clear that large areas of the atria *activated simultaneously* during AF, which was being driven by macro-reentrant circuits in the atria.[7] This finding was in direct contrast to Moe's computer model that proposed a "random motion" of activation during AF. A fundamental flaw in Moe's computer model of simulated AF was that specific effective refractory periods (ERPs) were randomly assigned to individual cells in the model. In reality, although the ERPs of cells can be inhomogeneous, they are not random because they do form patterns. Although Moe's "multiple wavelet theory" has been challenged by numerous other studies, our finding of macro-reentrant drivers and large areas of the atrium being activated passively, simultaneously, and irregularly in human AF unequivocally refuted Moe's hypothesis.

Although the random multiple wavelet theory has now been thoroughly debunked, confusion still exists some 60 years later regarding the difference between the random multiple wavelet hypothesis and the simultaneous presence of multiple macro-reentrant circuits in the atria that drive atrial flutter and AF. For example, a recent statement suggesting that reentrant circuits *"almost never manifest what we call head-tail interaction or circus movement"*[8] directly contradicts overwhelming evidence to the contrary. The purveyors of such misconceptions are left with the unenviable task of trying to explain how the Maze procedure can be successful if AF is not sustained by multiple macro-reentrant circuits. Even these respected electrophysiologic experts seem to stumble into incoherent and erroneous preconceived notions such as the following:

> *"The original MAZE surgical procedure to cure AF was postulated on the basis . . . that if you made a whole bunch of incisions in the atria they would heal the fibrosis, and these multiple reentrant wavelets couldn't conduct through the fibrosis so they would stop. When the MAZE procedure had some success [some?], they thought it was indirect confirmation of this theory."*[8]

They go on to hypothesize that the reason the Maze procedure works is simply because it includes pulmonary vein isolation (PVI) as a part of every procedure. This is precisely the type of misunderstanding of how AF is sustained that has resulted in the persistent practice of performing PVI alone in patients with long-standing persistent AF, the large majority of whom will not benefit from the procedure.

The only available experimental models of AF before 1980 consisted of Langendorf perfusion models with excised animal atria, simulated computer models, or the topical application of the irritant Aconitine to the atrium to make it fibrillate. We decided to develop a more clinically relevant animal model of AF in which under sterile operative conditions, a high-fidelity Millar pressure catheter and a Cope biopsy needle were passed into the left atrium through a purse-string suture placed in the *extrapericardial portion* of the left superior pulmonary vein (Fig. 5.2).[9] This extrapericardial approach specifically avoided the pericardial space in order to preclude the later formation of pericardial adhesions that could theoretically affect the characteristics of AF. In addition, it avoided the necessity of placing incisions in the atria for the same reason. The biopsy needle was used

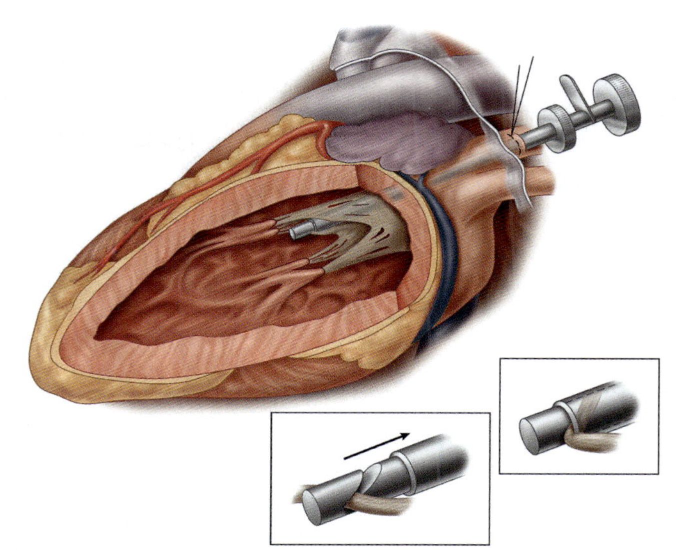

Fig. 5.2 Animal model of atrial fibrillation (AF). Mitral valve regurgitation was created by transecting the chordae tendineae until the left atrial pressure exceeded 20 mm Hg. The pericardium was not entered to preclude pericardial adhesions, and no scars were placed on or in the left atrium. After left atrial enlargement occurred at least 3 months later, AF could be easily induced by simple atrial pacing. This was a more clinically relevant model in which to study AF than previous animal models that used such artificial stimulants as topical aconitine and/or hyperstimulation of the vagus nerves.

to transect the chordae tendineae of the mitral valve sequentially until the left atrial pressure increased from its normal levels of 2 to 3 mm Hg to above 20 mm Hg, and then both the Millar catheter and the biopsy device were removed. The dogs were allowed to recuperate from surgery, and over the ensuing 3 months to 3 years, the left atrium enlarged from the mitral regurgitation as expected. AF was then easily induced with a single premature beat, and it was usually sustained indefinitely thereafter.

Between 1980 and 1983, the atria could be mapped only with analogue systems that were inadequate to perform global mapping of the atria. However, in 1983, a computerized mapping system was developed by Frank Witkowski and Peter Corr (Fig. 5.3, *upper panel*) that allowed multiple atrial electrodes to be recorded simultaneously.[10] This provided a means of performing multipoint digital global mapping of both atrial flutter (Fig. 5.4) and AF (Fig. 5.5) for the first time in humans. It soon became possible to reconstruct the atria in three dimensions using gated magnetic resonance imaging (MRI) scans, a method developed specifically for this purpose by Michael Vanier at the Mallinckrodt Institute of Radiology at Washington University in St. Louis (see Fig. 5.3). John Boineau and Richard Schuessler (Fig. 5.6), had already developed a three-dimensional (3D) electrode array with 256 bipolar electrodes for experimental 3D atrial mapping. Barry Branham (see Fig. 5.3 and Fig. 1.14), a computer scientist working in our laboratory, developed a computer program that allowed the 3D maps to be superimposed on the MRI-reconstructed 3D atrial anatomy that for the first time ever, provided anatomically accurate 3D maps of AF in animals (Fig. 5.7) (Video 5.1). Boineau and Schuessler then developed electrode arrays with 156 bipolar electrodes that form fit the epicardial surfaces of the atria in patients undergoing surgery for Wolff-Parkinson-White (WPW) syndrome, 30% of whom had associated AF (Fig. 5.8). Now, for the first time ever, human AF could be mapped in three dimensions.

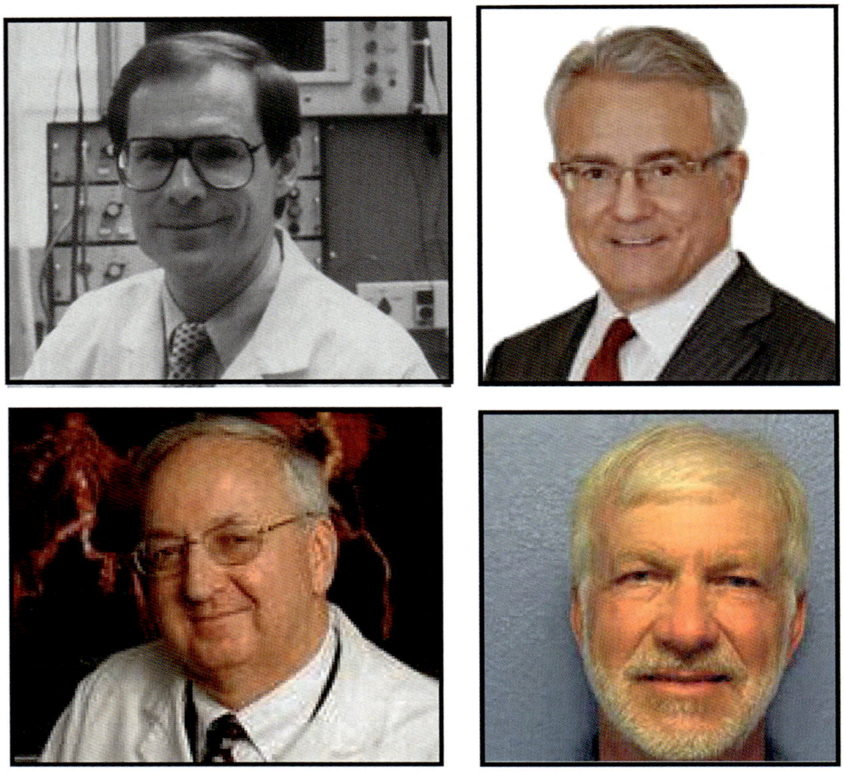

Fig. 5.3 Drs. Frank Witkowski (top left) and Peter Corr (top right) built the first multipoint computerized mapping system for humans that originally recorded data from 58 individual bipolar electrodes simultaneously and stored on a digital tape recorder. The system was later expanded to 256 channels. Dr. Michael Vanier (bottom left) developed the first three-dimensional (3D) reconstructions of the atria using "stacked" electrocardiography-gated magnetic resonance imaging scans. Barry Branham (bottom right) developed computer programs that allowed the recorded 3D electrical maps to be superimposed on the 3D atrial anatomy of the specific animal being mapped so that the first accurate anatomic-electrophysiologic maps of atrial fibrillation could be studied in animals.

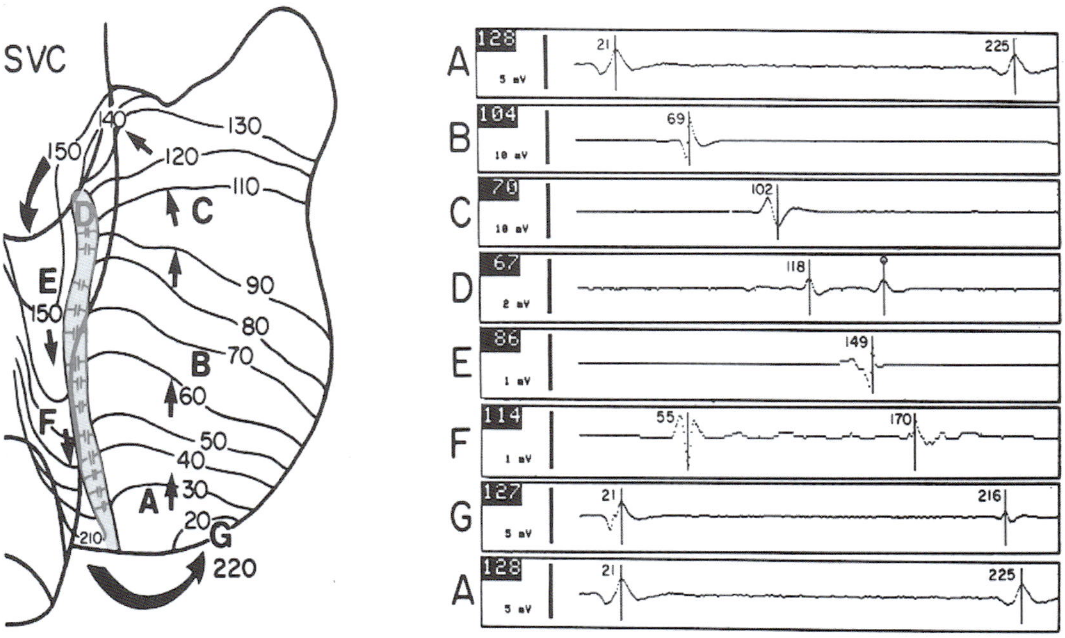

Fig. 5.4 Human atrial flutter. This is the first multipoint computerized activation-time map of human atrial flutter ever constructed. A total of 156 bipolar electrodes were imbedded into three silastic electrode plaques designed to form fit on the epicardial surfaces of both atria. The map shows a large macro-reentrant circuit in the right atrium rotating around a linear area of functional conduction block in the crista terminalis *(gray zone)*. The cycle length of this macro-reentrant driver ("flutter wave") is precisely 200 ms, meaning that electrical activity spins around the circuit five times per second (1000 ms) or 300 times per minute. Thus the atrial rate during atrial flutter is 300 beats/min (beats/min). (See text for further discussion.) *SVC,* Superior vena cava.

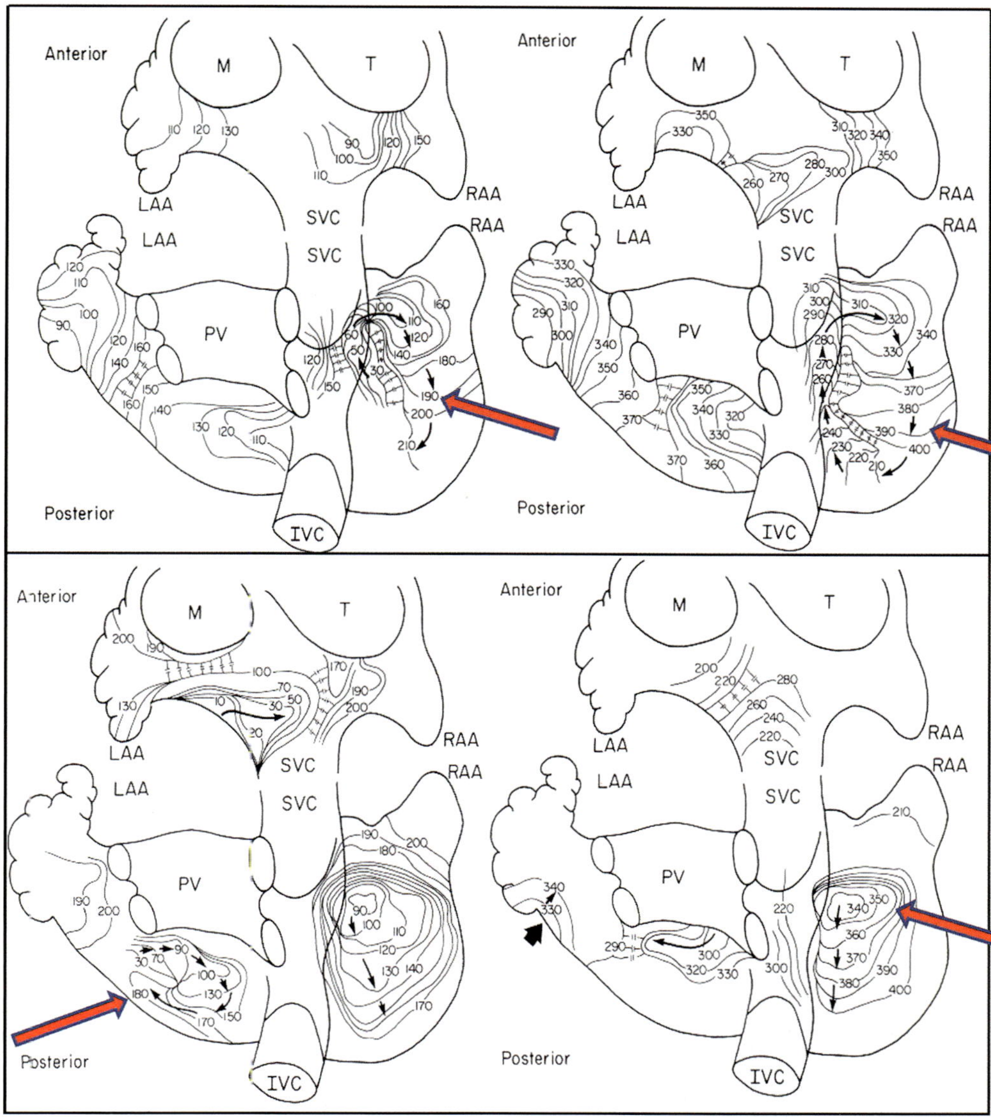

Fig. 5.5 **Human atrial fibrillation (AF).** This is the first multipoint computerized activation-time map of human AF ever constructed. The posterior and anterior surfaces of the atria are displayed as if the atria had been opened in the midsagittal plane and the anterior surface had been reflected upwards. A total of 156 bipolar electrodes were imbedded into three electrode plaques designed to form fit on the epicardial surfaces of both atria (see Fig. 5.10). The *map* shows the presence of multiple macro-reentrant circuits involving both atria *(red arrows)*. No atrial septal data were available because there were no septal electrodes in place. However, septal activity can be deduced from the pattern and timing of wavefront activation in the other areas of the atria. LAA *LAA,* Left atrial appendage; *M, mitral Valve*; *PV,* pulmonary vein; *RAA,* right atrial appendage; *T,* tricuspid valve.

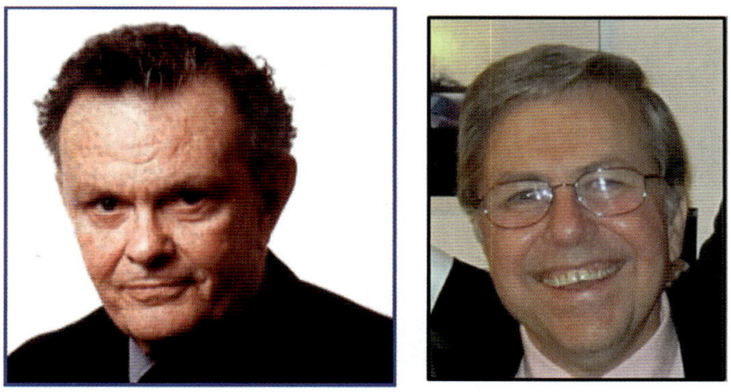

Fig. 5.6 Drs. John Boineau (left) and Richard Schuessler (right) were the first to map experimental atrial fibrillation (AF) in three dimensions. They developed special "target" bipolar electrode arrays for the study of anatomically accurate three-dimensional (3D) video maps of AF. Each bipolar electrode was constructed like a target with the anode in the center surrounded by the cathode. This eliminated any effect on the local bipolar electrogram that might be caused by the direction of the wavefront being recorded. They then studied the 3D video maps of AF and documented that AF is "driven" by at least two macro-reentrant circuits in the atria simultaneously.

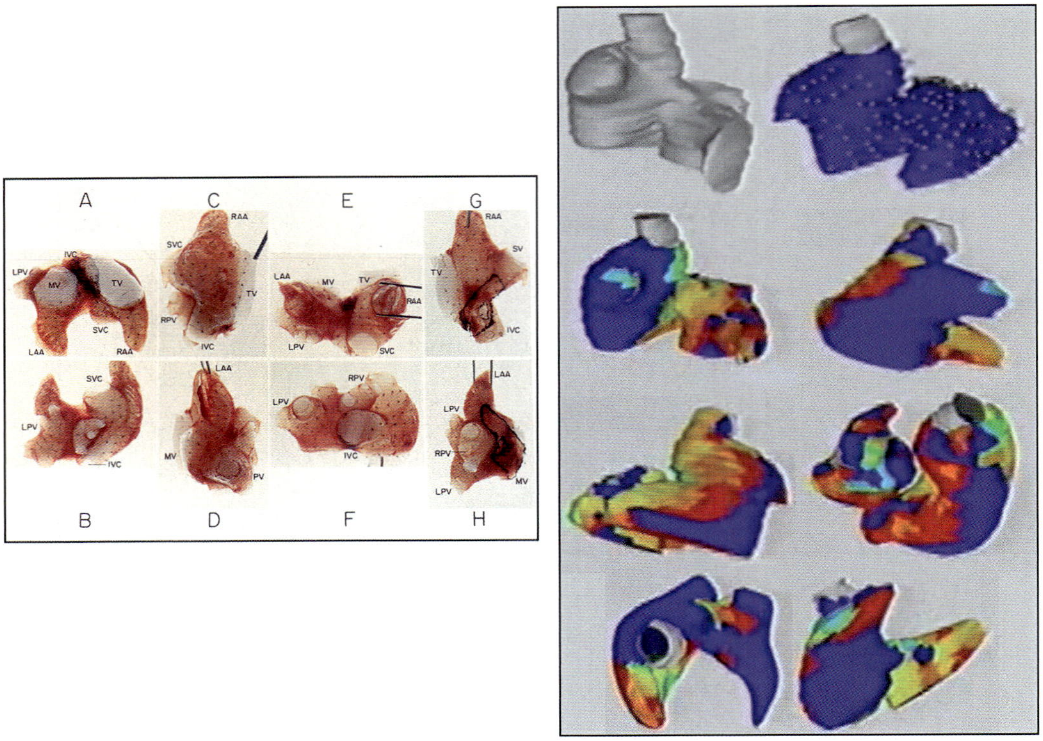

Fig. 5.7 *Left panel:* Silastic endocardial electrode arrays developed by Boineau and Schuessler that form fit inside canine atria during atrial fibrillation (AF). *Right panel:* Multiple snapshots from a three-dimensional video of canine AF recorded in early 1987. The ability to visualize such video maps of AF left no doubt that the underlying mechanism of AF was macro-reentry. *IVC,* Inferior vena cava; *LAA,* left atrial appendage; *LPV,* left pulmonary vein; *MV,* mitral valve; *RAA,* right atrial appendage; *RPV,* right pulmonary vein; *SVC,* superior vena cava; *TV,* tricuspid valve.

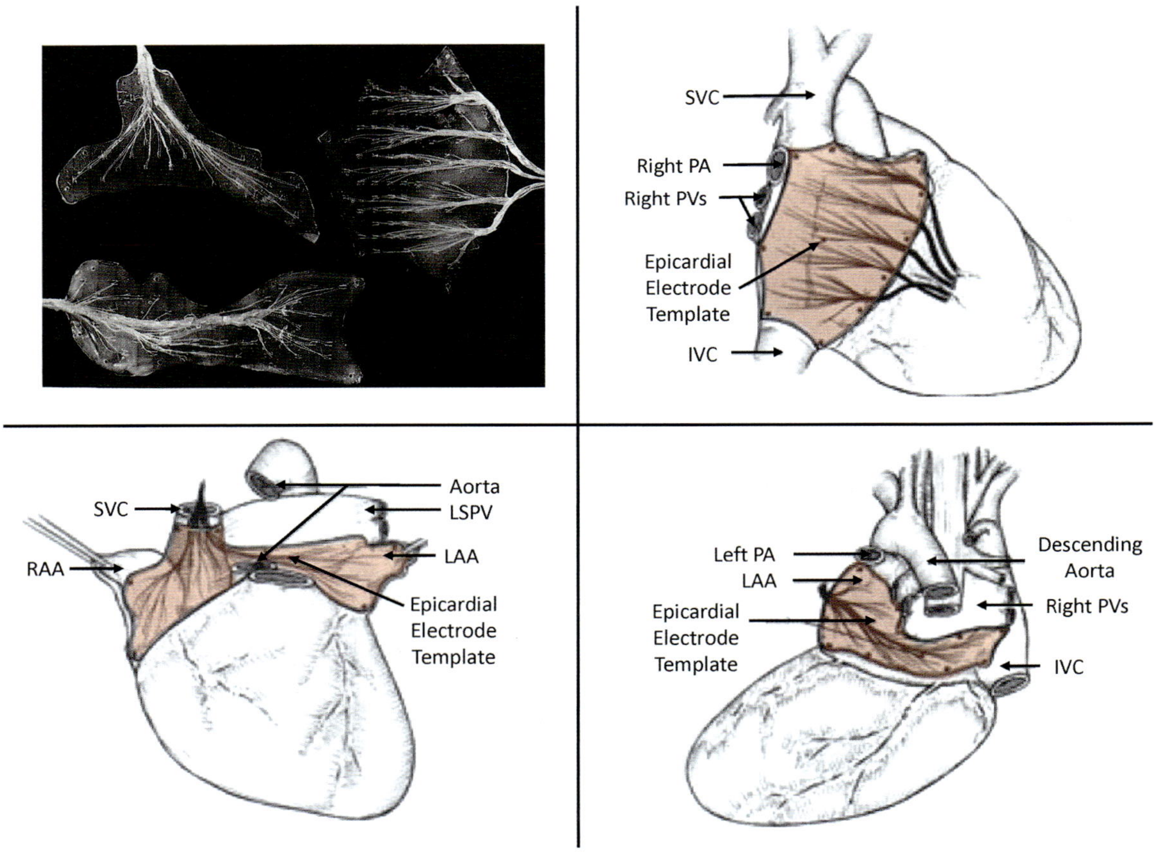

Fig. 5.8 Silastic epicardial electrode arrays also developed by Boineau and Schuessler for mapping human atrial fibrillation *(left upper panel).* The form-fitting electrode arrays were positioned on the exposed epicardial surfaces of both atria as illustrated. *IVC,* Inferior vena cava; *LAA,* left atrial appendage; *LSPV,* left superior pulmonary vein; *PA,* pulmonary artery; *PV,* pulmonary vein; *RAA,* right atrial appendage; *SVC,* superior vena cava.

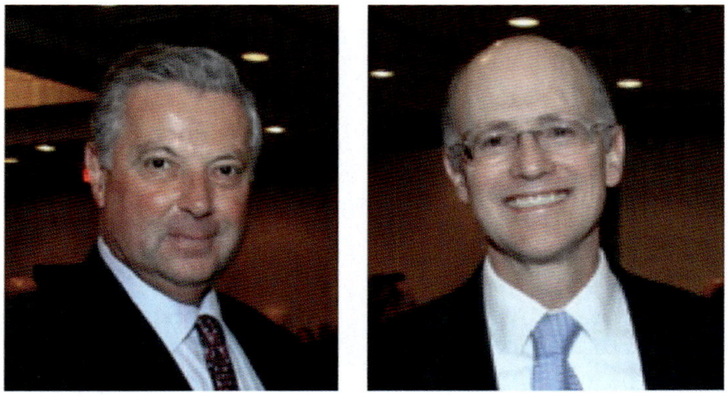

Fig. 5.9 Drs. Michael Cain (left) and Bruce Lindsay (right) were the first clinical electrophysiologists to map human atrial fibrillation (AF) using a digital computer system developed by Witkowski, Corr, and Branham and using epicardial electrode arrays developed by Boineau and Schuessler. With Barnes Hospital institutional review board approval, patients undergoing surgery for Wolff-Parkinson-White syndrome who also had a history of AF (~30%) were the subjects for mapping. The three silastic electrode arrays shown in Fig. 5.8 were sutured to the exposed epicardial surfaces of both atria, and AF was induced by atrial pacing. Several seconds of AF were recorded for later analysis.

Over the ensuing years and with the cooperation of clinical electrophysiologists Michael Cain and Bruce Lindsay (Fig. 5.9), AF was routinely mapped three dimensionally using the multi-point computerized mapping system in the operating room and studied extensively in hundreds of patients.

Our experimental and clinical studies confirmed by direct measurement that *after initiation*, AF maintenance depends on the presence of two or more active macro-reentrant circuits (drivers) in the atria simultaneously (Fig. 5.10).[7,11] The Maze procedure was conceived in 1987 on the basis that in order for macro-reentrant circuits to develop, a relatively large area of the atrium must be available to support the macro-reentrant circuit and that there was a relationship between the local conduction velocity, refractory period, and area of atrium available to participate in the macro-reentry. That concept was documented again in 2005 (Fig. 5.11),[12] and the relationship between the area of atrium available and the local atrial refractory period was further confirmed in 2013 (Fig. 5.12).[13] These fundamental anatomic-electrophysiologic characteristics of AF are not only consistent with the reentry concept of atrial arrhythmias described in Chapter 4, but they also confirm that once initiated, AF is sustained by macro-reentrant drivers, not by focal triggers.

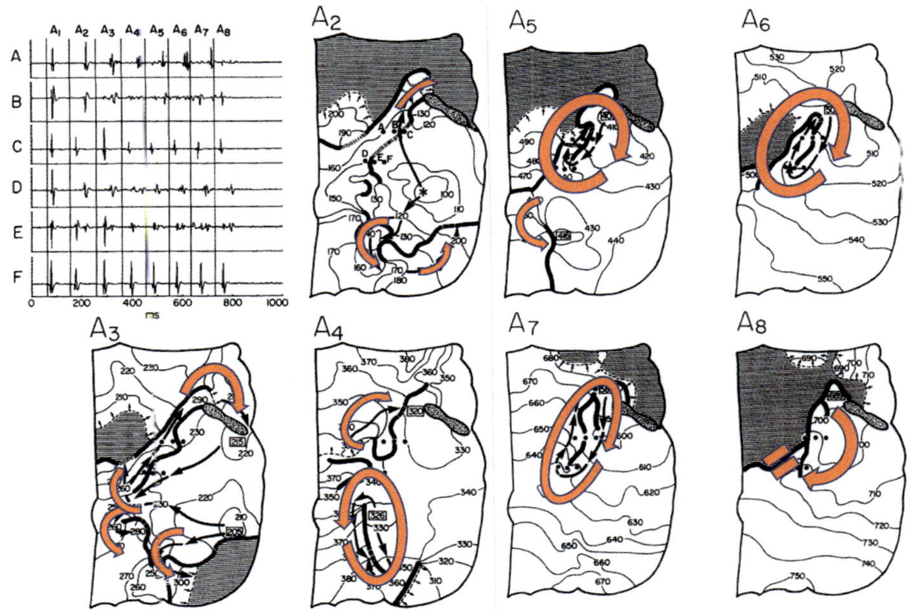

Fig. 5.10 Every map recorded of either experimental or human atrial fibrillation using the computerized three-dimensional mapping system showed the presence of two or more macro-reentrant circuits in the atria *(red circles)*. The macro-reentrant circuits typically rotated around anatomic structures where there was no electrical activity (anatomic orifices of the pulmonary veins or vena cavae or around areas of functional conduction block such as along the crista terminalis; see Fig. 5.4). (Reproduced from Schuessler RB, Grayson TM, Bromberg BI, Cox JL, Boineau JP. Cholinergically mediated tachyarrhythmias induced by a single extrastimulus in the isolated canine right atrium. *Circ Res.* 1992;71;1254–1267.)

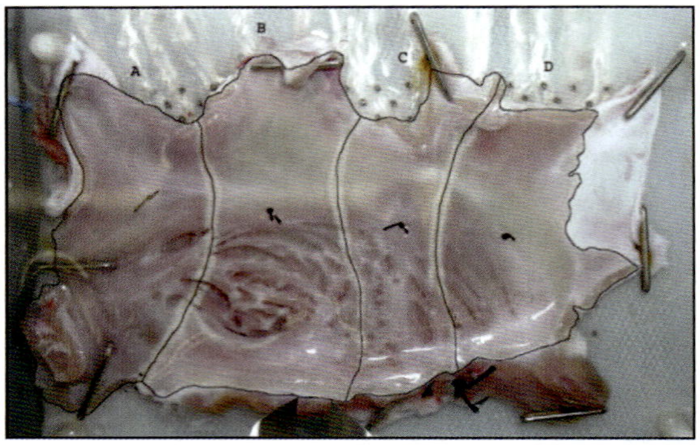

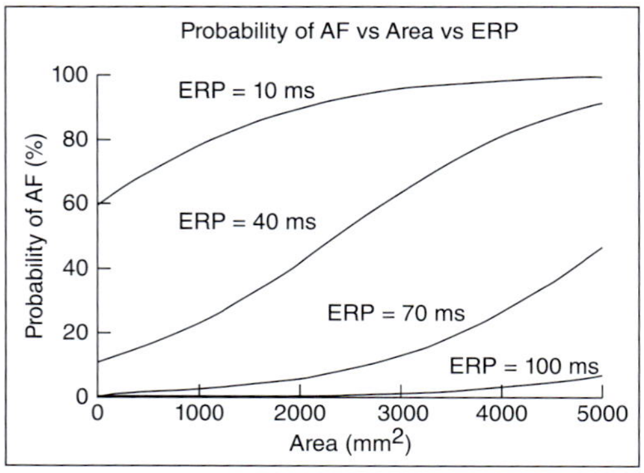

Fig. 5.11 _Upper Panel:_ Under experimental conditions, atrial fibrillation (AF) was induced by atrial pacing in isolated canine atria. The area of each isolated segment was measured as was the effective refractory period (ERP) of the local myocardium in each segment. The atrium was then divided into sequentially smaller isolated segments and the area and ERP were measured after each segmentation. _Lower Panel:_ Eventually, the relationship between the atrial segment size and its local ERP would no longer support AF. The graph shows that shorter ERPs promote the development of AF. (Reproduced from Byrd GD, Prasad SM, Ripplinger CM, et al. Importance of geometry and refractory period in sustaining atrial fibrillation: testing the critical mass hypothesis. *Circulation.* 2005;112(9):I-7–I-13.)

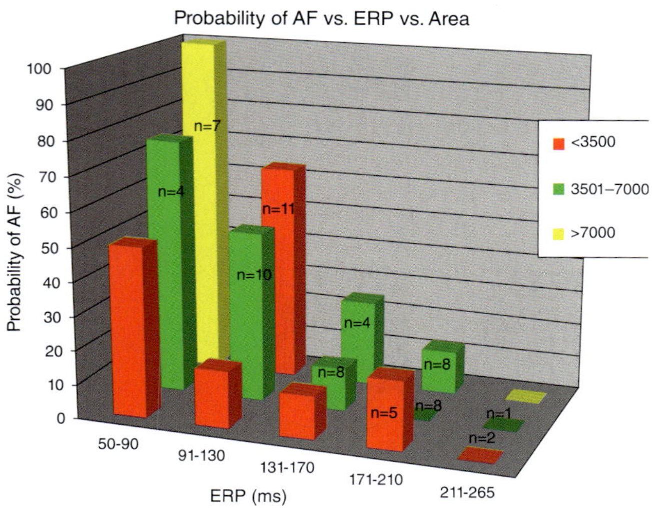

Fig. 5.12 The relationship between the local effective refractory period (ERP), the area of atrium available to support atrial fibrillation (AF), and the probability of developing AF. Both short ERPs and large areas of available atrium promote the maintenance of AF. These anatomic-electrophysiologic data document that although episodes of AF are usually *induced* by focal atrial triggers, they are *not sustained* by focal atrial triggers. (Reproduced from Byrd GD, Prasad SM, Ripplinger CM, et al. Importance of geometry and refractory period in sustaining atrial fibrillation: testing the critical mass hypothesis. *Circulation.* 2005;112(9):I-7–I-13.)

It was at this point that we realized we needed to crystallize our understanding of the relationship between the electrophysiology and *atrial anatomy* pertinent to AF. We leaned on the wisdom of one of our pediatric cardiology predecessors, Dr. Helen Tausig, to do so by turning to her experience during the development of congenital heart surgery.

CLARIFICATION AND SIMPLIFICATION OF THE ANATOMIC-ELECTROPHYSIOLOGIC RELATIONSHIPS IN ATRIAL FIBRILLATION

In the 1950s, the renowned pediatric cardiologist at Johns Hopkins University Dr. Helen Taussig developed an elegant and simple method to explain the various congenital heart anomalies so that their basic anatomy and pathophysiology could be better understood. She sketched the abnormal anatomy of each congenital heart anomaly and then superimposed the disrupted physiology of each anomaly onto the anatomic diagram.[14] We used similar simplistic anatomic diagrams to represent the anatomy of the atria and then superimposed the observed electrophysiology on that schematic anatomy. We started with a simple box as a two-dimensional representation of the atria, arbitrarily designating one side of the box as the right atrium and the other as the left atrium with the atrial septum lying between the two (Fig. 5.13).[15] "Atrial appendages" were added to both the right and left atrium, and the large "holes" in the right atrium caused by the superior vena cava (SVC) and inferior vena cava (IVC) orifices were illustrated as well. The four pulmonary veins were represented as a contiguous box within the left atrium. At the "top" of the atrial septum was the sinoatrial (SA) node, and at its bottom was the AV node, which tapered into the bundle of His, the bundle branches, and the ventricular myocardium.

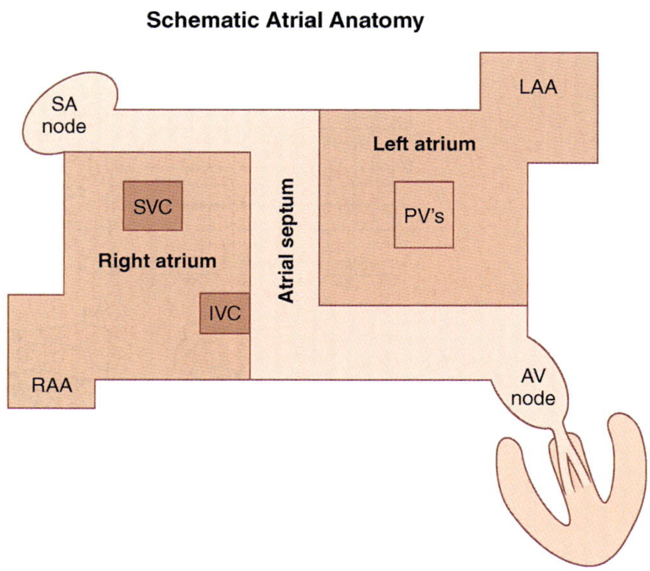

Fig. 5.13 Two-dimensional schematic representation of atrial anatomy that is pertinent to understanding the mechanisms of atrial flutter and atrial fibrillation. (See text for further discussion.) *AV,* Atrioventricular; *IVC,* inferior vena cava; *LAA,* left atrial appendage; *PV,* pulmonary vein; *RAA,* right atrial appendage; *SA,* sinoatrial. (Reproduced from Cox JL, Schuessler RB, D'Agostino HJ Jr, et al. The surgical treatment of atrial fibrillation: III. Development of a definitive surgical procedure. *J Thorac Cardiovasc Surg.* 1991;101:569–583.)

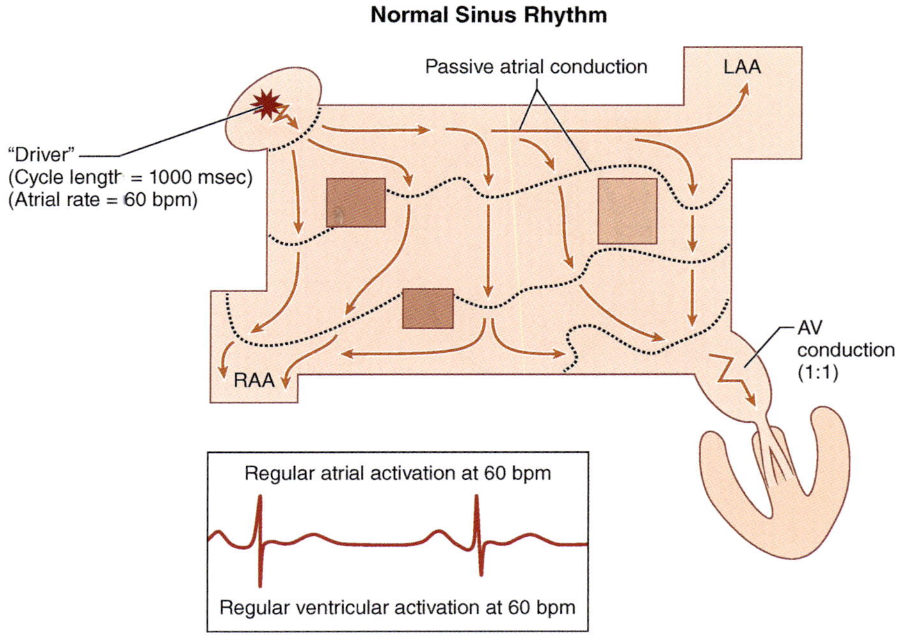

Fig. 5.14 Electrical activation of the atria during normal sinus rhythm (NSR) is superimposed on the two-dimensional anatomic diagram of the atria. NSR is driven by an impulse that arises spontaneously in the sino-atrial (SA) node and is passively conducted to the rest of the atrial myocardium. The impulse is then delayed 100 ms in the atrioventricular node and passes into the ventricles, which are also passively activated. The regularity of impulse generation in the SA node, in this case at a rate of 60 beats/min (cycle length of 1000 ms, or 1 s), results in a regular p-wave and QRS complex on the standard electrocardiogram. *AV,* Atrioventricular; *LAA,* left atrial appendage; *RAA,* right atrial appendage. (Modified and reproduced from Cox JL, Schuessler RB, D'Agostino HJ Jr, et al. The surgical treatment of atrial fibrillation: III. Development of a definitive surgical procedure. *J Thorac Cardiovasc Surg.* 1991;101:569–583.)

Normal Sinus Rhythm

The SA node and perinodal right atrial tissue is the "driver" for normal sinus rhythm because this is where each electrical impulse usually originates (Fig. 5.14). The SA node, normally fires regularly and the impulse is conducted away from the SA node passively to the rest of the atrial myocardium. If the driver fires once per second (i.e., every 1000 ms), the atrial heart rate will be 60 beats/min. After the SA node driver fires, both atria are subsequently activated by passive conduction of the sinus impulse away from the SA node across both atria. Conduction from the SA node, located near the top of the right atrium, to the top of the left atrium occurs quickly because of rapid conduction across Bachmann's bundle (see Chapter 3). The wavefront propagates passively across both atria and down the atrial septum until it reaches the AV groove, where it is blocked everywhere except at the site of the AV node–His bundle complex. This coordinated activation of the atria gives rise to a normal "p-wave" on the standard electrocardiogram (ECG). The impulse is normally delayed approximately 100 ms (0.1 s) in the AV node and is then conducted rapidly down the His bundle, bundle branches, and Purkinje system to the ventricular myocardium. Assuming that the conduction through the AV node is stable, a ventricular response will follow each sinus beat. Activation of the ventricle results in a regular QRS complex after each P wave on the standard ECG. Thus the ventricular rate ("heart rate") depends on the rate at which the SA node driver is firing.

Atrial Flutter

The anatomic-electrophysiologic basis of atrial flutter can also be described by superimposing its observed electrophysiology on the same anatomic diagram of the atria (Fig. 5.15). However, the driver during atrial flutter is not the SA node; rather, it is a single large macro-reentrant circuit (the so-called "flutter wave") that resides in the right atrium (see Fig. 5.4). This is a large macro-reentrant circuit because the refractory periods in the right atrium are relatively long (see Chapter 4). In fact, a normal right atrium is capable of harboring only this single macro-reentrant circuit because of the long refractory periods and the area of the right atrium available to participate in the reentrant circuit. The flutter wave is particularly stable because it has a large excitable gap, so changes in the ERP caused by variations in the autonomic tone do not affect the anatomic circuit or the time it takes to travel around it (see Chapter 4). The flutter wave (of which there are three possible locations) always uses the cavotricuspid isthmus (CTI) between the orifice of the IVC and the tricuspid valve, which explains why a CTI lesion is so successful for the treatment of atrial flutter.

Electrical activity during atrial flutter typically completes one trip around the circumference of this flutter wave every 200 ms, which is called the "cycle length" of the macro-reentrant circuit. One complete cycle every 200 ms is 5 cycles per second or 300 cycles per minute. With each trip around the macro-reentrant flutter-wave circuit, electrical activity exits the main circuit to activate the remainder of the atrium passively (see Chapter 4). Therefore, the atria are activated 300 times per minute during atrial flutter by this single macro-reentrant driver in the right atrium. Activation of the atrial myocardium outside the driver occurs by passive atrial conduction just as it does during sinus rhythm. Each coordinated activation of the atria causes a p-wave on the ECG, so the classic ECG characteristic of atrial flutter is a clear and discernible p-wave that occurs regularly at 300 times per minute.

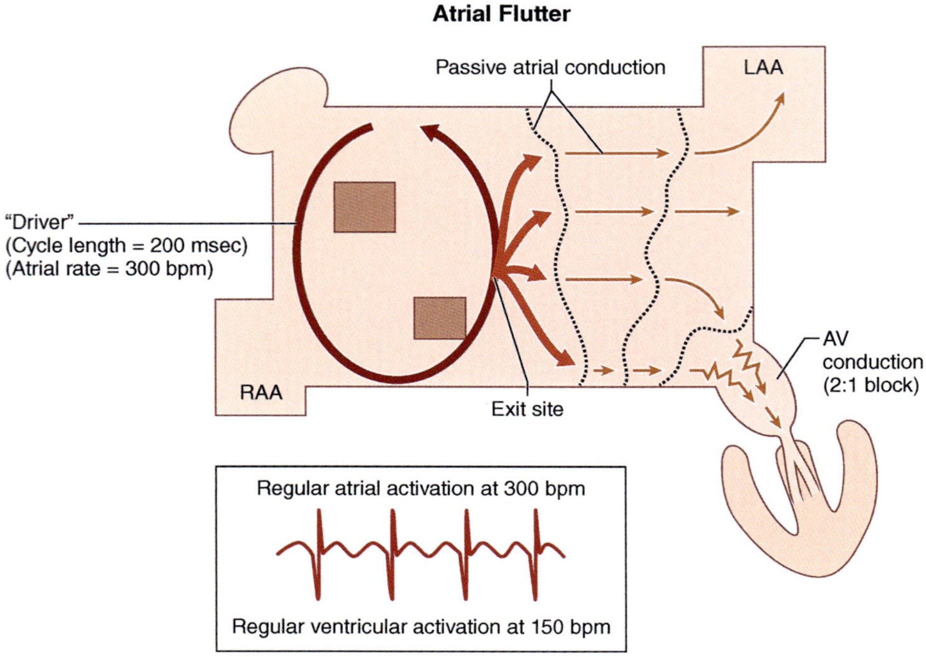

Fig. 5.15 Atrial flutter is driven by a large macro-reentrant circuit in the right atrium called the "flutter wave." It takes 200 ms for the electrical impulse to complete one cycle around this macro-reentrant circuit ("cycle length"), meaning that the impulse completes 5 cycles per second (1000 ms/200 ms) or 300 cycles per minute (5 cycles/second × 60 seconds). The electrical impulse exits the cycle with each circumvention and is conducted passively to the rest of the atrial myocardium, resulting in a regular atrial rate of 300 beats/min. Each of the 300 passively conducted atrial impulses enters the atrioventricular (AV) node, which is incapable of conducting activity at that high rate. Thus every other atrial impulse (rate, 300 beats/min) is blocked in the AV node, allowing 150 impulses to reach the ventricles. This electrophysiology results in a peripheral electrocardiogram that shows a regular p-wave at 300 beats/min and a regular QRS complex at 150 beats/min. *LAA,* Left atrial appendage; *RAA,* right atrial appendage.

The AV node is normally incapable of conducting 300 impulses per minute, so when the passive wavefront reaches the AV node 300 times per minute, every second impulse is blocked, resulting in only 150 impulses reaching the ventricles per minute. Because the passive atrial wavefronts are reaching the AV node on a regular basis of 300 beats/min and because the 2:1 AV nodal block is stable, the ventricular response to atrial flutter is regular at a ventricular rate of 150 beats/min. Thus the ECG during classic atrial flutter shows a regular p-wave at 300 beats/min and a regular ventricular rate of 150 beats/min.

Atrial Fibrillation

The electrophysiologic events that take place during AF are more complex but can be understood using the same anatomic-electrophysiologic framework as described for normal sinus rhythm and atrial flutter. Although there is general agreement that individual episodes of AF are *induced* by triggers in the atria, usually in or around the pulmonary vein orifices (see below), there is considerable controversy over what *sustains* AF after it has been induced. However, our studies clearly show that the drivers that *sustain* AF are the self-sustaining macro-reentrant circuits themselves.[11–13] Just as atrial flutter is sustained by a single self-perpetuating macro-reentrant circuit in the right atrium (see Figs. 5.4 and 5.15), AF is sustained by multiple self-sustaining macro-reentrant circuits that are usually, but not always, located in the left atrium (Fig. 5.16).

Because the multiple drivers cause disorganized passive atrial conduction in both atria, the ECG records a p-wave that, if present at all, is irregularly irregular and has a varying morphology. As a result of the irregular manner in which the passive wavefronts strike the AV node, the conduction through the AV node to the ventricles is also irregularly irregular (Fig. 5.17). The maximum *rate* at which these irregular impulses can be conducted through a normal AV node is approximately 150 per minute. Thus the ECG will show an irregular p-wave of varying morphology and an irregularly irregular QRS complex, the classic ECG findings of AF. It seems apparent that AF is an arrhythmia that is most commonly sustained by atrial macro-reentrant drivers that result in multiple wavefronts that are conducted passively to the rest of the atrium. Because 70% of these macro-reentrant drivers are located in the left atrium, the right atrium is usually activated passively in a random fashion. Theoretically, such random activation of the right atrium can induce a stable right atrial flutter wave so that the left atrium is fibrillating and the right atrium is in a regular atrial flutter that can be induced in the right atrium by the AF in the left atrium (Fig. 5.18). In the latter case, the right atrial flutter wave remains passive and is not a "driver" of AF. Obviously, if the AF is being "driven" by multiple left atrial macro-reentrant circuits, it would be essential to ablate or interrupt those circuits to cure AF. There are other instances in which the primary problem may be right atrial flutter that can induce left atrial macro-reentry circuits so that the latter are passive. If the right atrial flutter wave were the primary "driver" of the AF, an exceedingly rare event, simple interruption of the right atrial flutter wave would eliminate the AF.

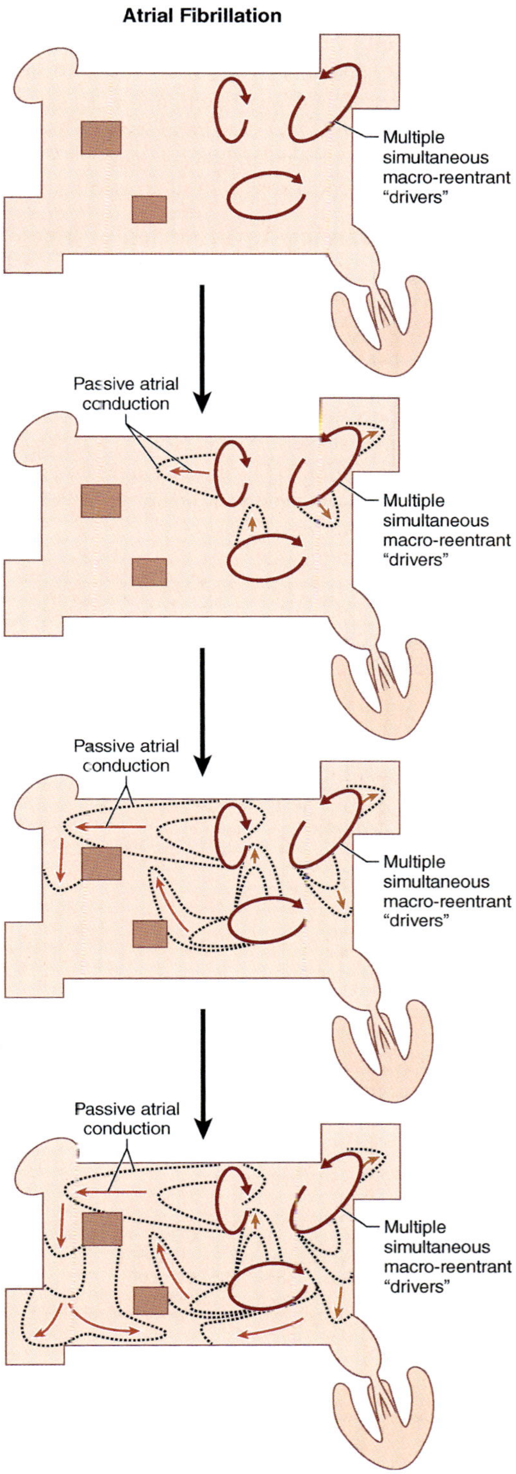

Fig. 5.16 Atrial fibrillation (AF) is typically driven by multiple macro-reentrant circuits, most of which are in the left atrium. Each of these macro-reentrant circuits acts as an individual driver because of natural "exit sites" in each circuit. All other electrical activity in the atria is passive. The passive atrial conduction of each of these impulses results in the inability to activate the atria in a regular, uniform fashion because of colliding wavefronts coming from each of the macro-reentrant circuits and the persistence of the circuits themselves. Although activation of the atria during AF at times appears to be chaotic, it is simply a case of the local atrial myocardium responding normally by passively conducting the repeated electrical impulses generated by the macro-reentrant circuits.

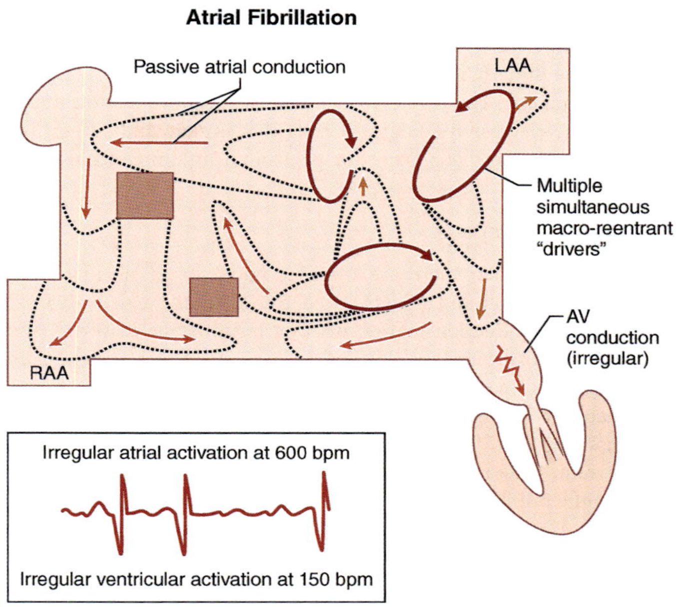

Fig. 5.17 Atrial fibrillation. Because of the competing macro-reentrant drivers, the atrial myocardium is activated non-synchronously in an irregularly irregular fashion. This results in an irregular or imperceptible p-wave and an irregularly irregular QRS complex on the electrocardiogram, and the atria are correctly diagnosed to be fibrillating. *AV,* Atrioventricular; *LAA,* left atrial appendage; *RAA,* right atrial appendage.

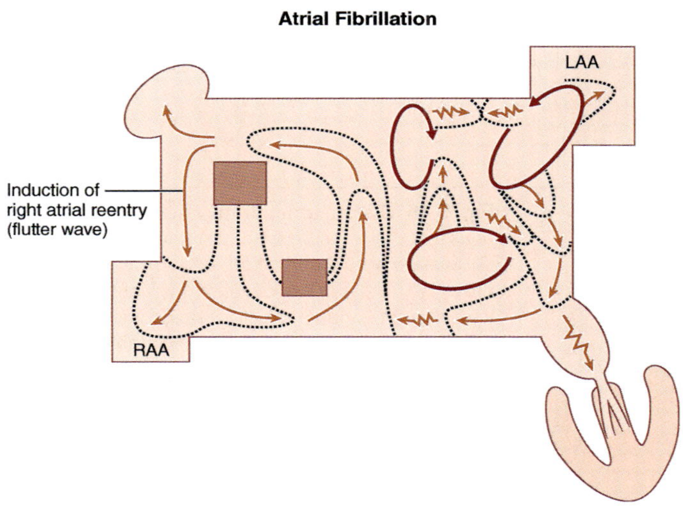

Fig. 5.18 In instances when the right atrium is completely normal, the disorganized impulses coming from left atrial reentrant circuits may be more organized when it reaches the right atrium. This can result in the development of a stable macro-reentrant circuit in the right atrium ("flutter wave"). The electrocardiogram will still show atrial fibrillation (AF) because there will be an irregular p-wave and QRS complex, but viewed by a surgeon in the operating room, one can see atrial flutter in the right atrium and AF in the left atrium. *AV,* Atrioventricular; *LAA,* left atrial appendage; *RAA,* right atrial appendage.

THE SPECTRUM FROM ATRIAL FLUTTER TO ATRIAL FIBRILLATION

It is important to recognize that the terms "atrial flutter" and "atrial fibrillation" describe arrhythmias that cause certain abnormalities on the standard ECG. They are descriptive names that have been applied to *clinical* events that in no way elucidate the electrophysiology that underlies either of them. When these arrhythmias could be mapped in detail, the underlying electrophysiologic events responsible for the ECG abnormalities could be delineated. Thus, it is now possible to understand the electrophysiological events that initiate and sustain the clinical arrhythmias that occupy the spectrum from simple atrial flutter to complex AF.

Classic Atrial Flutter

As explained earlier, there are three components of normal sinus rhythm, atrial flutter and AF: (1) the "driver(s)" of the arrhythmia, (2) passive atrial conduction that occurs as a result of the driver(s), and (3) conduction through the AV node (Fig. 5.19). Slight variations in one or more of these three components result in the clinical arrhythmias that cover the spectrum between simple atrial flutter and complex AF. Classic *atrial flutter* is caused by a single, stable flutter wave in the right atrium. Unless the left atrium is severely abnormal, the passive atrial conduction that results from a stable right atrial flutter wave will be regular. The stable atrial flutter wave (driver) combined with stable passive atrial conduction to the right and left atria results in a regular p-wave on the standard ECG. Because the flutter wave is also driving impulses into the AV node on a regular basis, if the AV node is normal, it will block every second beat resulting in a regular ventricular response. Thus the ECG will show a regular p-wave (at 300 beats/min) with a 2:1 block resulting in a regular QRS complex (at 150 beats/min), and classic atrial flutter is the correct clinical diagnosis.

Atrial Flutter With Varying Atrioventricular Block

A slight change in any of the three electrophysiologic components can cause a different clinical diagnosis. For example, if AV node conduction becomes unstable without any change in the atrial components, one of the "transitional" types of atrial flutter called *atrial flutter with varying AV block* occurs (Fig. 5.20). In this situation, the p-wave on the ECG remains regular because both the flutter wave driver and passive atrial conduction remain stable and regular. However, despite the stability of the flutter wave, unstable AV conduction results in an irregular QRS complex, so the clinical diagnosis is no longer "Atrial Flutter" but rather *atrial flutter with varying AV block*.

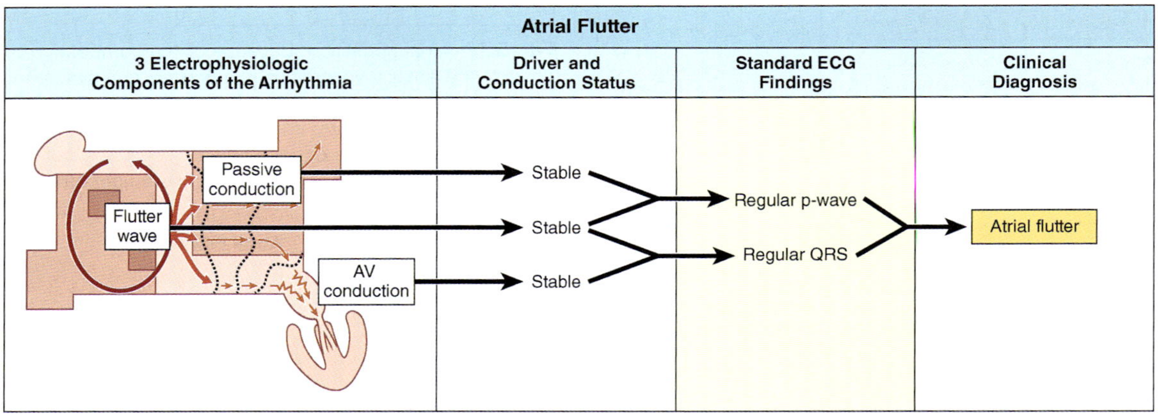

Fig. 5.19 **Classic atrial flutter.** There are three electrophysiologic components of each of the clinical arrhythmias that make up the spectrum from atrial flutter to complex atrial fibrillation: (1) atrial macro-reentrant driver(s), (2) passive atrial conduction, and (3) atrioventricular (AV) node conduction. When the atrial macro-reentrant driver is a single stable circuit in the right atrium ("flutter wave") and the passive atrial conduction to the right and left atria is stable, atrial activation will be regular, and a regular p-wave will appear on the electrocardiogram (ECG). If AV node conduction is also stable, then the QRS complex on the ECG will occur at half the rate of the p-wave, and the patient will have typical atrial flutter diagnosed on the ECG.

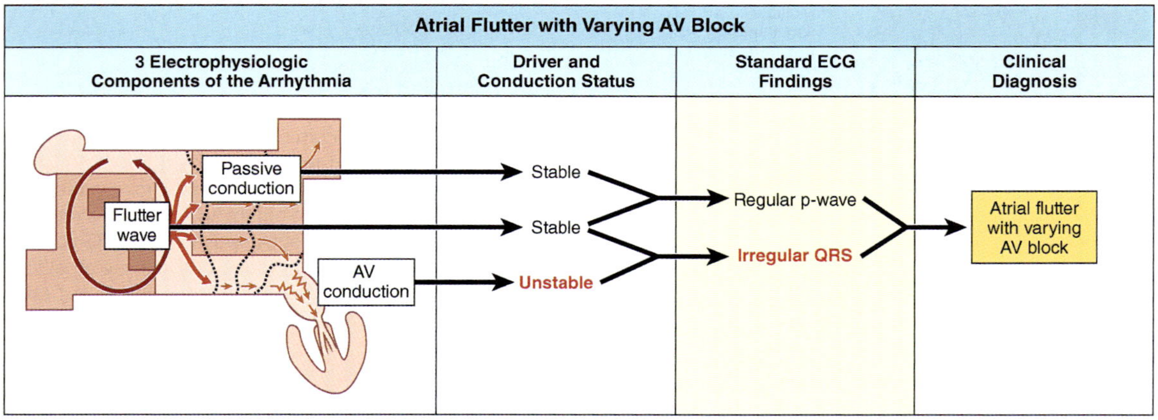

Fig. 5.20 **Atrial flutter with varying atrioventricular (AV) block.** In the presence of a stable flutter wave and stable passive atrial conduction, the electrocardiogram (ECG) will show a regular p-wave at 300 beats/min. This establishes that the clinical arrhythmia is atrial flutter. However, if AV node conduction in these patients is unstable, the combination of a stable flutter wave and unstable AV node conduction will result in an irregular QRS complex on the ECG, and the arrhythmia will be correctly diagnosed as atrial flutter with varying AV block.

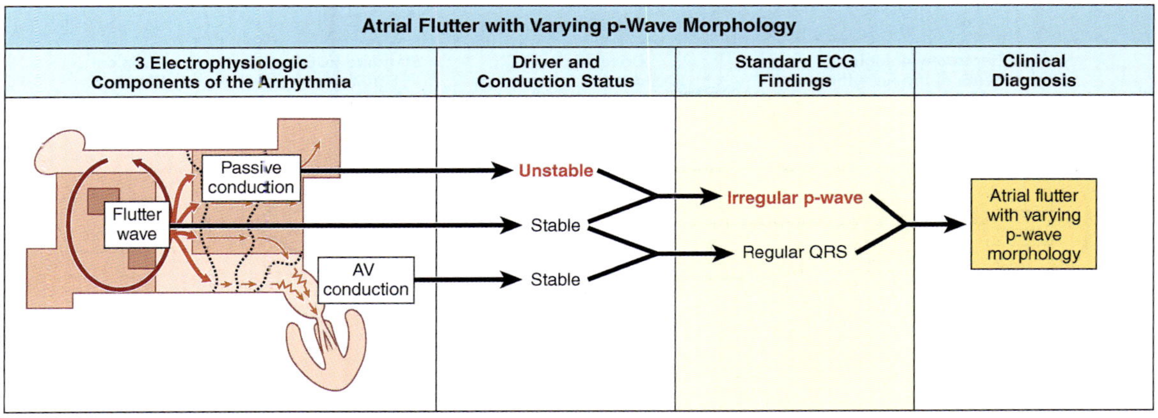

Fig. 5.21 Atrial flutter with varying p-wave morphology. If the flutter wave and atrioventricular (AV) node conduction are both stable, the QRS complex will be regular on the electrocardiogram (ECG). However, if passive atrial conduction is unstable, the p-wave will be irregular and may vary in amplitude on the ECG, and the arrhythmia will be correctly diagnosed as atrial flutter with varying P-wave morphology.

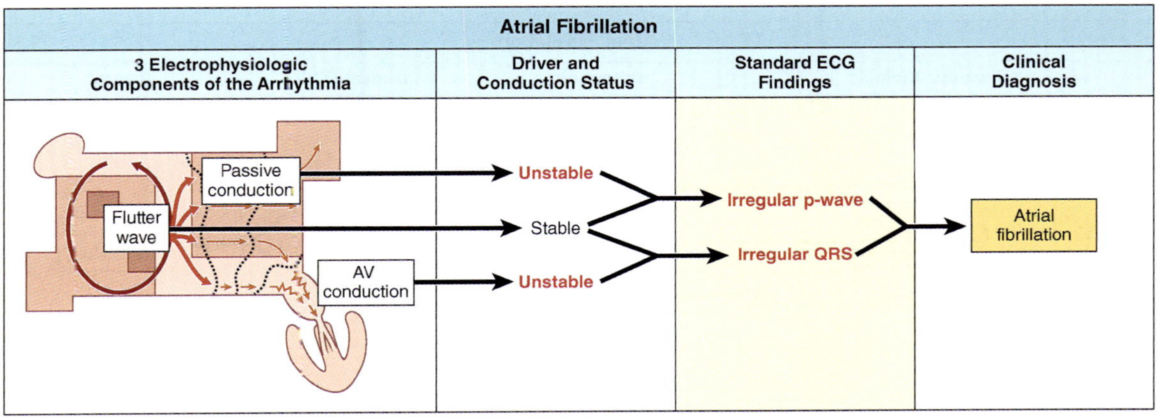

Fig. 5.22 Atrial fibrillation (AF)? If the atrial flutter wave is stable and passive atrial conduction is unstable, the p-wave will be irregular on the electrocardiogram (ECG). If atrioventricular (AV) node conduction is also unstable, the QRS complex will be irregular on the ECG even though the atria and ventricles are all being driven by a stable atrial flutter wave. The combination of an irregular p-wave and an irregular QRS complex on the ECG results in the diagnosis of AF even though the atria are not really fibrillating.

Atrial Flutter With Varying P-Wave Morphology

As long as the flutter wave driver is stable, it is unlikely that passive conduction to the left atrium will be unstable. However, under circumstances of left atrial fibrosis or stretch, such a situation may occur, leading to an irregular p-wave on the ECG. The stable, regular flutter wave driver, combined with stable AV conduction, results in a regular QRS complex. Thus the clinical diagnosis would be *atrial flutter with varying p-wave morphology* (Fig. 5.21).

Atrial Fibrillation Caused by a Single Right Atrial Macro-reentrant Circuit

Our multipoint computerized intraoperative mapping studies of the 1980's,[7,9,15-18] subsequent mapping studies using non-contact intracavitary catheters,[19] and more recent body surface mapping studies[20,21] have all shown that after being established, AF is characterized by the presence of *multiple* macro-reentrant circuits that occur in the atria simultaneously. As mentioned earlier, however, AF is a *clinical* diagnosis made solely on the basis of ECG findings. Rarely, AF (always defined by the standard ECG findings) can be caused by the presence of only *one* macro-reentrant circuit in the right atrium, the so-called "flutter wave."

Suppose that a right atrial flutter wave is stable, but because of scarring or stretch in the atrium, the passive conduction across the atria is unstable. As noted earlier, this combination will lead to an irregular p-wave on the ECG. Now add to that unstable passive atrial conduction unstable conduction through the AV node (Fig. 5.22), which, of course, causes an irregular QRS on the ECG. Under these circumstances, the ECG shows an irregular p-wave (unstable passive atrial conduction) and an irregular QRS complex (unstable AV node conduction), and the clinical diagnosis is atrial fibrillation. However, in this case, the only macro-reentrant circuit in either atrium is the classic flutter wave in the right atrium. Perhaps it might be more accurate to call this arrhythmia *atrial flutter with varying p-wave morphology and varying AV block,* but as mentioned earlier, arrhythmias are named on the basis of their ECG findings, not on the basis of their actual underlying electrophysiology. Thus, although this arrhythmia is actually a subtype of atrial flutter, its clinical diagnosis would be atrial fibrillation. This represents the rare example of AF that can be cured by simply interrupting the single macro-reentrant circuit in the right atrium. This explains one scenario that explains how the so-called "right atrial Maze procedure" alone might cure a case of AF. In addition, like classic atrial flutter, this type of AF could also be ablated by placing a simple lesion across the CTI with a catheter to interrupt the flutter wave.

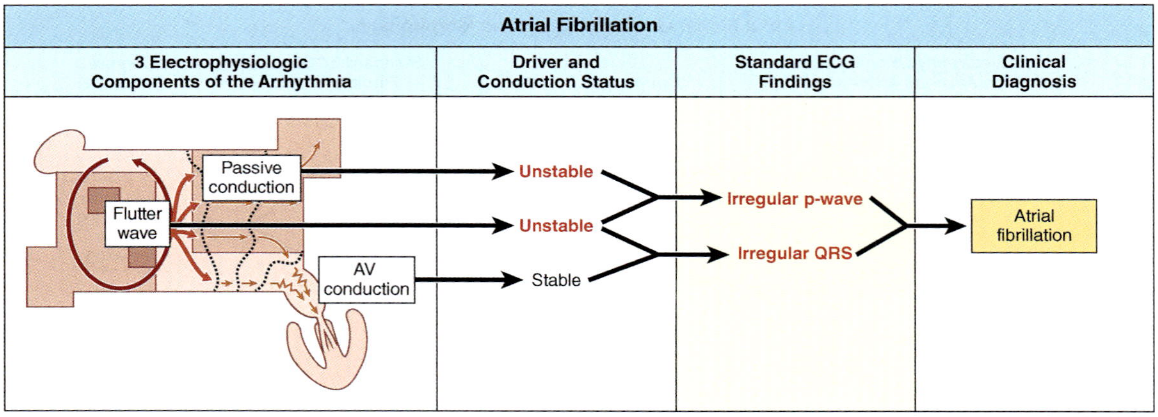

Fig. 5.23 Atrial fibrillation (AF)? If the flutter wave driver itself is unstable, the passive atrial conduction will almost certainly be unstable and irregular, leading to an irregular p-wave on the electrocardiogram (ECG). Despite normal atrioventricular (AV) node conduction, the QRS complex will be irregular on the ECG, and a diagnosis of AF is mandatory even though the atria are not fibrillating.

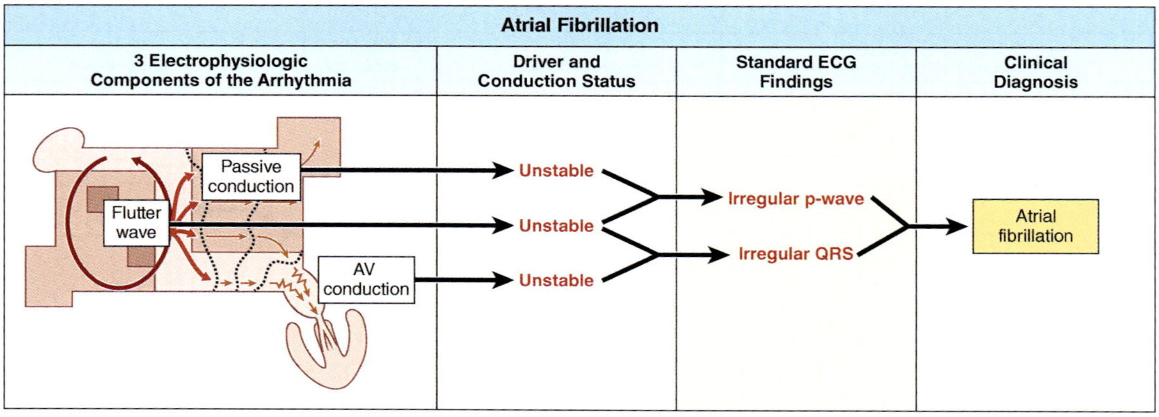

Fig. 5.24 Atrial fibrillation (AF). If the flutter wave driver is unstable, the passive atrial conduction will almost certainly be unstable and irregular, leading to an irregular p-wave on the electrocardiogram (ECG). If atrioventricular (AV) node conduction is also unstable, the QRS complex will be irregular on the ECG, and a diagnosis of AF is again obligatory even though the atria are not fibrillating.

Another scenario in which a single flutter wave in the right atrium can lead to a clinical diagnosis of AF is one in which the right atrial flutter wave itself is unstable (Fig. 5.23). In this situation, the cycle length of the flutter wave is not fixed at 200 ms; rather, it varies so that one cycle might take only 180 ms, but the next one takes 220 ms. This variability in the cycle length of the unstable flutter wave would almost certainly result in erratic (unstable) passive atrial conduction, the two components leading to an irregular p-wave on the ECG. In this case, whether conduction through the AV node is stable (see Fig. 5.23) or unstable (Fig. 5.24), the QRS complex on a standard ECG will be irregular. Again, it is the combination of an irregular p-wave and an irregular QRS complex on the ECG that dictates the clinical diagnosis of atrial fibrillation.

By far the most common type of AF is characterized by the presence of multiple macro-reentrant circuits in the left atrium that drive the remainder of the atria and the ventricles (Fig. 5.25). Because the macro-reentrant drivers do not stimulate the atria in a synchronous manner, the drivers of the arrhythmia are unstable and irregular. This causes unstable and irregular passive atrial conduction and an irregular or non-discernible p-wave on the ECG. In addition, regardless of the functional integrity of the AV node, the ventricular response will be highly irregular as well, so there is no question that the clinical diagnosis is AF. The passive atrial conduction that occurs in the right atrium in response to the left atrial macro-reentrant drivers is irregular in most cases but not necessarily so. Recall that the refractory periods in the right atrium are usually so long that the right atrium cannot normally support multiple macro-reentrant circuits simultaneously (see Chapter 4). Therefore, large portions of the right atrium may not even be activated by each successive passive wavefront coming from the left atrial macro-reentrant drivers, so even though the right atrium appears to be fibrillating as well, there may be no reentry per se within the right atrium. However, this passive activity in the right atrium may also become organized during AF so that the left atrial drivers effectively give rise to stable macro-reentry in the right atrium as well (Fig. 5.26). Because the normal right atrium is capable of harboring only one macro-reentrant circuit due to its long local refractory periods, the "induced" macro-reentrant circuit in the right atrium will have the same characteristics and be in the same location as the classic flutter wave of atrial flutter. The major difference between such "induced" right atrial flutter waves and flutter waves of classic atrial flutter is that the "induced" right atrial flutter waves are entirely *passive* and do not serve as one of the drivers of AF. Therefore, right atrial interventional procedures alone have absolutely no effect on this arrhythmia. Also, this explains the seemingly strange observation that cardiac surgeons have made for years when they see that "the left atrium is fibrillating but the right atrium is fluttering"!

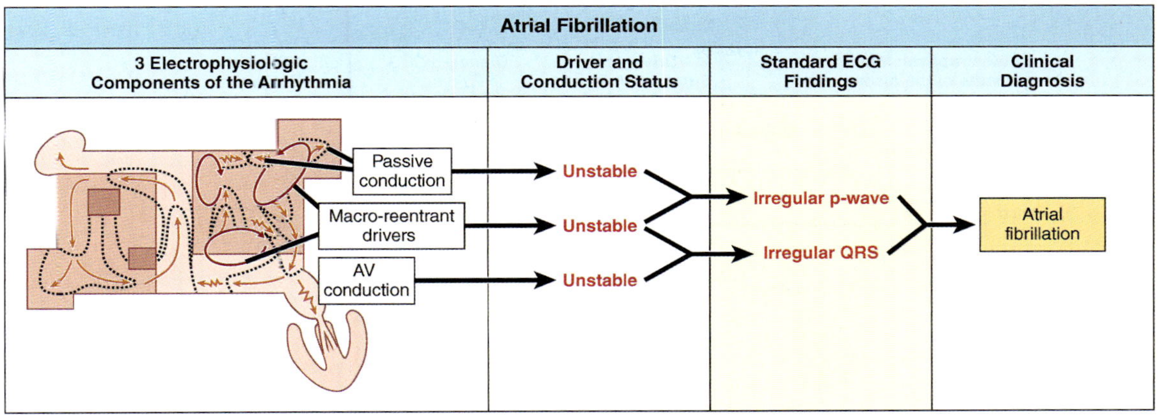

Fig. 5.25 Atrial fibrillation. When the multiple macro-reentrant drivers of AF are present, all three components of the arrhythmia are unstable and irregular, and both the p-wave and the QRS complex are irregular on the electrocardiogram. In this case, there is no doubt that the patient is experiencing AF. *AV,* Atrioventricular.

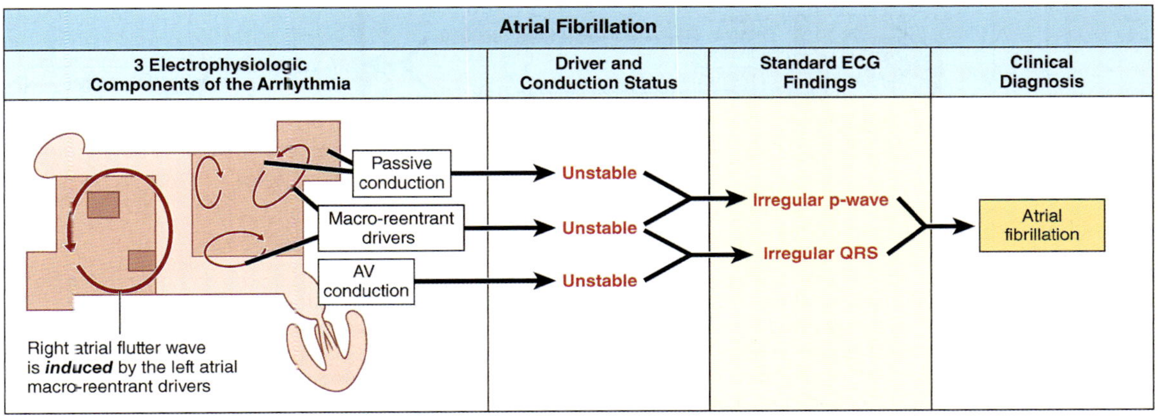

Fig. 5.26 Atrial Fibrillation. As shown in Fig 5.18, when the macro-reentrant drivers of atrial fibrillation (AF) are confined to the left atrium (LA), the passive conduction to the right atrium (RA) may become organized enough to form a single large macro-reentrant in the RA ("flutter wave"). In this case, the RA can exhibit right atrial flutter while the LA is fibrillating. In patients with long-standing persistent AF, approximately 70% of the macro-reentrant drivers are located in the LA and 30% in the RA. This means that interventional procedures for this type of AF that are confined to left atrial ablation alone have an obligatory 30% failure rate. *AV,* Atrioventricular.

Atrial Flutter/Fibrillation

Finally, one interesting clinical problem that falls within this spectrum of arrhythmias is what clinicians call "atrial flutter/fib" (Fig. 5.27). This is an especially common occurrence in the immediate postoperative period after cardiac surgery. This hybrid "diagnosis" refers to the situation when the ECG shows short runs of regular atrial flutter interspersed with short runs of irregular AF, as if the heart rhythm were "flipping" from one arrhythmia to the other. Although the actual electrophysiological mechanism for this situation has never been documented by mapping, it is highly unlikely that the classic form of AF with multiple drivers and disorganized passive atrial conduction shown in Fig. 5.25 would suddenly and intermittently break spontaneously to leave only a single stable right atrial flutter wave driving the atrium in a regular fashion like that shown in Fig. 5.19. Although this notion implies too drastic a change in too many of the components of this spectrum of arrhythmias, it is theoretically possible. However, it is far more likely that the underlying mechanism in "atrial flutter/fib" depends on the presence of a single flutter wave in the right atrium. Why does it matter? It matters because a single reentrant circuit in the right atrium can often be interrupted by atrial pacing, and complex AF cannot.

In classic right atrial flutter, the flutter wave is stable, and it drives activation of the rest of the atria and ventricles in a regular fashion (see Fig. 5.27, *left upper panel*). Surgical irritation, rewarming of the atrium, the trauma of surgery, elevated circulating catecholamines, and perioperative drugs can all cause the stable flutter wave to suddenly and intermittently become unstable, and what we would call "AF" (based on the ECG findings) would occur instantaneously (see Fig. 5.27, *lower right panel*). If the flutter wave then restabilizes for several beats, the ECG findings would instantaneously revert to those of classic atrial flutter. This scenario requires only a slight and transient change to occur in the cycle length of the right atrial flutter wave to result in the clinical picture of atrial flutter/fib. Because "atrial flutter/fib" is likely caused by a single flutter wave in the right atrium that alternates between being stable and unstable, the atria can frequently be captured and terminated by rapid atrial pacing.

In summary, classic atrial flutter and the most common type of atrial fibrillation occupy the two ends of a spectrum of clinical arrhythmias (Fig. 5.28). The specific clinical arrhythmia that occurs within

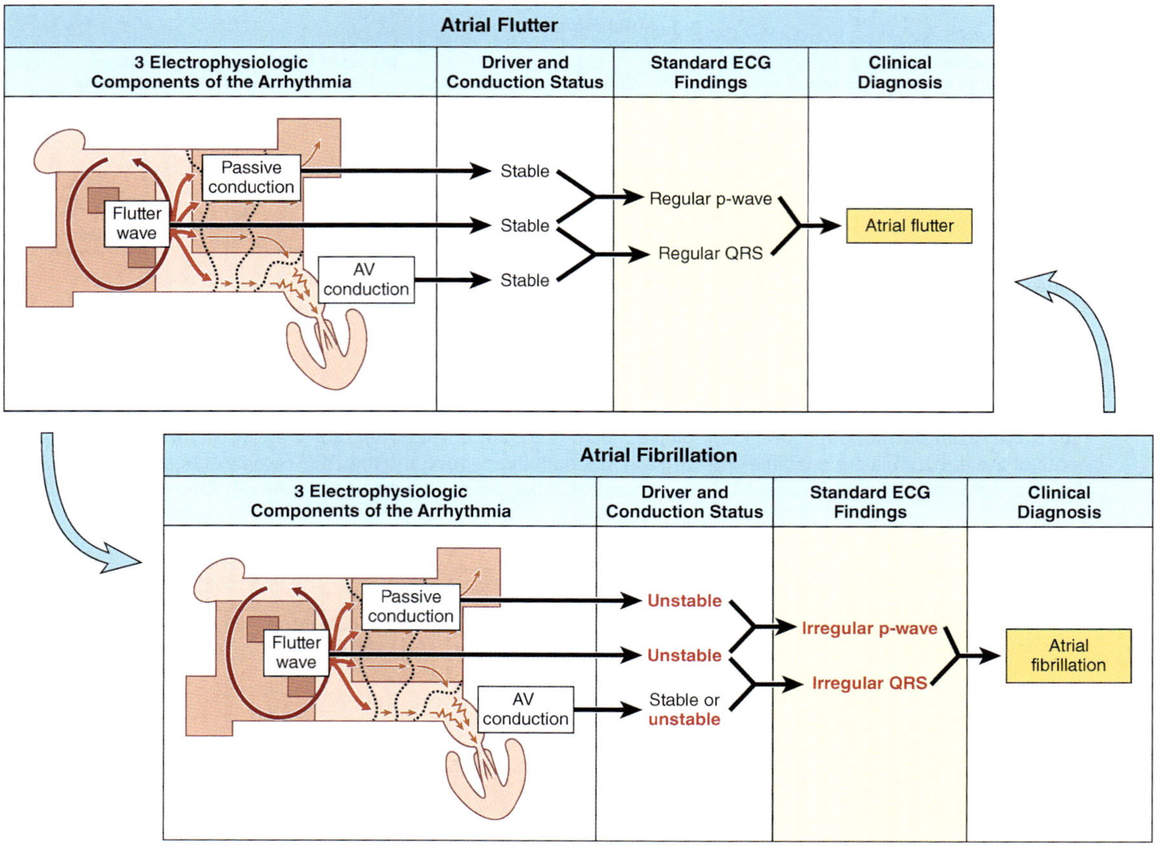

Fig. 5.27 Atrial flutter/fibrillation. In the immediate postoperative period after cardiac surgery, patients are often found to be in what is called "atrial flutter/fib." This does not necessarily mean that they are alternating between typical atrial flutter with one "flutter wave" in the right atrium and complex atrial fibrillation with multiple macro-reentrant circuits, though it is a possibility. More likely, the postoperative arrhythmia is being driven by a single flutter wave in the right atrium that alternates between being stable *(left upper panel)* and unstable *(right lower panel)*. This explains why early postoperative "atrial flutter/fib" can often be terminated by first capturing the atria with rapid atrial pacing and then continuing to pace the atrium at the highest tolerable rate until the heart fully rewarms and recovers from surgery. *AV,* Atrioventricular; *ECG,* electrocardiogram.

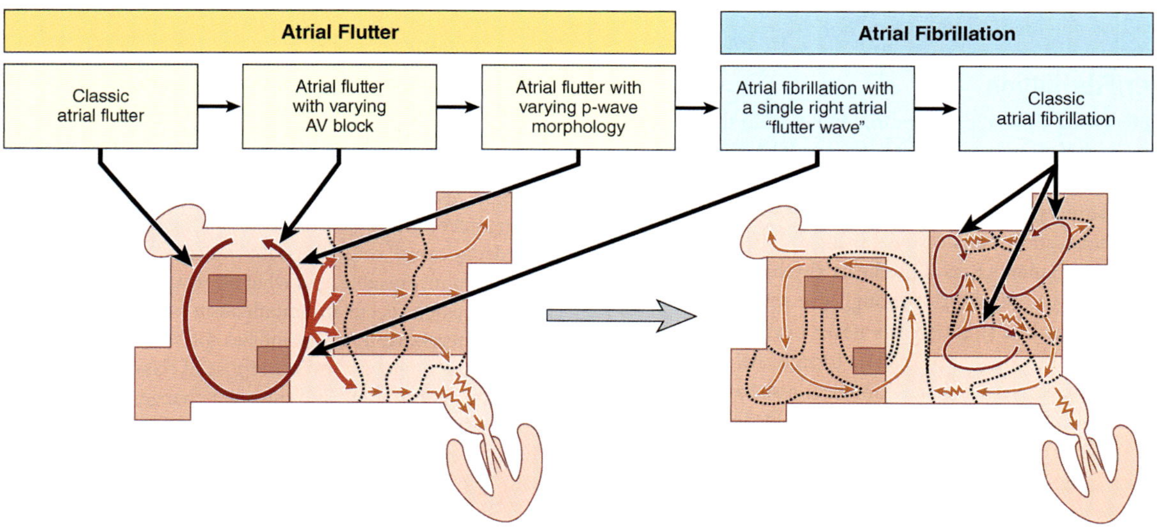

Fig. 5.28 A summary of the electrophysiology underlying the spectrum of clinical arrhythmias from typical atrial flutter to complex atrial fibrillation. The *black arrows* point to the "drivers" of each of the arrhythmias. (See text for further discussion.) *AV,* Atrioventricular.

this spectrum depends on interactions between the driver of the arrhythmia, passive atrial conduction, and conduction through the AV node–His bundle complex. The success of a specific catheter or surgical procedure in abolishing one of the specific arrhythmias within this spectrum depends on placing lesions in the appropriate places in the atrium to abolish or isolate the driver(s) of that specific arrhythmia. In some cases, this requires only a left atrial procedure. Rarely, it requires only a right atrial procedure. In most cases it requires that lesions be placed in both atria. However, one sure way to ablate any and all of the arrhythmias in this spectrum is to preclude the possibility of the development of macro-reentry in *either* atrium by placing the appropriate lesions in both.

TRIGGERS: THE INDUCTION OF ATRIAL FIBRILLATION

As mentioned earlier, our intraoperative mapping studies and experimental studies in the 1980s documented that when AF is established, it is characterized by the presence of multiple, fleeting macro-reentrant circuits that might appear in one position in the atria for only a few hundred milliseconds before moving to another area, much like eddies in a stream. However, our studies did not demonstrate how AF is *induced*. That revelation awaited the seminal paper by Haissaguerre and associates in 1998 in which they documented that AF is induced by atrial triggers, more than 90% of which are located in or around the orifices of the pulmonary veins in the left atrium.[22] Haissaguerre and colleagues' observation was reported after nearly a decade of electrophysiologists being able to treat arrhythmias other than AF (WPW syndrome, AV node reentry, and so on) by radiofrequency catheter ablation with a high rate of success. Their article provided the basis of a new interventional approach specifically for the treatment of patients with AF, PVI that ignited an immediate and explosive growth in catheter PVI for AF. In addition, it resulted in an increase in concomitant surgical ablation in patients with a history of AF who were undergoing coronary artery bypass grafting and/or valve surgery.

As important as Haissaguerre and coworkers' article was to the interventional treatment of patients with AF, as with many seminal medical advances, the responses of the medical and surgical communities to that article led to certain undesirable consequences through no fault of its authors. The most important misconception was that PVI alone was an adequate procedure for *all* types of AF, a notion that was not stated anywhere in Haissaguerre's article. Nevertheless, interventional electrophysiologists began to perform PVI routinely not only for paroxysmal AF but also for persistent AF and long-standing persistent AF. Likewise, cardiac surgeons who had been reluctant to add a Maze procedure to CABG and/or valve surgery now had a much simpler procedure (PVI) that they could perform for all types of AF. In turn, this led to the development of numerous new ablative energy sources and to the manufacture of surgical devices designed specifically to isolate the pulmonary veins. It has taken many years for both interventional electrophysiologists and arrhythmia surgeons to realize that whether performed with a catheter or by surgery, PVI alone is an excellent procedure for paroxysmal AF (as Haissaguerre and colleagues' article suggested), but PVI alone is an inadequate interventional procedure for persistent and long-standing persistent AF, which was not recommended in Haissaguerre and colleagues' article.

Induction of Atrial Fibrillation by "Arrhythmia Triggers"

Little attention has been given to the nature of the triggers that induce episodes of AF or to the fact that we have known about non-pulmonary vein "triggers" for decades but simply have not given them that name. Thus, it is instructive to think in terms of the multiple ways that AF can be induced and then to place pulmonary vein triggers within that context. Physicians have long recognized that atrial flutter can "deteriorate" into AF. As just described, typical *atrial flutter* can induce what appears to be AF on an ECG in multiple ways depending on the stability of the flutter wave, passive atrial conduction, and AV node conduction (Figs. 5.19 through 5.24). In addition, a right atrial flutter wave can lead to the induction of multiple macro-reentrant circuits, especially in the left atrium, that constitutes true AF (see Fig. 5.25).

During the 1970s and 1980s when surgery was frequently performed for patients with WPW syndrome, we noted that approximately 30% of the patients with WPW syndrome also had preoperative AF. These were the patients in whom we initially mapped AF intraoperatively in our clinical studies during the 1980s.[23] Surprisingly, after the accessory AV pathway responsible for WPW syndrome was surgically divided, only about 5% of the patients experienced AF thereafter.[24] This indicated that the accessory pathway was somehow causing AF to be induced in 25% of patients with WPW syndrome. This occurred because of the retrograde (ventricular-to-atrial) conduction of electrical impulses across the accessory pathway allowed electrical impulses to be intermittently conducted into the atrium without inducing reciprocating tachycardia but rather inducing AF instead (Fig. 5.29). Similarly, AV node reentry tachycardia (AVNRT) can also induce AF in some patients (Fig. 5.30).[25] Because patients with atrial flutter, the WPW syndrome, and AVNRT can now be treated successfully by radiofrequency catheter ablation, no surgical or catheter intervention specifically for AF is necessary in patients who have it induced by any of these "arrhythmia triggers."

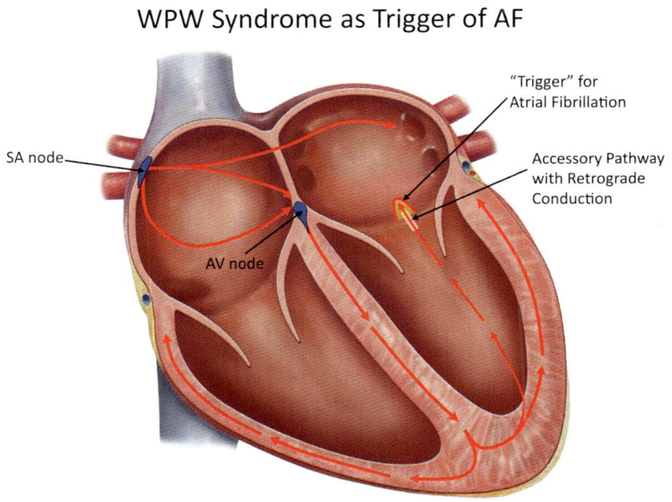

Fig. 5.29 Wolff-Parkinson-White syndrome. This is a congenital abnormality in which there is an accessory atrioventricular (AV) connection that can conduct electrical impulses from the atrium to the ventricles (antegrade) during sinus rhythm and usually from the ventricles to the atrium (retrograde) during the reciprocating tachycardia. If antegrade conduction of an atrial impulse is blocked in the accessory atrioventricular (AV) connection, the next ventricular wavefront can conduct retrograde from the ventricle to the atrium across the accessory AV connection and cause an atrial premature beat. This premature beat can act as a trigger to induce AF. In such patients, permanent interruption of conduction across the accessory AV connection by surgery or catheter ablation can cure the patient's AF.

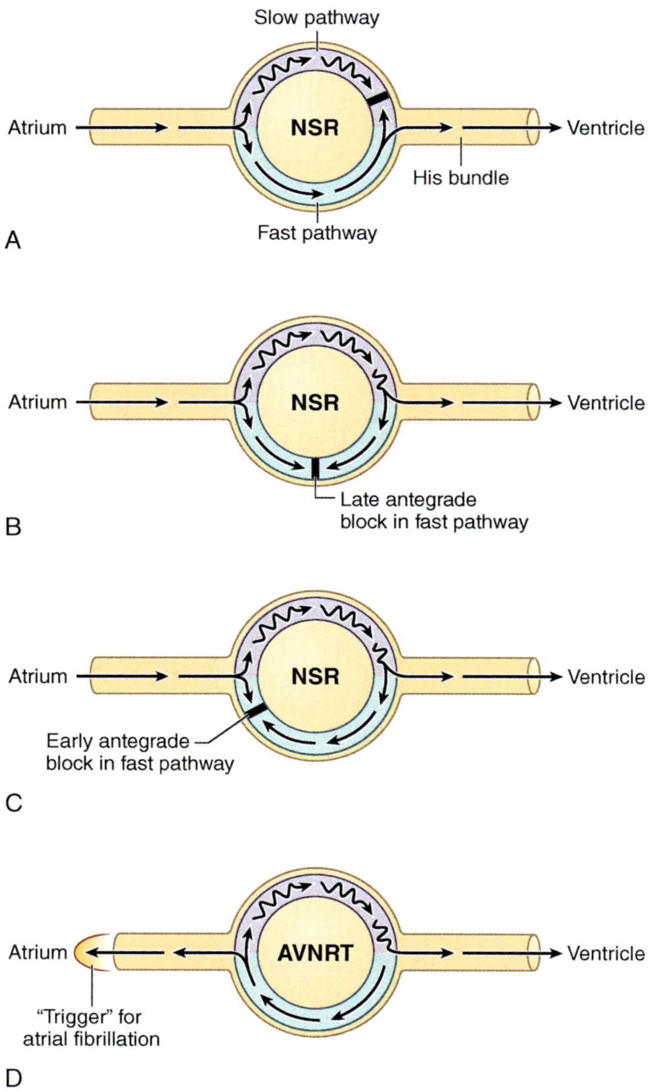

Fig. 5.30 Atrioventricular node reentry tachycardia (AVNRT) can also trigger atrial fibrillation (AF). AVNRT occurs because of dual conduction pathways within the atrioventricular (AV) node, one slow *(purple)* and one fast *(blue)*. (A) During normal sinus rhythm (NSR), atrial impulses are conducted preferentially via the fast pathway to the His bundle and ventricles. (B) If a conduction block occurs late in the fast pathway, the atrial impulse is conducted to the ventricles with a slight prolongation of the P-R interval on the electrocardiogram. (C) If a conduction block occurs early in the fast pathway, the atrial impulse traveling through the slow pathway can propagate retrograde up the fast pathway. (D) If the early conduction block is unidirectional, it can establish a reentrant circuit within the AV node that can conduct retrograde to the atrium. This retrograde impulse from the AV node back into the atria during AVNRT can act as a trigger to induce AF.

Induction of Atrial Fibrillation by "Atrial Triggers"

The triggers that induce AF, first described by Haissaguerre and coworkers[22] in 1998, are focal in origin and therefore, they must be either automatic foci or micro-reentrant foci or the result of afterdepolarizations ("triggered automaticity"). There are no other electrophysiologic options. Most clinical arrhythmias are either automatic or reentrant, but some authorities have suggested that "triggered automaticity," primarily in the ganglionic plexi, may be one of the underlying electrophysiologic events that give rise to the triggers that induce AF. Wit and Boyden describe triggered automaticity as follows:

> *"Triggered automaticity is a term used to describe impulse initiation in cardiac fibers that is dependent on afterdepolarizations. Afterdepolarizations are oscillations in membrane potential that follow the upstroke of an action potential. . . . However, the demonstration that triggered activity is a cause of arrhythmias in vivo, such as atrial fibrillation, is a major problem that is not completely resolved."*[26]

Thus it seems likely that most of the triggers responsible for the induction of AF episodes are either automatic foci or micro-reentrant foci, and most of them are in the region of the pulmonary veins.

Micro-reentrant circuits typically occur in areas of the heart where there is a transition from one cell type to another. For example, we have known for more than 50 years that there are multiple sites of transition between normal, ischemic, and dead myocardial cells in the ischemic border zone of acute myocardial infarctions[27] and that micro-reentry is prevalent in these areas (see Fig. 4.8 in Chapter 4).[28,29] Similar cellular transition zones are present near the orifices of the pulmonary veins where the pulmonary vein endothelium transitions into the left atrial endocardium. This transition is most prominent within the pulmonary veins themselves because "sleeves" of atrial endocardium commonly extend well up into the pulmonary veins (Fig. 5.31).[30] Thus focal micro-reentrant circuits can develop within this pulmonary vein cellular transition zone, representing one type, probably the most common type, of "pulmonary vein trigger."

Automatic foci caused by abnormally rapid spontaneous phase 4 depolarization of individual cells in and around the pulmonary veins can also act as AF triggers, and interestingly, automatic atrial tachycardias have been shown previously to originate from actual "cell rests" in the left atrium.[31] These cell rests are found most commonly near the orifice of the left superior pulmonary vein in a mirror-image position to the normal site of the anatomic SA node in the right atrium. A focal pulmonary vein trigger caused by automaticity cannot be differentiated from one caused by micro-reentry by simple atrial mapping (see Chapter 4), and both result in the premature atrial beats originating within and around the pulmonary veins that induce AF in susceptible patients.

Some of the main routes taken to the heart by the parasympathetic fibers of the vagus nerve are along the four pulmonary veins. These vagal fibers form *ganglionic plexi* on the epicardial surface of the atria

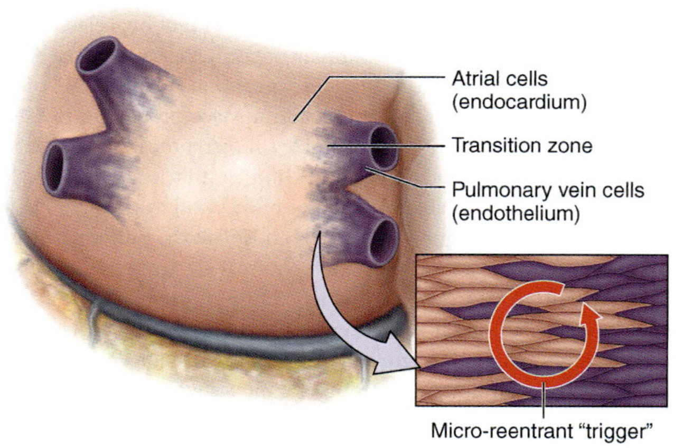

Fig. 5.31 The sleeve of left atrial (LA) endocardium that extends up into the pulmonary veins results in a cellular transition zone of LA endocardial cells and pulmonary vein endothelium located in the distal portion of all four pulmonary veins. These transition cellular zones in the distal pulmonary veins are excellent substrates for the formation of focal micro-reentrant circuits *(inset)*.

near the junction of the pulmonary veins with the left atrium. Some investigators believe that these ganglia play an important role in inducing, and perhaps even maintaining, AF.[32,33] As implied earlier, the exact mechanism by which these ganglia produce premature stimuli is unknown, though triggered automaticity as the result of afterdepolarizations and high-frequency driver regions have been suggested as possible mechanisms. Regardless of the precise mechanism involved in their genesis, triggered automaticity originating in the vagal plexi can theoretically give rise to premature stimuli that would appear on an atrial map to be a pulmonary vein trigger. Efforts to treat patients with AF by ganglionic plexus ablation are mixed at best (see Chapter 30).

In summary, triggers that induce episodes of AF can involve several different electrophysiologic mechanisms (Fig. 5.32). The most common triggers for AF are those that occur in and around the pulmonary veins, and the most common of these is *probably* a micro-reentrant circuit in the cellular transition zone of a distal pulmonary vein, although the micro-reentrant basis for these triggers has not been proven. Regardless of the specific mechanism involved, these triggers are only capable of *inducing* AF, not of *sustaining* it.

Most authorities agree that the atrium has to be "vulnerable" to the development of AF, or else the trigger will produce only a premature atrial beat, not atrial fibrillation (Fig. 5.33). There is some

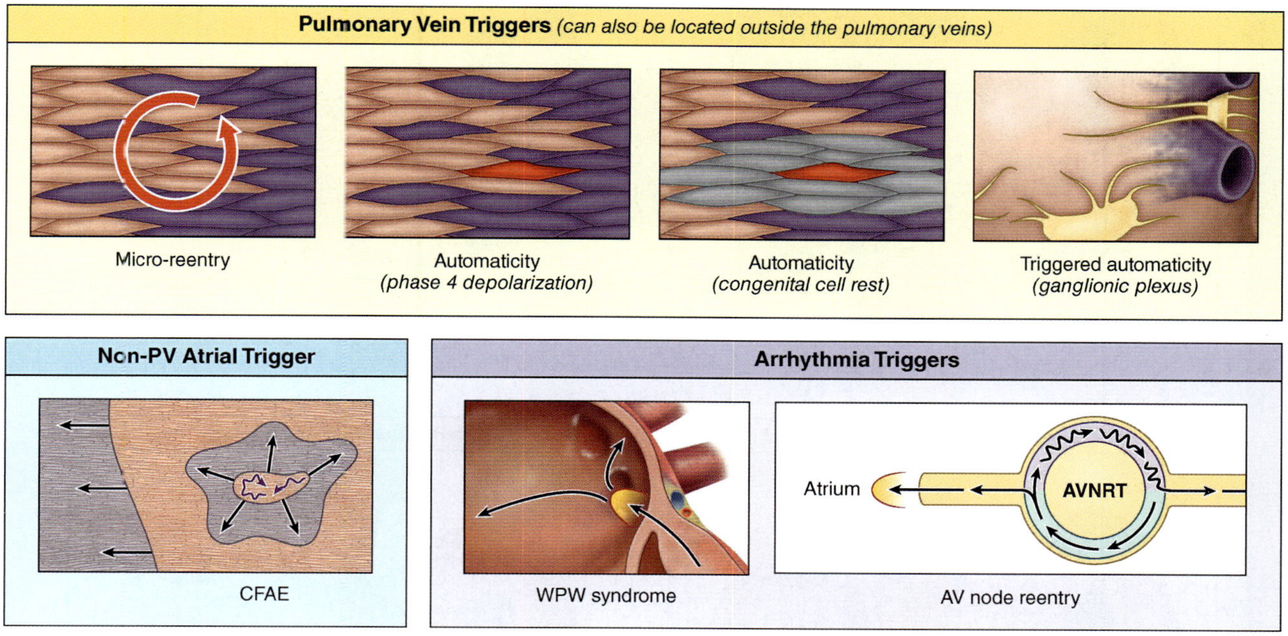

Fig. 5.32 *Upper panel*, The four main types of pulmonary vein triggers. All four types can also be located *outside* the pulmonary veins in the right or left atrium. *Left lower panel*, Areas of continuous fractionated atrial electrograms (CFAE) can serve as atrial triggers, but they are typically located outside the pulmonary veins. Such areas of CFAE can *induce*, but not *sustain*, atrial fibrillation (AF). *Middle and right lower panels*, Arrhythmia triggers such as Wolff-Parkinson-White (WPW) syndrome and atrioventricular (AV) node reentry tachycardia (AVNRT) can also function as atrial triggers that induce AF. Atrial flutter, not shown here, is also a frequent precursor to AF.

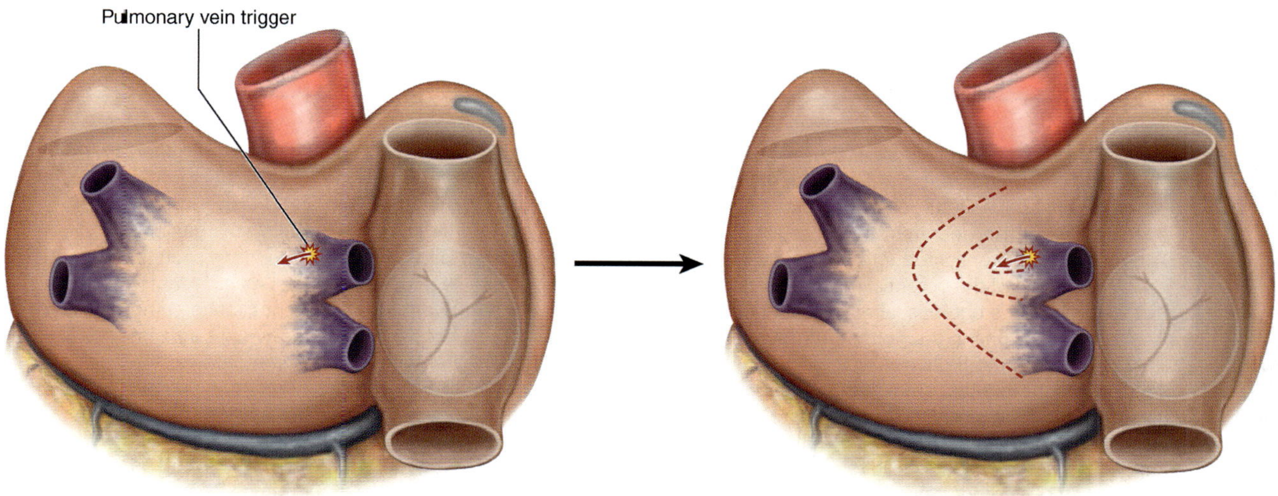

Fig. 5.33 When an electrically normal left atrium that is incapable of sustaining a macro-reentrant circuit is suddenly stimulated by any type of trigger, including pulmonary vein (PV) triggers *(left panel)*, the result will be a simple premature atrial contraction (PAC, *right panel*).

disagreement on exactly what constitutes atrial "vulnerability," but whatever anatomic-electrophysiologic-biochemical substrate is responsible, triggers induce AF only in those patients who have the *potential* to develop macro-reentrant circuits in the atria (Fig. 5.34). Potential atrial macro-reentry requires an area of atrial tissue of sufficient size to develop a complete circuit, the presence of unidirectional conduction block at some point in the potential circuit, and a combination of local conduction velocity and refractory period that allows for a constant excitable gap to exist within the potential circuit (see Chapter 4). When an atrium with this "vulnerability" is suddenly

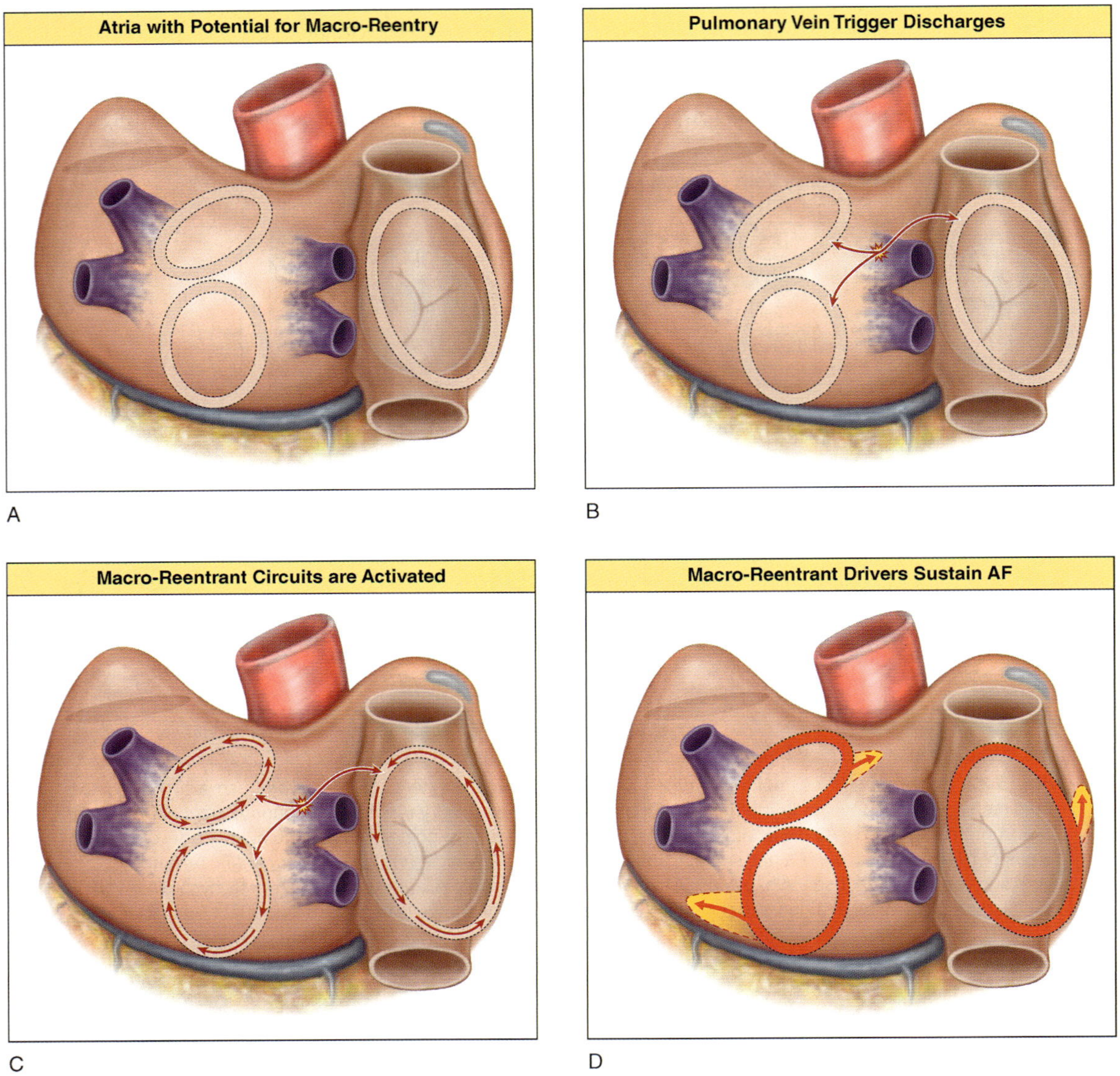

Fig. 5.34 The induction of atrial fibrillation (AF) by a micro-reentrant pulmonary vein trigger in a patient vulnerable to the development of AF. (A) Patient vulnerable to the development of AF because of three sites in the atria that are capable of developing and sustaining macro-reentry, two in the left atrium and one in the right atrium. (B) A micro-reentrant trigger or automatic trigger in the right superior pulmonary vein discharges and the impulse is propagated into both atria, which combined, harbor three potential macro-reentrant circuits. (C) Stimulation of the potential macro-reentrant circuits by the pulmonary vein trigger activates macro-reentry at all three of the potential sites in the atrium. (D) AF being driven by the two macro-reentrant circuits in the left atrium and one in the right atrium. Any one of these macro-reentrant circuits can be passive but at least two of them must be active drivers. If only one of the circuits is active and the other two are passive, the patient will have either atrial flutter or "atrial tachycardia", but not atrial fibrillation. The duration of the induced episode of AF depends on the length of time that the macro-reentrant circuits can sustain themselves. If they are self-perpetuating for less than 7 days, meaning that the patient has episodes of AF each of which lasts less than 7 days, the patient is said to have *paroxysmal AF*. In such patients, subsequent episodes of AF have to be reinduced by another trigger, also usually in the pulmonary veins. If the AF episode lasts more than 7 days but less than 1 year, the patient is said to have *persistent AF*. If the AF episode lasts more than 1 year, the patient is said to have *long-standing persistent AF*. Although no longer a part of the contemporary classification of AF, older classification systems also include a fourth category of *permanent AF* that referred to patients with long-standing persistent AF who could not be successfully cardioverted either electrically or pharmacologically.

triggered, macro-reentrant circuits are established in the vulnerable areas of the atria. If two or more such macro-reentrant circuits are induced and become sustained for any period, the patient has AF.

It is clear that certain factors, particularly advancing age, atrial fibrosis, and enlarged atria, make patients more vulnerable to the development of AF. In addition, a phenomenon called "electrical remodeling" occurs with AF in which the more episodes of AF a patient has, the more AF that patient is likely to have in the future[34] (see Chapter 8).

MACRO-REENTRANT DRIVERS: THE MAINTENANCE OF ATRIAL FIBRILLATION

Haissaguerre and coworkers'[22] seminal article in 1998 established that most individual episodes of AF are *induced* by triggers in and around the pulmonary vein orifices. Since that time, their observation has provided a sound scientific rationale for isolating the pulmonary veins for paroxysmal AF, thereby decreasing the *likelihood* of AF induction. However, after a PVI, most atria are still *capable of fibrillating* if stimulated by non-pulmonary vein triggers or arrhythmia triggers. However, two very different theories of how AF is *sustained* emerged following the publication of Haissaguerre and coworkers [22] article, and they have different connotations regarding how to treat non-paroxysmal types of AF (persistent AF, long-standing persistent AF).

Self-Perpetuating Atrial Macro-reentrant Circuits

In our opinion, AF is sustained by macro-reentrant circuits (drivers) in the atria that are usually induced by atrial triggers located in and around the orifices of the pulmonary veins. The macro-reentrant drivers can become self-perpetuating, depending on the complex interplay between wavefront conduction velocity, local refractory periods, and the area of atrium available to support the circuit.[12,13] If the macro-reentrant drivers remain self-sustaining for a relatively short period, say for a few hours or days, then the clinical diagnosis will be *paroxysmal AF* with episodes lasting for less than 7 days. However, because of electrical remodeling and associated age and morbidity, the macro-reentrant drivers can ultimately become stable enough to sustain themselves indefinitely, resulting in the clinical diagnosis of *persistent AF* (more than 1 week and less than 1 year) or *long-standing persistent AF* (more than 1 year).

It is important to recognize that once an episode of AF has been initiated, the underlying electrophysiology is the same *during the episode of AF* in paroxysmal AF and nonparoxysmal AF. The triggers that *induce* AF have little or nothing to do with the *maintenance* of AF because the maintenance of AF depends entirely on the ability of the macro-reentrant drivers to become self-perpetuating. This concept of the underlying mechanisms of AF has profound implications regarding its interventional treatment. It explains why isolation of the pulmonary veins (PVI) is effective for paroxysmal AF by isolating most of the AF triggers even though the atria can still fibrillate after the procedure. This concept also explains why PVI is an inadequate operation for nonparoxysmal AF because it does little to interrupt the macro-reentrant circuits responsible for sustaining persistent and long-standing persistent AF.

The phenomenon of "electrical remodeling" that promotes atrial macro-reentrant drivers to become more stable with time was first described by Maurits Allessie and coworkers at the University of Limburg in Maastricht, The Netherlands.[34] They documented that the more a patient experiences AF, the more AF that patient is likely to experience in the future. As Allessie and coworkers' instructive phrase states, *"Atrial fibrillation begats atrial fibrillation."* Although there may be several explanations for why this occurs, the only explanation that is important to the *interventional* treatment of AF is that electrical remodeling promotes the stabilization of atrial macro-reentrant drivers. This "stabilization" means that the delicate interplay between the physical size of the macro-reentrant circuits, the conduction velocity of the local atrial tissue within these circuits, and the refractory period of that tissue interact in such a fashion that it becomes possible for the circuits to last for several hours, several days, or indefinitely (see Fig. 4.13). We know that macro-reentrant circuits can become self-perpetuating because it happens clinically in classic right atrial flutter, during the reciprocating tachycardia of WPW syndrome, and even in iatrogenic rhythms such as atypical left atrial flutter (aka, "perimitral flutter") because after being initiated, these macro-reentrant arrhythmias require no further input from the initiating trigger(s). Thus there is no reason to doubt the ability of the macro-reentrant circuits of AF to become self-perpetuating just because they may be slightly smaller in size due to of the left atrium's shorter refractory periods (see Figs. 4.14 and 4.15).

In summary, the electrophysiology of AF that is important to interventional cardiologists and arrhythmia surgeons is easy to understand, and interventional treatment based solely on this concept has been extremely successful for more than 3 decades.[35] Episodes of AF are usually induced by focal triggers caused by a localized focus of either automaticity (including triggered automaticity) or by a localized focus of micro-reentry. Because these triggers are located in the area of the pulmonary veins in approximately 90% of patients with stand-alone paroxysmal AF (70% in concomitant AF), excellent results can be attained by simply isolating the pulmonary veins and the intervening posterior wall of the LA ("pulmonary vein cuff") in patients with paroxysmal AF. When AF becomes persistent, however, these pulmonary vein triggers become largely irrelevant because the AF is being maintained by self-perpetuating macro-reentrant circuits that are usually located outside the confines of the pulmonary vein cuff. Thus catheter and surgical interventional procedures for continuous AF should be directed at interrupting these atrial macro-reentrant drivers and precluding the possibility that they can form anywhere in the atria.

The Focal Driver or "Rotor" Theory

For several years after Haissaguerre and colleagues'[22] article, many interventional electrophysiologists believed that *focal* drivers of either automatic foci, micro-reentrant circuits or "triggered activity" continuously stimulated the atrium, causing persistent and long-standing persistent AF. This alternative concept of the mechanisms responsible for sustaining AF has had a profoundly negative effect on the lesion patterns that have been applied during catheter ablation and surgical therapy for the persistent forms of AF. The single misconception that AF is sustained by focal drivers is perhaps the primary factor contributing to the suboptimal results of catheter ablation for all forms of AF except the simplest type of paroxysmal AF that require only isolation of the pulmonary veins.

The concept that AF is sustained by focal drivers is problematic enough, but the problem is compounded by the notion that these drivers are located or anchored solely in and around the pulmonary veins.[36] This controversy is of more than academic importance because many interventional cardiologists and novice arrhythmia surgeons who believe in the "focal driver" theory perform simple PVI not only for paroxysmal AF but also for persistent and long-standing persistent AF with dismal results.[37,38] This controversy over exactly what drives AF in patients with non-paroxysmal AF has resulted in surgical approaches with no logical scientific basis, such as PVI + left atrial appendage isolation or PVI + autonomic denervation for persistent and long-standing persistent AF.[39] This controversy remains important because even today, some of the most revered icons in basic electrophysiology[8] still deny the concept of AF being sustained by macro-reentrant drivers and ignore the vast disparity between the clinical results of surgical intervention that is based on that concept[35] and catheter ablation based on the concept that AF is sustained by focal triggers.[40]

Just as the triggers for episodes of AF must be attributable to either automaticity or micro-reentry, so would the focal drivers suspected of being responsible for sustaining AF under this theory. However, for these same electrophysiologic mechanisms to be the drivers that *sustain* AF episodes, they would have to be capable of firing continuously for many years at a time. With extremely rare exceptions, no automatic focus, no micro-reentrant circuit, and no triggered automaticity activity has ever been shown to fire continuously over a period of years at a time. In our own personal experience, we have seen only one near instance, that of a 14-year-old male who had an automatic left atrial focus emanating from the LA appendage that fired continuously for more than 2 years. Interestingly, this incessantly firing focal stimulus did not cause AF but rather an absolutely recalcitrant, stable, and regular atrial tachycardia (see Fig. 4.11 in Chapter 4). Nevertheless, there is no question that in rare instances, persistent AF can be cured by ablating a specific focus in the atrium that is driving the macro-reentrant circuits. However, such occasional occurrences do not warrant focal ablation being the primary objective of interventional therapy for patients with nonparoxysmal AF.

Some interventional electrophysiologists have hypothesized that focal sites of continuous fractionated electrical activity (CFAE) are important in sustaining non-paroxysmal AF and they have performed "fractionation maps" specifically to identify these local CFAE sites in the atria for ablation.[41] Unfortunately, this interventional approach to non-paroxysmal AF has failed largely because it was based on a misunderstanding of exactly what areas of CFAE are (see Figs. 4.6 to 4.9 in Chapter 4).[42]

It is clear that some mechanism other than "continuous focal stimulation" must be at work in patients who have remained in AF continuously for, say, 10 years. Interestingly, the only electrophysiologic abnormality that has ever been shown to persist for such prolonged periods of time is atrial macro-reentry. This observation makes it even more puzzling to proclaim that less stable types of abnormal electrophysiology (focal automaticity, focal micro-reentry, focal triggered automaticity) are the underlying drivers that sustain long-term atrial macro-reentry.[8,36,37] Perhaps some of the confusion stems from equating small-diameter macro-reentrant circuits to micro-reentrant circuits simply because they can appear to be focal on electrophysiologic maps. However, small-diameter reentrant drivers produce an entirely different pattern of atrial activity than true micro-reentrant foci (Fig. 5.35). If a spiral pattern of any size is present on a map of AF (see Fig. 5.35, *lower panel*), the driver cannot be micro-reentrant because if it were, it would produce a radial activation pattern with the electrical impulse spreading outward from the micro-reentrant circuit (see Fig. 5.35, *upper panel*).

True micro-reentrant circuits and small-diameter macro-reentrant circuits are often seen during sustained AF, but this does not necessarily mean that they are actively sustaining the AF. Indeed, they are far more likely to be simple bystanders that are caused by macro-reentrant drivers. This is analogous to seeing local tornados (analagous to small-diameter macro-reentrant circuits, a.k.a., "rotors") in the vicinity of hurricanes (analagous to large-diameter macro-reentrant circuits). The tornados do not drive the hurricanes; rather, the hurricanes drive the tornados. Similarly, large-diameter macro-reentrant circuits are the drivers of AF, and they often "spin off" the smaller-diameter macro-reentrant circuits that have nothing to do with sustaining the AF.

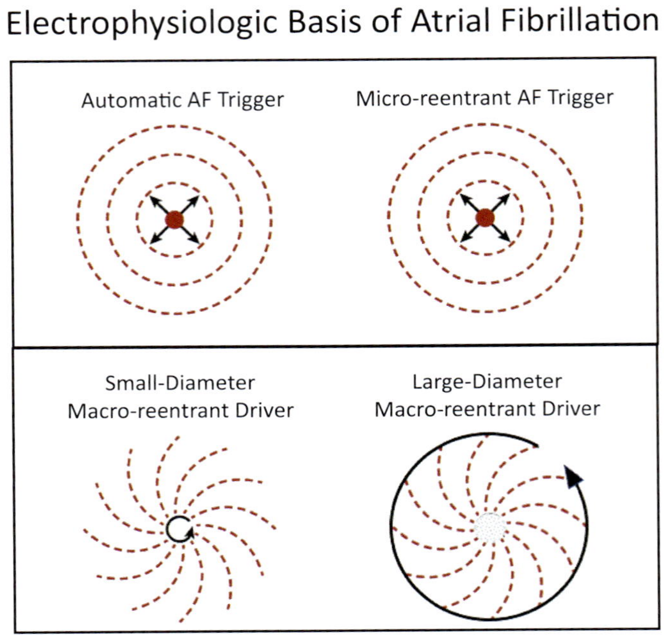

Fig. 5.35 Atrial fibrillation (AF) is induced by triggers and sustained by drivers. *Upper panel,* Both automatic and micro-reentrant triggers that induce AF originate at the cellular level; therefore, they always cause a radial pattern of outward wavefront propagation from the automatic or micro-reentrant focus. *Lower panel,* Any time a spiral pattern of wavefront propagation is mapped and shown to produce a spiral pattern, it is by definition macro-reentry. It may be a small-diameter macro-reentrant circuit (also called "rotors" or a large-diameter macro-reentrant circuit). The Maze procedure was conceived and designed on the basis of AF drivers being large macro-reentrant circuits.

Clinical Observations Impacting the Two Theories

One might fairly ask the question, "Why do we so readily accept that classic right atrial flutter and atypical left atrial perimitral flutter are sustained by large self-perpetuating macro-reentrant circuits but doubt that slightly smaller self-perpetuating macro-reentrant circuits in areas of the atria with known shorter refractory periods can sustain AF?" After all, interventional electrophysiologists routinely cure atrial flutter by interrupting the culprit right atrial macro-reentrant circuit at one site, the CTI.[43] Why is it so hard then to accept that AF can be cured similarly by interrupting the responsible macro-reentrant circuit(s) in the left (and right) atrium? In fairness, most interventional electrophysiologists have finally "come around" on this issue, but it took several years and consistently poor clinical results for them to accept the fact that in addition to isolating the pulmonary veins, they needed to add other lesions in all but the simplest types of paroxysmal AF. Here is how that evolution was described by my long-time clinical electrophysiology colleague in St. Louis, Bruce Lindsay[44]:

> *"Methods for ablation of AF have evolved from elimination of triggers, to segmental pulmonary vein isolation, to wide circumferential ablation incorporating a larger mass of atrial tissue. The evolution of ablation techniques recognizes that triggered mechanisms alone may account for AF in some patients, but in most there is a need to modify the substrate that sustains AF."*

Electrophysiologists use the term "substrate modification" as a euphemism for interrupting atrial macro-reentrant drivers outside the immediate pulmonary vein area. It is worth noting that this "substrate modification" was the basis of the first Maze procedure performed in 1987.[45]

Finally, when an electrophysiologist chooses to induce AF during a clinical electrophysiology study, one of the pacing protocols used is called "burst pacing" in which rapid atrial pacing is performed for short periods in an effort to induce AF. When the patient develops AF, the burst pacing is immediately stopped . . . but the atria continue to fibrillate. If the "AF trigger" is burst pacing, what is sustaining the AF after termination of the pacing? Clearly, the AF is being sustained by something other than the rapid atrial pacing. The point here is that the lack of importance of focal AF triggers in the *maintenance* of AF is analogous to the lack of importance of rapid atrial pacing in the maintenance of AF. Here are some examples of established facts (1a, 2a, and 3a) followed by observations (1b, 2b, and 3b) that differ only in the replacement of the term "rapid atrial pacing" with the term "focal atrial triggers":

1a. *Rapid atrial pacing* will not induce AF in a normal atrium.
1b. *Focal atrial triggers* will not induce AF in a normal atrium.
2a. *Rapid atrial pacing* can induce AF in an atrium that is susceptible to forming macro-reentrant circuits.
2b. *Focal atrial triggers* can induce AF in an atrium that is susceptible to forming macro-reentrant circuits.
3a. If *rapid atrial pacing* induces AF and the stimulation is stopped after AF has been induced, it is clear that the AF is being sustained by some self-perpetuating mechanism other than *rapid atrial pacing.*
3b. If *focal atrial triggers* induce AF and they are not continuously firing, it is clear that the AF is being sustained by some self-perpetuating mechanism other than the *focal atrial triggers.*
4a. If global activation mapping of the atria is performed during an episode of AF that was induced by *rapid atrial pacing*, multiple macro-reentrant circuits are the dominant electrophysiologic mechanism present in the atria.
4b. If global activation mapping of the atria is performed during an episode of AF that was induced by *focal atrial triggers*, multiple macro-reentrant circuits are the dominant electrophysiologic mechanism present in the atria.

To better appreciate the notion that AF is sustained by self-perpetuating macro-reentrant drivers, it is helpful to recall that the terms *atrial fibrillation* and *atrial macro-reentry* are different terms for the same event. The term *fibrillation* simply describes the *physical appearance* of the atria during the arrhythmia, and the term "macro-reentry" describes the *electrophysiologic events* that are occurring during the arrhythmia.

Regardless of our opinions, the question of exactly what sustains established AF can be answered definitively by simply placing multiple linear lesions in the atria during an episode of atrial macro-reentry and observing the results. Walter Garrey did this more than a century ago in his experimental studies, and we did it clinically more than 35 years ago with the Maze procedure. In both instances, multiple relatively widely spaced linear lesions in the atria completely abolished the AF. If the atrial macro-reentrant circuits had been only a passive response to continuously firing focal micro-reentrant circuits or small-diameter macro-reentrant circuits, the Maze procedure would still have been capable of terminating the atrial macro-reentry (AF), but postoperatively, the patients would have continued to experience supraventricular tachycardia because of the continued activity of the microscopic micro-reentrant foci (or small, focal macro-reentrant rotors) that would not have been eliminated or isolated by the Maze lesions. This simply did not happen in the patients who were operated on for persistent and long-standing persistent AF, which represented approximately 40% of the entire series.

Interestingly, approximately 10% of patients who underwent the Maze procedure for *paroxysmal* AF in our original series had occasional bouts (though, not continuous) of premature atrial beats after surgery. We understood that these bouts were caused by the spontaneous and intermittent activity of nonpulmonary vein triggers that were not isolated by the Maze procedure. We know that they were "nonpulmonary vein" triggers because the entire pulmonary vein cuff had been surgically separated from the left atrium during the Maze procedure, so they could not have been originating within that cuff. This clinical observation supports Haissaguerre and coworkers'[22] finding that approximately 10% of the triggers for paroxysmal AF are found outside the pulmonary vein region.[22] It also confirms that the AF triggers in these patients were not continuously firing and therefore could not have been responsible for sustaining AF even during finite episodes of paroxysmal AF lasting only a few days. These occasional random postoperative clusters of multiple premature atrial beats were almost certainly caused by the original *non-pulmonary vein triggers* because the common refrain in those patients months and even years after surgery was, *"I still feel the funny beats that I used to feel just before going into AF, but now I don't go into AF."* Clearly, they were feeling occasional bursts of activity from their non-pulmonary vein AF triggers that had not been isolated by the Maze procedure, but because macro-reentrant circuits could no longer form in the atria after the Maze procedure, these "funny beats" were not followed by AF. Few clinical observations are more supportive of Haissaguerre and coworkers'[22] demonstration that most episodes of paroxysmal AF are initiated by focal pulmonary vein triggers and of our notion that after being initiated, the AF episodes are sustained by self-perpetuating atrial macro-reentrant circuits, whether the episodes last hours, days, or years.

REFERENCES

1. Garrey WE. The nature of fibrillary contraction of the heart—its relation to tissue mass and form. *Am J Physiol.* 1914;33(3):397–414.
2. Mines GR. On circulating excitations in heart muscle and their possible relation to tachycardia and fibrillation. *Trans Roy Soc Can.* 1914;8:43–52.
3. Lewis T, Gilder MDD. XI. The human electrocardiogram: a preliminary investigation of young male adults, to form a basis for pathological study. *Philos Trans Royal Soc London.* 1912;202(292):351–376.
4. Moe GK. On the multiple wavelet hypothesis of atrial fibrillation. *Arch Int Pharmacodyn.* 1962;140:183–188.
5. Moe GK, Rheinboldt WC, Abildskov JA. A computer model of atrial fibrillation. *Am Heart J.* 1964;67:200–220.
6. Allessie MA, Bonker FI, Schopman FJ. Circus movement in rabbit atrial muscle as a mechanism of tachycardia. *Circ Res.* 1973;33(1):54–62.
7. Cox JL, Canavan TE, Schuessler RB, et al. The surgical treatment of atrial fibrillation: II. Intraoperative electrophysiologic mapping and description of the electrophysiologic basis of atrial flutter and atrial fibrillation. *J Thorac Cardiovasc Surg.* 1991;101:406–426.
8. Waldo A. The Moe model disproved: what next? AF Symposium 2022, Program Archive.
9. D'Agostino Jr HJ, Harada A, Eisenberg SB, Schuessler RB, Boineau JP, Cox JL. Surgical ablation of atrial fibrillation in a canine model of chronic mitral regurgitation. *Surg Forum.* 1986;XXXVII:302–303.

10. Kramer JB, Corr PB, Cox JL, Witkowski FX, Cain ME. Simultaneous computer mapping to facilitate intraoperative localization of accessory pathways in patients with Wolff-Parkinson-White syndrome. *Am J Cardiol.* 1985;56(10):571–576.
11. Schuessler RB, Grayson TM, Bromberg BI, Cox JL, Boineau JP. Cholinergically mediated tachyarrhythmias induced by a single extrastimulus in the isolated canine right atrium. *Circ Res.* 1992;71:1254–1267.
12. Byrd GD, Prasad SM, Ripplinger CM, et al. Importance of geometry and refractory period in sustaining atrial fibrillation: testing the critical mass hypothesis. *Circulation.* 2005;112(9):I-7-I-13.
13. Lee AM, Aziz A, Didesch J, Clark KL, Schuessler RB, Damiano Jr RJ. Importance of atrial surface area and refractory period in sustaining atrial fibrillation: testing the critical mass hypothesis. *J Thorac Cardiovasc Surg.* 2013;146(3):593–598.
14. Taussig HB. *Congenital Malformations of the Heart.* Harvard University Press; 1960.
15. Cox JL, Schuessler RB, D'Agostino Jr HJ, et al. The surgical treatment of atrial fibrillation: III. Development of a definitive surgical procedure. *J Thorac Cardiovasc Surg.* 1991;101:569–583.
16. Cox JL, Schuessler RB, Boineau JP. The surgical treatment of atrial fibrillation: I. Summary of the current concepts of the mechanisms of atrial flutter and atrial fibrillation. *J Thorac Cardiovasc Surg.* 1991;101:402–405.
17. D'Agostino Jr HJ, Harada A, Schuessler RB, Boineau JP, Cox JL. Global epicardial mapping of atrial fibrillation in a canine model of chronic mitral regurgitation. *Circulation.* 1987;76(Supp. IV):IV 165.
18. Canavan TE, Schuessler RB, Boineau JP, Corr PB, Cain ME, Cox JL. Simultaneous 156 point activation mapping during induced atrial fibrillation in patients with Wolff Parkinson White syndrome. *Circulation.* 1987;76(Supp. IV):IV 138.
19. Weber S, Ndrepepa G, Schneider M, et al. Characterization of onset mechanism and waveform analysis in patients with atrial fibrillation using a high-resolution noncontact mapping system. *J. Cardiovasc Electrophysiol.* 2003;14:176–181.
20. Ramanathan C, Jia P, Ghanem RN, Ryu K, Rudy Y. Activation and repolarization of the normal human heart under complete physiological conditions. *Proc Nat Acad Sci USA.* 2006;103: 6309–6314.
21. Wang Y, Cuculich PS, Woodard PK, Lindsay BD, Rudy Y. Focal atrial tachycardia after pulmonary vein isolation: noninvasive mapping with electrocardiographic imaging (ECGI). *Heart Rhythm.* 2007;4(8):1081–1084.
22. Haissaguerre M, Jais P, Shah DC, et al. Spontaneous initiation of atrial fibrillation by ectopic beats originating in the pulmonary veins. *N Eng J Med.* 1998;339(10):659–666.
23. Canavan TE, Schuessler RB, Boineau JP, Corr PB, Cain ME, Cox JL. Computerized global electrophysiological mapping of the atrium in patients with Wolff Parkinson White syndrome. *Ann Thorac Surg.* 1988;46:223–231.
24. Cox JL, Williams JM, Smith PK, Sabiston Jr DC. The surgical treatment of atrial fibrillation. In: Kulbertus HE, Olsson SB, Schlepper M, eds. *Atrial Fibrillation.* AB Hassle Publisher; 1982:321–333.
25. Brugada J, Mont L, Matas M, Navarro-Lopez F. Atrial fibrillation induced by atrioventricular nodal reentrant tachycardia. *Am J Cardiol.* 1997;79:681–682.
26. Wit AL, Boyden PA. Triggered activity and atrial fibrillation. *Heart Rhythm.* 2007;4:S517–S523.
27. Cox JL, McLaughlin VW, Flowers NC, Horan LG. The ischemic zone surrounding acute myocardial infarction. its morphology as detected by dehydrogenase staining. *Am Heart J.* 1968;76:650.
28. Cox JL, Daniel TM, Sabiston Jr DC, Boineau JP. De Synchronized activation in myocardial infarction: a re entry basis for ventricular arrhythmias. *Circulation.* 1969;40:III 63.
29. Boineau JP, Cox JL. Slow ventricular activation in acute myocardial infarction: a source of re entrant premature ventricular contractions. *Circulation.* 1973;48:702–713.
30. Saito T, Waki K, Becker A. Left atrial myocardial extension onto pulmonary veins in humans: anatomic observations relevant for atrial arrhythmias. *J Cardiovasc Elecrophysiol.* 2000;11(8):888–894.
31. Iwa T, Ichihashi T, Hashizume Y, Ishida K, Okada R. Successful surgical treatment of left atrial tachycardia. *Am Heart J.* 1985;109(1):160–162.
32. Sherlag BJ, Nakagawa H, Jackman WM, et al. Electrical stimulation to identify neural elements on the heart: their role in atrial fibrillation. *J Interventional Card Electrophysiol.* 2005;2005(Suppl 1):37–42.
33. Lemola K, Chartier D, Yeh YH, et al. Pulmonary vein region ablation in experimental vagal atrial fibrillation: role of pulmonary veins versus autonomic ganglia. *Circulation.* 2008;117(4):470–477.
34. Allessie MA. Atrial fibrillation-induced electrical remodeling in humans: what is the next step? *Cardiovasc Res.* 1999;44(1):10–12.
35. Prasad SM, Maniar HS, Camillo CJ, et al. The cox maze III procedure for atrial fibrillation: long-term efficacy in patients undergoing lone versus concomitant procedures. *J Thorac Cardiovasc Surg.* 2003;126:1822–1827.
36. Paponne C, Rosanio S, Oreto G, et al. Circumferential radiofrequency ablation of pulmonary vein ostia: a new anatomic approach for curing atrial fibrillation. *Circulation.* 2000;102:2619–2628.
37. Oral H, Knight BP, Tada H, et al. Pulmonary vein isolation for paroxysmal and persistent atrial fibrillation. *Circulation.* 2002;105:1077–1081.
38. Wolf RK. Minimally invasive surgical treatment of atrial fibrillation. *Sem Thorac Cardiovasc Surg.* 2007;19(4):311–318.
39. Cox JL. The central controversy surrounding the interventional-surgical treatment of atrial fibrillation. *J Thorac Cardiovasc Surg.* 2005;129(1):1–4.
40. Tilz RR, Rillig A, Thum AM, et al. Catheter ablation of long-standing persistent atrial fibrillation: 5-year outcomes of the Hamburg sequential ablation strategy. *J Am Coll Cardiol.* 2012;60(19):1921–1929.
41. Wu J, Estner H, Luik A, et al. Automatic 3D mapping of complex fractionated atrial electrograms (CFAE) in patients with paroxysmal and persistent atrial fibrillation. *J Cardiovasc Electrophysiol.* 2008;19(9):897–903.
42. Waranugraha Y, Rizal A, Setiaway D, Asis IJ. Additional complex fractionated atrial electrogram ablation does not improve the outcomes of non-paroxysmal atrial fibrillation: a systematic review and meta-analysis of randomized controlled trials. *Indian Heart J.* 2021;73(1):63–73.
43. Kottkamp H, Hindricks G. Catheter ablation of atrial flutter. *Thorac Cardiovasc Surg.* 1999;47(3):357–361.
44. Lindsay BD. Is pulmonary vein antrum isolation a critical determinant of recurrent arrhythmias after ablation of atrial fibrillation? *J Am Coll Cardiol.* 2007;50(9):875–876.
45. Cox JL. The first Maze procedure. *J Thorac Cardiovasc Surg.* 2011;141(5):1093–1097.

6

Intraoperative Mapping of Atrial Fibrillation

James L. Cox, Emilio Osorio-Jaramillo, Marek P. Ehrlich

CHAPTER OUTLINE

The development of surgical techniques for the treatment of patients with cardiac arrhythmias was paralleled by the development of intraoperative electrophysiologic mapping systems to determine precisely where to place the lesions of conduction block in a surgical procedure (i.e., to "guide" the surgical procedure). Specific surgical procedures to treat patients with Wolff-Parkinson-White syndrome,[1] elective His bundle ablation,[2] automatic left atrial tachycardias,[3] atrioventricular node reentry tachycardia,[4] automatic right atrial tachycardias,[5] ischemic ventricular tachcycardia,[6–8] and non-ischemic ventricular tachycardia[9] were all "map-guided" surgical procedures.

Because of this long and successful experience with map-guided arrhythmia surgery, when it was decided to develop a surgical procedure to treat atrial fibrillation (AF) in the 1980s, it was assumed that whatever surgical procedure we might develop would also have to be map guided. However, extensive experimental and clinical mapping of AF confirmed that it would be necessary to interrupt multiple macro-reentrant circuits that were fleeting in nature and constantly changing locations. Thus it was obvious that AF surgery could not be map-guided. Efforts were refocused on the development of a surgical procedure based on anatomy that could be performed the same way in all patients with AF. This new approach culminated in the Maze procedure.[10–12] Although intraoperative mapping was not used to guide the placement of lesions in the Maze procedure, we routinely mapped all patients who had AF surgery with a 156-channel computerized mapping system intraoperatively both before and after the Maze procedure. However, after a few dozen patients, it was apparent that the mapping was unnecessary, so we stopped performing intraoperative mapping. Even today, successful surgery for AF does not require intraoperative mapping.

The only two interventional procedures for the treatment of AF that have withstood the test of time over the past 40 years are pulmonary vein isolation (PVI) for paroxysmal AF[13] and the Maze procedure for all types of AF.[14–17] Both of these procedures are based on atrial anatomy, and neither of them requires electrophysiologic mapping to be successful. Nevertheless, sophisticated and expensive mapping systems are routinely used in all catheter ablation procedures for AF, though they are used primarily as a tool to confirm lesion integrity, not as a tool to guide the placement of catheter lesions in the atrium. Thus, the catheter ablation of AF is not actually "map-guided" because the procedures are all based on isolation of the pulmonary veins (PVI), which does not depend on AF mapping. In addition, the term "catheter ablation" itself is a misnomer because the objective of a PVI is not to ablate the AF but to isolate as many of its triggers as possible in hopes of decreasing the likelihood of having AF induced in the future.

Some interventional electrophysiologists do actually map AF during some catheter ablation procedures to locate and ablate extrapulmonary vein electrical and/or anatomic phenomena such as complex fragmented atrial electrogram spots, "rotors," and ganglionic plexi. Unfortunately, the identification and ablation of these abnormalities have not significantly improved the results of catheter ablation for AF.[18–20] Surgeons who treat AF also often use what is rather euphemistically called a "mapping system," but again, this system is used primarily to confirm lesion integrity by simple pacing techniques, not to guide the placement of lesions in the surgical procedure.

When computerized mapping was first developed, reconstruction of activation maps was unusually time-consuming and laborious. In addition, data could be recorded only from the specific sites where electrodes were located. This was a particular problem during the mapping of ventricular tachycardia (VT) because it often originated in the mid-myocardium of the ventricular septum. Therefore, with only endocardial and epicardial electrode arrays in place, activation mapping could not identify the true earliest activity ("site of origin") of such septal VT. As a result, "potential distribution mapping" (now called "voltage mapping") of the amplitude of unipolar or bipolar deflections was developed in hopes of determining the site of VT origination more accurately.[21] In addition, when three-dimensional (3D) mapping became available, 3D voltage maps of arrhythmias proved to be far easier to construct than were 3D activation maps. Few developments in all of cardiology compare with the monumental progress made in the development of arrhythmia mapping since that time.

Even though most surgeons are unfamiliar with preoperative or intraoperative mapping systems and techniques, it is important for them to understand some of the fundamentals of electrophysiologic mapping to optimally treat their patients with arrhythmia. A good starting point is to understand the difference between *activation mapping* and *voltage mapping*.

ACTIVATION MAPPING

Electrophysiologic maps based on the *sequence of electrical activation* of the heart are called "activation time maps," "sequential maps," "isochronous maps," or simply "activation maps." Activation maps record *dynamic* electrical activity, that is, the generation of an electrical impulse and its subsequent propagation as a wavefront (Fig. 6.1). Thus, activation maps are uniquely helpful in delineating the length and position of a line of conduction block. Even though a lesion is contiguous (has no "gaps") and is uniformly transmural, if it is positioned incorrectly, electrical activity will simply be rerouted around the lesion (Fig. 6.2). If the objective of an operation dependent on such a

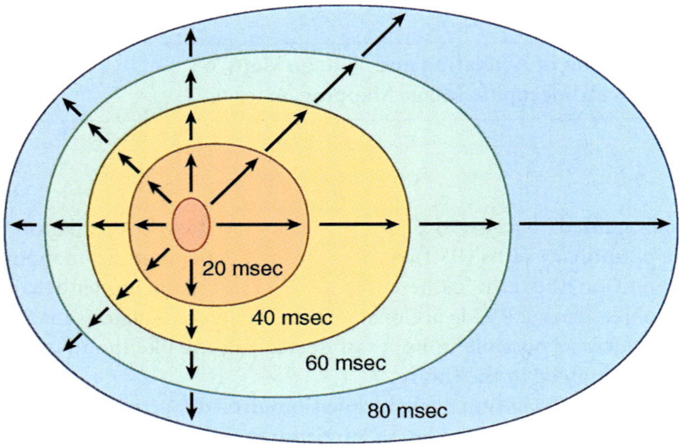

Fig. 6.1 Activation map. The *small red circle* represents the site of origin of an electrical impulse. The location of that impulse is designated every 20 ms as it propagates radially from the site of origin. These are *isochronous* lines (i.e., the tissue along each isochronous line is all activated at the same time in relation to the origin of the impulse). The tissue incorporated between successive 20-ms isochronous lines is color coded to show the sequential radial spread of the impulse away from its site of origin.

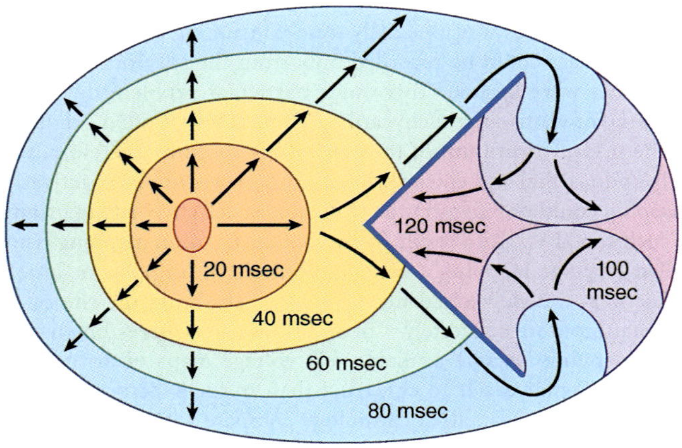

Fig. 6.2 Effect of an incomplete line of conduction block as seen on an activation map. Note that the line of conduction block *(heavy blue line)* has no "gaps," indicating that it is contiguous and uniformly transmural. This line of conduction block is not anchored on nonconductive tissue, so the wavefront is able to curl around both ends of the lesion. This disruption in the pattern of sequential tissue activation recorded on an activation map precisely identifies the location, shape, and length of the line of conduction block.

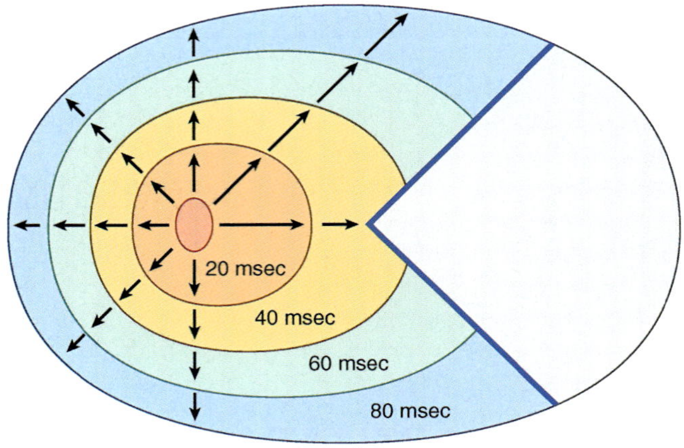

Fig. 6.3 Effect of a complete line of conduction block that is anchored at both ends to nonconductive tissue. Because the external extent of the tissue in this sketch is also nonconductive, the area beyond the line of conduction block is not activated and is therefore isolated from the rest of the atrium.

lesion is to isolate a portion of the atrium, say, the pulmonary veins, the procedure would fail. However, the ability to place such lesions in critical areas of the atrium is the basis of the Maze procedure because this is how one controls the direction of wavefront propagation postoperatively so that a sinus rhythm can activate both atria.

To attain complete isolation of a portion of the atrium with a lesion (Fig. 6.3), it must be anchored to nonconducting tissue such as a valve annulus or the orifice of a cardiac structure like the superior vena cava. Surgical isolation can also be accomplished by enclosing tissue entirely within the lesion itself, as is done with the "box lesion" in the Maze procedure that encircles all four pulmonary vein orifices and the intervening posterior left atrial wall. In either case, an activation map defines the precise length and location of lesions of conduction block and also of areas of the atrium that are completely isolated.

VOLTAGE MAPPING

Unlike activation maps in which *isochronous* lines are drawn at selected intervals of wavefront propagation, voltage maps are based on the amplitude of the local unipolar or bipolar complexes in which *isopotential* lines are drawn at selected amplitude intervals (Fig. 6.4). Even though a lesion is contiguous (has no "gaps") and is uniformly transmural, if it is positioned incorrectly, a voltage map can be quite misleading (Fig. 6.5). Because atrial activation continues beyond the incomplete atrial lesion, there are still local electrograms in these regions, and they have amplitudes that can be measured. The presence of local electrograms on both sides of the incomplete lesion means that there is no way to identify the precise location, shape, or length of that lesion. In fact, a previously placed contiguous, uniformly transmural atrial lesion may be entirely invisible on a voltage map if it is incomplete and does not isolate a portion of the atrium. Thus, it is important to recognize whether one is looking at an activation map or a voltage map, and it is especially important if one is trying to determine the integrity of a previously placed lesion of conduction block. Fortunately, when lesions of conduction block are placed in the correct position to completely isolate a region of the atrium, a voltage map is as valuable as an activation map (Fig. 6.6).

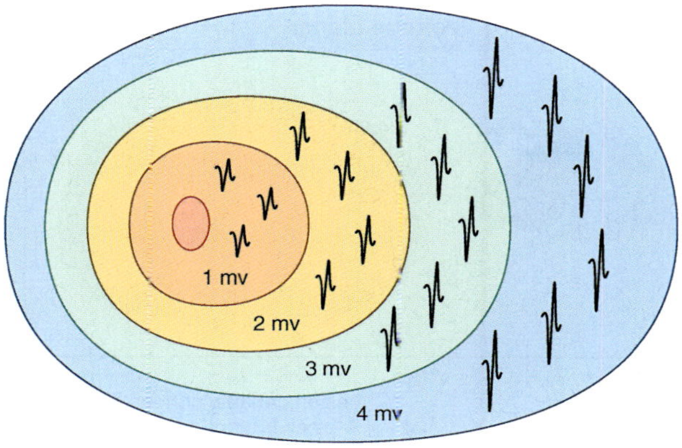

Fig. 6.4 Voltage maps represent the difference in local electrogram amplitudes as an impulse propagates away from its site of origin *(red circle)*. Propagation of the wavefront away from its site of origin is illustrated in this example by placing lines of the same voltage with every change of 1-mV amplitude in the electrograms. Thus these are *isopotential* lines (i.e., the tissue along each line all has the same local electrogram amplitude). The tissue incorporated between successive 1-mV isopotential lines is color coded and shows radial spreading of the impulse away from its site of origin.

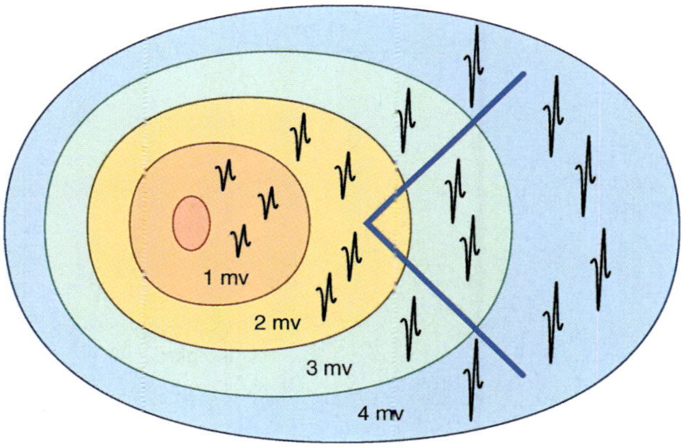

Fig. 6.5 A line of conduction block is placed in the same position on this voltage map as it was in the activation map shown in Fig. 6.2. In this case, however, electrical activation of the tissue beyond the line of block results in the ability to measure the amplitudes of persistent local electrograms on both sides of the block. This makes it virtually impossible to detect the location, shape, or length of an incomplete line of conduction block with voltage mapping.

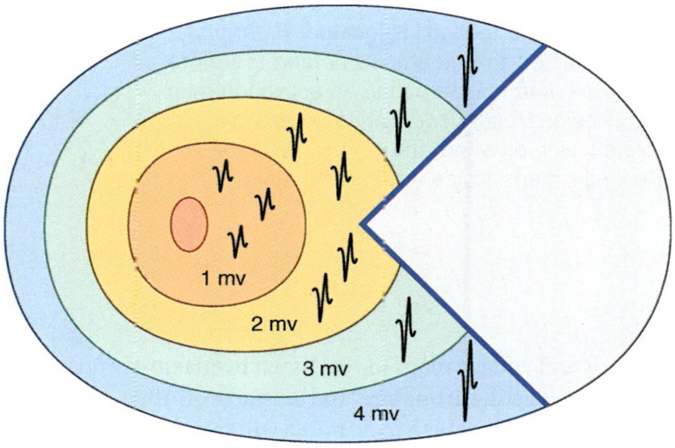

Fig. 6.6 Voltage map of a linear line of conduction block that is anchored to nonconductive tissue. This demonstrates that voltage maps are equally as effective as activation maps in documenting areas that are completely isolated.

COMPARISON OF ACTIVATION AND VOLTAGE MAPS

The fundamental difference between an activation map and a voltage map is analogous to the difference between a terrain map and topographical map. For example, a terrain map of an active volcano would show the volcano and the flow of lava from its peak. If a large structure were blocking the lava from flowing down the mountainside in a certain area, the lava would be forced to skirt around the edges of the wall to continue its flow to the bottom of the mountain (Fig. 6.7, *left upper panel*). On the contrary, a topographical map of that same active volcano would be unaffected by the presence of the large structure on the mountainside (Fig. 6.7, *right upper panel*).

As opposed to the clear identification of the position and length of a line of conduction block identified by activation maps (Fig. 6.7, *left middle panel*), the line of conduction block is completely invisible on a voltage map of the same area of atrium (Fig. 6.7, *right middle panel*). On the other hand, if the line of conduction block completely isolates a portion of the atrium, activation maps and voltage maps are of equal value in identifying the isolated segment (Fig. 6.7, *lower panels*).

These differences between activation maps and voltage maps are important in the evaluation of clinical failures. For example, in a patient who has previously undergone a successful PVI, a voltage map will delineate the isolated area because there is no electrical activity inside the isolated area, so there will be no local electrograms to measure (Fig. 6.8A). An activation map in this same patient would show the same isolation of the pulmonary veins. However, a PVI often fails because after having time to heal, the atrial lesions can develop a "gap" that allows electrical activity to enter the supposedly isolated area of atrial myocardium (Fig. 6.8B). In this situation, the deflection amplitudes of the local electrograms both inside and outside the supposedly isolated segment can be measured. This can render the previous PVI lesion completely invisible, and certainly the voltage map cannot determine the location of the "gap" (Fig. 6.8C). In this case, an activation map has to be performed to delineate the exact location of the PVI lesion and more important to localize the "gap" in that lesion that has caused the procedure to fail.

Another factor that leads to confusion is that activation maps and voltage maps look very similar in illustrations (Fig. 6.9). The only practical method for illustrating the sequence of propagation of an electrical impulse across the heart (activation map) is to designate "isochronous" regions by means of lines drawn through sites that activate at the same time and adding color coding to enhance the perception of wavefront propagation. Unfortunately, this is also the only practical method for illustrating changes in voltage across a given region of myocardium (voltage maps). The color schemes can be different for the maps, but voltage maps are still easily mistaken for activation maps, and vice versa. One of the advantages of activation mapping over voltage mapping is that atrial macro-reentrant circuits can be mapped and illustrated on activation maps (Fig. 6.9, *right upper panel*), but they are usually undetectable with voltage mapping.

ELECTROCARDIOGRAPHIC IMAGE MAPPING

As mentioned earlier, it was learned in the mid-1980s that it was impossible to "chase" the macro-reentrant circuits responsible for sustaining AF by first mapping them and then placing an incision across their path to ablate them. Not only were the mapping systems at the time incapable of providing global maps of AF in real time as they can today, but the macro-reentrant drivers also usually stayed in a given area of the atrium for only a few hundred milliseconds before moving elsewhere.

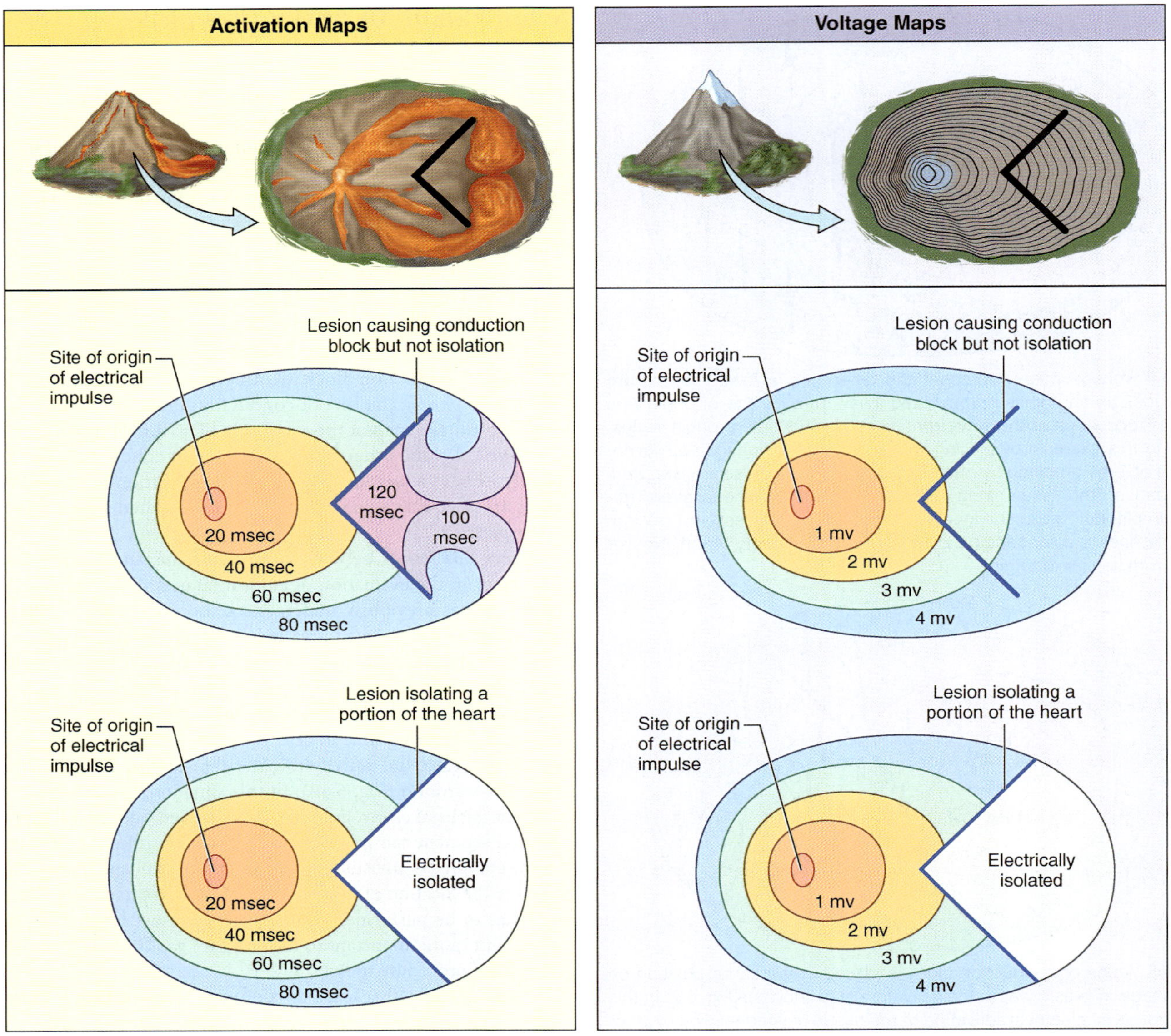

Fig. 6.7 Comparison of activation maps and voltage maps when mapping incomplete lines of conduction block and completely isolating lesions. The most critical difference is that voltage maps are inadequate for determining the precise location of incomplete lesions. The differences are essentially the same as the differences in terrain maps and topographical maps. *Left upper panel,* A terrain map of an active volcano with lava *(orange)* flowing down the mountainside. The flow of the lava is diverted by the presence of a large wall on the mountainside, and because of that diversion, we know precisely where the wall is located. *Right upper panel,* A topographic map is unaffected by the presence the large wall on the mountainside and therefore is of no value in determining the location or completeness of the wall. *Left middle panel,* An activation map shows the precise location of a lesion and identifies any gaps in the lesion. *Right middle panel,* A voltage map is incapable of accurately determining the location of an incomplete lesion or where the gaps in such a lesion are located. *Lower panels,* The ability of activation maps and voltage maps to identify completely isolated areas are equivalent.

It was for this reason that we were forced to take a "fall-back" position in our surgical approach to AF by focusing on the development of a procedure that would *prevent macro-reentry from developing anywhere in either atrium*, reasoning that if atrial macro-reentry could not occur, the atria could not fibrillate. Although mapping capabilities have dramatically improved since that time, the electrophysiology of AF has not changed. Thus, even with the current ability to construct accurate activation maps and voltage maps in real time, the macro-reentrant drivers of AF are still fleeting in nature and unstable in their location. This raises the question of whether or not it will ever be possible to guide an interventional procedure for persistent AF even using the real-time, 3D, anatomically accurate maps that are available today.

Many authorities continue to use intraprocedure mapping to guide the placement of lesions in some patients with AF, but this

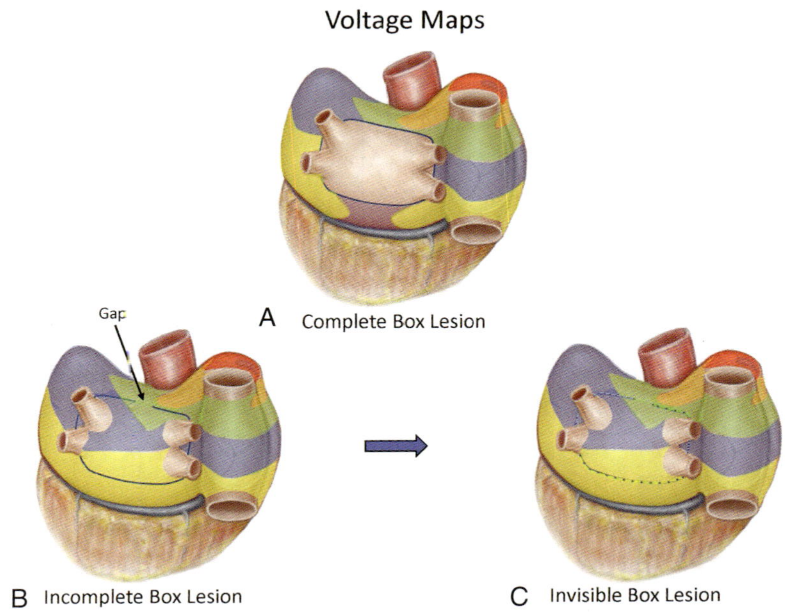

Fig. 6.8 The inability of voltage maps to accurately identify the location, shape, and length of incomplete lines of conduction block is most important when testing lesion integrity in patients who have had a previous pulmonary vein isolation (PVI) or box lesion that encompasses all four pulmonary veins and the posterior left atrial wall. For example, after a complete box lesion (A), both activation maps and voltage maps can document the isolation of the pulmonary veins and posterior left atrial wall. However, if the box lesion is incomplete (B), a voltage map will show the presence of electrical activity in the supposedly isolated area. Because the voltage inside the box lesion is unchanged by the incomplete lesion, this map is indistinguishable from a map in which no lesion at all was performed. Essentially, this makes the box lesion completely invisible (C). In such instances, it is necessary to perform an activation map to determine the location of the gap in the box lesion.

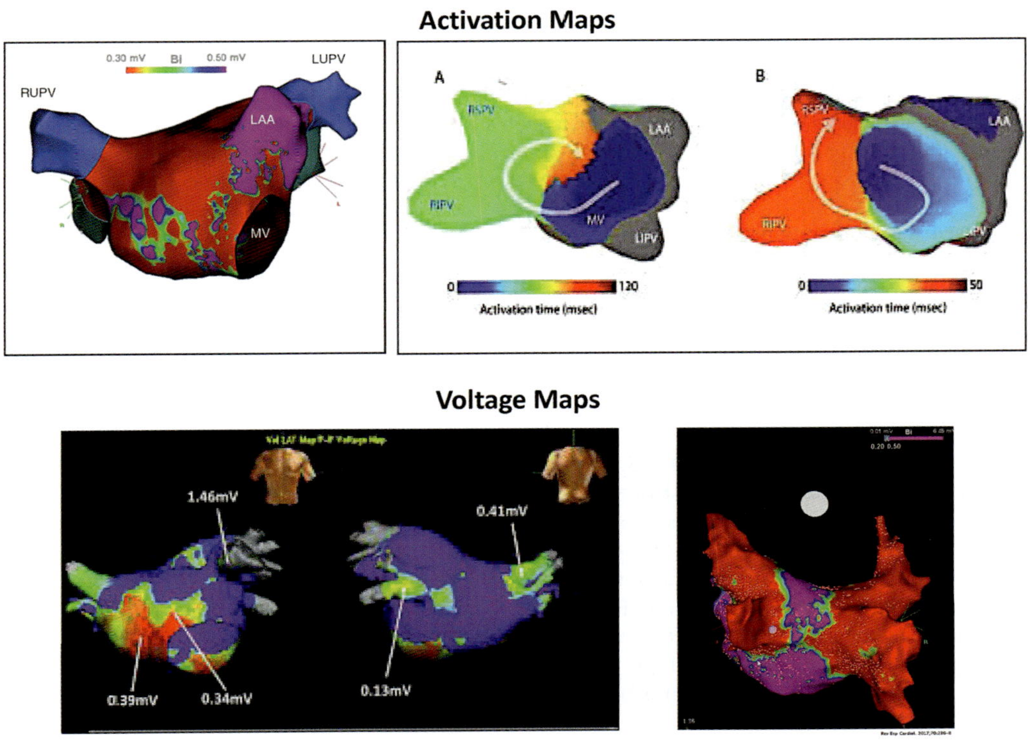

Fig. 6.9 Because of the limitations in how electrophysiologic data can be illustrated for visualization and study, activation maps *(upper panels)* and voltage maps *(lower panels)* can look very similar, though they contain different information. One advantage of activation maps over voltage maps is that the macro-reentrant circuits that drive atrial fibrillation can be detected by isochronous activation mapping *(right upper panel)* but not by isopotential voltage mapping.

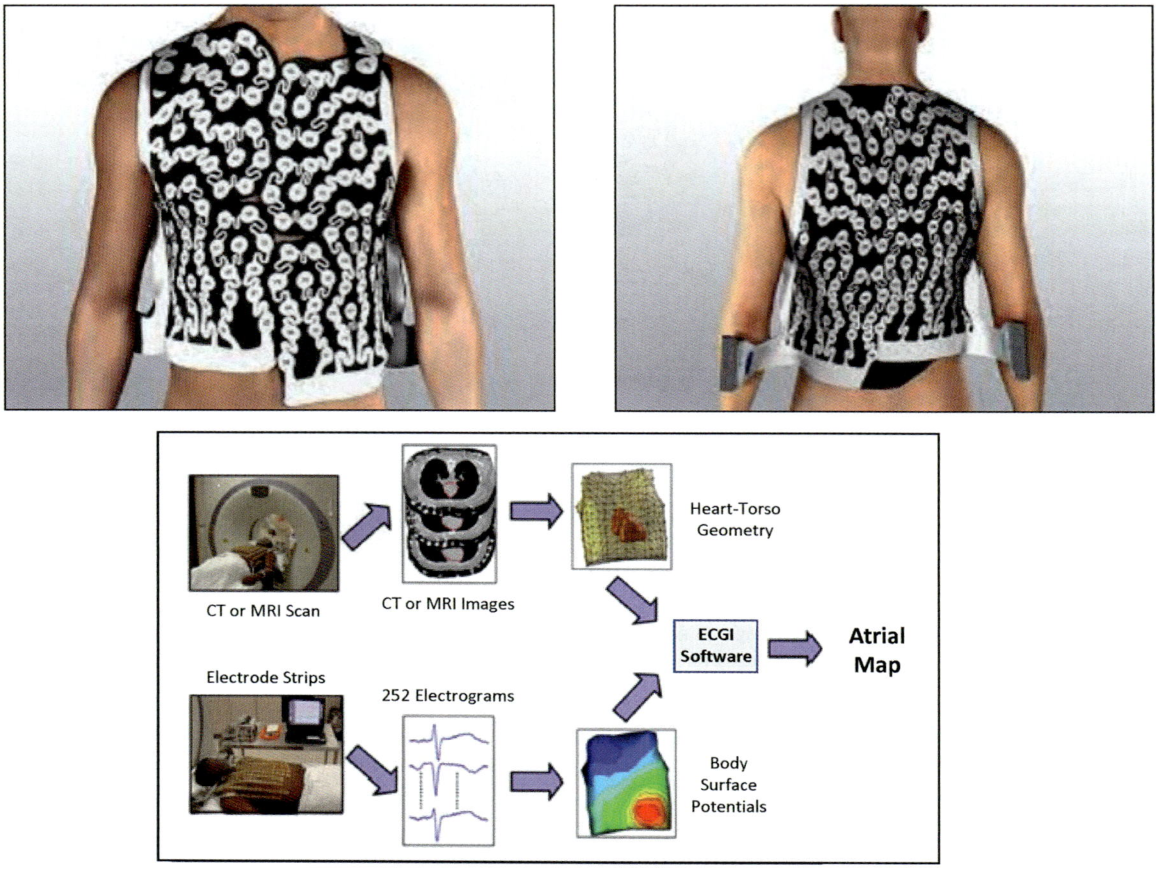

Fig. 6.10 *Upper panels,* The CardioInsight vest containing 252 electrodes for (ECGI) mapping body-surface mapping. *Lower panel,* Body-surface potentials are recorded from the electrodes imbedded in the vest and the heart-torso geometry is obtained from the computed tomography (CT) or magnetic resonance imaging (MRI). Mathematical algorithms are used to reconstruct epicardial potentials and unipolar electrograms on the heart's surface. (Reproduced from Osorio-Jaramillo E, Cox JL, Klenk S, et al. Dynamic electrophysiological mechanism in patients with long-standing persistent atrial fibrillation. *Front Cardiovasc Med.* 2022;9:1–13.)

approach has not improved the interventional results significantly. Their failures are not because of inadequate maps or inadequate tools for ablation, but rather they are attributable to the underlying electrophysiologic characteristics of AF. Thus, one must be skeptical when reports appear of new and improved interventional procedures that are "tailored" to each patient based on the intraprocedure mapping of the patient. Although the ability to tailor catheter ablation and surgical procedures for individual patients is a laudable goal, such tailored procedures have not improved the treatment of patients with late persistent and long-standing persistent AF. The use of AF maps to guide catheter or surgical ablation assumes that the lesions that are necessary to ablate AF will be the same on one day as another. In other words, this approach is based on the assumption that the drivers of AF are stable and do not change locations over time. That is an invalid assumption. The only way to prove or disprove the validity of that assumption is to map AF in the same patient multiple times to establish whether the electrophysiology specific to that patient's AF stays the same or changes over time.

Sequential atrial mapping at different times in the same patient is not feasible with endocardial catheters because they are too invasive for such a clinical experiment. However, that problem was overcome with the introduction of electrocardiographic image (ECGI) mapping by Rudy and colleagues.[22–24] ECGI mapping is performed using an array of multiple electrodes incorporated into a 252-electrode vest that holds the electrodes firmly against the body surface (Fig. 6.10, *upper panels*). With the vest in place, a computed tomography or magnetic resonance imaging scan of the torso is performed so that cardiac anatomy can be reconstructed in three dimensions (Fig. 6.10, *lower panel*). The body-surface potentials are recorded either immediately before or after the scan. A special software program then reconstructs cardiac surface activation maps that are anatomically accurate (Fig. 6.11) as well as voltage maps and repolarization maps. This mapping technique is completely noninvasive and as a result, it provides the opportunity to map patients with AF sequentially without any intervention between the two mappings. This ability to map AF sequentially in the same patient allows us to determine whether the small drivers ("rotors") that sometimes sustain AF are fixed in their positions or change locations over time. If they remain fixed, then electrophysiologic mapping would be capable of guiding catheter ablation and surgical procedures for the treatment of patients with AF. However, if the drivers do not remain in the same positions with time and the pattern of a given patient's AF changes with time, then trying to ablate AF on the basis of real-time mapping would be futile.

A recent study reported on 10 patients who underwent two separate body-surface mappings of their long-standing persistent AF

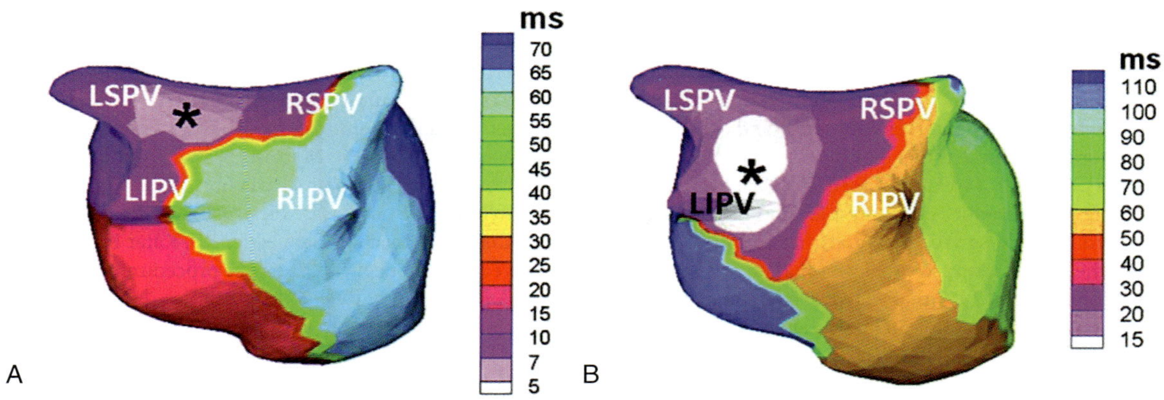

Fig. 6.11 A posterior view of an electrocardiographic image map of the atria. Note the focal trigger near the orifice of the left pulmonary veins *(asterisk)* in this patient with paroxysmal atrial fibrillation that gives rise to radial spread of the wavefront. *LIPV,* Left inferior pulmonary vein; *LSPV,* left superior pulmonary vein; *RIPV,* right inferior pulmonary vein; *RSPV,* right superior pulmonary vein. (Reproduced from Osorio-Jaramillo E, Cox JL, Klenk S, et al. Dynamic electrophysiological mechanism in patients with long-standing persistent atrial fibrillation. *Front Cardiovasc Med.* 2022;9:1–13.)

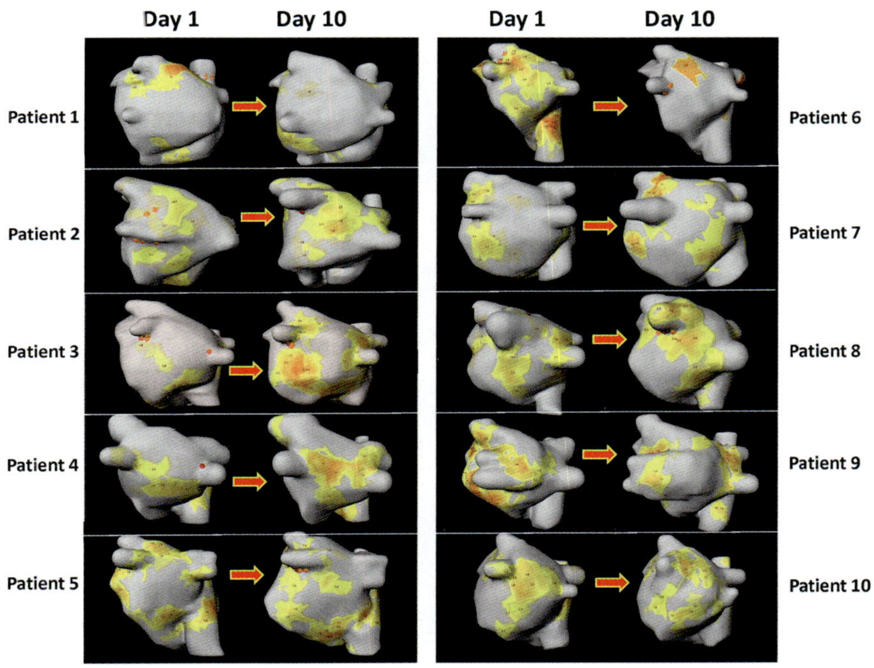

Fig. 6.12 Posteroanterior (PA) views of electrocardiographic image maps showing the distribution of focal and rotor activity of 10 patients with long-standing persistent atrial fibrillation (AF) who were mapped on day 1 and again on day 10. Note the change in location of the AF drivers between the sequential mapping of AF in the same patient on different days. If focal ablation had been based on the intraoperative map on day 1, the AF drivers would simply be located elsewhere in the atria by day 10. This is the primary reason that it is so difficult to "tailor" ablation procedures for individual patients with persistent AF using intraoperative maps to guide the placement of the lesions. (Reproduced from Osorio-Jaramillo E, Cox JL, Klenk S, et al. Dynamic electrophysiological mechanism in patients with long-standing persistent atrial fibrillation. *Front Cardiovasc Med.* 2022;9:1–13.)

with a median time interval of approximately 10 days.[25] The initial ECGI body-surface map in each of the 10 patients showed that AF "rotors" (i.e., the drivers that can sustain the AF) were more numerous in the left atrium, with approximately 30% being located in the right. The second ECGI body-surface map in patients 10 or 11 days later showed that although the number of rotors in the left atrium and right atrium had not changed, *the location of those rotors had changed to different locations in every patient* (Fig. 6.12). This means that if each patient had received ablative lesions based on the original maps ("map guided"), all of them would have had persistent AF drivers elsewhere in the atria several days later. These findings argue strongly against the use of intraprocedure maps to guide the placement of ablative lesions for the treatment of long-standing persistent AF.

In summary, ECGI mapping is a useful tool for studying the dynamic characteristics of AF by virtue of its non invasiveness. The ability to construct activation maps and voltage maps of AF at different time intervals in the same patient has provided new information and a better understanding of why some AF interventions work and some do not. An interesting historical anecdote is that on my first day of work in John Boineau's laboratory on July 1, 1969, Jack Kasell (see Chapter 1, Fig. 1.9) was lying on a table with a multielectrode vest around his upper torso. Boineau was recording body-surface potentials from him in hopes of being able to map the heart less invasively. However, there were problems with body-surface mapping in 1969 that were not overcome until Rudy and associates were able to do so some 30 to 40 years later.

REFERENCES

1. Cobb FR, Sealy WC, Boineau JP, Wagner GS, Wallace AG. Successful surgical interruption of the bundle of Kent in a patient with Wolff-Parkinson-White syndrome. *Circulation.* 1968;38:1018–1029.
2. Harrison L, Gallagher JJ, Kasell J, et al. Cryosurgical ablation of the A-V node-His bundle: a new method for producing A-V block. *Circulation.* 1977;55(3):463–470.
3. Williams JM, Ungerleider RM, Lofland GK, Cox JL. Left Atrial isolation: new technique for the treatment of supraventricular arrhythmias. *J Thorac Cardiovasc Surg.* 1980;80:373.
4. Cox JL, Ferguson Jr TB, Lindsay BD, Cain ME. Peri-nodal cryosurgery for AV node reentry tachycardia in 23 patients. *J Thorac Cardiovasc Surg.* 1990;99:440–450.
5. Harada A, D'Agostino Jr HJ, Boineau JP, Cox JL. Right atrial isolation: a new surgical treatment for supraventricular tachycardia. I. Surgical technique and electrophysiologic effects. *J Thorac Cardiovasc Surg.* 1988;95:643650.
6. Guiraudon G, Fontaine G, Frank R, Escande G, Etievent P, Cabrol C. Encircling endocardial ventriculotomy: a new surgical treatment for life-threatening ventricular tachycardias resistant to medical treatment following myocardial infarction. *Ann Thorac Surg.* 1978;26:438–444.
7. Josephson ME, Harken AH, Horowitz LN. Endocardial excision: a new surgical technique for the treatment of recurrent ventricular tachycardia. *Circulation.* 1979;60:1430–1439.
8. Boineau JP, Cox JL. Rationale for a direct surgical approach to control ventricular arrhythmias. *Am J Cardiol.* 1982;49:381.
9. Cox JL, Bardy GH, Damiano RJ, et al. Right ventricular isolation procedures for nonischemic ventricular tachycardia. *J Thorac Cardiovasc Surg.* 1985;90:212.
10. Cox JL, Canavan TE, Schuessler RB, et al. The surgical treatment of atrial fibrillation: II. Intraoperative electrophysiologic mapping and description of the electrophysiologic basis of atrial flutter and atrial fibrillation. *J Thorac Cardiovasc Surg.* 1991;101:406–426.
11. Cox JL, Schuessler RB, D'Agostino Jr HJ, et al. The surgical treatment of atrial fibrillation: III. Development of a definitive surgical procedure. *J Thorac Cardiovasc Surg.* 1991;101:569–583.
12. Cox JL. The surgical treatment of atrial fibrillation: IV. Surgical technique. *J Thorac Cardiovasc Surg.* 1991;101:584–592.
13. Medi C, Sparks PB, Morton JB, et al. Pulmonary vein antral isolation for paroxysmal aria fibrillation: results from long-term follow-up. *J Cardiovasc Electrophysiol.* 2011;22(2):37–141.
14. Cox JL, Boineau JP, Schuessler RB, Kater KM, Lappas DG. Five-year experience with the maze procedure for atrial fibrillation. *Ann Thor Surg.* 1994;56:814–824.
15. Prasad SM, Maniar HS, Camillo CJ, et al. The cox maze III procedure for atrial fibrillation: long-term efficacy in patients undergoing lone versus concomitant procedures. *J Thorac Cardiovasc Surg.* 2003;126(6):1822–1828.
16. Ad N, Holmes SD, Friehling T. Minimally invasive stand-alone cox maze procedure for persistent and long-standing persistent atrial fibrillation. *Circ Arrhythm Electrophysiol.* 2017;96(3):792–799.
17. Ad N, Holmes SD, Rongione AJ, et al. The long-term safety and efficacy of concomitant cox maze procedure for atrial fibrillation in patients without mitral valve disease. *J Thorac Cardiovasc Surg.* 2019;157(4):1505–1514.
18. Verma A, Jiang C-Y, Betts TR, et al. Approaches to catheter ablation for persistent atrial fibrillation. *N Engl J Med.* 2015;372(19):1812–1822.
19. Doshi RN. Highlights from heart rhythm 2019: Atrial fibrillation. *J Innov Card Rhythm Manag.* 2019;10(8):3793–3795.
20. Driessen AH, Berger WR, Krul SP, et al. Ganglionic plexus ablation in advanced atrial fibrillation: the AFACT study. *J Am Coll Cardiol.* 2016;68(11):1155–1165.
21. Harada A, D'Agostino Jr HJ, Schuessler RB, Boineau JP, Cox JL. Potential distribution mapping. New method for precise localization of intramural septal origin of ventricular tachycardia. *Circulation.* 1988;78(5):III137–147.
22. Oster HS, Taccardi B, Lux RL, Ershler PR, Rudy Y. Noninvasive electrocardiographic imaging: reconstruction of epicardial potentials, electrograms, and isochrones and localization of single and multiple electrocardiac events. *Circulation.* 1997;96:1012–1024.
23. Cuculich PS, Wang Y, Lindsay BD, et al. Noninvasive ECG imaging (ECGI): mapping the arrhythmic substrate of the human heart. *Int J Cardiol.* 2017;237:13–14.
24. Rudy Y. Noninvasive ECG imaging (ECGI): mapping the arrhythmic substrate of the human heart. *Int J Cardiol.* 2017;237:13–14.
25. Osorio-Jaramillo E, Cox JL, Klenk S, et al. Dynamic electrophysiological mechanism in patients with long-standing persistent atrial fibrillation. *Front Cardiovasc Med.* 2022;9:1–13.

7

The Basics of Myocardial Strain and Its Relationship to Atrial Fibrillation

Olga N. Kislitsina

CHAPTER OUTLINE

Evaluating myocardial contractile function by echocardiography has traditionally centered on volume-based assessments such as ejection fraction and regional evaluations of wall motion and visual estimation of regional thickening. However, these conventional methods present challenges related to reproducibility, standardization, and a high sensitivity to loading conditions. These limitations have spurred interest in more objective and reproducible techniques for assessing myocardial contractile function, leading to the development of deformation imaging techniques, including myocardial strain.[1] Speckle-tracking echocardiography (STE) has emerged as a valuable tool in the evaluation of myocardial strain, particularly longitudinal strain. This technique uses ultrasound to generate interference, reflection, and scattering as the ultrasound beam passes through myocardial tissue, creating acoustic markers called "speckles" on a standard B-mode echocardiographic image (Fig. 7.1).[2] Regional myocardial function can be assessed by tracking the movement of these speckles throughout the cardiac cycle.[3]

An organ's gross and/or histologic structure dictates its function. In the heart, differences in cavitary pressure between the pulmonary and systemic circulations drive several structural distinctions between the ventricles. The left ventricle (LV), with its thick walls and conical shape, propels blood into the high-pressure systemic circulation. In contrast, the right ventricle (RV), characterized by thin walls and a crescent shape, directs blood into the low-resistance pulmonary circulation. Despite the dynamic nature of the circulation, the RV is adept at maintaining low pressure, even under conditions of varying volume. At both the cellular and tissue levels, the ventricles adapt to meet the physiological demands of the entire body, continuing to develop into adulthood to fulfill the heart's function.[4] The myocardial architecture of the ventricles supports these distinct roles. In the RV, the majority of muscle fibers are transverse fibers with a smaller proportion of subendocardial longitudinal fibers. The LV, on the other hand, comprises endocardial and epicardial fibers arranged in a helical structure with circumferential fibers located at the mid-wall creating a more complex myocardial architecture.[5–7] The structural organization of myocardial muscle fibers in the ventricles and atria underscores the heart's mechanical efficiency (Fig. 7.2). Each myocardial bundle spirals around the heart chambers in a helical arrangement, enabling coordinated contraction and relaxation. This intricate fiber architecture highlights the heart's evolutionary optimization for mechanical efficiency and forms the foundation for advanced imaging and therapeutic strategies. Insights into myocardial fiber orientation are critical for interpreting strain imaging and identifying pathologies such as ischemia, cardiomyopathies, and arrhythmias. Given these distinct structural differences and functional roles, STE offers a noninvasive method for assessing the unique strain patterns of both ventricles.

The right atrium (RA) and left atrium (LA) also exhibit distinct myocardial functions. Emerging evidence suggests that the LA serves a far more dynamic role than simply acting as a conduit for left ventricular filling. Embryologically, most of the left atrial myocardium evolves from the primitive pulmonary vein (PV), and the RA is formed from the primitive RA and the sinus venosus that contributes to their smooth-walled endocardium.[8,9] This structural development makes both the LA and RA more susceptible to volume overloading due to mitral regurgitation (MR) or tricuspid regurgitation (TR), respectively, because of the thinner myocardial fibers oriented primarily in the longitudinal direction.[10,11] In addition, these thinner fibers allow the aria to expand more easily when exposed to increased volume stress. Echocardiographically, the strain patterns of the LA and RA differ from those of the ventricles. Whereas the LV and RV exhibit longitudinal, circumferential, and radial strain, the atria show primarily longitudinal strain because of their simpler myocardial structure. These differences in strain patterns reflect the embryologic and structural distinctions between the chambers and their corresponding roles in cardiac physiology (see Fig. 7.2C).

Strain imaging provides a comprehensive, noninvasive tool for assessing the unique functional roles of the atria and ventricles, offering crucial insights into both normal and pathological myocardial mechanics. This advanced imaging modality is particularly valuable in detecting subtle, early changes in myocardial function that may not yet manifest in traditional measures such as ejection fraction or atrial volumes.[12] By

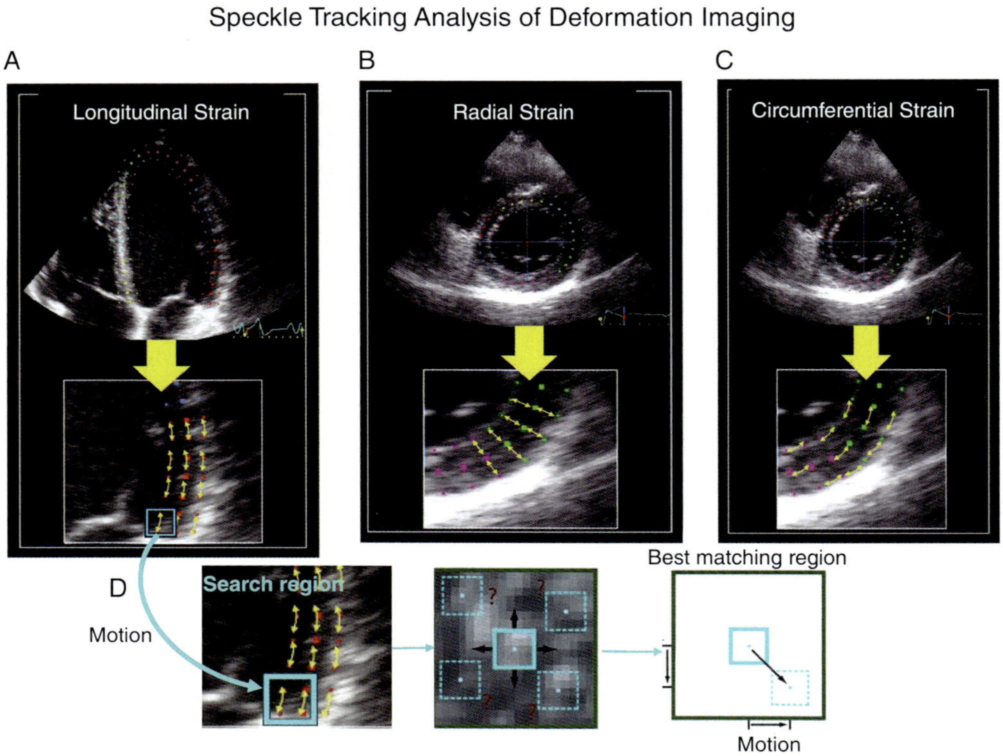

Fig. 7.1 The key components of speckle-tracking analysis used to assess myocardial deformation. (A) to (C) The three principal directions of myocardial strain in which a standard echocardiogram of the left ventricle (LV) shows acoustic "speckles" that result from the interaction between the ultrasound beam and myocardial tissue. These speckles are the foundation of strain calculation. (A) Longitudinal strain, tracking speckle movement in the long axis of the LV. (B) Radial strain, showing myocardial thickening (inward motion) during ventricular systole. (C) Circumferential strain, representing myocardial shortening around the circumference of the LV. (D) Depiction of the process of "block matching," an important part of the speckle-tracking technique in which the speckle pattern within a region of interest is identified in one frame and tracked across successive frames. The search regions *(dotted blocks)* are analyzed to find the optimal matching region. The displacement of the matching block determines tissue motion. This method, repeated across multiple regions of interest, allows estimation of regional myocardial deformation throughout the cardiac cycle. (Modified and reproduced from Badano LP, Visentin S, Palermo C, et al. Echocardiographic techniques of deformation imaging in the evaluation of maternal cardiovascular system in patients with complicated pregnancies. *Biomed Res Int*. 2017;1:1–10.)

identifying these early changes, strain imaging plays a pivotal role in diagnosing arrhythmias such as atrial fibrillation (AF) at a stage when structural or functional alterations in the atrial myocardium are just beginning to develop.[13] For example, reduced atrial strain can indicate impaired atrial compliance and/or contractile function, which often precede the onset of AF.[14,15] Similarly, strain imaging can detect early ventricular abnormalities, including regional strain impairments, that may signal ischemia, cardiomyopathy, or even subclinical fibrosis. These capabilities make strain imaging an indispensable tool in modern cardiology and cardiac surgery, enabling earlier interventions that can improve patient outcomes and prevent the progression of disease.

LEFT VENTRICULAR STRAIN

Historically, the assessment of left ventricular systolic function in AF has been challenging because of beat-to-beat variations. However, research has demonstrated that using the index beat to measure left ventricular global longitudinal strain (LV-GLS) in patients with AF is as accurate as averaging multiple cardiac cycles. Thus LV-GLS derived from the index beat serves as a definitive parameter for evaluating systolic function, even in patients with an irregular rhythm caused by AF.[16,17] Beyond its role in defining heart failure at earlier stages, LV-GLS also has significant predictive value in identifying patients at risk of developing AF.[16] Studies suggest that impaired LV-GLS may reflect subtle myocardial changes such as fibrosis or remodeling, which are precursors to the onset or progression of AF.[18,19] Moreover, a reduction in the LV-GLS in AF patients with preserved left ventricular ejection fractions (LVEF) often indicates underlying subclinical dysfunction, emphasizing the utility of LV-GLS as a sensitive biomarker.[20]

During ventricular systole, the ventricular myocardium shortens longitudinally and circumferentially while thickening radially. These changes reverse during diastole. As mentioned, strain measures the percentage change in myocardial fiber length from diastole to systole and is expressed as a negative percentage.[21,22] Specifically, longitudinal strain quantifies the shortening of myocardial fibers along the long axis of the heart. It is calculated using the following formula:

$$\text{Strain} = [(L_1 - L_0)/L_0] \times 100$$

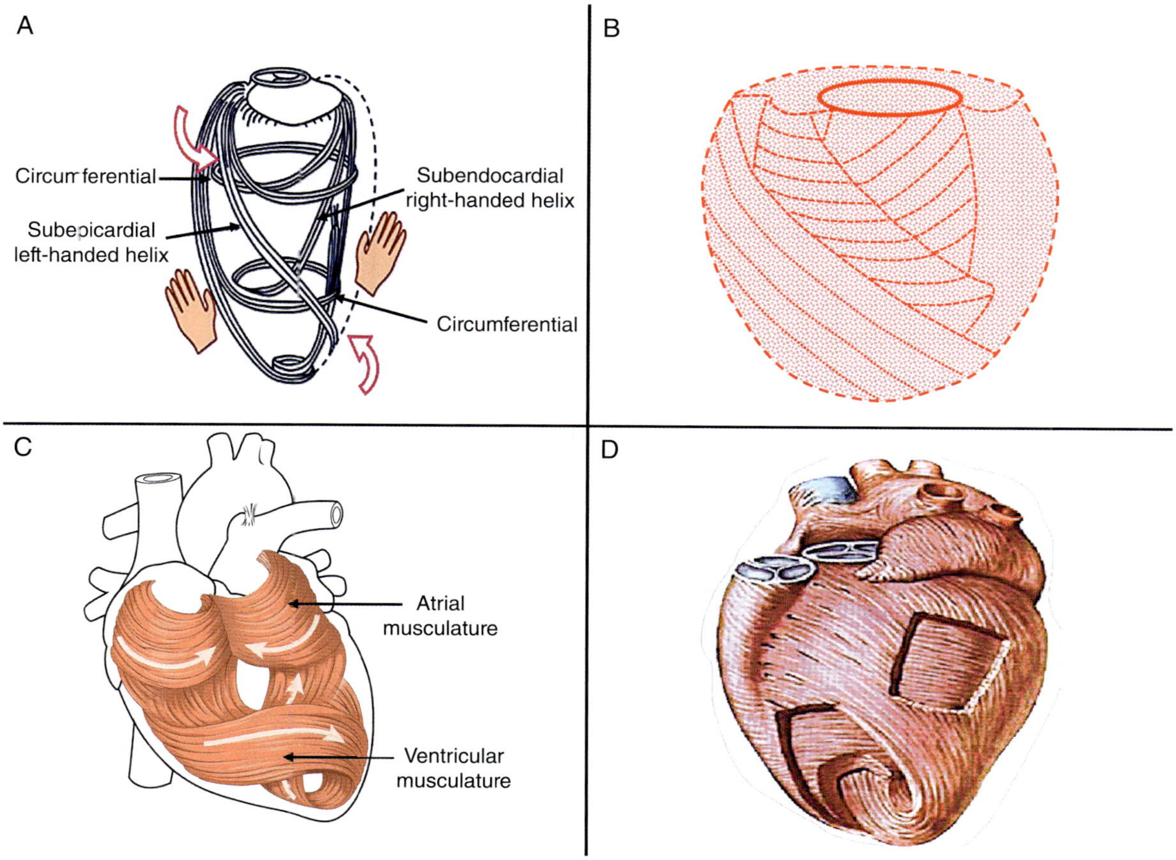

Fig. 7.2 (A) **Helical fiber arrangement.** The heart's muscle fibers are organized in a double-helical structure that facilitates the coordinated rotation of the base and apex during systole, optimizing blood ejection and diastolic filling. Subepicardial fibers adopt a left-handed spiral, and subendocardial fibers form a right-handed spiral. This arrangement creates a chiral fiber system that enables twisting (systole) and untwisting (diastole) motions, enhancing torsional mechanics. Circumferential fibers in the mid-myocardial layer contribute to radial thickening and support efficient ventricular pumping. (Reproduced from Nakatani S. Left ventricular rotation and twist: why should we learn? *J Cardiovasc Ultrasound.* 2011;19(1):1–6.) (B) **Anatomic fiber structure.** Anatomically, the myocardial fibers spiral continuously from the apex to the base. This configuration ensures uniform contraction, generating torsion for effective ejection of blood into the aorta and pulmonary artery. The twisting motion also optimizes diastolic filling. (C) **Atrial muscle fibers.** Atrial muscle fibers also exhibit a helical arrangement, supporting atrial contraction and reservoir functions. This structure plays a critical role in atrial efficiency, particularly in the context of arrhythmias such as atrial fibrillation. (Reproduced from Opdahl A, Helle-Valle T, Skulstad H, Smiseth OA. Strain, strain rate, torsion, and twist: echocardiographic evaluation. *Curr Cardiol Rep.* 2015;17(3):568.) (D) **Fiber interaction and functional implications.** The complex organization of fibers supports torsional mechanics, allowing for coordinated clockwise rotation of the base of the heart and counterclockwise rotation of the apex during systole. This interaction ensures energy-efficient contractions and optimal blood ejection.

in which L_0 is the diastolic (resting) fiber length and L_1 is the systolic (shortened) fiber length. For example, if the myocardial fibers shorten from 2 cm at end-diastole to 1.6 cm at end-systole, the strain value would be

$$\text{Strain} = [(1.6\ \text{cm} - 2\ \text{cm})/2\ \text{cm}] \times 100 = -20\%$$

This formula highlights the relationship between fiber shortening and myocardial performance, with negative values reflecting contraction. Longitudinal and circumferential strain values are typically negative because the fibers shorten during systole, but radial thickening produces positive strain values caused by fiber expansion.[23,24] For example, a 20% shortening corresponds to a strain value of minus 20% (−20%). Importantly, more negative strain values indicate better myocardial contraction and function (Fig. 7.3).

Myocardial Fiber Orientation and Mechanics

Understanding myocardial fiber orientation is fundamental to interpreting strain. As mentioned, subepicardial fiber contraction rotates the LV base clockwise and the apex counterclockwise, and subendocardial contraction produces the opposite effect.[5,21,25] This interplay results in torsion, a twisting motion that enhances ventricular ejection during systole and facilitates diastolic filling (Figs. 7.2A, 7.4, and 7.5). The torsional mechanics are critical for efficient cardiac performance, with subepicardial fibers dominating because of their larger radius of rotation.[25] Clinically, evaluating the balance between subepicardial and subendocardial function is essential for diagnosing and managing conditions such as myocardial ischemia, heart failure, and valvular diseases.

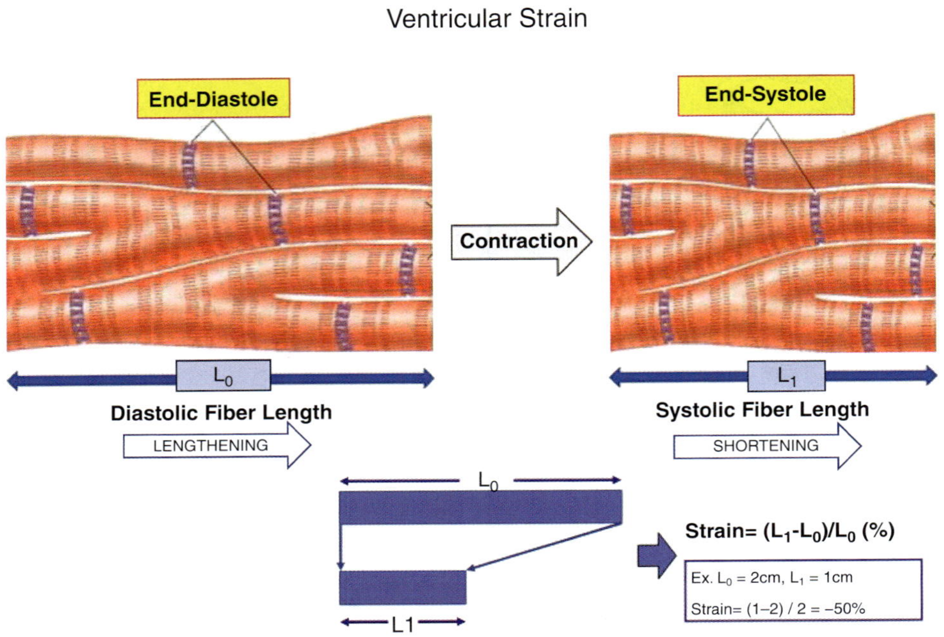

Fig. 7.3 The term "strain" fundamentally means "deformation." In the context of ventricular function, it provides a quantitative measure of how much the myocardial fibers stretch or contract during the cardiac cycle. Ventricular strain is defined as the percentage change in myocardial fiber length between the end-diastole (resting phase) and end-systole (contractile phase). *Left upper panel,* The state of myocardial fibers at their longest, corresponding to the heart's relaxation phase or end-diastole. *Right upper panel,* The state of myocardial fibers after shortening, corresponding to the heart's contraction phase or ventricular systole *Lower panel,* Strain is calculated using a formula in which L_0 represents the diastolic fiber length, and L_1 represents the systolic fiber length. Because the fibers shorten during contraction, L_1 is less than L_0, making strain a *negative percentage,* which reflects the reduction in fiber length during ventricular systole.

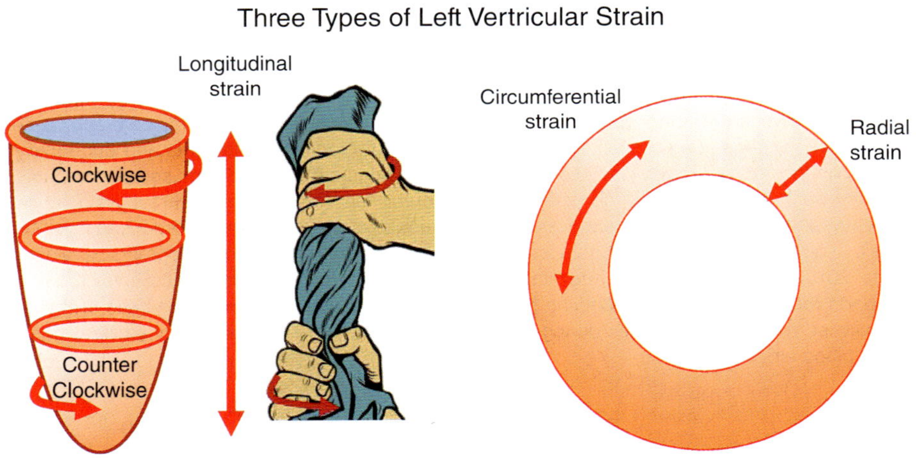

Fig. 7.4 *Left panel,* Left ventricular longitudinal strain represents the shortening of the long axis of the left ventricle (LV) during systole. This strain reflects the downward movement of the base toward the apex during contraction. In addition to longitudinal strain, the LV undergoes a rotational or torsional motion around its long axis during systole. When viewed from the apex, the apex rotates counterclockwise, and the base rotates clockwise. This opposing rotation creates a wringing or twisting motion of the LV, which enhances the efficiency of blood ejection during systole. During diastole, the LV untwists, generating an active suction force that promotes its early diastolic filling. *Right panel,* Left ventricular circumferential strain represents the reduction in the circumference of the left ventricular cross-section during contraction. This strain is a key indicator of the LV's ability to reduce its diameter and effectively eject blood. Radial strain, on the other hand, measures the thickening of the left ventricular wall along its radius during contraction. These two types of strain work in harmony to ensure efficient myocardial function and are complementary with longitudinal strain in maintaining overall cardiac performance. Radial strain predominantly reflects the contractility of the mid-myocardial fibers, whereas circumferential strain highlights the role of the subendocardial and subepicardial fiber layers in ventricular contraction. (Modified from Kislitsina ON, Thomas JD, Crawford E, et al. Predictors of left ventricular dysfunction after surgery for degenerative mitral regurgitation. *Ann Thor Surg.* 2020;109:669–677.)

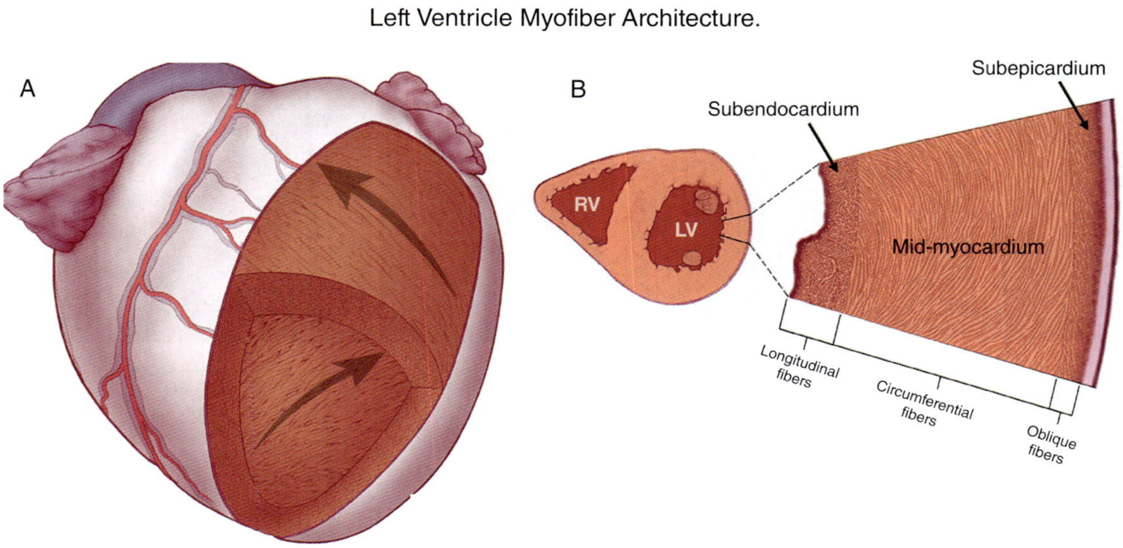

Fig. 7.5 (A) The helical arrangement of myocardial fibers within the left ventricle (LV). The transition of the myocardial fibers begins with a right-handed spiral pattern in the epicardium and gradually shifts to an orthogonal left-handed spiral in the subendocardium. This unique architecture supports the efficient torsional mechanics required for ventricular contraction and relaxation. (B) This is a cross-sectional view of the LV showing the orientation of myocardial fibers at different layers of the left ventricular wall. The *subendocardium* has longitudinal fibers that run from the base to the apex of the LV. They are responsible for longitudinal strain and are sensitive to early ischemia and other pathological processes. The *mid-myocardial* layer has circumferential fibers arranged around the circumference of the left ventricular cavity that contribute to circumferential strain, which plays a critical role in overall systolic function. The *subepicardium* has fibers that are arranged obliquely in a helical configuration that provide rotational and torsional motion. They ensure efficient cavitary blood ejection during systole and facilitate ventricular filling during diastole. This unique fiber architecture allows for the synchronized contraction and relaxation of the heart, which is critical for its efficient function as a pump. *RV,* Right ventricle. (Modified from Luis SA, Chan J, Pellikka PA. Echocardiographic assessment of left ventricular systolic function: an overview of contemporary techniques, including speckle-tracking echocardiography. *Mayo Clin Proc.* 2019;94(1):125–138; used with permission of Mayo Foundation for Medical Education and Research. All rights reserved.)

Longitudinal Strain: A Sensitive Marker

Longitudinal strain is often the first strain parameter to show impairment in early cardiac dysfunction. This is primarily because the subendocardial fibers, which are most vulnerable to ischemia, fibrosis, and increased wall stress, contribute predominantly to longitudinal contraction. Longitudinal strain is less affected by loading conditions (e.g., preload and afterload) compared with traditional measures of left ventricular function such as LVEF, making it a sensitive and reliable marker of intrinsic myocardial function. It is particularly valuable for the early detection of cardiotoxicity in patients undergoing chemotherapy and predicting outcomes in heart failure and ischemic heart disease.[21,24,25] The normal range for LV-GLS is generally accepted to be −18% to −22%, with less negative values (e.g., −16%) indicating abnormal function. Although vendor variability and hemodynamic factors such as heart rate and blood pressure can influence strain values, LV-GLS remains a robust and reproducible metric for determining left ventricular systolic function.

Atrial Fibrillation and Left Ventricular Strain

AF significantly impacts left ventricular function because of the loss of atrial compliance and booster function, which impairs left ventricular filling and compromises hemodynamics. Rapid ventricular rates resulting from AF can further exacerbate left ventricular dysfunction by promoting ventricular cardiomyopathy. Even with optimal ventricular rate control, the absence of the atrial compliance and booster pump functions may impair left ventricular systolic performance. Several studies confirm that AF independently affects LV-GLS, even after adjusting for factors such as blood pressure, heart rate, diabetes, left atrial volume index, and left ventricular mass index.[19,20] Compared with age-matched and LVEF-matched control participants without AF, AF patients consistently demonstrate impaired LV-GLS, underscoring its role as a major determinant of LV systolic function.

Global and Regional Strain Analysis

Left ventricular strain analysis includes both global longitudinal strain (LV-GLS) and regional (segmental) strain assessments, which are critical for evaluating myocardial function. Using the 16-, 17-, or 18-segment models recommended by the American Society of Echocardiography, left ventricular segmental strain provides an in-depth assessment of left ventricular performance. Whereas LV-GLS provides an overall measurement of left ventricular function, regional (segmental) strain analysis allows for the identification of localized dysfunction such as ischemia, fibrosis, or mechanical dyssynchrony, all of which are often associated with regional ischemia within specific coronary artery territories.[26]

Global Longitudinal Strain

For LV-GLS analysis, two-dimensional grayscale images are acquired from standard echocardiographic views, including the parasternal long

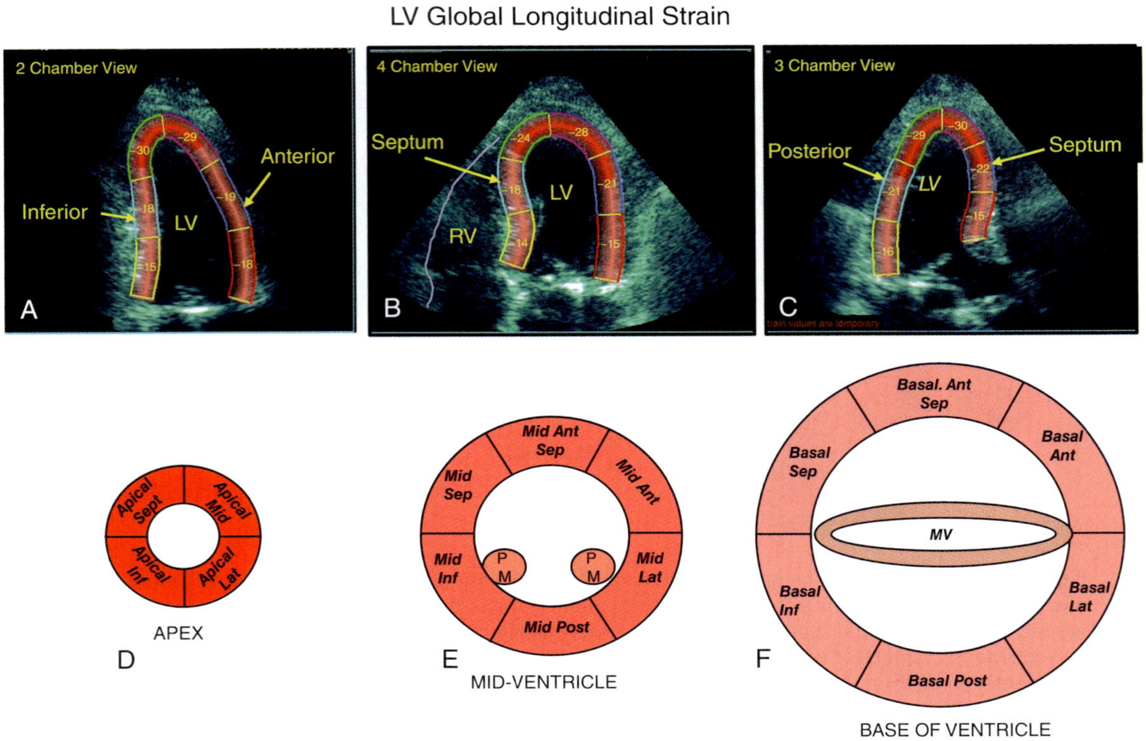

Fig. 7.6 (A–C) The echocardiographic views used to evaluate left ventricular global longitudinal strain (LV-GLS). Each panel corresponds to a standard imaging plane. (A) The "two-chamber view" shows the anterior and inferior walls of the left ventricle (LV). Strain values are calculated for specific myocardial segments along the left ventricular long axis. (B) The "four-chamber view" displays the septal and lateral walls of both the LV and the adjacent right ventricle (RV). This view is crucial for measuring strain in the septal and LV lateral wall segments. (C) The "three-chamber view" highlights the left ventricular posterior and septal walls. Each myocardial segment is color coded with strain values to provide a quantitative assessment of regional left ventricular function. (D–F) The three cross-sectional levels of the LV. (D) The left ventricular apex is divided into four myocardial segments representing the most distal part of the LV. (B) The cross-section of the LV at the mid-ventricular level is divided into six segments and passes through both papillary muscles. (C) The base of the LV also includes six segments and is aligned in the plane of the mitral valve. LV-GLS represents the average strain across all 17 left ventricular segments, capturing the overall deformation of the LV during systole. LV-GLS is particularly valuable for early detection of left ventricular dysfunction, even when the left ventricular ejection fraction appears to be normal. Left ventricular segmental strain provides for the functional analysis of individual myocardial segments, thus identifying regional dysfunction in the LV. (Modified from Kislitsina ON, Thomas JD, Crawford E, et al. Predictors of left ventricular dysfunction after surgery for degenerative mitral regurgitation. *Ann Thor Surg.* 2020;109:669–677.)

axis and apical four-, three-, and two-chamber views (Figs. 7.6 and 7.7). LV- GLS is computed using advanced speckle-tracking software that automatically constructs strain curves by analyzing myocardial deformation across cardiac cycles. The short-axis views of the apical, midlevel, and basal portions of the LV are then stacked to create a "bullseye map" to show the global longitudinal strain distribution across the entire left ventricular myocardium (Fig. 7.8).[21,25] Left ventricular strain imaging, including longitudinal, circumferential, and radial motion, has shown unparalleled sensitivity in detecting subclinical left ventricular dysfunction, often preceding detectable changes in the LVEF by other means, which leads to earlier treatment in asymptomatic patients.

Left Ventricular Regional (Segmental) Strain

An analysis of left ventricular segmental strain is particularly valuable for identifying localized areas of myocardial dysfunction in diseases such as ischemic cardiomyopathy, mitral valve (MV) prolapse, and degenerative MR (DMR).[27,28] For example, we have recently shown that in DMR, preoperative left ventricular segmental strain analysis can identify hypocontractility in the left ventricular wall segments subjacent to papillary muscles that is predictive of the late recurrence of MR after successful MV repair.[29] Our study found that for every 1% decrease in strain in the critical subpapillary left ventricular segments, there is a 6.2% increase the odds of developing late moderate-to-severe MR (odds ratio, 1.062). The early detection of left ventricular segmental strain abnormalities in patients with DMR and subsequent earlier MV repair can preclude the development of AF and irreversible left atrial remodeling (Fig. 7.9).

Restoration of atrial function after conversion from AF to normal sinus rhythm is impacted by patient comorbidities and the duration of AF. The recovery of atrial function is usually rapid in patients after isolated coronary artery bypass grafting (CABG) with a concomitant Maze procedure or after the Maze procedure alone.[30–32] However, in patients with long-standing DMR, both global and regional atrial dysfunction are often worsened by preexisting conditions.[21,33] The replacement of healthy atrial tissue with fibrotic tissue leads to irreversible remodeling of the LA, placing these patients at a higher risk for recurrent AF and stroke (see Chapter 8). Therefore the early detection of

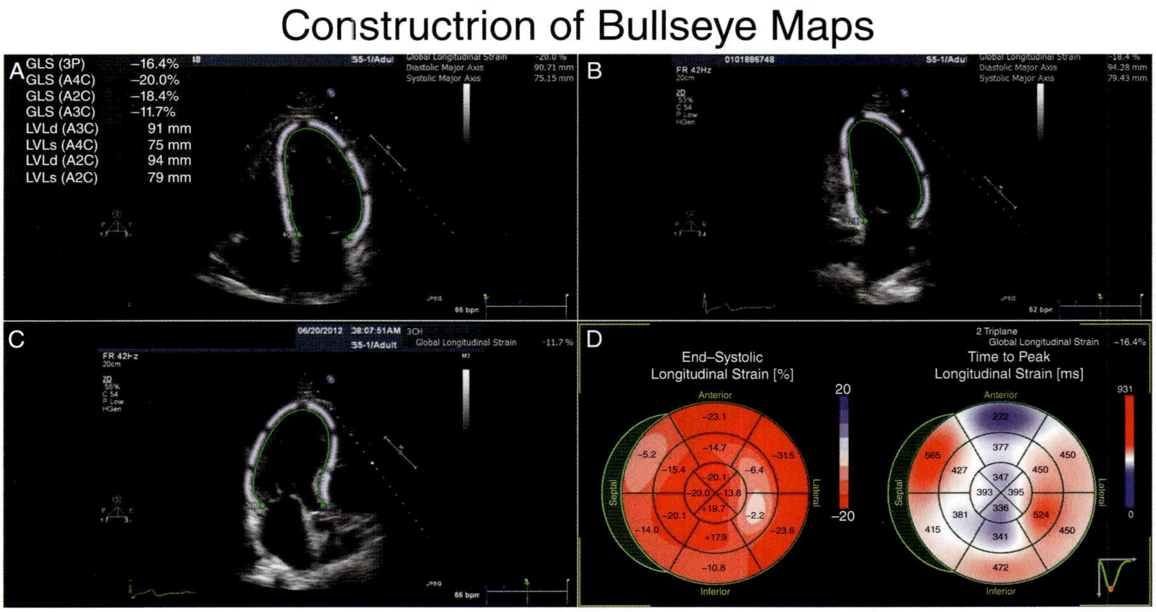

Fig. 7.7 Longitudinal echocardiographic views of the left ventricle in the three standard planes. Each echocardiographic image demonstrates myocardial deformation as determined by speckle-tracking echocardiography. (A) The three-chamber view shows the anterior, posterior, and septal left ventricular walls. (B) The four-chamber view highlights the left ventricular septal and lateral walls. (C) The two-chamber view focuses on the left ventricular anterior and inferior walls. (D) Bullseye maps provide a visual representation of left ventricular strain across all of its 17 standard segments, divided into apex, mid-ventricle, and basal levels. The color-coded myocardial segments and associated strain values indicate regional left ventricular function. *Left bullseye map*: Normal left ventricular segments are represented by *red hues*, indicating strong contraction, and segments with impaired strain are shown in *lighter shades* and abnormal strain values. *Right bullseye map*: This map is based not on the strength of left ventricular segmental contraction but rather on the time it takes each segment to reach its peak strain value. The *blue segments* show areas of delayed contraction suggesting mechanical dyssynchrony, which is often seen in such conditions as left bundle branch block or cardiomyopathies.

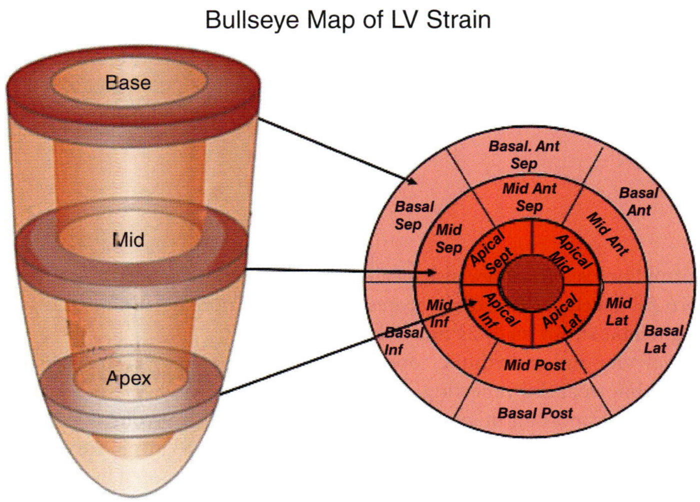

Fig. 7.8 Left ventricular strain across its three primary segments: the apex, mid-ventricle, and base, illustrating how the left ventricle (LV) is functionally divided for global and segmental strain analysis. *Left panel,* The left ventricular apical plane is the narrowest portion of the LV and represents only the most distal region of the LV involved in contraction and relaxation during the cardiac cycle. The mid-ventricular plane contributes to overall left ventricular function by coordinating strain dynamics with the apex and base. The basal plane is the section of the LV and is located near the level of the mitral valve plane. It plays a critical role in tethering the ventricular wall to ensure synchronized myocardial function. *Right panel,* The bullseye map is a two-dimensional representation of left ventricular strain data divided into 17 myocardial segments. Each segment corresponds to specific regions of the apex, mid-ventricle, and base, helping clinicians assess regional strain patterns and detect functional abnormalities. (Modified from Kislitsina ON, Thomas JD, Crawford E, et al. Predictors of left ventricular dysfunction after surgery for degenerative mitral regurgitation. *Ann Thor Surg.* 2020;109:669–677.)

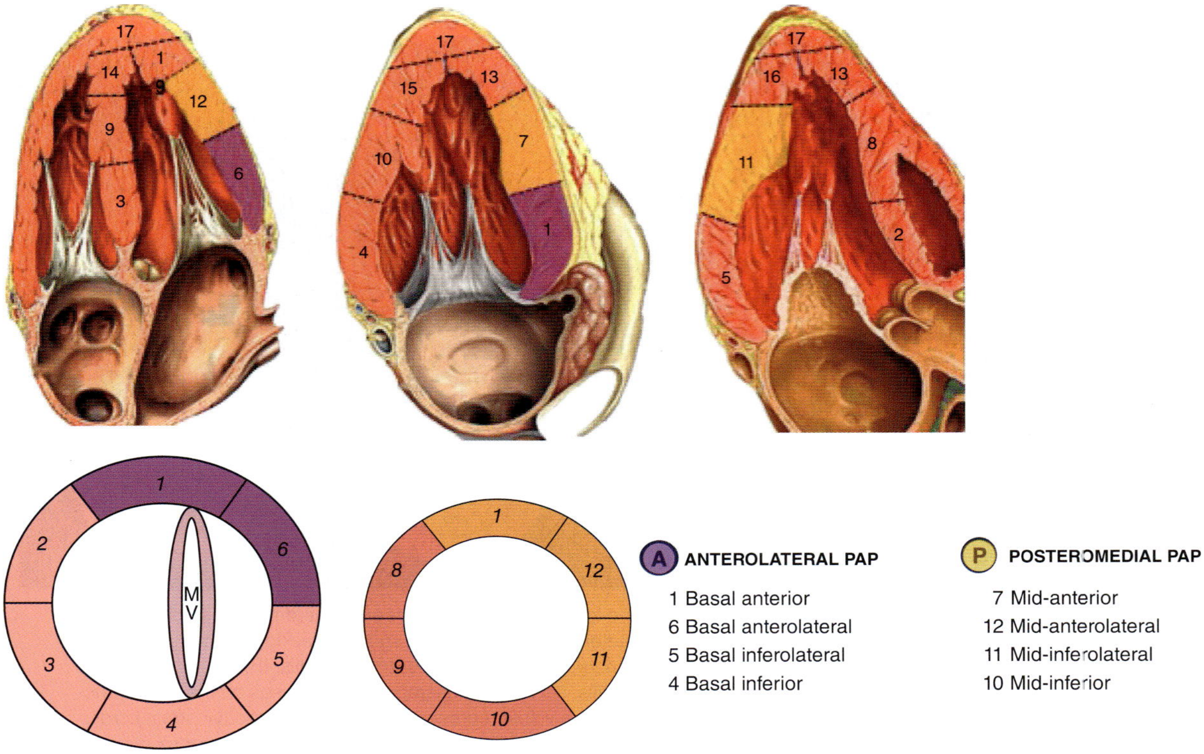

Fig. 7.9 *Upper panels,* Left ventricular segments 1 and 6 *(purple)* are located in the basal anterior and basal anterolateral regions and are subjacent to the anterolateral papillary muscle. We recently documented that abnormal *preoperative* strain in these left ventricular segments correlates with late recurrent mitral regurgitation (MR) after mitral valve (MV) repair for degenerative mitral regurgitation (DMR).[29] We also found that abnormal *preoperative* strain in left ventricular segments 7, 11, and 12 *(orange),* which are subjacent to the posteromedial papillary muscle in the mid-anterior, mid-anterolateral, and mid-inferolateral regions, is also predictive of late recurrent MR in these patients. *Lower panels,* The identification of these critical subpapillary left ventricular segments in our study is consistent with the current literature that associates segments 7, 12, 11, and 10 with the posteromedial papillary muscle and segments 1, 6, 5, and 4 with the anterolateral papillary muscle. The purple segments and orange segments are the ones we found to be predictive of late recurrent MR in DMR patients undergoing MV repair. These findings suggest that reinforcement of the anterior MV commissure during MV repair for DMR may be helpful in preventing long-term late recurrent MR. *LV,* Left ventricle.

left ventricular segmental strain abnormalities is critical because it can help identify changes in the LA before AF develops. This underscores the importance of left ventricular segmental strain analysis not only in ischemic heart disease but also in valvular and arrhythmic conditions.[29] Regional left ventricular strain abnormalities reflecting early mechanical dysfunction may be particularly important in guiding the timing of MV repair in asymptomatic patients. Early detection of left ventricular segmental changes allows clinicians to intervene before AF or irreversible remodeling occurs.

In summary, global and regional left ventricular strain imaging enhances diagnostic precision, aids in risk stratification, and provides a foundation for personalized treatment strategies. By combining LV-GLS and left ventricular segmental strain analysis, clinicians can assess both diffuse and localized myocardial dysfunction, offering a comprehensive view of left ventricular performance and guiding earlier, more targeted surgical interventions. The integration of regional and global strain data allows clinicians to assess both diffuse and focal myocardial dysfunction comprehensively, making strain imaging a cornerstone of modern cardiac diagnostics. Emerging techniques, such as myocardial work analysis, integrate strain with pressure-volume loops to provide an even more detailed evaluation of myocardial function.

RIGHT VENTRICULAR STRAIN

The RV plays a pivotal role in maintaining hemodynamic balance, particularly as it adapts to variations in preload and afterload from the pulmonary circulation. Unlike the LV, the RV is more sensitive to changes in afterload because of its thin wall and unique geometry. This sensitivity makes the RV prone to dysfunction in conditions such as pulmonary hypertension, TR, and chronic volume or pressure overload.[34,35] These hemodynamic disturbances can trigger right atrial dilatation, ultimately predisposing patients to AF.[36] TR and volume overload increase RV diastolic volume, stretching the myocardium and transiently enhancing contraction via the Frank-Starling mechanism. However, chronic volume overload eventually leads to right ventricular dilatation and impaired systolic function. Pulmonary hypertension increases right ventricular systolic pressure, which can result in right ventricular hypertrophy and strain on the free wall.[37]

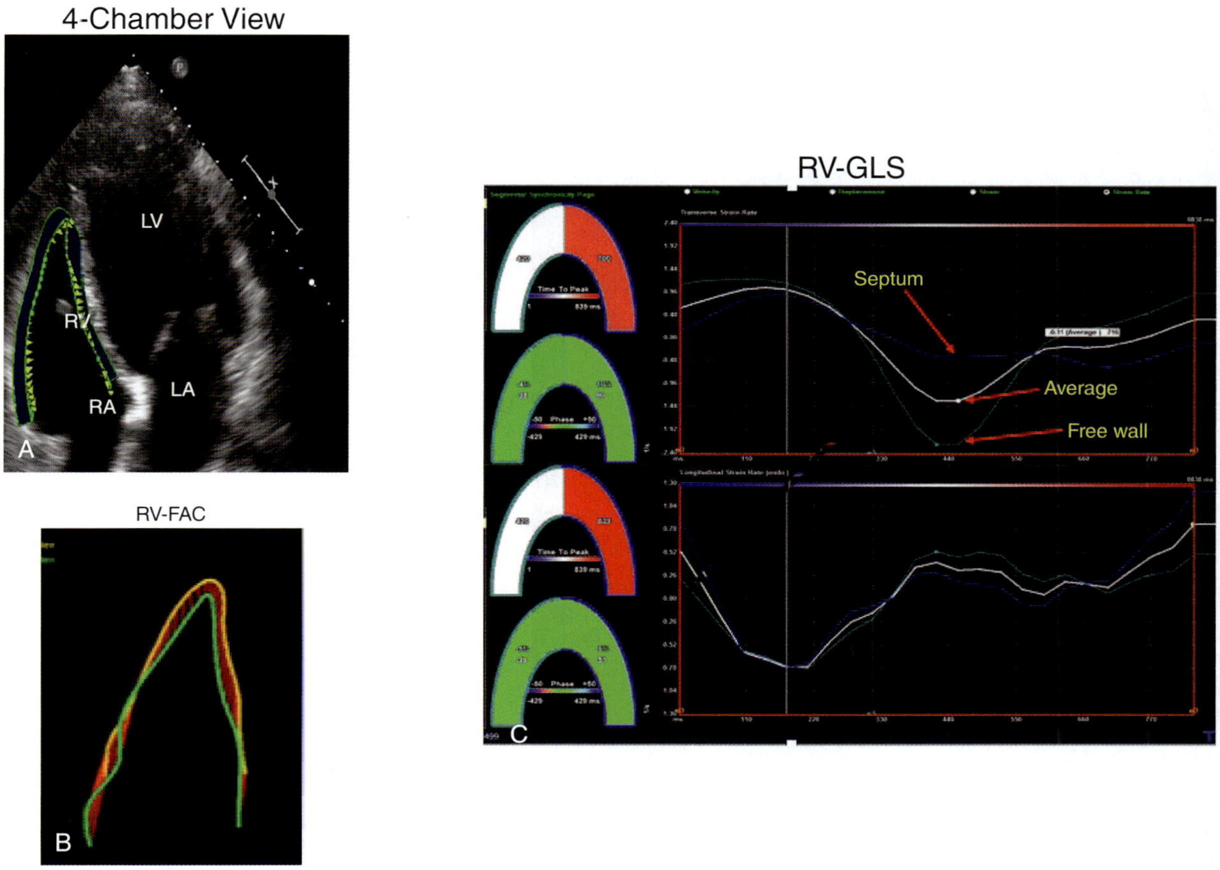

Fig. 7.10 (A) Four-chamber echocardiographic view with speckle-tracking echocardiography of the right ventricle (RV) outlined in *green*. The view simultaneously highlights the left ventricle (LV), left atrium (LA), and right atrium (RA), offering a comprehensive evaluation of all cardiac chambers. (B) Right ventricular fractional area change (RV-FAC) measures the percentage difference in the RV area between end-diastole *(orange)* and end-systole *(green)*. A reduced RV-FAC indicates impaired right ventricular contraction and function. (C) Right ventricular global longitudinal strain (RV-GLS) is calculated as the average strain value of the right ventricular free-wall and the right ventricular septal segments. The strain curve illustrates the deformation of the right ventricular myocardium throughout the cardiac cycle. Specific annotations identify the septal and free-wall strain, along with the averaged global strain value. RV-GLS is a sensitive marker for right ventricular systolic function and is particularly valuable in conditions such as pulmonary hypertension and heart failure.

In the past, right ventricular function was determined primarily by tricuspid annular plane systolic excursion (TAPSE) measured on standard echocardiography and by tissue Doppler imaging. The main limitations of those two techniques for assessing RV function is that they are both angle dependent. Speckle-tracking analysis is not angle-dependent and therefore has become the most important and accurate tool for the assessment of right ventricular function.[38,39]

Right ventricular global longitudinal strain (RV-GLS) is calculated as the average value of the longitudinal strain in the right ventricular free wall and the right ventricular septum (Fig. 7.10). Normal ranges for RV-GLS are −20% to −25%. Right ventricular fractional area change (RV-FAC) is calculated from the end-diastolic and end-systolic areas of the RV (see Fig. 7.10B) as follows, in which FAC is the right ventricular fractional area change, EDA is the end-diastolic area of the RV, and ESA is the end-systolic area of the RV:

$$\text{FAC} = \frac{\text{EDA} - \text{ESA}}{\text{EDA}} \times 100$$

Unlike ejection fraction, RV-FAC reflects area change and has a normal threshold of greater than 35%.[40] RV-FAC is particularly valuable for assessing right ventricular performance in conditions such as pulmonary hypertension, valvular heart disease, and heart failure. Its prognostic capability extends to predicting outcomes such as mortality after pulmonary embolectomy and the progression of heart failure.

Right ventricular free-wall strain (RV-FWS) measures the percentage change in the length of the RV free-wall during systole, providing a regional assessment of right ventricular function.[41] The normal range for RV-FWS in healthy individuals is approximately −29%, with negative values indicating myocardial shortening and contraction. As shown in Fig. 7.11, strain analysis allows for the visualization of segmental strain and highlights regional abnormalities in the right ventricular free-wall.[41,42]

RV-FWS is considered a better indicator of right ventricular function than RV-GLS because it isolates deformation of the free wall, which is most sensitive to pressure and volume overload. In contrast, RV-GLS incorporates septal strain, which may be influenced by left

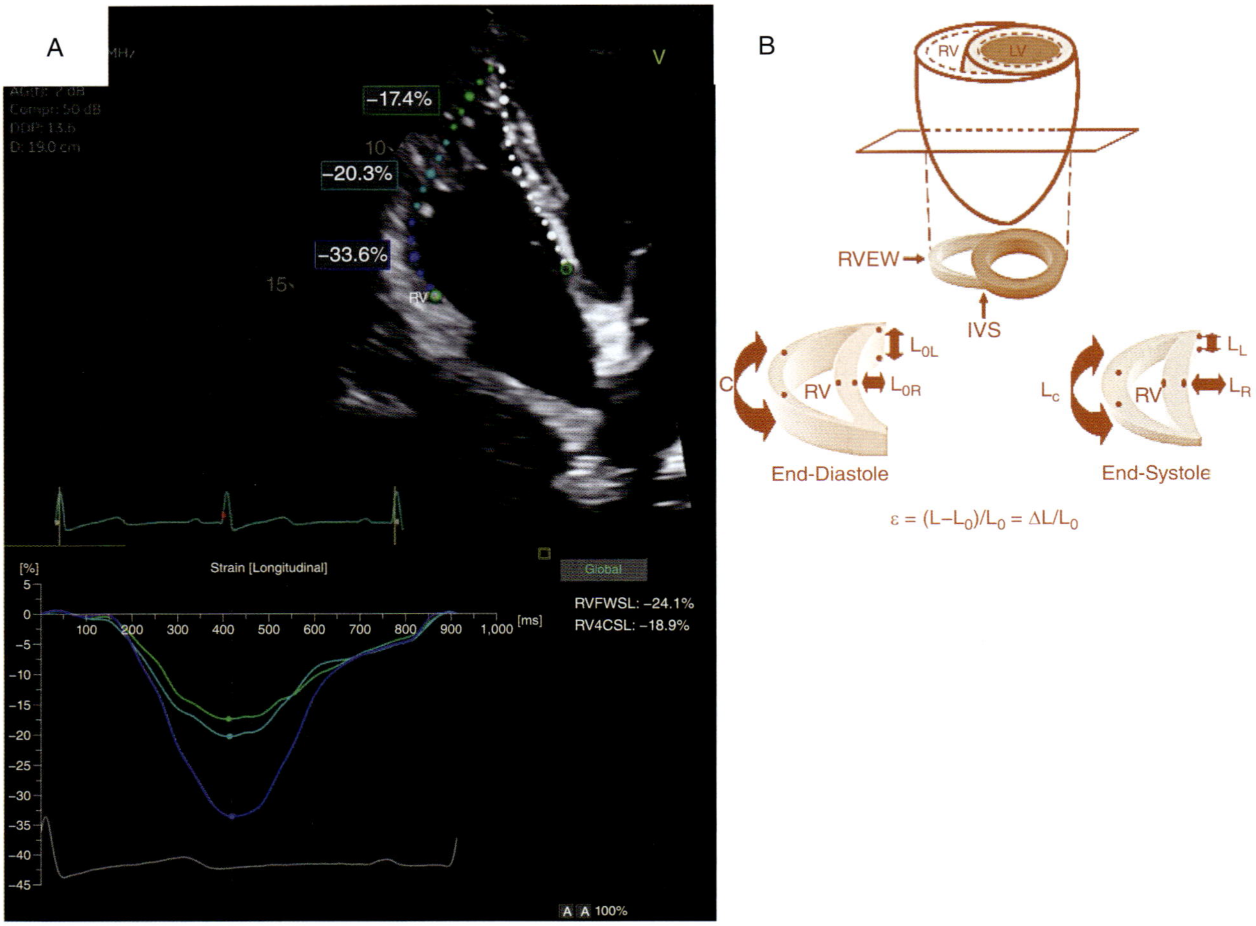

Fig. 7.11 (A) The apical four-chamber view shows strain measurements in the right ventricular free-wall (RV-FWS) and interventricular septum (IVS). Each segment's longitudinal strain value is noted, with the basal (−17.4%), mid (−20.3%), and apical (−33.6%) segments illustrating varying degrees of deformation. The strain curve below tracks segmental deformation over time, with distinct curves for the free-wall and septum. These values are averaged to calculate the free-RV-FWS and the right ventricular global longitudinal strain (RV-GLS). Notably, the RV-FWS (−24.1%) is more sensitive to early right ventricular dysfunction than the septal strain (−18.9%), highlighting its utility in clinical evaluation. (B) The three primary components of right ventricular deformation are illustrated: longitudinal strain (L_l), circumferential strain (L_a), and radial strain (L_r). This diagram underscores the unique contributions of the right ventricular free wall and IVS to overall right ventricular function and highlights the mechanical interplay necessary for effective ventricular performance. *RVEW*, Right Ventricular Endocardial Wall. (Modified from Cho EJ, Jiamsripong P, Calleja AM, et al. Right ventricular free wall circumferential strain reflects graded elevation in acute right ventricular afterload. *Am J Physiol Heart Circ Physiol.* 2009;296(2):H413–420.)

ventricular function and interventricular interactions, thereby limiting its specificity for right ventricular performance.[43]

In conditions such as pulmonary hypertension, significant TR, and RV pressure overload, RV-FWS detects early RV dysfunction even when conventional parameters like TAPSE and fractional area change (RV-FAC) remain normal. This is particularly relevant in patients with severe isolated TR, in whom RV-FWS can reveal subclinical impairment and guide the timing of interventions such as transcatheter tricuspid valve replacement. Severe functional TR, often associated with AF, contributes to right ventricular volume overload, right atrial dilatation, and AF progression.[44,45] As TR worsens, the increased preload stretches the RV, and the RV free-wall compensates by increasing contractility, which is reflected in RV-FWS measurements. However, prolonged overload eventually leads to reduced RV-FWS, right ventricular decompensation, and irreversible remodeling. Studies have shown that reduced RV-FWS is associated with worse outcomes in patients with significant TR, including higher rates of right heart failure, AF recurrence, and mortality. Our investigations have demonstrated that patients with DMR and paroxysmal AF (PAF) exhibit significantly worse RV-FWS than those without AF. This highlights the role of right ventricular dysfunction as both a consequence and contributor to atrial remodeling and AF.[46,47]

Chronic volume or pressure overload of the RA caused by TR or pulmonary hypertension leads to right atrial stretch and fibrosis, promoting the development of AF. In turn, the AF usually exacerbates TR because of the loss of atrial function, further increasing right ventricular preload and perpetuating the cycle of right ventricular dysfunction.[48] RV-FWS, as a load-sensitive yet highly reproducible parameter, is uniquely positioned to detect these dynamics early, enabling timely management to break this cycle.[41]

In summary, right ventricular strain analysis, particularly RV-FWS, represents a paradigm shift in the ability to evaluate right ventricular function accurately. By isolating free-wall deformation, RV-FWS provides a more specific and sensitive measure of right ventricular performance than traditional parameters. It plays a critical role in the early detection of right ventricular dysfunction, guiding risk stratification and the timing of interventions in patients with such conditions as TR, pulmonary hypertension, and AF. As the role of the RV in systemic processes becomes clearer, right ventricular strain analysis will continue to shape clinical decision-making processes and improve outcomes.

LEFT ATRIAL STRAIN

The left atrium (LA) is a complex structure consisting of three distinct components, each originating from different embryologic sources: the anterior LA, the posterior (venous) LA, and the LA appendage (LAA). The LA plays an active and dynamic role throughout the cardiac cycle, coordinating closely with the LV (see Fig. 7.2C).

The atria are far more than simply passive chambers positioned between their venous inlets and respective ventricles. Instead, they function in an interdependent relationship with the ventricles to optimize cardiac performance. Synchronized phasic changes within the atria are crucial to ensuring effective ventricular filling, whether on the left or right side of the heart.[13,49] Beyond their mechanical function, the atria also respond to stretching by releasing atrial natriuretic peptide, a hormone with potent diuretic, natriuretic, and vasorelaxant effects.[50]

Unlike ventricular strain, which is typically expressed as a negative percentage because of myocardial shortening during systole, atrial strain is expressed as a positive percentage. This distinction arises from their primary role as capacitance chambers, deforming passively in response to intracavitary pressure and volume rather than through active muscle contraction. However, depending on the chosen methodology and reference points (e.g., R-R or P-P intervals), atrial strain values, particularly during the contractile or conduit phases, may sometimes be negative because of the tracking system's coordinate setup or analysis of tissue displacement in opposing directions.[51] When using the speckle-tracking method, the analysis examines changes in the position of points on the tissue, which can result in negative values. This is because the system tracks deformation relative to the initial position of the point during contraction and relaxation. In such cases, negative values may indicate that tissue deformation occurs in the opposite direction (e.g., a compressive effect during contraction phases). Negative values can also be associated with the chosen method for analyzing distal tissue deformation. For example, if tissue contraction or tissue displacement is measured in the opposite direction relative to its normal functional position (e.g., opposite in the context of volume increase), it can produce negative results (Fig. 7.12).

Embryologically, the LAA originates from the primordial atrial tube, and the LA develops from the PVs.[52] These separate and distinct embryologic origins lead to histologic differences between the LAA

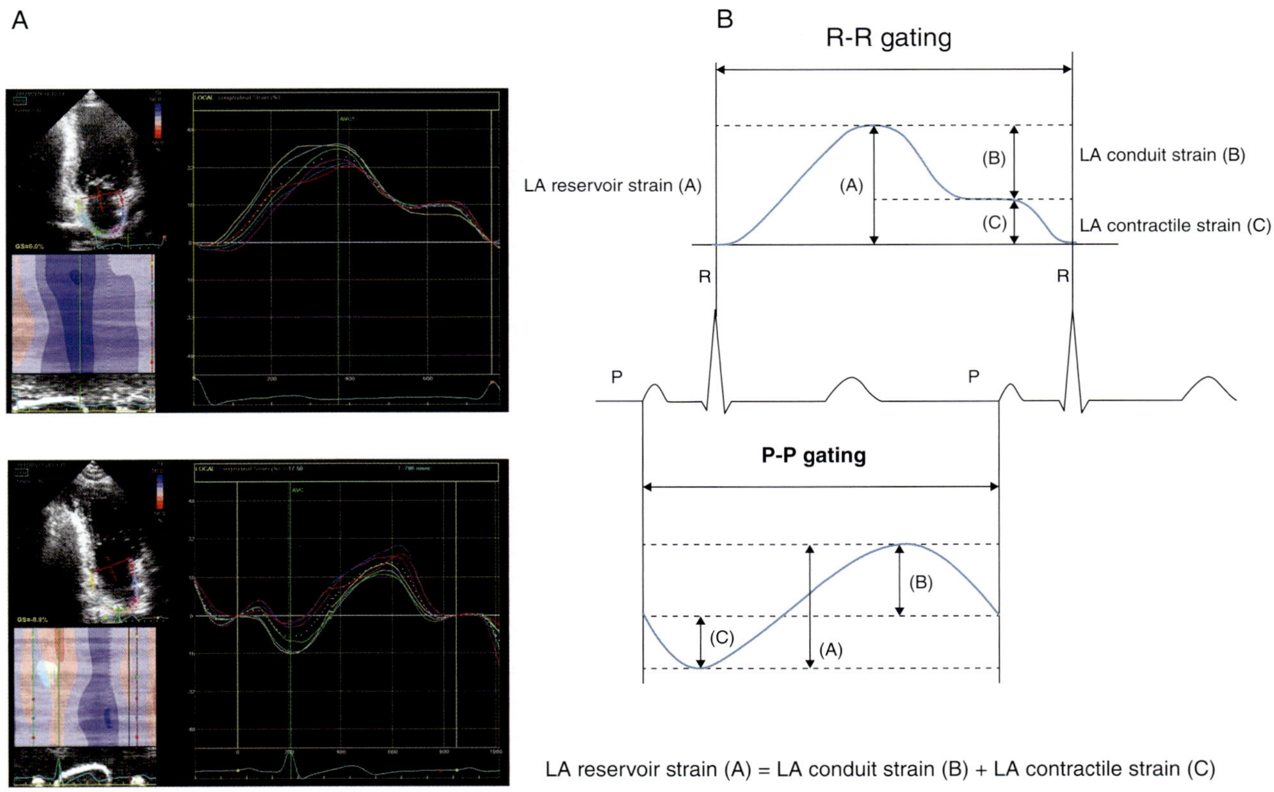

Fig. 7.12 (A) The reservoir, conduit, and contractile phases of left atrial function are highlighted on the strain curve to reflect its contribution during the different phases of the cardiac cycle. The images depict the speckle-tracking process used to record strain measurements and quantitatively evaluate LA deformation. (B) The left atrial strain curve is further analyzed by two different gating methods. R-R gating *(top panel)* adjusts left atrial strain measurements to align with the R-R interval, and P-P gating *(bottom panel)* adjusts left atrial strain measurements to align with the P-P interval, emphasizing atrial mechanical function during the complete cardiac cycle. The definitions of (A), (B), and (C) in the R-R gating method and the P-P gating method remain consistent, but the timing of the measurements during the cardiac cycle is different. (Modified from Sun BJ, Park JH. Echocardiographic measurement of left atrial strain- a key requirement in clinical practice. *Circ J.* 2021;86(1):6–13.)

and LA. The myocardial discontinuity observed at the transition from the LA to the LAA has been suggested as a potential substrate for the generation of arrhythmias.[53]

The contribution of LAA contraction to overall left atrial contraction has been reported in studies to be approximately 20% during sinus rhythm. Although the exact percentage can vary based on the population studied and the methodology used, studies have shown that the LAA's contractile activity is greater than that of the LA body.[52,54,55] However, since both the LA and the LAA are primarily capacitance chambers, the force of contraction in both is relatively unimportant in comparison to their roles as capacitance chambers. Dobutamine stimulation enhances LAA contraction in both sinus rhythm and AF, indicating its active participation in atrial mechanics (Fig. 7.13).[56]

In patients with restrictive cardiomyopathy, the LA plays a crucial role in compensating for heart failure by expanding to accommodate additional volume. The LAA contributes significantly to left atrial function, particularly in its reservoir and contractile phases. Surgical exclusion of the LAA has been shown to impact left atrial function, with studies indicating a reduction in left atrial reservoir and contractile functions after exclusion, although those studies did not address the potential off-setting positive effects on overall LA function following removal of the LAA due to decreasing the overall diameter of the remaining chamber in accordance with LaPlace's Law.[57]

In the context of hypertrophic cardiomyopathy (HOCM), LAA closure is a potential treatment option for patients experiencing heart failure, particularly those with concomitant AF.[58,59] LAA closure can significantly reduce the risk of stroke by preventing blood clots from forming in the LAA, a major source of emboli in AF patients with HOCM.[60] However, the effectiveness of LAA closure in patients with HOCM and heart failure remains under investigation and should be carefully evaluated with a cardiologist based on individual circumstances. Given the prevalence of diastolic dysfunction in HOCM, the compensatory mechanisms of the LA are crucial. The removal or clipping of the LAA in these patients could potentially diminish the LA's compensatory capacity, leading to adverse outcomes.[61] Specific studies directly linking LAA removal to poor outcomes in patients with HOCM are limited, emphasizing the need for further research to elucidate the precise impact of LAA exclusion in this patient population.

In patients with long-standing MV disease, the atria often exhibit significant remodeling (see Chapter 8). In patients undergoing isolated CABG and a concomitant Maze procedure or solely the Maze procedure, there is evidence of rapid recuperation of atrial pump function. Conversely, in cases of long-standing DMR, both global and regional atrial dysfunction are exacerbated by preexisting structural and functional changes, further complicating recovery.[30,31,62,63]

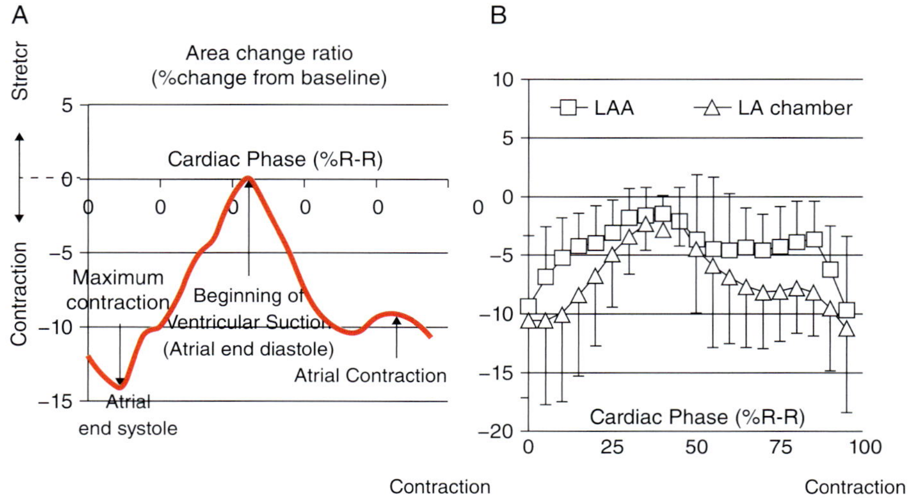

Fig. 7.13 (A) Graph demonstrating the area change ratio percent change from baseline across the cardiac cycle (R-R gating), specifically focusing on the left atrium (LA) and the left atrial appendage (LAA). The curve illustrates the three key components of left atrial strain that define overall left atrial function.

- Atrial end-systole: The point at which atrial contraction reaches its maximum, representing the atrial "pump" function that aids ventricular filling during late diastole.
- Beginning of ventricular suction: Occurs during early ventricular diastole, when the atrium passively transfers blood to the ventricle, indicating the conduit phase.
- Maximum contraction: Reflects the left atrial reservoir function, which occurs during ventricular systole when the LA collects pulmonary venous return while the mitral valve remains closed.

The passive filling of the LA (reservoir phase) and passive emptying of the LA (conduit phase), coupled with the brief muscular contraction of the LA just at the end or ventricular filling, optimize ventricular filling and overall cardiac output when it is synchronous with the left ventricle and with the right atrium (see Chapter 9). This figure highlights the importance of left atrial contractile function, however weak it is relative to ventricular contraction, that some believe can be compromised by interventions such as LAA closure or removal. It also confirms that the LA is primarily a capacitance chamber, not a pumping chamber (see Chapters 9 and 43). (B) Simultaneous plots of left atrial and LAA function showing how both the LA and LAA passively expand to accommodate incoming blood during ventricular systole and then passively allow blood from the LA and LAA to be sucked into the left ventricle by the ventricular dynamics of ventricular diastole. Finally, the brief "pump" phase of left atrial function shows active contraction of both the LA and LAA contributing to ventricular filling. Note that the LAA contributes additional reservoir capacity in the LA. Importantly, the conduit phases of the LA and LAA differentiate because the volume in the LAA tends to plateau and remain elevated in comparison to that of the LA until just at the onset of the "pump" phase.

During ventricular systole, each atrium serves as a reservoir when both atrioventricular (AV) valves are closed as they receive venous flow from the PVs. Atrial filling by PV flow is influenced by ventricular contraction, the descent of the ventricular base, systemic and pulmonary venous systolic pressure, and atrial properties (i.e., relaxation and chamber stiffness). The conduit function of the atria begins in early diastole when blood passively flows from the atrium to the ventricle. Left ventricular relaxation, compliance, stiffness, and early diastolic pressures are major determinants of LA conduit function. Late diastolic atrial contractility actively pumps the remaining blood into the ventricles. The atrial pressure–volume relationship consists of two loops: the A loop, representing atrial pump function; and the V loop, representing atrial reservoir function (Fig. 7.14).[64,65]

Atrial reservoir and booster functions increase with exercise, but conduit function does not.[56–68] Enhancement of reservoir function supports ventricular filling by creating a higher AV pressure gradient that favors diastolic flow and increases atrial pump function through preload augmentation. Any pressure and/or volume-loading conditions, such as AF, ischemic heart disease, heart failure, valvular disease, hypertension, and diabetes, lead to atrial remodeling. Atrial remodeling is driven by electrical, mechanical, and metabolic stressors over time, and it can be structural, functional, or electrical (see Chapter 8).[69–71] Prolonged stress (>5 weeks) may cause irreversible atrial damage, such as apoptosis and fibrosis. Whereas structural remodeling manifests as atrial dilatation, functional remodeling results in decreased function with or without a change in atrial size. Atrial arrhythmias, especially AF, are hallmarks of electrical remodeling.[72]

During AF, left atrial function depends on the harmony of wall compliance, preload (pulmonary venous flow), afterload (left ventricular filling pressure), and electromechanical synchrony. In contrast, a diseased LA, as observed in left atrial remodeling, represents structural and functional alterations caused by cumulative hemodynamic stress. The intensity and duration of this stress determine the phenotype of left atrial remodeling. Substrate changes, such as cardiomyocyte atrophy and replacement by fibrotic tissue, lead to wall thinning and progressive left atrial deterioration, stiffening, and dilatation.[13,69,71,72] LA dilatation, directly related to left ventricular filling pressure during diastole, is a potent indicator of left ventricular diastolic dysfunction and a prognostic marker in heart failure and AF (Fig. 7.15 and 7.16).[70,71]

Left atrial strain analysis by STE can detect functional abnormalities even in the absence of visible left atrial dilatation. For example, Hirose et al.[72] demonstrated that reduced booster pump function, measured by strain rate (SR), predicted newly developed AF in patients without prior arrhythmia history. Similarly, decreased left atrial strain has shown predictive value for thromboembolic events, emphasizing the need for careful evaluation even when sinus rhythm is restored. Studies on surgical AF ablation have reported variable incidences of both sinus rhythm restoration and atrial contraction recovery, ranging from 21% to 87%. Despite successful sinus rhythm restoration, progressive loss of left atrial function is observed, particularly in patients with rheumatic MV disease.[72–77]

Recent studies show disparities in left atrial functional recovery based on ablation protocols. For example, Loardi et al.[77] found that 76% of patients undergoing limited left atrial ablation had normal atrial function at 3 months, increasing to 98% at 2 years. However, other studies, such as the Heart Strain Evaluation and Recovery (HESTER) trial, report persistent reductions in left atrial function despite sinus rhythm restoration. These findings underscore the importance of comprehensive preoperative and postoperative left atrial function evaluation, particularly when considering anticoagulation withdrawal.[78]

Our retrospective analysis of strain in 821 patients undergoing surgical AF ablation revealed key preoperative predictors of postoperative outcomes. Lower preoperative left atrial and right atrial reservoir strain, larger atrial volumes, and severe TR were independently associated with postoperative AF recurrence. Biatrial Maze procedures were particularly effective in reducing recurrence in patients with impaired right atrial function.[62]

Although patients who were selected to undergo biatrial Maze procedures tended to be older and have more preoperative comorbidities, their left atrial reservoir function was restored to near-normal levels as opposed to patients who received only left atrial ablation lesions. However, variability in outcomes persist because of differences in lesion sets and the extent of underlying myocardial disease. Biatrial Maze procedures remain more effective in preventing AF recurrence, especially in patients with reduced preoperative right atrial strain.[36,62,63]

Preoperative strain analysis, encompassing both left atrial and right atrial reservoir strain, serves as a reliable tool for predicting outcomes and guiding procedural selection. Despite the restoration of sinus rhythm, left atrial strain often remains suboptimal in patients with

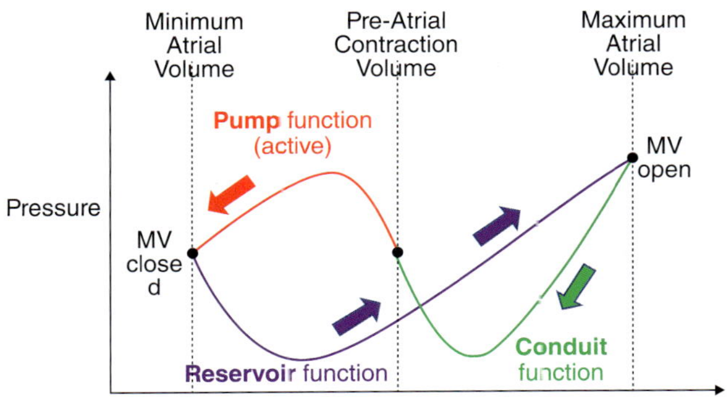

Fig. 7.14 The pressure–volume loop provides a visual representation of the left atrial function through its three phases: reservoir function, conduit function, and pump function. These phases correspond to different stages of the cardiac cycle:

1. Reservoir function *(purple line)*
   - Phase: This occurs during ventricular systole when the mitral valve (MV) is closed.
   - Mechanism: The left atrium (LA) serves as a reservoir, collecting blood from the pulmonary veins while the left ventricle (LV) contracts.
   - Volume dynamics: The atrial volume gradually increases, reaching its maximum atrial volume by the end of ventricular systole.
   - Pressure dynamics: Left atrial pressure slightly rises as blood accumulates.
2. Conduit function *(green line)*
   - Phase: This begins when the MV opens at the start of ventricular diastole.
   - Mechanism: Blood flows passively from the LA into the LV, driven by the pressure gradient between the two chambers.
   - Volume dynamics: The atrial volume decreases as the LA serves as a conduit for blood.
   - Pressure dynamics: LA pressure remains relatively low during this phase.
3. Pump function *(red line)*
   - Phase: This occurs just before ventricular systole when the LA contracts (atrial systole).
   - Mechanism: The atrium actively contracts to "pump" the remaining blood into the LV, enhancing ventricular filling.
   - Volume dynamics: The atrial volume decreases further, reaching its minimum atrial volume at the end of this phase.
   - Pressure dynamics: Left atrial pressure rises significantly during atrial contraction.

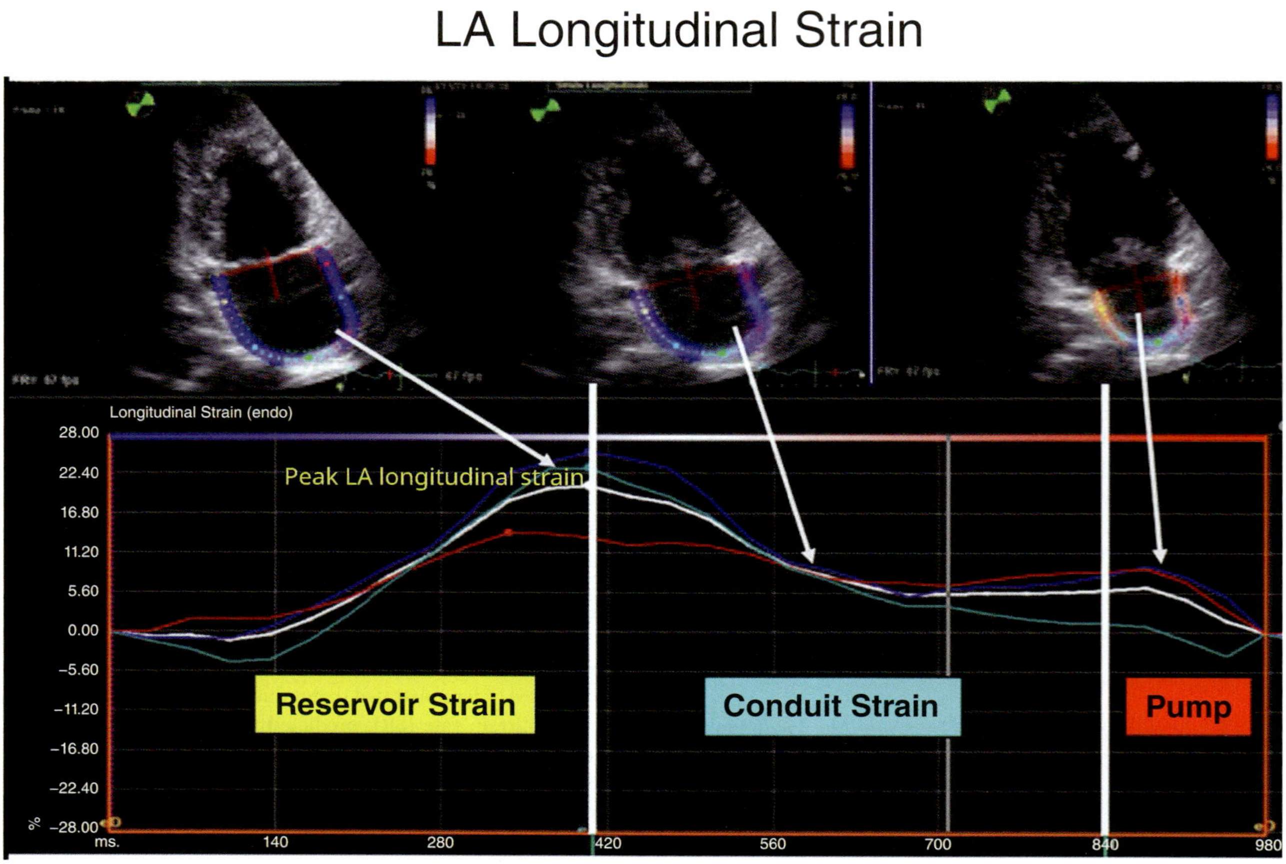

Fig. 7.15 The phasic functions of the left atrium as represented by left atrial longitudinal strain curves. Strain analysis provides a detailed assessment of left atrial mechanical function. The peak left atrial longitudinal strain (maximum positive strain value) is identified during the reservoir phase, highlighting left atrial stretch and storage of blood. Segmenting left atrial strain into distinct phases allows for a comprehensive evaluation of atrial function and identification of dysfunctions linked to various cardiac pathologies. Left atrial reservoir strain *(yellow)* represents left atrial function during ventricular systole and reflects left atrial compliance and the ability to accommodate blood during systole. Reduced reservoir strain can indicate atrial stiffening or fibrosis. Left atrial conduit strain *(blue)* represents left atrial function during early ventricular diastole and therefore is dependent on left ventricular relaxation and left atrial–left ventricular pressure gradients. Abnormal conduit strain may signal diastolic dysfunction. Left atrial pump function *(red)* represents left atrial active contraction during late ventricular diastole. It indicates left atrial contractility, which is essential in conditions such as heart failure with preserved ejection fraction in which atrial contraction compensates for reduced ventricular compliance.

extensive atrial remodeling or underlying MV disease. Similar findings were published by Parwani et al. in 2012.[79] In patients with persistent AF, those with preoperative left atrial strain of less than 10% exhibited significantly higher recurrence rates after catheter ablation. This emphasizes the critical importance of strain-guided patient selection for AF ablation procedures. Such patients should be considered strongly for anticoagulant therapy to mitigate thromboembolic risk.

Our group also demonstrated the prognostic value of left atrial reservoir strain (LASr) in assessing stroke risk after surgical AF ablation. For example, a low reservoir strain 1 year after surgery is strongly associated with an increased stroke risk even in patients with restored sinus rhythm. For every 1% reduction in LASr, the odds of postoperative stroke increased by approximately 6%. For patients with LASr below 12%, the risk of stroke is as high as 60%, warranting anticoagulation therapy and close follow-up to monitor left atrial functional recovery. It seems clear that quantifying atrial strain parameters allows clinicians to refine anticoagulation decisions, balancing hemorrhagic and thromboembolic risks.[36,62,63]

In summary, conventional parameters such as left atrial volume and left atrial diameter fail to capture the full extent of atrial remodeling in patients with atrial fibrillation, making atrial strain analysis indispensable. The interplay between preload, afterload, and left atrial strain provides crucial insights into cardiac mechanics. Left atrial strain is sensitive to changes in volume status. Chronic MR or left-sided heart failure increases left atrial preload, leading to progressive dilation and impaired strain. Elevated left ventricular filling pressures reduce reservoir strain, highlighting diastolic dysfunction. This serves as an early indicator of adverse hemodynamic conditions, guiding therapeutic interventions. Left atrial strain analysis has transformed the evaluation of atrial mechanics, offering unparalleled sensitivity for detecting dysfunction and predicting outcomes. By quantifying reservoir, conduit, and pump strain, clinicians gain insights into atrial compliance, remodeling, and thromboembolic risk. These parameters are invaluable in managing AF, guiding surgical and catheter-based interventions, and optimizing anticoagulation strategies.

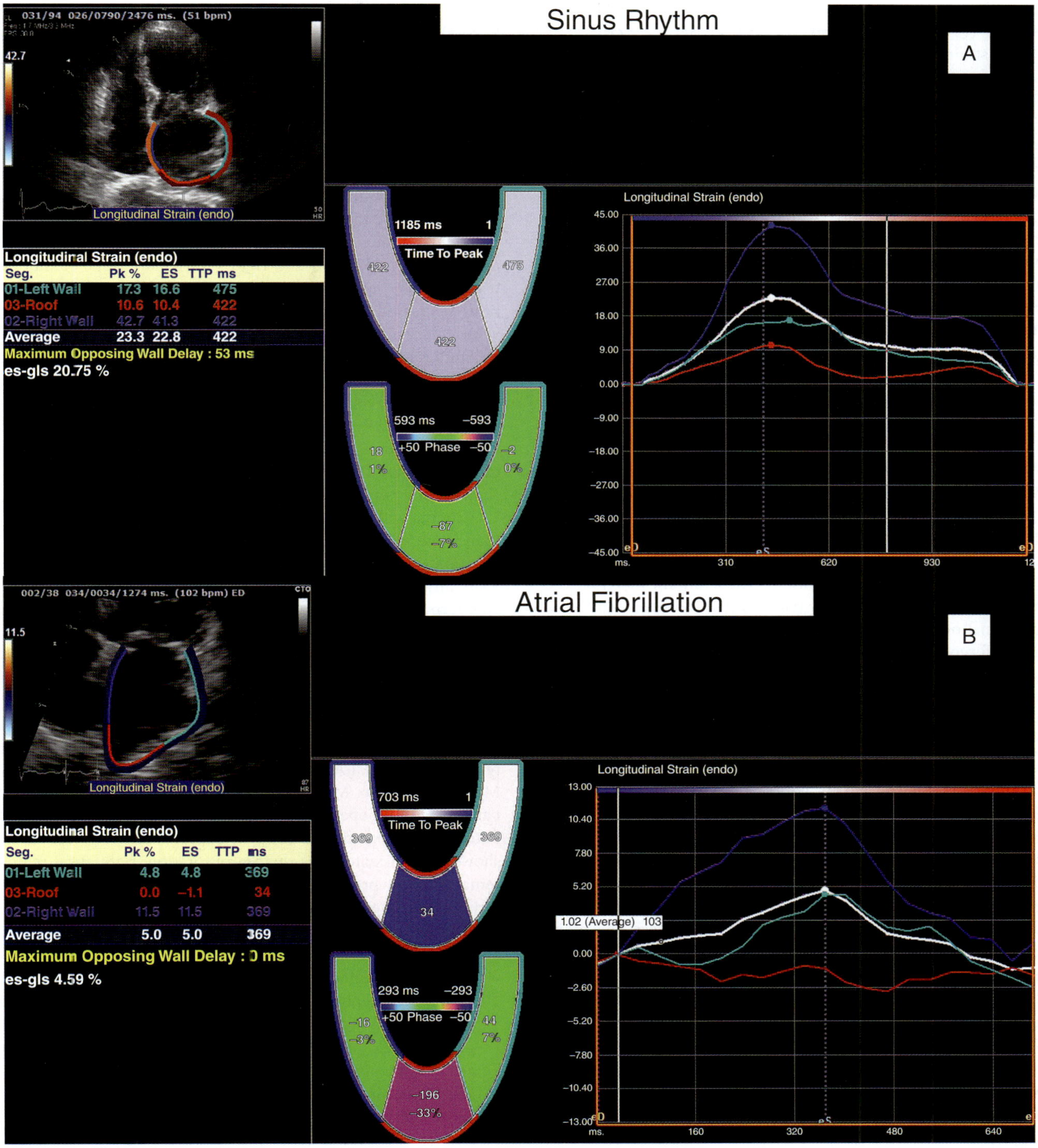

Fig. 7.16 Comparison of the different left atrial strain patterns during sinus rhythm (SR) and atrial fibrillation (AF). (A) During *sinus rhythm*, normal phasic strain reflects healthy left atrial function. Reservoir, conduit, and pump components can be independently assessed to identify subtle left atrial dysfunction in conditions such as heart failure or diastolic dysfunction. (B) During AF, the loss of atrial pump function and reduced reservoir strain indicate impaired left atrial mechanics. *Seg*, Segment, *Pk*, peak strain, *ES*, End systolic strain, *TTP*, Time to peak strain, *Endo*, Endocardial. Persistent low strain values in AF may correlate with atrial remodeling, fibrosis, and thromboembolic risk. Left atrial strain analysis is useful for preoperative evaluation, especially in patients undergoing rhythm control strategies (e.g., catheter ablation). Reduced left atrial strain during AF is associated with higher AF recurrence rates after ablation.

RIGHT ATRIAL STRAIN

Right atrial strain is measured in a similar manner to left atrial strain and is characterized by reservoir, conduit, and booster phases. However, its longitudinal strain pattern differs slightly from that of the LA (Fig. 7.17). Right atrial strain has emerged as a crucial predictor of adverse outcomes, particularly in conditions such as pulmonary artery hypertension (PAH) and chronic thromboembolic pulmonary hypertension (CTEPH).[37,80] Moreover, preoperative right atrial strain parameters in patients with PAF can aid in determining the optimal surgical approach, such as whether to perform biatrial or LA-only ablation procedures.[62,63,81]

The quantification of right atrial function has traditionally been challenging because of the lack of standardized parameters. However, recent advances in strain imaging have provided valuable insights into right atrial dynamics and their interactions with the RV and pulmonary vasculature.[80] RA strain encompasses several components, including peak atrial longitudinal strain (PALS), peak atrial contraction strain (PACS), and SR, which are measured during different phases of the cardiac cycle.[81,82] For example, PALS reflects right atrial reservoir function, PACS represents booster function, and conduit strain quantifies the passive transfer of blood from the RA to the RV during early RV diastole (see Fig. 7.17).

Recent studies demonstrate that right atrial reservoir function is predictive of clinical outcomes and hemodynamic parameters in patients with pulmonary hypertension.[80,82] These findings suggest that earlier diagnosis and treatment in patients with reduced right atrial reservoir function may prevent significant right heart remodeling. No longer the "forgotten chamber," the RA is now receiving increasing attention in the echocardiography literature. Several studies underscore the prognostic importance of right atrial size and function in this population. Haddad et al.[83] demonstrated that severe right atrial enlargement, defined as a more than 40% increase in volume above reference values, independently predicts adverse outcomes in PAH. Brunner et al.[84] found that reduced right atrial total emptying fraction (reservoir function) and active emptying fraction (pump function) were associated with higher mortality rates. Fukuda et al.[85] reported that the sum of right atrial strain components (reservoir, conduit, and pump strain) enhanced the prediction of clinical outcomes in pulmonary hypertension when added to a Cox regression model based on hemodynamic parameters and right ventricular free-wall strain. However, this model did not include right atrial volume.

These studies highlight the correlation between right atrial strain and right atrial volume, emphasizing the importance of both parameters in the evaluation of PAH. Furthermore, it remains unclear whether reduced right atrial reservoir and pump function could serve as early markers for PAH in asymptomatic patients with ostensibly normal right ventricular size and systolic function. If confirmed, the analysis of right atrial mechanics could become a critical tool in screening at-risk populations for PAH.

A meta-analysis of right atrial strain data in healthy individuals revealed the following normal ranges:[86]

- Right atrial reservoir strain (PALS): 25% to 63% (mean, 44%)
- Right atrial conduit strain: 7% to 28% (mean, 18%)
- Right atrial contractile strain (PACS): 2% to 32% (mean, 17%)
- Right atrial systolic SR: 0.9 to 3.4 s^{-1} (mean, 2.1 s^{-1})
- Right atrial diastolic SR: early diastolic SR ranges from −3.3 to −0.8 s^{-1} (mean, 2.0 s^{-1}), and late diastolic SR ranges from −2.4 to −1.3 s^{-1} (mean, −1.9 s^{-1}).

Age, body mass index, systolic and diastolic blood pressure, and heart rate are known to influence variability in right atrial strain values. Additionally, vendor and software differences in strain analysis contribute to interstudy heterogeneity, underscoring the need for standardization.[87]

The RA plays a vital role in the cardiac cycle by optimizing right ventricular filling while maintaining low right-sided pressures. Its reservoir function accommodates systemic venous return during tricuspid valve closure, its conduit function passively transfers blood during early diastole, and its booster function actively facilitates right ventricular filling during late diastole. Notably, the RA contributes approximately 6% to 10% to right ventricular stroke volume, a contribution that becomes critical in cases of right ventricular dysfunction. Decreased right atrial function therefore poses a risk for right ventricular failure and reduced cardiac output.[88]

Studies have also highlighted the influence of right atrial strain on outcomes in specific patient populations. Our group has shown that right atrial reservoir and contraction strain are significantly reduced in patients with PAF, indicating right atrial dysfunction. This dysfunction is strongly associated with a higher recurrence rate of AF after surgical or catheter-based ablation procedures, underscoring the critical role of right atrial strain in preoperative planning.[62,63]

Patients with DMR and PAF exhibit worse right atrial mechanics than those without PAF. We demonstrated that this right atrial dysfunction can persist for up to 1 year after a surgical Maze procedure. Right atrial strain and volume recovery are slower than their left atrial counterparts, highlighting the prolonged remodeling process of the right atrium after AF ablation. Similar to left atrial strain, right atrial strain analysis predicts AF recurrence rates and long-term thromboembolic risk. Patients with impaired right atrial strain and volume often require extended anticoagulation therapy.

In cases involving biatrial Maze procedures, the predictive power of preoperative right atrial strain is comparable to left atrial strain for AF recurrence. Biatrial AF ablation procedures, including the classic Cox Maze-III and Cox Maze-IV procedures, are especially beneficial for patients with preoperative right atrial dysfunction, offering improved outcomes compared with LA-only procedures. However, our studies showed that despite sinus rhythm restoration, right atrial remodeling remains a slow process, necessitating prolonged follow-up and monitoring of strain parameters.

Additionally, the anatomic and procedural factors influencing right atrial function warrant consideration. For example:

- **Cannulation site:** RA function may be affected by the use of cannulas in the right atrial appendage (RAA) during surgery. Comparisons between bicaval cannulation and RAA cannulation in CABG patients indicate that the choice of cannulation site influences right atrial functional recovery.[88]
- **Pericardial integrity:** Studies suggest that leaving the pericardium open after surgery can impair right atrial and right ventricular function because of a loss of pericardial support. This observation has implications for surgical planning, particularly in cases involving the right heart.[43,89] Right atrial strain analysis holds significant potential for early detection, prognostication, and management of right-sided cardiac conditions. By incorporating right atrial strain into routine echocardiographic assessment, clinicians can better stratify risk, optimize therapeutic strategies, and improve patient outcomes. Further research is needed to establish definitive reference ranges and evaluate the impact of right atrial strain on long-term cardiac health across diverse patient populations.

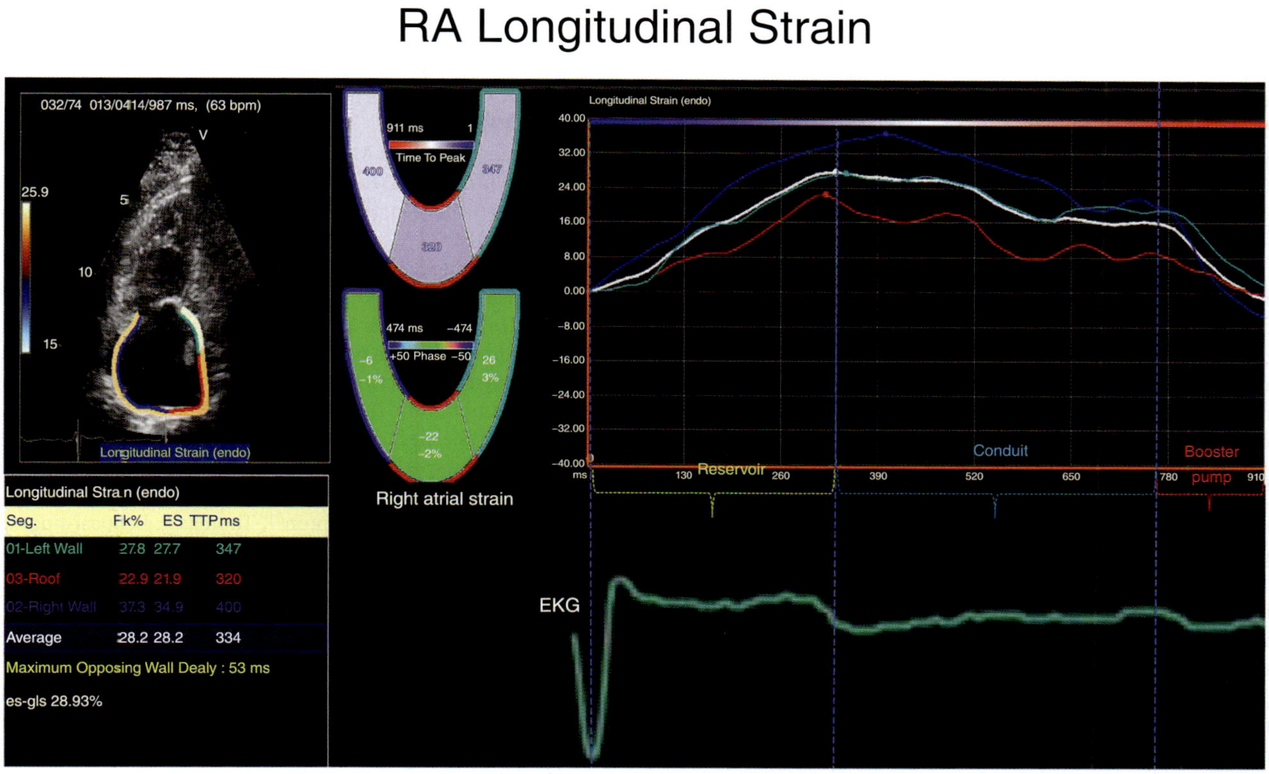

Fig. 7.17 An example of recording right atrial longitudinal strain, which is recorded and reported in much the same manner as it is for left atrial strain. The reservoir, conduit, and pump phases of right atrial function correspond to the same three phases for left atrial function and have similar connotations for the right side of the heart. *Left panel*, Right atrial strain analysis in the apical four-chamber view. The color-coded strain values for individual segments of the right atrium (RA) are shown, including: Left right atrial wall: peak strain, 27.8% Roof of the RA: peak strain, 22.9% Right atrial wall: peak strain, 37.3% The average right atrial strain is calculated at 28.2%. The strain delay between opposing right atrial walls in this patient is also provided (53 ms), indicative of possible dyssynchrony. *Seg*, Segment, *Pk*, Peak strain, *Es*, End-systolic strain, *TTP*, Time to peak strain, *Endo*, Endocardial border. *Right panel*, Recording of the right atrial strain curve representing the three phases of right atrial function during the cardiac cycle as indicated.

SUMMARY

Myocardial strain analysis represents a transformative advance in cardiac imaging, providing a sensitive, noninvasive measure of regional and global myocardial function across all four cardiac chambers. By leveraging speckle-tracking echocardiography (STE), clinicians can quantify myocardial deformation with precision, offering insights that surpass traditional metrics such as ejection fraction and atrial volumes. Strain imaging is particularly valuable for the early detection of subclinical dysfunction, risk stratification, and guiding therapeutic interventions.

This chapter highlights the growing clinical utility of strain imaging in both atrial and ventricular assessments. For the LV, LV-GLS has emerged as a critical marker for detecting subtle dysfunction, even in patients with preserved ejection fraction. It provides robust prognostic value for managing conditions such as heart failure, ischemic cardiomyopathy, and chemotherapy-induced cardiotoxicity. LV segmental strain analysis further localizes mechanical abnormalities, promoting earlier interventions in diseases like MR.

Atrial strain imaging has transformed the evaluation of left and right atrial mechanics. Left atrial strain parameters, including reservoir, conduit, and contractile strain, have proven invaluable in assessing compliance, remodeling, and thromboembolic risk. Reduced left atrial strain is a sensitive predictor of AF onset, recurrence, and associated thromboembolic events, underscoring its role in patient selection and follow-up for catheter and surgical ablation procedures. Similarly, right atrial strain has emerged as a powerful prognostic tool, particularly in patients with PAH and CTEPH. Right atrial strain parameters predict adverse outcomes and guide procedural decisions, such as the choice between biatrial and LA-only surgical AF ablation.

Despite these advances, significant challenges remain. Variability in strain measurements attributable to differences in imaging protocols, equipment, and software underscores the need for standardization. Furthermore, the interplay between atrial and ventricular function, as well as the influence of anatomic and procedural factors, warrants a more detailed investigation. For instance, the impact of right atrial cannulation sites and pericardial integrity on strain recovery highlights the complexity of integrating strain imaging into routine practice. As imaging technologies evolve, incorporating strain analysis into broader clinical workflows will undoubtedly refine patient management and improve outcomes. Future research should focus on establishing universal reference ranges, expanding strain applications to diverse cardiac pathologies, and integrating strain imaging with other advanced modalities such as myocardial work analysis and cardiac magnetic resonance imaging.

In conclusion, myocardial strain imaging provides unparalleled insights into cardiac mechanics, empowering clinicians to make informed decisions across a spectrum of cardiovascular conditions. Its adoption into routine practice marks a significant step forward in personalized cardiology and cardiac surgery, enabling earlier interventions, improved prognostication, and enhanced quality of care.

REFERENCES

1. Shah AM, Solomon SD. Myocardial deformation imaging: current status and future directions. *Circulation*. 2012;125(2):e244–e248.
2. Badano LP, Visentin S, Palermo C, et al. Echocardiographic techniques of deformation imaging in the evaluation of maternal cardiovascular system in patients with complicated pregnancies. *Biomed Res Int*. 2017;1:1–10.
3. Mondillo S, Galderisi M, Mele D, et al. Speckle-tracking echocardiography: a new technique for assessing myocardial function. *J Ultrasound Med*. 2011;30:71–83.
4. Bernal-Ramirez J, MC Díaz-Vesga, Talamilla M, et al. Exploring functional differences between the right and left ventricles to better understand right ventricular dysfunction. *Oxid Med Cell Longev*. 2021;1:9993060.
5. Nakatani S. Left ventricular rotation and twist: why should we learn? *J Cardiovasc Ultrasound*. 2011;19(1):1–6.
6. Opdahl A, Helle-Valle T, Skulstad H, Smiseth OA. Strain, strain rate, torsion, and twist: echocardiographic evaluation. *Curr Cardiol Rep*. 2015;17(3):568.
7. Akhan O, Demir E, Dogdus M, Cakan FO, Nalbantgil S. Speckle tracking echocardiography and left ventricular twist mechanics: predictive capabilities for noncompaction cardiomyopathy in the first degree relatives. *Int J Cardiovasc Imaging*. 2021;37(2):429–438.
8. Buijtendijk MFJ, Barnett P, van den Hoff MJB. Development of the human heart. *Am J Med Genet C Semin Med Genet*. 2020;184(1):7–22.
9. Combémorel N, Cavell N, Tyser RCV. Early heart development: examining the dynamics of function-form emergence. *Biochem Soc Trans*. 2024;28(4):1579–1589 52.
10. Muraru D, Badano LP, Hahn RT, et al. Atrial secondary tricuspid regurgitation: pathophysiology, definition, diagnosis, and treatment. *Eur Heart J*. 2024;45(11):895–911.
11. Deferm S, Bertrand PB, Verbrugge FH, et al. Atrial functional mitral regurgitation: JACC review topic of the week. *J Am Coll Cardiol*. 2019;73(19):2465–2476.
12. Smiseth OA, Torp H, Opdahl A, Haugaa KH. Urheim S: Myocardial strain imaging: how useful is it in clinical decision making? *Eur Heart J*. 2016;37(15):1196–1207.
13. Kislitsina ON, Cox JL, Shah SJ, et al. Preoperative left atrial strain abnormalities are associated with the development of postoperative atrial fibrillation following isolated coronary artery bypass surgery. *J Thorac Cardiovasc Surg*. 2022;164(3):917–924.
14. Mannina C, Ito K, Jin Z, et al. Left atrial strain and incident atrial fibrillation in older adults. *Am J Cardiol*. 2023;206:161–167.
15. Baman JR, Cox JL, McCarthy PM, et al. Atrial fibrillation and atrial cardiomyopathies. *J Cardiovasc Electrophysiol*. 2021;32(10):2845–2853.
16. Lee CS, Lin TH, Hsu PC, et al. Measuring left ventricular peak longitudinal systolic strain from a single beat in atrial fibrillation: validation of the index beat method. *J Am Soc Echocardiogr*. 2012;25(9):945–952.
17. Motoki H, Borowski AG, Shrestha K, et al. Incremental prognostic value of assessing left ventricular myocardial mechanics in patients with chronic systolic heart failure. *J Am Coll Cardiol*. 2012;60(20):2074–2081.
18. Puls M, Beuthner BE, Topci R, et al. Impact of myocardial fibrosis on left ventricular remodeling, recovery, and outcome after transcatheter aortic valve implantation in different haemodynamic subtypes of severe aortic stenosis. *Eur Heart J*. 2020;41(20):1903–1914.
19. Ross Agner BF, Katz MG, Williams ZR, et al. Left ventricular systolic function assessed by global longitudinal strain is impaired in atrial fibrillation compared to sinus rhythm. *J Atr Fibrillation*. 2017;10(4):1437.
20. Kuo JY, Chang SH, Sung KT, et al. Left ventricular dysfunction in atrial fibrillation and heart failure risk. *ESC Heart Fail*. 2020;7(6):3694–3706.
21. Kislitsina ON, Thomas JD, Crawford E, et al. Predictors of left ventricular dysfunction after surgery for degenerative mitral regurgitation. *Ann Thor Surg*. 2020;109:669–677.
22. Collier P, Phelan D, Klein A. A test in context: myocardial strain measured by speckle-tracking echocardiography. *J Am Coll Cardiol*. 2017;69:1043–1056.
23. Trivedi SJ, Altman M, Stanton T, Thomas L. Echocardiographic strain in clinical practice. *Heart Lung Circ*. 2019;28(9):1320–1330.
24. Zhang K, Sheu R, Zimmerman NM, et al. A Comparison of global longitudinal, circumferential, and radial strain to predict outcomes after cardiac surgery. *J Cardiothorac Vasc Anesth*. 2019;33(5):1315–1322.
25. Luis SA, Chan J, Pellikka PA. Echocardiographic assessment of left ventricular systolic function: an overview of contemporary techniques, including speckle-tracking echocardiography. *Mayo Clin Proc*. 2019;94(1):125–138.
26. Lang RM, Badano LP, Mor-Avi V, et al. Recommendations for cardiac chamber quantification by echocardiography in adults: an update from the American Society of Echocardiography and the European Association of Cardiovascular Imaging. *J Am Soc Echocardiogr*. 2015;28(1):1–39.
27. Cupps BP, Taggar AK, Reynolds LM, Lawton JS, Pasque MK. Regional myocardial contractile function: multiparametric strain mapping. *Interac Cardiovasc Thorac Surg*. 2010;10(6):953–957.
28. Lancaster TS, Kar J, Cupps BP, et al. Topographic mapping of left ventricular regional contractile injury in ischemic mitral regurgitation. *J Thorac Cardiovasc Surg*. 2017;154(1):149–158.
29. Kislitsina ON, Cox JL, Johnston DR, et al. Impact of left ventricular global and segmental dysfunction on early residual and late recurrent mitral regurgitation following mitral valve repair for degenerative disease. *Ann Thorac Surg*. Submitted May 2025.
30. Buber J, Luria D, Sternik L, et al. Left atrial contractile function following a successful modified Maze procedure at surgery and the risk for subsequent thromboembolic stroke. *J Am Coll Cardiol*. 2011;58(15):1614–1621.
31. Yamanaka K, Fujita M, Doi K, et al. Multi-slice computed tomography accurately quantifies left atrial size and function after the MAZE procedure. *Circulation*. 2006;114(1):I5–19.
32. Witkowski TG, Thomas JD, Debonnaire JMR, et al. Global longitudinal strain predicts left ventricular dysfunction after mitral valve repair. *Eur Heart J Cardiovasc Imag*. 2013;14(1):69–76.
33. Kim HM, Cho GY, Hwang IC, et al. Myocardial strain in prediction of outcomes after surgery for severe mitral regurgitation. *JACC Cardiovasc Imaging*. 2018;11:1235–1244.
34. Bernal-Ramirez J, MC Díaz-Vesga, Talamilla M, et al. Exploring functional differences between the right and left ventricles to better understand right ventricular dysfunction. *Oxid Med Cell Longev*. 2021(1):9993060.
35. Sun X, Ellis J, Kanda L, Corso PJ. The role of right ventricular function in mitral valve surgery. *Heart Surg Forum*. 2013;16(3):E170–E176.

36. Kislitsina O, Thomas J, Malaisrie S, et al. Preoperative left and right strain in surgical patients with atrial fibrillation after left atrial vs bi-atrial Maze procedure. *J Am Coll Cardiol*. 2022;79(9):1260.
37. Peters AC, Madhan AS, Kislitsina CN, et al. Temporal trends in right heart strain in patients undergoing pulmonary thromboendarterectomy for chronic thromboembolic pulmonary hypertension. *Echocardiography*. 2021;38(11):1932–1940.
38. Ji M, Wu W, He L, et al. Right ventricular longitudinal strain in patients with heart failure. *Diagnostics (Basel)*. 2022;12:445.
39. Kislitsina ON, Rich JD, Wilcox JE, et al. Propensity score-matched comparison of right ventricular strain in women and men before and after left ventricular assist device implantation. *Innovations*. 2022;17(2):102–110.
40. Arrigo M, Huber LC, Winnik S, Mikulicic F, Guidetti F, Frank M, Flammer AJ, Ruschitzka F. Right Ventricular Failure: Pathophysiology, Diagnosis and Treatment. *Card Fail Rev*. 2019;5(3):140–146.
41. Cho EJ, Jiamsripong P, Calleja AM, et al. Right ventricular free wall circumferential strain reflects graded elevation in acute right ventricular afterload. *Am J Physiol Heart Circ Physiol*. 2009;296(2):H413–H420.
42. Saha SK, Kiotsekoglou A, Gopal AS. Lindqvist P: Biatrial and right ventricular deformation imaging: implications of the recent EACVI consensus document in the clinics and beyond. *Echocardiography*. 2019;36:1910–1918.
43. Kislitsina ON, Kane B, Andrei A-C, et al. Subclinical changes in left and right ventricular strain as determined by speckle-tracking echocardiographic analysis after transcatheter or surgical aortic valve replacement. *J Am Coll Cardiol*. 2021;77(18):1178.
44. Scotti A, Curio J, Leone PP, et al. Management of volume overload in severe atrial-functional tricuspid regurgitation: improved feasibility of transcatheter edge-to-edge repair. *JACC Case Rep*. 2023;12:101776 19.
45. Utsunomiya H, Itabashi Y, Mihara H, et al. Functional tricuspid regurgitation caused by chronic atrial fibrillation: a real-time 3-dimensional transesophageal echocardiography study. *Circ Cardiovasc Imaging*. 2017;10(1):e004897.
46. Kislitsina O, Kane B, Maganti K, et al. Impact of paroxysmal atrial fibrillation on right ventricular function in patients undergoing mitral valve surgery for degenerative mitral regurgitation. *J Am Coll Cardiol*. 2020;75(11):2180.
47. Kislitsina O, Thomas J, Rigolin V, et al. Impact of preoperative paroxysmal atrial fibrillation on postoperative strain in patients with degenerative mitral regurgitation following mitral valve surgery. *J Am Coll Cardiol*. 2021;77(18):1777.
48. Arrigo M, Huber LC, Winnik S, et al. Right ventricular failure: pathophysiology, diagnosis and treatment. *Cardiol Fail Rev*. 2019;5(3):140–146.
49. Alfuhied A, Kanagala P, McCann GP, Singh A. Multi-modality assessment and role of left atrial function as an imaging biomarker in cardiovascular disease. *Int J Cardiovasc Imaging*. 2021;37(11):3355–3369.
50. Rao S, Pena C, Shurmur S, Nugent K. Atrial natriuretic peptide: structure, function, and physiological effects: a narrative review. *Curr Cardiol Rev*. 2021;17(6):e051121191003.
51. Sun BJ, Park JH. Echocardiographic measurement of left atrial strain- a key requirement in clinical practice. *Circ J*. 2021;86(1):6–13.
52. Al-Saady NM, Obel OA, Camm AJ. Left atrial appendage: structure, function, and role in thromboembolism. *Heart*. 1999;82:547–554.
53. Douglas YL, Jongbloed MRM, Groot A-D, et al. Histology of vascular myocardial wall of left atrial body after pulmonary venous incorporation. *Am J Cardiol*. 2006;97:662–670.
54. Pollick C, Taylor D. Assessment of left atrial appendage function by transesophageal echocardiography. Implications for the development of thrombus. *Circulation*. 1991;84:223–231.
55. Karim N, Ho SY, Nicol E, et al. The left atrial appendage in humans: structure, physiology, and pathogenesis, EP. *Europace*. 2020;22(1):5–18.
56. Kamalesh M, Copeland TB, Sawada S. Effect of inotropic stimulation on left atrial appendage function in atrial myopathy of chronic atrial fibrillation. *Echocardiography*. 2000;17:313–318.
57. Kamohara K, Popović ZB, Daimon M, et al. Impact of left atrial appendage exclusion on left atrial function. *J Thorac Cardiovasc Surg*. 2007;133(1):174–181.
58. Liu Y, Chen C, Chen Y, Su X, Li Z, Chen Y. Percutaneous left atrial appendage closure in patients with hypertrophic cardiomyopathy and persistent atrial fibrillation: 3-year-followed case series. *Medicine (Baltimore)*. 2023;102(17):333646.
59. Maron BJ, Desai MY, Nishimura RA, et al. Management of hypertrophic cardiomyopathy: JACC state-of-the-art review. *J Am Coll Cardiol*. 2022;79(4):390–414.
60. Aglan A, Fath AR, Maron BJ, et al. Percutaneous left atrial appendage closure for stroke prevention in hypertrophic cardiomyopathy patients with atrial fibrillation. *Heart Rhythm*. 2024;21(9):1677–1683.
61. Essayagh B, Resseguier N, Michel N, et al. Left atrial dysfunction as marker of poor outcome in patients with hypertrophic cardiomyopathy. *Arch Cardiovasc Dis*. 2021;114(2):96–104.
62. Kislitsina ON, Jankowski M, Rigolin VH, et al. The impact of preoperative four-chamber strain on failure of the maze IV procedure for atrial fibrillation: insights from conventional and speckle-tracking echocardiography. *Eur Heart J*. 2024;45 (Suppl 1):ehae666.041.
63. Kislitsina ON, Rigolin VH, Thomas J, et al. Failure of the surgical ablation of paroxysmal atrial fibrillation: the importance of preoperative left atrial and right atrial function estimated by conventional and speckle-tracking echocardiography. *J Am Coll Cardiol*. 2022;79(9):74.
64. Kojima T, Kawasaki M, Tanaka R, et al. Left atrial global and regional function in patients with paroxysmal atrial fibrillation has already been impaired before enlargement of left atrium: velocity vector imaging echocardiography study. *Eur Heart J Cardiovasc Imaging*. 2012;13(3):227–234.
65. Abhayaratna WP, Fatema K, Barnes ME, et al. Left atrial reservoir function as a potent marker for first atrial fibrillation or flutter in persons ≥ years of age. *Am J Cardiol*. 2008;101(11):1626–1629.
66. Baysan O, Ocaklı EP, Altuner TK, Kocaman SA. Atria: a comprehensive evaluation with echocardiography. *Heart Vessels Transpl*. 2017;1:11–19.
67. Nishikawa Y, Roberts JP, Tan P, et al. Effect of dynamic exercise on left atrial function in conscious dogs. *J Physiol*. 1994;481(2):457–468.
68. Zanaboni J, Panizza A, Marino PN. Left atrial conduit function modulates right ventricular afterload, exercise capacity and survival in heart failure patients. *J Cardiovasc Med*. 2021;22(5):396–404.
69. Gan GCH, Ferkh A, Boyd A, Thomas L. Left atrial function: evaluation by strain analysis. *Cardiovasc Diagn Ther*. 2018;8(1):29–46.
70. Chung M, Refaat M, Shen W, et al. Atrial fibrillation: JACC council perspectives. *J Am Coll Cardiol*. 2020;75(14):1689–1713.
71. Thomas L, Abhayaratna WP. Left atrial reverse remodeling: mechanisms, evaluation, and clinical significance. *JACC Cardiovasc Imaging*. 2017;10(1):65–77.
72. Hirose T, Kawasaki M, Tanaka R, et al. Left atrial function assessed by speckle tracking echocardiography as a predictor of

new-onset non-valvular atrial fibrillation: results from a prospective study in 580 adults. *Eur Heart J Cardiovasc Imaging.* 2012;13:243–250.
73. Al Ghamdi B, Hassan W. Atrial remodeling and atrial fibrillation: mechanistic interactions and clinical implications. *J Atr Fibrillation.* 2009;2(1):125.
74. Santos AB, Roca GQ, Claggett B, et al. Prognostic relevance of left atrial dysfunction in heart failure with preserved ejection fraction. *Circ Heart Fail.* 2016;9:e002763.
75. Morris DA, Belyavskiy E, Aravind-Kumar R, et al. Potential usefulness and clinical relevance of adding left atrial strain to left atrial volume index in the detection of left ventricular diastolic dysfunction. *JACC Cardiovasc Imaging.* 2018;11: 1405–1415.
76. Mondillo S, Cameli M, Caputo ML, et al. Early detection of left atrial strain abnormalities by speckle-tracking in hypertensive and diabetic patients with normal left atrial size. *J Am Soc Echocardiogr.* 2011;24:898–908.
77. Loardi C, Alamanni F, Galli C, et al. Surgical treatment of concomitant atrial fibrillation: focus onto atrial contractility. *Biomed Res Int.* 2015:274817.
78. Abu-Omar Y, Thorpe BS, Freeman C, et al. Recovery of left atrial contractile function after maze surgery in persistent longstanding atrial fibrillation. *J Am Coll Cardiol.* 2017;70:2309–2311.
79. Parwani AS, Morris DA, Blaschke F, et al. Left atrial strain predicts recurrence of atrial arrhythmias after catheter ablation of persistent atrial fibrillation. *Open Heart.* 2017;28: 4(1) e000572.
80. Bhave NM, Visovatti SH, Kulick B, et al. Right atrial strain is predictive of clinical outcomes and invasive hemodynamic data in group 1 pulmonary arterial hypertension. *Int J Cardiovasc Imaging.* 2017;33:847–855.
81. Tomaselli M, Badano LP, Cannone V, et al. Incremental value of right atrial strain analysis to predict atrial fibrillation recurrence after electrical cardioversion. *J Am Soc Echocardiogr.* 2023;36(9):945–955.
82. Olsen FJ, Biering-Sørensen T. Right atrial strain: tapping into a new reservoir of hemodynamic information. *Int J Cardiol.* 2021;326:226–228.
83. Haddad F, Spruijt OA, Denault AY, et al. Right heart score for predicting outcome in patients with idiopathic, familial or drug and toxin associated pulmonary arterial hypertension. *JACC Cardiovasc Imaging.* 2015;8:627–638.
84. Brunner NW, Haddad F, Kobayashi Y, et al. Prognostic utility of right atrial emptying fractions in pulmonary arterial hypertension. *Pulm Circ.* 2015;5:473–480.
85. Fukuda Y, Tanaka H, Ryo-Koriyama K, et al. Comprehensive functional assessment of right-sided heart using speckle tracking strain for patients with pulmonary hypertension. *Echocardiography.* 2016;33:1001–1008.
86. Krittanawong C, Maitra NS, Hassan Virk HU, et al. Normal ranges of right atrial strain: a systematic review and meta-analysis. *JACC Cardiovasc Imaging.* 2023;16(3):282–294.
87. Voeller RK, Aziz A, Maniar HS, et al. Differential modulation of right ventricular strain and right atrial mechanics in mild vs. severe pressure overload. *Am J Physiol Heart Circ Physiol.* 2011;301(6):H2362–H2371.
88. Tyberg JV, Taichman GC, Smith ER, et al. The relationship between pericardial pressure and right atrial pressure: an intraoperative study. *Circulation.* 1986;73(3):428–432.
89. Zanobini M, Saccocci M, Tamborini G, et al. Postoperative echocardiographic reduction of right ventricular function: is pericardial opening modality the main culprit? *BioMed Res Int.* 2017:4808757. https://doi.org/10.1155/2017/4808757.

8

Atrial Remodeling in Atrial Fibrillation: Atrial Fibrillation Begets Atrial Fibrillation

Niv Ad

CHAPTER OUTLINE

Atrial fibrillation (AF) is a potentially lethal arrhythmia, and unfortunately, its prevalence in the general population is increasing annually (see Chapter 2). From an interventional therapy standpoint, the two critical components of AF are the "triggers" that induce it and the "substrate" that sustains it. The types of AF triggers and their characteristics are discussed in detail in other chapters of this book, so this chapter focuses on the electrical and anatomic components of the substrate that sustains AF and how that substrate can change over time through a process called "atrial remodeling." Atrial remodeling can include changes in both the electrical characteristics of the atria (electrical remodeling) and changes in atrial anatomy such as enlargement, hypertrophy, and scarring (anatomic remodeling).

ATRIAL MYOPATHY AND THE CHANGING ATRIAL SUBSTRATE

Unlike sustained ventricular arrhythmias that are life-threatening if not addressed immediately, AF usually does not pose an imminent threat to a patient's life. The normal atrial substrate in patients without AF can evolve over time into a form of atrial cardiomyopathy, or atrial myopathy,[1] that is capable of sustaining AF. Patients with structural heart disease, such as severe mitral insufficiency, often develop atrial myopathy before they experience AF,[2] which can impact the decision on how to treat the AF. In addition, multiple episodes of AF and prolonged periods of AF can themselves aggravate atrial myopathy, leading to a spiraling of the entire pathophysiologic process.

Atrial stretch, inflammation, oxidative stress, and neurohumoral influences can initiate the development of atrial myopathy even in patients without structural heart disease. Atrial myopathies can result in electrical, functional, structural, and autonomic remodeling of the atrial substrate. In addition, the natural aging process and acquired structural heart disease can also lead to significant degenerative and fibrotic alterations of the atrial tissue, predisposing patients to develop AF. Natural aging and structural heart disease can also be associated. This may lead to significant degenerative, fibrotic, and other cellular and subcellular changes of the atrial tissue, predisposing patients to develop AF. In patients with advanced atrial tissue changes, the type of AF may "skip" the usual natural history of the arrhythmia from paroxysmal through persistent to long-standing persistent AF (LSpAF) with a significant burden of AF from its first event. Therefore, relating the type of AF to a certain pattern of ablation lesions may be too simplistic and can result in the potential for much higher failure.

Atrial fibrosis is an important component of atrial remodeling and is not only the result of the natural progression of AF; it is also a consequence of multiple catheter-based ablation procedures that leave scars throughout the atrial tissue. Thus, it is necessary to distinguish between the different precursors of atrial fibrosis. Changes in the atrial substrate related to the natural history of AF should be assessed in relation to potential interventions that may attenuate or modify the progression of the disease. One of the most significant pathophysiological processes in the development and progression of AF substrate change is the infiltration of fibrous tissue into the intermuscular atrial muscle space, a condition that is referred to as "endomysial" fibrosis.

Endomysial fibrosis is associated with atrial muscle dissociation and may exert its most important impact on the development of AF by promoting endocardial–epicardial dissociation that can modify atrial electrical activity[3,4] by facilitating three-dimensional reconfiguration of the atrial substrate. This enables the electrical waves to travel from one muscle layer to the other and increases the possible pathways for fibrillating waves, electrical fractionation, and dissociation.[5,6] The endomysial fibrosis phenomenon is especially significant in atrial areas with an abundance of atrial muscle fiber with clear orientation such as the posterior wall of the left atrium (LA). In the 1960s, the "multiple wavelet theory" was proposed by Gordon Moe,[7] describing how multiple wavefronts intersect with each other, leading to the breakdown of fibrillation wavefronts and the formation of new wavefronts. Later, de Groot and associates[8] showed that in many instances of AF, the atrial mass becomes large enough and the wavelengths short enough to allow "electrical triggers" to propagate and facilitate the formation of new reentrant wavelets. However, Cox and his group[9] showed the presence of multiple macro-reentrant circuits in the atria during AF that they believed to be the mechanism by which AF is sustained, and their findings served as the basis for the surgical Maze procedure and some catheter ablation procedures.

It is important to use caution when analyzing patients with AF after failed catheter ablations, especially when attempting to explain the mechanism of failure based on information that was gathered in patients with no prior catheter or surgical ablation procedures. The scar tissue created by catheter or surgical procedures themselves can modify the atrial substrate in a way that, if incomplete, can lead to AF. Subsequent electrophysiological mapping will then demonstrate only the mechanism of the recurrent AF secondary to failed ablation because it is no longer mapping the natural history and the pathophysiologic evolution of the original clinical AF. These types of findings may have ramifications related to treatment option decisions.

ATRIAL REMODELING

The LA serves as a reservoir, conduit, and volume booster and is not primarily a contractile chamber (see Chapter 43). Normal function of the atria is fundamental to maintaining optimal blood flow and allowing for adaptation to certain changes in ventricular function such as diastolic dysfunction.[10] Normal function of the LA is also paramount in reducing the risk of clot formation and systemic thromboembolism. AF is associated with a significant disruption of normal atrial function, but it also results in the induction of atrial remodeling. Atrial remodeling is a progressive process, and its severity is not always directly associated with the type of AF, the duration of AF, or the size of the atria. The dynamic and progressive nature of atrial remodeling leads to more frequent and widespread electrophysiologic abnormalities that further promote the perpetuation of AF,[1] leading to the phrase "AF begets AF."[11] The three types of atrial remodeling are electrical remodeling, functional remodeling, and structural remodeling.

Electrical Remodeling

The first signs of electrical remodeling can be identified within hours to several days after the onset of AF. The primary indicator of electrical remodeling during the early stages of AF is a shorter action potential duration that occurs as the result of acutely modified ion channels.[12] Acute electrical remodeling early on in the course of AF with rapid ventricular response plays a seminal role in compensating and achieving Ca^{2+} homeostasis.[1] The rapid atrial rate ultimately leads to intracellular calcium overload.[13] High intracellular calcium levels are cytotoxic. Therefore, autoprotective cellular mechanisms are activated to target and control the excess Ca^{2+}. These adaptive mechanisms lead to hyperpolarization and shortened action potentials.

Gap junction modification and alteration also occur early in the course of AF and play a major role in the development of macro-reentrant circuits. This process involves alteration in the function of connexins composing the gap junction channels that facilitate the electrical coupling of atrial cells. In general, the process results in dysfunctional gap junctions, varying in severity, throughout the atrial tissue and reduced conduction velocity.[14] The combination of a shorter refractory period and reduced atrial conduction velocities leads to significantly shorter atrial wavelengths, making them much more likely to become self-perpetuating. These changes become even more arrhythmogenic when there is a large enough atrial mass (or area) to allow multiple macro-reentrant circuits to exist simultaneously in the atria, the very definition of AF (see Chapters 4 and 5). What starts as an autoregulation process to control the excessive Ca^{2+} influx results in a self-perpetuating process that drives AF.[11]

Functional Remodeling

Functional remodeling is most often associated with an elevated risk for thromboembolic events and stroke caused by the loss of synchronized atrial contraction in patients with AF. However, the importance of reduced atrial function goes beyond the increased risk of embolic events. To understand the role of functional remodeling in patients with AF, attention should be directed toward the impaired atrial emptying function that occurs during an episode of AF and that may or may not be restored when patients either spontaneously revert or are converted back into sinus rhythm. The severity and the duration of atrial capacitance abnormalities and contractile dysfunction varies and is somewhat dependent on the duration of AF.[15] Therefore, the risk of thrombus formation secondary to atrial dysfunction during AF has to be monitored carefully in patients with AF.[16,17] The functional remodeling process can be defined as a total loss or diminished capacity of the atrial muscle's ability to stretch and contract normally. It is obvious that there is no effective atrial contraction during AF, but functional remodeling is often associated with reduced contractility function even when sinus rhythm is restored. Functional remodeling cannot be dissociated from electrical remodeling because it too is involved in the cellular processes that occur after Ca^{2+} influx into the cells as a result of AF and atrial tachycardia. The compensatory process to autoregulate the calcium levels occurs from, among other things, the activation of specific proteases that lead to the destruction of the Ca^{2+} channels and sarcomeres.[12] A brief period of AF allows recovery of the atrial myocardium, but a longer period of AF leads to irreversible damage and significant sarcomere destruction and loss.[17]

It is challenging to define the precise contribution of each component of atrial tachycardia-induced ventricular dysfunction because it may vary with the duration of the atrial arrhythmia, coexisting heart disease, drug therapy, and other potential factors. Therefore, the treatment of the underlying cause of the atrial tachycardia that is causing the ventricular cardiomyopathy may be more effective than treatments that address downstream consequences in the ventricle. It is important to recognize that in many patients, other coexisting cardiac conditions may have preceded the tachycardia-induced cardiomyopathy such as chronic volume overload associated with mitral valve disease or systolic and/or diastolic ventricular dysfunction. Volume overload leads to atrial dilatation and atrial stretch, causing increased atrial wall stiffness and reduced atrial compliance.[18]

Structural Remodeling

Like electrical and functional remodeling, structural remodeling is tightly linked to the progression of AF and is considered to be the consequence of multiple episodes of AF with varied durations. However, the notion that AF is more complex and persistent because of time-dependent structural remodeling alone should be viewed with caution, especially in surgical patients undergoing concomitant cardiac surgical procedures. The associated structural heart anomalies, such as mitral valve insufficiency, can cause structural remodeling of the atria before the first AF episode has occurred, so that the remodeling may not be directly related to the number of AF episodes and their duration.[1] Atrial structural remodeling is usually a combination of atrial dilatation and changes in atrial tissue architecture caused by the destruction of cardiomyocytes from enzymatic or apoptotic activity, modification in extracellular matrix function, and increased production of fibroblasts, leading to fibrosis and, in extreme situations, calcification.[19] In advanced states of atrial structural remodeling, dissociation of atrial muscle is observed because of a phenomenon that was mentioned earlier this chapter, endomysial fibrosis.[3,20]

Increased epicardial fat or adipose tissue is another significant aspect of structural remodeling. As surgeons, we often see a large amount of epicardial fat when operating on patients with AF, but the fat becomes more significant when it infiltrates the atrial myocardium. This can lead to electrical instability, which may impede the ability to ablate the atrium adequately as part of the treatment of AF.[21] Adipose tissue accumulation can also be detrimental to tissue energy consumption, inflammation, and fibrosis.[22] As mentioned, epicardial adipose tissue accumulation is more prominent in patients with persistent and LSpAF than in most patients with paroxysmal AF (PAF). This observation is consistent with the observation that patients with persistent AF usually exhibit more advanced structural remodeling than patients with PAF.[22,23]

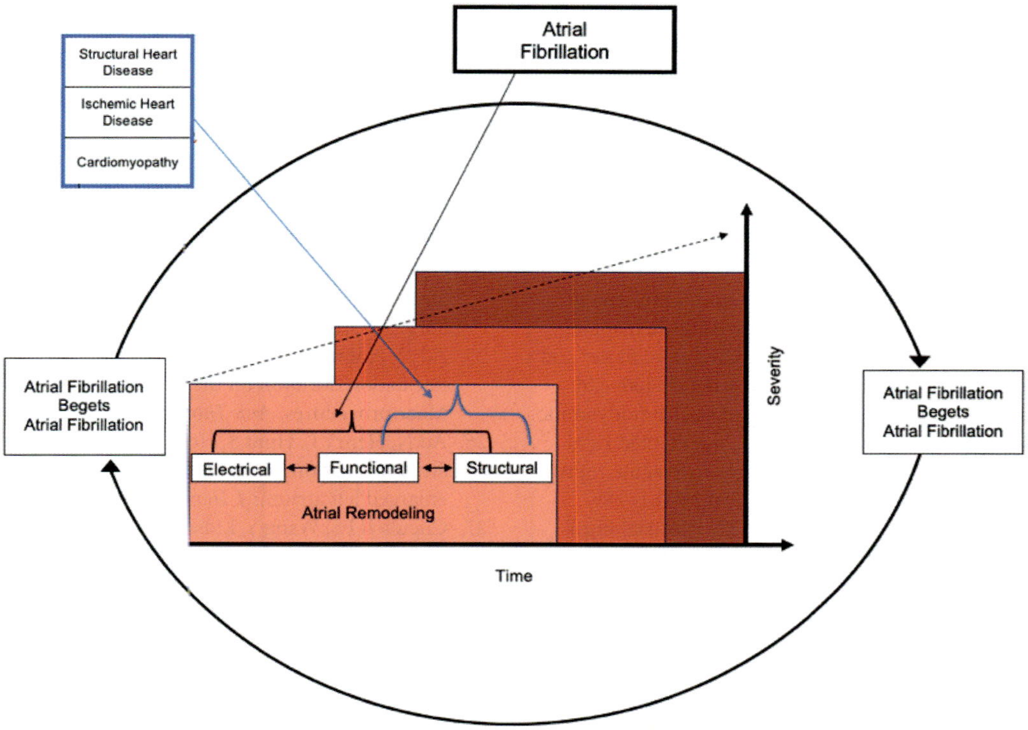

Fig. 8.1 Atrial remodeling (electrical, functional, and structural) gets more severe over time, and each component contributes to the pathophysiology of atrial fibrillation (AF). Nonarrhythmia triggers for atrial myopathy and remodeling exist in patients with structural heart disease, ischemic heart disease, and cardiomyopathy. In such instances, the degree of atrial remodeling is usually more severe with the events of AF. Therefore, the type and duration of AF would not correlate with the significance of atrial remodeling.

THE IMPORTANCE OF ATRIAL REMODELING

The surgical literature is clear regarding the factors associated with higher failure rates after the surgical ablation of AF. They include longer duration of AF, increased left atrial size, and more persistent types of AF,[24–26] all of which can be directly associated with the atrial remodeling process. The more advanced and chronic AF is, the harder it is to treat. This includes the ability to create contiguous, uniformly transmural ablation lesions and the number and the extent of lesions required to ablate the AF.

There is a clear difference between the complexity of the underlying electrophysiologic patterns of AF and the type of AF.[27] Thus, it is not surprising that global atrial mapping has consistently documented that both the right atrium and the LA are involved in sustaining persistent and LSpAF.[28] Other factors such as mitral valve disease that may itself cause atrial myopathy and remodeling should be approached as if the patient has associated advanced atrial remodeling when deciding on which lesion set and surgical ablation devices are to be used. Unfortunately, this principle has not been consistently observed clinically because many surgeons opt for a simpler pulmonary vein isolation procedure with or without ablation of the posterior left atrial wall for all types of AF. This suggests that the objective of the procedure is not the application of the best possible operation for the patient but rather the quickest and least invasive procedure that can be performed.[29–31] This approach largely disregards atrial myopathy and remodeling and can lead to inferior long-term success rates[32] (Fig. 8.1).

In many instances, the long duration of AF and enlarged left atria drive surgeons to the decision not to perform surgical ablation at all. Significant atrial remodeling combined with lower success rates when an ablation is not performed leads to unnecessary patient suffering with severe consequences as a result of remaining in AF with an atrial myopathy. A more collaborative approach between surgeons and electrophysiologists can lead to further improvement in overall decision-making and patient outcomes by selecting the optimal surgical approach and by performing a follow-up electrophysiological study within 6 months of the index procedure.

Atrial myopathy or remodeling is a critically important process that should always be considered when planning to treat patients with AF. New imaging platforms such as magnetic resonance imaging and photon-counting computed tomography scans and better assessments of atrial tissue remodeling via F-wave analysis and cellular signaling pathway analysis may further improve our understanding of atrial remodeling and our ability to deliver better patient care.[33–35]

REFERENCES

1. Schotten U, Verheule S, Kirchhof P, et al. Pathophysiological mechanisms of atrial fibrillation: a transitional appraisal. *Physiologic Rev.* 2011;91:265–325.
2. Vandervoort PM, Deferm S. The course of atrial functional mitral regurgitation: the atrium dictate the path. *Am J Cardiol.* 2024;83(16):1508–1510.
3. Massen B, Verheule S, Zeemering S, et al. Endomysial fibrosis, rather than overall connective tissue content is the main determinant of conduction disturbances in human atrial fibrillation. *EP Europace.* 2022;24:1015–1024.
4. Verheule S, Tuyis E, Gharaviri A, et al. Loss of continuity in the thin epicardial layer because of endomysial fibrosis increase the complexity of atrial fibrillatory conduction. *Circ Arrhyth Electrophys.* 2013;6:202–211.

5. Allessie MA, de Groot NM, Huben RP, et al. Electrophysiological substrate of long standing persistent atrial fibrillation in patients with structural heart disease: longitudinal dissociation. *Circ Arrhyth Electrophys.* 2010;3:606–615.
6. Iwasaki YK, Nishida K, Kato T, et al. Atrial fibrillation pathophysiology: implications for management. *Circ.* 2011;124:2264–2274.
7. Moe GK. On the multiple wavelet hypothesis of atrial fibrillation. *Arch Int Pharmacodyn Ther.* 1962;140:183.
8. de Groot NM, Allessie MA. Mapping of atrial fibrillation. *Ann Ist Super Sanita.* 2001;37:383–392.
9. Cox JL, Canavan TE, Schuessler RB, et al. The surgical treatment of atrial fibrillation. II. Intraoperative electrophysiologic mapping, and description of the electrophysiological basis of atrial flutter and atrial fibrillation. *J Thorac Cardiovac Surg.* 1991;101(3):406–426.
10. Goldstein JA, Harada A, Yagi Y, Barzilai B, Cox JL. Hemodynamic importance of systolic ventricular interaction, augmented right atrial contractility and atrioventricular synchrony in acute right ventricular dysfunction. *J Am Coll Cardiol.* 1990;16:181–189.
11. Wijffels MC, Kirchhof CJ, Dorland R, Allessie MA. Atrial fibrillation begets atrial fibrillation. A study in awake instrumented goats. *Circ.* 1995;92:1954–1968.
12. Allesie MA, Ausma J, Schotten U. Electrical, contractile, and structural remodeling during atrial fibrillation. *Cardiovasc Res.* 2002;54:230–246.
13. Ausma J, Dipersyn GD, Duimel H, et al. Changes in ultrastructural calcium distribution in goat atria during atrial fibrillation. *J Mol Cell Cardiol.* 2000;32:355–364.
14. Polontchouk L, Haefliger J, Ebelt B, et al. Effects of chronic atrial fibrillation on gap junction distribution in human and rat atria. *J Am Coll Cardiol.* 2001;38:883–891.
15. Schotten U, Verheule S, Kirchhof CJ, et al. Pathophysiological mechanisms of atrial fibrillation: a translational appraisal. *Physiol Rev.* 2011;91:265–325.
16. Wakili R, Yeh Y-H, Yan Qi X, et al. Multiple potential molecular contributors to atrial hypocontractility caused by atrial tachycardia remodeling in dogs. *Circ Arrhythm Elctrophysiol.* 2010;3:530–541.
17. Schotten U, Duytschaever M, Ausma J, et al. Electrical and contractile remodeling during the first days of atrial fibrillation go hand in hand. *Circ.* 2003;107:1433–1439.
18. Scotten U, de Haan S, Neuberger HR, et al. Loss of atrial contractility is primary cause for atrial dilatation in first days of atrial fibrillation. *Am J Physiol.* 2004;287:H2324–H2331.
19. Nattel S, Burstein B, Dobrev D. Atrial remodeling and atrial fibrillation: mechanisms and implications. *Circ Arrhyth Electrophysiol.* 2008;1:62–73.
20. Kharbanda RK, Garcia-Izquierdo E, Borgers AJ, et al. Focal activation patterns: breaking news grounds in the pathophysiology of atrial fibrillation. *Exp Rev Cardiovasc Ther.* 2018;16:479–488.
21. Gaeta M, Bandera F, Tassinari F, et al. Is special fat depot associated with atrial fibrillation? A systemic review and meta analysis. *Europace.* 2017;19:747–752.
22. Wong CX, Ganesan AN, Selvanayagam JB. Epicardial fat and atrial fibrillation: current evidence, potential mechanisms, clinical implications, and future directions. *Eur Heart J.* 2016;38:1294–1302.
23. Lin YK, Chen YJ, Chen SA. Potential atrial arrhythmogenicity of adipocytes: implications for the genesis of atrial fibrillation. *Med Hypotheses.* 2010;74:1026–1029.
24. Gaynor SL, Schuessler RB, Bally MS, et al. Surgical treatment of atrial fibrillation: predictors of late recurrence. *J Thor Cardiovasc Surg.* 2005;129:104–111.
25. Ad N, Holmes SD, Schuman DJ, Pritchard G. Impact of atrial fibrillation duration on the success of first-time concomitant Cox Maze procedures. *Ann Thorac Surg.* 2015;100:1613–1618.
26. Ad N, Henry L, Hunt S, Holmes SD. Should surgical ablation for atrial fibrillation be performed in patients with a significantly enlarged left atrium? *J Thor Cardiovasc Surg.* 2014;147:236–241.
27. Cuculich PS, Wang Y, Lidsay BD, et al. Noninvasive characterization of epicardial activation in humans with diverse atrial fibrillation patterns. *Circ.* 2010;122:364–372.
28. Ehrlich MP, Laufer G, Coti L, Peter M, Andreas M, Stix G, Ad N. Noninvasive mapping before surgical ablation for persistent, long-standing atrial fibrillation. *J Thor Cardiovasc Surg.* 2019;157:248–256.
29. Ad N, Suri R, Gammie JS, et al. Surgical ablation of atrial fibrillation trends and outcomes in North America. *J Thor Cardiovasc Surg.* 2012;144:1051–1060.
30. Ad N, Kang JK, Chinedozi IRD, et al. Statewide data on surgical ablation for atrial fibrillation: the data provide a path forward. *J Thor Cardiovasc Surg.* 2024;167:1766–1775.
31. Mehaffey JH, Charles EJ, Berens M, et al. Barriers to atrial fibrillation ablation during mitral valve surgery. *J Thor Cardiovasc Surg.* 2023;165:650–658.
32. Boyalla V, Haldar S, Khan H, et al. Long-term clinical outcomes and cost-effectiveness of catheter vs thoracoscopic surgical ablation in long-standing persistent atrial fibrillation using continuous cardiac monitoring: CASA-AF randomized controlled trial. *Heart Rhythm.* 2024;21:1562–1569.
33. Aquino GJ, Mastrodicasa D, Alabed S, et al. Radiology: cardiothoracic imaging highlights. *Radiol Cardiothorac Imag.* 2024;6:e240020.
34. Goudazi M, Ross MM, Zhou W, et al. Development of a novel proteomic approach for mitochondrial proteomics from cardiac tissue from patients with atrial fibrillation. *J Proteom Res.* 2011;10:3484–3492.
35. Kakuta T, Fukushima S, Minami K, et al. Novel risk score for predicting recurrence of atrial fibrillation after the Cryo-Maze procedure. *Eur J Cardio-Thorac Surg.* 2021;59:1218–1225.

9

Arrhythmia Surgery Prior to Atrial Fibrillation Surgery

James L. Cox

CHAPTER OUTLINE

As mentioned in Chapter 1, the first successful surgical procedure for a cardiac arrhythmia, the Wolff-Parkinson-White (WPW) syndrome, was performed in 1968.[1] The only new surgical procedure developed over the next 10 years was elective ablation of the atrioventricular (AV) node–His bundle complex[2] for various types of recalcitrant supraventricular arrhythmias that occasionally included intractable, medically refractory, highly symptomatic atrial fibrillation (AF).

In 1978, several groups developed direct surgical approaches for ischemic ventricular tachycardia (VT).[3–5] During the next 5 years, we modified the surgical technique for WPW syndrome[6] and developed new surgical procedures for the treatment of patients with non-ischemic VT,[7] automatic left atrial and right atrial tachycardias,[8,9] and AV node reentry tachycardia.[10] This chapter describes the surgical procedures developed for patients with "non-AF" arrhythmias, though surgery for them is considered to be obsolete today because they can be treated quite successfully with catheter ablation. Occasionally, however, neither drugs nor catheter ablation is successful in treating patients with non-AF arrhythmias, and surgical therapy is warranted. Such rare instances are problematic today because there are not many clinically active cardiac surgeons remaining who know how to perform the surgical procedures for non-AF arrhythmias. However, several principles of arrhythmia surgery were learned during the development of surgery for non-AF arrhythmias that were critical to the later development of the Maze procedure for AF, and these principles remain important for arrhythmia surgeons today.

WOLFF-PARKINSON-WHITE SYNDROME

Accessory AV connections (accessory pathways) are remnants of atrial myocardium in the AV groove that failed to resorb when the atria and ventricles were partitioning and separating during embryonic development. Most accessory pathways are capable of conducting electrical activity both *antegrade* from the atrium to the ventricle and *retrograde* from the ventricle to the atrium. However, there is no slowing of the speed of electrical propagation across accessory pathways like there is through the AV node where there is a delay of approximately 100 ms from the atria to the ventricles that appears as the "P-R interval" on a standard electrocardiogram (ECG). Therefore, during normal sinus rhythm (NSR), the atrial wavefront propagates across the accessory pathway faster and arrives in the ventricle earlier than it does through the AV node (Fig. 9.1). This early arrival of the atrial impulse in the ventricle is called "ventricular preexcitation," and it causes an early deflection of the QRS complex off the baseline that results in a "delta wave" appearing on the ECG and with resultant shortening of the P-R interval. Fusion of the two sites of activation in the ventricles from the impulse arriving both through the AV node and across the accessory pathway results in a widened QRS complex.

As long as the patient remains in sinus rhythm, heart function remains normal despite the abnormal sequence of ventricular activation (Fig. 9.2, *left panel*). The problem arises when an atrial impulse is blocked from crossing the accessory pathway antegrade (Fig. 9.2, *middle panel*), which can be caused by factors such as a premature atrial beat, a sudden change in the vagal nerve input to the heart, or sudden exposure of the heart to hot, cold, or irritating agents in the esophagus. The lack of *antegrade* conduction across the accessory pathway results in a normal ECG for that single beat. Because the accessory pathway was not activated during that cardiac cycle, it is not refractory, and the electrical activity in

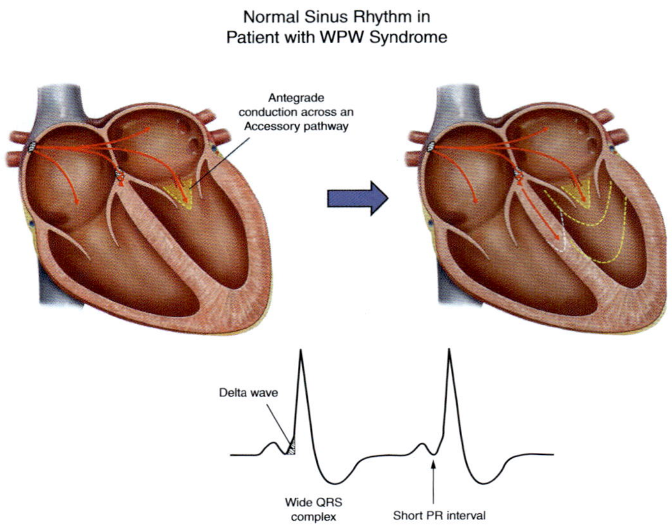

Fig. 9.1 Wolff-Parkinson-White (WPW) syndrome during normal sinus rhythm (NSR). *Left upper panel,* Antegrade conduction across both the atrioventricular (AV) node and the accessory pathway results in the wavefront reaching the ventricles earlier across the accessory pathway than through the AV node, where there is a normal slowing of conduction by about 100 ms. This results in "preexcitation" of the ventricles causing an early deflection off baseline on the standard electrocardiogram (ECG) ("delta wave") and an obligatory shortening of the P-R interval. *Right upper panel,* As the wavefront continues to propagate, the velocity of conduction in the His bundle and bundle branches becomes faster than the velocity of conduction through the ventricular myocardium, and the wavefront becomes fused, resulting in a widened QRS complex on the ECG. *Lower panel,* The combination of a delta wave, a shortened P-R interval, and a widened QRS complex on a standard ECG during normal sinus rhythm identifies the problem as WPW syndrome because no other abnormality causes these specific ECG findings.

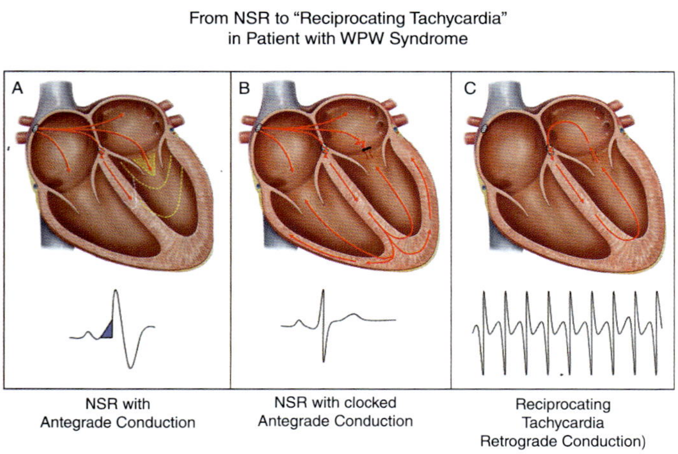

Fig. 9.2 Reciprocating tachycardia caused by Wolff-Parkinson-White (WPW) syndrome. (A) As long as a patient with WPW syndrome is in a normal sinus rhythm, there is no tachycardia. (B) If antegrade conduction of atrial activity across the accessory pathway is blocked for a single beat, the electrocardiogram for that one heartbeat will be normal. (C) However, when the ventricular activation reaches the base of the ventricle, it can propagate retrograde across the nonrefractory accessory pathway and establish a stable reciprocating tachycardia with antegrade atrioventricular node conduction and retrograde accessory pathway conduction. This is the classic "reciprocating tachycardia" associated with the WPW syndrome.

the ventricles can conduct retrograde across the pathway, resulting in a reciprocating tachycardia (Fig. 9.2, *right panel*). Some patients have what is called a "concealed" accessory pathway, which is one that conducts in the retrograde direction only. The lack of antegrade conduction across these accessory pathway means that these patients have an entirely normal ECG during NSR, hence the designation as a "concealed pathway."

Ventricular fibrillation with sudden death can occur in patients with the WPW syndrome who have the unfortunate combination of an antegrade-conducting accessory pathway with an abnormally short refractory period and who then develop an episode of atrial fibrillation (AF). In this case, the ventricles are no longer protected from the rapid and irregular bombardment of the AV node during AF, so the AF can be conducted from the atrium across the accessory pathway and cause the ventricles to fibrillate. One would expect this life-threatening combination to occur more often in older adult patients because of the higher incidence of AF associated with advancing age. However, most patients in our series who experienced this particular problem and were successfully resuscitated were young, perhaps because older patients with the condition experienced sudden death without successful resuscitation. Over the years, we operated on 14 patients with the WPW syndrome who had had a prior ventricular fibrillation cardiac arrest. Their average age was 21 years and included a 14-year-old male who was in the lead entering the final lap of the US Junior Amateur Indoor Bicycle Championship race. As he crossed the finish line with one lap to go (the "pistol lap"), the starter fired a pistol near his left ear, and he developed sudden AF that fibrillated his ventricles. He immediately collapsed on the track with sudden cardiac arrest. Fortunately, he was successfully resuscitated and subsequently underwent successful surgery for a left free-wall accessory pathway.

For purposes of WPW surgery, the AV groove was divided into four arbitrary anatomic spaces, the left free-wall space, right free-wall space, posterior septal space, and anterior septal space (Fig. 9.3). Accessory pathways are located in the left free-wall space in approximately 70% of patients with the WPW syndrome, the posterior septal space in 15%, the right free-wall space in 10%, and the anterior septal space in 5%. The objective of surgery is to divide the accessory pathway, which can been accomplished by dividing it at its atrial end or its ventricular end. Originally, intraoperative epicardial mapping of the atrium and ventricles was conducted with a single handheld electrode (Fig. 9.4A) to identify the precise location of the accessory pathway within one of the four anatomic spaces of the AV groove. The AV groove fat pad was then dissected away from the epicardial surface of the ventricle at the site of the accessory pathway and for 1 to 2 cm on either side of that site. This intentionally limited dissection left open the possibility that other nearby and unsuspected accessory pathways could be present that could become functional after surgery (Fig. 9.4B). In the first 200 patients who had this procedure between 1968 and 1980, the success rate for the initial operation was 61%. The overall success rate was 87% after approximately 25% of patients had a second, third, or fourth surgical procedure, and the incidence of heart block was 10.5%.[11] In the majority of these patients, the accessory pathways were divided via the endocardial approach with limited dissection, although epicardial dissection and cryoablation were used occasionally.

In 1980, we changed the surgical technique to a more anatomy-based procedure so that surgical dissection in the AV groove was no longer confined to the immediate site of the accessory pathway (Fig. 9.5A). In addition, a more expeditious way to localize the accessory pathway during surgery was created in 1983 using a "band electrode" array (Fig. 9.5B and C). After the accessory pathway was localized by preoperative and intraoperative mapping to one of the four anatomic

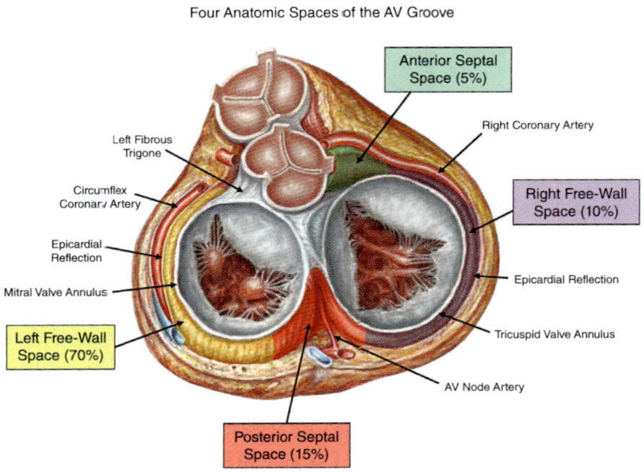

Fig. 9.3 Four anatomic spaces of the atrioventricular (AV) groove. The locations of accessory pathways in patients with Wolff-Parkinson-White syndrome are categorized as being located in one (or more) of four anatomic spaces in the AV groove. The most common site (70%) for accessory pathways to be located is in the *left free-wall space (yellow shading)* that is bordered by the mitral valve annulus and the epicardial reflection off the left ventricle (LV) and extends from the left fibrous trigone to the posterior superior process of the LV. The second most common site (15%) is the *posterior septal space (red shading)* that is bordered by the mitral and tricuspid valve annuli and the posterior portions of each ventricle and extends from the central fibrous body to the epicardial reflection off both posterior ventricles. In this space, the AV node artery penetrates the posterior ventricular septum and travels to the AV node in the atrial septum. (See text for further discussion.) The *right free-wall space (purple shading)* is the next most common site for accessory pathways to occur (10%) and is bordered by the tricuspid valve annulus and the epicardial reflection off the right ventricle (RV) and extends around the complete free wall of the RV. The least common site for accessory pathways (5%) is in the *anterior septal space (green shading)*, which is bordered by the tricuspid annulus, aortic root, and epicardial reflection off the anterior right ventricle.

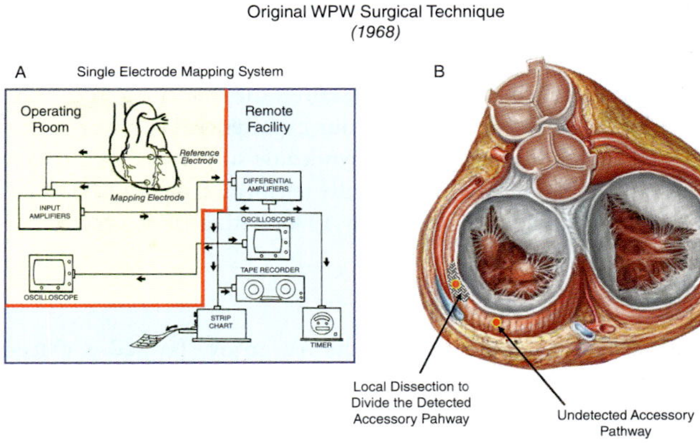

Fig. 9.4 (A) The original single-point, analog mapping system used to map patients with Wolff-Parkinson-White syndrome. One fixed reference electrode was sutured onto the epicardial surface of the right ventricle and a roving handheld exploring electrode was used to determine the activation sequence of the ventricles and the precise site of ventricular preexcitation. After documenting the insertion site of the accessory pathway in the ventricle, reciprocating tachycardia was induced if possible. If not, ventricular pacing near the pathway was performed. Both of these cause retrograde conduction across the accessory pathway. The atrial side of the atrioventricular (AV) groove was then mapped to confirm that site of atrial insertion of the pathway corresponded anatomically with the ventricular insertion site, and the subsequent surgical dissection was carried out in that vicinity of the AV groove. (B) The AV groove was exposed either from the endocardium or the epicardium at the mapped site of the accessory pathway and a plane of dissection was established between the AV groove fat pad and the top of the ventricle. This dissection plane was extended for 1 to 2 cm on each side of the pathway as determined by the intreoperative mapping. This limited dissection resulted in other unknown nearby accessory pathways sometimes being missed with the initial surgical procedure, requiring repeat surgery in approximately 25% of patients.

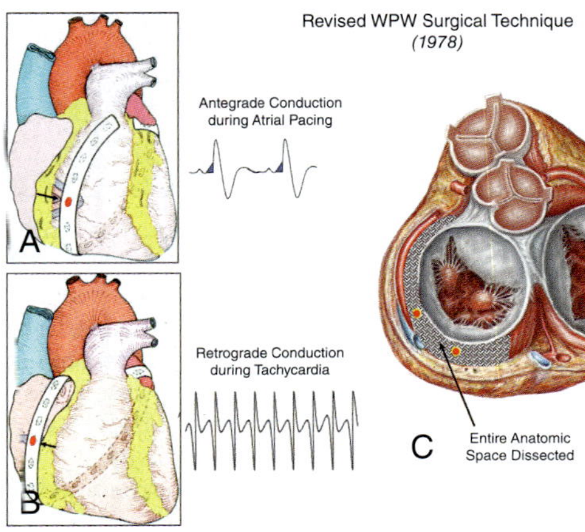

Fig. 9.5 (A) In 1980, we changed the surgical approach to dividing accessory pathways in patients with the Wolff-Parkinson-White (WPW) syndrome. Rather than continuing the practice of limited dissection in the atrioventricular (AV) groove based on the precise site of the accessory pathway (see Fig. 9.4), all pathways within a specific anatomic space received the same complete surgical dissection of that space based on its anatomic boundaries. Thus, intraoperative mapping was used primarily to confirm the findings of preoperative mapping in identifying the correct anatomic space harboring the pathway. In this example (new anatomic approach) and that in Fig. 9.4 (previous map-based approach), the accessory pathways were in the left free-wall space. (See text for further discussion.) (B and (C) In 1983, a new method for performing intraoperative mapping in patients with WPW syndrome employed the "band electrode" array in which 16 separate bipolar electrodes were imbedded in a cloth band that could be placed around the ventricular side of the AV groove to localize the site of ventricular preexcitation during normal sinus rhythm or atrial pacing (B) and around the atrial side of the AV groove to localize the atrial end of the accessory pathway during induced reciprocating tachycardia (C). This "band electrode" greatly decreased the time required for intraoperative mapping in patients with the WPW syndrome. (Modified from Cox JL, Gallagher JJ, Cain ME. Experience with 118 consecutive patients undergoing surgery for the Wolff-Parkinson-White syndrome. *J Thorac Cardiovasc Surg*. 1985;90:490–501.)

spaces, the AV groove fat pad in that *entire anatomic space* was dissected free of the epicardial surface of the ventricle. As a result, the only way we could fail surgically was for a previously undetected second accessory pathway to be located in an entirely different anatomic space. Fortunately, that rarely happened in our experience. We reported the first 118 patients undergoing WPW syndrome surgery using this new surgical approach,[6] and we subsequently performed nearly 1,000 such procedures during the 1980s and early 1990s with a 100% success rate after the initial operation.

Left Free-Wall Pathways

An endocardial incision to expose the AV groove fat pad is placed 2 mm above the posterior mitral valve annulus from the left fibrous trigone to the posterior atrial septum (Fig. 9.6A) Video 9-1. A plane of dissection is developed between the AV groove fat pad and the ventricular surface throughout the length of this incision (Fig. 9.6B). The anatomic boundaries of the left free-wall space are the mitral annulus, the epicardial reflection off the ventricle, the left fibrous trigone, and the posterior superior process of the left ventricle (LV). The dissection plane is developed in the entire space within those boundaries. Even though surgery for the WPW syndrome became an anatomy-based procedure after 1980, we continued to perform intraoperative mapping primarily to confirm that the preoperative mapping had correctly identified the anatomic space in the AV groove harboring the accessory pathway.

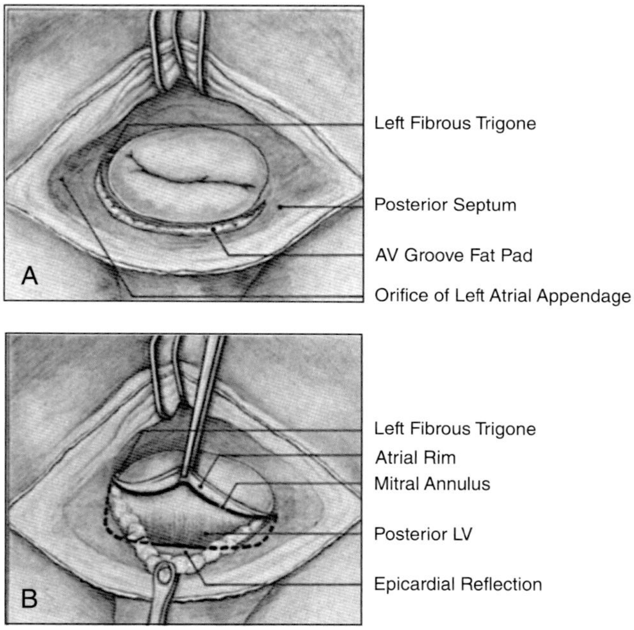

Fig. 9.6 Surgical technique for left free-wall accessory pathways. (A) The atrioventricular (AV) groove fat pad is exposed through a supra-annular incision placed 2 mm above and parallel to the mitral valve annulus extending from the left fibrous trigone to the posterior superior process of the left ventricle. As an added safety measure against residual A-V fibers crossing the mitral annulus, the two ends of this supra-annular incision were "squared off" to the mitral annulus to isolate the supra-annular strip of atrial myocardium from the rest of the heart.
(B) A plane of dissection is then established between the AV groove fat pad and the top of the posterior left ventricle throughout the length of the supraannular incision. The mitral valve annulus is meticulously freed of any visible fibers between the atrium and ventricle, and the dissection is extended all the way to the epicardial reflection off the ventricle. (Modified from Cox JL, Gallagher JJ, Cain ME. Experience with 118 consecutive patients undergoing surgery for the Wolff-Parkinson-White syndrome. *J Thorac Cardiovasc Surg.* 1985;90:490–501.)

Posterior Septal Pathways

An endocardial incision to expose the fat pad in the posterior septal space is placed 2 mm above the tricuspid valve annulus beginning well posterior to the membranous atrial septum and extending counterclockwise onto the posterior right atrial free-wall (Fig. 9.7A). The boundaries of the posterior septal space are the central fibrous body, the posteromedial mitral valve annulus, the epicardial reflection off the posterior ventricles, and the posterior right ventricular free wall, and the dissection plane is developed in the entire space within these boundaries (Fig. 9.7B). The floor of the posterior septal space is the posterosuperior ventricular septum, and it is often penetrated by the AV node artery. Prior to 1980, every effort was expended to avoid

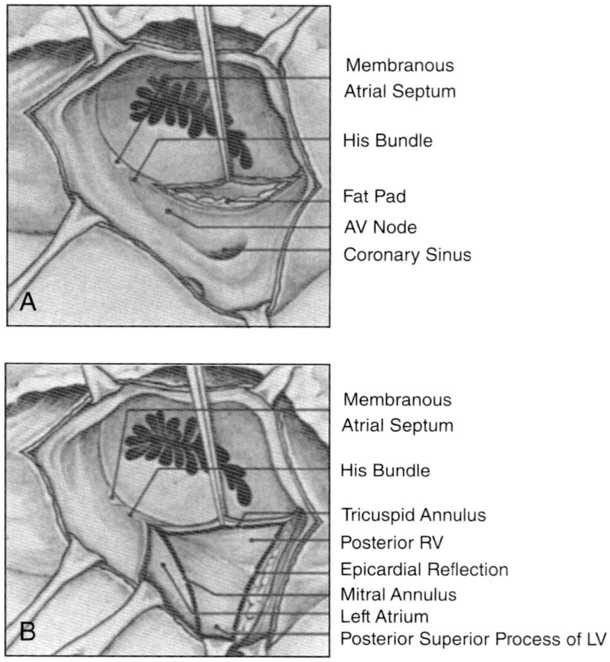

Fig. 9.7 Surgical technique for posterior septal accessory pathways: (A) The atrioventricular (AV) groove fat pad in the posterior septal space was exposed by a supra-annular incision placed 2 mm above and parallel to the tricuspid valve annulus extending from the posterior central fibrous body to the posterior free-wall of the right ventricle.
(B) A plane of dissection was then established between the fat pad and the top of the posterior ventricular septum, and the dissection was extended throughout the boundaries of the posterior septal space, including the posteromedial mitral valve annulus and the posteromedial tricuspid valve annulus and the epicardial reflection off the posterior left and right ventricles. The AV node artery penetrates the posterior ventricular septum in the mid-portion of this space and prior to 1980, it was spared for fear of creating heart block. However, the failure rate of the approach was excessively high. In the revised more anatomic approach, the AV node artery was specifically identified and purposely divided between two vascular clips because of a suspicion that the accessory pathway was accompanying the AV node artery between the ventricular septum and the atrial septum where the AV node is located. Elective division of the AV node artery was performed in 114 consecutive patients with posterior septal pathways, and not one case of heart block occurred. (See text for further discussion.) (Modified from Cox JL, Gallagher JJ, Cain ME. Experience with 118 consecutive patients undergoing surgery for the Wolff-Parkinson-White syndrome. *J Thorac Cardiovasc Surg.* 1985;90:490–501.)

dividing the AV node artery out of fear of creating heart block. However, that approach resulted in an exceptionally high failure rate. We subsequently reasoned that because accessory pathways often travel in one bundle with an artery, the AV node artery should be identified, skeletonized, and purposely divided in all patients with a posterior septal pathway. Division of the AV node artery did not cause heart block because it is not an end artery. I purposely divided the AV node artery in 114 consecutive patients with posterior septal accessory pathways without a single case of postoperative heart block.

Right Free-Wall Pathways

An endocardial incision to expose the right AV groove fat pad is placed 3 mm above the tricuspid valve annulus throughout the length of the right atrial free-wall. The boundaries of the right free-wall space are the tricuspid annulus and the epicardial reflection off the right ventricle (RV) throughout the extent of the right ventricular free wall. The dissection plane is developed in the entire space within these boundaries. The right coronary resides in this fat pad and must be protected from injury during dissection. In addition, the free walls of the right atrium (RA) and RV "foldover" one another, so the accessory pathway can be missed if only the fat pad is separated from the ventricular epicardium (see Chapter 3, Fig. 3.22). To overcome this potential problem, it is wise to place a cryolesion at each end of the supraannular incision to isolate the intervening 2-mm strip of atrial muscle from the rest of the heart in case there is an accessory pathway within the folded-over portion of the RA–RV free wall.

Anterior Septal Pathways

An endocardial incision to expose the AV groove fat pad is placed 3 mm above the tricuspid annulus from the membranous atrial septum to the anterior right atrial free wall. The boundaries of the anterior septal space are the tricuspid annulus, the root of the aorta, the epicardial reflection off the ventricle that is immediately under the proximal right coronary artery, and the free wall of the RV. The dissection plane is developed in the entire space within those boundaries. The first 1 to 2 cm of the right coronary artery is not in the actual AV groove, and the dissection plane is safest in this area, though it is still beneath the right coronary artery after the latter joins the right AV groove.

This anatomic approach for dividing accessory pathways in all four anatomic spaces resulted in an improvement of the success rate of the *initial* operation for the WPW syndrome from 61% to 100%, and there were no instances of permanent heart block.

ATRIOVENTRICULAR NODE REENTRY TACHYCARDIA

AV node reentry tachycardia (AVNRT) results from the presence of two pathways of conduction through the AV node, a fast pathway and a slow pathway. During NSR, antegrade conduction travels down both pathways, but because it reaches the His bundle earlier through the fast pathway, antegrade conduction in the slow pathway is blocked at its distal end (Fig. 9.8A). However, if antegrade block occurs halfway through the fast pathway, the impulse in the slow pathway will not only activate the ventricles, but it can also conduct retrograde in the fast pathway to the site of block (Fig. 9.8B). Normally, this will not cause reentry because the refractory period in the fast pathway is not short enough to allow it to develop. However, if antegrade conduction block occurs in the *proximal* end of the fast pathway (Fig. 9.8C), the retrograde conduction coming from the slow pathway can cause reentry within the AV node (Fig. 9.8D). This AV node reentrant circuit then activates both the ventricles and the atria, and it does so quite rapidly because of the relatively small size of the reentrant circuit.

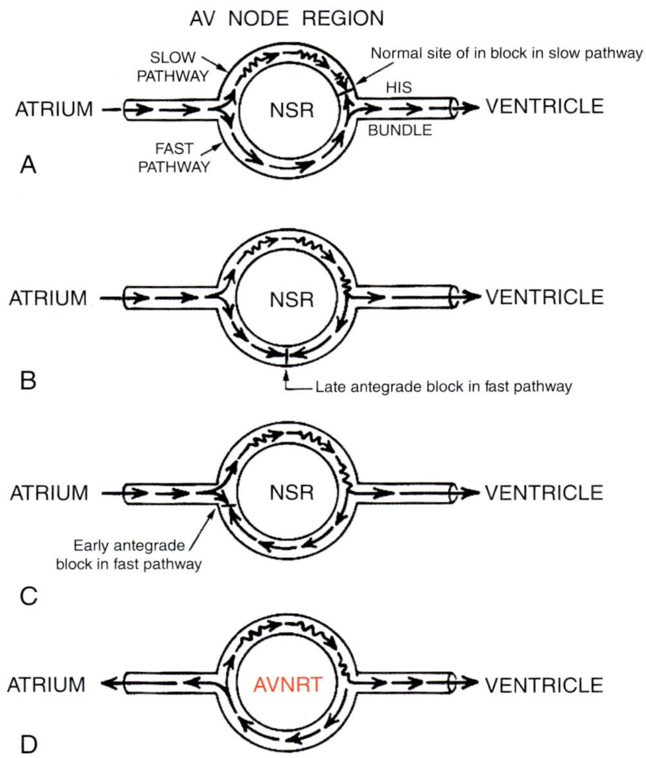

Fig. 9.8 (A) Atrioventricular node reentry tachycardia (AVNRT) is caused by the presence of two separate conduction pathways through the atrioventricular (AV) node, one fast pathway and one slow pathway. Because conduction is faster through the fast pathway, conduction is normally blocked at the distal end of the slow pathway. (B) If antegrade block occurs in the distal or middle portion of the fast pathway, there are no adverse sequelae because most of the fast pathway is refractory even though it is also blocked. (C) However, if antegrade block occurs in the proximal portion of the fast pathway, this entire pathway will not be refractory, and the impulse conducted through the slow pathway can reenter it in the retrograde direction. (D) This can result in a reentrant circuit forming within the AV node and a tachycardia that activates the atria and the ventricles simultaneously.

In 1979, Dr. Sealy and I were performing an elective open His bundle ablation in a patient with intractable AVNRT. As described in Chapter 11, it was surprisingly difficult to block the His bundle surgically in these cases, so surgical dissection in the region of the AV node–His bundle complex was routinely more extensive than one might expect. During the dissection, the patient's AVNRT suddenly terminated *but without heart block*. The sudden AVNRT termination with restoration of NSR, rather than heart block, suggested that we had inadvertently blocked only one of the two conduction pathways in the AV node. This meant that the two conduction pathways were *physically separated* by enough distance that one of them could be divided without injuring the other.

This singular fortuitous event could not be repeated in subsequent patients despite all efforts to do so, but it stimulated me to try to develop a reproduceable way to block only one of AV node conduction pathways in patients with AVNRT while leaving the second pathway intact. I believed that our best option was to use a small-tipped cryoprobe, rather than a scalpel, to "sneak up" on the AV node and selectively block only one of the pathways while leaving the other pathway intact. Frigitronics, Inc. made us a special small cryoprobe with a 2-mm active

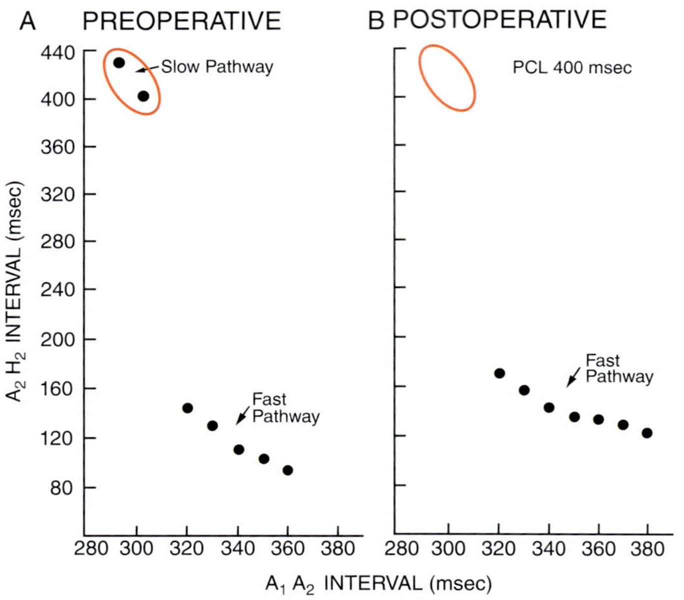

Fig. 9.9 Specific pacing studies can identify the two atrioventricular (AV) node pathways in a patient with AV node reentry tachycardia. (A) By plotting the A_1A_2 interval against the A_2H_2 interval, the slow pathway and fast pathway are easily distinguishable. In this particular study, the pacing studies were performed in a dog with dual AV conduction pathways. (B) After performing the discrete cryosurgery procedure around the AV node (see Fig. 9.10), the fast pathway is no longer present. *A,* Atrium; *H,* His bundle; *PCL,* pacing cycle length. (Reproduced from Cox JL. Surgery for cardiac arrhythmias. *Cur Prob Cardiol.* 1983;8(4):1–60.)

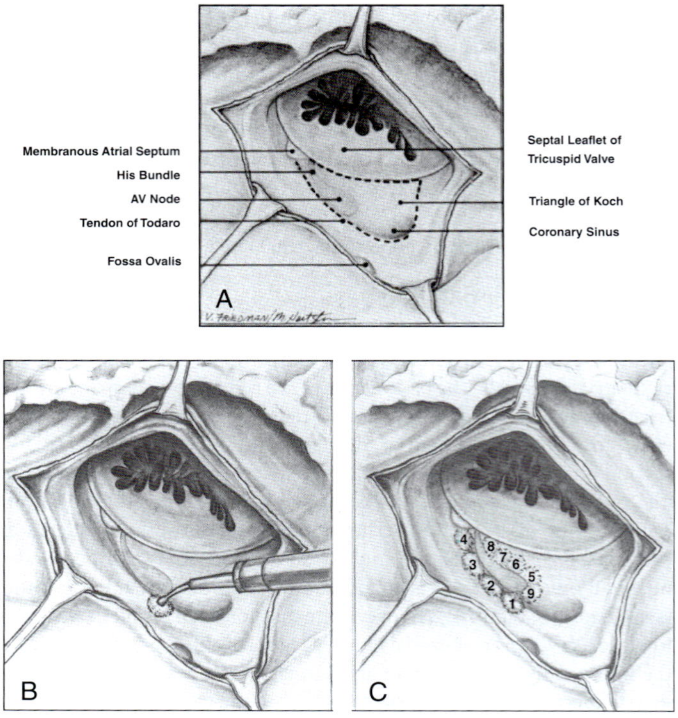

Fig. 9.10 **Discrete cryosurgical procedure for atrioventricular node reentry tachycardia.** (A) The boundaries and contents of the triangle of Koch in the atrial septum from the surgeon's view. (B) The discrete cryosurgical procedure begins by creating a small cryolesion at the lateral end of the tendon of Todaro with a 2-mm cryoprobe. (C) Sequential overlapping cryolesions are placed around the borders of the triangle of Koch while the A-V interval is monitored on a beat-to-beat basis. (Reproduced from Cox JL, Holman WL, Cain ME. Cryosurgical treatment of atrio-ventricular node reentry tachycardia. *Circulation.* 1987;76:1329–1336.)

tip, and I assigned the task of trying to block a single pathway to Drs. William Holman and Masatoshi Ikeshita, who had joined our research laboratory in the summer of 1980. The problem was that dogs do not have AVNRT, but by performing pacing studies on every animal entering our laboratory, Holman was able to find three dogs that had dual AV node conduction pathways. The procedure that we had envisioned of "sneaking up" on the AV node using a small cryoprobe was successful in blocking only one of the pathways in all three of those dogs while leaving the second pathway intact, thereby negating the need for a postoperative pacemaker (Fig. 9.9).[12]

After institutional review board approval in August 1982, we performed the first "discrete cryosurgery procedure" for AVNRT in a 35-year-old female patient in whom we successfully divided the slow pathway in the AV node while leaving the fast pathway intact. Dynamic teamwork between the surgeon and the electrophysiologist was required during the surgical procedure because of the close monitoring of the A-V interval required during application of the cryosurgery. We started the procedure by placing a series of overlapping cryolesions around the borders of the triangle of Koch (Fig. 9.10).[10] Electrical signals were recorded on a storage oscilloscope from leads I, aVF, and V_5R and from epicardial electrodes on the surfaces of the RA and RV (Fig. 9.11). Each sweep of the signals was triggered on the RA electrogram and stored on the oscilloscope screen so that with each heartbeat, the A-V interval could be visualized and compared with the A-V interval of the previous heartbeat. After encircling the triangle of Koch, 2-minute cryolesions were placed inside the triangle beginning in the region closest to the os of the coronary and working toward the apex of the triangle. During that time, if the patient suddenly developed complete heart block (i.e., the ventricular deflection disappeared), the cryothermia was immediately stopped. Within a few seconds, the ventricular deflection would reappear, and the

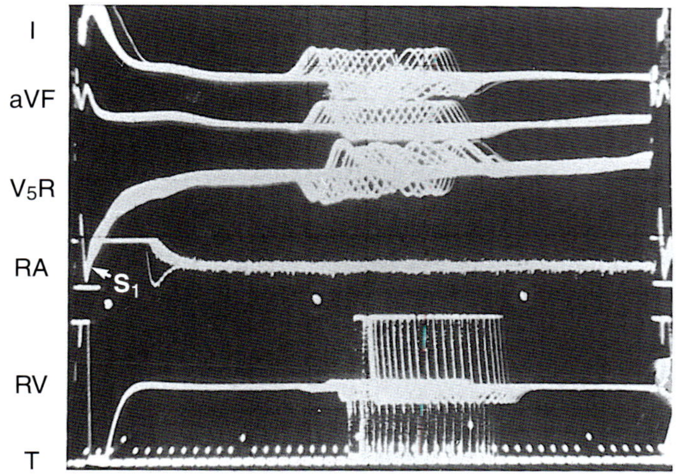

Fig. 9.11 During the discrete cryosurgical procedure, the A-V interval is monitored on a beat-to-beat basis using a storage oscilloscope with a screen sweep on every heartbeat that is triggered on the atrial pacing spike. This not only allows the A-V interval to be stored, but it also graphically demonstrates any prolongation of the A-V interval with every heartbeat. (See text for details.) (Reproduced from Cox JL, Holman WL, Cain ME. Cryosurgical treatment of atrio-ventricular node reentry tachycardia. *Circulation.* 1987;76:1329–1336.)

A-V interval would start to shorten with each heartbeat. The endpoint of the surgical procedure was the inability to place a cryolesion anywhere within the triangle of Koch for at least 2 minutes without causing complete heart block.

During the remainder of the decade, we had a 100% success rate for this cryosurgical technique for AVNRT and Dr. David Johnson from Westmead in Sydney, Australia, attained a 92% success rate using a surgical dissection technique rather than discrete cryosurgery.[13] When radiofrequency (RF) catheter ablation became possible around 1990, the interventional electrophysiologists used our surgical procedure as a model for their RF catheter procedure with essentially the same success rates.[14]

AUTOMATIC LEFT ATRIAL TACHYCARDIA

Automatic atrial tachycardias in the left atrium (LA) tend to be singular in origin, stable in location, and regular in rhythm and they can occur anywhere in the LA (Fig. 9.12). Most automatic left atrial tachycardias are believed to be caused by abnormal phase 4 depolarization in a few localized atrial cells, but some have been shown to arise from cell rests near the orifice of the left superior pulmonary vein, which is a mirror image of the location of the anatomic sinoatrial (SA) node in the RA.[15] In the 1970s, preoperative mapping could localize the automatic focus generally to the LA but not to a precise site in the atrium. Therefore, intraoperative mapping was very important in localizing the automatic focus so that it could then be either surgically isolated or ablated. Unfortunately, automatic tachycardias are quite susceptible to being suppressed by general anesthesia, so it was common to operate on these patients with the intention of mapping them and ablating the focus only to have the arrhythmia disappear just before the mapping procedure could be performed. Because automatic arrhythmias do not respond to programmed electrical stimulation techniques, the left atrial tachycardia could not be induced for mapping in the operating room. The only surgical alternative was to electively ablate the His bundle and insert a permanent ventricular pacemaker. Unfortunately, most of the patients referred to us with automatic left atrial tachycardia were in their teens or early 20s, making the life-long dependency on a permanent pacemaker even more undesirable.

After just such a case in a 16-year-old otherwise healthy male in 1978, it occurred to me that it should be possible to cure these patients without resorting to a His bundle ablation and permanent pacemaker implantation. We knew from preoperative mapping that the automatic focus was located somewhere in the LA, so if we could not map it intraoperatively because of the general anesthesia, we might be able to simply confine it to the LA. Because the SA node is in the RA and the AV node–His bundle complex is in the atrial septum, it should be possible to isolate the entire body of the LA from the rest of the heart while leaving the specialized conduction system intact. This would mean that even though the tachycardia persisted in the LA, the RA and the ventricles would be in a sinus rhythm (Fig. 9.13).

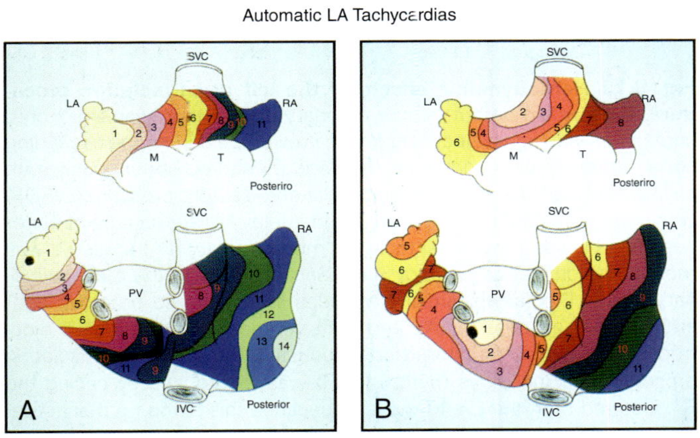

Fig. 9.12 (A) Automatic left atrial tachycardia originating in the left atrial appendage. This automatic focus was permanently ablated during the tachycardia with one application of a 2.5-cm cryoprobe at the site of the black dot. (B) Automatic left atrial tachycardia in a different patient apparently located just beneath the inferior pulmonary veins on the posterior wall of the left atrium (LA). This site was cryoablated with a 2.5-cm cryoprobe during the tachycardia *(black dot)*, the tachycardia terminated, and the patient was returned to the postoperative intensive care unit. Approximately 1 hour later, the tachycardia reappeared, and the patient was immediately returned to the operating room. This time we mapped between the two sets of pulmonary veins (PVs), which had not been done earlier, and found a site that was even earlier that the one we had ablated. This true site of origin of the automatic arrhythmia was then permanently cryoablated. The problem was that we had not "bracketed" the apparent earliest site of activation in the first map. (Note the upper border of the *yellow area number 1*) This area appeared to be the earliest site of activation, but it actually was not. We had made the same mapping error that was made by Sealy on the second patient he operated on in 1968 for the Wolff-Parkinson-White syndrome who had an anterior septal accessory pathway, not a right free-wall pathway, and on both of Guiraudon's patients with non-ischemic ventricular tachycardia in 1979 (see below), who likely had arrhythmias that originated from sites in the supracristal ventricular septum. IVC, Inferior vena cava; *M*, mitral valve; *RA*, right atrium; *SVC*, superior vena cava; *T*, tricuspid valve.

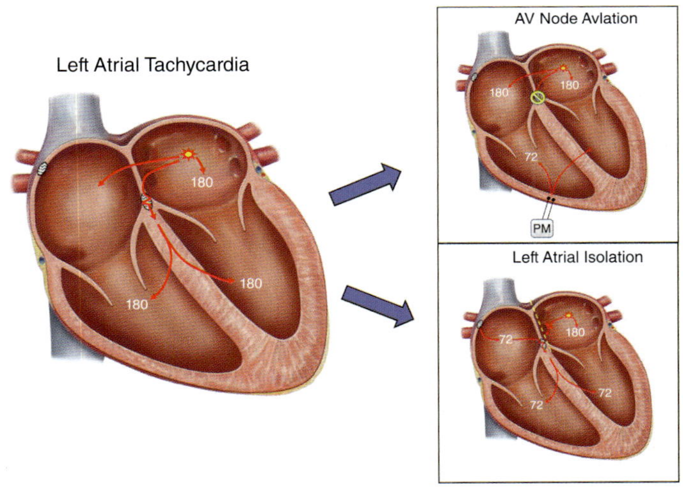

Fig. 9.13 Rationale for the left atrial isolation procedure. *Left panel,* Preoperative mapping showed the automatic tachycardia to be arising in the left atrium (LA). However, the precise location of the automatic focus could not be determined intraoperatively because the general anesthesia suppressed the arrhythmia, and it could not be mapped. The numbers represent rates of activation in each of the four heart chambers. In this case, the automatic left atrial tachycardia of 180 beats/min is driving the entire heart at the same rate. *Right upper panel,* The traditional way to treat this problem was to electively ablate the His bundle and insert a permanent ventricular pacemaker. This confined the automatic driver to the atria and allowed the ventricular rate to be controlled with a pacemaker. *Right lower panel,* Because the sinoatrial node is in the right atrium and the atrioventricular node–His bundle complex is in the atrial septum, if the body of the LA that is known to harbor the automatic focus could be separated (isolated) from the rest of the heart, the arrhythmia could be confined to the LA, the other three cardiac chambers could remain in a sinus rhythm, and a permanent pacemaker could be avoided. *PM*, pacemaker.

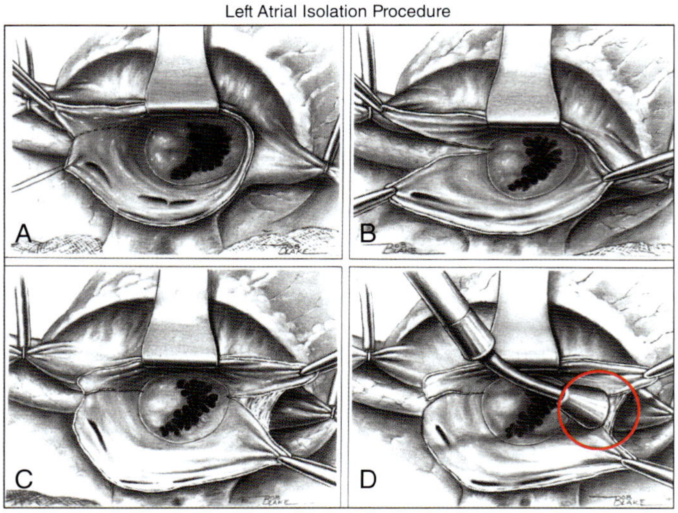

Fig. 9.14 Left atrial isolation procedure. (A) The left atrium is entered via a standard atriotomy in Waterston's groove. The mitral valve in dogs is not oriented precisely the same as in humans, whose mitral valves would be more counterclockwise than illustrated in this figure. (B) The atriotomy that is just to the left of the atrial septum and is extended anteriorly down to the level of the anterior mitral annulus. This exposes the underlying aortic root and proximal ascending aorta. (C) The atriotomy is then extended posteriorly to the level of the posterior mitral annulus remaining just to the left of the atrial septum. When the level of the atrioventricular (AV) groove is reached posteriorly, the atriotomy remains transmural and fully exposes the AV groove fat pad (containing the circumflex coronary artery) and the coronary sinus. (D) The final step is to isolate and ablate the coronary sinus circumferentially in the plane of the atriotomy *(red circle)*. This was the first time that the coronary sinus was shown to be capable of conducting electrical activity and that its ablation was essential to stop electrical conduction across what was later designated as the "Left Atrial isthmus" between the inferior pulmonary veins and the posterior mitral valve annulus. See text for further discussion. (Reproduced from Williams JM, Ungerleider RM, Lofland GK, Cox JL. Left atrial isolation: new technique for the treatment of supraventricular arrhythmias. *J Thorac Cardiovasc Surg.* 1980;80:373.)

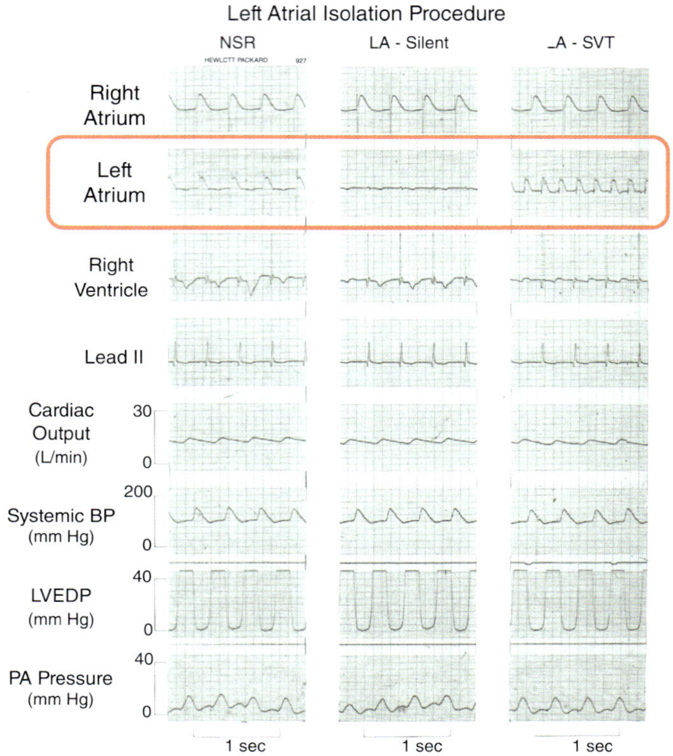

Fig. 9.15 Hemodynamic effects of the left atrial isolation procedure. The cardiac output (minus coronary artery flow) was monitored continuously using an electromagnetic flow probe around the ascending aorta. Systemic blood pressure (BP) was monitored continuously with an indwelling arterial line. Left ventricular end-diastolic pressure (LVEDP) was monitored continuously with a high-fidelity Millar pressure catheter positioned inside the left ventricle. Pulmonary artery (PA) pressure was monitored continuously with a Swan-Ganz catheter in the main pulmonary artery. Bipolar epicardial electrodes were sutured onto the right atrium (RA), left atrium (LA), and right ventricle, and the lead II electrocardiogram was monitored continuously. After a left atrial isolation procedure, normal sinus rhythm (NSR) was reproduced by pacing the RA first and then the LA 40 ms later because this is the normal activation time difference between the two atria. All of the baseline measurements were recorded during NSR *(left panel)*. The pacing wire to the LA was then suddenly disconnected from the pacemaker, leaving the LA electrically silent *(middle panel)*. No change occurred in any of the hemodynamic parameters. The left atrial wire was then connected to a separate rapid atrial pacemaker, and automatic left atrial tachycardia was simulated by rapidly pacing the LA *(right panel)*. Again, there was no measurable effect on systemic or PA blood pressure, LVEDP, or cardiac output from loss of left atrial function. (Reproduced from Williams JM, Ungerleider RM, Lofland GK, Cox JL. Left atrial isolation: new technique for the treatment of supraventricular arrhythmias. *J Thorac Cardiovasc Surg.* 1980;80:373.)

In 1978, we began a series of canine experiments in which every effort was made to electrically isolate the LA from the rest of the heart. It was not particularly difficult to separate the LA from the RA surgically, but despite their complete physical separation (Fig. 9.14A–C), they remained connected electrically. Because all of the atrial muscle around the coronary sinus had been dissected free, it finally became apparent that the only possible way for electrical activity to be getting from its pacing site in the LA to the rest of the heart was *through the coronary sinus itself* that had been left intact for survival purposes. Therefore, as a last step in the procedure, I cryoablated the coronary sinus while the heart was being paced from a site in the LA (Fig. 9.14D). Within a few seconds of applying the cryothermia to the coronary sinus, all conduction from the LA to the rest of the heart suddenly stopped. This was irrefutable evidence that the coronary sinus was capable of conducting electrical activity. A surgical research fellow in my laboratory at the time, Dr. Mark Williams, was subsequently assigned the task of evaluating the hemodynamic impact of this "left atrial isolation procedure" that allowed the LA to be in one rhythm and the rest of the heart in another (Fig. 9.15).[8] Surprisingly, we learned that as long as the RA and RV are in synchrony and the LV is normal, the LA has no effect on forward cardiac output. After performing the first left atrial isolation procedure clinically on December 4, 1982, an electrophysiologic study was performed several months after surgery. It confirmed complete electrical isolation of the LA and also showed that on the standard ECG, the "P wave" follows the activation of the LA, not the RA (Fig. 9.16).

We also learned that AF can be confined to the LA after a left atrial isolation procedure (Fig. 9.17). This opened one avenue of treating patients with AF surgically several years before the Maze procedure. However, we chose not to apply this procedure for the treatment of those with AF because it did not eliminate the problems of systemic embolism and loss of left-sided A-V synchrony. Despite our own reluctance to use LA isolation as a surgical treatment of patients with AF, Vigano's group in Italy reported on 100 left atrial isolation procedures performed for AF in patients under-

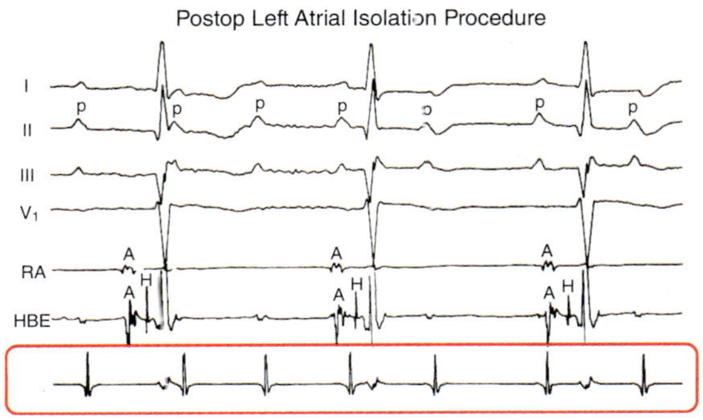

Fig. 9.16 First left atrial isolation procedure in a patient. After the left atrial isolation procedure, the tachycardia is confined to the left atrium (LA; *red box*) and is independent of electrical activation in the remainder of the heart. The right atrium (RA), His bundle (HBE), and ventricles are in perfect sinus rhythm with normal activation sequences. However, the p-wave on the standard electrocardiogram (ECG) leads I, II, III, and V1 is being generated by activity in the isolated LA, not in the normal RA. This causes the standard ECG to have the pattern of complete heart block, which is clearly not the case as documented on the His Bundle electrogram (HBE) tracing showing sequential activation of the right atrium (A), His bundle (H), and ventricles.

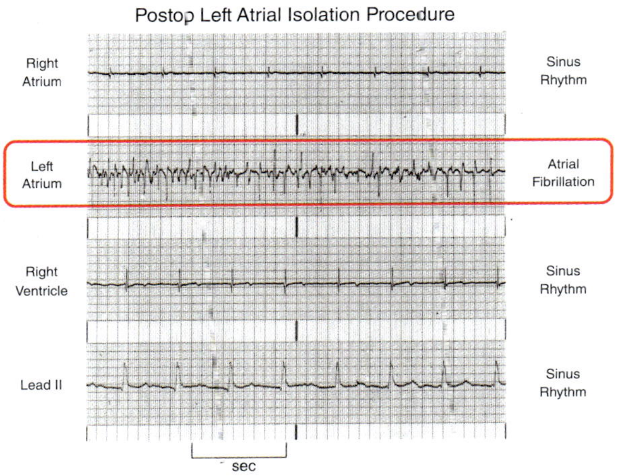

Fig. 9.17 After the left atrial isolation procedure, atrial fibrillation can be confined to the left atrium while the remainder of the heart remains in a sinus rhythm. (Reproduced from Williams JM, Ungerleider RM, Lofland GK, Cox JL. Left atrial isolation: new technique for the treatment of supraventricular arrhythmias. *J Thorac Cardiovasc Surg.* 1980;80:373.)

going mitral valve operations with a long-term success rate of restoring sinus rhythm in the other three heart chambers in 73%.[16]

It is noteworthy that several lessons were learned from our experience in developing the left atrial isolation procedure that were critical to the later development of the Maze procedure for AF. Demonstration that the coronary sinus could conduct electrical activity was critically important to the Maze procedure and can account for up to a 15% failure rate if ignored. Likewise, we demonstrated that the LA is not primarily a contractile chamber and that decreasing or even eliminating its contractile contribution is irrelevant to the cardiac output as long as there is right-sided A-V synchrony and the LV is normal.

AUTOMATIC RIGHT ATRIAL TACHYCARDIA

Automatic atrial tachycardias in the RA tend to be multiple in origin, variable but stable in location, and regular in rhythm, and they can occur anywhere in the RA. Because of their multifocal origin, they are more difficult to map and focally ablate, so we developed the right atrial isolation procedure (Fig. 9.18) to isolate the multiple sites of origin to the body of the RA and leave the rest of the heart in a sinus rhythm. The objective in this case is to isolate as much of the RA as possible while leaving the anatomic SA node in continuity with the atrial septum and therefore with the AV node–His bundle complex. It is also preferable, though not essential, to avoid interrupting a branch of the right coronary artery that courses across the mid-right atrial free-wall if possible. We developed this procedure in 1984 and then evaluated its safety (Fig. 9.19) and efficacy (Fig. 9.20) in several labora-

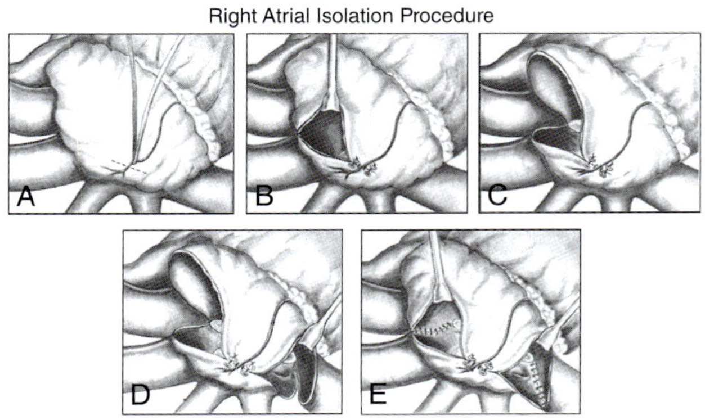

Fig. 9.18 (A–E) Right atrial isolation procedure. See text for description. (Reproduced from Harada A, D'Agostino Jr. HJ, Boineau JP, Cox JL. Right atrial isolation: a new surgical treatment for supraventricular tachycardia. I. Surgical technique and electrophysiologic effects. *J Thorac Cardiovasc Surg.* 1988;95:643–650.)

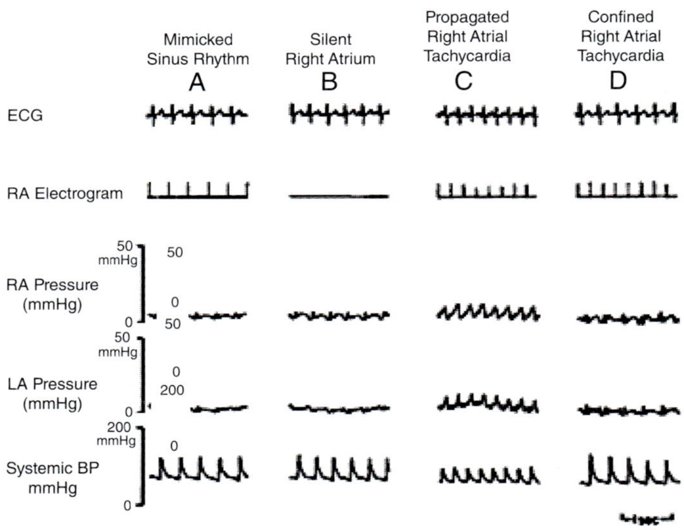

Fig. 9.19 *Panels A* and *B* show the hemodynamic effects of loss of right atrial synchrony after a right atrial isolation procedure. Postoperative lead II, the local right atrial (RA) electrogram, RA pressure, left atrial (LA) pressure, and systemic blood pressure (BP) are recorded during simulated sinus rhythm and silent right atrium. There is no difference in RA pressure, LA pressure, of systemic BP with and without RA synchrony. *Panels C* and *D* show beneficial hemodynamic effects of confining tachycardia to the isolated RA by RA isolation in the same animal. Conversion from propagated to confined RA tachycardia results in decrease in RA pressure and LA pressure with concomitant increase in systemic BP. Therefore, RA isolation prevents hemodynamic deterioration caused by automatic RA tachycardias. (Reproduced from Harada A, D'Agostino Jr. HJ, Boineau JP, Cox JL. Right atrial isolation: a new surgical treatment for supraventricular tachycardia. I. Surgical technique and electrophysiologic effects. *J Thorac Cardiovasc Surg.* 1988;95:643–650.)

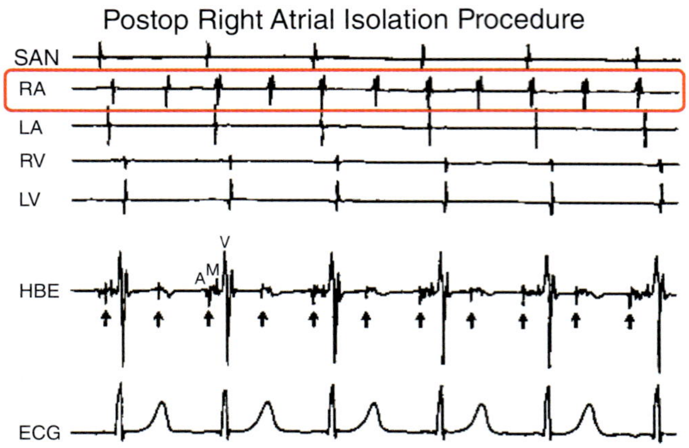

Fig. 9.20 Postoperative electrograms recorded from the same animal as in Fig. 9.19 during simulated tachycardia in the isolated right atrium. Tachycardia is simulated by rapid right atrial pacing at a cycle length of 200 ms and is confined to the isolated right atrium. The simulated right atrial tachycardia does not affect sinus rhythm or the normal conduction sequence in the remainder of the heart. *Arrows* mark right atrial pacing spikes reflected in the His bundle electrogram (HBE). *LA,* Left atrium; *LV,* left ventricle; *RA,* right atrium; *RV,* right ventricle; *SAN,* sinoatrial node. (Reproduced from Harada A, D'Agostino Jr. HJ, Boineau JP, Cox JL. Right atrial isolation: a new surgical treatment for supraventricular tachycardia. I. Surgical technique and electrophysiologic effects. *J Thorac Cardiovasc Surg.* 1988;95:643–650.)

tory experiments.[9] We first isolated the RA clinically with Drs. Sidney Levitsky and Harold Roberts in a patient at the University of Illinois in Chicago in 1986. Guiraudon later isolated the RA clinically when he combined the right atrial isolation procedure with the left atrial isolation procedure to create the corridor procedure (see Chapter 9).[17]

ISCHEMIC VENTRICULAR TACHYCARDIA

By the late 1970s, the most intense interest in arrhythmia therapy worldwide was in trying to develop a satisfactory surgical treatment for VT associated with myocardial infarction and left ventricular aneurysms. It was believed by the authorities that the success of surgery for ischemic VT was largely dependent on intraoperative mapping, so the number of centers with the ability to develop ischemic VT surgery was limited. Two surgical cardiology teams were the leaders in the effort to develop a surgical procedure for ischemic VT, Gerard Guiraudon and Guy Fontaine in Paris and Alden Harken and Mark Josephson in Philadelphia. Josephson's group was particularly adept at mapping and discerning the pathophysiology of ischemic VT. They documented that ischemic VT originated from sites at the edges of old myocardial infarcts and particularly around the endocardial borders of left ventricular aneurysms.[18] Therefore, when a standard left ventricular aneurysm resection was performed in which 1 to 2 cm of aneurysm tissue was purposely left behind to close the ventricle more securely, the endocardial sites at the junction of normal and scarred myocardium that generate VT were also left behind (Fig. 9.21A and B).

Guiraudon was the first to perform a procedure specifically designed to treat patients with ischemic VT. He developed the "encircling endocardial ventriculotomy" in which a transmural endocardial-to-epicardial incision that spared only the epicardial peel was placed all the way around the base of an left ventricular aneurysm in the normal myocardium just outside the endocardial scar (Fig. 9.21C). Although this procedure was effective in ablating ischemic VT, it decreased myocardial blood flow to the encompassed portion of the left ventricular,[19] decreased systolic and diastolic function left ventricular function,[20] and was associated with such a high operative mortality rate that it was soon abandoned clinically. At approximately the same time, Harken started

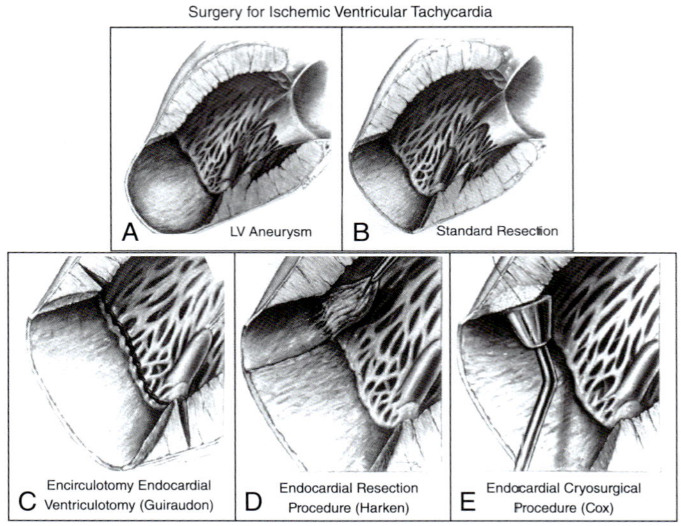

Fig. 9.21 (A) and (B) Appearance and standard resection of a left ventricular aneurysm. Note that approximately 2 cm of the scarred aneurysm cuff was routinely left unresected so that it could be used to close the left ventricular aneurysm defect after resection. Unfortunately, this left the associated endocardial scar/normal myocardium border unmolested, and this is where the reentrant origins and drivers of ischemic ventricular tachycardia (VT) originate. (C) The encircling endocardial ventriculotomy developed by Guiraudon and Fontaine to isolate or interrupt the reentrant circuits responsible for ischemic VT associated with left ventricular aneurysms. (D) The local subendocardial resection procedure developed by Harkin and Josephson for ischemic VT associated with left ventricular aneurysms. The site of origin of the VT was first located by single-point endocardial mapping, and then the endocardial scar in that area was peeled away and resected. (E) The endocardial cryosurgical procedure developed by the author and John Gallagher for ischemic VT associated with left ventricular aneurysms. We used transmural needle electrodes for identifying the site of origin of the VT, which was often intramural. We then resected the endocardial scar in that area and applied endocardial cryoablation afterward to destroy potential mid-myocardial sites. (Modified from Cox JL. Anatomic-electrophysiologic basis for the surgical treatment of refractory ischemic ventricular tachycardia, *Ann Surg.* 1983;198:119.)

performing the subendocardial resection (SER) procedure in which a localized area of the endocardial scar was resected, the specific area being identified by Josephson's intraoperative mapping[4,18] (Fig. 9.21D). This procedure became the standard of care for treating patients with ischemic VT surgically for several years thereafter.

At Duke we initially mapped the ventricles epicardially with the "sock electrode" that contained 64 bipolar electrodes (Fig. 9.22) Video 9-2. We

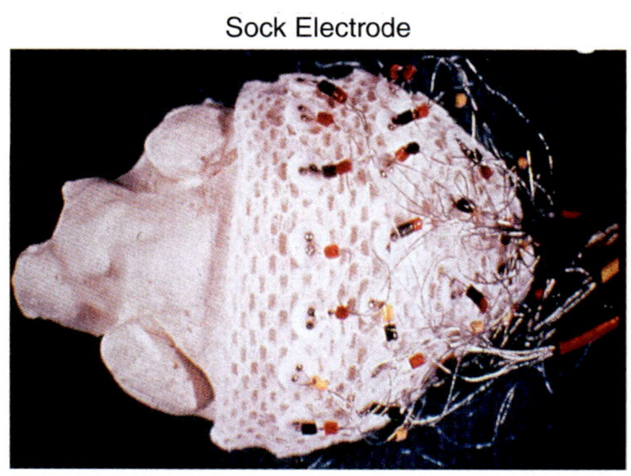

Fig. 9.22 The "sock electrode" was made of a fiber mesh used in pantyhose, and up to 64 bipolar electrodes were imbedded into the material, which kept the electrodes in contact with the epicardial surface of both ventricles without functionally constricting the ventricles.

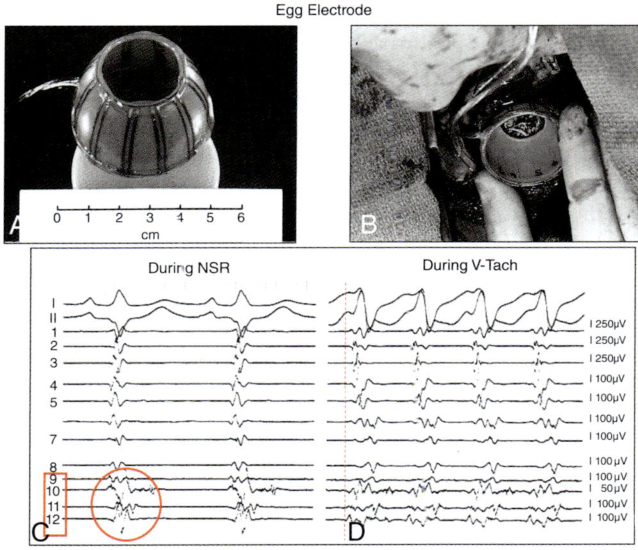

Fig. 9.23 (A) The "egg electrode" used to map the endocardium at the base of left ventricular aneurysms. Twelve longitudinal bipolar electrodes were placed around the surface of a portion of a plastic egg for analogue recordings. (B) The egg electrode was positioned directly into the opening of an LV aneurysm to obtain circumferential endocardial information. (C) and (D) During normal sinus rhythm (NSR), continuous fractionated electrical activity was recorded at electrodes 9 to 12. These same electrodes activated earliest during induced ventricular tachycardia (V-Tach), indicating that the endocardial scar in that area represented the site of origin of the V-Tach and should be resected.

then identified which area of the endocardial scar gave rise to the ischemic VT by using the "egg electrode," so called because it was constructed from a plastic Easter egg (Fig. 9.23A). Twelve separate strips of bipolar electrodes were fixed on the outer half of a plastic egg with the tip cut off so we could better visualize the inside of the LV. The egg electrode was then inserted directly into the open left ventricular aneurysm (Fig. 9.23B), and activation times at each of the 12 bipolar electrodes were recorded during NSR. The culprit site usually showed fractionated electrical activity during NSR (Fig. 9.23C). When VT was then induced by programmed electrical stimulation, the area of fractionation was consistently the earliest site to activate during VT (Fig. 9.23D). We then performed intramural mapping with multiple needle electrodes placed transmurally from the epicardium in the region of the site of VT origin. These 0.23-gauge needles had bipolar electrodes embedded every millimeter, or in some cases every half millimeter, along their shaft (Fig. 9.24). Endocardial cryosurgery was then performed at the site or sites of origin of the VT[5] (see Fig. 9.21E).

The subendocardial resection (SER) procedure and the endocardial cryoablation procedure continued to be used worldwide for the next several years, but in 1985 Adib Jatene in Sao Paulo, Brazil and Vincent Dor in Monte Carlo, Monaco independently introduced the concept of *repairing* left ventricular aneurysms rather than resecting them.[21,22] Although their individual operative procedures differed slightly, both included techniques that "tightened" the base of the aneurysm, thereby altering the tension forces on the endocardial scar associated with the left ventricular aneurysm (Fig. 9.25).[23] When combined with unguided endocardial scar resection and cryoablation, the Dor procedure resulted in the virtual disappearance of ischemic VT associated with left ventricular aneurysms.[24] Thus the extensive mapping techniques and the direct surgical procedures for ischemic VT were rendered

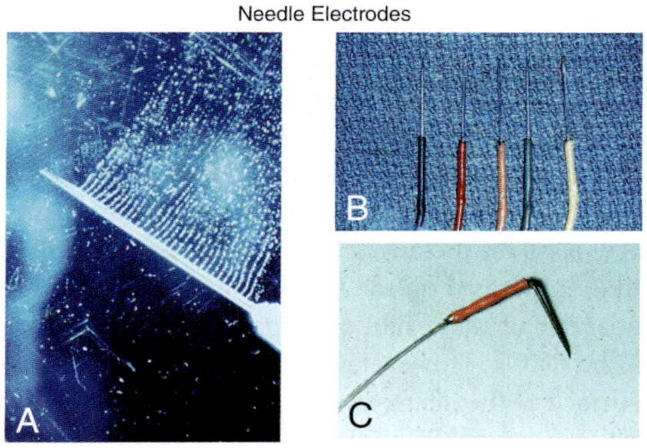

Fig. 9.24 Needle electrodes for intramural mapping of the ventricles. (A) A 0.23-guage needle with electrodes imbedded every half millimeter along its shaft. (B) Up to 40 needles at a time were used to map ischemic ventricular tachycardia (VT). Each of these clinical mapping needles had four electrodes imbedded in their shaft to record epicardial, subepicardial, subendocardial and endocardial electrograms in patients with ischemic VT. (C) A right-angle needle electrode that made it easier to map the intramural posterior left ventricular wall.

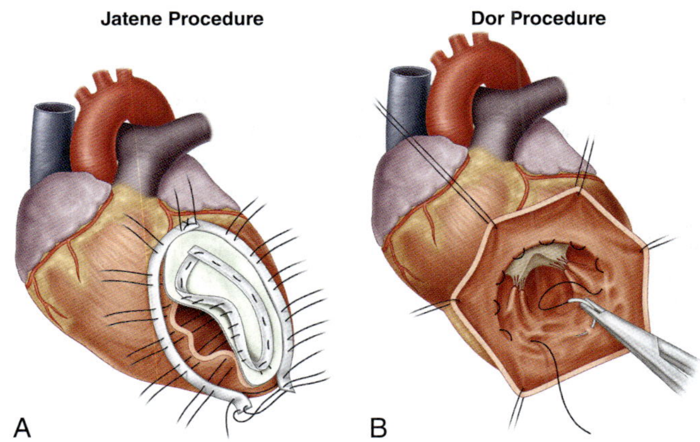

Fig. 9.25 (A) The Jatene approach to repairing anteroseptal left ventricular aneurysms. Before this stage of the operation, the septal part of the aneurysm had been imbricated. (B) The Dor approach to repairing anteroseptal left ventricular aneurysms. Rather than imbricating the septal part of the aneurysm, it is excluded by the circumferential endocardial pursestring suture shown here. The major difference in the two procedures from an anatomic standpoint is that the Jatene procedure leaves the left ventricular apex in the same position relative to the septum, and the Dor procedure moves the apex slightly to the left relative the septum. Both are excellent operations that revolutionized surgery for left ventricular aneurysms, and both resulted in the virtual disappearance of ischemic ventricular tachycardia. (Modified from Jatene A. Left ventricular aneurysmectomy: resection or reconstruction. *J Thorac Cardiovasc Surg.* 1985;37:11–19 and Dor V, Saab M, Coste P, Kornaszewska M, Montiglio F. Left ventricular aneurysm: a new surgical approach. *J Thorac Cardiovasc Surg.* 1989;37(1):11–19.)

obsolete by the Dor procedure and to a lesser extent by the Jatene procedure.

NON-ISCHEMIC VENTRICULAR TACHYCARDIA

Whereas the LV is most commonly involved in ischemic VT, the RV is the source of most non-ischemic VT. The two most common types of non-ischemic VT seen clinically are idiopathic VT and VT associated with arrhythmogenic right ventricular dysplasia (ARVD).

Idiopathic Ventricular Tachycardia

This term describes VT that occurs in patients in whom the only clinical manifestation of cardiac disease is the arrhythmia itself. There is no evidence of either gross or microscopic anatomic disease, and the only abnormality is global dilatation of the heart associated with tachycardia-induced heart failure. Most idiopathic VTs originate in the RV outflow tract (RVOT), including the supracristal portion of the septum. Guiraudon operated on the first two patients with idiopathic VT in 1979, and both of them had an apparent site of VT origin in the free-wall of the RVOT. However, Fontaine and he could map only the epicardial surface of the heart, and in retrospect, they were likely misled about the true site of VT origin in both cases, neither of which was successful. A few months later we operated on a 16-year-old female patient with idiopathic VT and an ejection fraction of 16%. During the initial mapping phase, the epicardial map with the sock electrode array indicated that, as in Guiraudon and Fontaine's two cases, the earliest site of activation during VT appeared to be on the free-wall of the RVOT. However, Gallagher suspected that the true site of origin of the idiopathic VT in both of their patients and in ours as well was in the supracristal RV septum. Therefore, we inserted a needle electrode into the right ventricular septum and immediately documented that his suspicion was correct. The site of origin of the VT was in the supracristal septum of the RVOT.

A vertical atriotomy was placed in the free wall of the RVOT to expose the supracristal ventricular septum. Several attempts were made to cryoablate the site in the supracristal septum that appeared to be the site of origin, all to no avail. As a result, the free-wall ventriculotomy was extended across the nonconducting pulmonary valve annulus for 2 to 3 mm into the main pulmonary artery. A vertical counterincision was placed in the supracristal septum directly across from the free-wall incision, and the proximal ends of both vertical incisions were connected with a horizontal incision halfway around the RVOT. This effectively isolated the site of origin of the VT from the remainder of the heart (Fig. 9.26).[7] After surgery the patient remained free of any episodes of VT, and her ejection fraction had increased from 16% to 61% by postoperative day 7. The patient went on to become a cheerleader in her high school and several years later had two healthy children.

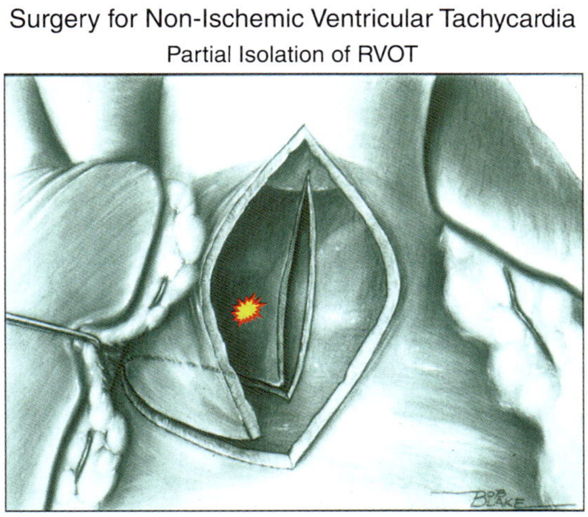

Fig. 9.26 Regional isolation of the lateral half of the supracristal right ventricular outflow tract for idiopathic non-ischemic ventricular tachycardia (VT) arising in the supracristal portion of the septum. The site of origin of the non-ischemic V is designated by the *yellow starburst*. (Reproduced from Cox JL, Bardy GH, Damiano RJ, et al. Right ventricular isolation procedures for non-ischemic ventricular tachycardia. *J Thorac Cardiovasc Surg*. 1985;90:212.)

Arrhythmogenic Right Ventricular Dysplasia

This non-ischemic VT is also called arrhythmogenic RV cardiomyopathy and was first described by Guy Fontaine in 1977 (Fig. 9.27).[25] In ARVD three primary areas of the right ventricular free-wall are thin and arrhythmogenic—the posterior base, the distal RV near the apex, and the RVOT. VT can arise from any or all of these sites, making focal ablation of their site of origin difficult. We also used regional isolation of the RV free-wall in most of these patients, including our first patient with ARVD in 1979. He was a 66-year-old male patient who had VT that upon mapping appeared to be originating in at least three different sites in the RV free-wall. We isolated a large portion of the right ventricular free wall based on the right coronary artery and its right ventricular branches and extended an incision through a small aneurysm near the right ventricular apex (Fig. 9.28) that resulted in no further episodes of VT.

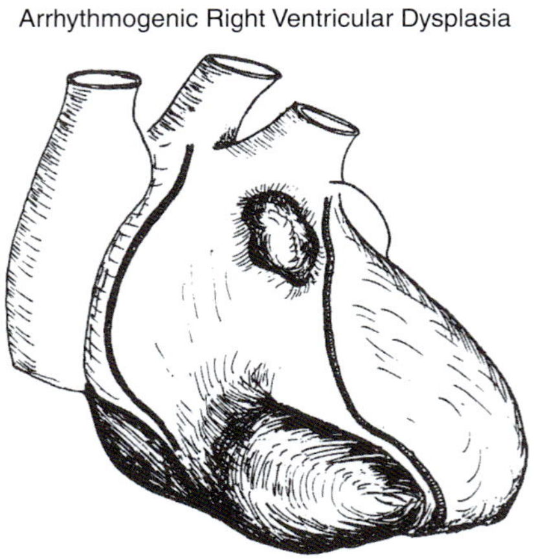

Fig. 9.27 Arrhythmogenic right ventricular dysplasia. The three areas of the right ventricle that are locally aneurysmal and arrhythmogenic are designated. (Courtesy Dr. G. Fontaine).

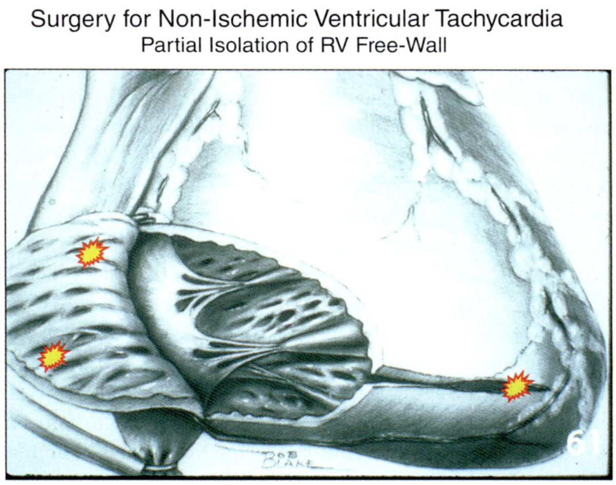

Fig. 9.28 Localized right ventricular isolation in a patient with arrhythmogenic right ventricular dysplasia. The patient had multifocal non-ischemic ventricular tachycardia (VT) originating in the sites indicated with *yellow starbursts*. A flap of right ventricular free-wall based on the right coronary artery was isolated. In addition, a linear incision was placed from the flap through a small aneurysm located in the right ventricular apex that gave rise to one of the three morphologic types of VT in this patient. (Reproduced from Cox JL, Bardy GH, Damiano RJ, et al. Right ventricular isolation procedures for non-ischemic ventricular tachycardia. *J Thorac Cardiovasc Surg*. 1985;90:212.)

In 1982, we operated on two young patients with ARVD, one of whom had gone through more than 250 individual episodes of cardiopulmonary resuscitation by the age of 16 years. He was the second patient to ever receive an automatic defibrillator that was implanted by Drs. Levi Watkins and Phil Reed at Johns Hopkins University. Unfortunately, his fibrillation episodes were so frequent that the automatic defibrillator proved to be of little help. Mapping had shown that he had numerous separate VTs, all originating in the RV free-wall. Watkins and Reed brought the patient down to Duke, where we removed the automatic defibrillator and disconnected (isolated) his entire right ventricular free-wall from the rest of the heart (Fig. 9.29). This total right ventricular disconnection procedure was actually an extension of the two regional right ventricular isolation procedures that we had performed in the previous patients described in Figs. 9.26 and 9.28. The total right ventricular disconnection did not stop the VT in the RV, but it did confine it to the RV, thereby protecting the rest of the heart from its effects (Fig. 9.30).

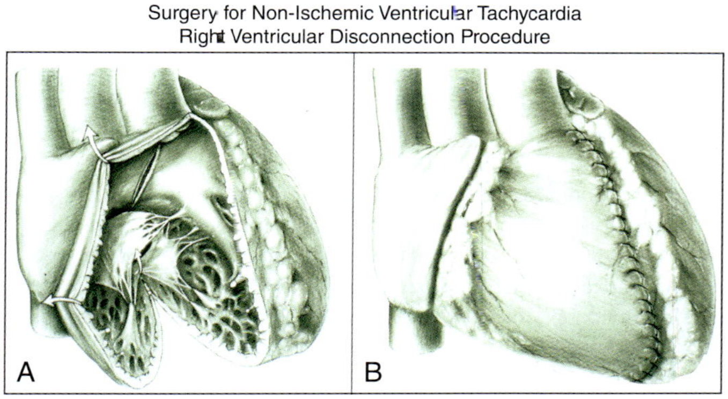

Fig. 9.29 (A) and (B) Total disconnection of the right ventricle from the rest of the heart. Two of these procedures were performed for severe arrhythmogenic right ventricular dysplasia in 1982. (Reproduced from Cox JL. Surgery for cardiac arrhythmias. *Curr Probl Cardiol.* 1983;8(4):1–60.)

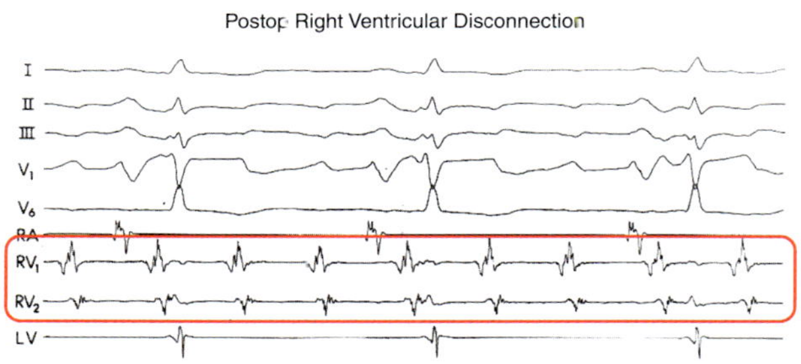

Fig. 9.30 Recordings after total disconnection of the right ventricle (RV) for multifocal non-ischemic right ventricular tachycardia caused by arrhythmogenic right ventricular dysplasia. Note that the ventricular tachycardia persists in the RV while the rest of the heart is in normal sinus rhythm. (Reproduced from Reproduced from Cox JL, Bardy GH, Damiano RJ, et al. Right ventricular isolation procedures for non-ischemic ventricular tachycardia. *J Thorac Cardiovasc Surg.* 1985;90:212.)

LESSONS LEARNED FROM NON–ATRIAL FIBRILLATION SURGERY THAT WERE CRITICAL TO THE DEVELOPMENT OF THE MAZE PROCEDURE

As already mentioned, the experience that we and others gained during the development of surgical procedures for patients with non-AF arrhythmias provided us with a wealth of information and several seminal observations that were critical to the development of the Maze procedure for AF.

Wolff-Parkinson-White Syndrome

- Retrograde conduction (V-to-A) across an accessory pathway in WPW syndrome usually results in classic "reciprocating tachycardia," but it can also serve as a *trigger* for the induction of AF. Therefore, the WPW syndrome or the presence of an accessory AV connection (pathway) that conducts in only the retrograde direction must be ruled out as a potential trigger for AF before performing a pulmonary vein isolation (PVI), Maze procedure, or any other interventional procedure to treat a patient with AF. So-called concealed pathways do not cause the typical findings of the WPW syndrome on a standard ECG because they cannot conduct antegrade (A-to-V), but they can still serve as a trigger for AF.
- Special attention should be paid to atrial lesions that terminate at a valve annulus, particularly the tricuspid annulus where the RA and RV "overlap" at their junction. This can lead to a lesion that appears to terminate at the valve annulus and is therefore complete when it is actually incomplete and will fail. This potential problem is best handled by placing a cryolesion at the end of any atrial lesion that terminates on either valve annulus.
- The pressure in AV groove hematomas is always greater than the central venous pressure. Therefore, hematomas in the left AV groove can safely be decompressed into the coronary sinus, which has the same pressure as the RA.
- WPW syndrome is caused by a strand of residual atrial myocardium the size of a human hair that conducts electrical activity. Therefore, if a gap occurs in an ablation lesion for AF that is the size of a human hair or larger, it may not function as a line of complete conduction block, and the procedure can potentially fail. Each atrial lesion in the Maze procedure must be contiguous (no gaps) and uniformly transmural.

Left Atrial Isolation Procedure

- The coronary sinus itself is capable of conducting electrical activity; therefore, it must be ablated along with the mitral line to prevent conduction across the left atrial isthmus, which is essential to the development of postoperative peri-mitral flutter (see Chapter 48).
- Left atrial function alone does not contribute to forward cardiac output if the RA and RV are normal and in synchrony and the LV is normal. Therefore, a slight decrease in left atrial transport function after a Maze procedure should have little or no effect on forward cardiac output if there is AV synchrony on both sides of the heart.
- The p-wave on a standard ECG is caused by activation of the LA, not the RA. Therefore, after atrial procedures such as the Maze procedure, what seems to be clear heart block on a standard 12-lead ECG may not be actual heart block in the AV node.

Focal Isolation or Ablation of Automatic Atrial Tachycardias

- When attempting to localize the site of origin of any focal arrhythmia, it is essential to "bracket" the potential site of origin of the arrhythmia with electrode arrays to determine its location accurately. Otherwise, it is impossible to identify the earliest activation site during the tachycardia. If the potential site of origin is not "bracketed," the electrodes located on the "edge" of the array will be activated first even though they are not the actual earliest site of activation. Ablation at this erroneous site of origin will result in failure (see Chapter 4, Fig. 4.11).

His Bundle Ablation for Supraventricular Tachycardia and Discrete Cryosurgery for Atrioventricular Node Reentry Tachycardia

- Retrograde conduction (V-to-A) during AVNRT can serve as a trigger for the induction of AF. Therefore, AVNRT must be ruled out as a potential trigger for AF before performing a PVI, Maze procedure, or any other interventional procedure to treat a patient with AF. This is especially important in younger patients and in patients who develop AF late in life but have a history of non-AF arrhythmias since childhood or early adulthood.
- Cryosurgery can be used as if the cryoprobe is a reversible knife. This allows the surgeon to temporarily block electrical conduction to (1) observe its effect and then discontinue the cryothermia application to allow normal electrical conduction to resume or (2) further decrease the temperature to permanently ablate conduction.

Right Atrial Isolation Procedure

- Right atrial function alone does not contribute to forward cardiac output if the other three heart chambers are normal and in synchrony.

Ischemic Ventricular Tachycardia Surgery

- Continuous fractionated electrical activity can act as a *trigger* for the induction of AF but not as a *driver* to sustain AF (see Chapter 49, Figs. 4.5 to 4.9).
- Many arrhythmias that occur in association with scars are not caused by the scar itself but rather by abnormal stresses placed on the surrounding normal myocardium (see Fig. 9.25). This is the reason that even heavily scarred left atria that are enlarged are "downsized" as a part of the Maze procedure(see Chapter 18).

REFERENCES

1. Cobb FR, Blumenschein SD, Sealy WC, Boineau JP, Wagner GS, Wallace AG. Successful surgical interruption of the bundle of Kent in a patient with Wolff-Parkinson-White syndrome. *Circulation.* 1968;38:1018.
2. Harrison L, Gallagher JJ, Sadell J, et al. Cryosurgical ablation of the A-V node-His bundle: a new method for producing A-V block. *Circulation.* 1997;55(3):463–470.
3. Guiraudon G, Fontaine G, Frank R, Escande G, Etievent P, Cabrol C. Encircling endocardial ventriculotomy: a new surgical treatment for life-threatening ventricular tachycardias resistant to medical treatment following myocardial infarction. *Ann Thor Surg.* 1978;26(5):438–444.
4. Harken AH, Horowitz LN, Josephson ME. The surgical treatment of ventricular tachycardia. *Ann Thor Surg.* 1980;30(5):499–508.
5. Gallagher JJ, Cox JL. Status of surgery for ventricular arrhythmias (editorial). *Circulation.* 1979;60:1440.
6. Cox JL, Gallagher JJ, Cain ME. Experience with 118 consecutive patients undergoing surgery for the Wolff-Parkinson-White Syndrome. *J Thorac Cardiovasc Surg.* 1985;90:490–501.
7. Cox JL, Bardy GH, Damiano RJ, et al. Right ventricular isolation procedures for non-ischemic ventricular tachycardia. *J Thorac Cardiovasc Surg.* 1985;90:212.
8. Williams JM, Ungerleider RM, Lofland GK, Cox JL. Left atrial isolation: new technique for the treatment of supraventricular arrhythmias. *J Thorac Cardiovasc Surg.* 1980;80:373.
9. Harada A, D'Agostino Jr HJ, Boineau JP, Cox JL. Right Atrial isolation: a new surgical treatment for supraventricular tachycardia. I. Surgical technique and electrophysiologic effects. *J Thorac Cardiovasc Surg.* 1988;95:643–650.
10. Cox JL, Holman WL, Cain ME. Cryosurgical treatment of atrioventricular node reentry tachycardia. *Circulation.* 1987;76:1329–1336.
11. Gallagher JJ, Sealy WC, Cox JL, Kasell JH. Results of surgery for pre-excitation in 200 cases (abst). *In: Circulation.* 1981;64(4):146.
12. Cox JL. Surgery for cardiac arrhythmias. *Cur Prob Cardiol, Yearbook Medical Publishers.* 1983;VIII(4).
13. Johnson DC, Nunn GR, Meldrum-Hanna W. Surgry for atrioventricular node reentry tachycardia: the surgical dissection technique. *Semin Thorac Cardiovasc Surg.* 1989;1(1):53–57.
14. Jackman WM, Beckman KJ, McClelland JH, et al. Treatment of supraventricular tachycardia due to atrioventricular nodal reentry by radiofrequency catheter ablation of slow-pathway conduction. *N Engl J Med.* 1992;327:313–318.
15. Iwa T, Ichihashi T, Hashizuma Y, Ishida K, Okada R. Successful surgical treatment of left atrial tachycardia. *Am Heart J.* 1985;109(1):160–162.
16. Graffigna A, Pagani F, Minzioni G, Salerno J, Vigano M. Left atrial isolation associated with mitral valve operations. *Ann Thorac Surg.* 1992;54(6):1093–1097.
17. Guiraudon GM, Campbell CS, Jones DL, McLellan JL, MacDonald JL. Combined sino-atrial node atrio-ventricular node isolation: a surgical alternative to his bundle ablation in patients with atrial fibrillation. *Circulation.* 1985;72:111–220.
18. Horowitz LN, Josephson ME, Harken AH. Epicardial and endocardial activation during sustained ventricular tachycardia in man. *Circulation.* 1980;61(6):1227–1238.
19. Ungerleider RM, Holman WL, Stanley TE, et al. Encircling endocardial ventriculotomy (EEV) for refractory ischemic ventricular tachycardia: II: effects on regional myocardial blood flow. *J Thorac Cardiovasc Surg.* 1982;83:850.
20. Ungerleider RM, Holman WL, Calcagno D, et al. Encircling endocardial ventriculotomy (EEV) for refractory ischemic ventricular tachycardia: III: effects on regional left ventricular function. *J Thorac Cardiovasc Surg.* 1982;83:857.
21. Jatene A. Left ventricular aneurysmectomy: resection or reconstruction. *J Thorac Cardiovasc Surg.* 1985;37:11–19.
22. Dor V, Saab M, Coste P, Kornaszewska M, Montiglio F. Left ventricular aneurysm: a new surgical approach. *J Thorac Cardiovasc Surg.* 1989;37(1):11–19.
23. Cox JL. Surgical management of left ventricular aneurysms: a clarification of the similarities and differences between the Jatene and Dor techniques. *Semin Thorac Cardiovasc Surg.* 1997;9(2):131–138.
24. Sartipy U, Albage A, Straat E, Insulander P, Lindblom D. Surgery for ventricular tachycardia in patients undergoing left ventricular reconstruction by the Dor procedure. *Ann Thorac Surg.* 2006;81(1):65–71.
25. Fontaine G. Arrhythmogenic right ventricular dysplasia. *Br Heart J.* 1993;70(3):293–294.
26. Cox JL. Anatomic-electrophysiologic basis for the surgical treatment of refractory ischemic ventricular tachycardia. *Ann Surg.* 1983;198:119.
27. Cox JL. Surgery for cardiac arrhythmias. In: Harvey WP, ed. *Cur Prob Cardiol.* 1983; VIII.
28. Gallagher JJ, Cox JL, German LD, Kasell JH. Non-pharmacologic treatment of supraventricular tachycardia. In: Josephson ME, Wellens HJJ, eds. *Tachycardias: Mechanisms, Diagnosis, Treatment.* Lea & Febiger; 1984.

10

Principles and Goals That Govern the Interventional Treatment of Atrial Fibrillation

James L. Cox

CHAPTER OUTLINE

THE STUDY OF ARRHYTHMIAS USING SURGICAL SCARS

All tissue, including myocardium, subjected to irreversible damage heals by forming scars that consist of fibrocytes that do not conduct electrical activity. From GR Mines'[1] first description of reentry in 1914 to Will Sealy's[2] first surgical procedure to interrupt an accessory pathway responsible for the Wolff-Parkinson-White syndrome in 1968 (54 years between the procedures), scars were used exclusively to *study* arrhythmias. Sealy's operation marked the first time that a surgical scar had ever been used to *treat* an arrhythmia, though it was also important in establishing the mechanism of the arrhythmia. Until that successful surgical procedure, many prominent cardiologists of the day believed that longitudinal dissociation of the His bundle was the underlying electrophysiologic abnormality responsible for WPW syndrome. Although Sealy's successful WPW operation was crucial to the final documentation of the underlying electrophysiology of WPW syndrome, it was also the basis for all subsequent interventional therapy for cardiac arrhythmias.

The Maze procedure served a similar function in elucidating the underlying mechanisms responsible for sustained atrial fibrillation (AF). Although AF is infinitely more complex than WPW syndrome, the Maze procedure's success in the treatment of patients with paroxysmal, persistent, and long-standing persistent AF has provided several undeniable facts regarding the electrophysiology of AF. For example, if AF were sustained by the continuous firing of focal triggers in the atrium, the Maze procedure would simply not work because the focal triggers located between the lesions of the Maze procedure would continue to cause the atria to fibrillate (see Chapter 4, Fig. 4.21). Indeed, this was the basis of Gordon Moe's original experiments in the early 1960s.[3]

Isolation of the focal triggers in and around the pulmonary veins *decreases the likelihood* that an AF episode will occur,[4] but it does not make the atria incapable of fibrillating. Thus the focal triggers are largely irrelevant in the more sustained types of AF. As a result, their isolation or ablation has a salutary effect on paroxysmal AF but a suboptimal effect on persistent AF and long-standing persistent AF.[5] The occasional successful ablation of persistent and long-standing persistent AF by pulmonary vein isolation (PVI) is not because the PVI isolates the triggers that induce AF but rather because the PVI has inadvertently interrupted the macro-reentrant circuits sustaining AF in that particular patient.

THE CONCEPT OF ABLATION AND ISOLATION PROCEDURES

Regardless of whether the cause of an arrhythmia is automatic, micro-reentrant, macro-reentrant, or some combination of these mechanisms, the interventional approach to its treatment follows certain principles that should be understood by all arrhythmia surgeons and interventional electrophysiologists. We have found it helpful to categorize interventional procedures for cardiac arrhythmias into either isolation procedures or ablation procedures.[6] *Isolation procedures* do not actually ablate arrhythmias; rather, they confine them and/or their triggers to a specific region of the heart that minimizes their adverse effects in the remainder of the heart. Examples of isolation procedures are elective His bundle ablation, the left atrial (LA) isolation procedure, and PVI.

On the other hand, *ablation procedures* preclude arrhythmias from developing either by destroying their trigger mechanisms or by altering (or removing) the substrate that allows the arrhythmia to be induced and sustained. Examples of ablation procedures are the interruption of accessory pathways responsible for WPW syndrome, discrete cryosurgery of the atrioventricular node for atrioventricular node reentry tachycardia, and the Maze procedure for AF.

ADOPTABILITY OF INTERVENTIONAL PROCEDURES

The adoption of a new interventional procedure is inversely related to its complexity; that is, as the complexity of a procedure increases, its adoptability decreases (Fig. 10.1). The impact of the procedure's efficacy (success rate) on its adoptability is negligible (Fig. 10.2). Despite the high success rate of the Maze procedure in ablating AF, the complexity of the procedure has prevented its widespread adoption by surgeons (Fig. 10.3). On the contrary, despite the known lower success rate of catheter ablation for AF, its lower complexity and lower degree of invasiveness have resulted in its widespread adoption by interventional electrophysiologists (Fig. 10.4). Procedures that are deemed to be too complex or that have too many failures are not widely adopted (Fig. 10.5).

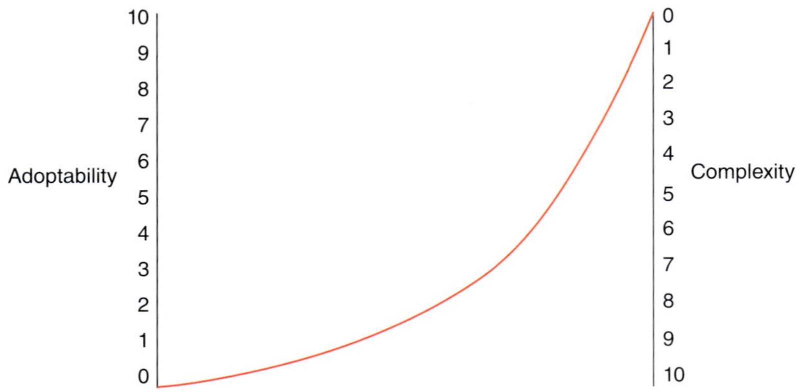

Fig. 10.1 There is an inverse relationship between the complexity of an interventional procedure and its adoption by physicians and surgeons.

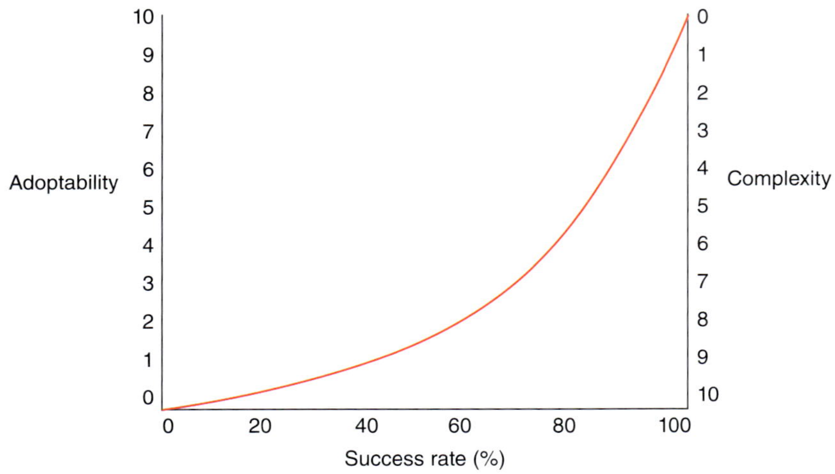

Fig. 10.2 The efficacy of an interventional procedure has little or no effect on its adoption by physicians and surgeons.

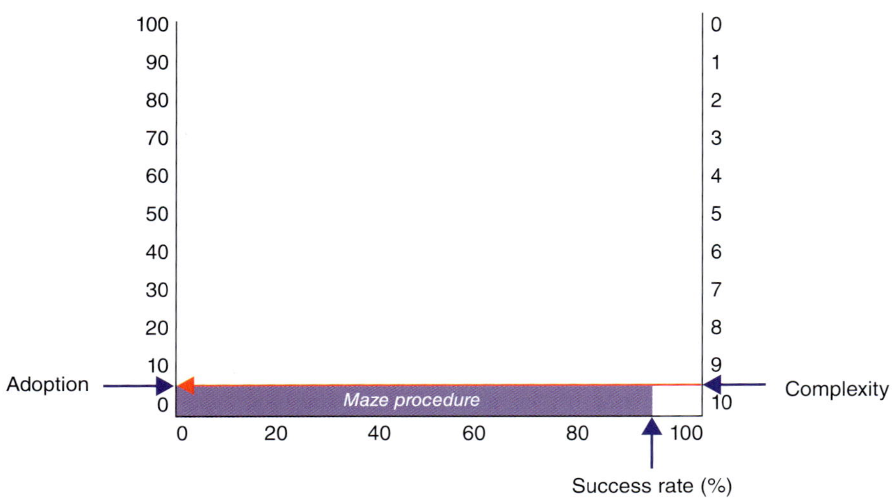

Fig. 10.3 Because of the complexity of the Maze procedure, it has not been widely adopted despite its outstanding efficacy. As a result, the absolute number of patients treated successfully for atrial fibrillation by the Maze procedure is relatively small.

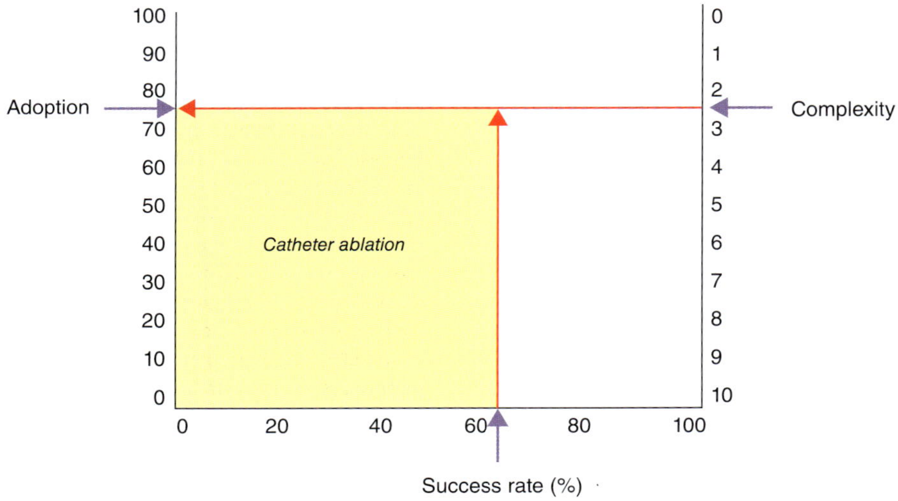

Fig. 10.4 Because the complexity and degree of invasiveness of catheter ablation is relatively low, it has been widely adopted despite its suboptimal efficacy compared with a Maze procedure. As a result, the absolute number of patients treated successfully for atrial fibrillation by catheter ablation is relatively large and far exceeds the absolute number of patients treated successfully by the Maze procedure.

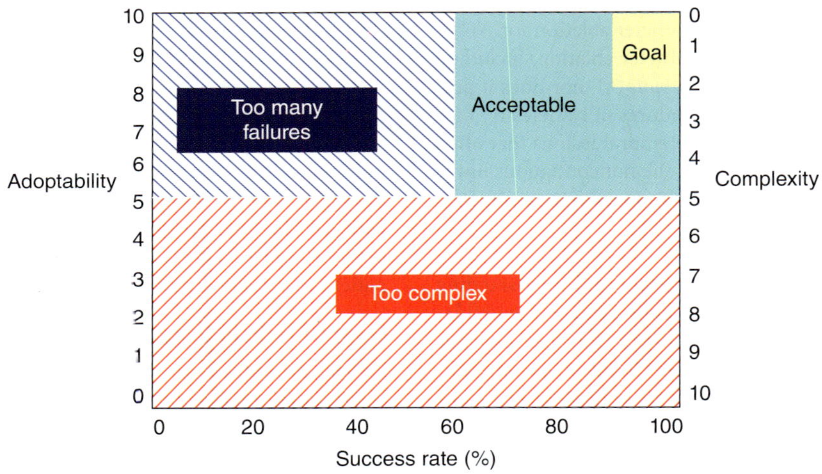

Fig. 10.5 Currently, highly complex interventional procedures such as the Maze procedure are considered to be too complex to be widely adopted. Less complex surgical and catheter procedures with low success rates are not widely adopted because of too many failures. The *turquoise block* defines the approximate current parameters for an acceptable interventional procedure for atrial fibrillation. The *yellow block* defines the parameters that should be attainable in the future.

Because of the wider acceptance of catheter ablation for AF, the absolute number of patients successfully treated by catheter ablation is far greater than the absolute number successfully treated by Maze procedures despite the substantially higher efficacy of the latter. Surgeons who are reluctant to perform a Maze procedure have substituted other simpler "non-Maze" surgical procedures in hopes of attaining success rates similar to those of the Maze procedure. Because most of those procedures have no sound scientific basis, they are far less effective than the Maze procedure for the treatment of patients with AF (see Chapter 19). Unfortunately, the term "Maze procedure" has become a generic term for any surgical procedure done in the atrium to treat patients with AF. This has led to confusing and inaccurate results being reported for the Maze procedure because some of these operations have nothing to do with the Maze procedure,[7] and others were called "Maze procedures" but were performed improperly.[8] This logic of "less is better" has also led interventional electrophysiologists to extend the only procedure that they are capable of doing reliably, PVI, to complex forms of AF that have no relationship whatsoever to pulmonary vein triggers. Again, as expected, these procedures have also had dismal results.[9]

GOALS OF INTERVENTIONAL TREATMENT OF PATIENTS WITH ATRIAL FIBRILLATION

Three things can cause catheter ablation or surgical ablation for AF to fail:

1. Incomplete lesions ("gaps")
    - These occur because an inadequate energy source was used or because the operator used an acceptable energy source improperly.

2. Incorrect operation
   - This is the result of creating complete lesions of conduction block but placing them in the wrong location (i.e., when non-Maze procedures are performed for AF or when PVI is used to treat long-standing persistent AF).
3. Incomplete lesions and incorrect operation
   - These include creating incomplete lesions of conduction block and placing them in the wrong location.

Goals of Catheter Ablation

Paroxysmal Atrial Fibrillation

In patients with paroxysmal atrial fibrillation (PAF), the goal of catheter ablation is to isolate the pulmonary veins (PVI) and ablate or isolate as much of the posterior LA wall as possible. If PVI is combined with posterior LA wall isolation, the resultant lines of conduction block create a so-called "box lesion" around all four pulmonary veins and include the intervening posterior LA wall. The objective of PVI ± posterior LA wall isolation (the box lesion) is to separate as many of the triggers that induce episodes of AF as possible from the rest of the heart. Thus PVI is not an *ablation* procedure; rather, as its name implies, it is an *isolation* procedure. As such, catheter ablation does not ablate PAF, and the atria can still fibrillate if a premature atrial beat is generated by triggers elsewhere in the atria. AF can also still occur after a PVI for PAF as the result of neural stimulation or esophageal irritation from hot or cold drinks, caffeine, alcohol, and so on. Thus the term "catheter ablation for AF" is a misnomer when applied to PAF because catheter ablation, including PVI ± posterior LA wall isolation, does not *ablate* AF nor does it preclude the atria from being able to fibrillate. Failures of catheter PVI for PAF are most commonly the result of nontransmural lesions that often result from unipolar radiofrequency ablation, the noncontiguous linear lesions (gaps) used for box lesions, and nonpulmonary vein triggers.

Nonparoxysmal Atrial Fibrillation

Nonparoxysmal AF (non-PAF) includes persistent and long-standing persistent AF. In these patients, catheter intervention can be a true ablation procedure, though the results are suboptimal. Non-PAF depends primarily on the ability of atrial macro-reentrant circuits to become self-perpetuating drivers of long episodes of AF. Because these macro-reentrant drivers are not located within the pulmonary veins, as many focal triggers are, isolation of only the pulmonary veins has a limited effect. Some small-diameter macro-reentrant drivers are located close enough to the pulmonary veins that PVI can inadvertently interrupt them, but this is rare. On the other hand, these small-diameter macro-reentrant drivers are sometimes located in the posterior LA wall between the right and left pulmonary veins and therefore can be isolated with a box lesion. In addition, perhaps 30% of the large-diameter macro-reentrant drivers of AF use the posterior LA wall as a part of their reentrant circuit, and either a single roof lesion or a box lesion can interrupt them. The most effective catheter intervention for non-PAF is a PVI plus posterior LA wall isolation in the form of a box lesion, but the success rate is well below 50% even with multiple catheter ablation sessions.[9]

Failures of catheter ablation for non-PAF are most commonly the result of performing the wrong operation because PVI is simply not an adequate operation for non-PAF. The combination of potentially incomplete individual lesions coupled with the wrong operation explains the dismal results that are routinely reported after PVI for non-PAF.

Goals of the Maze Procedure

The Maze procedure is a true ablation procedure in that it either interrupts or precludes the development of the macro-reentrant drivers that sustain AF. Therefore, it is equally successful for PAF and non-PAF. It is probable that much of its success in patients with PAF results from the fact that a part of the operation is the creation of a box lesion around the pulmonary veins and the intervening posterior LA wall (PVI + posterior LA wall isolation). At the time the Maze procedure was first performed (1987), the importance of pulmonary veins triggers was unknown because they were first described by Haissaguerre some 11 years later. John Boineau had some suspicion that the pulmonary vein cuff played a role in AF, but we did not know exactly what that role was. Thus the reason we included a box lesion in the Maze procedure was not to isolate the triggers but to make the Maze procedure easier technically. Regardless, the objective of the Maze procedure was to render the atria incapable of fibrillating whether or not it was stimulated by atrial or other triggers.

It is interesting that when Haissaguerre demonstrated that 90% of the atrial triggers that induce AF are located in the region of the pulmonary veins in stand-alone PAF, it immediately explained a complaint we had experienced after successful Maze procedures for stand-alone PAF. Approximately 10% of patients of our patients who had successful Maze procedures for stand-alone AF reported that they still experienced the "feeling of a fast heartbeat that I used to get just before atrial fibrillation started, but the atrial fibrillation no longer follows that feeling." This is clearly consistent with the periodic rapid firing of nonpulmonary vein triggers that can still be felt by the patient because they had not been isolated but that can no longer induce AF because the Maze procedure had precluded the ability of the atria to fibrillate by preventing the possibility of large-diameter macro-reentrant circuits (drivers) from forming.

The objective of the Maze procedure is to create every atrial lesion that is necessary to prevent the development of any macro-reentrant circuits anywhere in either atria. This includes the mitral line and coronary sinus cryolesion in the posterior LA isthmus between the inferior pulmonary veins and the posterior mitral valve annulus. This is done in every case even though it is essential in only 10% to 15% of patients with AF. However, we don't know who that 10% to 15% of patients are before surgery, so it is necessary to create the lesions in every surgical patient to prevent a 10% to 15% failure rate.

Goal of Hybrid Procedures

Hybrid procedures are interventions for AF in which surgeons and electrophysiologists combine their expertise to treat patients with AF. There are several different hybrid procedures, but they all include an initial off-pump thoracoscopic or subxiphoid procedure followed by an obligatory catheter ablation either during the same setting ("joint hybrid") or at intervals separated from 6 to 12 weeks ("staged hybrid"). Because catheter ablation is successful for PAF, hybrid procedures are used almost exclusively for patients with non-PAF, especially those with long-standing persistent AF. These procedures are described in detail in subsequent chapters, but they are mentioned here to emphasize that the surgical goals of the initial thoracoscopic or subxiphoid procedures are not the same as the goals of a Maze procedure or even a non-Maze open surgical procedure. In these on-pump procedures, everything is done to ablate the AF so that a second procedure will not be necessary. This is why the mitral line–coronary sinus lesion is performed in every patient. However, in hybrid procedures, the purpose of the initial procedure is to modify the atrium enough to make the follow-up catheter procedure easier and more effective. It is impossible to create the mitral line and coronary sinus lesions off pump with a thoracoscopic or subxiphoid procedure, so they are not a part of the initial surgical portion of a hybrid procedure. However, after an epicardial box lesion has been created thoracoscopically, the electrophysiologist can check the integrity of the lesions and ablate any "gaps" during the follow-up catheter procedure. In addition, if an atrial arrhythmia such as perimitral flutter can be induced, the mitral line and coronary sinus lesions can be performed during the catheter procedure.

Summary of Interventional Goals

In summary, the goal of *catheter ablation* is to isolate as many of the triggers of AF as possible der to decrease the likelihood that episodes of AF will be induced. This is best accomplished in patients with PAF by performing a PVI plus posterior LA wall isolation ("box lesion"). Catheter ablation is only marginally successful for the treatment of patients with non-PAF.

The goal of the *Maze procedure* and other on-pump surgical interventions is to ablate the AF with one operation to avoid the need for another procedure. After all, if you're going to open a person's chest, place them on cardiopulmonary bypass, and arrest their heart, you need to be as certain as possible that you have cured their problem. The best way to do this is to perform a full biatrial Maze procedure to preclude the development of macro-reentrant circuits (drivers) anywhere in either atrium.

The surgical goal of *hybrid procedures* is to make it easier for the interventional electrophysiologist to place the necessary "finishing touches" to complete the lesions necessary to cure AF in the particular patient.

REFERENCES

1. Mines GR. On circulating excitations in heart muscle and their possible relation to tachycardia and fibrillation. *Trans Roy Soc Can*. 1914;8:43–52.
2. Cobb FR, Blumenschein SD, Sealy WC, Boineau JP, Wagner GS, Wallace AG. Successful surgical interruption of the bundle of Kent in a patient with Wolff-Parkinson-White syndrome. *Circulation*. 1968;38:1018.
3. Moe GK. On the multiple wavelet hypothesis of atrial fibrillation. *Arch Int Pharmacodyn*. 1962;140:183–188.
4. Haissaguerre M, Jais P, Shah DC, et al. Spontaneous initiation of atrial fibrillation by ectopic beats originating in the pulmonary veins. *N Eng J Med*. 1998;339(10):659–666.
5. Oral H, Knight BP, Tada H, et al. Pulmonary vein isolation for paroxysmal and persistent atrial fibrillation. *Circulation*. 2002;105:1077–1081.
6. Cox JL. Atrial fibrillation II: rationale for surgical treatment. *J Thorac Cardiovasc Surg*. 2003;126:1693–1699.
7. Wolf RK, Schneeberger EW, Osterday R, et al. Video-assisted bilateral pulmonary vein isolation and left atrial appendage exclusion for atrial fibrillation. *J Thorac Cardiovasc Surg*. 2005;130(3):797–802.
8. Gillinov AM, Gelijns AC, Parides MK, et al. Surgical ablation of atrial fibrillation during mitral-valve surgery. *N Eng J Med*. 2015;372(15):1399–1409.
9. Tilz RR, Rillig A, Thum AM, et al. Catheter ablation of long-standing persistent atrial fibrillation: 5-year outcomes of the Hamburg sequential ablation strategy. *J Am Coll Cardiol*. 2012;60(19):1921–1929.

11

Atrial Fibrillation Surgery Prior to the Maze Procedure

James L. Cox

CHAPTER OUTLINE

As described in Chapter 9, a number of lessons were learned from surgery for other arrhythmias that were critical to the development of surgery for atrial fibrillation (AF). The treatment of patients with the Wolff-Parkinson-White (WPW) syndrome and ischemic ventricular tachycardia dominated clinical arrhythmia surgery in the 1970s, but by the early 1980s, surgical procedures had been developed for essentially all clinically important arrhythmias except AF (see Chapter 9). Arrhythmia surgery reached its peak during the decade of the 1980s with frequent operations being performed in some centers for the WPW syndrome, ischemic and non ischemic ventricular tachycardia, automatic atrial arrhythmias, and atrioventricular node reentry tachycardia (AVNRT). The most active period in the development of surgery for AF was also in that decade, especially from 1980 to 1987.

SURGICAL ISOLATION PROCEDURES FOR ATRIAL FIBRILLATION

His Bundle Ablation

The first interventional procedure used clinically for the treatment of patients with AF was surgical His bundle ablation, though it was not developed specifically for the treatment of those with AF.[1] Obviously, successful His bundle ablation necessitated the implantation of a permanent ventricular pacemaker (Fig. 11.1) Elective His bundle ablation was first performed for patients with WPW syndrome whose accessory pathways could not be divided successfully[2] (Fig. 11.2A). Although the primary objective of WPW surgery was always to divide the accessory atrioventricular (AV) connection responsible for the arrhythmia (see

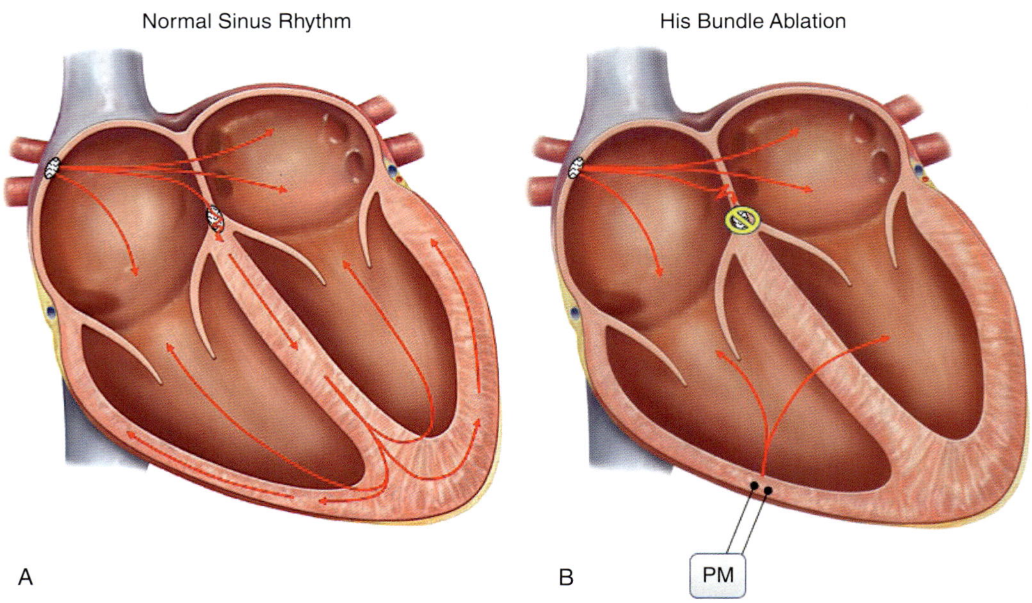

Fig. 11.1 (A) Diagram of the four chambers of the heart and propagation of a normal sinus rhythm impulse *(red arrows)* through the heart. (B) Ablation of the His bundle confines the sinus-generated impulse to the two atria, which continue to be activated in a normal manner. However, ventricular activation must be maintained by a permanent ventricular pacemaker after His bundle ablation. *PM,* pacemaker.

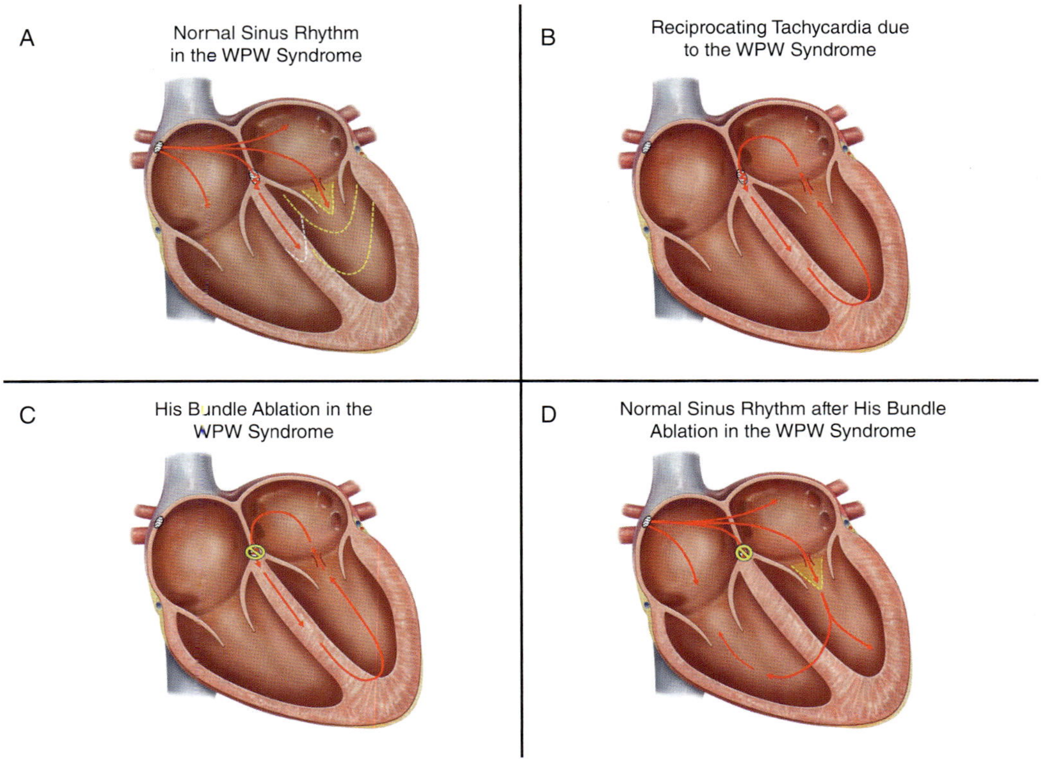

Fig. 11.2 (A) In patients with the Wolff-Parkinson-White (WPW) syndrome, antegrade conduction across the accessory atrioventricular connection (yellow area) causes ventricular preexcitation, resulting in a "delta wave" on the standard electrocardiogram. (B) If antegrade conduction across the accessory pathway is blocked, the following beat will conduct retrograde and result in the reciprocating tachycardia characteristic of WPW syndrome. (C) The primary objective in WPW surgery is to divide the accessory pathway, but when this cannot be accomplished, the reciprocating tachycardia can be terminated permanently by ablating the His bundle as a last resort. (D) Ablation of the His bundle in patients with WPW syndrome results in abnormal, but effective, ventricular conduction postoperatively and does not require a permanent ventricular pacemaker.

Chapter 9), it was sometimes impossible to do so, especially in the earliest days of arrhythmia surgery.[3] Because the macro-reentrant circuit responsible for the reciprocating tachycardia of the WPW syndrome includes antegrade conduction through the AV node and retrograde conduction across the accessory pathway (Fig. 11.2B), the reentrant circuit can be interrupted by ablating the His bundle but only as a last resort if the accessory pathway cannot be successfully divided (Fig. 11.2C). His bundle ablation in patients with the WPW syndrome ablates the reciprocating tachycardia but leaves the patient with an abnormal ventricular activation pattern postoperatively because the ventricles are activated across the accessory pathway, not through the AV node (Fig. 11.2D). However, there is no need for a postoperative ventricular pacemaker.

Fortunately, it was rarely necessary to ablate the His bundle as a last resort in patients with WPW syndrome. More commonly, His bundle ablation was used to treat patients with other medically refractory supraventricular tachycardias that could not be adequately localized by intraoperative mapping to allow for focal ablation. These arrhythmias included automatic atrial tachycardias in either atrium and occasionally poorly defined refractory atrial reentrant tachycardias.[1] The intraoperative localization of automatic atrial tachycardias was especially problematic because the general anesthesia required for surgery usually suppressed the automatic focus, making it impossible to localize. Because automatic foci do not respond to programmed electrical stimulation, the automatic atrial arrhythmias could not be induced intraoperatively. In these cases, the surgeon frequently had no choice but to resort to His bundle ablation for both automatic right atrial tachycardia, which was usually multifocal in origin (Fig. 11.3A), and automatic left atrial tachycardia, which was usually unifocal in origin (Fig. 11.3B). At that time, atrial flutter and AF were poorly understood, and if either could not be controlled by medical therapy and was sufficiently symptomatic, His bundle ablation with pacemaker implantation was performed to confine the arrhythmia to the atria, thus protecting the ventricles[1] (Fig. 11.3C and 11.3D).

The first lesson we learned when trying to create heart block by elective ablation of the AV node–His bundle complex was that it was surprisingly difficult to accomplish surgically. This observation seems paradoxical in view of the ease with which heart block can be caused inadvertently when performing surgery at or below the tricuspid valve annulus such as tricuspid valve repair or replacement and closure of membranous ventricular septal defects in tetralogy of Fallot. Elective His bundle ablation was performed through an incision identical to that described in Chapter 9 for dividing posterior septal accessory pathways in patients with the WPW syndrome (see Fig. 9.7), and the fat pad in the anterior portion of the posterior septal space was dissected free of the ventricular septum. In addition, the AV node artery was originally identified and divided in hopes of creating heart block by that maneuver alone, but as described in Chapters 3 and 9, the AV node is not an end artery, and its division does not result in heart block (see Figs. 3.19 and 3.20).

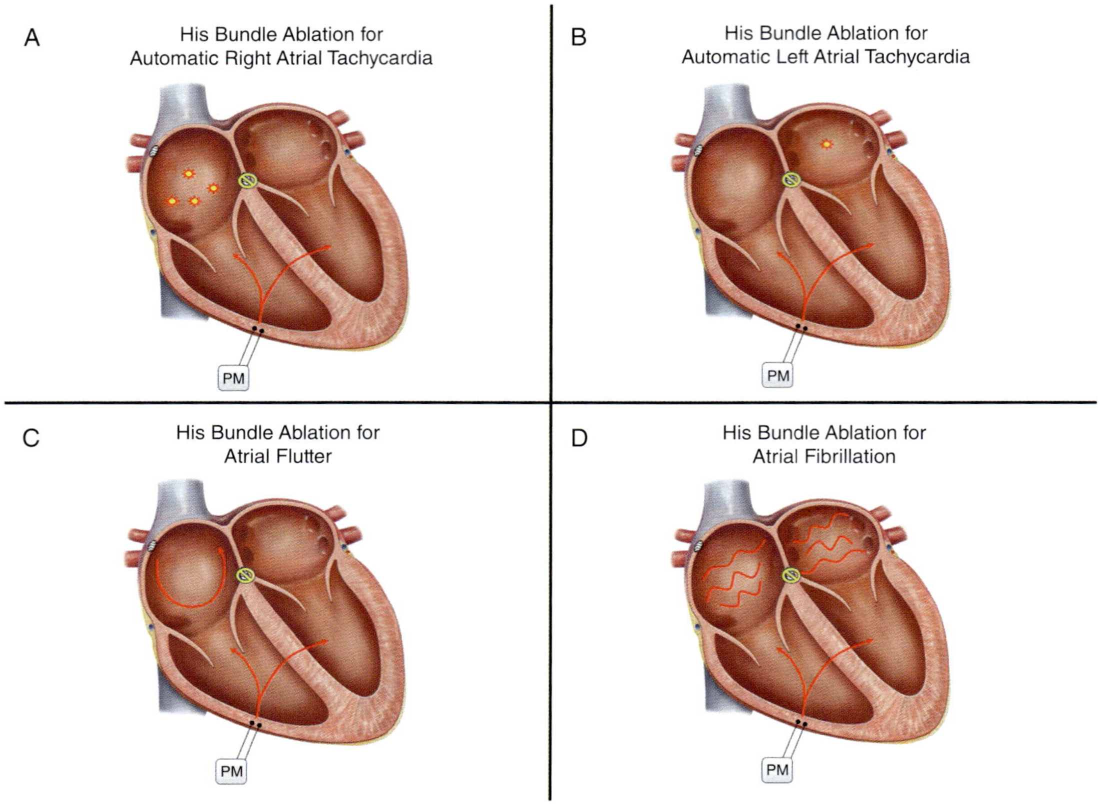

Fig. 11.3 (A) Elective His bundle ablation is an effective therapy for automatic right atrial tachycardia in which the specific site(s) of origin of the tachycardia cannot be identified by intraoperative mapping. Automatic right atrial tachycardia is typically multifocal in origin. A ventricular pacemaker is required after surgery. (B) Elective His bundle ablation is also an effective therapy for automatic left atrial tachycardia in which the specific site(s) of origin of the tachycardia cannot be identified by intraoperative mapping. Automatic left atrial tachycardia is typically unifocal in origin. A ventricular pacemaker is required after surgery. (C) Elective His bundle ablation was an effective therapy for refractory atrial flutter before learning that its macro-reentrant driver (the "atrial flutter wave") uses the cavotricuspid isthmus as a part of its circuit. When elective His bundle ablation was used to treat patients with atrial flutter, a ventricular pacemaker was required after surgery. (D) Before identifying the electrical events that occur during atrial fibrillation (AF), elective His bundle ablation was used to treat patients with refractory AF. A ventricular pacemaker was required after surgery.

Even extensive surgical dissection in this region proved to be an unreliable method for creating heart block. Therefore cryoablation of the His bundle replaced surgical dissection as the technique of choice in the mid-1970s.[4] The right atrium (RA) was opened in the usual manner, but no incision was made inside the atrium. The only clinical cryoprobes available at the time were non disposable nitrous oxide probes of varying sizes. Nitrous oxide cooled the cryoprobes to −60°C, but the temperature of the cryoprobe could be held at any level above 0°C if so desired. We took advantage of that feature to "ice map" for the location of the His bundle just above the tricuspid valve annulus and immediately posterior to the membranous atrial septum by first cooling the cryoprobe to only 0°C. After the exact location of the His bundle was identified, conduction through it was temporarily blocked, but conduction returned a few seconds after stopping the freeze. By moving the probe to slightly different positions in the known region of the His bundle, it was possible to find a single spot where 0°C caused temporary heart block. After that position was found, we cooled to 0°C to cause temporary heart block, stopped the freeze without moving the probe tip, waited for the return of AV conduction, and then cooled down to −60°C for 2 minutes. Cryoablation of the His bundle proved to be far easier and more reliable than surgical dissection and remained the procedure of choice for elective His bundle ablation until Scheinman developed the catheter fulguration technique for His bundle ablation in 1982.[5]

Left Atrial Isolation Procedure

A disproportionate number of the patients with automatic atrial tachycardias in whom we had to ablate the His bundle and implant permanent pacemakers were younger than 30 years of age and included several teenagers. This was stimulation enough to try to devise some better way to treat un mappable automatic atrial tachycardias that would not necessitate lifelong pacemaker dependence. Because the sinoatrial (SA) node is in the upper lateral RA and the AV node–His bundle complex is in the atrial septum, it seemed rather obvious that if we could devise a way to separate the body of the left atrium (LA) from the rest of the heart surgically, it would isolate the automatic focus to the LA and allow the rest of the heart to stay in a normal sinus rhythm (Fig. 11.4 and Fig. 9.16).

In 1978, we initiated a series of surgical experiments designed to isolate the LA.[6] The project proved to be far more difficult than expected because we had no idea at the time that the coronary sinus was capable of conducting electrical activity. Thus, in one experiment after another, the LA was clearly physically separated from the rest

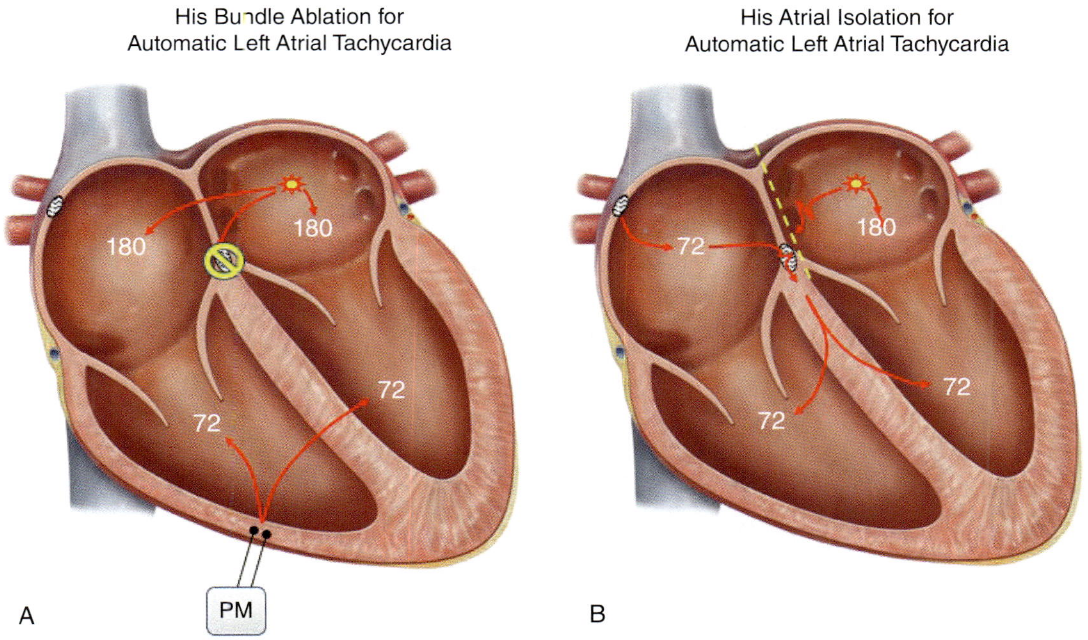

Fig. 11.4 (A) Automatic left atrial tachycardia could be confined to the atria by creating heart block. A ventricular pacemaker was required after surgery. (B) The left atrium (LA) is isolated from the remainder of the heart after a left atrial isolation procedure for an automatic left atrial tachycardia. Note that the sinoatrial node is capable of generating a normal sinus rhythm after isolation of the LA with normal activation of the right atrium, right ventricle, and left ventricle. *PM,* pacemaker.

of the heart, but LA appendage pacing still captured the whole heart. In these experiments, the coronary sinus was always skeletonized in a meticulous manner so that blood flowing inside it could clearly be seen with the naked eye. This was done with special care to remove all myocardial fibers along the coronary sinus that might be capable of conducting electrical activity. I finally deduced that there was simply no remaining structure that could possibly be conducting electrical activity other than the coronary sinus itself. Therefore, a cryoprobe was placed directly onto the exposed coronary sinus, and pressure was applied to collapse the walls of the sinus together so that a circumferential cryolesion could be created around the entire coronary sinus at that site. Approximately 10 seconds into the freeze, electrical conduction from the LA to the rest of the heart suddenly stopped. Thus, it was immediately clear that the coronary sinus had to be ablated, as well as the atrial myocardium, to stop conduction across the left atrial isthmus between the inferior pulmonary veins (PVs) and the posterior mitral valve annulus. This observation subsequently proved to be a critical part of the success of the Maze procedure that was developed nearly 10 years later.[7]

An unexpected finding during this series of experiments was that the left atrial isolation procedure was also capable of isolating atrial fibrillation to the LA while the remainder of the heart remained in sinus rhythm[6] (Fig. 11.5) (see Chapter 9). Despite this observation, we never used the LA isolation procedure to treat patients with AF ourselves because it did not restore left atrial function and it did not remove the danger of systemic thromboembolism associated with AF. However, Vigano's group[8] in Italy reported on 205 patients who had the left atrial isolation procedure for concomitant AF during mitral valve surgery with a return to normal sinus rhythm in 44% of the patients.

Shortly after developing the left atrial isolation procedure, we developed the right atrial isolation procedure to treat patients with

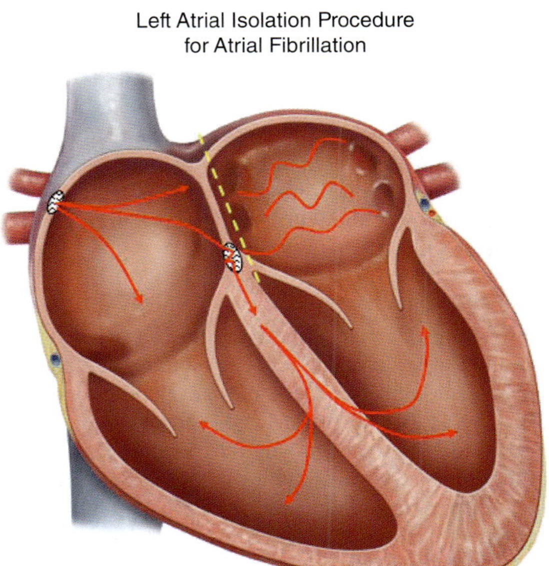

Fig. 11.5 The left atrial isolation procedure is also capable of confining atrial fibrillation to the left atrium only and allowing the remaining three chambers to be activated normally by sinus rhythm. However, the risk of systemic thromboembolism is not alleviated, and there is no left atrial transport function after surgery.

automatic right atrial tachycardias and occasionally atrial flutter, again to avoid the necessity of having to ablate the His bundle[9,10] (Fig. 11.6). Obviously, it was essential to leave the SA node in contiguity with the AV node and LA to obviate the need for a permanent ventricular

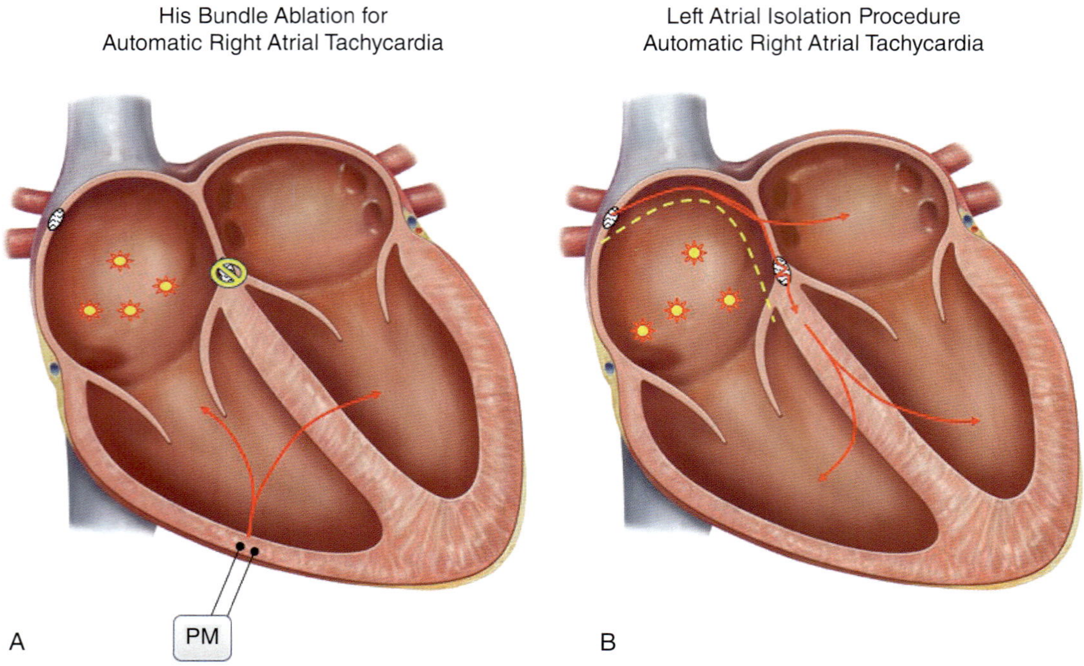

Fig. 11.6 (A) His bundle ablation for automatic right atrial tachycardia. (B) Right atrial isolation procedure for automatic right atrial tachycardia. Note that the sinoatrial (SA) node and atrial septum containing the atrioventricular (AV) node are not included in the portion of the right atrium that is isolated. This leaves the SA node and AV node–His bundle complex capable of generating and conducting normal sinus rhythm beats after isolation of the right atrium with normal activation of the left atrium, right ventricle, and left ventricle. *PM,* ***.

pacemaker (see Chapter 9). As with the LA isolation procedure, the right atrial isolation procedure was not developed primarily to treat patients with AF. Although we used it several times for patients with other refractory supraventricular arrhythmias, to our knowledge, neither we nor anyone else ever used the right atrial isolation procedure to treat patients with AF. However, in 1985 Guiraudon combined the left atrial isolation procedure with the right atrial isolation procedure to create the "corridor procedure" that was used specifically for the treatment of patients with AF.[11]

Corridor Procedure

The objective of the corridor procedure was to isolate AF to the RA and LA but to leave a "corridor" of contiguous atrial septal tissue between the SA node and AV node to obviate the need for a ventricular pacemaker (Fig. 11.7). Unfortunately, permanent pacemakers were required in 15% to 20% of patients after the corridor procedure,[12] largely negating the only theoretical advantage of the corridor procedure over His bundle ablation. In addition, both atria usually continued to fibrillate following the corridor procedure, so as with His bundle ablation, there was no A-V synchrony on either side of the heart, and the patient remained vulnerable to systemic thromboembolism from the left atrial appendage (LAA).

Summary

The first three surgical procedures that were used to treat patients with refractory AF were His bundle ablation, the left atrial isolation procedure, and the corridor procedure. All three of these were *isolation* procedures and none of them were designed to actually *ablate* AF. Up to this time, no attempt had been made to ablate AF because not enough was understood about its electrophysiology to design a reasonable approach to its ablation.

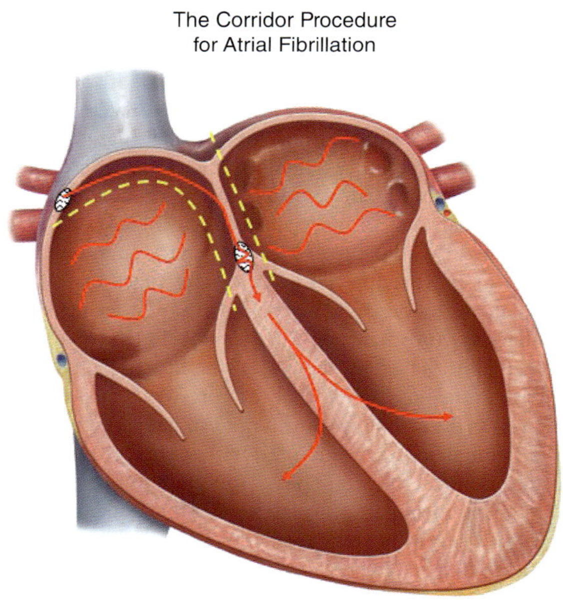

Fig. 11.7 The corridor procedure was developed by Guiraudon specifically for the treatment of patients with atrial fibrillation (AF). By combining the left atrial isolation procedure and the right atrial isolation procedure into one operation, the corridor procedure, AF could be confined to the two isolated atria, and a sinus-generated impulse could still be conducted through the remaining corridor of septal tissue containing the atrioventricular node into the ventricles. The objective was not to *ablate* AF but rather to isolate the ventricles from AF without creating the necessity of a postoperative ventricular pacemaker. However, the risk of systemic thromboembolism is not alleviated, and there is no left atrial or right atrial transport function after surgery.

SURGICAL ABLATION PROCEDURES FOR ATRIAL FIBRILLATION

Atrial Transection Procedure

Because we had a clinically relevant animal model of AF,[13] we initiated a series of experiments in 1985 to determine the AF ablation potential of several different surgical procedures. These were trial-and-error procedures because our mapping techniques had not yet been developed to the point that we adequately understood the electrical events taking place during AF.

The first surgical procedure that we tried was complete encirclement of all four PVs (including the posterior left atrial free wall), a technique that come to be known in future years as the "box lesion" (Fig. 11.8A). John Boineau suggested this as the initial trial procedure because of a vague suspicion that the PVs probably had something to do with AF. Unfortunately, the "box lesion" had no effect whatsoever on the sustained AF in our animal model. We then added a left lateral atrial lesion extending from the box lesion to the lateral mitral valve annulus (Fig. 11.8B, *red arrow*). Again, the addition of this lesion had no effect on AF. A septal lesion was then added (Fig. 11.8C, *red arrow*), and surprisingly, AF was prevented by this set of lesions in all animals. However, in each case in our animal model, atrial flutter could still be easily induced after the creation of these left atrial and septal lesions. As a result, we added a final lesion from the septal lesion laterally across the RA between the orifices of the superior vena cava (SVC) and inferior vena cava (IVC) (Fig. 11.8D, *red arrow*). After this set of lesions, neither AF nor atrial flutter could be induced by programmed electrical stimulation or burst pacing techniques.

These experimental observations suggested to us that AF might be caused by the presence of two large macro-reentrant circuits, one in the LA rotating around the orifices of the LAA and the PVs and a second in the RA rotating around the orifices of the SVC and IVC (Fig. 11.9). However, we had no confirmation of this hypothesis based on actual electrophysiological mapping. Nevertheless, we recognized that if this hypothesis were true, the two macro-reentrant circuits could be interrupted by creating one long atrial lesion from the left lateral

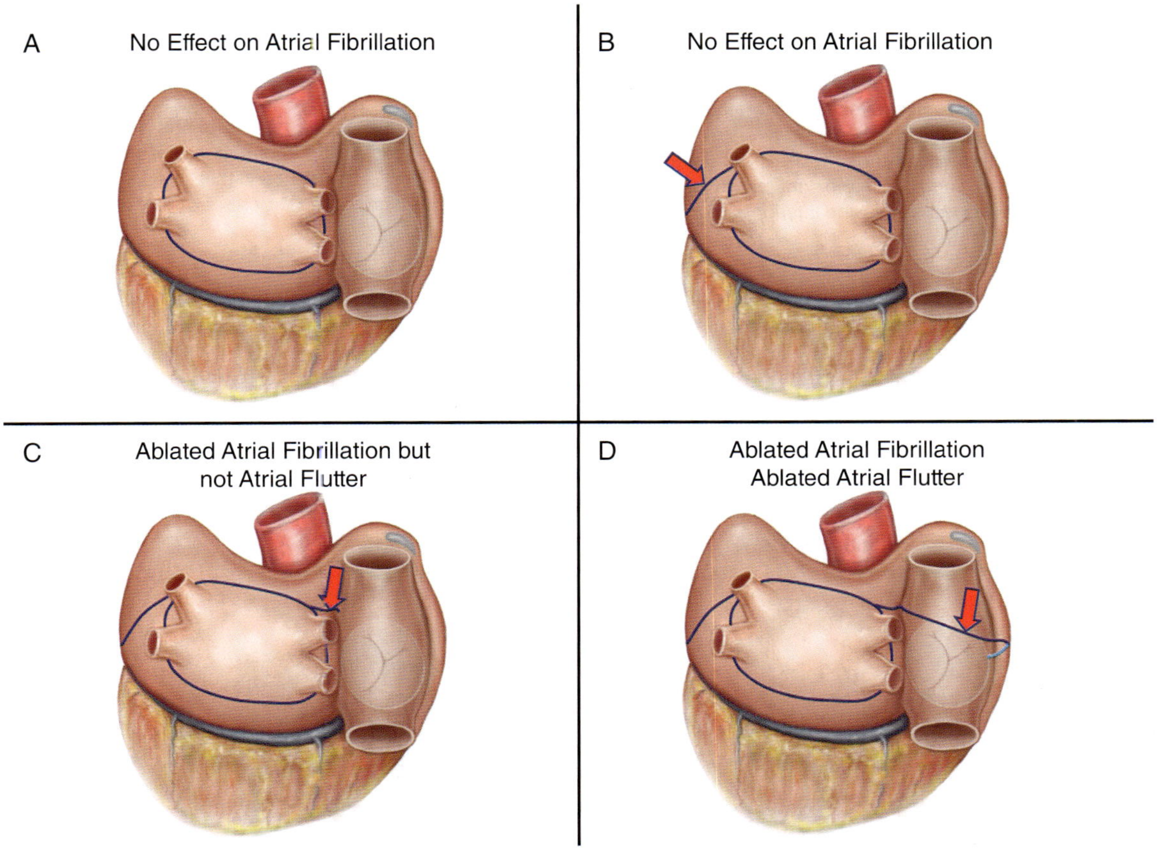

Fig. 11.8 Before the development of sophisticated multipoint mapping systems that elucidated the underlying electrophysiology of atrial fibrillation (AF), a series of trial-and-error surgical interventions was used in an effort to ablate AF in an experimental animal model. (A) The first surgical procedure tried was a circumferential "box lesion" encompassing all four pulmonary vein (PV) orifices and the intervening posterior left atrial wall between the right and left PVs. This procedure had no effect on the ability of the atria to fibrillate in our experimental model. (B) A lesion was then added from the PV box lesion across the lateral left atrium extending down to the lateral mitral valve annulus *(red arrow)*. The lesion was positioned between the orifices of the left atrial appendage and the PVs. This lesion set also had no effect on the ability of the atria to fibrillate. (C) An atrial septal lesion *(dashed line)* was then added, sparing only the lower septum that harbored the atrioventricular node–His bundle complex *(red arrow)*. This set of lesions resulted in the inability to induce AF despite using all programmed electrical stimulation and burst pacing techniques. Instead, these pacing techniques invariable resulted in atrial flutter. (D) A final lesion was added from the septal lesion across the right atrial free wall between the orifices of superior vena cava and inferior vena cava extending to the lateral tricuspid valve annulus *(red arrow)*. This lesion set rendered the atria incapable of developing either AF or atrial flutter.

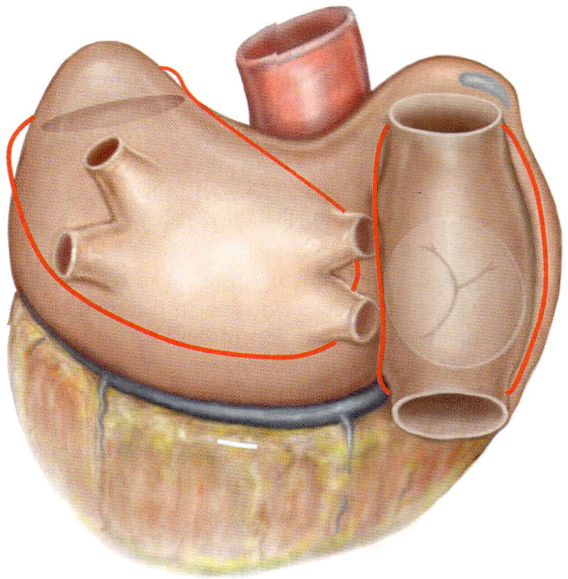

Fig. 11.9 The findings of the trial-and-error surgical procedures described in Fig. 11.8 suggested that the electrical events during atrial fibrillation might be due to the presence of two separate macro-reentrant drivers, one in the left atrium that rotated around the orifices of the left atrial appendage and the pulmonary veins, and one in the right atrium that rotated around the orifices of the superior vena cava and inferior vena cava.

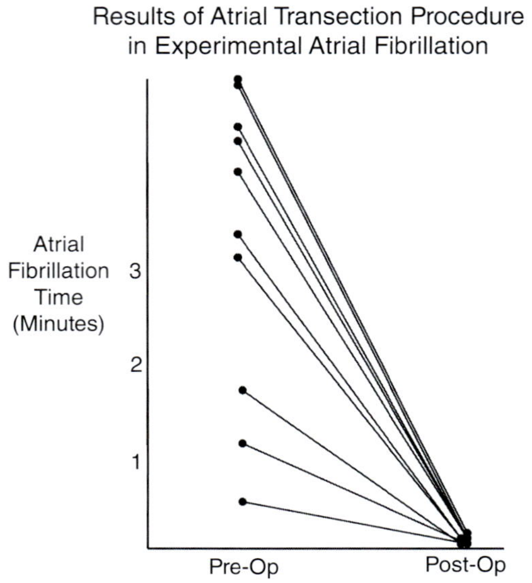

Fig. 11.11 Results of the atrial transection procedure in our animal model of atrial fibrillation (AF). The duration that AF was allowed to persist in 10 animals after preoperative induction is shown in the *left column*. The duration that AF lasted postoperatively in each animal is shown on the *right*. These results of the atrial transection procedure were highly suggestive that our concept of the electrophysiology of AF was correct (which it was not) and that this surgical procedure should be effective for the surgical treatment of AF in humans (which it was not).

mitral valve annulus, across the body of the LA between the orifices of the LAA and the PVs, across the atrial septum (sparing its lower portion containing the AV node), and extending across the body of the RA between the orifices of the SVC and IVC to the right lateral tricuspid valve annulus, an approach that we called the "atrial transection procedure" (Fig. 11.10). This surgical procedure was subsequently performed in our animal model of AF, and in all cases it resulted the prevention of AF and atrial flutter (Fig. 11.11).

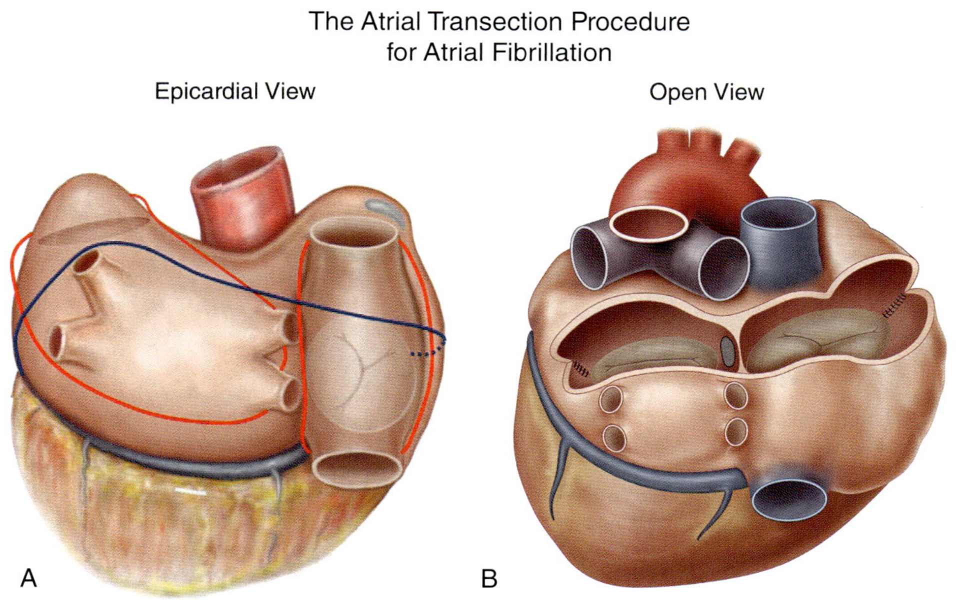

Fig. 11.10 (A) Suspecting that the drivers of atrial fibrillation were those illustrated in Fig. 11.9, we created a single incision that from the lateral mitral valve annulus, across the left atrium between the left atrial appendage and the pulmonary vein orifices, across the atrial septum *(dashed line)*, sparing its lower portion containing the atrioventricular node, across the right atrium between the orifices of the superior vena cava and inferior vena cava, and terminating at the lateral tricuspid valve annulus. We called this the atrial transection procedure. (B) A three-dimensional rendering of the atrial transection procedure.

Despite these observations, we were extremely reluctant to perform the atrial transection procedure clinically based entirely on these trial-and-error experiments. Nevertheless, an unusually persuasive young airline pilot from Cypress, Captain George Dheere, convinced us that it was worth trying in his particular case, so after institutional review board approval in September 1986, he underwent the atrial transection procedure, the first surgical procedure ever designed specifically to ablate AF. The details of that experience are discussed in Chapter 1 and are not repeated here except to say that the operation failed after approximately 5 months, and Captain Dheere eventually underwent the second Maze procedure ever performed in February 1988. After his Maze procedure, Captain Dheere developed the first known case of an iatrogenic arrhythmia that was originally called "atypical left atrial flutter" but is now known as "peri-mitral flutter" (see Chapter 48).

Maze Procedure

The second surgical procedure that was specifically designed to *ablate* AF was the Maze procedure, which is discussed in detail in subsequent chapters.

REFERENCES

1. Sealy WC, Gallagher JJ, Kasell J. His bundle interruption for control of inappropriate ventricular responses to atrial arrhythmias. *Ann Thor Surg*. 1981;32(5):429–438.
2. Sealy WC. His bundle interruption for reentry tachycardia in Wolff-Parkinson-White syndrome. *Ann Thor Surg*. 1983;36(3):345–352.
3. Gallagher JJ, Sealy WC, Cox JL, Kasell JH. Results of surgery for pre-excitation in 200 cases. *Circulation*. 1981;64(4):146.
4. Harrison L, Gallagher JJ, Kasell J, et al. Cryosurgical ablation of the AV node-His bundle: a new method for producing AV block. *Circulation*. 1977;55(3):463–470.
5. Scheinman MM, Morady F, Hess DS, Gonzalez R. Catheter-induced ablation of the atrioventricular junction to control refractory supraventricular arrhythmias. *JAMA*. 1982;248(7):851–855.
6. Williams JM, Ungerleider RM, Lofland GK, Cox JL. Left atrial isolation: new technique for the treatment of supraventricular arrhythmias. *J Thor Cardiocasc Surg*. 1980;80:373.
7. Cox JL. The surgical treatment of atrial fibrillation: IV. *J Thor Cardiovasc Surg*. 1991;101:584–592.
8. Vigano M, Graffigna A, Ll Ressia, et al. Surgery for atrial fibrillation. *Eur J Cardiothorac Surg*. 1996;10(7):490–497.
9. Harada A, D'Agostino Jr HJ, JP Boineau, JL Cox. Right atrial isolation with preservation of the sinoatrial node: electrophysiologic and hemodynamic effects. *Circulation*. 1986(Suppl.74):II–135.
10. Harada A, D'Agostino Jr HJ, RB Schuessler, JP Boineau, JL Cox. Biatrial isolation with preservation of normal sinus node function and sino-ventricular conduction: a surgical treatment for supraventricular tachycardias. *JACC*. 1987;9(2):100A.
11. Guiraudon GM, Campbell CS, Jones DL, McLellan JL, MacDonald JL. Combined sino-atrial node atrioventricular node isolation: a surgical alternative to His bundle ablation in patients with atrial fibrillation. *Circulation*. 1985;72:220.
12. Van Hemel NM, Defauw JJ, Kingma JH, et al. Long-term results of the corridor operation for atrial fibrillation. *Brit Heart J*. 1994;71(2):170–176.
13. D'Agostino Jr HJ, Harada A, Eisenberg SB, Schuessler RB, Boineau JP, Cox JL. Surgical ablation of atrial fibrillation in a canine model of chronic mitral regurgitation. *Surg Forum XXXVII*. 1986:302303.

12

Development and Evolution of the Maze Procedure for Atrial Fibrillation

James L. Cox

CHAPTER OUTLINE

The development of surgical techniques for the treatment of patients with cardiac arrhythmias was dependent on the availability of intraoperative electrophysiologic mapping systems that provided the ability to determine precisely where to place the lesions of conduction block in each patient. Intraoperative mapping was used to "guide" the surgical procedures for Wolff-Parkinson-White syndrome,[1] elective His bundle ablation,[2] automatic left atrial tachycardias,[3] atrioventricular (AV) node reentry tachycardia,[4] automatic right atrial tachycardias,[5] ischemic ventricular tachcycardia,[6–8] and nonischemic ventricular tachycardia.[9] Because of the success of map-guided arrhythmia surgery for those arrhythmias, we naturally assumed that any successful surgical procedure for atrial fibrillation (AF) would also be map-guided. Our extensive experimental and clinical mapping studies documented that during AF, multiple macro-reentrant circuits were present in both atria.[10–12] However, the maps also demonstrated that these macro-reentrant drivers of AF were fleeting in nature and frequently changed locations. It soon became clear that locating these ever-changing circuits by intraoperative mapping and then trying to ablate them with individual lesions (i.e., "chasing" them) was simply not feasible. We actually tried this approach experimentally, but as soon as one reentrant circuit was abolished surgically, another reentrant circuit would appear in a different location, and the AF persisted.

THE MAZE PROCEDURE CONCEPT

The inability to map-guide AF surgery suggested the need for a single surgical technique that was capable of ablating AF in all patients regardless of the specific electrophysiologic activation pattern present in each patient. Such a procedure would have to take advantage of the single common characteristic of all AF, the simultaneous presence of two or more large macro-reentrant circuits in the atria. We observed that macro-reentrant circuits (drivers) during AF frequently rotated around sites of normal conduction block in the atria (e.g., the orifices of various structures connecting to the atria such as the pulmonary veins, atrial appendages, vena cavae) and the mitral and tricuspid valve annuli.

Despite numerous earlier studies, AF at this time (c. 1986) was still widely considered to be a "chaotic arrhythmia" and as such, untreatable by surgical intervention. In early 1987, I had a conversation completely by chance with the recently retired chairman of the Department of Pure Mathematics and Mathematical Statistics of Cambridge University in the airport at Maastricht in the Netherlands. He asked if I did any research, and when I answered that I was working on a "chaotic" rhythm of the heart, he said, "Well, you know, my people in Cambridge are the world's experts on the chaos theory." This chance meeting resulted in my giving a lecture later to his mathematics department in Cambridge on what we knew about AF at the time. I also took multiple examples of our raw data (simple numbers representing the local activation times in the atria during AF) for his faculty to examine, and they confirmed that our data suggested specific patterns of activation that were indeed, not chaotic. This further strengthened our belief that AF was not a chaotic arrhythmia at all but rather one characterized by certain anatomic-electrophysiologic features that were common to all patients with AF. Furthermore, correlation of the normal anatomic structures with the observed interactions between local conduction velocity, local refractory periods, and the area of atrium necessary to sustain these reentrant circuits (i.e., their size) indicated that the number of potential locations in the atria that were capable of sustaining atrial macro-reentry was finite. This meant to us that it should be possible to treat atrial fibrillation surgically. The initial reasoning underlying the design of the Maze procedure that addressed these issues are discussed in other chapters and need not be repeated here. However, continuing experimental investigation and clinical experience further clarified why the Maze procedure was successful in ablating AF and confirmed that afterward, the atria could be activated by a sinus-generated impulse, thus restoring inter-atrial and AV synchrony.

Potential Left Atrial Drivers During Atrial Fibrillation

The local refractory periods were known to be shorter in the left atrium (LA) than in the right atrium (RA); therefore, the macro-reentrant circuits were potentially smaller in the LA (see Chapter 4, Figs. 4.14 and 4.15). Thus, atrial anatomy limited the potential sites where macro-reentry could develop to drive AF (Fig. 12.1A–C). We later learned that after pulmonary vein isolation, a new iatrogenic type of long cycle-length atrial flutter

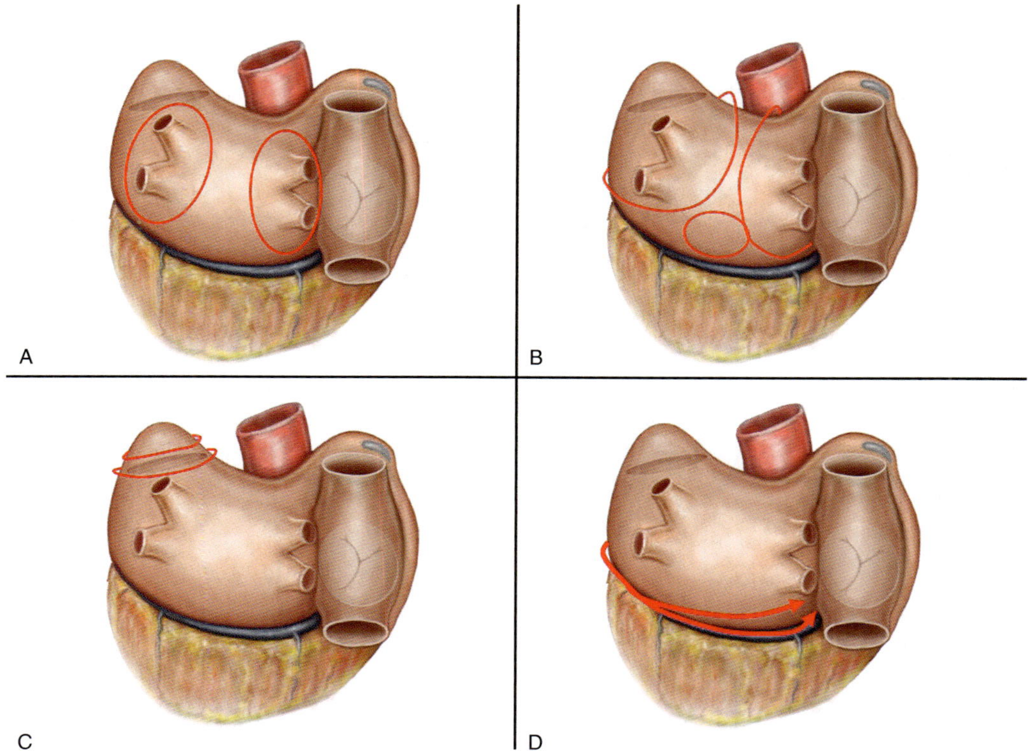

Fig. 12.1 The locations of left atrial macro-reentrant drivers fall into four general categories, which are as follows. (A) Those rotating around the two pairs of pulmonary veins that usually incorporate very little of the posterior left atrial wal' as a part of their circuits. (B) Those rotating around the one pair of pulmonary veins that use either the atrial septum or the lateral left atrial free well and incorporate the posterior left atrial wall as a part of their circuits. In addition, one smaller circuit is shown in the left atrial isthmus area because it was recorded in the first patient ever to be mapped with a multipoint computerized mapping system during atrial fibrillation (see Chapter 5, Fig. 5.5). (C) Those within the body of the left atrial appendage (rare) or just below the orifice of the appendage using the so-called "coumadin ridge" (more common). (D) The iatrogenic arrhythmia peri-mitral flutter, which uses the left atrial isthmus, including either the atrial myocardium or the coronary sinus as a part of its circuit (see Chapter 48).

often developed in the left atrium that uses the atrial myocardium and the coronary sinus in the left atrial isthmus between the inferior pulmonary vein orifices and the posterior mitral valve annulus (Fig. 12.1D). We called this iatrogenic arrhythmia "atypical left atrial flutter," but its name was later changed to "peri-mitral flutter," a troublesome arrhythmia that is addressed in greater detail in Chapter 48. Thus even though all of these left atrial macro-reentrant drivers of AF had not been specifically documented before our first attempt at the surgical ablation, it was clear where these left atrial drivers could potentially be located (Fig. 12.2).

Potential Right Atrial Drivers During Atrial Flutter and Atrial Fibrillation

Atrial Flutter

Because the macro-reentrant circuits in the RA require a larger area to develop and sustain themselves than macro-reentrant circuits in the LA. There are only a few RA sites where they can be located. Santucci et al.[13] published an excellent article in 2009 documenting that classic atrial flutter can be caused by one of three potential macro-reentrant circuits in the RA, the so-called atrial flutter waves (Fig. 12.3). All three of these potential RA drivers of atrial flutter use the cavo-tricuspid isthmus (CTI) between the inferior vena cava (IVC) orifice and the tricuspid valve annulus as a part of their macro-reentrant circuit. This explains why the isolated CTI lesion created by catheter ablation usually cures classic atrial flutter (Fig. 12.4).

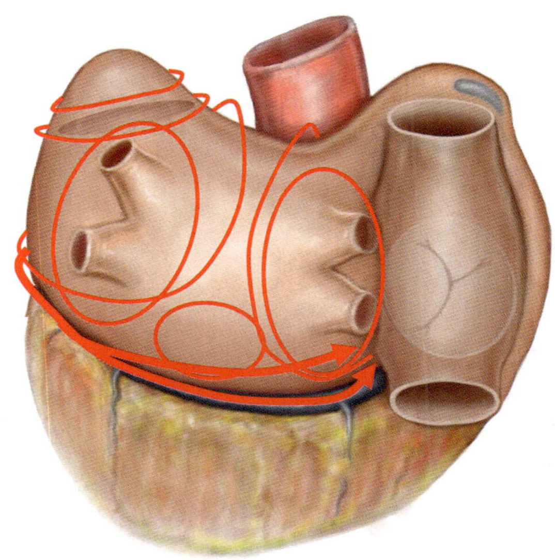

Fig. 12.2 Left atrial macro-reentrant drivers of atrial fibrillation (AF). This figure comprising all of the known left atrial macro-reentrant drivers of AF shows that some of them use the posterior wall of the left atrium (LA) as a part of their circuit and some do not. In long-standing persistent AF, these left atrial macro-reentrant circuits represent approximately 70% of the drivers of AF.

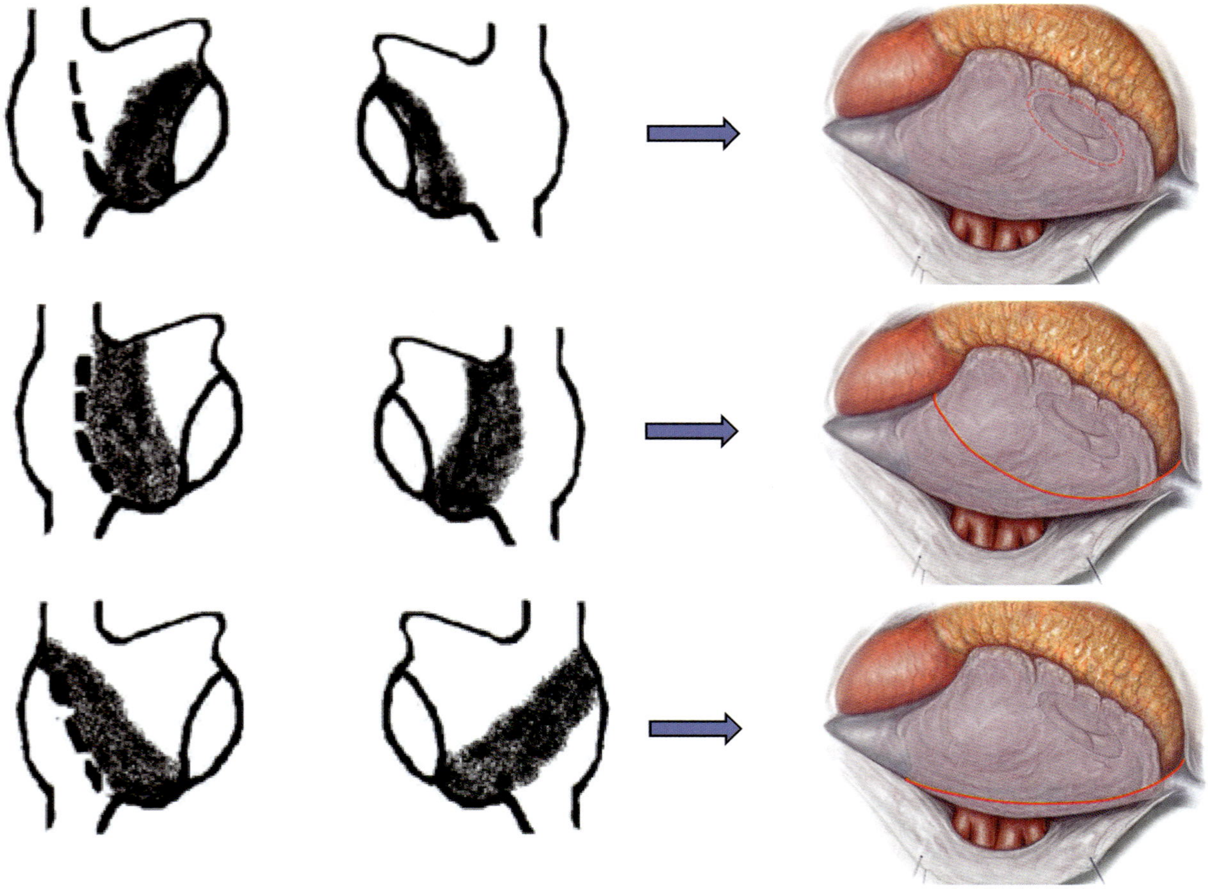

Fig. 12.3 Right atrial macro-reentrant drivers of atrial flutter. *Left panel,* Key figure from Santucci and coworkers' 2009 article[13] showing the locations of each of the three macro-reentrant circuits that can cause classic right atrial flutter. *Right panel,* Three-dimensional representation of the location of the three macro-reentrant circuits in the *left panel* that can drive classic right atrial flutter. Only one of these reentrant circuits is present at a time. They are (1) a single large circuit in the right atrium (RA) above the annulus of the tricuspid valve *(top panels)* that uses the cavotricuspid isthmus (CTI) inferiorly; (2) a single large circuit that uses the right atrial free wall and atrial septum, passing *anterior* to the superior vena cava (SVC) orifice superiorly and the CTI inferiorly *(middle panels)*; or (3) a single large circuit that uses the right atrial free wall and atrial septum, passing *posterior* to the SVC orifice superiorly and the CTI inferiorly *(lower panels)*. All three of these "atrial flutter waves" use the CTI. Therefore, a single lesion placed across the CTI with either a catheter or surgically is highly effective in the treatment of patients with atrial flutter. (Reproduced from Santucci PA, Varma N, Cytron J, et al. Electroanatomic mapping of postpacing intervals clarifies the complete active circuit and variants in atrial flutter. *Heart Rhythm.* 2009;6(11):1586–1595.)

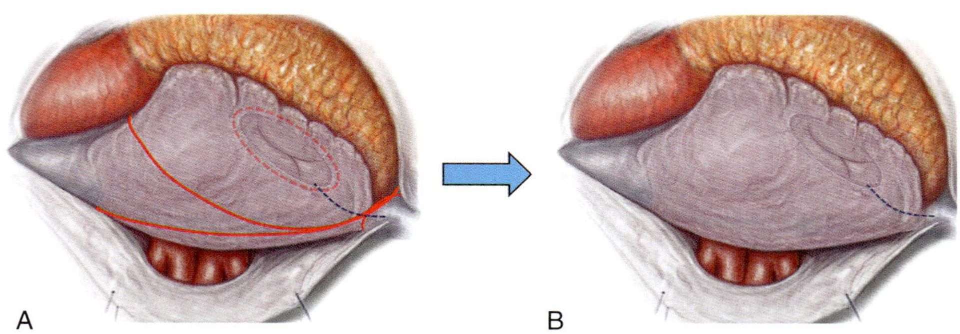

Fig. 12.4 Cavotricuspid isthmus (CTI) lesion for atrial flutter. An endocardial lesion placed across the CTI *(dashed blue line)* is extremely effective for the treatment of patients with *atrial flutter* because all three of the "flutter waves" that can potentially cause atrial flutter use the CTI as a part of their macro-reentrant circuit. (A) CTI lesion across the three "flutter waves" that can drive atrial flutter. (B) No remaining "flutter waves" after CTI lesion for atrial flutter.

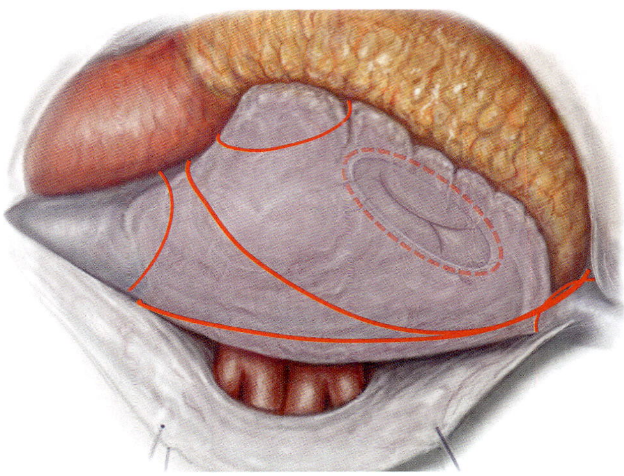

Fig. 12.5 Right atrial drivers of atrial fibrillation (AF). The locations of the three potential atrial flutter waves plus the other sites in the right atrium shown to be capable of sustaining macro-reentry and therefore of driving AF as well. The additional sites include reentrant circuits around the base of the right atrial appendage and around the orifices of the superior vena cava and inferior vena cava (IVC). In addition to the three atrial flutter waves that use the cavotricuspid isthmus (CTI) in their circuits, the reentrant circuit around the IVC also uses the CTI as a part of its circuit.

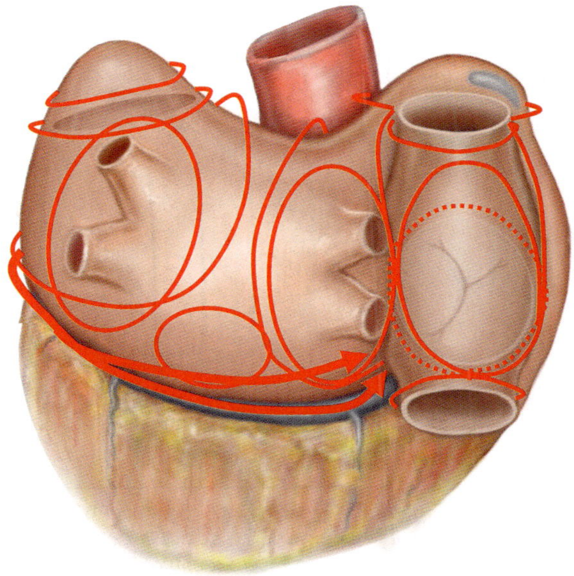

Fig. 12.7 Two-dimensional representation of the known macro-reentrant drivers of atrial fibrillation (AF) that were originally only theoretical but have since been documented by electrophysiological mapping. This method of illustrating the location of the drivers provides a basis for understanding the results of surgical and catheter ablation for persistent and long-standing persistent AF.

Atrial Fibrillation

The contribution of the RA to the maintenance of AF is finally beginning to get its due as a result of multiple mapping studies showing that up to 50% of patients with persistent and long-standing persistent AF have drivers in the RA.[14] In addition to the three "flutter waves," three additional sites of potential macro-reentrant drivers in the RA are (1) around the superior vena cava (SVC) orifice, (2) around the IVC orifice, and (3) around the base of the RA appendage (RAA; Fig. 12.5). This explains why, unlike atrial flutter, an isolated CTI lesion is inadequate to ablate all of the RA drivers of AF because it leaves the possibility of a macro-reentrant driver around the orifice of the SVC and around the base of the RAA (Fig. 12.6). The potential macro-reentrant drivers of AF in the RA are combined with the left atrial drivers to document the basis for the development of a biatrial surgical procedure for AF (Fig. 12.7).

Interruption of the Right and Left Atrial Drivers of Atrial Fibrillation

We knew that one way to ablate AF would be to "breadloaf" the atria into multiple separate compartments, as had been done experimentally some 25 years earlier (see Chapter 5, Fig. 5.11). Although breadloafing the atria would certainly ablate AF (Fig. 12.8, *left panel*), it was not feasible clinically. The two sequelae of atrial "breadloafing" that negated

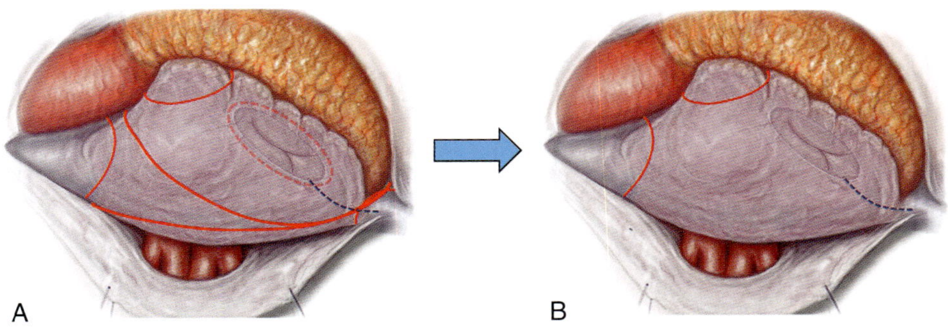

Fig. 12.6 Cavotricuspid isthmus (CTI) lesion for atrial fibrillation (AF). An endocardial lesion placed across the CTI (*dashed blue line*) is not as effective for the treatment of patients with AF as it is for those with atrial flutter because potential reentrant sites remain around the right atrial appendage and the superior vena cava (SVC), either of which can still participate (with left atrial reentrant circuits) in driving AF. However, combining a right atrial CTI lesion with the left atrial maze lesions in patients with AF significantly enhances the success rate in comparison with placing no lesions at all in the right atrium (RA). This is because macro-reentry around the right atrial appendage and SVC is quite rare, so most of the right atrial drivers that participate in AF are one of the three atrial flutter waves or the inferior vena cava reentrant circuit. (A) CTI lesion for atrial fibrillation. (B) Remaining potential RA macro-reentrant circuits after CTI lesion for atrial fibrillation.

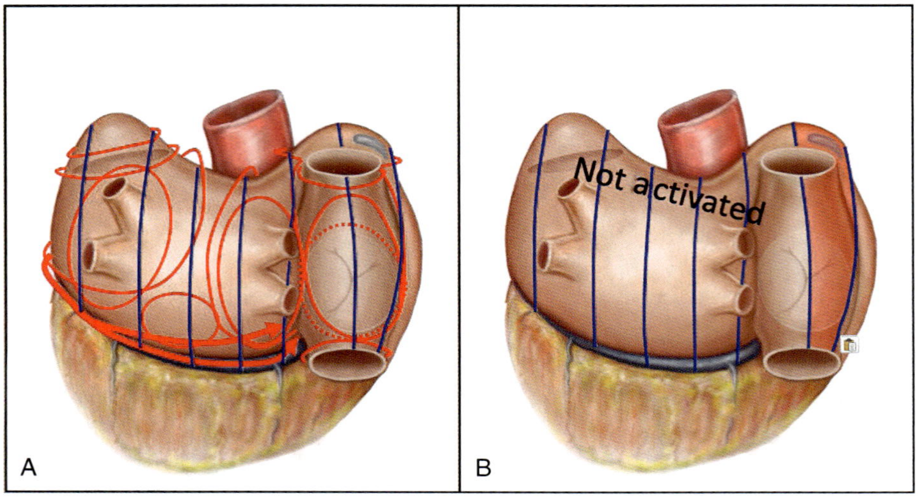

Fig. 12.8 "Breadloafing" the atria. (A) The creation of multiple parallel lines of conduction block that separate the atria into multiple electrically isolated compartments ablates atrial fibrillation if the compartments are too small to sustain macro-reentry. (B) However, compartmentalization of the atria means that there is only one compartment that can be activated by the sinus node postoperatively *(red shaded compartment)*. The rest of the atrium cannot be activated by a sinus-generated impulse.

its clinical feasibility were (1) the total isolation (compartmentalization) of individual segments of the atrium from one another, which precluded any subsequent synchronized activation of the atrial myocardium, and (2) the only part of the atrium that could resume a sinus rhythm postoperatively was the isolated compartment that contained the sinoatrial (SA) node (see Fig. 12.8).

Despite not being clinically applicable, the breadloafing experiments showed that the critical factor that determines the ability to develop atrial macro-reentry is the *area of contiguous atrium* available to participate in the macro-reentrant circuit. These studies also showed rather inadvertently that the critical area can be limited by placing atrial lesions close enough together to prevent the development of large macro-reentrant circuits. This suggested the possibility of ablating atrial macro-reentry (fibrillation) by avoiding the complete isolation (compartmentalization) of the individual segments and leaving them connected so that they remained a single unit of myocardium from an electrical standpoint. The obvious reasoning was that if the large macro-reentrant drivers could not form, then the atria could not fibrillate (Fig. 12.9). It then occurred to me that if instead of placing parallel lesions as is done with the breadloafing approach, we placed the lesions in a "maze" pattern, atrial macro-reentry (fibrillation) could still be surgically ablated, but in this case, the entire atrial myocardium could be activated by the SA node afterward. Thus the objective of such a "maze procedure" would be twofold: (1) to preclude the

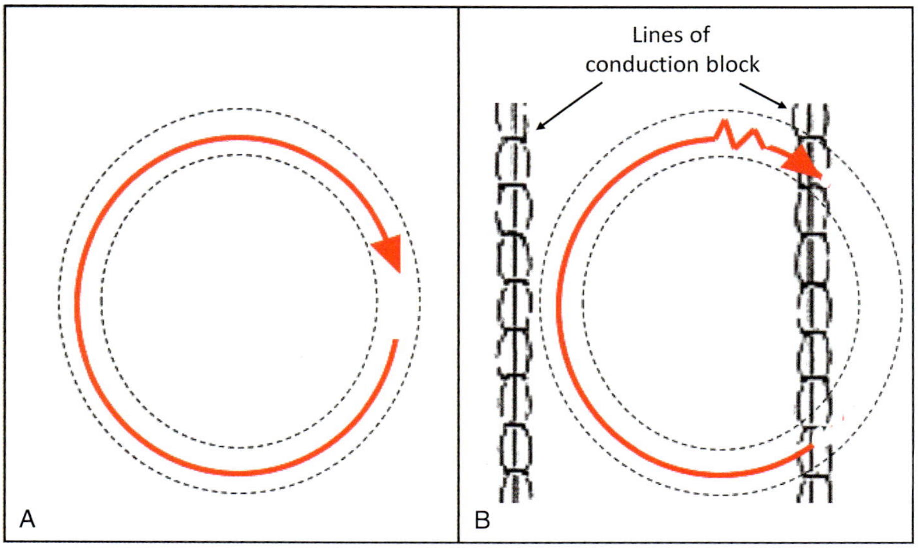

Fig. 12.9 (A) The *dotted circle* represents a potential macro-reentrant circuit. The *red arrow* within that *dotted circle* indicates that the potential circuit has been stimulated and is now active. (B) As mentioned in the text, these macro-reentrant drivers are relatively large and are therefore vulnerable to being ablated by placing lesions (lines of conduction block) close enough together in the atria to preclude their ability to form. The areas between these lesions do not have to be isolated (as with "breadloafing") and therefore can remain in continuity with the remainder of the atrium. If such macro-reentrant circuits cannot occur in the atrium, the atria cannot fibrillate.

development of atrial macro-reentry (fibrillation) and (2) to leave the atria capable of responding to a sinus-generated impulse that could activate both atria.

The next step was to figure out how to create an electrical "maze" in the atria.[15] It is critical to recognize the fact that the myocardium of the RA, atrial septum, and LA are all one piece of atrial muscle. We commonly think of the RA and LA as separate structures because they function on different sides of the cardiovascular system. However, from an electrophysiologic standpoint, they are a single unit of myocardium that is activated in a sequential manner irrespective of their individual hemodynamic functions. And exactly what is an "electrical maze"? It is a pattern of atrial lesions that has one entry site (the SA node), one exit site (the AV node), one route of conduction between the entrance and exit sites, and multiple "blind alleys" along that route. The "blind alleys" provide the means of activating the entire atrial muscle by the SA node. The story of how the Maze procedure came about is described in more detail in Chapter 1.

THE ORIGINAL MAZE-I PROCEDURE

Surgical Technique

The lesions of the original Maze procedure[16] satisfied both goals of a surgical procedure for AF: (1) ablation of the arrhythmia (Fig. 12.10, *left panel*), and (2) leaving the atria capable of responding to a sinus-generated impulse postoperatively (Fig. 12.10, *right panel*) (Video 12.1). The lesions were placed close enough together to preclude the development of macro-reentry anywhere in either atrium, thereby ablating AF. The so-called "box lesion" around the four pulmonary vein orifices and the intervening posterior left atrial wall isolated the encompassed portion of the LA from the rest of the atrial myocardium. Otherwise, the entire myocardium in both atria could be activated by a sinus-generated impulse. After the Maze-I procedure, the two atria were completely activated in approximately 140 ms compared with activation of normal atria within approximately 110 ms (Fig. 12.11). This 30 ms difference

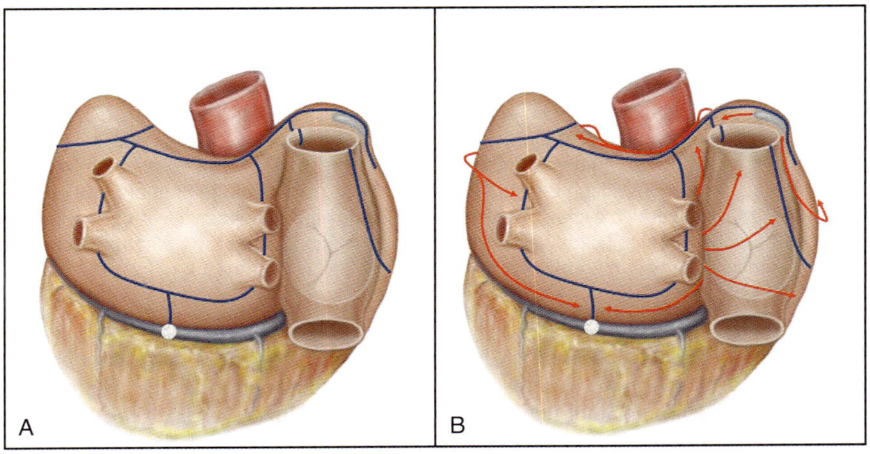

Fig. 12.10 Maze-I procedure. (A) The lesions of the Maze-I procedure precluded the ability of large macroreentrant circuits to form in the atria and therefore rendered the atria incapable of fibrillating. (B) Placing the lesions in the pattern of a maze provided the ability of a sinus-generated impulse to activate all of the myocardium of both atria except for the atrial appendages, which were removed, and the isolated pulmonary vein cuff that included the pulmonary vein orifices and the posterior left atrial wall between them.

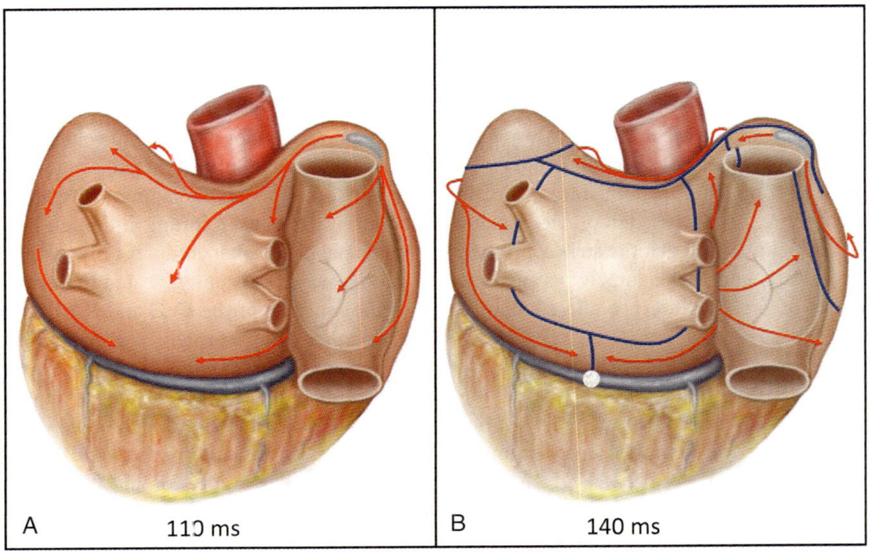

Fig. 12.11 Atrial activation time. (A) The entire myocardium of both atria is activated within approximately 110 ms in normal hearts. (B) After the Maze procedure, the entire myocardium of both atria (except the isolated pulmonary vein cuff) is activated in approximately 140 ms. In both cases, atrial activation is completed long before the atrial muscle contracts in response to the activation.

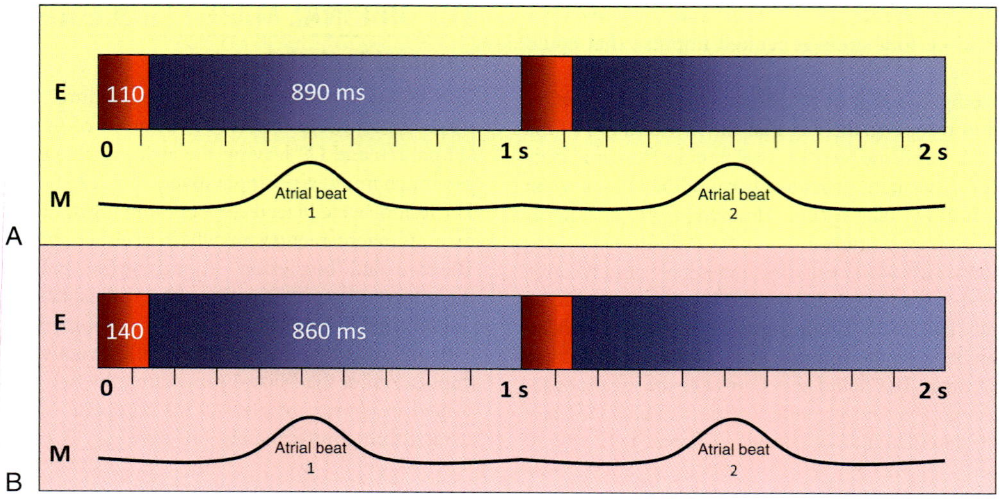

Fig. 12.12 Atrial electromechanical activity during normal sinus rhythm (NSR) (A) Normal heart. The temporal relationship between atrial electrical activation and atrial mechanical function is illustrated in a patient with a heart rate of 60 beats/min. At this heart rate, the heart beats every 1 second or every 1000 ms. The extremely rapid atrial electrical activation in a normal heart (110 ms, outlined in *red*) is over well before atrial mechanical function begins. This results in the atria being electrically silent for 89% of each cardiac cycle in a normal heart at a rate of 60 beats/min (890 ms, outlined in *blue*). (B) Post–Maze procedure heart. Atrial electrical activation in a patient with a heart rate of 60 beats/min after the Maze procedure (140 ms, outlined in *red*) is also over well before atrial mechanical contraction begins. In these post–Maze procedure patients, the atria are electrically silent for 86% of each cardiac cycle compared with 89% of the cardiac cycle in normal patients. Thus, the Maze procedure does not significantly alter the temporal relationships of the electro-mechanical activity of the atria. *E,* Electrical activity in the atria; *M,* mechanical activity in the atria.

in the total time required to activate the atria had no effect on the hemodynamics of the heart or on mechanical AV synchrony because electrical activation is well over before mechanical function of the atria is initiated (Fig. 12.12). For example, at a heart rate of 60 beats/min, the heart beats every 1 second or every 1000 ms. This means that in the normal heart with a rate of 60 beats/min, the atria are electrically silent for 890 ms (89%) of each heartbeat. After the Maze procedure, the atria are electrically silent for 860 ms (86%) of each heartbeat at a rate of 60 beats/min. In both normal and post-Maze hearts, the mechanical function of the atria occurs within this electrically silent portion of the heartbeat.

The same electro-mechanical relationship is present even when the heart is beating twice as fast in sinus rhythm (i.e., at 120 beats/min). In this case, the atria are electrically silent for 78% of each cardiac cycle in the normal heart and for 72% of each cardiac cycle after the Maze procedure (Fig. 12.13). Again, the atrial mechanical function occurs well after electrical activation has been completed in both normal hearts and in hearts after the Maze procedure. As discussed in previous chapters, great effort was expended in documenting that the atria continued to function after the Maze procedure, and this is largely because the electromechanical characteristics of the atria are not altered significantly by the Maze procedure.

Problems With the Maze-I Procedure

The two main postoperative problems that occurred in some, but not all, patients after the Maze-I procedure were chronotropic incompetence and interatrial conduction delay.[17]

Chronotropic Incompetence

The original Maze-I procedure was performed in some 35 patients, and several of them were athletes who competed in marathons and triathlons. These patients were especially attuned to their cardiovascular status, including their heart rates before, during, and after exercise. Some of them noted that after they had completely recovered from surgery and began to exercise again, they could not generate a normal chronotropic response to exercise as they had before surgery. Characteristically, they would begin exercising, and their heart rate would increase normally until it reached 100 to 110 beats/min and then would level off despite their continuing to exercise (Fig. 12.14). Interestingly, after they stopped exercising, the heart rate remained the same much longer than normal before eventually decreasing back to its resting level. If one plotted the expected normal sinus tachycardia resulting from this amount of exercise in individual patients, the abnormal extenuation of the heart rate at the same level after cessation of exercise and then its return to resting levels paralleled what would have occurred if the chronotropic response had been normal. Clearly, the atrial pacemaker was working normally except for its ability to generate a normal sinus tachycardia.

My colleague John Boineau, suggested that the surgical procedure might somehow be damaging a suspected "sinus tachycardia site" in an atrial pacemaker complex, though he had previously documented this atrial pacemaker complex only in dogs.[18] The sinus tachycardia site in dogs was consistently located in a small site in the RA just anterior to the junction of the SVC and RA. He suspected that such an atrial pacemaker complex might also exist in humans, but we were unaware of this possibility in humans when we began performing the first Maze procedures. We quickly studied a number of normal patients, and Boineau and Schuessler documented that indeed, humans had a similar atrial pacemaker complex,[19] and it also included a "sinus tachycardia site" similar in location and function to that in dogs (Fig. 12.15). The atrial pacemaker complex is discussed in more detail in Chapter 3.

The cause of the chronotropic incompetence was immediately clear because one of the lesions of the Maze-I procedure passed directly through this sinus tachycardia site and was almost certainly responsible for the fact that the patients could not generate an appropriate

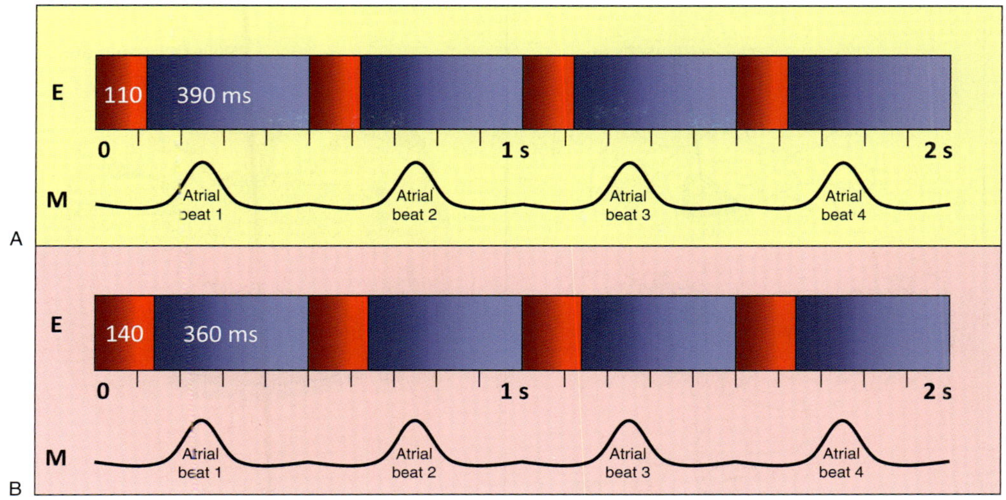

Fig. 12.13 Atrial electromechanical activity during normal sinus rhythm (NSR) (A) Normal heart. The temporal relationship between atrial electrical activation and atrial mechanical function is illustrated in a patient with a sinus tachycardia of 120 beats/min. At this heart rate, the heart is beating twice per second or every 500 ms. Even at this rate of sinus tachycardia, the atrial electrical activation is over well before atrial mechanical function begins. This results in the atria being electrically silent for 78% of each cardiac cycle in a normal heart at a heart rate of 120 beats/min (390 ms, outlined in *blue*). (B). Post–Maze procedure heart. Atrial electrical activation in a patient with a sinus tachycardia of 120 beats/min after the Maze procedure (140 ms, outlined in *red*) is also over well before atrial mechanical function begins. In these patients, the atria are electrically silent for 72% of each cardiac cycle compared with 78% of the cardiac cycle in normal patients. Thus, the Maze procedure does not significantly alter the electro-mechanical temporal relationships of the atria. *E,* Electrical activity in the atria; *M,* mechanical activity in the atria.

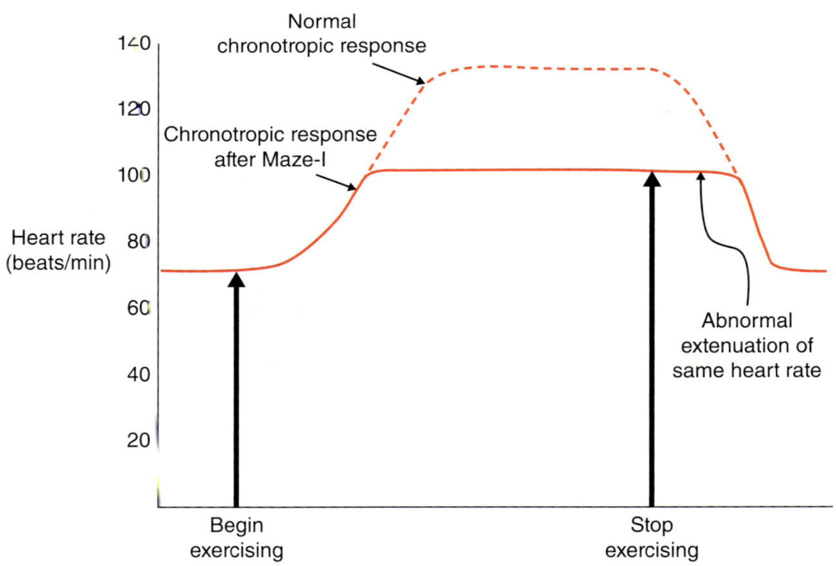

Fig. 12.14 After the Maze-I procedure, many patients could not generate a sinus tachycardia above 100 to 110 with exercise *(solid red line)*. In addition, the heart rate did not decelerate normally on cessation of exercise but rather remained stable at 100 to 110 beats/min for several minutes before starting its return to a normal resting rate. By plotting the expected chronotropic response to exercise and the observed response in individual patients (*dashed red line*), it was clear that the sinoatrial node was responding normally to physiological events except for its inability to generate a sinus tachycardia. This suggested that the Maze-I procedure was inadvertently destroying the sinus tachycardia site of the atrial pacemaker complex in some patients.

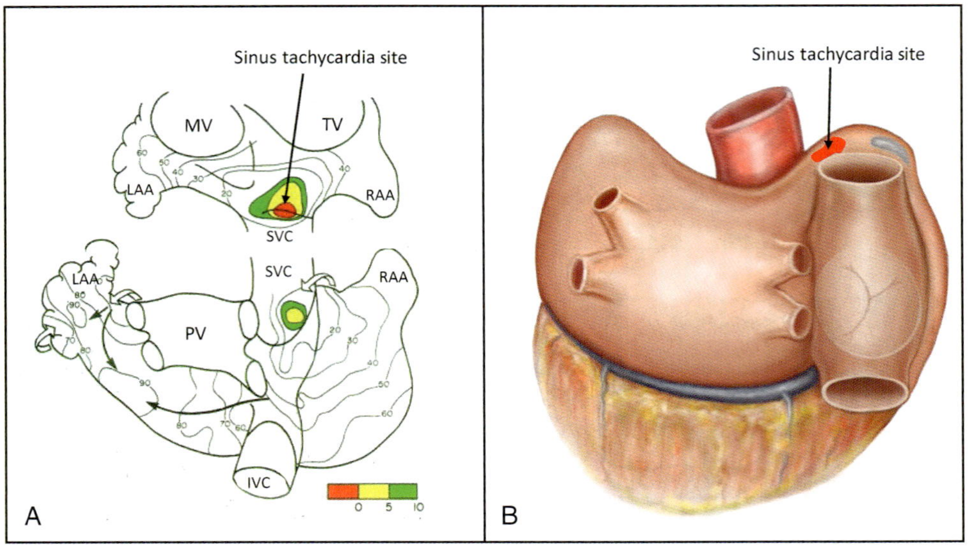

Fig. 12.15 *Left panel,* Two-dimensional illustration of the sinus tachycardia site in humans located at the top of the right atrium (RA) just anterior to the junction of the superior vena cava (SVC) and RA. The posterior surface of the atria is below, and the anterior surface is above, as if the atria had been bisected and the anterior portion flipped upward. *IVC,* Inferior vena cava; *MV,* mitral valve; *PV,* pulmonary vein; *RAA,* right atrial appendage; *TV,* tricuspid valve. *Right panel,* Clarification of the location of the sinus tachycardia site in humans *(red area).* (Reproduced from Boineau JP, Canavan TE, Schuessler RB, Cain M, Corr PB, Cox JL. Demonstration of a widely distributed atrial pacemaker complex in the human heart. *Circulation.* 1988;77:1221-1237).

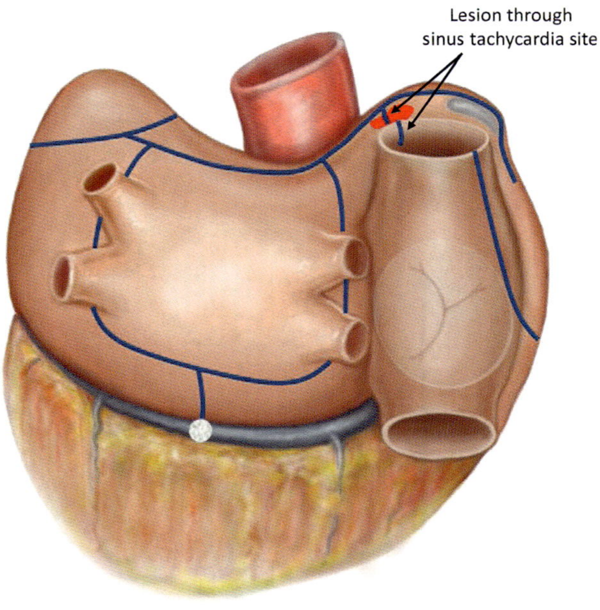

Fig. 12.16 Maze-I procedure. The Maze-I procedure included several lesions around the sinus tachycardia site and one lesion directly through it. Because this was a transmural surgical incision that required suture closure, it is not surprising that it essentially deactivated the sinus tachycardia site.

sinus tachycardia during strenuous exercise (Fig. 12.16). This observation was one of the main reasons that we modified the original lesion pattern of the Maze-I procedure. The other was the virtual simultaneous recognition that the Maze-I lesion pattern was causing a significant interatrial conduction block that resulted in an apparent lack of left atrial transport function postoperatively.

Interatrial Conduction Delay

In the Maze-I procedure, the inside of the LA was exposed via an anterior transseptal incision extending from the RA, across the septum down to the base of the fossa ovalis and the Tendon of Todaro, and across the top of the LA over to the base of the left atrial appendage (LAA; Fig. 12.17). An effort was made to place this transseptal atriotomy *anterior* to Bachmann's

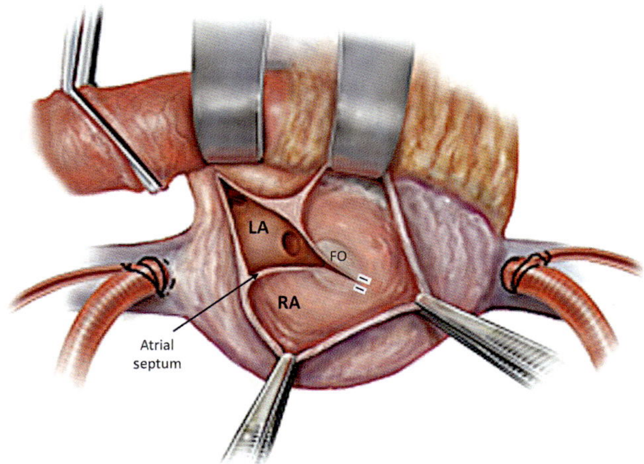

Fig. 12.17 Maze-I procedure. Anterior transseptal incision to expose the left atrium (LA). The incision extended down the atrial septum and across the limbus of the fossa ovalis and the fossa ovalis (FO) itself to the tendon of Todaro. Because of the thinness of the fossa ovalis, a pledgeted horizontal mattress suture was placed at the base of the FO to prevent it from tearing during the remaining surgery and extending across the tendon of Todaro. Superiorly, the transseptal incision was extended across the top of the LA to the base of the left atrial appendage. *RA,* Right atrium.

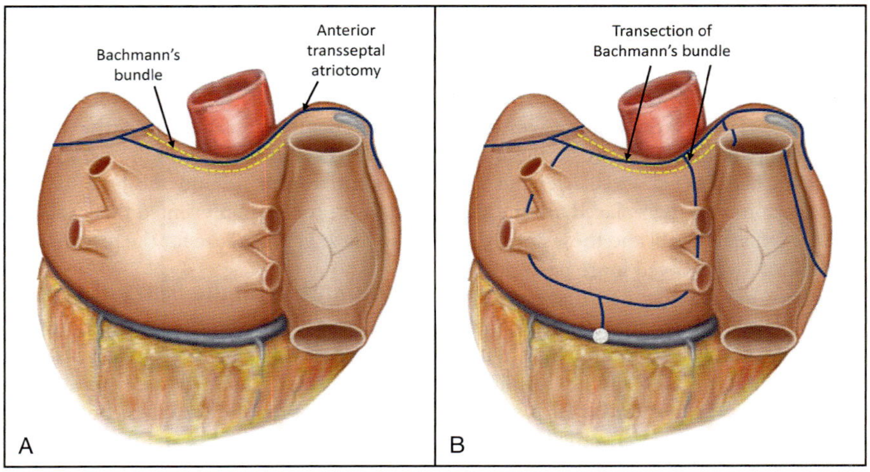

Fig. 12.18 Maze-I procedure. (A) The anterior transseptal atriotomy was placed anterior to Bachmann's bundle but the distal end of the atriotomy usually damaged or transected the bundle. This resulted in one of two options for completing the upper portion of the box lesion around the four pulmonary veins. Option one was to place the roof of the box lesion posterior to Bachmann's bundle, leaving a strip of left atrium (LA) between the box lesion and the transseptal lesion. However, this would establish an ideal scenario for the development of large macro-reentrant circuits involving the atrial septum and LA and fundamentally violated the concept of the maze pattern of lesions. Option two was to use the transseptal incision as the roof of the box lesion, which was our choice. (B) This decision was based on our lack of appreciation at that time of how important Bachmann's bundle was to the synchronous interatrial activation times between the right and left atria. Unfortunately, we soon realized that using the transseptal lesion that was anterior to Bachmann's bundle as the roof of the box lesion necessitated the extension of the medial and lateral portions of the box lesion directly across the bundle. The combination of lateral damage or transsection and proximal transection of Bachmann's bundle resulted in severely delayed conduction from the right atrium to the LA during sinus rhythm.

bundle but its distal portion often crossed Bachmann's bundle (Fig. 12.18, *left panel*). The "box lesion" encompassing the four pulmonary vein orifices and the posterior wall of the LA was completed by extending its medial and lateral components superiorly to the anterior transseptal atriotomy, which served as the roof of the box lesion (Fig. 12.18, *right panel*). This invariably resulted in transection of Bachmann's bundle. Transection of the bundle *laterally* by either the transseptal lesion or the lateral box lesion probably caused little or no problem because it was near enough to the base of the LAA that the fibers of the bundle had essentially dissipated by that point. However, the lesion that divided Bachmann's bundle *medially* (i.e., more proximal on the bundle), as well as the anterior transseptal atriotomy, and the lesion that transected the sinus tachycardia site all prevented a sinus-generated impulse from propagating across Bachmann's bundle from the SA node to the top of the LA in its customary 40 ms. The resultant severe conduction delay between the right and left atria (140–150 ms) caused the LA to be activated simultaneously (at 150 ms) with the left ventricle in approximately 30% of patients after the Maze-I procedure (Fig. 12.19). This resulted in the LA passively emptying and actively contracting against a closed mitral valve and on echocardiography, there appeared to be no emptying or contraction of the LA. The fact that the apparent loss of left atrial transport function in these cases was due to the interatrial conduction delay rather than to atrial structural injury was confirmed by pacing the LA with an endocardial catheter, which immediately resulted in the LA's emptying and contracting normally.

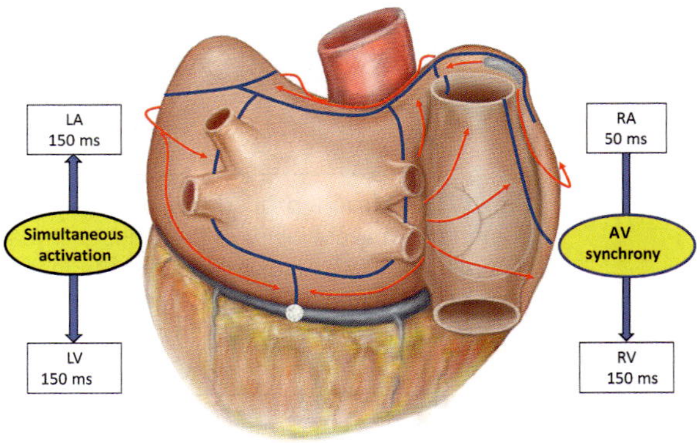

Fig. 12.19 Maze-I procedure. Normally, it takes approximately 40 ms for a sinus-generated impulse in the right atrium (RA) to arrive in the left atrium (LA). This virtual simultaneous activation of the two atria is possible because of the rapidity of impulse propagation across Bachmann's bundle because its muscle fibers are parallel with the direction of wavefront propagation (see Anisotropy of Conduction, Fig. 3.13). After the Maze-I procedure, which completely interrupted conduction across Bachmann's bundle in roughly one-third of our patients, it took approximately 150 ms to activate the LA. Because the sinus-generated impulse is normally delayed approximately 100 ms in the atrioventricular (AV) node, the ventricles are also activated normally approximately 150 ms after the sinus impulse is generated. This means that the RA and right ventricle (RV) remain in normal AV synchrony, but the LA and left ventricle (LV) are activated simultaneously. As a result, they contract simultaneously, which leads to emptying (conduit phase) and contraction of the LA against a closed mitral valve and there being no apparent LA function on echocardiography. However, when the LA itself was paced, normal AV synchrony of the LA and LV was restored immediately, proving that the apparent loss of LA transport function after the Maze-I procedure in one-third of our patients was due to a severe interatrial conduction delay and not to surgical injury of the LA.

THE MAZE-II PROCEDURE

Surgical Technique

The combination of postoperative chronotropic incompetence and interatrial conduction delay caused by the original Maze procedure (Maze-I) in roughly one-third of our patients dictated that some of the anterior lesions would have to be moved to more posterior locations.

This required that the SVC be transected approximately 2 cm above its junction with the RA to provide enough exposure of the LA. The first step was to move the anterior transseptal atriotomy to a more posterior position *behind* Bachmann's bundle. However, this meant that its proximal end extended into the SVC. The atrial septum was then opened through the SVC stump to keep the lesion well posterior to the sinus tachycardia site and Bachmann's bundle (Fig. 12.20, *left panel*). A single circumferential lesion (box lesion) was then placed around the four pulmonary veins and posterior left atrial wall, and the lesion from the box lesion to the orifice of the LAA was moved more posterior to avoid the distal portion of Bachmann's bundle (Fig. 12.20, *right panel*).

Two other modifications of the Maze-I pattern were made to finalize the Maze-II procedure. First, in the Maze-I procedure, the longitudinal lateral right atriotomy originating in the SVC did not terminate in the IVC but rather was curved in its lower portion to terminate at the tricuspid valve annulus (Fig. 12.21). In the Maze-II procedure, this lesion was extended to the IVC to prevent reentry around the IVC. A right lateral "T" lesion was then placed from this intercaval lesion, diagonally across the lower lateral RA to the tricuspid valve annulus. Second, a "counterlesion" was added from the tip of the RAA down the medial wall of the RA to the level of the tricuspid annulus just anterior to the membranous portion of the interatrial septum (see Chapter 13, Fig. 13.13). This lesion had to be added to the Maze-II procedure to prevent reentry around the base of the RAA. Other lesions in the Maze-I procedure prevented this problem but they were eliminated in the Maze-II procedure for the reasons described.

Problems With the Maze-II Procedure

The Maze-II procedure was just as effective in ablating AF as was the Maze-I procedure,[20] and fortunately, the problems of chronotropic incompetence and interatrial conduction delay were eliminated. The only problem with the Maze-II procedure was its technical difficulty. The combination of having to transect the SVC and then having two lesions extending into the stump of the SVC (see Fig. 12.21, *right panel*) caused the closure and repair

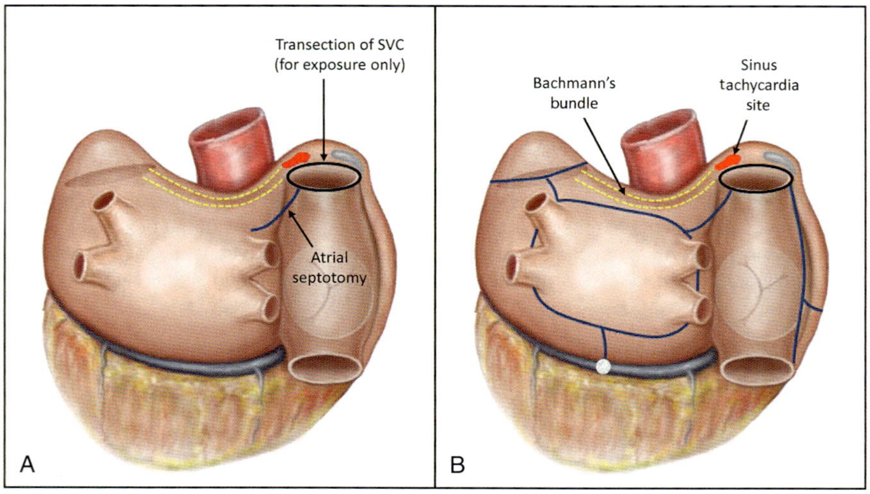

Fig. 12.20 Maze-II procedure. In the Maze-II procedure, the anterior transseptal incision was moved more posteriorly to avoid injury of the sinus tachycardia site and transection of Bachmann's bundle. Unfortunately, this resulted in the proximal end of the incision being within the orifice of the superior vena cava (SVC). In addition, it was necessary to transect the SVC 1 to 2 cm above its orifice to gain enough exposure of the left atrium to perform the operation.

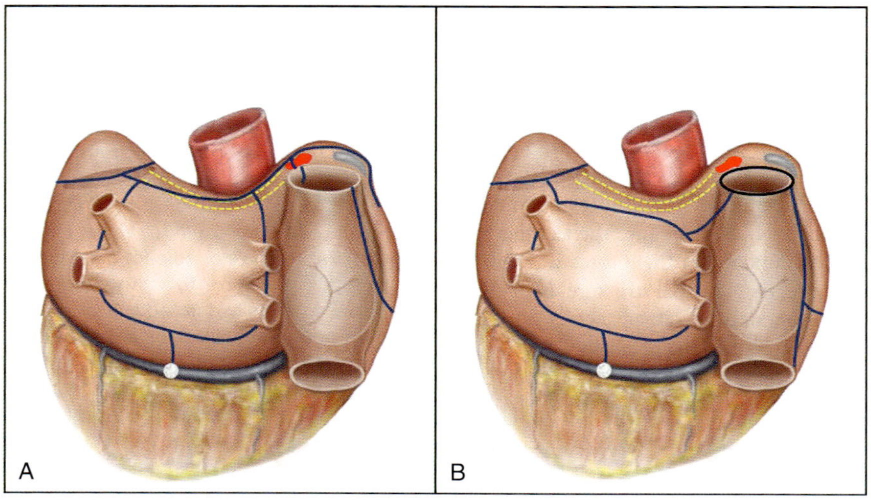

Fig. 12.21 A side-by-side comparison of the lesion patterns of the Maze-I (A) and Maze-II procedures demonstrates how several lesions of the Maze-I procedure were moved more posterior in the Maze-II procedure to avoid the problems of chronotropic incompetence and interatrial conduction delay after the Maze-I procedure. See text for further discussion.

of the SVC to be technically difficult. Indeed, it was necessary to place a pericardial patch in this area in most patients, further complicating the SVC repair. After performing the Maze-II procedure in some 14 patients, it was further modified into the Maze-III procedure in hopes of making it technically easier.[21] The Maze-III surgical technique was developed and again studied extensively in the experimental laboratory before the first clinical Maze-III procedure was finally performed in April 1992.

THE CUT-AND-SEW MAZE-III PROCEDURE

Since 1992, the Maze-III lesion pattern has been the basis of subsequent Maze iterations regardless of the energy source used, including the cut-and-sew Maze-III procedure (knife and scissors), the minimally invasive CryoMaze-III procedure (cryosurgery), the Maze-IV procedure (radiofrequency and cryosurgery), and the McCarthy modification of the CryoMaze-III procedure for concomitant AF surgery. The Maze-III procedure was based primarily on the decision to move the atrial septal incision even farther posterior than it was in the Maze-II so that its upper end would not terminate in the SVC. The SVC-IVC lesion in the RA was performed first, and then a standard left atriotomy in Waterston's groove was added to leave only the atrial septum between the parallel RA and LA longitudinal atriotomies. It was then quite simple to place the septal lesion posterior to the orifice of the SVC and across the fossa ovalis down to the tendon of Todaro (Fig. 12.22). Thus the critical difference in the Maze-I, Maze-II, and Maze-III lesion patterns was the position of the atrial septotomy (Fig. 12.23). The primary

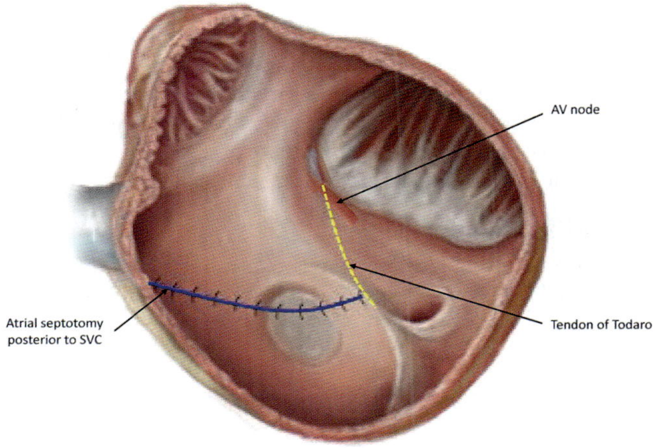

Fig. 12.22 Atrial septotomy in the Maze-III procedure. The combination of the longitudinal superior vena cava–inferior vena cava (SVC-IVC) incision in the right atrium and a standard left atriotomy in Waterston's groove leaves the atrial septum between the two atriotomies. The atrial septotomy of the cut-and-sew Maze-III procedure was placed posterior to the orifice of the SVC and extended diagonally across the fossa ovalis to terminate at the level of the tendon of Todaro. Under no circumstances should the atrial septotomy ever extend across the tendon of Todaro so that injury of the atrioventricular (AV) node within the triangle of Koch can be avoided (see Chapter 3, Fig. 3.18).

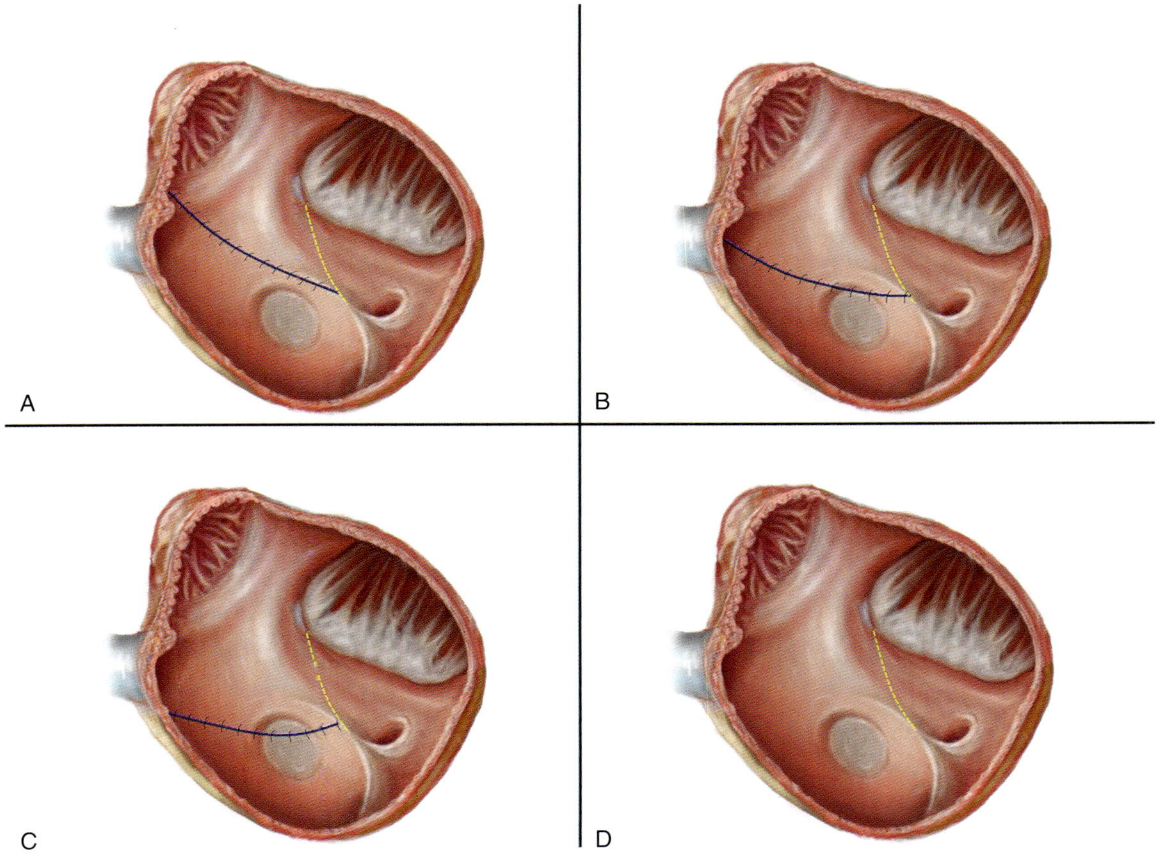

Fig. 12.23 The upper end of the atrial septotomy was located anterior to the superior vena cava (SVC) orifice in the cut-and-sew Maze-I procedure (A) and within the SVC orifice in the cut-and-sew Maze-II procedure (B). It is posterior to the SVC orifice in the cut-and-sew Maze-III procedure (C). The septotomies in all three Maze iterations ended at or above the tendon of Todaro *(yellow dashed line)*. There is no atrial septal lesion in either the CryoMaze-III procedure or the Maze-IV procedure (D).

purpose of the atrial septal incision in all three procedures was to gain better exposure of the inside of the LA. Whether or not the septal lesion contributes to the ablation of AF is unknown, though there is no septal lesion at all in the CryoMaze-III procedure or in Maze-IV procedure developed by Ralph Damiano, yet the success rate is equivalent to that of the first three iterations of the Maze procedure.[22] Dr. Damiano discusses the Maze-IV procedure in detail in Chapter 17.

Surgical Technique

The cannulation technique for venous return in all Maze procedures was designed to maximize exposure for lesion placement in both atria. The SVC is cannulated with a right-angle venous return cannula placed approximately 2 cm above its junction with the RA. The IVC is cannulated separately with a right-angle venous return cannula placed as low and anterior as possible in the RA.

The location of the lesions and the surgical technique of the original "cut-and-sew" Maze-III procedure are illustrated in Figs. 12.24 to 12.37. Each step of the procedure is explained in the accompanying figure legends and need not be repeated here (Video 12.2). The Maze-III proved to be the easiest to perform technically of the first three Maze procedure iterations, and placing the atrial septotomy posterior to the orifice of the SVC provided superb exposure of the inside of the LA.

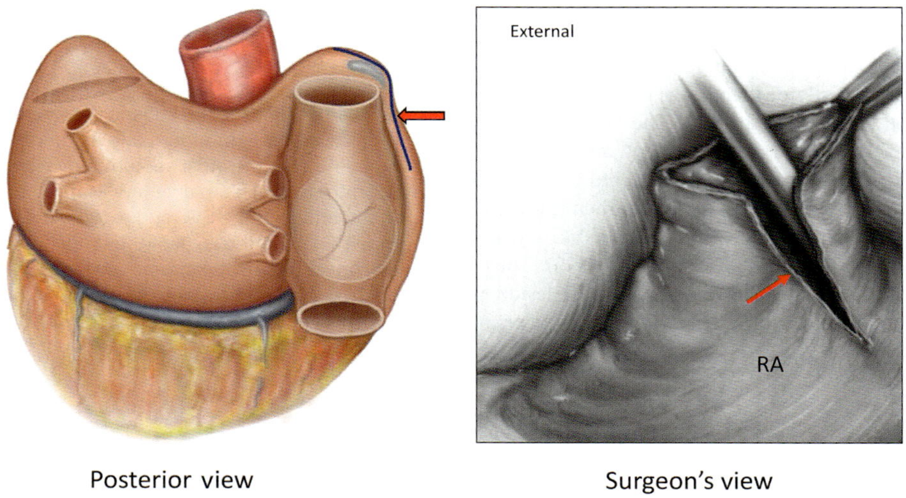

Fig. 12.24 The cut-and-sew Maze-III procedure: lateral right atrial lesion. *Left panel,* Posterior view of the heart to illustrate the location of the initial lateral right atrial (RA) lesion *(red arrow). Right panel,* Surgeon's view of the corresponding lesion *(red arrow).* The cut-and-sew Maze-III procedure begins with a short lateral RA lesion from the tip of the RA appendage a few centimeters down the RA free wall. Only the tip of the RA appendage (RAA) is excised, or alternatively, this incision can be performed through a small stab wound in the RAA.

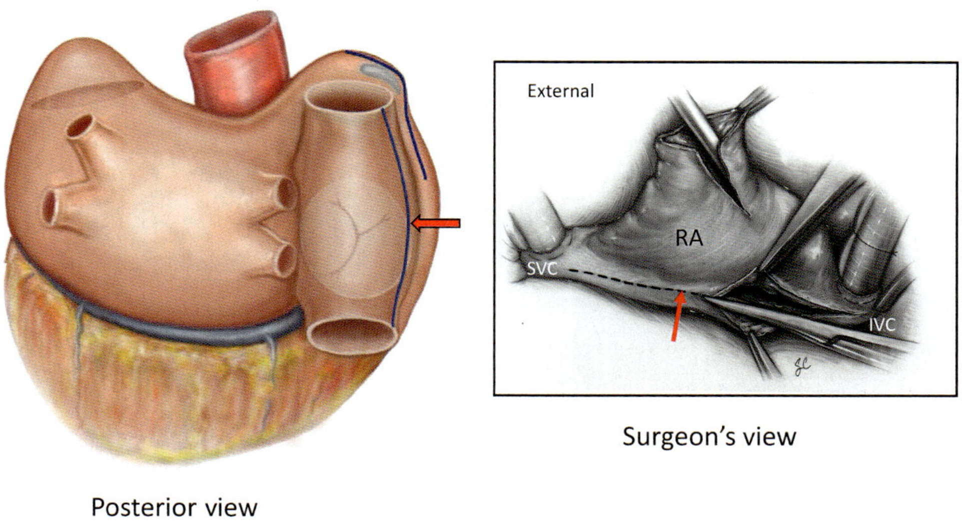

Fig. 12.25 The cut-and-sew Maze-III procedure: intercaval lesion. *Left panel,* Posterior view of the heart to illustrate the location of the intercaval lesion *(red arrow)* in the right the atrium (RA). *Right panel,* Surgeon's view of the intercaval lesion. The intercaval lesion from the superior vena cava to the inferior vena cava is placed immediately anterior to the crista terminalis where the RA begins to thin *(red arrow).* Its upper end is curved slightly in the posterior direction to keep it as far away as possible from the anatomic sinoatrial node.

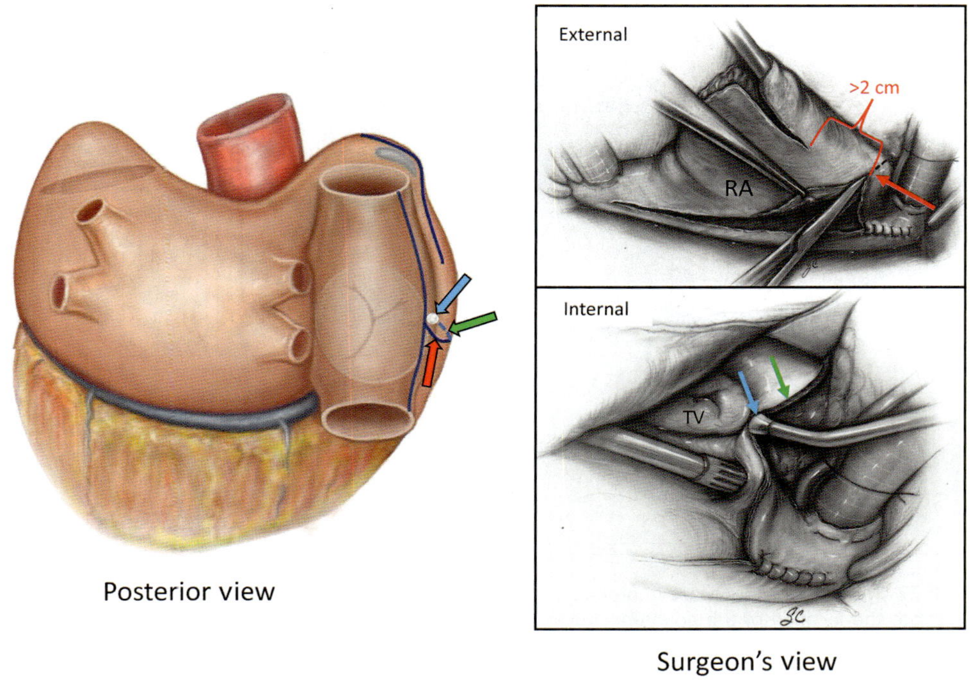

Fig. 12.26 The cut-and-sew Maze-III procedure: "T" lesion. *Left panel,* Posterior view of the heart to illustrate the location of the "T" lesion *(red arrow)* in the right atrium (RA). The *dotted line* represents the extension of the "T" lesion down to the tricuspid valve (TV) annulus *(green arrow).* A cryolesion is placed at the distal end of the "T" lesion to ensure that all conduction across the lesion is blocked *(blue arrow). Right upper panel,* Surgeon's view of the "T" lesion, which is started from the lower portion of the intercaval lesion approximately two-thirds of the way between the superior vena cava orifice and the inferior vena cava orifice. This should be a *diagonal* incision so that it parallels the orientation of the myocardial fibers of the RA in this region (see Chapter 3, Fig. 3.8). The "T" lesion is placed low in the RA to avoid injury of the atrial pacemaker complex (see Chapter 3, Fig. 3.9). In addition, in the original Maze-III it was placed low to leave a 2-cm or more bridge of tissue between the distal end of the lateral RA lesion and the "T" lesion to assure normal impulse propagation from the upper RA to the rest of the RA and left atrium. However, in later modifications of the RA lesion patterns of the Maze-III procedure, no lateral RA lesion is performed, so the 2-cm requirement is no longer a consideration (see Chapter 13). *Right lower panel,* To extend the "T" lesion to the tricuspid annulus, it is necessary to perform the distal part of the lesion with a scalpel from inside the RA to divide the atrial myocardium without involving the atrioventricular groove fat pad or the right coronary artery *(green arrow).* After it is completed, a final cryolesion is placed at the distal end of the incision *(blue arrow).* This cryolesion is essential because of the "folding over" of the RA and right ventricular walls at the level of the tricuspid annulus (see Chapter 3, Fig. 3.22).

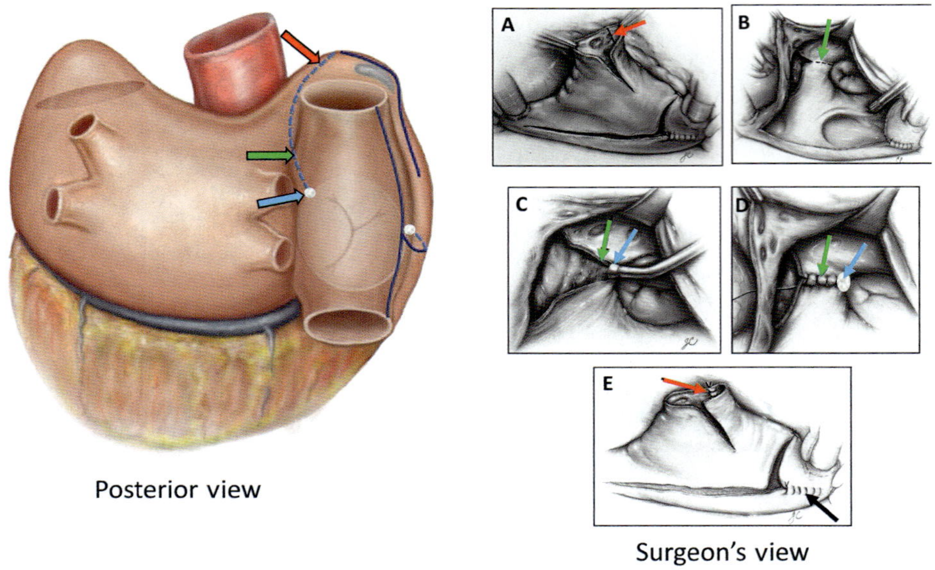

Fig. 12.27 The cut-and-sew Maze-III procedure: the "counterlesion." *Left panel,* Posterior view of the heart to illustrate the location of the counterlesion in the right atrium (RA; *dotted light blue line).* The *dotted line* represents the extension of the counterlesion from the tip of the right atrial appendage (RAA; *red arrow*) medially down to the tricuspid valve annulus *(green arrow).* A cryolesions is placed at the termination of the counterlesion at the tricuspid valve annulus. The counterlesion prevents reentry around the base of the RAA. However, later modifications in the RA lesions of the Maze-III eliminate the need for a counterlesion (see Chapter 13). *Right panel,* Surgeon's view of the "counterlesion". The counterlesion was added to the Maze-II and Maze-III procedures but was not necessary in the Maze-I procedure. It begins at the tip of the RAA medially (A, *red arrow*) and is extended to the tricuspid valve annulus (B, *green arrow*). After the incision has been completed, a small cryolesion is placed at the level of the tricuspid valve annulus (C, *blue arrow*), again to overcome the "folding over" of the RA and right ventricular free walls at the annulus. The counterlesion is then closed to avoid tearing during the remainder of the surgical procedure (D and E). The lower end of the intercaval lesion is also partially closed for the same reason (E, *black arrow*).

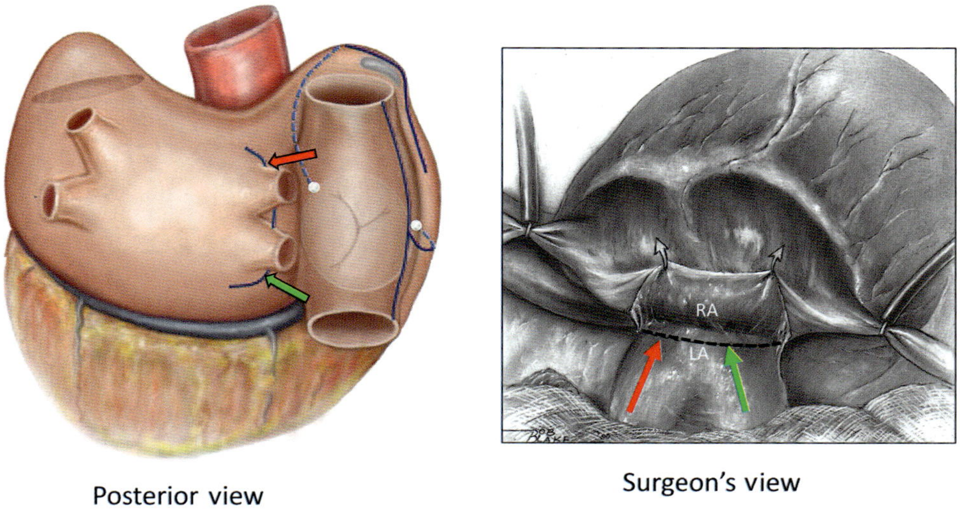

Fig. 12.28 The cut-and-sew Maze-III procedure: left atriotomy. *Left panel,* Posterior view of the heart to illustrate the location of the standard left atriotomy in Waterston's groove (superior end, *red arrow*; inferior end, *green arrow*). *Right panel,* Surgeon's view of the standard left atriotomy in Waterston's groove (superior end, *red arrow*; inferior end, *green arrow*).

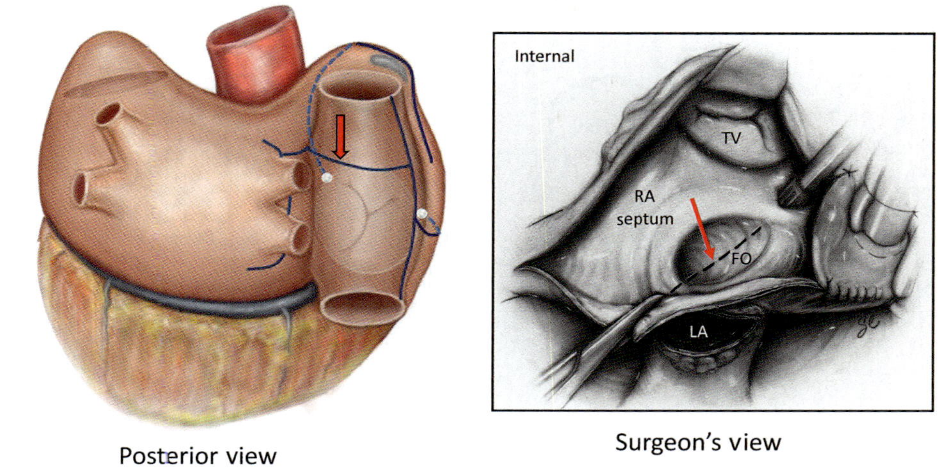

Fig. 12.29 The cut-and-sew Maze-III procedure: atrial septotomy. *Left panel,* Posterior view of the heart illustrating the location of the atrial septotomy posterior to the orifice of the superior vena cava (SVC; *red arrow*). *Right panel,* Surgeon's view of the atrial septotomy *(red arrow).* Note that the septotomy of the Maze-III procedure is *posterior* to the orifice of the SVC. See further description in the legend for Fig. 12.22. *FO,* Fossa ovalis; *TV,* tricuspid valve.

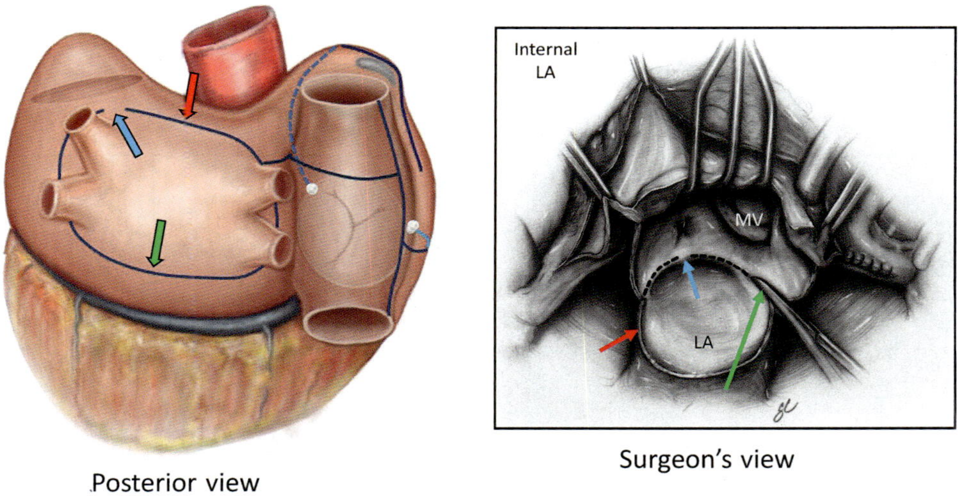

Fig. 12.30 The cut-and-sew Maze-III procedure: box lesion. *Left panel,* Posterior view of the heart illustrating the extensions of the box lesion across the roof *(red arrow)* and floor *(green arrow)* of the posterior left atrium (LA) while preserving a "tissue bridge" (*blue arrow*) to assist in later closure. *Right panel,* Surgeon's view of the corresponding lesions. The roof and floor portions of the box lesion are extended between the orifice of the left atrial appendage and the left pulmonary veins to encompass all four pulmonary veins and the posterior LA wall between the right and left pulmonary veins. *MV,* Mitral valve.

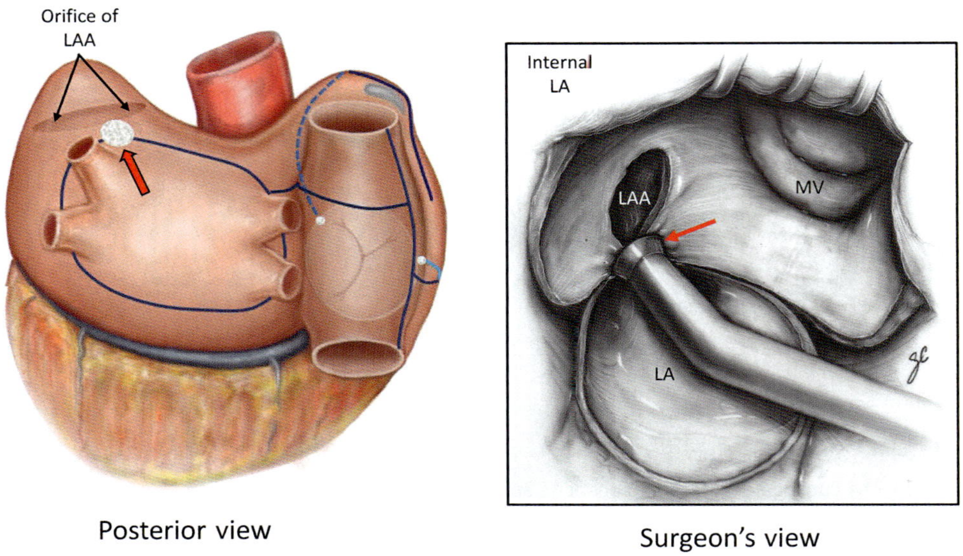

Fig. 12.31 The cut-and-sew Maze-III procedure: completion of the box lesion. *Left panel,* Posterior view of the heart showing that the box lesion is completed with a cryolesion *(red arrow)* that spans the tissue bridge between the roof and floor lesions and the orifice of the left atrial appendage (LAA). *Right panel,* Surgeon's view of creation of the cryolesion to complete the box lesion *(red arrow).* This bridge of tissue was necessary in the cut-and-sew Maze-III procedure because complete surgical separation of the boxed-in tissue from the rest of the heart resulted in the entire box dropping deep within the chest. This made it very difficult to subsequently align the box properly with its surrounding tissue when reattaching it with sutures. By maintaining a bridge of tissue in this manner, the problem of accurately realigning the box with its surrounding tissues was eliminated.

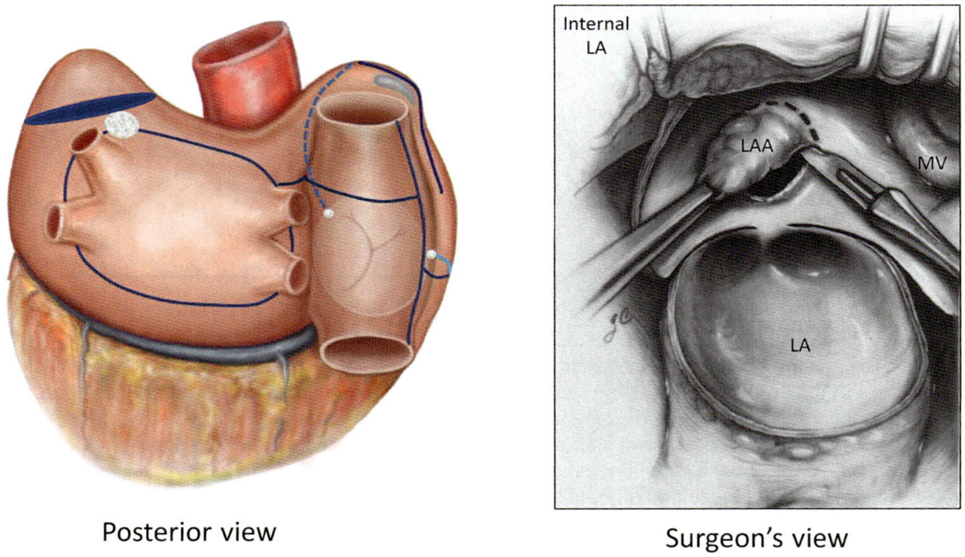

Fig. 12.32 The cut-and-sew Maze-III procedure: left atrial appendage (LAA) amputation and closure. *Left panel,* Approximate location of the orifice of the LAA *(blue oval). Right panel,* Amputation of the LAA from inside the left atrium (LA). The entire appendage was inverted so that there could be no doubt about the level of its base. A scalpel was then used to carefully amputate the appendage from within the LA. Special care was taken when dissecting in the area illustrated here because it is the area where the circumflex coronary artery is closest to the base of the appendage. After this area was carefully freed, the rest of the appendage was amputated and closed.

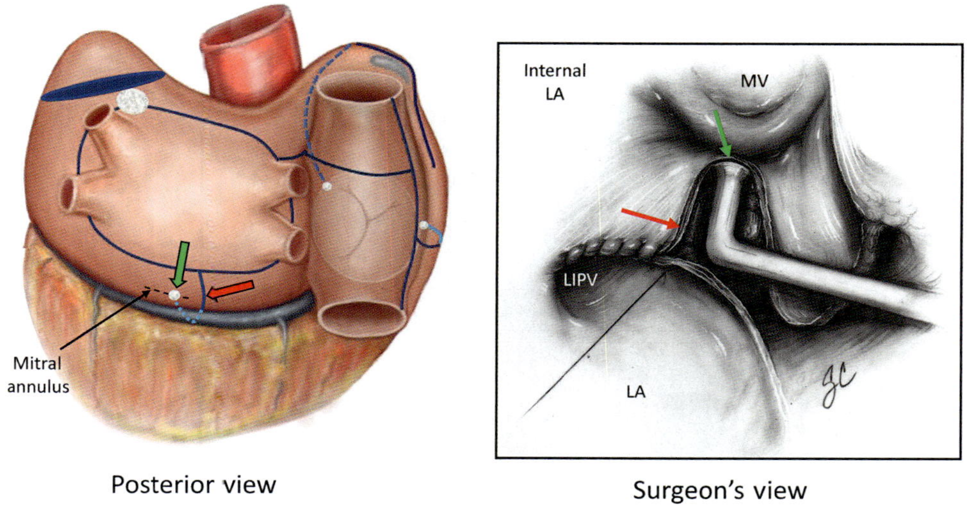

Fig. 12.33 The cut-and-sew Maze-III procedure: mitral line. *Left panel,* The mitral line *(red arrow)* extends from the box lesion to the posterior mitral valve (MV) annulus *(green arrow)* to prevent electrical conduction across the myocardium of the left atrial isthmus causing postoperative peri-mitral flutter (see Chapter 48). *Right panel,* The atrioventricular groove fat pad containing the coronary sinus and circumflex coronary artery lies immediately beneath the posteroinferior atrial wall, so it is exposed immediately after creating the transmural mitral line. A cryolesion is placed at the end of the mitral line (*red arrow*) on the mitral annulus to ablate any potential small muscle fibers that might still be connecting the two sides of the mitral line *(green arrow)*. *LA,* Left atrium.

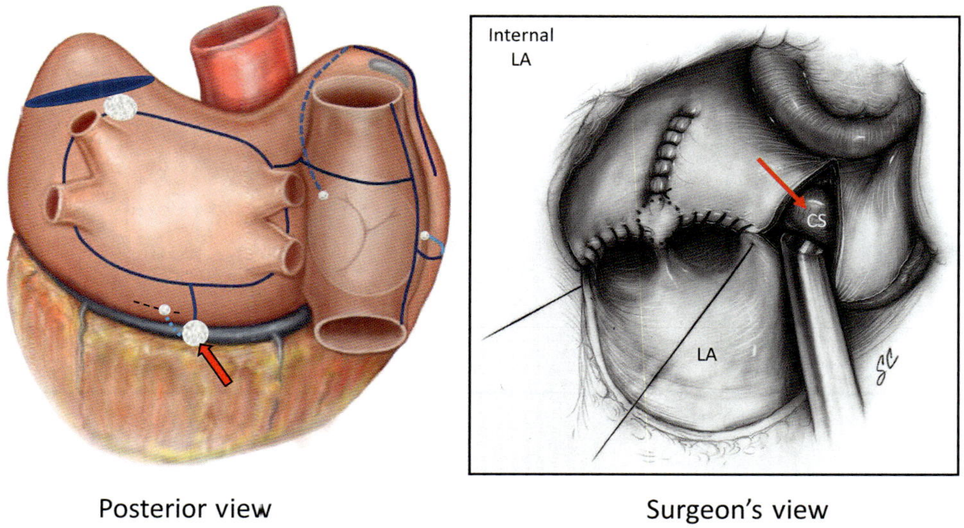

Fig. 12.34 The cut-and-sew Maze-III procedure: coronary sinus (CS) lesion. *Left panel,* A circumferential cryolesion is created on the CS *(red arrow)* in the same plane as the mitral line to prevent conduction across the left atrial isthmus, causing postoperative peri-mitral flutter. *Right panel,* After the mitral line has been completed and the underlying atrioventricular groove fad pad has been exposed, the CS *(red arrow)* is dissected free of surrounding tissues, encircled, and then cryoablated. *LA,* Left atrium.

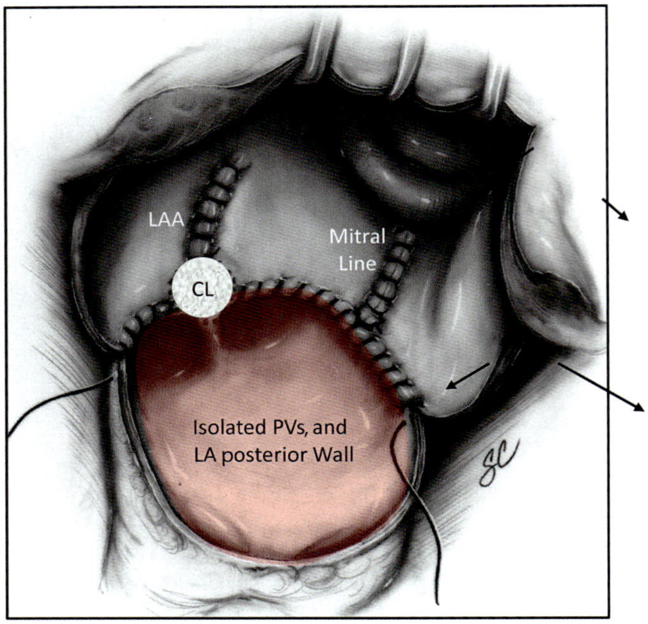

Fig. 12.35 The cut-and-sew Maze-III procedure: all incisions and the defect created by amputation of the left atrial appendage (LAA), are closed with running sutures. The *red shaded area* shows the isolated portion of the left atrium (LA) created by the box lesion. *CL*, Cryolesion; *PV*, pulmonary vein.

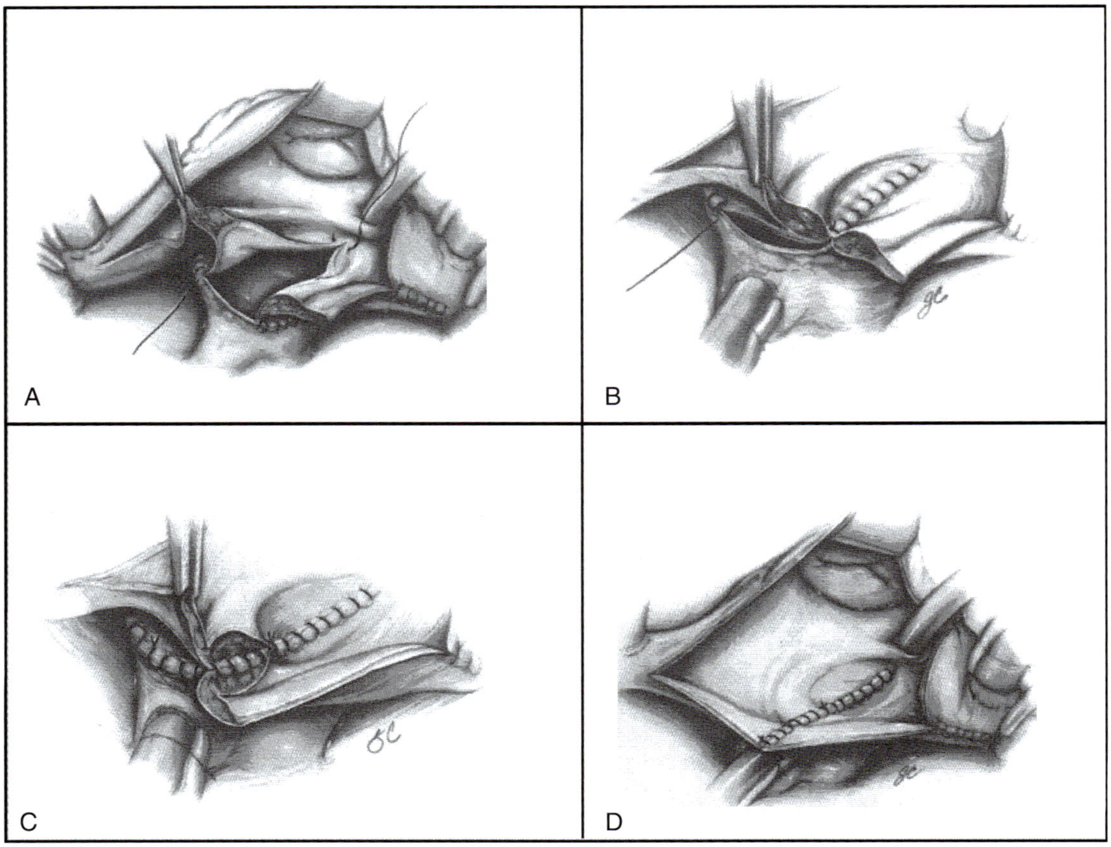

Fig. 12.36 The cut-and-sew Maze-III procedure: closure of the left atrium. After most of the box lesion has been closed, a suture is placed at the bottom of the septotomy just above the tendon of Todaro (A), and the fossa ovalis is closed (B). Because the septotomy suture line is in the same plane as the suture line of the left atriotomy in Waterston's groove, they are closed together as a single suture line (C). This leaves the limbus of the fossa ovalis and the posterior free wall of the right atrium (RA) to close. After that has been completed (D), attention is directed to closing the remaining RA incisions.

The Cut-and-Sew Maze-III Procedure

Closure of Right Atrium

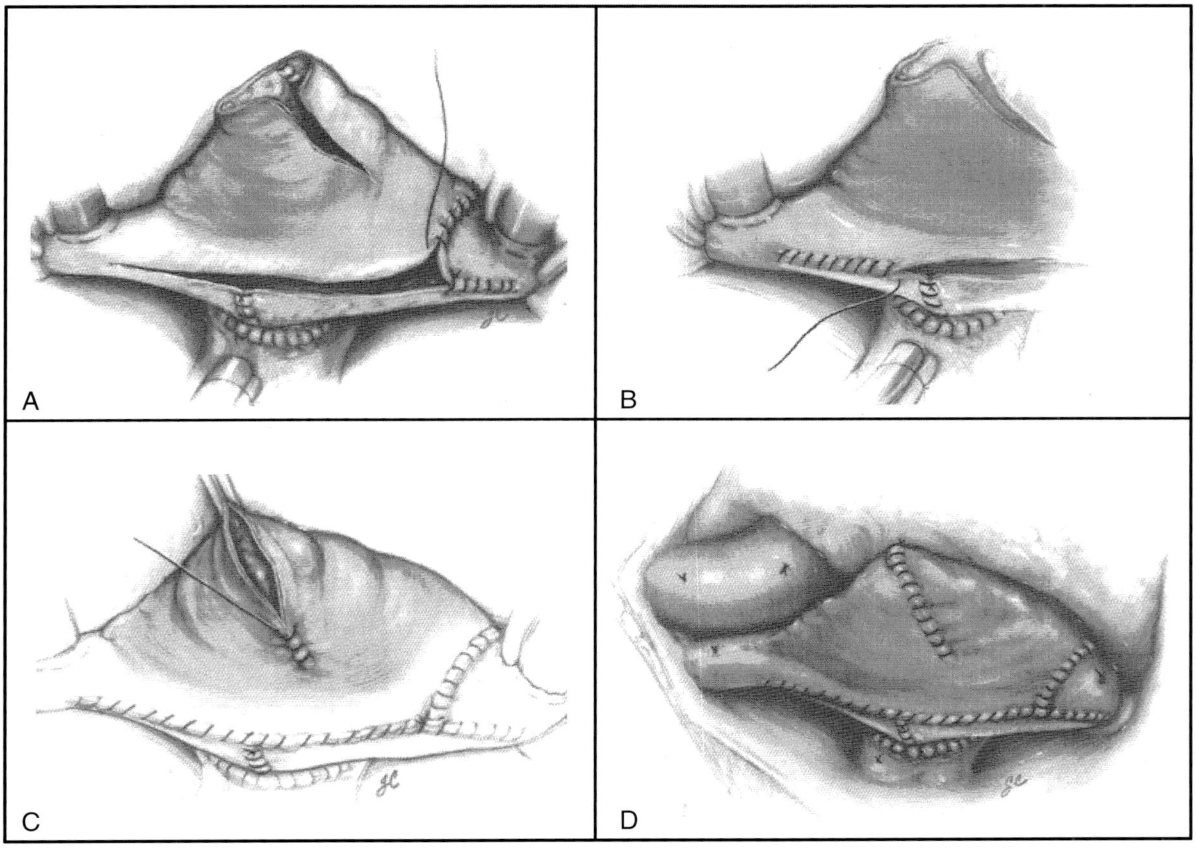

Fig. 12.37 The cut-and-sew Maze-III procedure: closure of the right atrium (RA). Sequential closure of the right atrial incisions is illustrated as seen by the surgeon. (A) Closure of the "T" lesion. (B) Closure of the superior portion of the intercaval lesion. (C) Closure of the lateral lesion in the right atrium. (D) The final appearance of the heart from the surgeon's view after a completed cut-and-sew Maze-III procedure.

REFERENCES

1. Cox JL, Gallagher JJ, Cain ME. Experience with 118 consecutive patients undergoing surgery for the WolffParkinsonWhite syndrome. *J Thor Cardiovasc Surg*. 1985;90:490–501.
2. Harrison L, Gallagher JJ, Sadell J, et al. Cryosurgical ablation of the A-V node-His bundle: a new method for producing A-V block. *Circulation*. 1977;55(3):463–470.
3. Williams JM, Ungerleider RM, Lofland GK, Cox JL. Left atrial isolation: new technique for the treatment of supraventricular arrhythmias. *J Thorac Cardiovasc Surg*. 1980;80:373.
4. Cox JL, Holman WL, Cain ME. Cryosurgical treatment of atrioventricular node reentry tachycardia. *Circulation*. 1987;76: 1329–1336.
5. Harada A, D'Agostino Jr HJ, Boineau JP, Cox JL. Right atrial isolation with preservation of the sinoatrial node: electrophysiologic and hemodynamic effects. *Circulation*. 1986;74:II–135.
6. Guiraudon G, Fontaine G, Frank R, Escande G, Etievent P, Cabrol C. Encircling endocardial ventriculotomy: a new surgical treatment for life-threatening ventricular tachycardias resistant to medical treatment following myocardial infarction. *Ann Thor Surg*. 1978;26(5):438–444.
7. Harken AH, Horowitz LN, Josephson ME. The surgical treatment of ventricular tachycardia. *Ann Thor Surg*. 1980;30(5): 499–508.
8. Gallagher JJ, Cox JL. Status of surgery for ventricular arrhythmias. *Circulation*. 1979;60:1440.
9. Cox JL, Bardy GH, Damiano RJ, et al. Right ventricular isolation procedures for nonischemic ventricular tachycardia. *J Thorac Cardiovasc Surg*. 1985;90:212.
10. D'Agostino HJ Jr, Harada A, Schuessler RB, Boineau JP, Cox JL. Global epicardial mapping of atrial fibrillation in a canine model of chronic mitral regurgitation. *Circulation*. 1987;76(Supp. IV): IV–165.
11. Canavan TE, Schuessler RB, Cain ME, et al. Computerized global electrophysiological mapping of the atrium in a patient with multiple supraventricular tachyarrhythmias. *Ann Thor Surg*. 1988;46:232–235.

12. Cox JL, Canavan TE, Schuessler RB, et al. The surgical treatment of atrial fibrillation: II. Intraoperative electrophysiologic mapping and description of the electrophysiologic basis of atrial flutter and atrial fibrillation. *J Thorac Cardiovasc Surg*. 1991;101:406–426.
13. Santucci PA, Varma N, Cytron J, et al. Electroanatomic mapping of postpacing intervals clarifies the complete active circuit and variants in atrial flutter. *Heart Rhythm*. 2009;6(11):1586–1595.
14. Lim HS, Hocini M, Dubois R, et al. Complexity and distribution of drivers in relation to duration of persistent atrial fibrillation. *J Am Coll Cardiol*. 2017;69(10):1257–1269.
15. Cox JL. The first Maze procedure. *J Thorac Cardiovasc Surg*. 2011;141(5):1093–1097.
16. Cox JL. The surgical treatment of atrial fibrillation: IV. Surgical technique. *J Thorac Cardiovasc Surg*. 1991;101:584–592.
17. Cox JL, Boineau JP, Schuessler RB, Lappas DG. Modification of the Maze procedure for atrial flutter and atrial fibrillation. I-rationale and surgical results. *J Thorac Cardiovasc Surg*. 1995;110:473–484.
18. Boineau JP, Schuessler RB, Mooney CR, et al. Multicentric origin of the atrial depolarization wave: the pacemaker complex. Relation to dynamics of atrial conduction, P-wave changes and heart rate control. *Circulation*. 1978;58(6):1036–1048.
19. Boineau JP, Canavan TE, Schuessler RB, Cain M, Corr PB, Cox JL. Demonstration of a widely distributed atrial pacemaker complex in the human heart. *Circulation*. 1988;77:1221–1237.
20. Cox JL, Boineau JP, Schuessler RB, Kater KM, Lappas DG. Five-year experience with the maze procedure for atrial fibrillation. *Ann Thor Surg*. 1994;56:814–824.
21. Cox JL, Jaquiss RD, Schuessler RB, Boineau JP. Modification of the Maze procedure for atrial flutter and atrial fibrillation. II. Surgical technique of the Maze III procedure. *J Thorac Cardiovasc Surg*. 1995;110:(2):485–495.
22. Ruaengsri C, Schill MR, Khiabani AJ, Schuessler RB, Melby SJ, Damiano, RJ Jr. The Cox-Maze IV procedure in its second decade: still the gold standard? Eur *J Cardiothorac Surg*. 2018;53(1):i19–i25.

13

Importance of the Right Atrial Lesions in the Maze Procedure

James L. Cox, Harold G. Roberts, Jr.

CHAPTER OUTLINE

The confusion among cardiac surgeons regarding whether or not to include the right atrial lesions of the Maze procedure for the treatment of atrial fibrillation (AF) is understandable. Our literature includes publications stating that right atrial lesions are essential to attaining optimal outcomes,[1–4] a few suggest that right atrial lesions contribute nothing to the outcomes,[5,6] and still others argue that the right atrial lesions are helpful in some patients but not in others.[7,8] Many surgeons are convinced that inclusion of the right atrial lesions in a Maze procedure results in damage of the sinoatrial (SA) node and/or the atrioventricular (AV) node and that therefore right atrial lesions result in an increased need for new permanent pacemakers after surgery. Some also believe that including the right atrial lesions adds to cardiopulmonary bypass time and aortic cross-clamp time and that therefore, they add to perioperative morbidity and mortality.

One reason for this confusion is that we are accustomed to thinking of the right atrium (RA) and left atrium (LA) as separate anatomic structures because they provide different hemodynamic roles. However, atrial myocardium is one contiguous muscle mass, and the fact that it is partitioned into two separate chambers by the atrial septum is irrelevant to it being a single electrophysiological entity (Fig. 13.1). The presence of

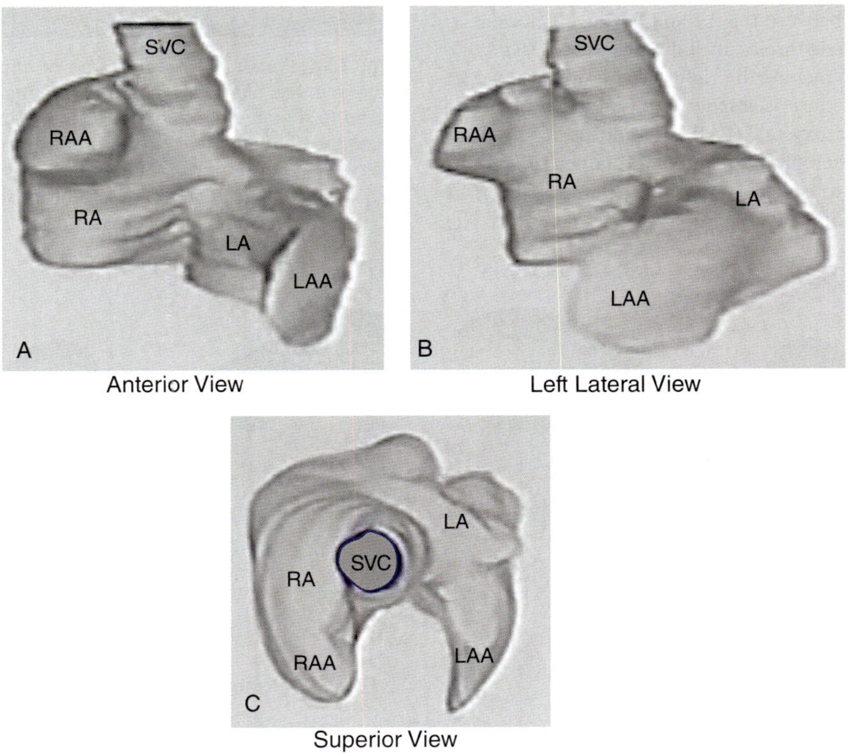

Fig. 13.1 Early electrocardiography-gated magnetic resonance scans from 1986 that allowed three-dimensional reconstruction of the atria demonstrating that the myocardium of the two atria is one muscle mass (A) Anterior view. (B) Left lateral view. (C) Superior view. *LA*, Left atrium; *LAA*, left atrial appendage; *RA*, right atrium; *RAA*, right atrial appendage; *SVC*, superior vena cava.

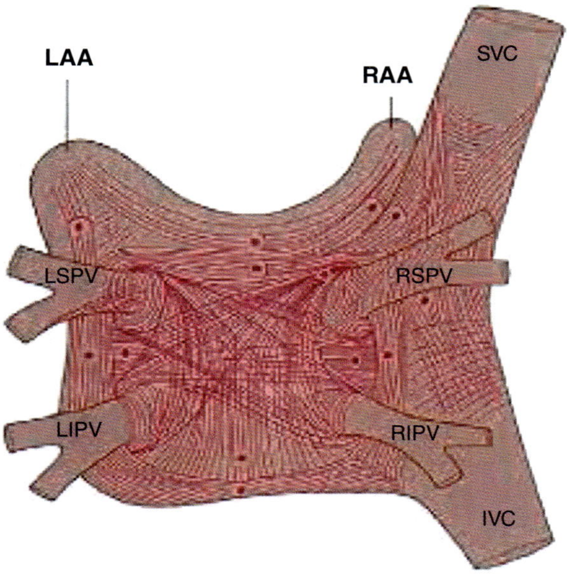

Fig. 13.2 Interconnecting muscle fibers *(dark red lines)* in the vicinity of the pulmonary veins and between the left atrium and right atrium emphasizing their electrical continuity. *IVC,* Inferior vena cava; *LAA,* Left atrial appendage; *LIPV,* left inferior pulmonary vein; *LSPV,* left superior pulmonary vein; *RAA,* right atrial appendage; *RIPV,* right inferior pulmonary vein; *RSPV,* right superior pulmonary vein; *SVC,* superior vena cava.

multiple interatrial muscle bands with preferential routes of conduction further emphasizes the singular nature of electrical activity involving the myocardium of the two atria (Fig. 13.2). Global electrophysiologic maps of the atria confirm that the two atria act as one mass of myocardium with no electrical distinction between the RA and LA during normal sinus rhythm or during atrial arrhythmias, including AF (Fig. 13.3).

This dilemma of when to include the right atrial lesions as part of a surgical AF ablation procedure is further confounded by the fact that the treatment goals in paroxysmal (PAF) and non-paroxysmal AF (non-PAF) are completely different as explained in Chapter 10. The objective of surgery for PAF is to isolate as many of the atrial triggers as possible to decrease the likelihood of an AF episode being induced. The objective of surgery for non-PAF is to interrupt the macro-reentrant circuits (drivers) that sustain AF, thereby rendering the atria incapable of fibrillating.

BIATRIAL LESIONS VERSUS LEFT ATRIAL–ONLY LESIONS

The first meta-analysis comparing biatrial versus left atrial–only lesions was published in 2006 by Barnett and Ad.[1] Their meta-analysis included 69 studies comprising 5885 patients who had undergone concomitant AF ablation at the time of coronary artery bypass graft or valve surgery. The study showed that biatrial lesions were more successful in ablating AF at 3 months, 1 year, 2 years, and 3 years (Fig. 13.4). Their findings were confirmed by subsequent reports from Burnett et al.[2] in 2014 and Gelsomino et al.[3] in 2016. However, in 2013, Soni et al.[6] reported that in 325 patients, a complete LA lesion set was better than pulmonary vein isolation (PVI) alone and that adding the

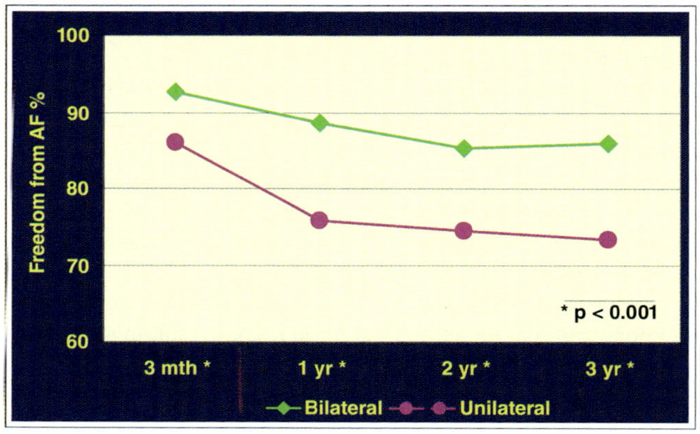

Fig. 13.4 Percent of patients free of atrial fibrillation (AF) at indicated time intervals after surgery for AF. The results for biatrial ablation procedures (bilateral) were superior to those for procedures that did not include the right atrial lesions (unilateral). These data are from a metaanalysis of 69 reports totaling 5885 patients. (Reproduced from Barnett SD, Ad N. Surgical ablation as treatment for the elimination of atrial fibrillation: a meta-analysis. *J Thorac Cardiovasc Surg.* 2006;131(5):1029–1035.)

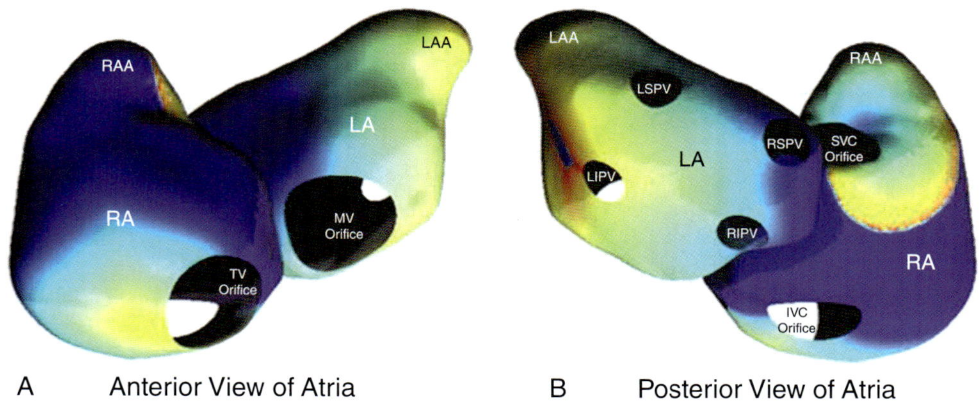

Fig. 13.3 A single frame from the video of a phase map of the atria during atrial fibrillation. Note that the electrical activity between the two atria is contiguous and uninterrupted. (A) Anterior view of the atria. (B) Posterior view of the atria. *IVC,* Inferior vena cava; *LA,* left atrium; *LAA,* left atrial appendage; *LIPV,* left inferior pulmonary vein; *LSPV,* left superior pulmonary vein; *MV,* mitral valve; *RA,* right atrium; *RAA,* right atrial appendage; *RIPV,* right inferior pulmonary vein; *RSPV,* right superior pulmonary vein; *SVC,* superior vena cava; *TV,* tricuspid valve.

right atrial lesions to a complete left atrial lesion set did not improve the success rate for AF ablation.[6] Two years later, the cardiothoracic surgical trials network (CTSN) Clinical Trials Investigators reported the results of the first multicenter randomized controlled trial (RCT) showing that surgical AF ablation in patients with persistent forms of AF undergoing mitral valve surgery had better outcomes than patients in whom the AF was left untreated.[5] They then did an *inadequately powered* comparison between PVI and what they called a "biatrial Maze" procedure and showed that at 1 year, 61% of the PVI group had no recurrent AF versus 66% of the "biatrial Maze" group with no recurrent AF. As discussed in the article, this suggested that PVI was as effective as a "biatrial Maze" procedure for the treatment of patients with persistent forms of AF associated with mitral valve disease. However, in 2019, Blackstone et al.[4] published a follow-up study of the same cohort of patients using more sophisticated statistical analysis and showed that in fact, the "biatrial Maze" group had less recurrent AF than did the PVI group. In 2017, Ad et al.[7] reported their personal experience in 800 patients undergoing AF ablation between 2005 and 2015, 110 of whom had LA-only ablation. Their conclusions were that LA-only ablation yielded "acceptable" success rates in patients with shorter AF duration and smaller left atria, but the success rate for LA-only ablation was not as effective as biatrial Maze procedures in patients with traditional predictors of failure. Finally, the group at Northwestern University published results suggesting that in their 836 patients with AF undergoing mitral valve surgery, adding the right atrial lesions did not affect the outcomes.[8] Because everything that is known about the electrophysiology of AF indicates this to be impossible, there must be some alternate explanation.

One possibility that affected the Northwestern study is that there are a few cardiac surgeons who are recognized for their expertise in mitral valve surgery and who therefore receive more referrals for mitral surgery than do other surgeons. This higher volume of mitral valve patients is associated with earlier referrals as well. Earlier surgical intervention means patients undergo surgery at a less advanced stage of mitral valve disease with a greater likelihood of intervening before the RA has become actively involved in sustaining the AF. In such patients with early AF secondary to mitral valve disease, confining the Maze lesions to the LA would be expected to produce similar outcomes to those of a full biatrial Maze procedure.

Another possible explanation for surgeons getting similar outcomes after LA-only procedures and biatrial Maze procedures is that they perform the biatrial Maze procedure incorrectly so that an LA-only procedure becomes as successful as an incorrectly performed biatrial Maze. That was a problem in the CTSN RCT mentioned earlier in which the authors compared the results of the two different types of surgical procedures in the subgroup of surgically treated patients. They acknowledged that their study was not sufficiently powered to compare the LA-only procedure (PVI) with the biatrial Maze procedure, but they did so anyway. Despite the follow-up report by Blackstone showing the superiority of the biatrial procedure over the PVI, the fact remains that this oft-quoted RCT had one unfortunate consequence. Its unpowered comparison between PVI and a biatrial Maze procedure suggested that PVI was as effective as a biatrial Maze procedure (when imperfectly performed) for the treatment of patients with persistent AF. This misinformation subsequently led to an inadequate surgical procedure (PVI) being performed for concomitant persistent AF in patients all over the world.

In the biatrial Maze subgroup of the CTSN trial, the surgeons were apparently trying to perform a Maze-IV procedure, but not a single patient in the subgroup received a properly performed Maze procedure. That is why the 1-year success rate for a "biatrial Maze" procedure in the study was a dismal 66%, which, by definition, means that the procedure was being done incorrectly. Not only were no coronary sinus lesions performed in any of the patients (an obligatory 10–15% failure rate), but most of the left atrial lesions and all of the right atrial lesions were performed with unipolar ablation devices that are notoriously unreliable for creating complete (contiguous, uniformly transmural) atrial lesions. In addition, surgeons in the trial were allowed to perform all of the right atrial lesions of the Maze procedure even if a cavo-tricuspid isthmus (CTI) lesion had been performed previously by catheter ablation. As explained later, this combination of lesions in the RA results in complete isolation of the lower third of the RA where the sinus bradycardia region of the atrial pacemaker complex resides.

Another problem with the CTSN trial was that the requirements for new permanent pacemakers in the biatrial Maze arm of the study was more than 20%.[5] New pacemakers were required at this surprisingly high rate primarily because of postoperative *heart block*, not postoperative *SA node dysfunction*. However, it is anatomically impossible to create heart block with a surgical lesion that is not in the atrial septum because the AV node–His bundle complex resides exclusively within the atrial septum (see Chapter 3, Fig. 3.17). No patient in that study had a septal lesion performed as a part of their "biatrial Maze procedure," so the procedure itself could not possibly have caused the heart block. The actual reasons why a higher postoperative pacemaker requirement is common after a biatrial Maze procedure are discussed in more detail in Chapter 21.

Finally, global atrial mapping has documented that during episodes of sustained AF, up to 30% of the macro-reentrant circuits present in AF are located in the RA.[9,10] This means that failure to perform the right atrial lesions in patients with sustained AF dictates a potential failure rate of up to 30% unless there is some way to determine preoperatively if the RA is actively participating in the AF. Currently, short of a full preoperative electrophysiologic study or global intraoperative mapping, there is no reliable way to distinguish between passive right atrial involvement and active right atrial involvement (i.e., the RA is "driving" the AF). Therefore, it is impossible to be certain preoperatively whether the right atrial lesions are essential to surgical success. As a result, most experienced arrhythmia surgeons routinely perform both the left atrial lesions and the right atrial lesions in all patients with concomitant persistent or long-standing AF.

EVOLUTION OF THE RIGHT ATRIAL LESION PATTERN

Several different right atrial lesion sets have been used over the past 3 decades, depending on new knowledge gained with experience, individual surgeon preference, or untested surgical whims. Perhaps this explains why surgeons are consistently more perplexed by the right atrial lesions of the Maze procedure than by the left atrial lesions.

In the original Maze-I procedure, there was no intercaval lesion from the superior vena cava (SVC) to the inferior vena cava (IVC) and there was no "T" lesion from the intercaval line to the tricuspid annulus.[11] Instead, there was a lesion that extended from the SVC down the posterior right atrial wall two-thirds of the way toward the IVC, where it was then curved across the lower RA and extended down to the tricuspid annulus (Fig. 13.5, *left upper panel*). This lesion did not prevent potential macro-reentry around the orifice of the IVC; therefore, in the Maze-II and Maze-III procedures, the SVC lesion was extended to the IVC, and a separate "T" lesion was placed from the intercaval lesion to the tricuspid valve annulus (Fig. 13.5, *right lower panel*). The right atrial lesions in the Maze-IV procedure are only slightly different from the Maze-II and Maze-III procedures and are described below.

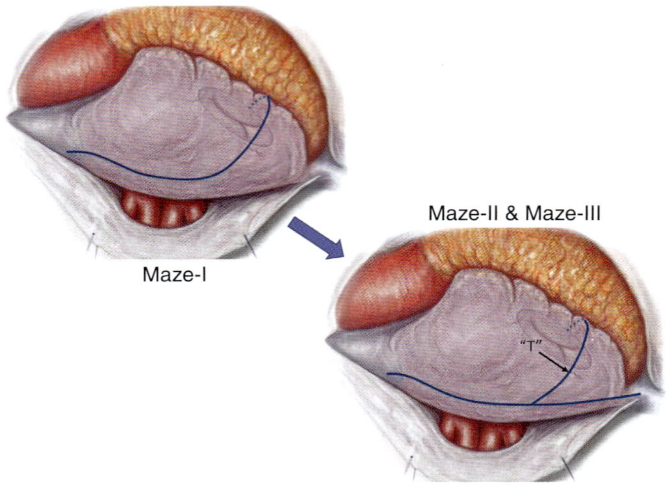

Fig. 13.5 *Left upper panel,* The original Maze-I procedure had no intercaval lesion from the superior vena cava (SVC) to the inferior vena cava (IVC) and therefore, offered no protection against postoperative reentry around the IVC orifice. Instead, a lesion was placed from the SVC down the posterior right atrial wall two-thirds of the way toward the IVC, where it was then curved across the lower right atrium and extended down to the tricuspid annulus. *Right lower panel,* In the Maze-II procedure, an intercaval lesion from the SVC to the IVC was added, and a separate "T" lesion was placed from the intercaval lesion to the tricuspid valve annulus. This combination of intercaval and "T" lesions were retained in the Maze-III and Maze-IV procedures. See text for further discussion.

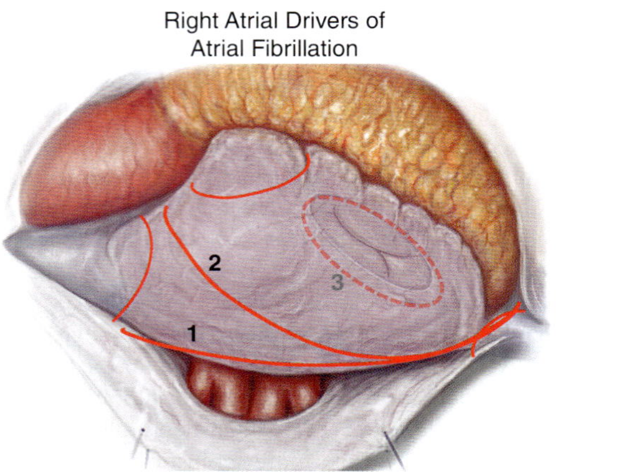

Fig. 13.6 Potential sites of right atrial drivers of atrial fibrillation (AF). The *red circles* represent the locations of the macro-reentrant circuits that can potentially serve as the right atrial drivers of AF. When present with no other macro-reentrant drivers in either atrium, driver 1, 2, or 3 is responsible for classic atrial flutter. Note that all three of these potential "flutter waves" use the cavotricuspid isthmus (CTI) between the orifices of the inferior vena cava (IVC) and the tricuspid valve, explaining why a CTI lesion is so effective in treating atrial flutter. In addition, the circuit around the orifice of the IVC also uses the CTI. See text for further discussion.

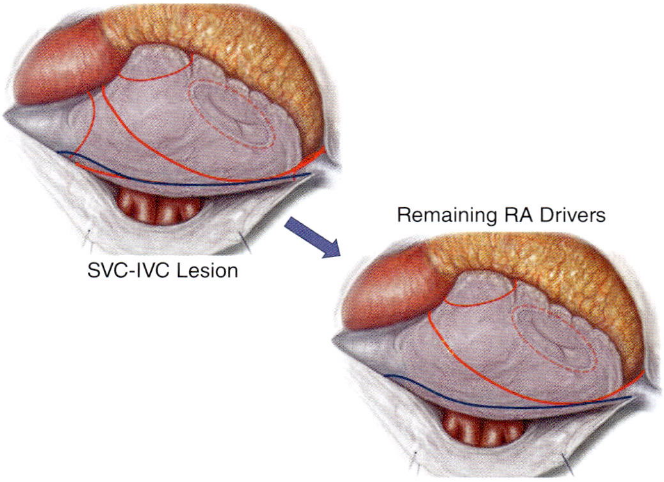

Fig. 13.7 *Left upper panel,* The right atrial lesions are represented as *blue lines*. The intercaval lesion between the superior vena cava (SVC) and inferior vena cava interrupts reentry around the orifices of these two structures as well as the potential "flutter wave" that passes posterior to the SVC. *Right lower panel,* This leaves two potential "flutter waves," one around the tricuspid valve annulus and one around the base of the right atrial appendage (RAA), as well as the potential for reentry around the base of the RAA. See text for further discussion.

CURRENTLY RECOMMENDED RIGHT ATRIAL LESION PATTERN

The potential locations of the right atrial macro-reentrant drivers of AF in a normal-sized atrium are illustrated in Fig. 13.6. As described in Chapter 12, three of these drivers (1, 2, or 3), when occurring alone, can drive classic atrial flutter (see Fig. 12.3).[12] Importantly, all three of these "flutter waves" use the CTI in the RA between the orifice of the IVC and the tricuspid valve annulus. This explains why a CTI lesion, which is easily created with endocardial catheters, is so effective for the treatment of classic atrial flutter. Unfortunately, a CTI lesion cannot be performed surgically without opening the RA.

There are three other sites in the RA where reentrant circuits have been documented to occur by endocardial mapping: (1) around the orifice of the SVC, (2) around the orifice of the IVC, and (3) around the base of the right atrial appendage (RAA). The right atrial lesions in the Maze procedure are designed to prevent the development of any of these documented macro-reentrant drivers of atrial flutter and/or AF. There are three right atrial lesions of the Maze procedure that accomplish that goal: the intercaval lesion, the "T" lesion, and the RAA lesion.

Intercaval Lesion

This lesion extends from the SVC to the IVC and is created primarily to prevent the development of macro-reentry around the orifice of both the SVC and the IVC. In addition, the intercaval lesion also interrupts one of the potential atrial "flutter waves" that passes posterior to the orifice of the SVC (Fig. 13.7).

Some interventional electrophysiologists, and indeed some surgeons, choose to place a transverse lesion across the lower end of the SVC to isolate so-called "SVC triggers" that they believe can induce episodes of AF. Interestingly, in the thousands of surgical Maze procedures that have been performed over the past 30+ years, "SVC triggers" have not been a significant problem postoperatively. Although the intercaval lesion of the Maze-III and Maze-IV procedures prevents *reentry* around the orifice of the SVC, it does not isolate the SVC from the heart. Therefore, the linear lesion extending into the SVC offers no protection against focal triggers that might be located in the lower SVC. The lack of active postoperative SVC triggers after a Maze procedure begs the question of whether such triggers actually exist. Our suspicion is that these so-called "SVC triggers" are actually far-field recordings of triggers within the right superior pulmonary vein (PV), which lies immediately against the posterior wall of the SVC just above its junction with the RA. Even though the right PVs may have been isolated by previous catheter ablation or surgery, the isolated PV triggers are still capable of spontaneously firing just as they did before isolation. If right superior PV triggers fire under such circumstances, the endocardial electrode that is nearest the SVC orifice would be the first to record the trigger's activity, but this might not be the actual site of origin of the impulse. Without electrodes in both the right superior PV and the SVC *simultaneously*, the possibility that these triggers are actually located in the right superior PV cannot be ruled out. In such a case, the triggers only appear to be in the SVC because the closest recording electrode is in the SVC. Our skepticism regarding the actual existence of "SVC triggers" that induce AF is the reason we have never recommended that the lower SVC be electrically isolated from the RA as a part of any surgical or catheter procedure for AF. This practice was justified by a 2016 metaanalysis of 526 patients by Sharma et al.[13] showing that empiric isolation of the SVC orifice did not add any benefit to PVI for the catheter ablation of AF.

"T" Lesion

Our preferred location of the *"T" lesion* has also remained unchanged since the Maze-II procedure. As described in previous chapters, the proximal end of the "T" lesion is connected to the intercaval lesion approximately two-thirds of the way down from the SVC to the IVC and is then directed diagonally across the RA to the tricuspid annulus (Fig. 13.8, *left upper panel*). This "T" lesion interrupts two of the potential atrial flutter waves, one that passes anterior to the orifice of the SVC and the one around the tricuspid valve (Fig. 13.8, *right lower panel*).

We believe that placing the "T" lesion relatively low in the RA wall and making it diagonal decreases the likelihood of damage to the atrial pacemaker complex (Fig. 13.9). However, Robertson et al.[14] prefer to place this lesion higher on the RA free wall and to make it more perpendicular to the intercaval line(Fig. 13.10). In their modification of the CryoMaze-III procedure, McCarthy and coworkers[15] expose the inside of the RA with a right atriotomy from near the tip of the RAA across the RA free wall toward the IVC. They then create the "T" lesion with a cryolesion from the SVC to the atriotomy combined with another cryolesion from the atriotomy to the tricuspid annulus[15] (Fig. 13.11). Although we do not prefer either of those RA lesion patterns, neither has been shown to increase the need for more postoperative pacemakers than a "T" lesion placed in the position that we advocate.

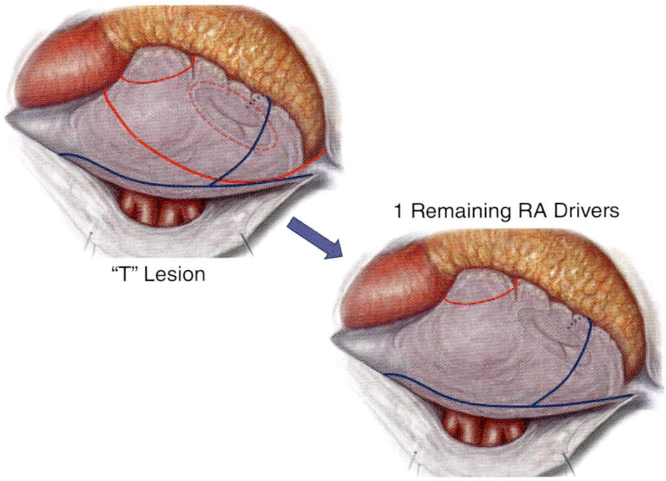

Fig. 13.8 *Left upper panel,* The so-called "T" lesion extends from the lower intercaval lesion diagonally across the lower right atrial wall to the tricuspid valve annulus and blocks the remaining two flutter waves around the tricuspid valve and anterior to the superior vena cava. *Right lower panel,* The combination of the intercaval lesion and the "T" lesion leaves only one site where right atrial reentry has been recorded previously (i.e., around the base of the right atrial appendage).

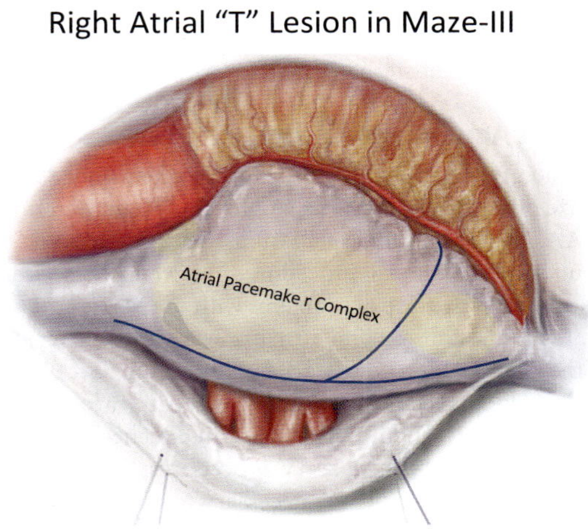

Fig. 13.9 Right atrial "T" lesion in the Maze-III procedure. The "T" lesion is placed in the lower portion of the right atrium (RA) to avoid the major portion of the atrial pacemaker complex *(yellow area)* that drives normal heart rates above 60 beats/min and the sinus bradycardia region of the complex in the lower RA that drives normal sinus rhythm at rates below 60 beats/min.

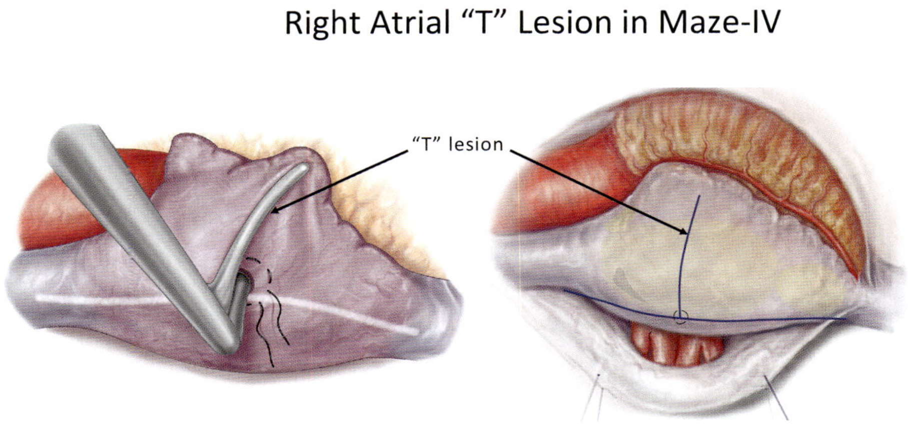

Fig. 13.10 Right atrial "T" lesion in the Maze-IV procedure. *Left panel,* In the Maze-IV procedure, the "T" lesion is created with a bipolar radiofrequency clamp placed through a pursestring suture at the *middle* of the intercaval line and then placed *perpendicular* to the intercaval line across the right atrial free wall. *Right panel,* We do not recommend that the "T" lesion be placed in this location or at the illustrated angle in relation to the intercaval lesion because it bisects the middle of the atrial pacemaker complex. However, this placement of the "T" lesion has not been shown to increase the need for more postoperative pacemakers.

Right Atrial "T" Lesion in Modified CryoMaze-III

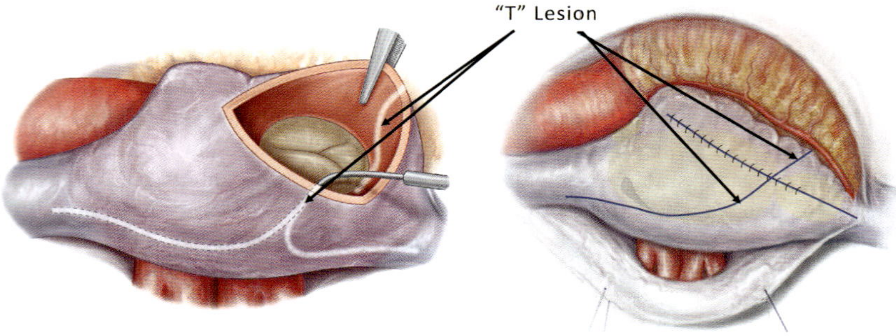

Fig. 13.11 Right atrial "T" lesion in the modified CryoMaze-III procedure. *Left panel,* In the modified CryoMaze-III procedure, an atriotomy is performed for exposure that extends from the right atrial appendage to just above the junction of the right atrium and inferior vena cava. The "T" lesion is created by combined cryolesions from the superior vena cava to the atriotomy and another from the atriotomy to the tricuspid annulus. The extension of the latter cryolesion along the tricuspid annulus and into the coronary sinus is not essential to the success of this procedure but neither does it detract from this success. *Right panel,* This combination of right atrial free-wall lesions should theoretically impact the atrial pacemaker complex less than the "T" lesion of the Maze-IV procedure, and like a properly performed Maze-IV procedure, it is not followed by an increase in the need for postoperative pacemakers.

Right Atrial Appendage Lesion

The RA lesion that has been modified most often since the early days of the Maze procedure is the one that prevents reentry around the base of the RAA. There were multiple lesions that prevented RAA reentry in the cut-and-sew Maze-I procedure, but when these lesions were moved posteriorly because of problems with the Maze-I procedure (see Chapter 12), no lesion remained that prevented RAA reentry. Therefore, in the Maze-II procedure, a new lesion, the so-called "counterlesion," was added specifically to prevent reentry around the base of the RAA (Fig. 13.12), and it was retained in the cut-and-sew Maze-III, the CryoMaze-III, and the Maze-IV procedures. To anchor this lesion to non-conducting tissue, it was necessary to extend its distal end all the way to the tricuspid valve annulus. The combination of the "counterlesion" and the "T" lesion results in two of the right atrial lesions reaching the tricuspid annulus, the counterlesion in the 10 o'clock position and the T lesion in the 2 o'clock" position (Fig. 13.13). However, because it is not necessary to interrupt the reentrant circuit around the tricuspid annulus in more than one place, the fact that the counterlesion has to be extended medially to the tricuspid annulus as an anchor is redundant.

The counterlesion is still preferred by many experienced arrhythmia surgeons, but less experienced surgeons have always been concerned about creating heart block with this lesion because of the close proximity of its distal end to the AV node–His bundle complex. As a result, many of these surgeons simply eliminated it from the right atrial lesion pattern, accepting a small additional failure rate. Fortunately, there is a simple maneuver to avoid placing the counterlesion too close to the AV node–His bundle, which is to place the left index finger (or a soft-tipped surgical instrument) between the RA and the proximal ascending aorta down to the tricuspid annulus. The only place where one can actually reach the tricuspid annulus externally is the exact location of the mem-

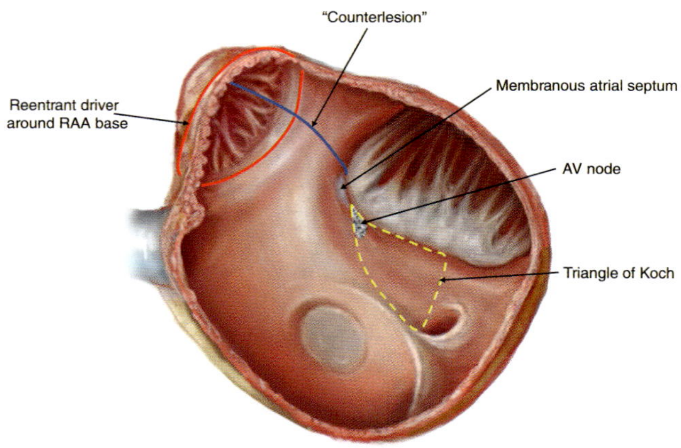

Fig. 13.12 When the Maze-I procedure was modified to the Maze-II procedure, it was necessary to add a "counterlesion" from the tip of the right atrial appendage (RAA) medially down to the tricuspid valve annulus to prevent reentry around the RAA. See text for further discussion. *AV,* Atrioventricular.

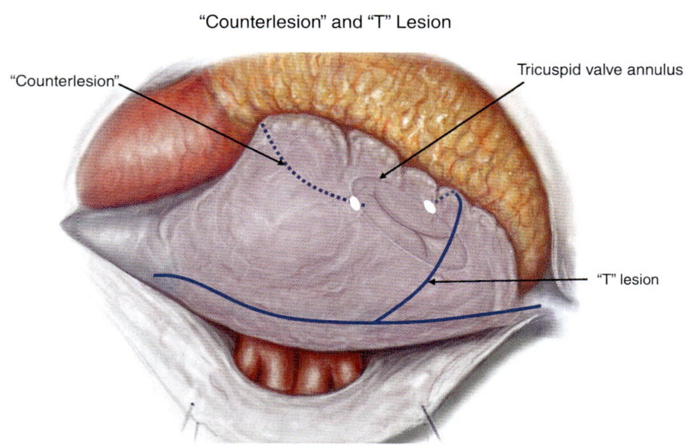

Fig. 13.13 "Counterlesion" and "T" lesion. Although the primary purpose of the "counterlesion" is to prevent reentry around the right atrial appendage, both the "counterlesion" and the "T" lesion terminate at the tricuspid valve annulus at the 10 o'clock and 2 o'clock positions, respectively, where focal cryolesions are created *(white dots).* Therefore, reentry around the tricuspid valve is prevented by both lesions. However, it is necessary to block a reentrant circuit in only one place, so these two lesions, although essential to block all potential RA reentrant drivers, are redundant in regard to the reentrant driver around the tricuspid valve.

branous portion of the interatrial septum. Because the AV node–His bundle complex is always posterior to the membranous septum, it can be avoided by placing the counterlesion anterior to one's index finger.

Because of the persistent reluctance of surgeons to create counterlesions in this position, it was suggested to me (JLC) almost simultaneously a few years ago by Dr. Antonius Driessen of Amsterdam University Medical Center (UMC) and Doug Seith and Rob Dickson of AtriCure, Inc., that perhaps it would be easier to delete this counterlesion and replace it with a lesion on the free wall of the RA from the "T" lesion up to the tip of the RAA (Fig. 13.14). This lesion accomplishes the same goal as the counterlesion (i.e., prevention of reentry around the RAA), but it is clearly much easier to perform (Fig. 13.15). Their independent suggestions were clearly an attractive alternative to the counterlesion, so I mentioned it to my coauthor, Dr. Harold Rob-

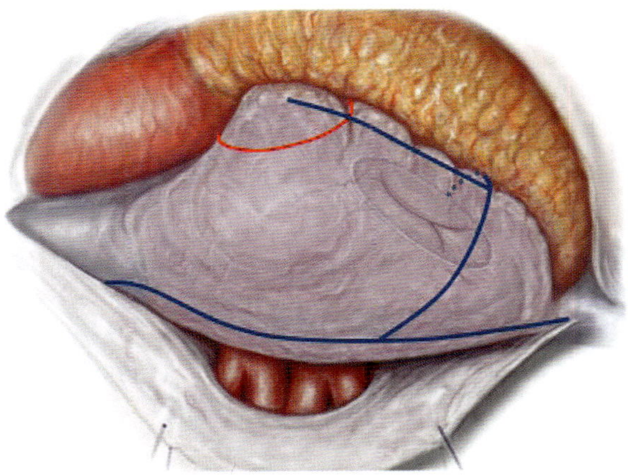

Fig. 13.14 Right atrial appendage (RAA) lesion. Because of the perceived difficulty of performing the "counterlesion," we replaced it with a lesion from the distal portion of the "T" lesion just above the atrioventricular groove to the tip of the RAA. The only purpose of this so-called "RAA lesion" is to prevent macro-reentry around the base of the RAA. See text for further discussion.

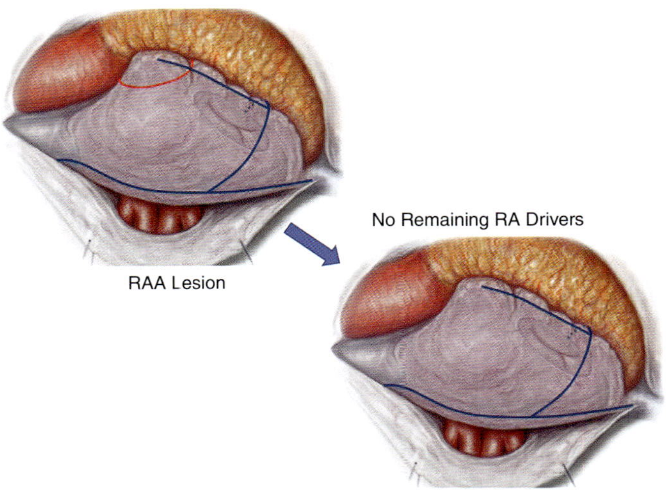

Fig. 13.15 *Left upper panel,* The right atrial appendage (RAA) lesion is the last right atrial lesion applied, and it prevents reentry around the base of the appendage. *Right lower panel,* The final pattern of currently recommended right atrial lesions prevents all know macro-reentrant drivers in the right atrium.

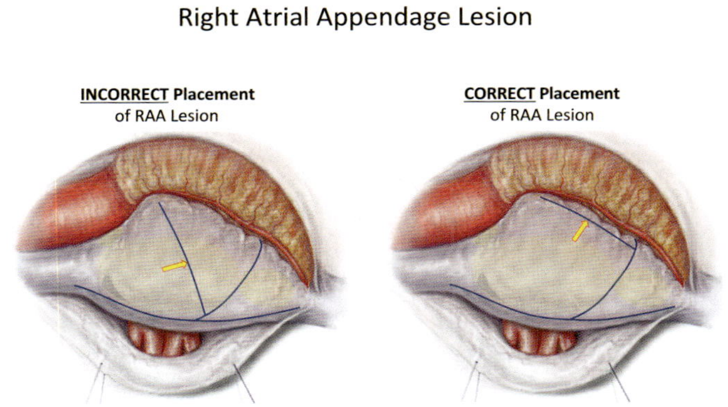

Fig. 13.16 Right atrial appendage (RAA) lesion. *Left panel,* Incorrect placement of the RAA lesion too far medially *(yellow arrow)* results in bisection of the atrial pacemaker complex *(yellow area)* and risks increasing the need for postoperative pacemakers. *Right panel,* Correct placement of the RAA lesion near the anterior edge of the right atrium *(yellow arrow)* does not interfere with the atrial pacemaker complex and does not result in the need for postoperative pacemakers.

erts, who soon accumulated a series of 112 patients using this new RA lesion pattern.[16] His clinical experience confirmed that the success rate with this repositioning of the RAA lesion was similar to that of the previous counterlesion in preventing reentry around the base of the RAA. However, the modified RAA lesion was initially placed too medially and actually bisected the atrial pacemaker complex (Fig. 13.16, *left panel*), which almost certainly explains the increased requirements for postoperative pacemakers in his series. Since that time, Dr. Roberts has moved the RAA lesion to its proper position at the front edge of the RA (Fig. 13.16, *right panel*) and has seen a substantial decrease in postoperative pacemaker requirements. When properly performed, there is no reason that postoperative pacemaker requirements would be increased with this RAA lesion, so we currently recommend that this pattern of right atrial lesions be used in all Maze-III and Maze-IV procedures.

A cardinal rule when creating the right atrial lesions of the Maze procedure is that one should avoid using forceps on the lateral wall of the RA encompassed by the intercaval lesion, the "T" lesion and the RAA lesion. All of these lesions can be created with scissors, bipolar radiofrequency clamps, or linear cryoprobes, but if possible, one should avoid using forceps or other surgical instruments on the encompassed right atrial wall to create the right atrial lesions. We call this portion of the RA the "no-touch" zone (Fig. 13.17) because it gives rise to all heart rates above 60 beats/min.

Another, perhaps even more important, cardinal rule when creating the right atrial lesions of the Maze procedure is that they should *never* be combined with the CTI lesion across the CTI. This combination of lesions completely isolates all of the RA wall below the level of the "T" lesion, which includes the sinus bradycardia area of the atrial pacemaker complex (Fig. 13.18). This complication would almost certainly result in one's inability to develop an appropriate bradycardia during sleep or in response to rate-reducing medications, although that potential problem has not been adequately studied.

The most common use of this combination of right atrial lesions occurs when a patient has had a previous CTI lesion created for the treatment of atrial flutter by endocardial catheter ablation and then presents for a Maze procedure for AF. The critical problem with combining the right atrial Maze lesions with a CTI lesion is that both the "T" lesion" and the CTI terminate at the tricuspid annulus and both also terminate in the IVC. Thus, rather than creating the normal RA lesion pattern in such patients, a right atriotomy should first be placed in the recommended position. The atriotomy creates the majority of the "T" lesion,

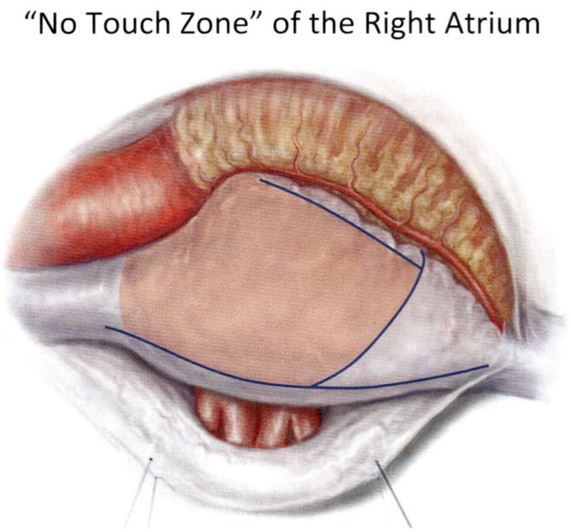

Fig. 13.17 "No-touch zone" of the right atrium. A good rule of thumb when creating the right atrial lesions of the Maze procedure is to avoid touching the area of right atrial free wall between the superior vena cava lesion, the "T" lesion, and the right atrial appendage lesion. It is especially important to avoid grasping this tissue with forceps or otherwise traumatizing it in any way if possible. We refer to this area of the right atrial free wall as the "no-touch zone" *(shaded red area).*

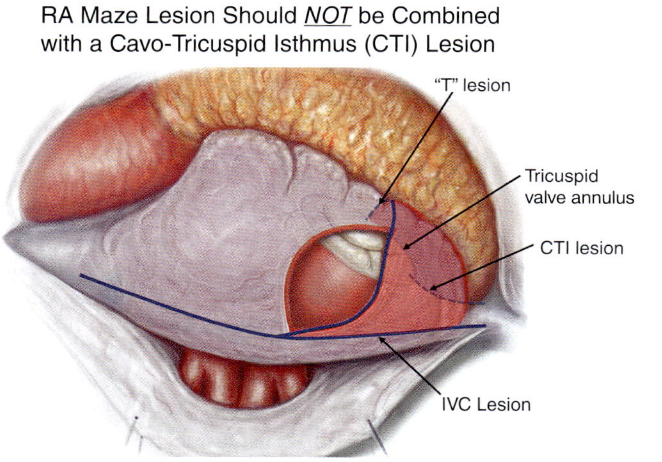

Fig. 13.18 If a patient already has a cavotricuspid isthmus (CTI) lesion from previous catheter ablation for atrial flutter and the right atrial lesions described earlier are then added during later surgery, the right atrium below the level of the "T" lesion will be completely isolated (shaded areas). Therefore, the right atrial Maze lesions and a CTI lesion should *never* be created in the same patient. *IVC,* Inferior vena cava.

but its distal end is *not* extended to the tricuspid annulus. The only right atrial lesions that need to be created after the atriotomy are from its proximal end up into the SVC and from its distal end up to the tip of the RAA (Fig. 13.19). This combination of right atrial Maze lesions with a CTI lesion still interrupts all of the potential macro-reentrant drivers in the RA than can contribute to sustaining AF; it also does not isolate the lower one-third of the RA containing the sinus bradycardia area of the atrial pacemaker complex (Fig. 13.20).

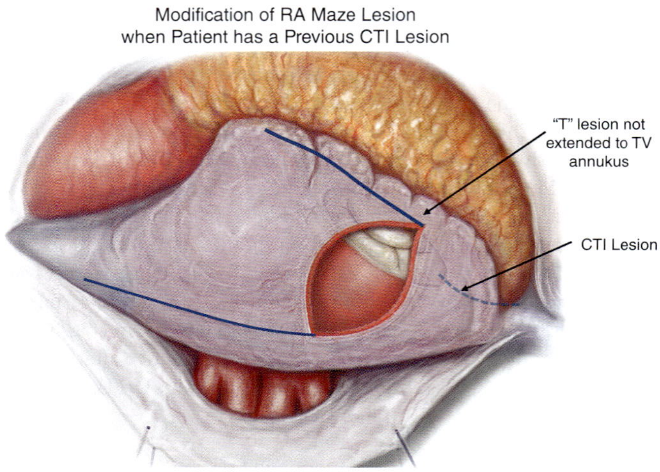

Fig. 13.19 Modification of right atrial Maze lesions when a patient has a previous cavotricuspid isthmus (CTI) lesion. In the presence of a previous CTI lesion, an atriotomy should be placed as diagrammed beginning two-thirds of the way down from the superior vena cava (SVC) toward the inferior vena cava (IVC) just anterior to the crista terminalis. This should be a diagonal atriotomy, and it should *not* be extended down to the tricuspid valve (TV) annulus. After the atriotomy has been created, only two right atrial lesions should be added to it: (1) the SVC lesion from the proximal end of the atriotomy to the SVC and (2) the right atrial appendage (RAA) lesion from the distal end of the atriotomy to the tip of the RAA.

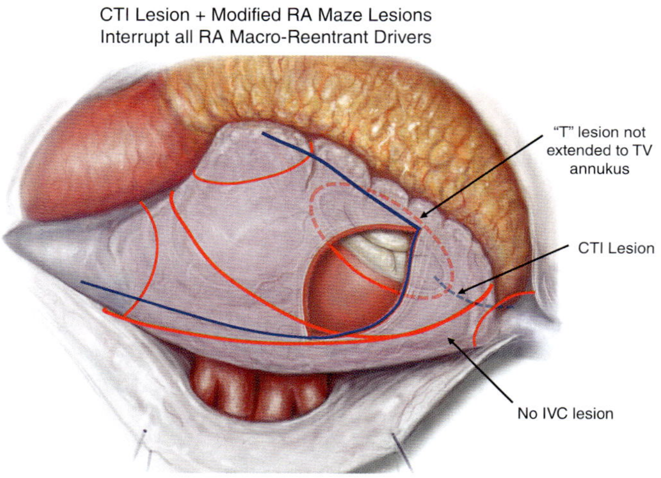

Fig. 13.20 A cavotricuspid isthmus (CTI) lesion plus modified right atrial Maze lesions interrupt all right atrial macro-reentrant drivers. The superior vena cava lesion, the right atrial appendage lesion, and the partial "T" lesion resulting from the atriotomy combined with the previous CTI lesion interrupts all of the right atrial drivers of atrial fibrillation just as effectively as the three right atrial Maze lesions without the CTI lesion. *IVC,* Inferior vena cava; *TV,* tricuspid valve.

REFERENCES

1. Barnett SD, Ad N. Surgical ablation as treatment for the elimination of atrial fibrillation: a meta-analysis. *J Thorac Cardiovasc Surg.* 2006;131(5):1029–1035.
2. Burnett LA, Kocheril AG. Putative role of right atrial ablation in atrial fibrillation. *J Atr Fibrillation.* 2014;6(6):1085–1087.

3. Gelsomino S, La Meir M, Van Breugel HN, et al. Surgical ablation in patients undergoing mitral valve surgery: impact of lesion set and surgical techniques on long-term success. *Europace*. 2016;18(10):1529–1537.
4. Blackstone EH, Chang HL, Rajeswaran J, et al. Biatrial Maze procedure versus pulmonary vein isolation for atrial fibrillation during mitral valve surgery: new analytical approaches and end points. *J Thorac Cardiovasc Surg*. 2019;157(1):234–243.
5. Gillinov AM, Gelijns AC, Parides MK, et al. Surgical ablation of atrial fibrillation during mitral-valve surgery. *N Eng J Med*. 2015;372(15):1399–1409.
6. Soni LK, Cedola SR, Cogan J, et al. Right atrial lesions do not improve the efficacy of a complete left atrial lesion set in the surgical treatment of atrial fibrillation but they do increase procedural morbidity. *J Thorac Cardiovasc Surg*. 2013;145(2):356–361.
7. Ad N, Holmes SD, Lamont D, Shuman DJ. Left-sided surgical ablation for patients with atrial fibrillation who are undergoing concomitant cardiac surgical procedures. *Ann Thorac Surg*. 2017;103:58–63.
8. Churyla A, Iddriss A, Andrei A-C, et al. Biatrial or left atrial lesion set for ablation during mitral surgery: risks and benefits. *Ann Thorac Surg*. 2017;103:1856–1865.
9. Lim HS, Hocini M, Dubois R, et al. Complexity and distribution of drivers in relation to duration of persistent atrial fibrillation. *J Am Coll Cardiol*. 2017;69(10):1257–1269.
10. Osorio-Jaramillo E, Cox JL, Klenk S, et al. Dynamic electrophysiological mechanism in patients with long-standing persistent atrial fibrillation. *Front Cardiovasc Med*. 2022;9:953622. https://doi.org/10.3389/fcvm.2022.953622.
11. Cox JL. The surgical treatment of atrial fibrillation: IV. Surgical technique. *J Thorac Cardiovasc Surg*. 1991;101:584–592.
12. Santucci PA, Varma N, Cytron J, et al. Electroanatomic mapping of postpacing intervals clarifies the complete active circuit and variants in atrial flutter. *Heart Rhythm*. 2009;6(11):1586–1595.
13. Sharma SP, Sangha RS, Dahal K, Krishnamoorthy P. The role of empiric superior vena cava isolation in atrial fibrillation: a systematic review and meta-analysis of randomized controlled trials. *J Interv Card Electrophysiol*. 2017;48(1):61–67.
14. Robertson JO, Saint LL, Leidenfrost JE, Jr Damiano. RJ: Illustrated techniques for performing the Cox-Maze IV procedure through a right mini-thoracotomy. *Ann Cardiothorac Surg*. 2014;3(1):105–116.
15. McCarthy PM, Cox JL, Kruse J, Elenbaas C, Andrei AC. One hundred percent utilization of a modified cryoMaze III procedure for atrial fibrillation with mitral surgery. *J Thorac Cadiovasc Surg*. 2024;167(4):1278–1289.e3. https://doi.org/10.1016/j.jtcvs.2022.08.028.
16. Cheema FH, Younus MA, Siddiqui OT, et al. Early results of the modified right atrial lesion set for the Cox-CryoMaze procedure. *Innovations*. 2016;11:342–348.

14

Conversion from the Cut-and-Sew Maze-III Procedure to the Minimally Invasive CryoMaze-III Procedure

James L. Cox

CHAPTER OUTLINE

In the mid-1990s, cardiac surgeons became increasingly interested in the development of minimally invasive surgery for patients with ischemic and valvular heart disease. Some efforts centered on exposing the heart for coronary artery bypass graft and valve surgery through smaller incisions while others focused on eliminating the need for cardiopulmonary bypass when performing coronary artery bypass surgery. Specialized instruments and devices were developed that enhanced surgical exposure, cannulation for cardiopulmonary bypass, occlusion of the ascending aorta for antegrade cardioplegic arrest, bypassing the coronary arteries, and repairing or replacing heart valves.

The limiting factor in the development of a minimally invasive surgical procedure to treat patients with atrial fibrillation (AF) was the obvious risk of trying to perform all of the atrial lesions of the cut-and-sew Maze-III procedure through a small thoracotomy rather than via the traditional median sternotomy. For example, the left atrial appendage (LAA) cannot be amputated safely through a small right anterolateral thoracotomy. In the cut-and-sew Maze-III procedure, the LAA was inverted into the left atrium (LA) and amputated at its base with a knife (see Fig. 12.32). LAA amputation typically results in the transection of a small atrial branch of the circumflex coronary artery located at the extreme lateral aspect of the base of the LAA. Control of this small arterial bleeder is simple through a median sternotomy but extremely difficult through a small right thoracotomy. We addressed this problem in the development of a minimally invasive Maze-III procedure by leaving the LAA intact and closing it endocardially. Another problem was potential bleeding from the multiple atrial incisions that were foundational to the success of the cut-and-sew Maze-III procedure. This barrier was overcome by replacing the cut-and-sew Maze-III incisions with linear *cryolesions*. Unfortunately, in the mid-1990s, there were no commercially available linear cryoprobes, so to create one, we removed the insulation from the shaft of a 2-mm cryoprobe previously designed for us by Frigitronics, Inc. to treat patients with atrioventricular node reentry tachycardia (AVNRT). This provided us with an excellent linear cryoprobe capable of creating all of the lesions of the Maze-III procedure (Fig. 14.1). We modified two such cryoprobes to freeze tissue

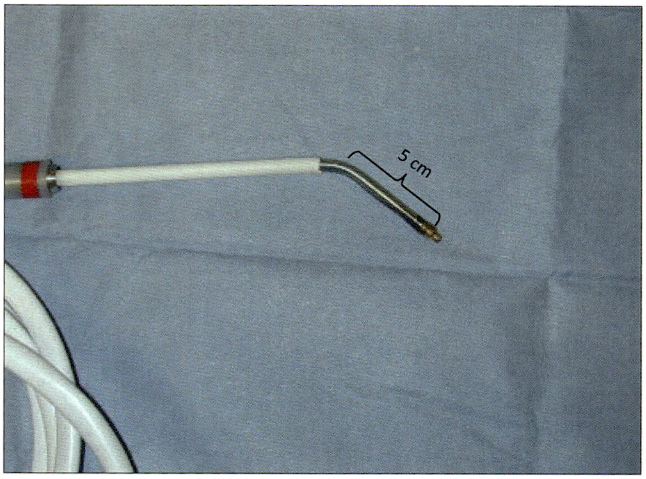

Fig. 14.1 This non-disposable cryoprobe was designed with a 2 mm active tip for the treatment of atrioventricular node reentry tachycardia (AVNRT). Because there were no commercially available linear cryoprobes at the time, we removed the insulation on the shaft of this cryoprobe to expose a 5-cm segment that could be used as a linear cryoprobe in the minimally invasive CryoMaze-III procedure. Two such "linear cryoprobes" were prepared in this manner so that they could be placed on both sides of the pulmonary veins for pulmonary vein isolation and on both sides of the atrial septum to create the atrial septal lesion. We called this technique a "floating cryoprobe clamp," which we used routinely to perform minimally invasive CryoMaze-III procedures after 1996.

from both sides simultaneously, which was made possible by the newly available (at the time) dual-channel Frigitronics console. The ability to freeze both sides of the tissue simultaneously simplified isolation of the pulmonary veins as well as creation of the atrial septal lesion. Fortunately, commercial disposable linear cryoprobes are now readily available and far superior to our homemade non-disposable probes, making it much easier to create the Maze-III cryolesions through a small chest incision (see Chapter 16).

PRINCIPLES OF CREATING A PERMANENT MYOCARDIAL CRYOLESION

Heat-based energy sources such as radiofrequency, microwave, laser, and high-intensity focused ultrasound kill myocardial cells by heating them to a critical lethal temperature of 61°C.[1] However, cryothermia creates lesions by *withdrawing* heat from the myocardium to freeze the cells to a critical lethal temperature. When performed properly, both heat-based lesions and cryosurgical lesions are as effective as surgical incisions in blocking electrical conduction in the atrium.

Cryobiology That Affects the Creation of a Cryolesion

Cryosurgery kills myocardial cells during both the freezing and thawing phases of the cryolesion.[2] The slower the frozen tissue thaws, the greater the volume of cell death,[3,4] and repeating the freeze–thaw cycle increases the size of the ultimate cryolesion.[2] Cell death during the freezing phase is caused by direct cellular injury from the formation of intracellular and extracellular ice crystals that destroy the cell membranes. During the thawing phase, cell death occurs because of microvascular stasis that develops around the edges of the cryolesion.

Plant cells and pancreatic cells have a critical lethal temperature of −20°C at which they literally "explode" with complete disruption of the cell wall and the escape of cellular contents into the surrounding intercellular tissues (Fig. 14.2). However, the seminal studies of John G. Baust,

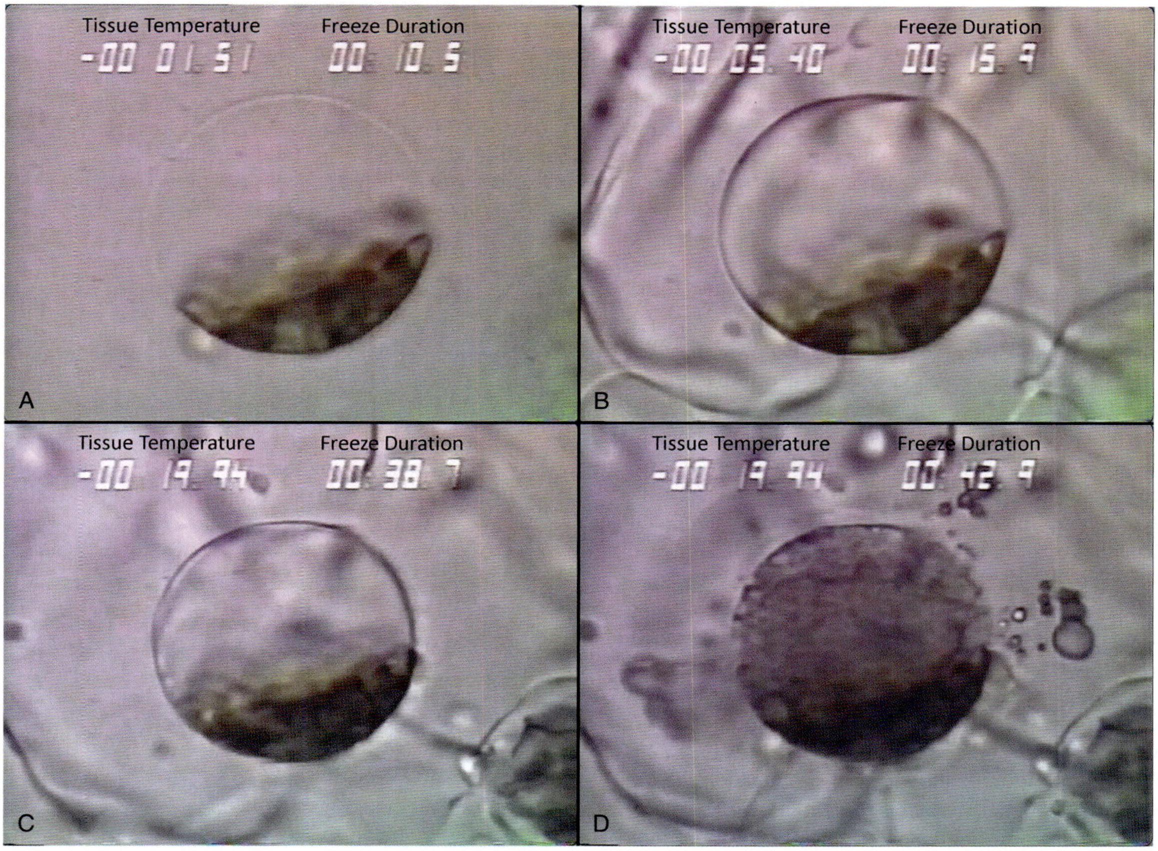

Fig. 14.2 Sequential photomicrographs from a video of a single pancreatic cell while being exposed to cryothermia. In each frame, the temperature of the cell and surrounding interstitial tissue is continuously displayed in the *left upper portion* of the frame, and the duration of the cryothermia application (freeze duration in seconds) is continuously displayed in the *right upper portion* of the frame. (A) After 10.5 seconds of cryothermia application, the tissue temperature is −1.51°C, and there is no evidence of either cellular or extracellular ice formation. (B) Extracellular and intracellular ice form almost simultaneously, though ice appears slightly earlier in the extracellular tissue. After 15.9 seconds of freezing, the tissue temperature is −5.4°C and intracellular and extracellular ice is apparent. (C). After 38.7 seconds of freezing, the tissue temperature is −19.94°C. Ice is prominent in both the cellular and extracellular tissues, and the cell wall is still intact. (D) 4.2 seconds later (42.9 seconds) at the same temperature of −19.94°C, the cell wall suddenly disrupts, and cellular contents are exposed to the extracellular tissues. The *small round circles* in this frame are fragments of the cell wall that have rolled into a ball much like a window shade suddenly wrapping up on itself. This is the histological hallmark of irreversible cellular injury. Whereas the lethal cryothermic temperature for this pancreatic cell and several other animal and plant cells is −20°C, the lethal cryothermic temperature for myocardial cells is −30°C. (Courtesy Dr. JG Baust).

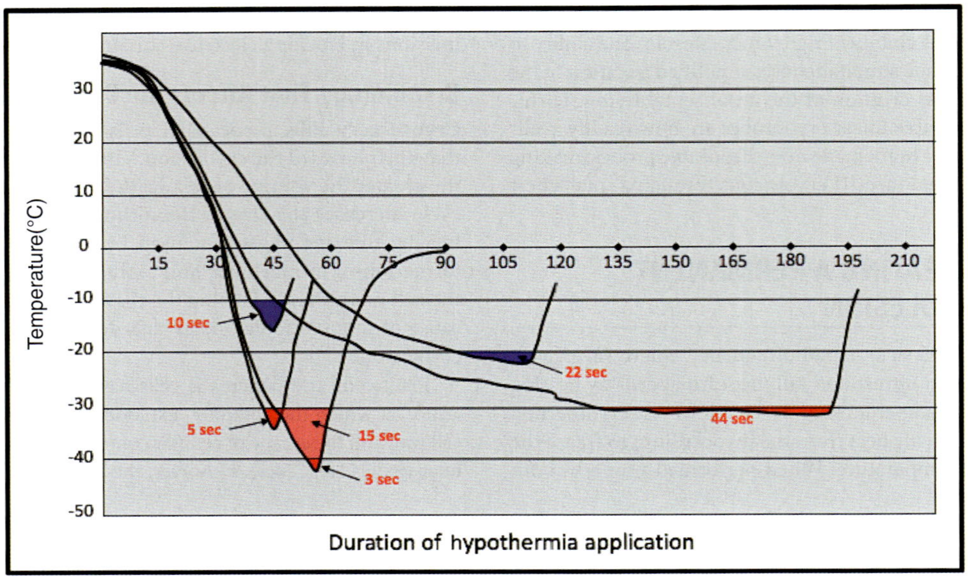

Fig. 14.3 Correlation of myocardial cell damage with tissue temperature and duration of cryothermia exposure (axis in seconds). These are five examples of continuous temperature curves recorded from five separate tissue sites where the myocardium was monitored continuously by thermocouples. Note that myocardial cells survived at sites that were exposed to tissue temperatures below –10°C for 10 seconds and below –20°C for 22 seconds *(blue shading)*. However, if the myocardial temperature reached –30°C *(red shading)*, even for only 5 seconds, the myocardial cells did not survive. (Reproduced from Cox JL, Malaisrie C, Churyla A, et al. Cryosurgery for atrial fibrillation: physiologic basis for creating optimal cryolesions. *Ann Thorac Surg*. 2021;112:354–362.)

John M. Baust, and Kristi K. Snyder documented that the critical lethal temperature of myocardial cells is −30°C. Sudden myocardial cell death that occurs at −30°C does not depend on the time the myocardial cell is kept at that temperature, only that the cell reaches that temperature. In the sequential images of a pancreatic islet cell being frozen that are shown in Fig. 14.2 (from a video by John G. Baust), sudden death occurred 4.2 seconds after the cell temperature reached −19.94°C. Likewise, our independent experimental studies confirmed that myocardial cells die within 5 seconds of reaching −30°C (Fig. 14.3).[5]

Although the freezing portion of the freeze–thaw cycle alone can kill myocardial cells if they reach the critical lethal temperature of −30°C during the freeze, it is often impossible to reach that temperature in all of the targeted tissue because of the "heat sink" effect of the surrounding tissues (see Chapter 20). This limitation results in a non-transmural cryolesion and procedural failure. The primary effect of prolonging the application of a cryoprobe is to increase the number of cells that reach −30°C, thereby resulting in a larger permanent cryolesion. Thus, the myocardial temperature scale pertinent to creating permanent lesions of conduction in the heart ranges from the critical lethal temperature of 61°C for heat-based ablative energies to the critical lethal termperature of −30°C for cryothermia-based ablative energy (Fig. 14.4).

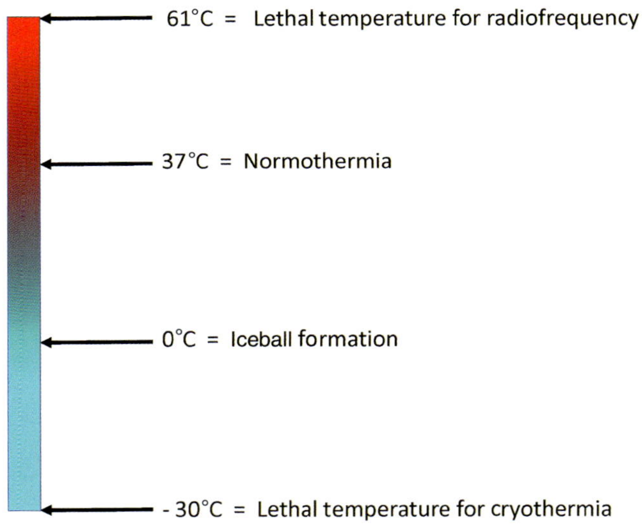

Fig. 14.4 Temperature scale for the critical lethal temperature of myocardial cells using heat-based ablation devices such as radiofrequency catheters and surgical devices (61°C) to the critical lethal temperature of myocardial cells using cryothermia-based ablation devices such as cryoballoon catheters and surgical cryoprobes (–30°C).

How to Create a Permanent Contiguous, Uniformly Transmural Cryolesion

Perhaps the most misunderstood aspect of cryosurgery for cardiac arrhythmias is the so-called "2-minute rule."[5] The traditional application of cryothermia for "2 minutes" has been variously interpreted as being:

1. Total cryoprobe application time of 2 minutes (Fig. 14.5, *left panel*)
   Applying a cryoprobe for a predetermined 2-minute period of time ignores the effects of varying clinical circumstances and is likely to fail as often as it succeeds. The temperature of the cryoprobe, the temperature of the targeted myocardium, the thickness of the atrial wall, and the heat-sink effect of cavitary blood all impact the size, depth, and integrity of the ultimate cryolesion. These factors can combine to make a simple 2-minute application of cryothermia completely ineffective.

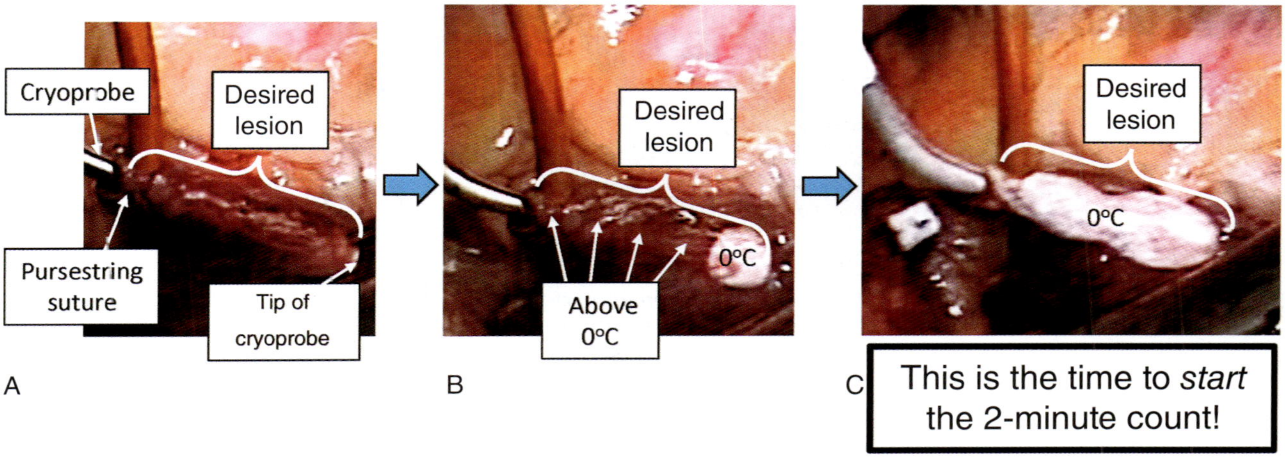

Fig. 14.5 This sequence of intraoperative photographs demonstrates how to apply the traditional "2-minute rule" of cryothermia exposure correctly to ensure that a permanent contiguous, transmural cryolesion will invariably be created. These operative photos were chosen for illustration because they allow the surgeon to visualize the creation of a transmural iceball on the opposite surface of the atrium (epicardium) from the surface of cryothermia application (endocardium). (A) Initiation of cryothermia. A stab wound was made inside a pursestring suture (secured by a Rumel tourniquet) so that a linear cryoprobe could be introduced into the right atrium and placed against the endocardial surface in the location of the desired linear cryolesion. The desired cryolesion extends from the pursestring suture to the tip of the cryoprobe. If cryothermia is initiated immediately after positioning the cryoprobe and continued for 2 minutes, much of the frozen myocardium in the desired linear lesion site will never reach the critical lethal temperature of –30°C, and the cryolesion will fail in a high percentage of patients. (B) First appearance of iceball. After the initiation of cryothermia, an epicardial iceball will appear shortly, almost always at the tip of the cryoprobe. This indicates that the epicardial surface at the site of the iceball has reached a temperature of 0°C, which is a sublethal temperature (see text). Moreover, note that the majority of the atrial muscle in the desired lesion site between the pursestring suture and the iceball has not yet reached even this sublethal temperature of 0°C as evidenced by the absence of an iceball in this segment of atrial wall. Therefore, if cryothermia is applied for an additional 2 minutes beginning at this stage, much of the frozen myocardium in the desired linear lesion site will recover, and the cryolesion will fail in a high percentage of patients. (C) Iceball throughout the length of the desired lesion. To ensure that a permanent linear cryolesion will be created in the desired location, it is essential that the 2-minute "counting period" for application of cryothermia begin only after the epicardial iceball has formed completely *throughout the length of the desired lesion*. This is the proper way to use the traditional "2-minute rule" for creating atrial cryolesions, and it has proven to be extremely successful over the past 4 decades. (Reproduced from Cox JL, Malaisrie C, Churyla A, et al. Cryosurgery for atrial fibrillation: physiologic basis for creating optimal cryolesions. *Ann Thorac Surg*. 2021;112:354–362.)

2. Two minutes from the first appearance of an iceball on the myocardial surface opposite the site of cryoprobe application (Fig. 14.5, *middle panel*)
   Likewise, applying a cryoprobe for 2 minutes after the first appearance of an iceball on the surface opposite the cryoprobe will not reliably result in an adequate permanent cryolesion because the myocardial fibers not included in the iceball remain above 0°, a non-lethal temperature.
3. Two minutes from the time an "iceball" is created throughout the length of the desired lesion (Fig. 14.5, *right panel*)
   The iceball must first be allowed to form *throughout the length of the desired lesion*. The surface iceball forms when the tissue temperature reaches 0°C as water vapor from the immediately adjacent air turns into ice crystals. However as noted earlier, 0°C is not a lethal temperature for myocardial cells, so despite the tissue being visibly frozen transmurally, it will recover if the lowest tissue temperature attained is 0°C (Fig. 14.6).

One should continue to freeze the tissue for an additional 2 minutes after the iceball has formed throughout the length of the desired lesion to be certain that all of the myocardial cells of the desired lesion have been destroyed. This probably represents a bit of "overkill" but is based on studies that were performed specifically to determine how long it takes for cryoablated tissue to decrease from 0°C (iceball formation) to –30°C (cell death) (Fig. 14.7). As mentioned earlier, this time varies depending on a variety of factors, but under experimental conditions, it was usually around 30 seconds. To be certain that every cryolesion is created perfectly under all conditions, we recommend that cryoablation be continued for 2 minutes after the formation of an iceball along the entire length of the desired lesion site. When the opposite side of the atrial wall cannot be seen, we routinely perform 3-minute cryloesions, the 3 minutes being from the time the cryothermia is initiated. If the atrial wall is thicker than normal, we occasionally freeze along the same lesion line on both sides of the atrial wall to be certain of permanent transmurality.

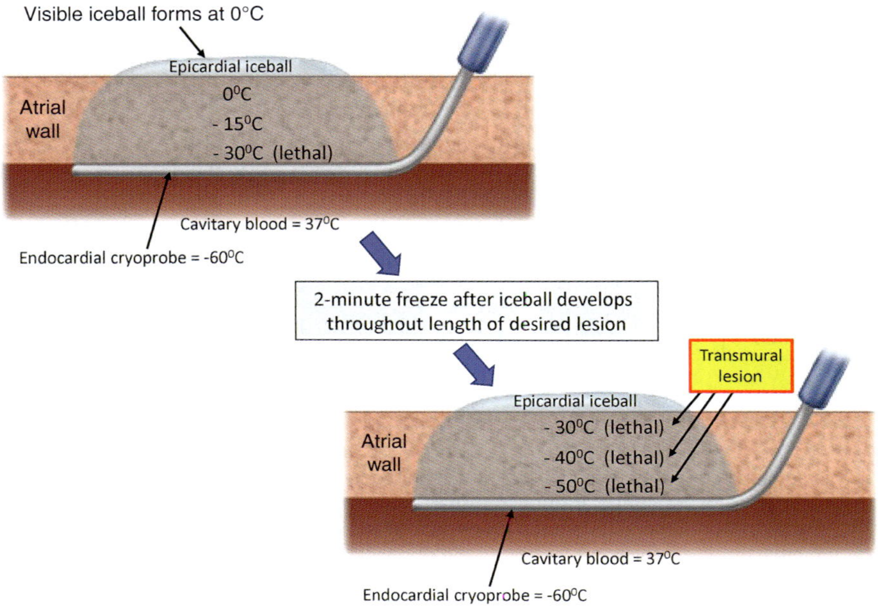

Fig. 14.6 *Left upper panel,* This diagram illustrates why the appearance of an iceball on the epicardial surface opposite an endocardial cryoprobe is not the time to stop freezing the myocardium. An iceball forms when the epicardial surface temperature reaches 0°C because it is the temperature at which water vapor in the adjacent air forms ice crystals. Even when the iceball has formed along the entire length of the desired lesion, the subepicardial temperature will still be well above the critical lethal temperature of –30°C because there is always a temperature gradient from the site nearest the cryoprobe to the site farthest away from the cryoprobe. Therefore, if freezing is stopped at this point, the subepicardial myocardium will recover, the permanent cryolesion will be nontransmural, and the ablation procedure will fail. The same principles and limitations are operative when freezing from the epicardial surface and when using cryoprobes that cool to lower temperatures. After an iceball has formed *throughout the length of the desired lesion*, an additional 2 minutes of freezing should be applied. *Right lower panel,* During the additional critical 2 minutes of freezing, the temperature of the tissue located farther away from the cryoprobe will continue to decrease until eventually, the tissue at the opposite surface of the cryoprobe will reach the critical lethal temperature of –30°C, although there will still be a temperature gradient within the frozen tissue. However, when the subepicardium (in this case) reaches –30°C, the eventual permanent lesion will be permanently transmural.

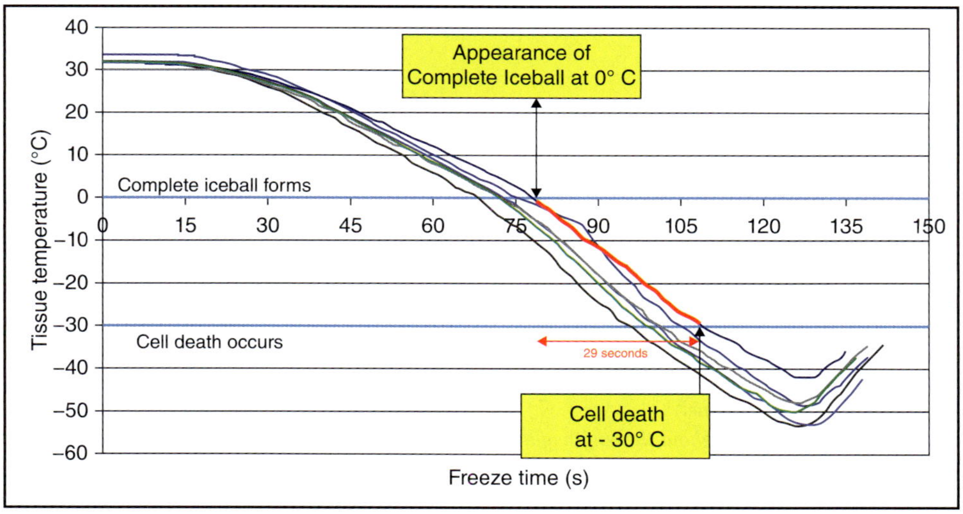

Fig. 14.7 Temporal relationship between iceball formation and myocardial cell death. These are continuous myocardial temperature curves recorded from the tissue surface opposite the cryoprobe in tissue slabs that were of varying thickness. Because iceballs form at 0°C and the critical lethal temperature for myocardial cells is -30°C, the additional freeze time needed for permanent transmurality after the appearance of a complete iceball can be determined. In normothermic tissue, the time from iceball formation to cell death is approximately 30 seconds *(red line)*. Thus, freezing for an additional 2 minutes after the formation of a complete iceball opposite the cryoprobe is more than adequate to create a permanent transmural cryolesion.

SURGICAL TECHNIQUE OF THE MINIMALLY INVASIVE CRYOMAZE-III PROCEDURE

The cannulation and exposure techniques for performing on-pump minimally invasive procedures vary widely and have evolved substantially since the mid-1990s because of cumulative surgical experience and the evolution of specifically designed minimally invasive tools and devices. Therefore, this aspect of the surgical technique of the minimally invasive CryoMaze-III procedure is not discussed here. My personal preference is to expose the heart through an anterolateral mini-thoracotomy in the right fourth intercostal space (Fig. 14.8),[6] but others prefer a more lateral mini-thoracotomy. We originally used the Heartport system[7] to occlude the ascending aorta to deliver antegrade cardioplegia but later switched to the Chitwood clamp[8] because of its ease of application and lower cost. The specific technique of the minimally invasive CryoMaze-III procedure that is currently used is discussed in more detail in Chapter 28 by Dr. Niv Ad. In addition, in Chapters 15 and 27, Dr. Patrick McCarthy describes his technique for performing all of the lesions of the CryoMaze-III procedure when ablating concomitant AF associated with other cardiac surgery by applying only three freezes in the LA and three freezes in the right atrium (RA). His recent modification of the CryoMaze-III procedure decreases the aortic cross-clamp time for AF ablation in patients undergoing coronary artery and/or valve surgery.[9]

Right Atrial Lesions

Creation of Right Atrial Lesions Off-Pump

The right atrial lesions of the minimally invasive CryoMaze-III procedure can be created entirely through two pursestring sutures in the RA without cardiopulmonary bypass if so desired. The first step is to place a pursestring suture approximately two-thirds of the way down from the superior vena cava SVC to the inferior vena cava (IVC) immediately anterior to the crista terminalis and secure it with a Rumel tourniquet. A linear cryoprobe is then inserted through the pursestring suture and passed well into the SVC, keeping it as lateral as possible to avoid directly freezing the anatomic sinoatrial (SA) node (Fig. 14.9). The cryoprobe is placed inside the RA and lifted upward to assure good contact with the endocardial surface. In addition, lifting the probe against the endocardium assures that there is no blood between the probe and the endocardium. Another advantage of this technique is that it allows visual confirmation of the epicardial iceball developing along the desired lesion. After the SVC lesion is completed as described, the probe is positioned into the IVC to complete the SVC–IVC intercaval lesion (Fig. 14.10). After this lesion is completed, the cryoprobe is removed, and the first pursestring suture is tied down.

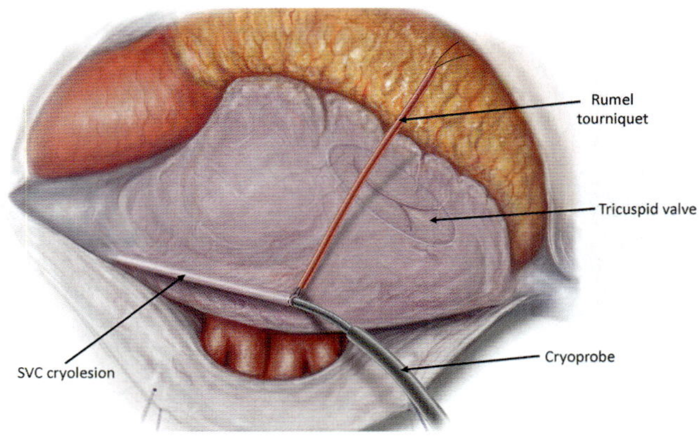

Fig. 14.9 Minimally invasive CryoMaze-III procedure: right atrial lesions off-pump. The first pursestring suture is place approximately two-thirds of the way down from the superior vena cava (SVC) to the inferior vena cava at the anterior edge of the crista terminalis and secured with a Rumel tourniquet. A linear cryoprobe is inserted through this pursestring suture and passed into the SVC to create the SVC lesion. See text for further discussion.

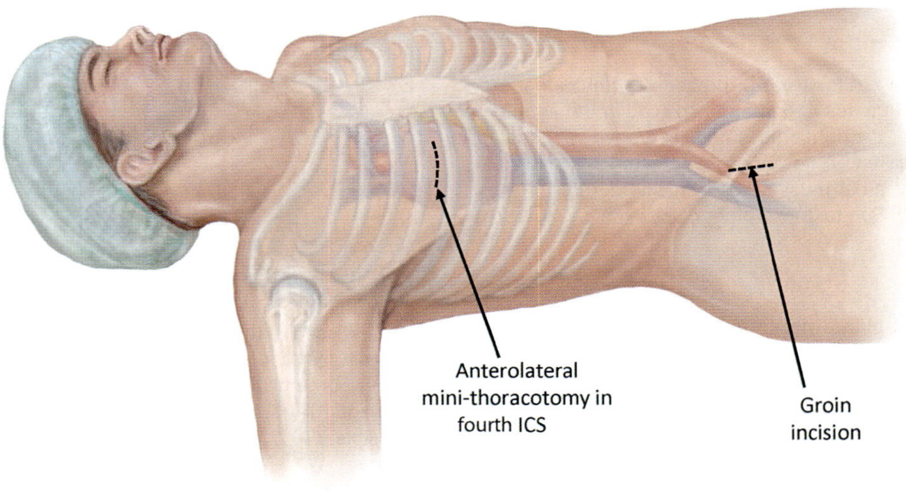

Fig. 14.8 Minimally invasive CryoMaze-III procedure: patient position and exposure. In the initial minimally invasive CryoMaze-III procedure, the heart is exposed through an anterolateral mini-thoracotomy in the right fourth intercostal space (ICS). Some surgeons prefer a more lateral mini-thoracotomy. The right femoral artery is cannulated for arterial inflow, though other arterial cannulation sites can be used. The right femoral vein is cannulated for venous return from the inferior vena cava. The superior vena cava can be cannulated directly with a right-angle cannula through a separate small stab wound below the mini-thoracotomy or via the right jugular vein.

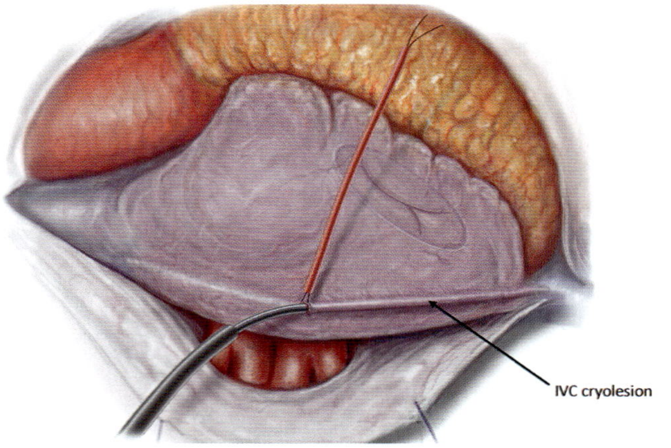

Fig. 14.10 Minimally invasive CryoMaze-III procedure: right atrial lesions off-pump. Through the same pursestring suture, the cryoprobe is turned and its tip is placed well into the inferior vena cava (IVC) to create the IVC lesion, thus completing the intercaval superior vena cava to inferior vena cava (SVC–IVC) lesion. It is often necessary to loosen the tape around the IVC during the creation of the IVC lesion.

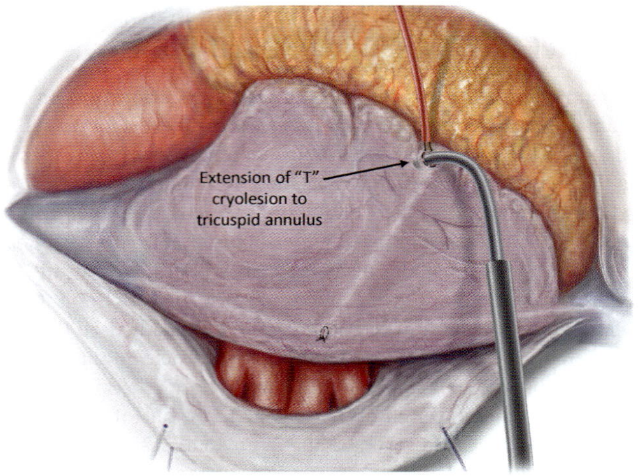

Fig. 14.12 Minimally invasive CryoMaze-III procedure: right atrial lesions off-pump. Through this second pursestring suture, the cryoprobe is positioned down to the level of the tricuspid valve to complete the "T" lesion. See text for further discussion. The combination of the intercaval lesion and the "T" lesion prevents the development of all three of the macro-reentrant drivers that can cause classic right atrial flutter. These lesions should never be performed in patients who have had a former cavotricuspid isthmus lesion performed because that combination of lesions will isolate all of the right atrium below the "T" lesion (see Figs. 14.13–14.18).

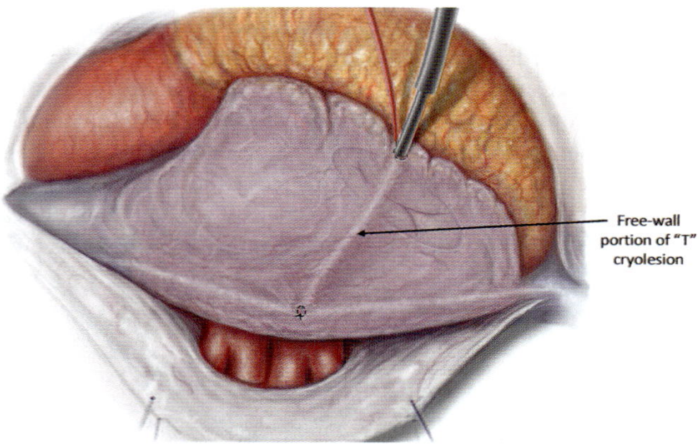

Fig. 14.11 Minimally invasive CryoMaze-III procedure: right atrial lesions off-pump. The second pursestring suture is placed in the anterior edge of the right atrium near the right atrioventricular groove so that the proximal portion of the so-called "T" lesion can be created in a diagonal fashion parallel to the right atrial muscle fibers in this portion of the atrium (see Figs. 14.3–14.8). See text for further discussion.

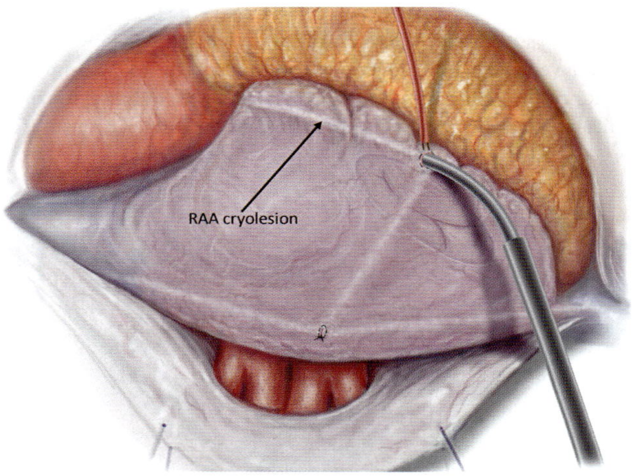

Fig. 14.13 Minimally invasive CryoMaze-III procedure: right atrial lesions off-pump. Through the second pursestring suture, the tip of the probe is passed to the tip of the right atrial appendage to create the final right atrial lesion of the CryoMaze-III procedure. This lesion prevents the development of macro-reentry around the base of the right atrial appendage (RAA). It should be placed as far anterior in the right atrium as possible.

A second pursestring is placed near the right AV groove fat pad and positioned diagonally downward in relation to the first pursestring suture. The linear cryoprobe is inserted through this second pursestring suture and placed against the right atrial endocardium from this pursestring suture back to the first pursestring suture (Fig. 14.11). This creates the right atrial free-wall portion of the so-called "T" lesion, which is then completed by extending it from this same pursestring suture down to the tricuspid valve annulus (Fig. 14.12). This is a blind lesion that can be performed easily by first palpating the tip of the probe through the upper right ventricular wall and then placing downward pressure on the intervening right AV groove to assure good contact of the cryoprobe. As the lesion is being created, an iceball will usually appear on the epicardial surface of the right ventricle at the tip of the cryoprobe, confirming that the tricuspid annulus has been crossed. Freezing the leaflet of the tricuspid valve has no adverse consequences. After the "T" lesion has been completed, the cryoprobe is directed from the second pursestring suture to the tip of the right atrial appendage (RAA) to create the final lesion in the RA (Fig. 14.13). This completes the right atrial lesions of the CryoMaze-III procedure (Fig. 14.14).

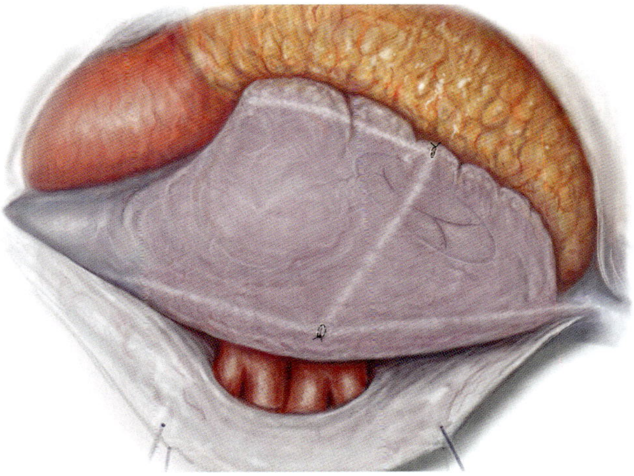

Fig. 14.14 Minimally invasive CryoMaze-III procedure: right atrial lesions off-pump. The complete right atrial lesion set of the CryoMaze-III procedure whether performed minimally invasively or as a concomitant procedure with other types of cardiac surgery. In this case, the entire right atrial lesion set was completed off-pump through two pursestring sutures in the right atrium (RA). There are three linear lesions in the right atrial lesion set of the CryoMaze-III procedure: (1) the intercaval lesion between the superior vena cava and inferior vena cava, (2) the "T" lesion from the intercaval lesion to the tricuspid valve annulus, and (3) the right atrial appendage (RAA) lesion from the "T" lesion to the tip of the RAA.

Creation of Right Atrial Lesions On-Pump

Because the extension of the "T" lesion from the second pursestring to the tricuspid annulus is a blind lesion, most surgeons prefer to create the right atrial lesions under direct vision through a right atriotomy rather than through pursestring sutures. If so, the right atriotomy should follow the course of the muscle fibers in the right atrial wall (see Chapter 3, Fig. 3.8) and extend *diagonally* from a point approximately two-thirds of the way down between the SVC and IVC to a point near the right AV groove (Fig. 14.15). A common mistake is to place this atriotomy straight across the wall of the RA rather than making it a diagonal atriotomy. This results in the atriotomy terminating too high on the anterior edge of the right atrial free wall and potentially interfering with an important part of the atrial pacemaker complex (see Chapter 3, Fig. 3.9). After the atriotomy is positioned properly (Fig. 14.16), it is quite simple to place a curved linear cryoprobe inside the atrium and complete the lesion from the distal end of the atriotomy down to the tricuspid valve annulus (Fig. 14.17). The SVC lesion is placed from the proximal end of the atriotomy up into the SVC, and the IVC lesion is then placed from the proximal end of the atriotomy to the IVC to complete the intercaval lesion (Fig. 14.18). The SVC portion of the intercaval lesion should be placed laterally where it extends into the SVC orifice to keep it away from the anatomic SA node.

The only remaining potential site for a macro-reentry circuit to form in the RA is around the base of the RAA. Therefore, a final lesion is placed from the distal end of the right atriotomy, along the anterior edge of the RA up to the tip of the RAA (Fig. 14.19). The right atriotomy is then closed (Fig. 14.20). It should be mentioned that all of these right atrial lesions can be created just as easily and effectively with a bipolar radiofrequency clamp except for the distal extension of the "T" lesion from the right atriotomy down to the tricuspid valve annulus, which can be created safely only with a cryoprobe. In addition, using

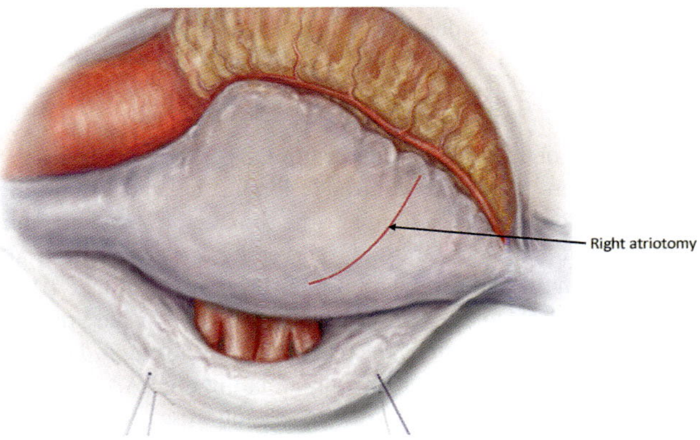

Fig. 14.15 Minimally invasive CryoMaze-III procedure: right atrial lesions on-pump. Most surgeons prefer to open the right atrium to perform the right atrial lesions of the CryoMaze-III procedure. If so, this lesion should start approximately two-thirds of the way down from the superior vena cava to the inferior vena cava and extend *diagonally* across the right atrial free wall to the anterior edge of the right atrium.

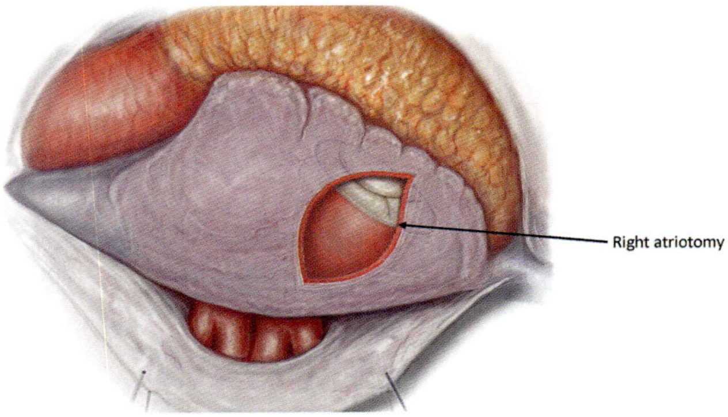

Fig. 14.16 Minimally invasive CryoMaze-III procedure: right atrial lesions on-pump. The right atriotomy serves as the proximal portion of the "T" lesion and provides better exposure of the inside of the right atrium. Some surgeons prefer to extend this atriotomy more proximally than is illustrated here to divide the crista terminalis. Whether or not this improves the effectiveness of the procedure has not been documented definitively.

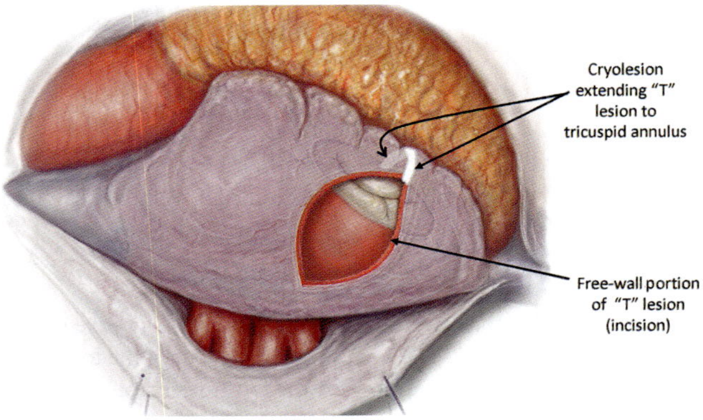

Fig. 14.17 Minimally invasive CryoMaze-III procedure: right atrial lesions on-pump. A curved linear cryoprobe is placed from the distal end of the atriotomy down to the level of the tricuspid valve to complete the "T" lesion.

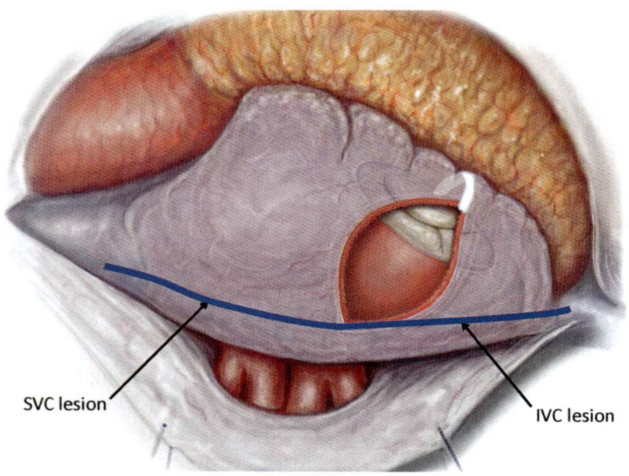

Fig. 14.18 Minimally invasive CryoMaze-III procedure: right atrial lesions on-pump. The superior vena cava (SVC) lesion is created from the proximal end of the right atriotomy to the SVC, and the inferior vena cava (IVC) lesion is created from the proximal end of the atriotomy to the IVC, thus completing the intercaval SVC–IVC lesion.

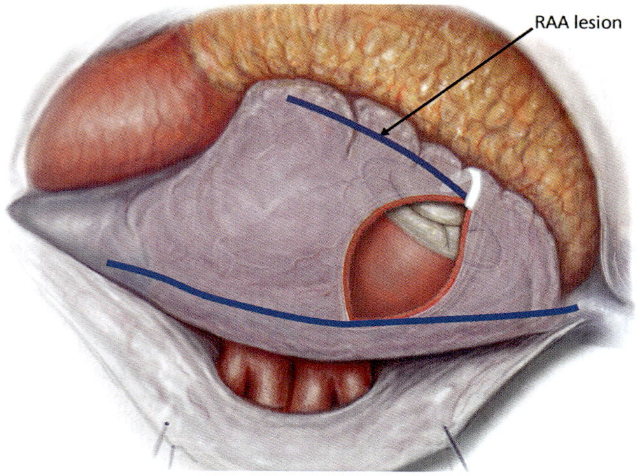

Fig. 14.19 Minimally invasive CryoMaze-III procedure: right atrial lesions on-pump. A lesion is created from the distal end of the atriotomy to the tip of the right atrial appendage (RAA) to prevent reentry around the base of the RAA. This completes the right atrial lesions of the CryoMaze-III procedure.

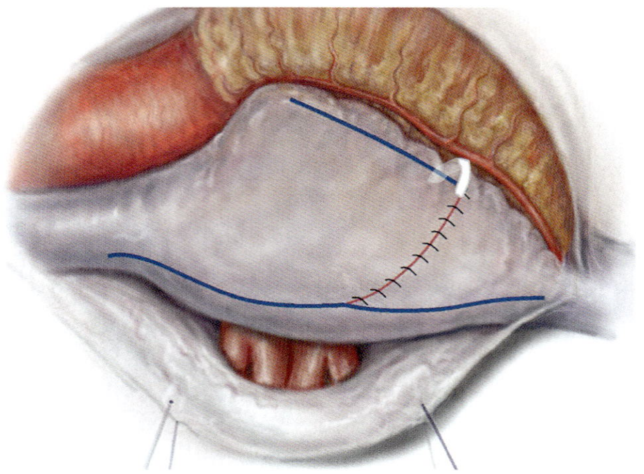

Fig. 14.20 Minimally invasive CryoMaze-III procedure: right atrial lesions on-pump. The atriotomy is closed in the usual fashion.

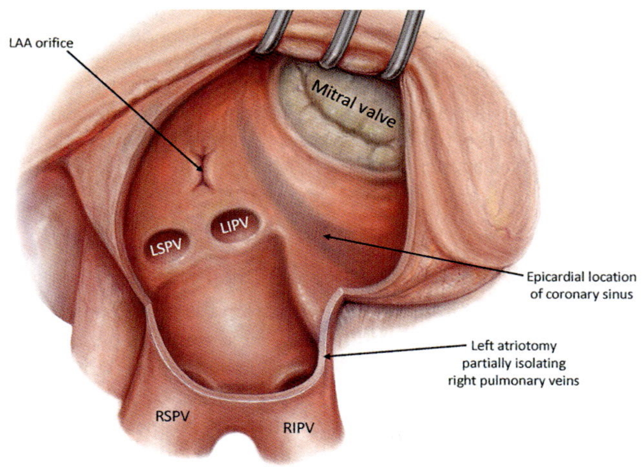

Fig. 14.21 Minimally invasive CryoMaze-III procedure: left atrial lesions. The inside of the left atrium is exposed through a standard left atriotomy in Waterston's groove. It is helpful to extend this atriotomy a few millimeters farther toward the left inferior pulmonary vein (LIPV) than normal to improve exposure of the left pulmonary veins and the orifice of the left atrial appendage (LAA). *LSPV,* Left superior pulmonary vein; *RIPV,* right inferior pulmonary vein; *RSPV,* right superior pulmonary vein.

a cryoprobe for this distal extension of the "T" lesion overcomes the problem of the "folding over" of the RA and right ventricle in this area (see Chapter 3, Fig. 3.22).

Left Atrial Lesions

A standard left atriotomy is performed in Waterston's groove to expose the inside of the LA (Fig. 14.21). It is helpful to curve the lower end of this incision and extend it up toward the left inferior pulmonary vein a bit more than one would for mitral valve surgery. A malleable linear cryoprobe is placed from the lower end of the left atriotomy, across the posterior left atrial wall, around the left inferior pulmonary vein orifice, and as far between the LAA orifice and pulmonary vein orifices as it will reach (Fig. 14.22). The linear cryoprobe is then shaped to extend from the upper end of the left atriotomy around the orifice of the left superior pulmonary vein to overlap with the lesion just created around the left inferior pulmonary vein to complete the "box lesion" that encompasses all four pulmonary veins and the intervening posterior left atrial wall (Fig. 14.23). In the first several minimally invasive CryoMaze-III procedures that we performed, we routinely cryoablated the base of the LAA circumferentially to isolate it electrically before closing it. However, in the late 1990s, we stopped electrically isolating the LAA and began to create a separate single longitudinal cryolesion from the box lesion into the LAA to prevent macro-reentry around the LAA base that uses the so-called "coumadin ridge" located between the LAA and the left pulmonary veins (Fig. 14.24). Unfortunately, at that time, we did not appreciate the importance of the LAA as a potential source of AF triggers and therefore, the importance of electrically isolating it. That was a mistake. If the LAA is left intact and simply closed with a suture endocardially,

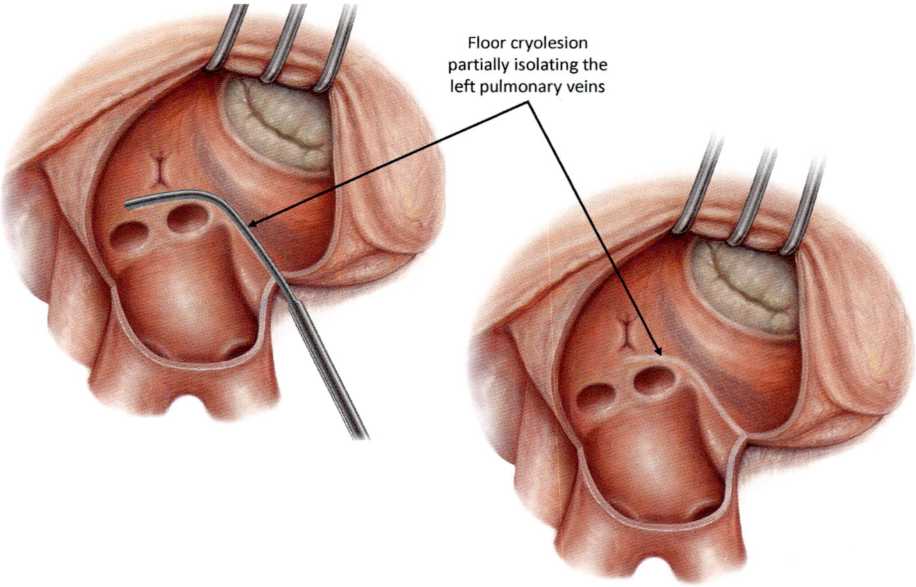

Fig. 14.22 Minimally invasive CryoMaze-III procedure: left atrial lesions. A linear cryoprobe is placed from the lower end of the left atriotomy, across the floor of the left atrium, and around the orifice of the left inferior pulmonary vein as far as possible. This lesion is placed between the left inferior pulmonary vein and the orifice of the left atrial appendage. Because an iceball cannot be seen on the opposite side of this lesion, it is recommended that the freeze be applied for a total of 3 minutes under cardioplegic arrest.

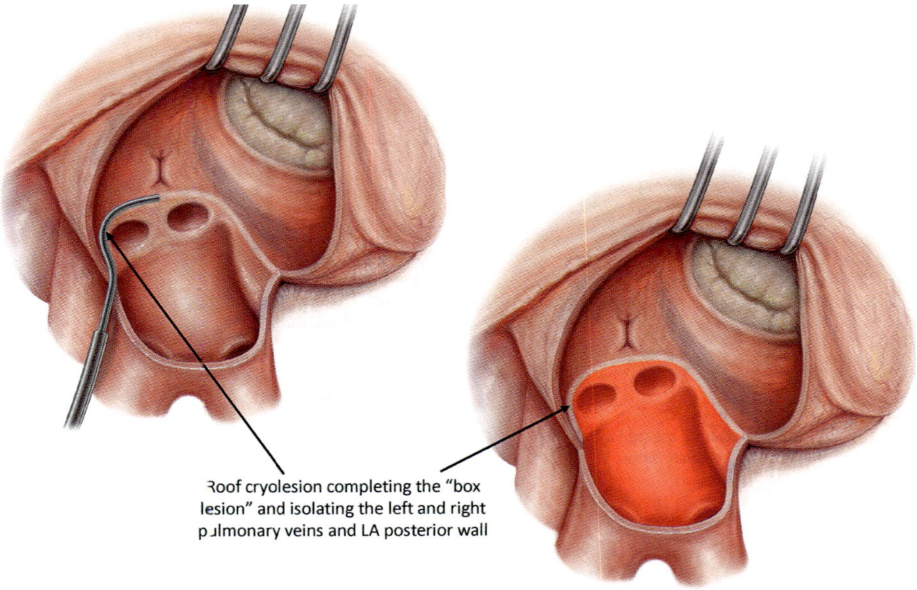

Fig. 14.23 Minimally invasive CryoMaze-III procedure: left atrial lesions. The linear cryoprobe is then reshaped and placed from the upper end of the left atriotomy, around the orifice of the left superior pulmonary vein to complete the "box lesion" that isolates all four pulmonary veins and the posterior wall of the left atrium (*red area in right panel*). Again, because an iceball cannot be seen on the opposite side of this lesion, it is recommended that the freeze be applied for a total of 3 minutes under cardioplegic arrest.

it should always be isolated electrically before closure. The simplest way to electrically isolate an intact LAA is to cryoablate the entire base of the appendage circumferentially from inside the heart.

At this stage of the procedure, the only remaining LA lesions are the coronary sinus lesion and the "mitral line" that in combination prevent conduction across the left atrial isthmus, an important arm of the reentrant circuit that causes postoperative peri-mitral flutter (see Chapter 48). The lower end of the atriotomy is grasped with forceps and retracted upward to expose the coronary sinus posteriorly near the epicardial surface of the AV groove. The tip of a malleable liner cryoprobe

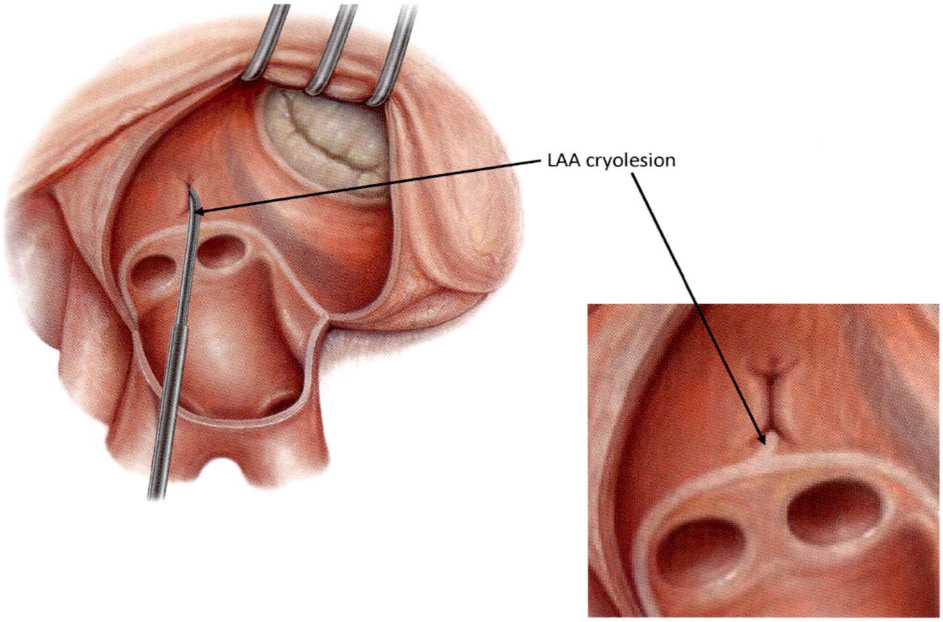

Fig. 14.24 Minimally invasive CryoMaze-III procedure: left atrial lesions. A linear lesion is created from the Box lesion into the left atrial appendage (LAA) to prevent reentry that uses the coumadin ridge between the LAA orifice and the left pulmonary veins. See text for further discussion.

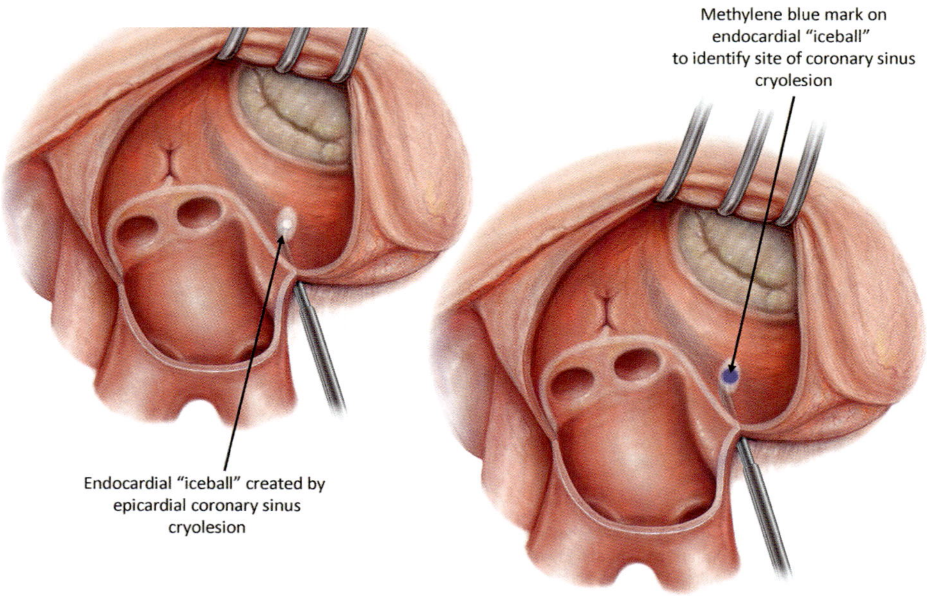

Fig. 14.25 Minimally invasive CryoMaze-III procedure: left atrial lesions. A cryoprobe is placed against the epicardial surface of the coronary sinus from outside the atrium and a circumferential coronary sinus cryolesion is created *(left upper panel)*. This results in an iceball appearing on the endocardium of the left atrium. Because the iceball will disappear when the coronary sinus freeze is terminated, it is helpful to mark the left atrial endocardial iceball with methylene blue so that after the iceball thaws, its precise location will be known. This is an important step because it is absolutely essential that the coronary sinus cryolesion and the "mitral line" that will be created next are aligned in the same plane (see Chapter 48). See text for further discussion.

is placed directly on the epicardial surface of the coronary sinus and the forceps are removed to allow this part of the LA to resume its normal position. With upward pressure on the tip of the epicardial cryoprobe, the coronary sinus is flattened, and during the epicardial freeze, an iceball invariable appears on the endocardial surface of the adjacent LA (Fig. 14.25, *left upper panel*). This indicates that the coronary sinus is being frozen circumferentially at an epicardial site that corresponds to this endocardial site in the LA. It is absolutely critical to align this coronary sinus cryolesion with the endocardial mitral line that is about to be created so that electrical conduction across this left atrial isthmus is blocked both in the coronary sinus and in the atrial myocardium. If these two lesions are not aligned precisely, neither of them will prevent

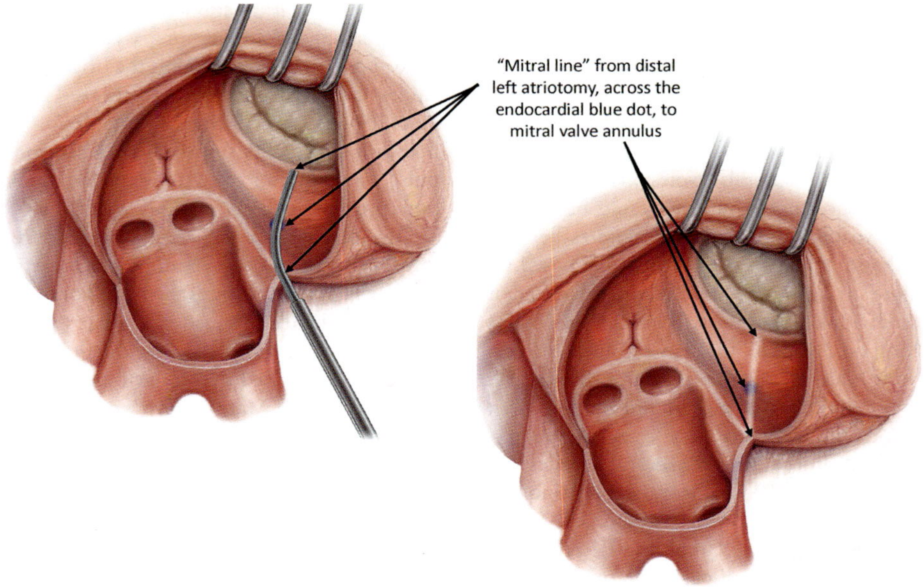

Fig. 14.26 Minimally invasive CryoMaze-III procedure: left atrial lesions. A linear lesion is created from the distal end of the left atriotomy, across the endocardial methylene blue mark, to the level of the mitral valve annulus to create the "mitral line." These two lesions, in combination, prevent the development of postoperative peri-mitral flutter (see Chapter 48).

conduction across the left atrial isthmus, and postoperative peri-mitral flutter can develop (see Chapter 48). Therefore, while the LA endocardial iceball is present, it is helpful to mark it with methylene blue so that when the iceball disappears after completion of the coronary sinus lesion, the surgeon can still identify the precise plane in which to create the mitral line (Fig. 14.25, *right lower panel*)

After creating the coronary sinus lesion and marking the left atrial endocardium, a linear cryoprobe is placed inside the LA from the lower end of the left atriotomy to the mitral valve annulus *directly across the endocardial methylene blue dot* (Fig. 14.26). This assures perfect alignment of the endocardial mitral line with the epicardial coronary sinus lesion. The LAA orifice is then closed in the with a two-layer endocardial suture closure (Fig. 14.27).

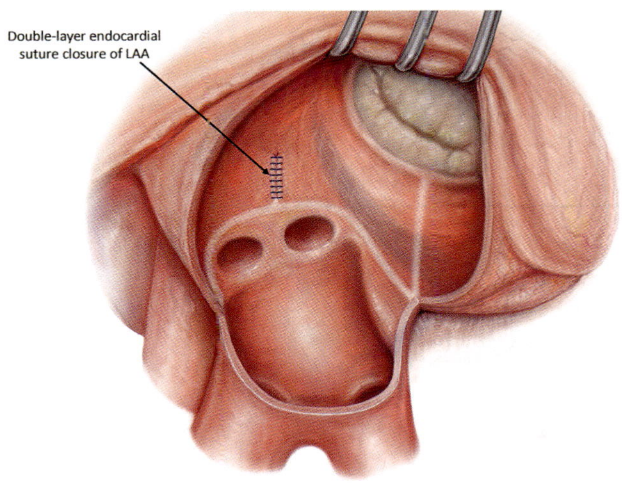

Fig. 14.27 Minimally invasive CryoMaze-III procedure: left atrial lesions. Final left atrial lesions of the CryoMaze-III procedure and closure of the left atrial appendage (LAA).

COMPARISON OF THE MINIMALLY INVASIVE CRYOMAZE-III PROCEDURE TO THE CUT-AND-SEW MAZE-III PROCEDURE

Between March 1, 1996 and July 1, 2000, we performed 65 minimally invasive CryoMaze-III procedures including 11 patients requiring mitral valve repair or replacement, 2 patients requiring both mitral valve and tricuspid valve repair, and 3 patients requiring closure of an atrial septal defect. There were no operative deaths or transient ischemic attacks (TIAs), but one patient had a mild stroke that resolved without residual sequelae within 48 hours. There were no late TIAs, strokes, or failures, and only 6% of patients (4 of 65) required permanent postoperative pacemakers. The dramatic decrease in postoperative pacemaker requirements with the minimally invasive CryoMaze-III approach compared with the cut-and-sew Maze-III procedure through a median sternotomy was attributed to the fact that far less extracardiac dissection was performed in the patients undergoing minimally invasive procedures, though there could have been other explanations.

One of the most persistent misconceptions in the arrhythmia literature is that the term "Maze-III" is used to refer only to the original cut-and-sew Maze-III procedure. However, as described in this chapter, the only difference between the cut-and-sew Maze-III procedure and the minimally invasive CryoMaze-III procedure was that the Maze-III lesions in the latter were created with cryoprobes rather than by surgical incisions in the latter. However, the *lesion patterns* of the two approaches were identical. Perhaps we should have designated this new cryosurgical procedure as the "Maze-IV" procedure, but I was concerned that a new Roman numeral designation would imply a new lesion pattern, which was not the case. The Maze-I, Maze-II, and original Maze-III procedures were all "cut-and-sew" procedures that had significantly different lesion patterns and therefore different postoperative atrial activation characteristics, so they were given separate Roman numeral designations. Because the lesion pattern of the CryoMaze-III procedure was identical to that of the "cut-and-sew" Maze-III procedure, postoperative atrial activation was also identical, so I did not give it a separate Roman numeral designation.

By the time we did the first Maze-III procedure using cryoablation alone on March 1, 1996, we had accrued more than 20 years of experience using cryosurgery for numerous other arrhythmias (see Chapters 9 and 11), so we had complete confidence in our ability to create permanently contiguous, uniformly transmural cryolesions reliably. We did not expect to see any differences in the surgical results of the cut-and-sew Maze-III and the cryosurgical Maze-III procedures because their lesion patterns were the same. Our expectations were based on the axiom that "The heart doesn't know how the lesions are created; it only knows whether each individual lesion is perfect and if the lesions are placed in the correct locations." Indeed, the only significant difference between the cut-and-sew Maze-III and the CryoMaze-III was that the latter resulted in fewer postoperative pacemaker implantations. Drs. Patrick McCarthy and Niv Ad, among others, have continued to perform thousands of CryoMaze-III procedures over several decades and have attained some of the best results in the world for the interventional treatment of patients with AF.[9,10] In the following chapter, Dr. McCarthy describes his recent modification of the CryoMaze-III procedure that decreases the aortic cross-clamp time and perfusion time required to perform the CryoMaze-III for AF concomitantly with other cardiac surgery. Dr. Ad describes his vast experience and excellent results with the minimally invasive CryoMaze-III procedure in Chapter 28.

COMPARISON OF THE MAZE-III LESION PATTERN WITH THE MAZE-IV LESION PATTERN

In 2002, Dr. Ralph Damiano and his group in St. Louis described the Maze-IV procedure in which he used both radiofrequency clamps and cryosurgery to decrease the time required to perform a typical Maze procedure.[11] This procedure was given a new Roman numeral primarily because of the types of energy sources used to create the atrial lesions, not because it resulted in different postoperative atrial activation characteristics. There is no difference in the functional lesion pattern between the Maze-III and the Maze-IV procedures (Fig. 14.28). Both procedures result functionally in a box lesion in the posterior LA that encompasses all four pulmonary vein orifices and the intervening posterior LA wall. Also, although the original Maze-III lesion pattern includes an atrial septal lesion, the Maze-IV pattern has no septal lesion at all. However, the lack of a septal lesion in the Maze-IV procedure does not alter the postoperative conduction of a sinus-generated impulse from anterior to posterior in the atrial septum that occurs after both procedures.

The advantage of the Maze-IV procedure over the Maze-III procedure is that the Maze-IV can be performed quicker by surgeons who are less experienced in arrhythmia surgery. However, this is not the case in the hands of most experienced arrhythmia surgeons and certainly not when compared with the modification of the CryoMaze-III procedure described by McCarthy in the following chapter. Another advantage of the Maze-IV procedure is that it is easier to teach and more readily accepted by surgeons who are less experienced with arrhythmia surgery because fewer lesions have to be performed *inside* the LA in the Maze-IV procedure than in the Maze-III procedure. Regardless of which technique one choses for the treatment of AF, both are safe and effective, and both should be applied more often for the treatment of concomitant AF associated with coronary artery and valvular heart disease requiring surgery. Dr. Damiano describes his vast experience and excellent results with the Maze-IV procedure in Chapter 17.

ADVANTAGES AND DISADVANTAGES OF CRYOSURGERY

Unlike all heat-based energy sources, cryothermia preserves tissue collagen because both fibroblasts and collagen are resistant to freeze injury.[2,3] This means that the structure and strength of the ablated tissue are preserved. This unique characteristic of cryosurgery allows tissue ablation to be safe anywhere in the heart. For example, valve leaflets, chordae tendineae, papillary muscles, and venous structures such as the coronary sinus can be ablated with impunity without affecting the critical function of these structures.[1,6,12,13] Thus, cryosurgery rarely causes a problem when used to ablate AF. However, there are at least two separate case

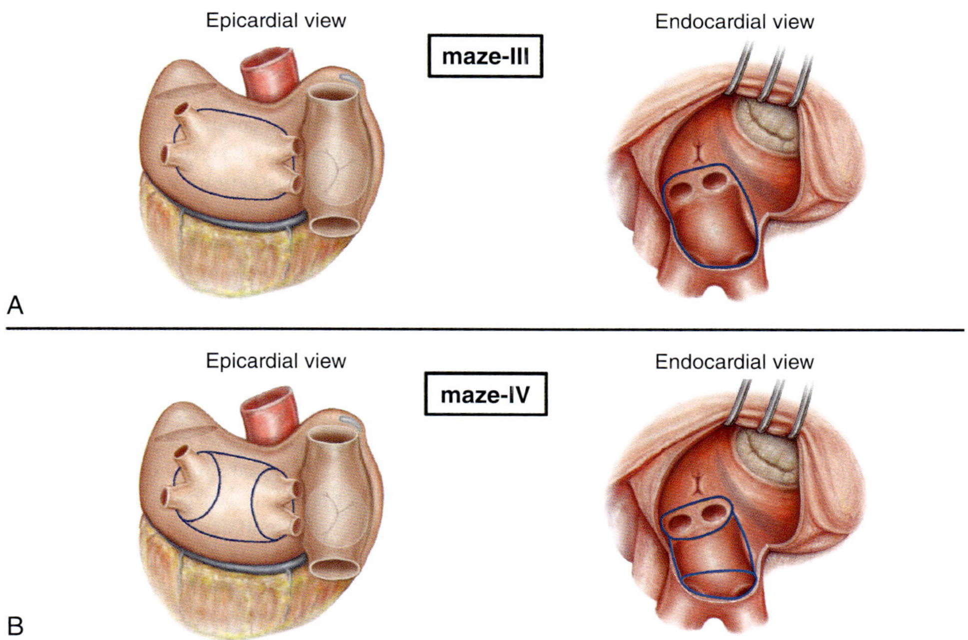

Fig. 14.28 A comparison of the "box lesion" of the Maze-III procedure (A) and the Maze-IV procedure (B). There is no electrophysiological difference in these two procedures. See text for further discussion.

reports of cryosurgery causing coronary artery spasm, and in one case, it was spasm of the circumflex coronary artery that led to a dissection of one of its posterior branches.[14] Another case report described reversible cryosurgery-induced right coronary artery spasm.[15] Fortunately, both patients recovered without significant negative consequences.

Whether or not direct freezing of the coronary arteries results in long-term coronary artery stenosis is unclear. Large blood vessels are quite resistant to structural change after freezing, and they continue to function as blood conduits after direct freezing.[2,16] Mikat et al[17] and Iida et al.[18] both demonstrated experimentally that direct freezing of major coronary arteries results in only minimal and transient arterial changes and that the vessels remain patent after freezing. Many years ago, we subjected the coronary arteries in dogs to direct cryosurgery using a N_20 cryoprobe and performed coronary angiography preoperatively, a few weeks after cryosurgery, and 6 months later.[19] Although the coronary angiograms were normal at 6 months, histologic examination revealed mild intimal hyperplasia at the frozen sites in the coronary arteries. Other studies in which the coronary arteries were subjected to even colder temperatures and followed for longer periods of time suggested that these intimal changes in the coronaries that appeared several months after cryosurgery were transient and eventually resolved with no significant long-term coronary stenosis.[2,20] A more recent clinical study by Cheema et al.[21] concluded that cryosurgery performed during the CryoMaze-III procedure did not damage the coronary arteries. Additionally, the fact remains that despite the tens of thousands of Maze procedures in which at least some of the coronary arteries must have been inadvertently frozen, there have been no convincing documented instances in which cryosurgery has resulted in significant coronary artery injury other than the one dissection mentioned earlier. Nevertheless, it is prudent to avoid direct freezing of the coronary arteries whenever possible.

REFERENCES

1. Wood M, Goldberg S, Lau M, et al. Direct measurement of the lethal isotherm for radiofrequency ablation of myocardial tissue. *Circ Arrhythm Electrophysiol.* 2011;4:373–378.
2. Gage AA, Baust JM, Baust JG. Experimental cryosurgery investigations in vivo. *Cryobiology.* 2009;59:229.
3. Gage AA, Baust J. Mechanisms of tissue injury in cryosurgery. *Cryobiology.* 1998;37:171–186.
4. Baust JG, Gage AA. The molecular basis of cryosurgery. *BJU Int.* 2005;95:1187–1191.
5. Cox JL, Malaisrie C, Churyla A, et al. Cryosurgery for atrial fibrillation: physiologic basis for creating optimal cryolesions. *Ann Thorac Surg.* 2021;112:354–362.
6. Cox JL. The minimally invasive Maze-III procedure. *Op Tech Thorac Cardiovasc Surg.* 2000;5:79–92.
7. Fann JI, Burdon TA, Pompili MF. Minimally invasive cardiac surgery using the heartport technique. *Asia Pacif Heart J.* 1999;8(1):19–26.
8. Chitwood Jr WR. Video-assisted mitral valve surgery: using the Chitwood clamp. *Op Tech Thorac Cardiovasc Surg.* 2000;5(3):190–202.
9. McCarthy PM, Cox JL, Kruse J, Elenbaas C, Andrei AC. One hundred percent utilization of a modified CryoMaze III procedure for atrial fibrillation with mitral surgery. *J Thorac Cardiovasc Surg.* 2024;167(4):1278–1289 2022.
10. Ad N, Holmes SD, Friehling T. Minimally invasive stand-alone Cox Maze procedure for persistent and long-standing persistent atrial fibrillation: perioperative safety and 5-year outcomes. *Circ Arrhyth Electrophysiol.* 2017;10(11):e005352.
11. Ruaengsri C, Schill MR, Khiabani AJ, Schuessler RB, Melby SJ, Damiano Jr RJ. The Cox-Maze IV procedure in its second decade: still the gold standard? *Eur J Cardiothorac Surg.* 2018;53(1):i19–i25.
12. Cox JL. Anatomicelectrophysiologic basis for the surgical treatment of refractory ischemic ventricular tachycardia. *Ann Surg.* 1983;198:119–129.
13. Cox JL, Bardy GH, Damiano RJ, et al. Right ventricular isolation procedures for non-ischemic ventricular tachycardia. *J Thorac Cardiovasc Surg.* 1985;90:212.
14. Doguet F, Le Guillou V, Litzler PY, et al. Coronary artery dissection after surgical cryoablation procedure. *Ann Thorac Surg.* 2008;87(6):1946–1948.
15. Rajbanshi BG, Rodrigues E, Lynch JJ, Gulati R, Sundt III TM. Coronary artery spasm after cryo Maze III procedure. *Ann Thorac Surg.* 2011;92(5):1884–1887.
16. Cooper IS, Samra K, Wisniewska K. Effects of freezing on major arteries. *Stroke.* 1971;2:471–482.
17. Mikat EM, Hackel DB, Harrison L, Gallagher JJ, Wallace AG. Reaction of the myocardium and coronary arteries to cryosurgery. *Lab Invest.* 1977;37:632–641.
18. Iida S, Misaki T, Iwa T. The histological effects of cryocoagulation on the myocardium and coronary arteries. *Jpn J Surg.* 1989;19:319–325.
19. Holman WL, Ikeshita M, Ungerleider RM, Smith PK, Ideker RE, Cox JL. Cryosurgery for cardiac arrhythmias: acute and chronic effects on coronary arteries. *Am J Cardiol.* 1983;51:149–155.
20. Gage AA, Fazekas G, Riley Jr EE. Freezing injury to large blood vessels in dogs. *Surgery.* 1967;61(5):748–754.
21. Cheema F, Pervez MG, Mehmood M, et al. Does CryoMaze injure the circumflex artery? A preliminary search for occult postprocedure stenoses. Innovations. 2013;8(1):56–66.

15

Rationale for Modification of the CryoMaze-III Procedure

Patrick M. McCarthy

CHAPTER OUTLINE

BACKGROUND

Following years of preclinical research, the Cox-Maze procedure was first performed clinically in 1987 to ablate all types of atrial fibrillation (AF) and reduce the risk of stroke.[1,2] The original procedure, which is now referred to as the Cox Maze-I procedure, went through several subsequent modifications to the Cox Maze-II procedure in 1990 and the Cox Maze-III procedure in 1992 (see Chapter 14). All three of these first iterations of the procedure were created using a "cut-and-sew" technique, and they all demonstrated early safety and great success as determined by freedom from AF (FFAF), reduction in stroke, and improvement in quality of life.[3–6] The Maze pattern of the lesions divided all potential macro-reentrant circuits (drivers) of AF and dictated that the subsequent sinus-generated impulse would activate both atria and traverse the atrioventricular (AV) node to activate the ventricles in a normal fashion.[7] In all three iterations of the cut-and-sew Cox Maze procedure, small cryolesions were placed at the end of all incisions that terminated at a valve annulus and to create conduction block across the coronary sinus.[7] Cryoablation has been shown to be very effective for a variety of arrhythmias, including the Wolff-Parkinson-White syndrome, ventricular tachycardia, and AV node reentry.[8–10] In 1997, the cut-and-sew Cox Maze-III procedure was replaced by the minimally invasive Cox CryoMaze-III procedure in which all of the lesions were created with linear cryoprobes rather than with a scalpel and scissors.[11,12]

Each of the lesions of the Cox Maze-III procedure is created to prevent the development of the macro-reentrant drivers that sustain AF as follows

Left Atrial Lesions

1. Box lesion
   - Isolates 70% of the triggers that *induce* concomitant paroxysmal AF (PAF; Fig. 15.1)
   - Prevents 30% of the macro-reentrant drivers of non-PAF that use the posterior left atrial wall between the right and left pulmonary veins (PVs) and serves as an anchor for the other lesions of the Maze procedure (Fig. 15.2)
2. Left atrial appendage (LAA)–left superior PV lesion across the coumadin ridge (Fig. 15.3)
   - Prevents reentry around the base of the LAA
3. LAA closure (Fig. 15.4)
   - Isolates triggers and reentry in musculature of the LAA
   - Protects against subsequent stroke

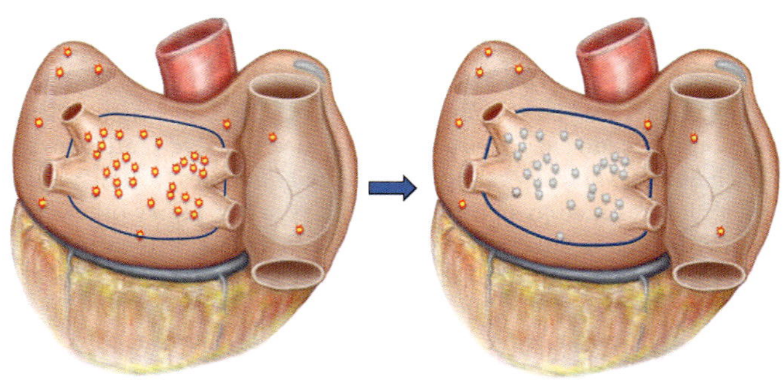

Fig. 15.1 **Box lesion for concomitant paroxysmal atrial fibrillation (PAF).** The left atrial box lesion of the Cox Maze-III procedure isolates 70% of the potential atrial triggers *(focal yellow starbursts)*responsible for inducing PAF that is associated with structural disorders of the left heart requiring surgery ("Concomitant PAF"). *Left panel,* Box lesion *(blue lines)* encompassing all four pulmonary veins and the intervening posterior left atrial wall between the right and left pulmonary veins. *Right panel,* After the creation of a box lesion, the isolated atrial triggers are still present but cannot induce AF *(gray starbursts).*

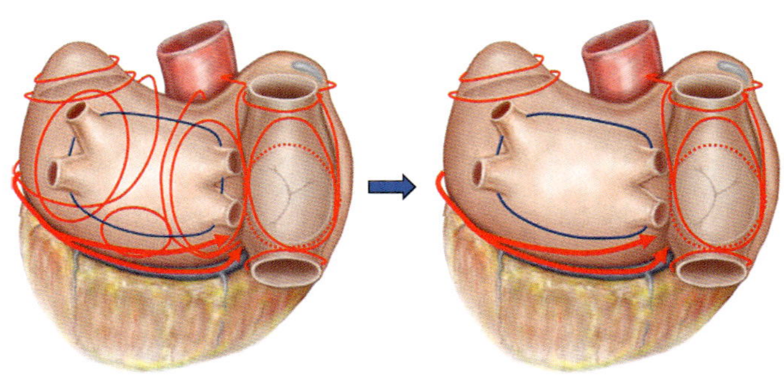

Fig. 15.2 **Box lesion for concomitant non-paroxysmal atrial fibrillation (non-PAF).** The *red circles* represent the potential macro-reentrant drivers of AF, and the *blue lines* represent surgical lesions. *Left panel,* A box lesion in patients with non-PAF interrupts approximately 30% of the macro-reentrant drivers using the posterior left atrial wall as a part of their circuit. *Right panel,* After the creation of a box lesion, multiple sites for potential macro-reentrant AF drivers remain in both atria.

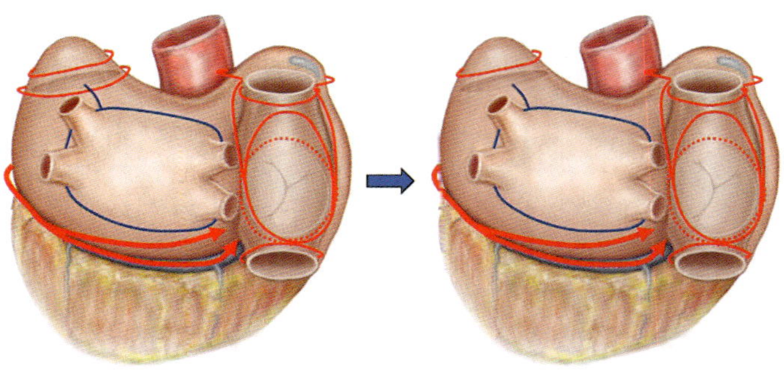

Fig. 15.3 Left atrial appendage (LAA)–left superior pulmonary vein (LSPV) lesion across the coumadin ridge. In the Cox Maze-III procedure, a lesion is created from the LSPV to the orifice of the LAA across the coumadin ridge to prevent macro-reentry around the base of the LAA, which often uses this ridge. *Left panel,* Location of the LAA–LSPV lesion in the Cox Maze-III procedure. *Right panel,* Elimination of macro-reentry around the base of the LAA using the coumadin ridge.

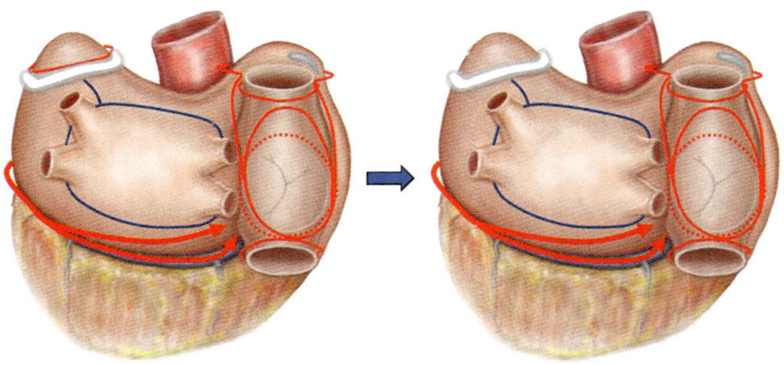

Fig. 15.4 Left atrial appendage (LAA) closure with an AtriClip. Application of an AtriClip to close the LAA eliminates any triggers and any macro-reentrant drivers that use the LAA as a part of their circuit.

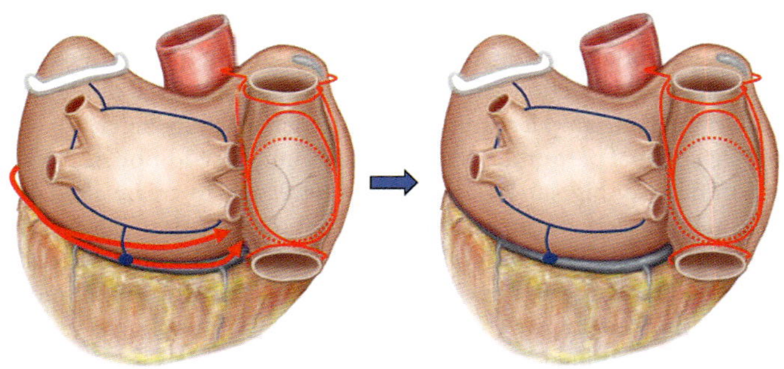

Fig. 15.5 Mitral line and coronary sinus lesions. A serious complication of performing a box lesion is peri-mitral atrial flutter caused by a large macro-reentrant circuit that uses the anterior, posterior, lateral, and medial (septal) areas of the left atrium. To prevent this iatrogenic postoperative arrhythmia, the Cox Maze-III procedure includes the creation of a "mitral line" across the left atrial isthmus between the box lesion and the posterior mitral valve annulus and a coronary sinus cryolesion in the same plane as the mitral line (see Chapter 48).

4. Mitral line and coronary sinus lesions (Fig. 15.5)
   - Prevent postoperative peri-mitral flutter

Right Atrial Lesions

1. Superior vena cava (SVC)–inferior vena cava (IVC) lesion (Fig. 15.6)
   - Prevents reentry around the SVC orifice and around the IVC orifice
   - Prevents on atrial flutter-wave that circles posterior to SVC orifice
   - Serves as an anchor for "T" lesion to tricuspid valve annulus
2. "T" lesion (Fig. 15.7)
   - Prevents atrial flutter-wave that circles anterior to the SVC orifice
   - Prevents atrial flutter wave around the tricuspid valve annulus
3. Right atrial appendage (RAA) lesion (Fig. 15.8)
   - Prevents reentry around base of RAA

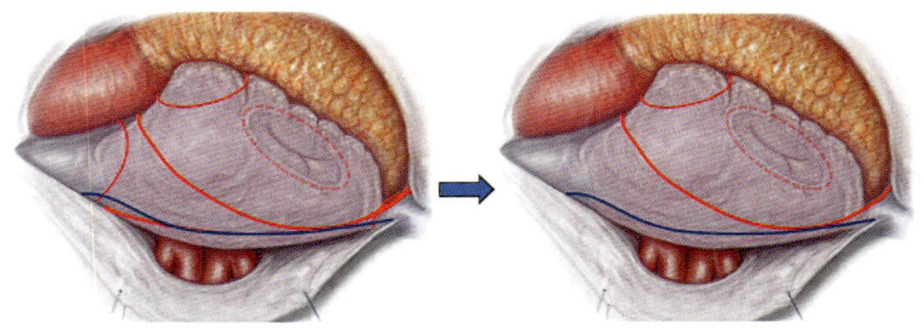

Fig. 15.6 Superior vena cava (SVC)–inferior vena cava (IVC) lesion. The right atrial lesions of a Cox Maze-III procedure include an intercaval lesion between the SVC and the IVC placed immediately anterior to the crista terminalis in the thin portion of the posterior right atrium. This lesion prevents macro-reentry around the orifices of both the SVC and IVC and prevents one of the three potential reentrant circuits of atrial flutter (i.e., the one that circles behind the SVC).

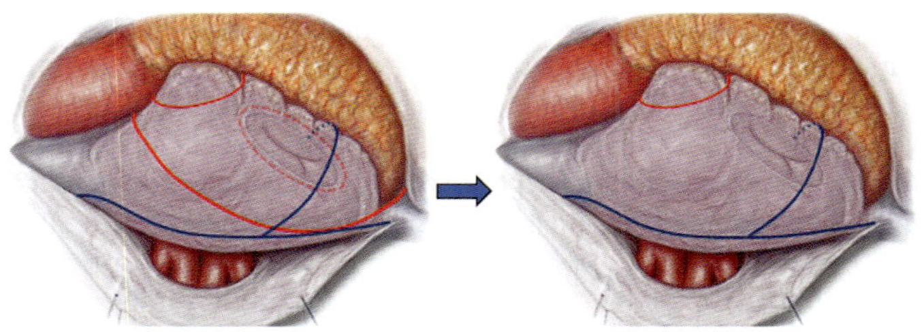

Fig. 15.7 "T" lesion. The "T" lesion of the Cox Maze-III procedure extends from the intercaval lesion across the lower third of the right atrium down to the tricuspid valve annulus at what is traditionally called the 2 o'clock position. The "T" lesion prevents reentry around the tricuspid annulus and also another reentrant circuit that can also cause atrial flutter that circles anterior to the superior vena.

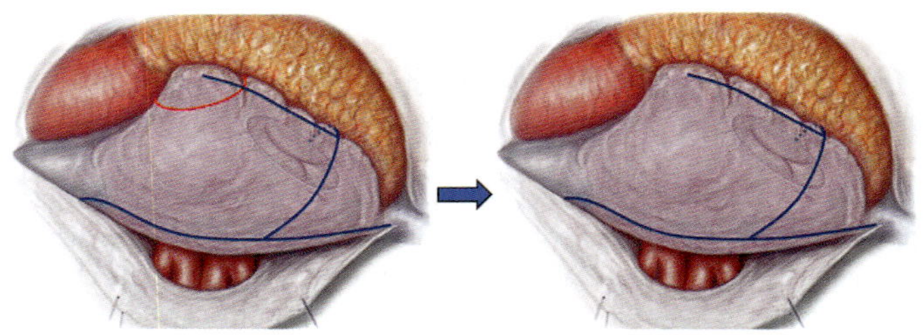

Fig. 15.8 Right atrial appendage (RAA) lesion. The final right atrial lesion in the Cox Maze-III procedure is a single lesion anchored on the "T" lesion that is created along the anterior edge of the right atrium from the "T" lesion to the tip of the RAA. This lesion prevents reentry around the base of the RAA.

Not many surgeons mastered the lesion set used for cut-and-sew operations. There were concerns by most surgeons, and there still are, about cross-clamp and cardiopulmonary bypass (CPB) time when adding a Maze procedure to other cardiac operations.[13] The Maze procedure was a natural fit with mitral valve (MV) operations because the left atriotomy was one of the Cox Maze-III incisions, and patients with MV disease have the highest incidence of AF before mitral surgery compared with other heart operations.[14,15] Combined MV repair and Maze surgery was first reported in 1993 from the Cleveland Clinic.[16] Still today, MV surgery is the most common concomitant operation with a Maze procedure.[14,15,17] The specific manner in which we modified the Cox CryoMaze-III procedure to create all of the cryolesions of the Cox CryoMaze-III procedure described above in less time is described in Chapter 27.

In the "Maze-IV" procedure, bipolar radiofrequency (RF) and cryoablation were used to replace the incisions of the cut-and-sew Cox Maze-III and the cryolesions of the CryoMaze-III procedures.[18,19] Although the lesions were created in a different manner, the ultimate lesion pattern was electrophysiologically identical to the Maze III procedure (see Chapter 17). After US Food and Drug Administration approval of the Synergy bipolar RF clamp (AtriCure Inc.) in November 2012,[20] it became easier to teach surgeons to perform the Cox Maze-IV lesion set than it had been trying to teach them the Cox Maze-III procedure.[21] This resulted in an increase in concomitant ablation and more standardization of the lesion set. Other technologies (microwave, laser, high-intensity-focused ultrasonography) appeared in practice and faded away because they did not consistently provide transmural lesions and effectiveness was not acceptable (see Chapter 20). However, the operation was still complex, so many violations of the basic principles of the Maze procedure followed[22] in an effort to simplify the procedure. Besides disagreement about the lesion set and which technology was best, there were also unanswered questions and strong opinions about which patients were candidates for AF surgery. The excessive limitation of ablation by excluding patients with a long AF duration, very large atria, and combination procedures such as multiple valves, valve and coronary bypass, and valve and aneurysm resulted in higher success rates but left the majority of patients untreated and therefore, deprived of the long-term benefits of the surgery. In addition, the Ablate-AF trial and similar studies that indicated an increased need for new pacemakers and prolonged hospitalization following AF ablation appeared just as "length of stay" was becoming a publicly reported quality metric.[13,15,23,24] Many surgeons hesitated. They needed more assurance that there were clinically important benefits to adding a Maze procedure to routine coronary artery bypass graft (CABG) procedures and valve surgery and that risks could be minimized, efficiency improved, and the lesion set made easier to understand.

RATIONALE FOR THE MODIFICATION OF THE COX CRYOMAZE-III PROCEDURE

At Northwestern University, we revamped the cardiac surgery program in 2004 into the Bluhm Cardiovascular Institute, which launched on Valentine's Day 2005. An important aspect of the change was to create a database to track the outcomes of our cardiac surgery operations, not for just 30 days as required by the Society of Thoracic Surgeons (STS) but annually for years after surgery. Surgery for AF was a particular focus of the database creation, and many "custom" fields with details about the type and duration of AF, ablation techniques, and detailed follow-up were added to the basic STS information. We also created a team of nurses and research staff to maintain high-quality tracking. Early in our experience, we used the "cut-and-sew" Cox Maze-III procedure for patients with a dilated left atrium (LA; >6 cm), for all stand-alone AF surgery, and in young patients in whom we wanted to maximize the chances of success. Results were similar to our published series from the Cleveland Clinic.[5] We had published an overview of the bipolar RF technology, and some of the operations included cryoablation using reusable probes.[19] The reusable cryoprobes were stiff and had limited surface areas for ablation (Fig. 15.9),[25] which was satisfactory for short applications but not efficient in replacing linear ablation lines. As a result, we began using the new disposable cryoprobes in patients undergoing reoperative MV surgery. We started with reoperations because the epicardial adhesions essentially eliminated the ability to use a bipolar RF clamp. The extensive dissection around the left PVs, the left atrial dome, and posterior left atrial wall required for placement of a bipolar clamp was not an essential part of the redo MV operation. In addition, the optimal number of bipolar RF applications necessary to create a reliable transmural lesion was an ongoing debate at the time. It took years for the current routine of multiple "doublets," clamping without release with two ablations, was developed, and even though this technique showed marked improvement experimentally,[26] the clinical results remained suboptimal.[27]

Reusable Cryoprobes

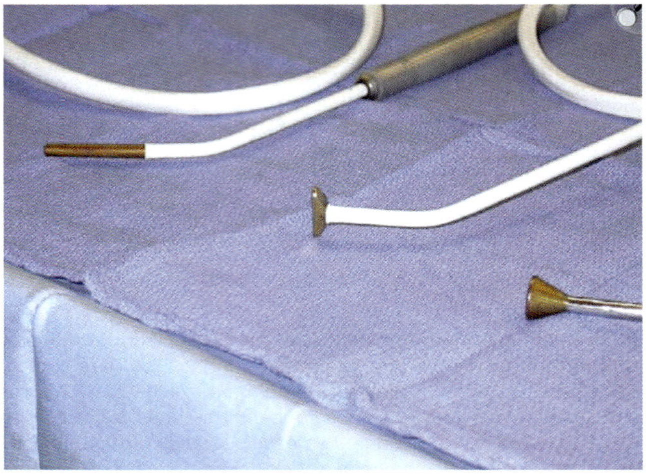

Fig. 15.9 Examples of some of the reusable cryoprobes that were available in the 1990s to create cryolesions in the heart. They were inflexible, and most were developed to perform focal cryolesions at specific sites in the atrium or ventricle. The cryoprobe on the left was the first linear cryoprobe ever developed (c. 1998), but it was quite cumbersome to use to create linear cryolesions. (Reproduced from Lee AM, Clark K, Bailey MS, Aziz A, Schuessler RB, Damiano Jr. RJ. A minimally invasive Cox Maze procedure: operative technique and results. *Innovations*. 2010;5(4):281–286.)

Instead, we began treating reoperative patients with endocardial cryoablation only using the new disposable commercially available devices (Fig. 15.10). These longer flexible probes allowed the surgeon to create long linear ablation lines with each application, which saved CPB time and aortic cross-clamp time. In addition, the disposable cryoprobes were malleable and therefore allowed for the creation of curved linear lesions, which was a major advantage when a lesion was placed across the dome of the LA, around the mitral annulus, and in other irregular areas (see Chapter 27). At that time, we were publishing our Northwestern Maze results regarding FFAF, and the number of patients undergoing reoperations

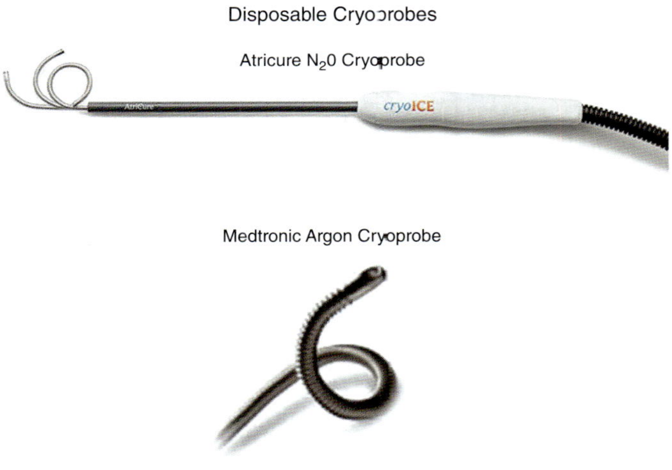

Fig. 15.10 Modern linear cryoprobes available for cardiac cryosurgery today. These cryoprobes are linear, flexible, light, and easy to use in any part of either atrium. The *upper panel* shows the AtriCure cryoprobe that uses nitrous oxide gas as the cryogen that cools the cryoprobe to approximately −60°C. The *lower panel* shows the Medtronic cryoprobe that uses argon gas as the cryogen that cools the cryoprobe to approximately −160°C. Used appropriately, the results of cryosurgery for atrial fibrillation with these two probes are equivalent because they are both excellent devices for creating permanent contiguous, uniformly transmural lesions in the atria.

who were treated with cryoablation was significantly less,[27] We had expected the results in the cryoablation group to be worse because cryosurgery was used only in reoperations, so we were surprised to find that in midterm follow-up, there was no difference in FFAF or stroke rate between the RF and cryosurgical groups. Therefore, we developed a standardized cryoablation lesion set that followed the Cox Maze-III pattern, which we knew was highly effective. In addition, the new cryoprobes allowed an efficient operation that minimized cross-clamp and bypass times to reduce renal dysfunction from prolonged bypass. In addition, proper placement of the cryoablation lesions minimized the risk of pacemakers.

As in most other centers, we initially ablated AF selectively in patients with concomitant AF ablation. However, several observational studies and randomized trials indicated improved FFAF[28–34] and late strokes[3–6] in CABG and valve surgery patients in whom the AF was treated concomitantly with the Maze procedure. In addition, quality of life (QoL) studies for patients with stand-alone AF treated with a Maze procedure showed improvement and even a return of QoL to normal in some patients.[35,36] However, an improved survival rate had not yet been shown for patients undergoing a concomitant Maze procedure during routine cardiac surgery.

At the Cleveland Clinic, we had demonstrated that coronary artery bypass patients with untreated preoperative AF had significantly lower survival rates than patients who did not have AF before surgery,[37] and others reported similar findings.[38,39] We studied our Northwestern patients using propensity score-matching of those who had concomitant AF surgical ablation either by a Maze procedure or by pulmonary vein isolation (PVI) compared with those with no AF treatment. In 2012, we published the results of that study of 3262 patients undergoing a variety of cardiac operations, including 25% (813) with preoperative AF and 75% (2449) without a history of AF.[26] For the patients with preoperative AF, there was a high rate of concomitant AF ablation (70%; $n = 565$). Propensity scores were used to match 744 patients. Survival was compared between those with surgical ablation versus those without surgical ablation and between those with FFAF at 1 year (success) compared with those with AF recurrence (failure). The survival rate for patients with untreated preoperative AF was lower than for those with no history of AF (Fig. 15.11), as had been demonstrated previously.[37–39] However, the early and late survival rates of patients with AF and surgical ablation were the same for patients who had never had AF, indicating that we had restored survival to normal in the surgical ablation–treated group (Fig. 15.12). At 1 year, FFAF was 78% in the surgical ablation group. The survival rate for patients with successful surgical ablation was significantly higher than for those with surgical ablation failure (Fig. 15.13).

The subgroup of patients with PAF was relatively underreported in the literature, and randomized trials focused primarily on patients with persistent or long-standing persistent AF. In 2013, we published a propensity score-matched study of 4947 patients undergoing cardiac surgery and after matching we compared 423 preoperative AF patients who received concomitant surgical ablation with 129 patients without surgical ablation.[40] The patients who had surgical ablation had fewer

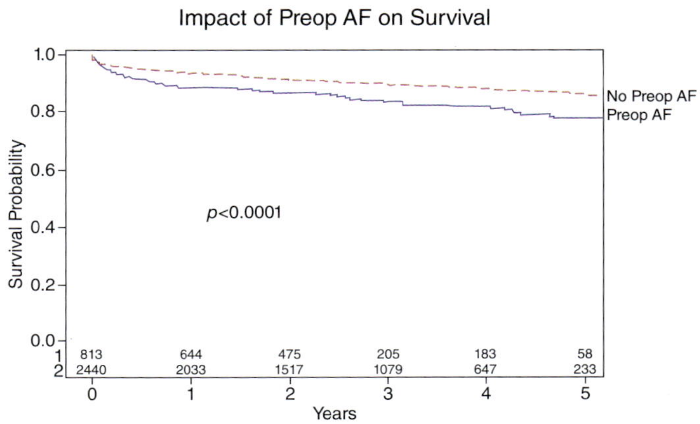

Fig. 15.11 Unadjusted survival in patients with a history of preoperative atrial fibrillation (AF) compared with no AF history. (Reproduced from Lee R, McCarthy PM, Wang EC, et al. Midterm survival in patients treated for atrial fibrillation: a propensity-matched comparison to patients without a history of atrial fibrillation. *J Thorac Cardiovasc Surg.* 2012;143(6):1341–1351; discussion 1350–1351.)

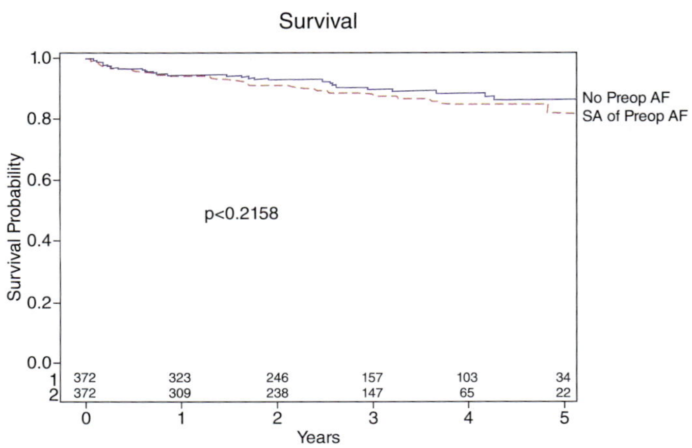

Fig. 15.12 Kaplan-Meier analysis of survival for propensity score-matched patients of atrial fibrillation (AF) ablated versus no AF shows no difference in survival. (Reproduced from Lee R, McCarthy PM, Wang EC, et al. Midterm survival in patients treated for atrial fibrillation: a propensity-matched comparison to patients without a history of atrial fibrillation. *J Thorac Cardiovasc Surg.* 2012;143(6):1341–1351; discussion 1350–1351.)

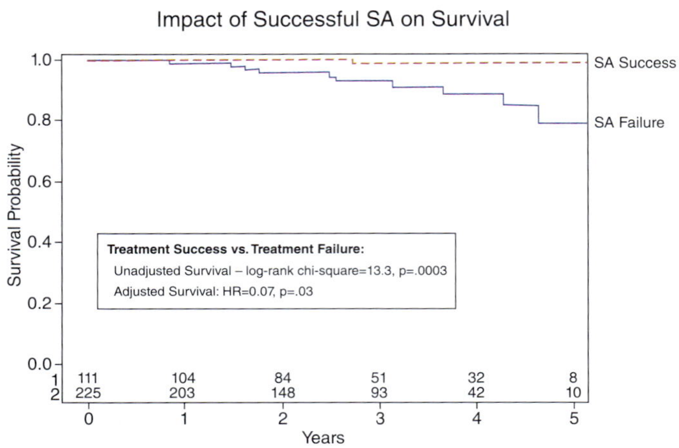

Fig. 15.13 Kaplan-Meier analysis of survival in atrial fibrillation (AF) ablated groups by "success" (freedom from AF and antiarrhythmic therapy at 1 year) versus "failure." *HR,* Hazard ratio. (Reproduced from Lee R, McCarthy PM, Wang EC, et al. Midterm survival in patients treated for atrial fibrillation: a propensity-matched comparison to patients without a history of atrial fibrillation. *J Thorac Cardiovasc Surg.* 2012;143(6):1341–1351; discussion 1350–1351.)

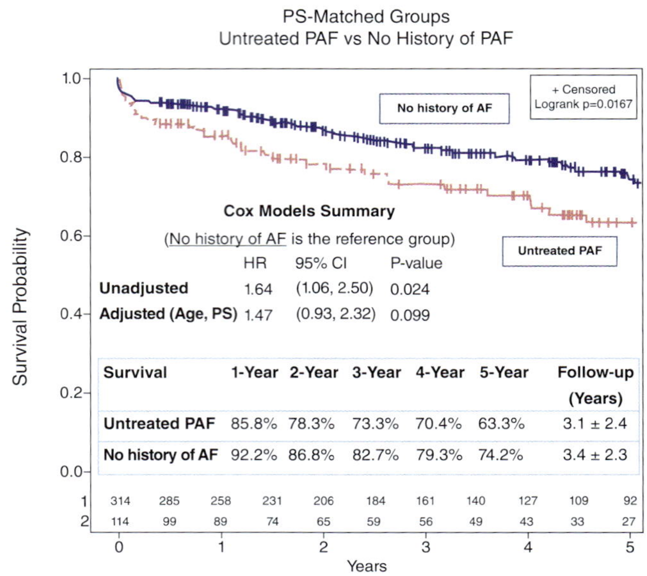

Fig. 15.15 Survival outcomes between propensity score (PS)-matched groups with no history of atrial fibrillation (AF) and those with untreated paroxysmal AF (PAF) when undergoing cardiac surgery. *CI,* Confidence interval; *HR,* hazard ratio. (Reproduced from McCarthy PM, Manjunath A, Kruse J, et al. Should paroxysmal atrial fibrillation be treated during cardiac surgery? *J Thorac Cardiovasc Surg.* 2013;146(4):810–823.)

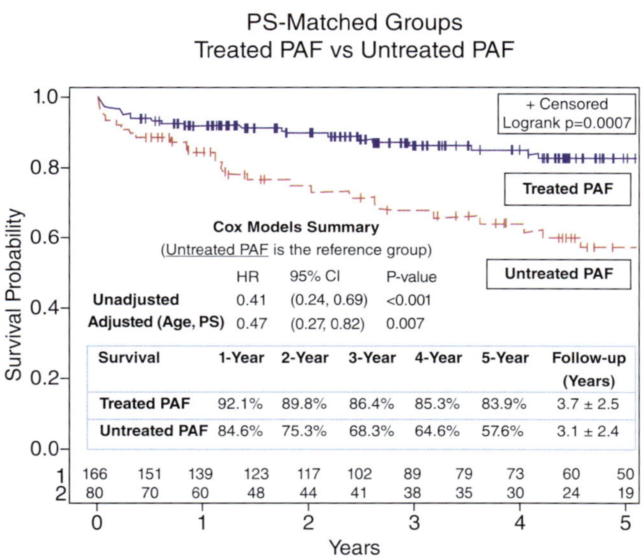

Fig. 15.14 Survival outcomes between propensity score (PS)-matched groups with treated paroxysmal atrial fibrillation (PAF) and those with untreated PAF when undergoing cardiac surgery. *CI,* Confidence interval; *HR,* hazard ratio. (Reproduced from McCarthy PM, Manjunath A, Kruse J, et al. Should paroxysmal atrial fibrillation be treated during cardiac surgery? *J Thorac Cardiovasc Surg.* 2013;146(4):810–823.)

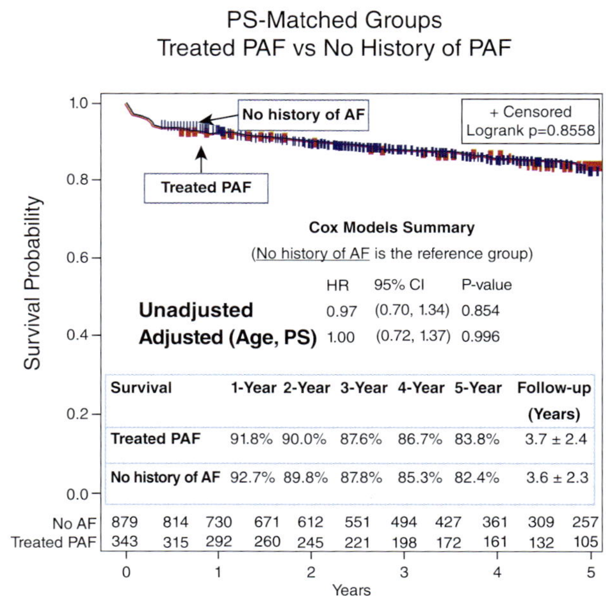

Fig. 15.16 Survival outcomes between propensity score (PS)-matched groups with no history of atrial fibrillation (AF) and those with treated paroxysmal AF (PAF) when undergoing cardiac surgery. *CI,* Confidence interval; *HR,* hazard ratio. (Reproduced from McCarthy PM, Manjunath A. Kruse J, et al. Should paroxysmal atrial fibrillation be treated during cardiac surgery? *J Thorac Cardiovasc Surg.* 2013;146(4):810–823.)

perioperative complications (26% versus 46%; $P = .001$), similar 30-day mortality rates, better FFAF at 12 months (81% versus 60%; $P = .007$), and better late survival rates (Fig. 15.14). Also, as in the larger study, the untreated PAF patients had an increased mortality rate compared with patients with no history of AF (Fig. 15.15), and for those treated with surgical ablation, survival the rates was restored to that of patients with no AF history (Fig. 15.16).

These two articles changed our practice because they documented a new important benefit to surgical ablation showing not just FFAF, stroke, and improved QoL but also improved late survival. In 2013 we began a series of mitral surgery patients who had the modified Cox CryoMaze-III procedure for AF ablation with the goal of performing concomitant surgical ablation in 100% of MV patients with preoperative AF. From our experience with reoperations, we knew we could achieve a high FFAF with minimal complications, and the modified Cox CryoMaze-III was an efficient procedure that added very little CPB or cross-clamp time. Importantly for our field, it was not complex, and most surgeons should be able to master the procedure quickly.

LEFT ATRIAL–ONLY ABLATION VERSUS BIATRIAL ABLATION

The earliest Maze operations were performed in patients with standalone AF, so of course, these operations were biatrial to eliminate all potential sources of macro-reentry in either atrium. As Maze procedures were added to other operations, some surgeons looked for ways to eliminate some of the Maze lesions to simplify the procedures, especially for patients with right-sided congenital heart lesions who were treated with right atrial ablation only.[41] When bipolar RF clamps became available, many surgeons began performing PVI only based on Haïssaguerre and colleagues' identification of PV AF triggers in 1998 and the fact that PVI alone could reduce the frequency of AF.[42]

For the modified Cox CryoMaze-III operation, we are selective about the lesion set that we choose. For patients with dilated right atria and/or in patients undergoing tricuspid valve repair, we include the right atrial lesions and have a complete biatrial lesions set.[43,44] However, many patients today are asymptomatic and referred very early in the course of mitral regurgitation without pulmonary hypertension, tricuspid regurgitation, or right atrial dilatation, so the right atrium (RA) is less likely to be actively involved in driving the AF in such patients. In other words, the RA may be fibrillating entirely as a passive response to the active AF drivers in the LA. Although these patients cannot be definitively identified preoperatively, we use these criteria to select the ones who will receive the left atrial lesions only, and there has been no statistically difference in FFAF between the group receiving LA-only lesions and those receiving biatrial lesions.[45] Also, even though surgeons may carefully avoid the sinus node and atrial pacemaker complex, traction from retractors and other right atrial trauma may contribute to the higher need for pacemakers when the right atrial lesions are performed, a problem that we would prefer to avoid.[46,47] Finally, we have rarely documented a failure of concomitant AF ablation resulting from omission of the right atrial lesions.[43] Recently, we summarized our practical approach to concomitant surgical ablation, including frequent use of the modified CryoMaze-III procedure, our most common procedure for concomitant surgical ablation.[48]

REFERENCES

1. Cox J. The surgical treatment of atrial fibrillation. IV. Surgical technique. *J Thorac Cardiovasc Surg*. 1991;101(4):584–592.
2. Cox JL, Schuessler RB, Boineau JP. The development of the Maze procedure for the treatment of atrial fibrillation. *Sem Thorac Cardiovasc Surg*. 2000;12(1):2–14.
3. Ad N, Cox JL. Stroke prevention as an indication for the Maze procedure in the treatment of atrial fibrillation. *Sem Thorac Cardiovasc Surg*. 2000;12(1):56–62.
4. Schaff HV, Dearani JA, Daly RC, Orszulak TA, Danielson GK. Cox-Maze procedure for atrial fibrillation: mayo clinic experience. *Sem Thorac Cardiovasc Surg*. 2000;12(1):30–37.
5. McCarthy PM, Gillinov AM, Castle L, Chung M, Cosgrove 3rd D. The cox-maze procedure: the Cleveland clinic experience. *Sem Thorac Cardiovasc Surg*. 2000;12(1):25–29.
6. Arcidi Jr JM, Doty DB, Millar RC. The Maze procedure: the LDS Hospital experience. *Sem Thorac Cardiovasc Surg*. 2000;12(1):38–43.
7. Cox JL, Schuessler RB, D'Agostino Jr HJ, et al. The surgical treatment of atrial fibrillation. III. Development of a definitive surgical procedure. *J Thorac Cardiovasc Surg*. 1991;101(4):569–583.
8. Holman WL, Ikeshita M, Douglas Jr JM, Smith PK, Cox JL. Cardiac cryosurgery: effects of myocardial temperature on cryolesion size. *Surgery*. 1983;93(2):268–272.
9. Cox JL, Ferguson Jr TB. Surgery for atrioventricular node reentry tachycardia: the discrete cryosurgical technique. *Sem Thorac Cardiovasc Surg*. 1989;1(1):47–52.
10. Cox JL, Ferguson Jr TB. Surgery for the Wolff-Parkinson-White syndrome: the endocardial approach. *Sem Thorac Cardiovasc Surg*. 1989;1(1):34–46.
11. Cox JL. The minimally invasive Maze-III procedure. *Op Tech Thorac Cardiovasc Surg*. 2000;5(1):79–92.
12. Ad N, Cox JL. The Maze procedure for the treatment of atrial fibrillation: a minimally invasive approach. *J Card Surg*. 2004;19(3):196–200.
13. Mehaffey JH, Charles EJ, Berens M, et al. Barriers to atrial fibrillation ablation during mitral valve surgery. *J Thorac Cardiovasc Surg*. 2021. https://doi.org/10.1016/j.jtcvs.2021.03.039.
14. McCarthy PM, Davidson CJ, Kruse J, et al. Prevalence of atrial fibrillation before cardiac surgery and factors associated with concomitant ablation. *J Thorac Cardiovasc Surg*. 2020;159(6):2245–2253.e15.
15. Badhwar V, Rankin JS, Ad N, et al. Surgical ablation of atrial fibrillation in the United States: trends and propensity matched outcomes. *Ann Thorac Surg*. 2017;104(2):493–500.
16. McCarthy PM, Cosgrove 3rd DM, Castle LW, White RD, Klein AL. Combined treatment of mitral regurgitation and atrial fibrillation with valvuloplasty and the Maze procedure. *Am J Cardiol*. 1993;71(5):483–486.
17. Wyler von Ballmoos MC, Hui DS, Mehaffey JH, et al. The society of thoracic surgeons 2023 clinical practice guidelines for the surgical treatment of atrial fibrillation. *Ann Thorac Surg*. 2024;118(2):291–310.
18. Gaynor SL, Diodato MD, Prasad SM, et al. A prospective, single-center clinical trial of a modified Cox Maze procedure with bipolar radiofrequency ablation. *J Thorac Cardiovasc Surg*. 2004;128(4):535–542.
19. Mokadam NA, McCarthy PM, Gillinov AM, et al. A prospective multicenter trial of bipolar radiofrequency ablation for atrial fibrillation: early results. *Ann Thorac Surg*. 2004;78(5):1665–1670.
20. Synergy clamp Premarket approval letter. Accessed June 3, 2024. https://www.atricure.com/sites/default/files/pdf-doc/P100046-S013.Letter.APPR__0.pdf.
21. McCarthy PM, Gerdisch M, Philpott J, et al. Three-year outcomes of the postapproval study of the atricure bipolar radiofrequency ablation of permanent atrial fibrillation trial. *J Thorac Cardiovasc Surg*. 2022;164(2):519–527 e4.
22. Cox JL, Churyla A, Malaisrie SC, et al. When is a Maze procedure a Maze procedure? *Can J Cardiol*. 2018;34(11):1482–1491.
23. Gillinov AM, Gelijns AC, Parides MK, et al. Surgical ablation of atrial fibrillation during mitral-valve surgery. *N Eng J Med*. 2015;372(15):1399–1409.
24. Philpott JM, Zemlin CW, Cox JL, et al. The ABLATE trial: safety and efficacy of Cox Maze-IV using a bipolar radiofrequency ablation system. *Ann Thorac Surg*. 2015;100(5):1541–1546 discussion 1547-8.
25. Lee AM, Clark K, Bailey MS, Aziz A, Schuessler RB, Jr Damiano. RJ: A minimally invasive Cox Maze procedure: operative technique and results. *Innovations*. 2010;5(4):281–286.
26. Khiabani AJ, MacGregor RM, Manghelli JL, et al. Bipolar radiofrequency ablation on explanted human hearts: how to ensure transmural lesions. *Ann Thorac Surg*. 2020;110(6):1933–1939.

27. Lee R, McCarthy PM, Wang EC, et al. Midterm survival in patients treated for atrial fibrillation: a propensity-matched comparison to patients without a history of atrial fibrillation. *J Thorac Cardiovasc Surg*. 2012;143(6):1341–1351 discussion 1350-1351.
28. Deneke T, Khargi K, Grewe PH, et al. Efficacy of an additional MAZE procedure using cooled-tip radiofrequency ablation in patients with chronic atrial fibrillation and mitral valve disease. A randomized, prospective trial. *Eur Heart J*. 2002;23(7):558–566.
29. Schuetz A, Schulze CJ, Sarvanakis KK, et al. Surgical treatment of permanent atrial fibrillation using microwave energy ablation: a prospective randomized clinical trial. *Eur J Cardiothorac Surg*. 2003;24(4):475–480 discussion 480.
30. Akpinar B, Guden M, Sagbas E, et al. Combined radiofrequency modified Maze and mitral valve procedure through a port access approach: early and mid-term results. *Eur J Cardiothorac Surg*. 2003;24(2):223–230.
31. Abreu Filho CA, Lisboa LA, Dallan LA, et al. Effectiveness of the Maze procedure using cooled-tip radiofrequency ablation in patients with permanent atrial fibrillation and rheumatic mitral valve disease. *Circulation*. 2005;112(9 Suppl):I20–I25.
32. Doukas G, Samani NJ, Alexiou C, et al. Left atrial radiofrequency ablation during mitral valve surgery for continuous atrial fibrillation: a randomized controlled trial. *J Am Med Assoc*. 2005;294(18):2323–2329.
33. Blomstrom-Lundqvist C, Johansson B, Berglin E, et al. A randomized double-blind study of epicardial left atrial cryoablation for permanent atrial fibrillation in patients undergoing mitral valve surgery: the Swedish multicentre atrial fibrillation study (SWEDMAF). *Eur Heart J*. 2007;28(23):2902–2908.
34. Chevalier P, Leizorovicz A, Maureira P, et al. Left atrial radiofrequency ablation during mitral valve surgery: a prospective randomized multicentre study (SAFIR). *Arch Cardiovasc Dis*. 2009;102(11):769–775.
35. Melby SJ, Zierer A, Lubahn JG, et al. Normal quality of life after the Cox maze procedure for atrial fibrillation. *Innovations*. 2008;3(3):142–146.
36. Lundberg C, Albage A, Carnlof C, Kenneback G. Long-term health-related quality of life after Maze surgery for atrial fibrillation. *Ann Thor Surg*. 2008;86(6):1878–1882.
37. Quader MA, McCarthy PM, Gillinov AM, et al. Does preoperative atrial fibrillation reduce survival after coronary artery bypass grafting? *Ann Thor Surg*. 2004;77(5):1514–1522 discussion 1522–1524.
38. Ngaage DL, Schaff HV, Mullany CJ, et al. Does preoperative atrial fibrillation influence early and late outcomes of coronary artery bypass grafting? *J Thorac Cardiovasc Surg*. 2007;133(1):182–189.
39. Ngaage DL, Schaff HV, Mullany CJ, et al. Influence of preoperative atrial fibrillation on late results of mitral repair: is concomitant ablation justified? *Ann Thor Surg*. 2007;84(2):434–442 discussion 442-443.
40. McCarthy PM, Manjunath A, Kruse J, et al. Should paroxysmal atrial fibrillation be treated during cardiac surgery? *The J Thorac Cardiovasc Surg*. 2013;146(4):810–823.
41. Theodoro DA, Danielson GK, Porter CJ, Warnes CA. Right-sided Maze procedure for right atrial arrhythmias in congenital heart disease. *Ann Thor Surg*. 1998;65(1):149–153 discussion 153-154.
42. Haissaguerre M, Jais P, Shah DC, et al. Spontaneous initiation of atrial fibrillation by ectopic beats originating in the pulmonary veins. *N Eng J Med*. 1998;339(10):659–666.
43. McCarthy PM, Cox JL, Kruse J, Elenbaas C, Andrei AC. One hundred percent utilization of a modified CryoMaze III procedure for atrial fibrillation with mitral surgery. *J Thorac Cardiovasc Surg*. 2024;167(4):1278–1289.e3.
44. McCarthy PM. Simple but effective modifications to the cox maze procedure using only cryoablation. *Op Tech Thorac Cardiovasc Surg*. 2024;29(2):134–148. https://doi.org/10.1053/j.optechstcvs.2023.05.006.
45. Churyla A, Iddriss A, Andrei AC, et al. Biatrial or left atrial lesion set for ablation during mitral surgery: risks and benefits. *Ann Thor Surg*. 2017;103(6):1858–1865.
46. Soni LK, Cedola SR, Cogan J, et al. Right atrial lesions do not improve the efficacy of a complete left atrial lesion set in the surgical treatment of atrial fibrillation, but they do increase procedural morbidity. *J Thorac Cardiovasc Surg*. 2013;145(2):356–361 discussion 361-3.
47. Cappabianca G, Ferrarese S, Tutino C, et al. Safety and efficacy of biatrial vs left atrial surgical ablation during concomitant cardiac surgery: a meta-analysis of clinical studies with a focus on the causes of pacemaker implantation. *J Cardiovasc Electrophysiol*. 2019;30(10):2150–2163.
48. McCarthy PM, Cox JL. Practical approaches to concomitant surgical ablation of atrial fibrillation: matching the ablation to the patient. *J Thorac Cardiovasc Surg*. 2024. https://doi.org/10.1016/j.jtcvs.2024.03.023.

16

Robotic CryoMaze-III Procedure

Vinay Badhwar, W. Randolph Chitwood, Jr.

CHAPTER OUTLINE

Surgical ablation of atrial fibrillation (AF) received multi-society guideline recommendations in 2017 that have been updated in 2024 for concomitant (Class I) and stand-alone therapy (Class II).[1] Despite increasing evidence supporting left atrial appendage (LAA) occlusion for patients with AF with or without the need of concomitant cardiac surgery, 3-year survival after surgical ablation plus LAA occlusion remains superior to LAA treatment alone.[2] Moreover, catheter-based ablation success in patients with persistent AF remains limited, and recent epicardial subxiphoid ablation techniques remain arrhythmically and anatomically incomplete.[3–7] Although recent years of robust contemporary evidence and guidelines in support of surgical ablation have resulted a modest increase adoption of concomitant surgical ablation, patients and referring cardiologists remain hesitant to undergo a stand-alone Cox CryoMaze-III procedure whether it is performed through a median sternotomy or minimally invasively via a mini-thoracotomy in the right anterior fourth intercostal space.

The Cox CryoMaze-III and Cox Maze-IV procedures have been shown to have similar results when they are performed minimally invasively compared with when they are performed through a median sternotomy.[8,9] These procedures are performed under direct vision by a tableside surgeon with or without videoscopic assistance. In addition to the need for potential rib spreading, occasional challenges may occur with the handling of cardiac tissues to avoid tissue gaps during the creation of a cryolesion. Chitwood and colleagues first introduced the robotic approach for AF ablation in 2003 using microwave technology and subsequently with cryothermia.[10,11] Chitwood's robotic approach was performed through a single working right minithoracotomy similar to the minimally invasive cryosurgical Maze-III procedure first performed by Cox in 1996. Minimally invasive and robotic ablation procedures enjoyed short-term excellent outcomes, but historically, they have lacked consistency of the lesion set and often do not conform to the classic Cox CryoMaze-III procedure. Although the long-term results of the minimally invasive cryosurgical Cox CryoMaze-III procedure have been well-documented (see Chapter 38), there has been a paucity of reports documenting the long-term clinical and electrophysiological outcomes of the robotic Cox CryoMaze-III procedure. Since 2016, the West Virginia University robotic program has performed robotic Cox CryoMaze-III procedures using the identical cryosurgical lesion pattern of the minimally invasive Cox CryoMaze-III procedure. We perform the robotic approach through a non–rib-spreading 3-cm right lateral mini-thoracotomy placed at the anterior axillary line that has provided consistently excellent clinical and electrophysiological results on long-term follow-up.[12] The objective of this chapter is to describe the current approach, technical details, and longitudinal results of the robotic Cox CryoMaze-III procedure.

PREOPERATIVE PREPARATION

After the presence of symptomatic AF has been confirmed and the patient has met guideline indications for surgical ablation, patients without prior cardiac surgery or a right thoracotomy are considered for a robotic approach, and preoperative anatomic imaging is performed. A history of prior catheter ablations is not a contraindication to robotic surgery. Coronary artery imaging for patients with significant risk factors is performed by radial cardiac catheterization or coronary computed tomography angiography (CTA). CTA of the chest, abdomen, and pelvis is obtained to detect occult stenoses that could potentially elevate the risk of peripheral cannulation for CPB. Preoperative transesophageal echocardiography (TEE) is performed if there is any concern for a thrombus in the LAA and if there is moderate or greater structural valve pathology on transthoracic echocardiography.

OPERATIVE PREPARATION AND SURGICAL TECHNIQUE

Patients receive a pre-induction intrathecal injection of 0.5 mg of morphine sulfate and an intercostal injection of 0.25% bupivacaine in the preoperative holding area to enhance rapid postoperative recovery and timely extubation. Patients also have double-lumen endotracheal intubation, a left brachial arterial line, left internal jugular large-bore intravenous (IV) access, and external defibrillator pads. The robotic-assisted Cox CryoMaze-III procedure is performed in the supine position via a 3-cm rib-sparing minimally invasive lateral thoracotomy at the level of the anterior axillary line and is facilitated by single lung ventilation. The superior vena cava (SVC) is cannulated percutaneously via the right internal jugular vein with an 18- to 20-Fr cannula (FemFlex II, Edwards Lifesciences) under TEE guidance that is flushed with heparinized saline. Folded towels are placed under the right side of the patient below the tip of the scapula to facilitate a slight drop of the right shoulder and opening of the rib spaces. The patient is then prepped and draped.

The cardiac structures are accessed via the fourth intercostal space, with the right superior pulmonary vein viewed under direct vision as the anatomic landmark to confirm the optimal level thoracic entry. A small soft tissue wound retractor is placed to facilitate exposure (Alexis, Applied Medical Resources). The pericardium is opened at least 3 cm anterior to the right phrenic nerve from the inferior vena cava (IVC) to the distal ascending aorta, and gentle retraction sutures are placed to facilitate exposure of the heart and aorta. Sharp dissection facilitates the mobilization of the SVC and IVC. The anterior surfaces of the right femoral vessels are exposed via a 1-cm skin incision, robotic port sites are prepared, and the patient is heparinized. The IVC is cannulated via the right common femoral vein with a 25-Fr multi'stage venous cannula that is positioned in the right atrium (RA) (Bio-Medicus, Medtronic). The right common femoral artery is cannulated with a 17- to 19-Fr arterial cannula (Bio-Medicus, Medtronic). A 5-Fr distal perfusion catheter is placed in the right superficial femoral artery (Micro-Introducer, Braun) and connected to the arterial line.

Robotic ports are inserted at the following locations: (1) the third intercostal space anterior axillary line for the first or left robotic arm, (2) the working incision is used for the robotic camera connected to the second robotic arm, (3) the fourth intercostal space mid-clavicular line for the dual blade left atrial retractor connected to the third robotic arm, and (4) the fifth intercostal space mid-axillary line for the fourth or right robotic arm. A stab incision in the second intercostal space at the posterior axillary line is made for passage of a transthoracic aortic cross-clamp and one at the same level in the fifth intercostal space for later passage of a left ventricular vent. After commencement of CPB, a cardioplegia cannula is inserted into the ascending aorta for the administration of antegrade cold cardioplegia, and a left ventricular vent is inserted via the right superior pulmonary vein. The Da Vinci Xi robotic system (Intuitive Surgical, Inc.) is then docked. The high-definition camera is positioned at the superior aspect of the working incision. The robotic instruments used are the DeBakey forceps via the first or left arm, the EndoWrist dual-blade atrial retractor in third arm, and the needle driver and curved scissors in the right or fourth arm (Fig. 16.1). Carbon dioxide is continuously infused via the third arm port at 2 L/min. A previously positioned transthoracic

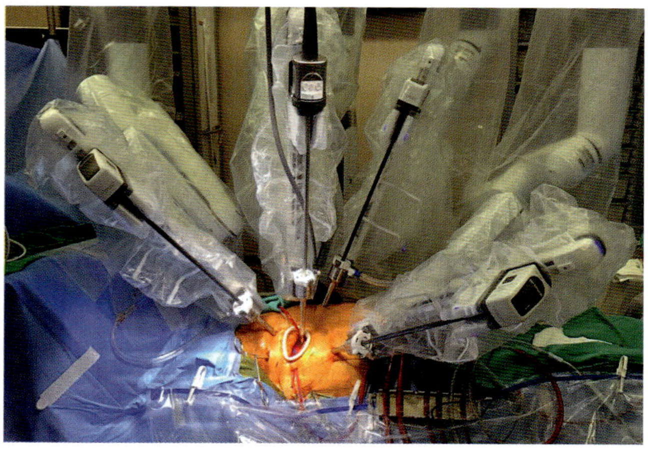

Fig. 16.1 Surgeon's view of the operative preparation for a robotic Maze procedure through a 3-cm right mini-thoracotomy.

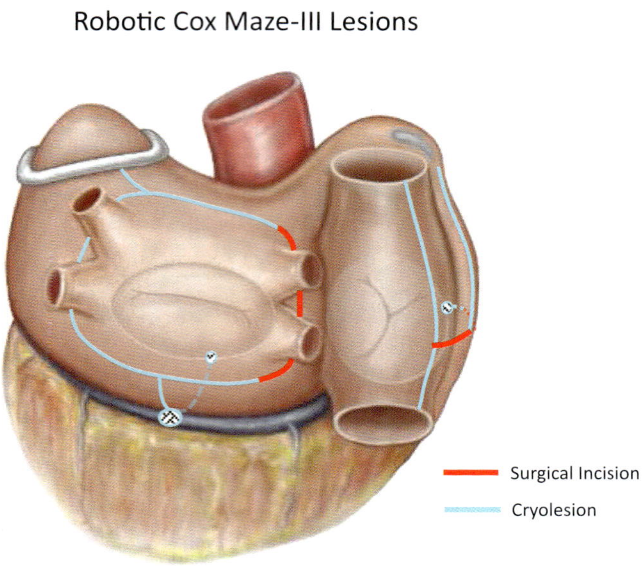

Fig. 16.2 Robotic Cox Maze-IIII lesions. The cryosurgical Cox Maze-III lesion setup performed robotically. While an AtriClip LAAO device is shown in this diagram, it is not always applied in the robotic procedures. *IVC*, Inferior vena cava; *LAA*, left atrial appendage; *RAA*, right atrial appendage; *SVC*, superior vena cava.

aortic cross-clamp is gently applied to the distal ascending aorta under full camera visualization. Intermittent antegrade cold blood cardioplegia is delivered at 20-minute intervals to maintain optimal myocardial protection throughout the operative procedure. Cardioplegia management may be tailored to institutional protocols, but it is important to avoid retrograde catheters in the coronary sinus that may impair lesion creation.

After robotically performed atriotomies, a nitrous oxide cryoprobe (AtriCure, Inc.) is used to create cryolesions in a prespecified manner consistent with the pattern of the minimally invasive Cox CryoMaze-III procedure while complete tissue contact is visually confirmed to avoid gaps in the lesions (Fig. 16.2). Left atrial lesions are each performed for 3 minutes, and right atrial lesions are performed for 2 minutes to assure complete transmurality. If at any time non-transmurality is suspected (e.g., thick or scarred atrial tissue), cryoablation time is extended until transmurality can be assured. In this situation, it is also helpful to apply the cryoprobe on the opposite side of the first cryolesion if possible so that the tissue is frozen from both sides of the atrial wall. After completion of the cryolesions, the LAA is surgically closed.

Left Atrial Lesions

After a robotically performed curvilinear standard left atriotomy is placed just beyond the left inferior pulmonary vein via the oblique sinus, the dual-blade atrial retractor is inserted to provide full exposure of the inside of the left atrium. A left ventricular vent is positioned into the left inferior pulmonary vein to create a relatively bloodless operative field. We begin by creating the coronary sinus cryolesion that is performed epicardially via the oblique sinus. An endocardial iceball occurs inside the left atrium during this coronay sinus freeze and its location is marked inside the LA with methylene blue so that we will know exactly where to place the mitral line later (Fig. 16.3). Next, the floor lesion of the left atrial box is created around the inferior half of the pulmonary veins with the tip of the probe extending into the LAA orifice, which simultaneously

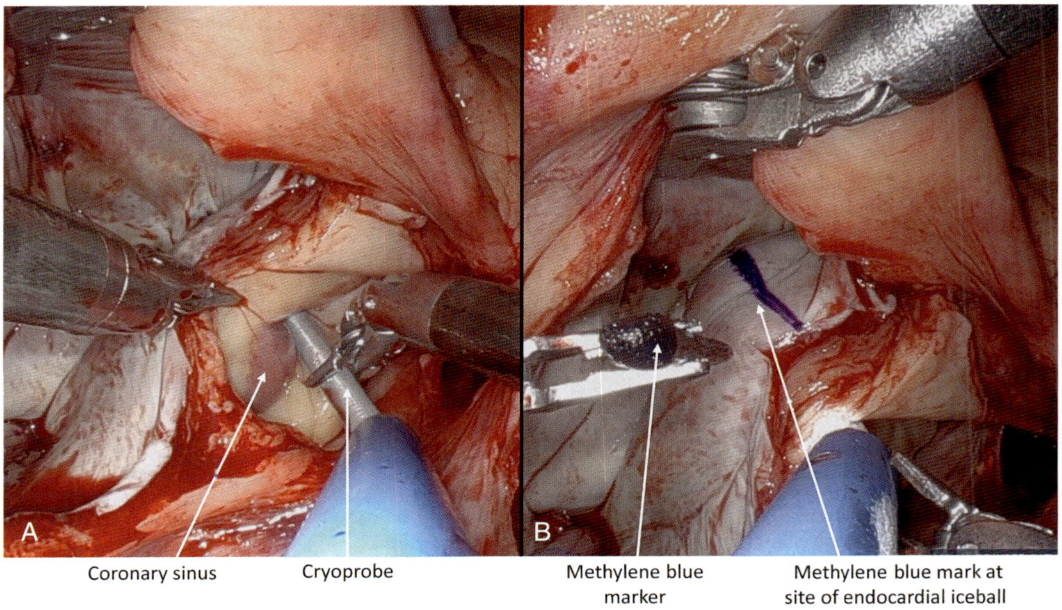

Fig. 16.3 Coronary sinus cryolesion. (A) The coronary sinus cryolesion is created epicardially just below the inferior end of the left atriotomy in Waterston's groove. (B) During creation of the epicardial coronary sinus lesion, an iceball appears on the endocardial surface of the left atrium (LA). The site of this endocardial iceball is marked with methylene blue to identify exactly where the endocardial mitral line will have to be placed. It is critical to position the endocardial mitral line and the epicardial coronary sinus cryolesion in exactly the same plane to prevent the possibility of postoperative peri-mitral flutter (see Chapter 48, Figs. 48.6 and 48.7).

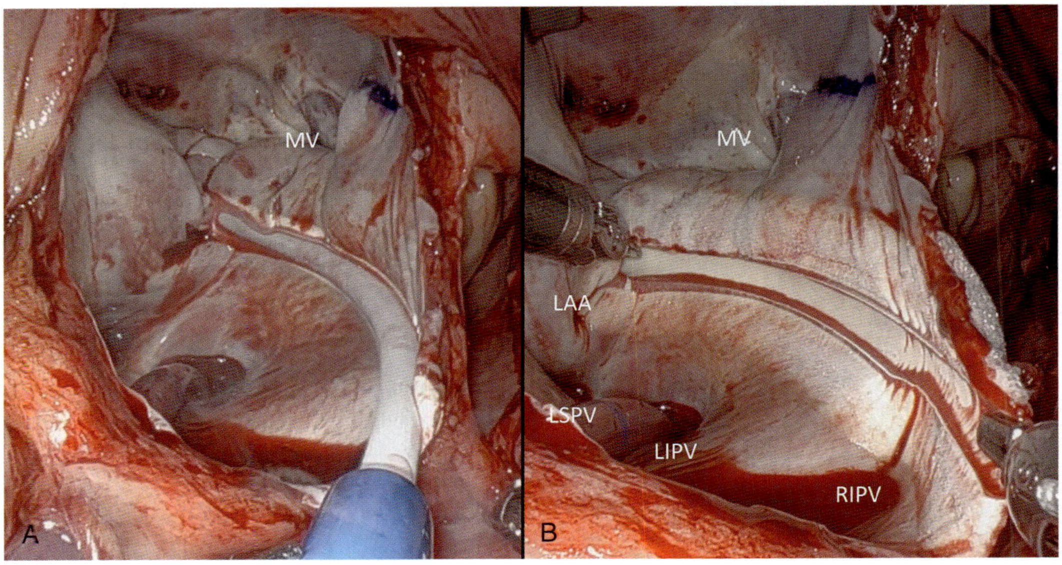

Fig. 16.4 Inferior (floor) lesion of the left atrial box and left atrial appendage (LAA) lesion across the coumadin ridge. (A) Creation of the endocardial floor lesion that extends from the inferior end of the left atriotomy across the posteroinferior left atrium (LA) to the orifice of the LAA. By extending this lesion to the LAA orifice, macro-reentrant circuits (drivers) that use the coumadin ridge are prevented. (B) Appearance of the floor lesion after removal of the cryoprobe documenting that the lesion is homogenous and free of tissue gaps. *LIPV,* Left inferior pulmonary vein; *LSPV,* left superior pulmonary vein; *MV,* mitral valve; *RIPV,* right inferior pulmonary vein.

creates the line across the coumadin ridge (Fig. 16.4). The roof lesion is then placed above the right and left superior pulmonary veins extending from the superior end of the left atriotomy to the end of the floor lesion where it overlaps with the floor lesion (Fig. 16.5). Importantly, the distal portion of this roof lesion is placed low and parallel to the right superior and left superior pulmonary veins to avoid inadvertent electrical interruption of Bachman's bundle. Finally, the endocardial mitral line is placed from the floor lesion to the posterior mitral annulus, and we usually end it toward the P3 mitral valve scallop. To avoid postoperative peri-mitral atrial flutter, this mitral line is placed in the same plane as the epicardial ablation of the coronary sinus, covering the previously placed methylene blue mark in the LA (Fig. 16.6).[12,13]

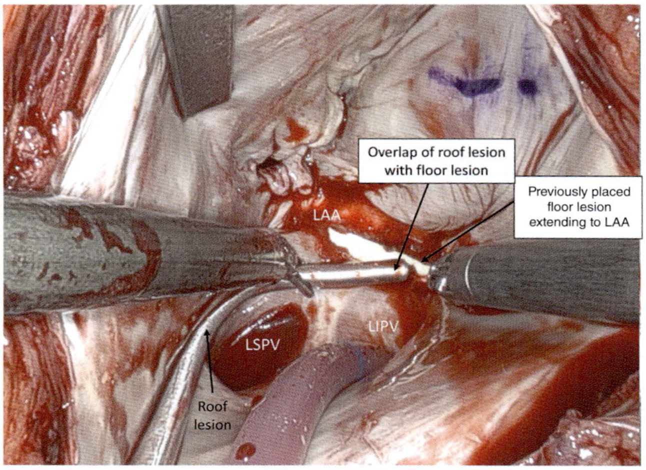

Fig. 16.5 Superior (roof) lesion of the left atrial box. The roof lesion circles around the left pulmonary veins and overlaps the floor lesion that was placed earlier. This completes the posterior left atrial box around all four pulmonary veins and the intervening posterior left atrial wall. The roof lesion is placed close to the orifices of the two superior pulmonary veins to avoid Bachmann's bundle. It also completes the lesion across the coumadin ridge. *LA,* Left atrium; *LIPV,* left inferior pulmonary vein; *LSPV,* left superior pulmonary vein.

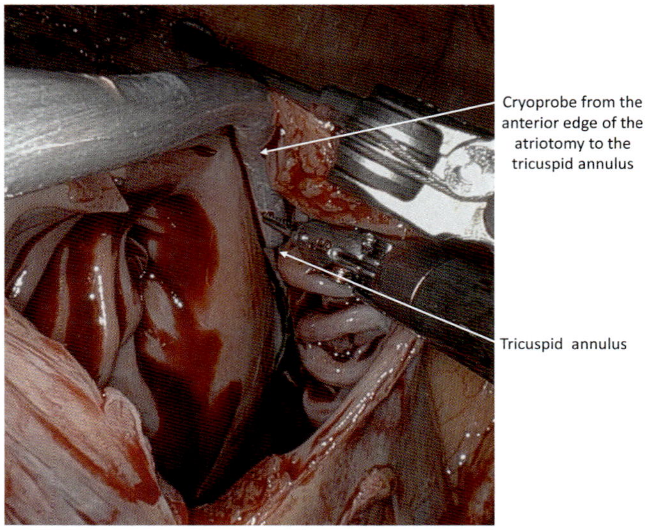

Fig. 16.7 Completion of the right atrial "T" lesion. After a diagonal atriotomy across the caudal third of the right atrium, a linear cryolesion is placed from the distal end of the atriotomy to the tricuspid annulus to extend and complete the so-called "T" lesion of the Cox Maze-III procedure.

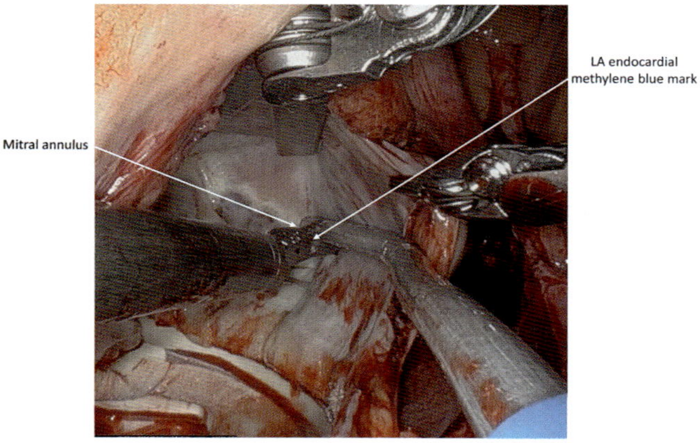

Fig. 16.6 Mitral line. The endocardial mitral line is placed opposite the epicardial coronary sinus cryolesion at the level of the prior methylene blue mark. This results in the coronary sinus cryolesion and the mitral line being in exactly the same plane so that together, they block all conduction across the left atrial isthmus and prevent the development of postoperative peri-mitral flutter.

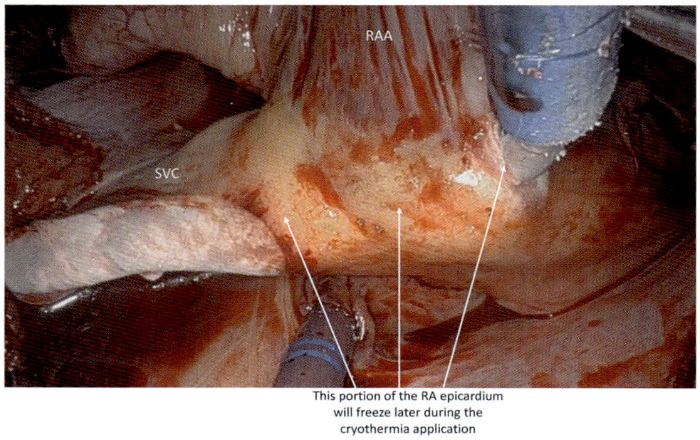

Fig. 16.8 Superior vena cava (SVC) line. The SVC line is placed from the posterior end of the right atriotomy up into the SVC just anterior and parallel to the crista terminalis. Care is taken to keep this lesion as lateral and posterior as possible to avoid injury of the anatomic sinoatrial node. *RAA,* Right atrial appendage.

Right Atrial Lesions

The right atrial lesions are performed following a right atriotomy placed across the caudal third of the right atrial free wall (see Chapter 13). This location avoids potential damage of the atrial pacemaker complex, and we believe it lessens the likelihood of requiring a new permanent pacemaker postoperatively. Vacuum-assisted venous drainage to control caval inflow makes snaring of the vena cavae unnecessary, thereby aiding the extension of right atrial lesions well into the SVC and IVC. A linear cryolesion is placed between the anterior end of the right atriotomy down to the tricuspid valve annulus to extend and complete what is commonly called the "T" lesion of the Cox CryoMaze-III procedure (Fig. 16.7). This is followed by creation of the SVC cryolesion that extends from the lower end of the atriotomy upward into the SVC orifice for approximately 2 cm. This lesion is placed just anterior and parallel to the crista terminalis and is placed as far posterior and lateral as possible to decrease the likelihood of injury of the anatomic sinoatrial (SA) node (Fig. 16.8). Next, the right atrial appendage (RAA) line is created perpendicular to the right atriotomy and as anterior in the right atrial free wall as possible so that all of the right atrial free wall above the "T" lesion and between the SVC lesion and the RAA lesion is completely avoided (Fig. 16.9).[14] The final lesion is the IVC line that extends from the proximal end of the "T" lesion down across the orifice and into the IVC (Fig. 16.10). The combination of the right atriotomy, the SVC lesion, and the RAA lesion leaves the majority of the free wall of the RA that contains the atrial pacemaker complex completely free of ablative lesions.

Finally, a few additional technical elements bear mentioning. When constructing the SVC line, it is important to stay posterior to the SVC–RA junction to avoid the SA node complex during ablation. During formation of the line to the SVC and IVC, care must be taken to ensure that the probe does not come in contact with the adjacent pericardium

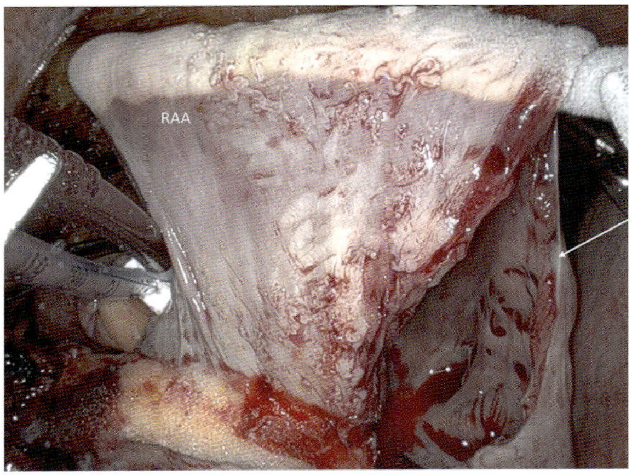

Fig. 16.9 Right atrial appendage (RAA) lesion. The lesion that prevents reentry around the base of the RAA is placed from the distal end of the right atriotomy up the anterior edge of the right atrial free-wall to the tip of the RAA. This leaves the majority of the right atrial free wall containing the atrial pacemaker complex completely free of ablative lesions.

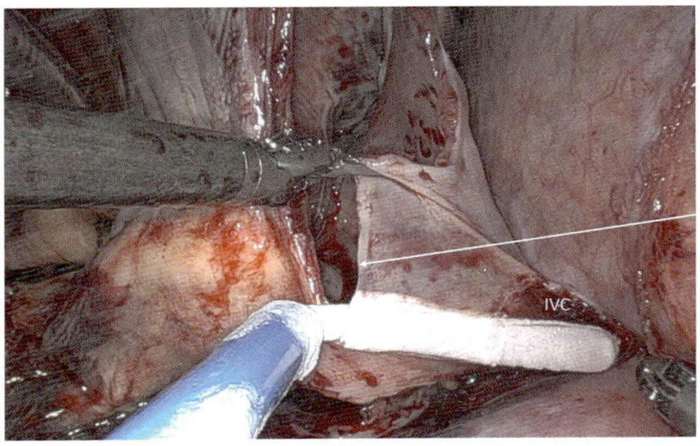

Fig. 16.10 Inferior vena cava (IVC) lesion. The IVC lesion is placed from the proximal end of the right atriotomy to the orifice of the IVC.

and the subjacent but protected right phrenic nerve. This is facilitated by confirming that the pericardial retraction sutures are firmly affixed outside of the chest. Also, when performing the line to the tip of the RAA, the probe is positioned within 5 mm of the atrioventricular groove to avoid injuring the paranodal region.[15] If these additional technical principles of RA lesion creation are followed, junctional rhythm after surgical ablation, the most common lesion-based reason for potential pacemaker requirement, is virtually always avoided.[12,13]

LEFT ATRIAL APPENDAGE OCCLUSION

Closing the LAA directly impacts subsequent stroke rate and long-term survival, and its occlusion is an essential component of the Cox CryoMaze-III procedure.[2,8,12,13,16] Contemporary exclusion of the appendage can be performed by LAA epicardial clipping or endocardial multilayer suture closure, and both methods can be effective when performed precisely.[17] In both open and robotic Cox CryoMaze-III/IV procedures, we prefer to close the LAA using a two-layer deep closure that incorporates the entire body of the LAA.[12,13,17] The first suture line across the orifice of the LAA incorporates the entire body of the LAA that is intussuscepted to collapse and obliterate the entire LAA space. The second suture line imbricates the first with a running Lembert suture that further plicates the LA wall and eliminates tension on the linear suture line. This leaves a smooth endocardial left atrial surface at least 1 to 2 cm away from the mitral annulus. After LAA closure, both the right and left atriotomies are closed with a running 4-0 suture, followed by the placement of temporary epicardial atrial and ventricular pacing wires before aortic cross-clamp release.

POSTOPERATIVE CARE

After the patient is separated from cardiopulmonary bypass (CPB), the pericardium is closed primarily after placement of a single soft silicone-based chest drain. Patients not previously loaded with amiodarone are given an IV amiodarone infusion at the commencement of CPB. Patients are most often in normal sinus rhythm or being atrially paced at the completion of the operative procedure. In our experience, it is exceedingly rare that a patient is in AF at the conclusion of the procedure. After incision closure and anesthetic reversal, the patient is usually extubated in the operating room and transferred to the intensive care unit. The intraoperative infusion of amiodarone is transitioned to oral dosing starting on postoperative day 1 and it is continued for 90 days. For the rare patient who is intolerant to amiodarone, it is replaced with sotalol, which is started on postoperative day 1 and continued for 90 days.

Patients are usually discharged by the fourth postoperative day. If they develop early postoperative AF, it may be necessary to cardiovert them electrically before hospital discharge. No patients are discharged from the hospital in AF. All patients receive clinical follow-up at 1, 3, 6, 9, 12, 18, and 24 months, with a 24-hour Holter monitor before every visit after 6 months.[13] Annual visits with Holter monitoring are obtained thereafter to 5 years. Unless there are specific indications (e.g., mechanical or bioprosthetic replacements, clotting diathesis, depressed left ventricular function), patients are not routinely anticoagulated.[13,18] However, the decision regarding the use of oral anticoagulation postoperatively can be based on institutional protocols as long as the decision making remains between the patient and surgeon and is consistent with current guidelines.

FOLLOW-UP AND RESULTS

We follow all robotic Cox CryoMaze-III patients with direct in-person surgical team clinic visits at the time intervals listed earlier. Patients without an existing implantable pacemaker after 6 months receive a 24-hour Holter monitor, and those who underwent concomitant valve repair receive annual echocardiography. If in-person follow-up is not geographically possible, the patients are mailed a 24-hour Holter and a remote televideo follow-up is performed. Freedom from AF, freedom from antiarrhythmic drugs, and freedom from oral anticoagulation is recorded for all patients at all time intervals.

From November 2016 to January 2022, 135 patients with persistent AF received robotic Cox CryoMaze-III procedures and were followed longitudinally.[13] Patients with paroxysmal AF who underwent the robotic Cox CryoMaze-III procedure, most often concomitant with valve operations, were excluded for rhythm homogeneity reasons for the purpose of this analysis. The median preoperative AF duration was 4 years, and nearly one-third of the patients had failed at least one catheter-based ablation. A stand-alone Cox CryoMaze-III procedure was performed in 25.2%, and concomitant robotic valve surgery was performed in 74.8%. The 30-day operative mortality rate was 2.2%, but there were no deaths in the stand-alone patients. Only one patient required catheter ablation at 8 months postoperatively, and there was one non-embolic stroke at 18 months, neither in stand-alone patients. Freedom from both atrial tachyarrhythmias by 24-hour Holter monitoring and freedom from antiarrhythmic drugs at 9, 12, 18, 24, 36, and 48 months were 97.0, 96.7, 98.1, 97.1, and 100%, respectively (Fig. 16.11).

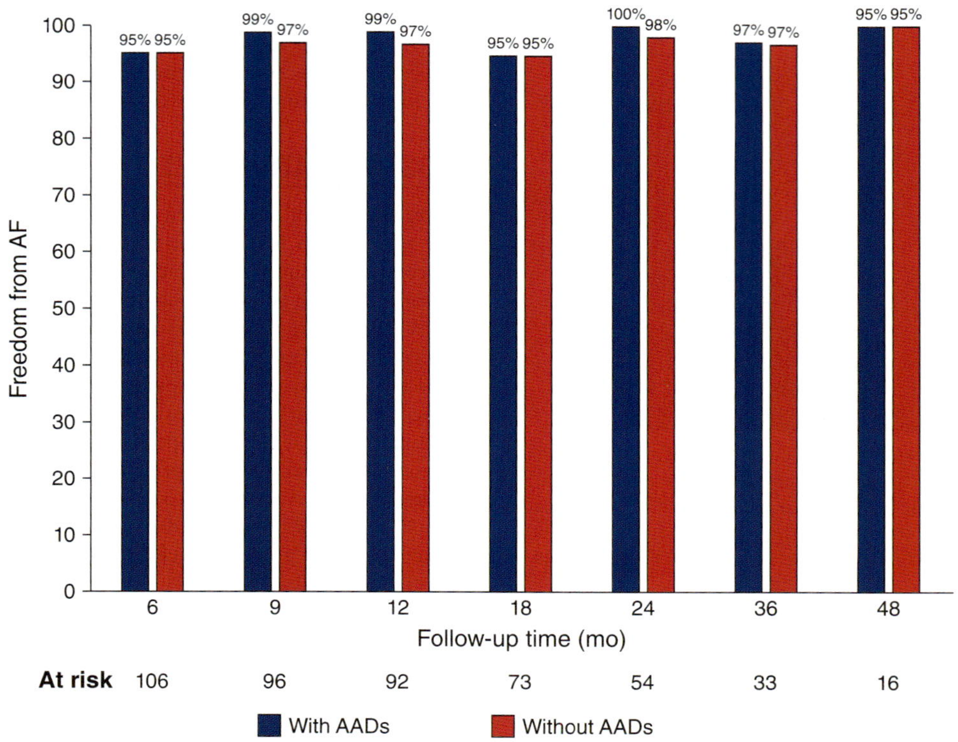

Fig. 16.11 Four-year freedom from atrial fibrillation (AF) with and without antiarrhythmic drugs (AADs) after the Cox CryoMaze-III procedure.

PERSPECTIVE

There has been a surge of interest in robotic cardiac surgery in recent years with more institutions launching successful programs. Recent expert consensus recommendations have stated that for robotic program sustainability, dedicated teams of surgeons, scrub assistants, anesthesiologists, nurses, and perfusionists with institutional commitment should be established.[19] Programs should perform a minimum of 250 open-heart cases per year for 3 consecutive years, and surgeons should have experience with a minimum of 50 intracardiac cases, 15 of which were performed via a mini-thoracotomy, within the 2 years before robotic commencement. After robotic cardiac programs have been established, the application of concomitant robotic surgical ablation is straightforward and scalable.

The robotic Cox CryoMaze-III procedure permits very clear visualization of each lesion and the related tissues, including the pectinate muscles. Unlike other open and minimally invasive surgical ablative techniques with a single operator, the robotic Cox CryoMaze-III procedure is performed not with two "hands" but with five. The tableside surgeon, who may be a physician assistant or equivalent, delivers the cryoprobe via the working incision and holds it steady as the robotic console surgeon controls its precise placement while simultaneously ensuring that all tissue gaps are eliminated by a combination of stretching out any atrial wall redundancy and providing excellent optics via the robotic camera. Because avoidance of tissue gaps in surgical ablation is likely the most important elements correlating to durable rhythm success, the precision, and extra "hands," make the robotic approach potentially the technique to facilitate the most accurately placed lesions possible.

REFERENCES

1. Wyler von Ballmoos MC, Hui DS, Mehaffey JH, et al. The society of thoracic surgeons 2023 clinical practice guidelines for the surgical treatment of atrial fibrillation. *Ann Thorac Surg*. 2024. S0003-4975(24)00057-2. https://doi.org/10.1016/j.athoracsur.2024.01.007.
2. Mehaffey JH, Hayanga JWA, Wei L, Mascio C, Rankin JS, Badhwar V. Surgical ablation of atrial fibrillation is associated with improved survival compared with appendage obliteration alone: an analysis of 100,000 Medicare beneficiaries. *J Thorac Cardiovasc Surg*. 2023. S0022-5223(23)00345-8. https://doi.org/10.1016/j.jtcvs.2023.04.021.
3. Weerasooriya R, Khairy P, Litalien J, et al. Catheter ablation for atrial fibrillation: are results maintained at 5 years of follow-up? *J Am Coll Cardiol*. 2011;57:160–166.
4. Packer DL, Mark DB, Robb RA, et al. Effect of catheter ablation vs antiarrhythmic drug therapy on mortality, stroke, bleeding, and cardiac arrest among patients with atrial fibrillation: the CABANA randomized clinical trial. *J Am Med Assoc*. 2019;321:1261–1274.
5. Khan Z, Hamandi M, Khan H, DiMaio JM, Evans M. Convergent epicardial-endocardial ablation for treatment of long-standing persistent atrial fibrillation: a review of literature. *J Card Surg*. 2020;35:1306–1313.
6. Larson J, Merchant FM, Patel A, et al. Outcomes of convergent atrial fibrillation ablation with continuous rhythm monitoring. *J Cardiovasc Electrophysiol*. 2020;31:1270–1276.
7. Luo X, Li B, Zhang D, Zhu J, Qi L, Tang Y. Efficacy and safety of the convergent atrial fibrillation procedure: a meta-analysis of observational studies. *Interact Cardiovasc Thorac Surg*. 2019;28:169–176.
8. Cox JL. The minimally invasive Maze-III procedure. *Oper Tech Thorac Cardiovasc Surg*. 2000;5:79–92.
9. Schill MR, Sinn LA, Greenberg JW, et al. A minimally invasive stand-alone Cox-Maze procedure is as effective as median sternotomy approach. *Innovations (Phila)*. 2017;12:186–191.
10. Bolotin G, Kypson AP, Nifong LW, Chitwood WR Jr. Robotically-assisted left atrial fibrillation ablation and mitral valve repair through a right mini-thoracotomy. *Ann Thorac Surg*. 2004;78:e63–e64.

11. Nifong LW, Rodriguez E, Chitwood WR J. 540 Consecutive robotic mitral valve repairs including concomitant atrial fibrillation cryoablation. *Ann Thorac Surg*. 2012;94:38–42.
12. Alreshidan M, Roberts HG, Rankin JS, Wei LM, Badhwar V. Current approach to surgical ablation for atrial fibrillation. *Semin Thorac Cardiovasc Surg*. 2019;31:141–145.
13. Almousa A, Mehaffey JH, Wei LM, et al. Robotic-assisted cryothermic Cox maze for persistent atrial fibrillation: longitudinal follow-up. *J Thorac Cardiovasc Surg*. 2023;165:1828–1836.e1.
14. Cheema FH, Younus MJ, Pasha A, Cox JL, Roberts HG. An effective modification to simplify the right atrial lesion set of the Cox-cryomaze. *Ann Thorac Surg*. 2013;96:330–332.
15. Chandler N, Aslanidi O, Buckley D, et al. Computer three-dimensional anatomical reconstruction of the human sinus node and a novel paranodal area. *Anat Rec Adv Integr Anat Evol Biol*. 2011;294:970–979.
16. Friedman DJ, Piccini JP, Wang T, et al. Association between left atrial appendage occlusion and readmission for thromboembolism among patients with atrial fibrillation undergoing concomitant cardiac surgery. *J Am Med Assoc*. 2018;319:365–374.
17. Badhwar V, Scott Rankin J, Lee R, McCarthy PM, Wei LM. Contemporary left atrial appendage management during adult cardiac surgery. *J Thorac Cardiovasc Surg*. 2023;165:1398–1404.
18. Murashita T, Rankin JS, Wei LM, Roberts HG, Alkhouli MA, Badhwar V. Oral anticoagulation may not be necessary for patients discharged in sinus rhythm after the Cox Maze IV procedure. *J Thorac Cardiovasc Surg*. 2018;155:997–1006.
19. Badhwar V, Wei LM, Geirsson A, et al. Contemporary robotic cardiac surgical training. *J Thorac Cardiovasc Surg*. 2023;165:779–783.

17

The Cox-Maze-IV Procedure for Atrial Fibrillation

Ralph J. Damiano, Jr., Taras Lysyy

CHAPTER OUTLINE

The management of atrial fibrillation (AF) was transformed with the introduction of the Maze procedure in 1987, successfully pioneered by Dr. James Cox at Washington University in St. Louis.[1] The lesions of the Cox-Maze I, -II, and -III procedures were created with a scalpel and/or scissors, so all three of them were "cut-and-sew" Maze procedures. Cryoablation was used around the valve annuli. They were all performed through a median sternotomy and included strategically placed incisions in both atria but with different lesion patterns. The Roman numerals were assigned to differentiate between the three different lesion patterns used in the three operations. The cut-and-sew Maze procedures created nonconducting scars in the atria that interrupted or precluded the development of macro-reentrant circuits (drivers) that were felt to be responsible for sustaining AF.[2,3] The success rates were outstanding and durable and were associated with a freedom from symptomatic AF exceeding 90%, even in challenging cases of long-standing persistent AF (LSpAF).[4] The optimal lesion set was determined to be the Cox-Maze-III pattern, but despite its proven effectiveness, widespread adoption of this approach was limited because of its technical complexity, a substantial increase in cardiopulmonary bypass (CPB) time, and associated morbidity and mortality.[5,6]

In 1996, Cox replaced the cut-and-sew Maze-III procedure with a minimally invasive totally cryosurgical procedure in which the only surgical incision was the left atriotomy that was necessary to gain entrance into the left atrium (LA).[7,8] All other lesions in this minimally invasive cryosurgical Maze-III procedure were created with nondisposable linear cryoprobes through a right anterolateral minithoracotomy in the fourth intercostal space. However, the lesion pattern of this minimally invasive "CryoMaze-III" procedure remained identical to the lesion pattern of the cut-and-sew Maze-III procedure; therefore, the procedure was not given a separate Roman numeral (see Chapter 14).[4]

In 2002, after extensive laboratory testing, our group introduced the Cox-Maze-IV, a procedure combining bipolar radiofreqency (RF) and cryoablation technologies, leveraging their complementary strengths. Bipolar RF excelled in creating precise lines quickly, and cryoablation ensured the lines were safe and transmural near the valve annuli, as had been the practice in all previous iterations of the Cox-Maze procedure. The combination of bipolar RF and cryosurgery to replace the surgical incisions of the cut-and-sew Cox-Maze-III and the linear cryolesions of the CryoMaze-III procedures reduced the complexity and duration of the procedure, expanding its adoption.[9] Since its introduction, more than 1500 Cox-Maze-IV procedures have been performed at our institution, with excellent long-term results for both stand-alone and concomitant surgical procedures.[10] As of now, tens of thousands of Cox-Maze-IV procedures have been performed globally with excellent success rates, and it remains the only surgical procedure that is approved by the US Food and Drug Administration for the surgical treatment of patients with AF.

Despite the Cox-Maze-IV procedure's having a well-established record of safety and effectiveness over the long term, the current use falls short of meeting the needs of all the patients who could benefit from it. Many patients with AF undergoing cardiac surgery for other pathologies are not offered a concomitant Cox-Maze-IV procedure, whereas other patients with lone AF are not offered surgical intervention at all. Recent studies indicate that approximately one-third of patients with a history of AF undergoing mitral valve (MV) surgery do not receive the Cox-Maze-IV procedure.[11] Reluctance to perform a concomitant Cox-Maze procedure is multifactorial and is primarily attributed to insufficient education, experience, and comfort among surgeons. Additionally, over the past 35 years, numerous variations of the Cox-Maze procedure have been described, and multiple ablation devices have become available. This has resulted in a lack of procedural standardization and a perception that performing a Cox-Maze procedure is exceptionally complex. This chapter provides an overview and a practical guide detailing the surgical technique of the Cox-Maze-IV procedure performed either via a median sternotomy or a minimally invasive right mini-thoracotomy.

INDICATIONS FOR SURGICAL ABLATION

The *absolute indications* for surgical ablation of AF have been outlined in a recent consensus statement and are recommended for three categories of surgical procedures.[12–14]

Concomitant Open Atrial Operations (Mitral Valve Surgery)

Surgical ablation for AF is recommended for all symptomatic patients with documented AF during concomitant MV surgery (Class I, Level A). This recommendation comes with no added risk of operative mortality and major morbidity.

Concomitant Closed Atrial Operations (Aortic Valve, Coronary Artery Bypass Graft, or Aortic Valve and Coronary Artery Bypass Graft Surgery)

Surgical ablation for AF is recommended for all symptomatic patients with documented AF during concomitant isolated aortic valve surgery, isolated coronary artery bypass graft (CABG) surgery, and aortic valve plus CABG surgery (Class I, Level B nonrandomized). This recommendation comes with no added risk of operative mortality and major morbidity.

Stand-Alone Operations (Without Structural Heart Disease)

Stand-alone surgical ablation for AF is recommended for all symptomatic patients who are refractory or intolerant to antiarrhythmic drug therapy and who have failed one or more attempts of catheter ablation, are not candidates for catheter ablation, or prefer a surgical approach. (paroxysmal AF [PAF]: Class IIB, Level B randomized; persistent AF and LSpAF: Class IIA, Level B nonrandomized).

In our opinion, there are also *relative indications* for the surgical ablation of AF that were not addressed or explicitly mentioned in the consensus statement:

1. Patients with AF who have a contraindication to long-term anticoagulation therapy and a high stroke risk (CHA_2DS_2-VASc Score ≥2) are excellent candidates for surgery. The Cox-Maze-IV procedure not only effectively eliminates AF in the majority of these patients but also completely removes or closes the left atrial appendage (LAA), a significant source of atrial thrombus formation. Notably, the incidence of stroke after the procedure without anticoagulation has been remarkably low, even among patients with high CHA_2DS_2-VASc scores.
2. Patients with persistent and LSpAF who have experienced a stroke despite receiving adequate anticoagulation are at high risk for recurrent neurologic events. In our experience with 236 patients who underwent a stand-alone Cox-Maze-IV procedure, only 3 patients have experienced a postoperative stroke. This is particularly noteworthy considering that roughly 15% of these patients had previously had at least one cerebrovascular accident before undergoing surgery.[15]
3. Patients with AF and with a thrombus in the LAA are unsuitable candidates for catheter ablation and should be evaluated for surgical ablation.

Finally, in the present era of minimally invasive approaches such as totally thoracoscopic procedures and hybrid procedures, it is crucial to establish a collaborative multidisciplinary team involving both electrophysiologists and surgeons to guarantee the proper selection and treatment of patients requiring stand-alone procedures.

FOUNDATIONS AND PRACTICAL STRATEGIES FOR SUCCESSFUL LESIONS

To create successful lesions, several specific criteria must be met (see Chapter 20). The accurate *positioning of each lesion* in both atria is crucial to achieving consistently successful clinical results. In addition, each lesion must extend completely through the *full thickness* of the atrial myocardium. Ensuring a *continuous connection* between lesions is critical, avoiding any gaps that might compromise their overall effectiveness. We and others have demonstrated that even tiny gaps in a lesion can permit the conduction of aberrant electrical impulses.[16] Moreover, these small gaps may be proarrhythmic because they often lead to slow conduction, heightening the probability of sustaining reentrant circuits.

The energy source (e.g., RF, cryoablation) must be applied to create the desired transmural lesion effectively. To ensure complete lesion transmurally with bipolar RF clamps, we recommend performing a minimum of two consecutive (double) ablations without unclamping using either irrigated or non-irrigated bipolar RF clamps.[17,18] We perform two sets of double ablations for each right-sided atrial lesion, making slight adjustments in clamp position between each set. Similarly, to isolate the posterior LA and pulmonary veins (PVs), we routinely perform three sets of two successive (double) ablations without unclamping, making slight adjustments in clamp position between each set. Importantly, when using a non-irrigated bipolar clamp, it is essential to clean the clamp's jaws of any residue or char after every set of ablations. For cryoablation, we recommend performing a 2- to 3-minute ablation at the target temperature and to have excellent and firm contact between the probe and the target tissue.

In general, each lesion must originate from or terminate in tissue that is not electrically conductive, which means either another lesion or anatomically nonconductive tissue such as a valve annulus or vena cava orifice. This *anchoring* of both ends of a given lesion is necessary to interrupt conduction and/or isolate the tissue. Lesions that are not anchored on at least one side by electrically nonconductive tissue can potentially act as a nidus for macro-reentrant circuits. This results in the rotation of iatrogenic macro-reentrant circuits around the lesion as occurs in postoperative peri-mitral atrial flutter (see Chapter 48).[19]

Surgeons should strive to *minimize collateral damage* to adjacent healthy tissue. For example, the superior vena cava (SVC) end of the intercaval ablation line in the right atrium (RA) is placed as laterally and posteriorly as possible to avoid harming the anatomic sino-atrial node and atrial pacemaker complex (see Chapter 13). To avoid potential phrenic nerve injury during creation of the left atrial isthmus lesion, a protective lap pad should be placed beneath the cryoprobe's shaft. To avoid circumflex artery injury in creating the left atrial isthmus lesion, the isthmus line should be directed toward P2 and P3 scallops in a right-dominant system and toward the posteromedial commissure in a left-dominant system.

Monitoring tools are used to test for *intraoperative exit and/or entrance block* to and from each isolated PV before and after surgical ablation to confirm the successful creation of transmural nonconducting lesions. Meeting these criteria enhances the likelihood of successful lesion creation and contributes to the ultimate efficacy of the procedure.

PREOPERATIVE EVALUATION AND PLANNING

When evaluating patients for AF ablation surgery, it is important to conduct a comprehensive assessment of their medical history, comorbidities, and current medications. This evaluation seeks to understand the nature and patient impact of AF to determine the need for surgical intervention. Factors such as symptom severity, previous treatment outcomes, and associated comorbidities should be carefully considered.

Several preoperative diagnostic tests are essential in evaluating patients for AF ablation surgery. Continuous Holter monitoring documents the AF burden, differentiates between paroxysmal and nonparoxysmal AF (non-PAF), and can correlate symptoms with episodes of PAF. Transthoracic echocardiography (TTE) assesses valvular disease, detects left atrial and/or LAA thrombosis, and determines left atrial size, which is inversely related to surgical success. Suspected preoperative left atrial thrombi seen on TTE should be confirmed with transesophageal echocardiography (TEE). Patients who have had failed catheter ablation should have contrast-enhanced chest computed tomography (CT) to rule out PV stenosis that might require surgical correction. Additionally, coronary angiography not only helps to identify significant coronary artery lesions, but it also defines coronary anatomy, which is crucial in patients with a left-dominant circulation where the circumflex artery can be vulnerable during the creation of left atrial isthmus lesions.[20]

When planning a right mini-thoracotomy approach, it is important to consider several factors. A thorough assessment of pulmonary health is crucial, and further evaluation may be needed if single-lung ventilation is suspected of posing a challenge during surgery. Historical elements should be documented, including risk factors such as prior right thoracotomy, pectus excavatum, and peripheral vascular disease. All patients should have CT angiography (CTA) of the thoracic and abdominal aorta, iliac, and femoral vessels to determine the feasibility of femoral cannulation for CPB. Patients with a small anteroposterior diameter of the chest (<10 cm) make a right thoracotomy approach difficult.

Patients typically continue their antiarrhythmic and rate-control medications until the morning of surgery. Warfarin is usually stopped 3 to 5 days before surgery, and non–vitamin K antagonist oral anticoagulants are discontinued 36 to 48 hours before surgery. For patients at high risk of thromboembolic stroke (CHA_2DS_2-VASc score ≥5), recent stroke, or a history of systemic embolism, an intravenous (IV) heparin or bivalirudin bridge before surgery is recommended.

CONDUCT OF THE SURGICAL PROCEDURE

The following section describes the Cox-Maze-IV lesion set and the management of the LAA. It is important to note that the sequence described may differ from the actual intraoperative sequence because of anatomic considerations and the chosen operative approach.

Selection of Surgical Approach

Three decades of research and clinical experience have shaped our clinical decision-making process, and the following description reflects our current practice pattern. The Cox-Maze-IV procedure can be performed through either a median sternotomy or a minimally invasive right mini-thoracotomy. The choice of approach is determined by the presence or absence of concomitant cardiac pathology, patient-specific anatomic characteristics, and the expertise of the operating surgeon.[21] In our institution, the preferred surgical approach for a Cox-Maze-IV procedure in patients undergoing stand-alone AF ablation or as a concomitant procedure to mitral or tricuspid valve surgery is a right mini-thoracotomy. Median sternotomy is reserved for patients with severe peripheral vascular disease that hinders femoral cannulation for CPB, patients with a history of a previous right thoracotomy, individuals with severe left ventricular dysfunction or chest wall deformities such as pectus excavatum,[20] or cases in which the Cox-Maze-IV procedure is combined with other concomitant procedures such as aortic valve replacement and coronary artery bypass grafting.[21] All Cox-Maze-IV patients should undergo preoperative echocardiography to assess ventricular function and to search for intracardiac thrombosis, patent foramen ovale (PFO) or atrial septal defect (ASD), and aortic insufficiency.

Cardiopulmonary Bypass

The Cox-Maze-IV procedure performed through a median sternotomy uses central cannulation of the aorta and bicaval cannulation or, rarely, femoral artery and vein cannulation for CPB. With a right mini-thoracotomy approach, peripheral cannulation is performed through a femoral cutdown (our preferred approach) or percutaneous cannulation of the femoral artery and vein.

Intraoperative Cardioversion and Pulmonary Vein Exit Block Testing

Patients who are in AF at the time of surgery receive a dose of IV amiodarone after initiation of CPB. If a left atrial thrombus can be ruled out by intraoperative TEE, electrical cardioversion is performed. All patients undergo intraoperative exit block testing from each pair of isolated PVs after surgical ablation. This testing involves standard sterilizable insulated bipolar forceps connected to pacing cables and a temporary pacemaker (100–120 ppm). Pacing thresholds are measured from the PVs. Using a bipolar RF ablation device, the PVs are isolated by ablating a cuff of surrounding atrial tissue. Confirmation of electrical isolation is achieved by demonstrating the exit block from each PV. Although all four PVs are usually tested when using a median sternotomy, only the right PVs can be tested during minimally invasive right mini-thoracotomy. This quick, efficient, and inexpensive technique for assessing lesion integrity is the sole intraoperative quality control method. It confirms the successful creation of transmural nonconductive lesions and complete isolation of the PVs immediately after surgical ablation.

SURGICAL TECHNIQUE

Right Atrial Lesions

The right atrial lesion set of the Cox-Maze-IV includes (1) a continuous line of block from the SVC to the inferior vena cava (IVC), (2) a separate line from this intercaval line to the nonconductive tissue of the tricuspid annulus, and (3) a third lesion from the base of the right atrial appendage (RAA) across the anterolateral RA, taking care not to damage the sinoatrial (SA) or atrioventricular (AV) nodes (Figs. 17.1 to 17.3). These RA lesions differ from those in the Cox-Maze-III procedure in that the lesion to prevent reentry around the base of the RAA in the Cox-Maze-III procedure is placed more anteriorly in the RA extending from lesion #3 up to the tip of the RAA (see Chapters 13 and 14).

Substantial evidence supports the significance of the RA in the maintenance of persistent AF and of the cavotricuspid isthmus in classic atrial flutter.[22,23] Previous studies, including our own, have shown that up to one-third of AF drivers are located in the RA.[23] This is why the best late outcomes of surgical ablation have been observed in patients who receive a biatrial lesion set rather than a LA-only lesion set.[24]

We prefer to perform the right atrial lesion set on CPB before aortic cross-clamping. A bipolar RF ablation clamp is used for most lesions (see Figs. 17.1 and 17.3). When there is no need to open the RA, the right atrial free-wall ablations are typically made through three

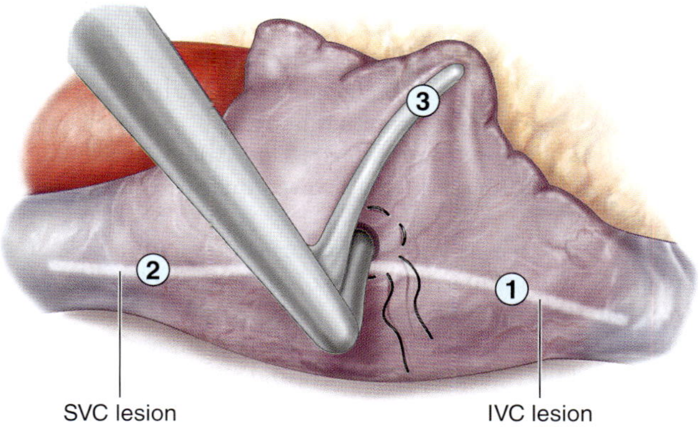

Fig. 17.1 Application of first pursestring suture and stab incision just above the interatrial septum, midway between the superior vena cava (SVC) and inferior vena cava (IVC), followed by radiofrequency ablations of the *(1)* IVC, *(2)* SVC, and *(3)* right atrial free wall directed toward the atrioventricular groove near the acute margin of the heart. This lesion is traditionally called the "T" lesion.

pursestring sutures (see Chapter 14). However, a single incision in the right atrial free wall is necessary if there is a need to repair the tricuspid valve or address a defect in the atrial septum (PFO or ASD). A small right atriotomy is also helpful for visualizing and cannulating the coronary sinus ostium for retrograde cardioplegia, and is used in all sternotomy cases.

The first pursestring suture is placed just above the interatrial septum, midway between the SVC and IVC. (It is placed two-thirds of the way down from the SVC to the IVC in the Cox-Maze-III procedure.) It is crucial to avoid the crista terminalis because of the thickness of the tissue in the area. One jaw of the bipolar RF clamp is introduced into the RA through a stab incision. Three separate ablation lines are performed through this first pursestring suture. These lines extend up into the SVC, down into the IVC, and across the right atrial free wall toward the AV groove near the acute margin of the heart (see Fig. 17.1). The IVC ablation line should extend as far as possible onto the IVC, and the SVC ablation line should be placed as lateral and posterior as possible to reduce the risk of injury to the anatomic SA node.

The second pursestring suture is placed at the superior end of the right atrial free wall ablation line near the AV groove. Temporarily filling the RA with volume can facilitate the placement of this pursestring suture. Care must be taken to avoid injuring the right coronary artery in this area. A linear cryoprobe is placed through this pursestring to extend the right atrial free-wall line (the "T" lesion) down to the tricuspid valve annulus, where it terminates at the 2 o'clock position (see Fig. 17.2). Before initiating freezing, it is important to palpate the cryoprobe in the right ventricle. Additionally, confirmation of correct placement is ensured when the beating heart deflects the probe. For nitrous oxide (N_2O) devices, cryoablations are performed at −60°C for 3 minutes each. For argon devices, the cryoablation is performed between −140°C and −160°C for 2 minutes each.

The third pursestring suture is placed at the base of the RAA. One jaw of the bipolar RF clamp is inserted through this pursestring into the RA, and a second right atrial free wall ablation is created, extending several centimeters toward the SVC. It is crucial to avoid the anatomic SA node, so we leave a minimum of 2 cm between the end of this ablation line and the SVC line (see Fig. 17.3). We now perform this ablation line down the aortic side of the RAA to avoid the area of the SA node complex. The right atrial lesion set is completed by performing another endocardial cryoablation down to the tricuspid valve annulus at approximately the 10 o'clock position (Fig. 17.4).

Left Atrial Lesions

The primary goals of the LA lesion set are (1) to establish a complete "box lesion" around all four PVs that electrically isolates not only the PVs but also the intervening posterior left atrial wall between the right and left PVs and (2) to block electrical conduction across the left atrial isthmus by connecting the box lesion to the mitral annulus, which is nonconductive.

Achieving complete isolation of the four PVs and the posterior LA with a box lesion is the single most important component of both the Cox-Maze-IV and Cox-Maze-III procedures (see Chapter 14, Fig. 14.28). The posterior LA, encompassing the PVs, has consistently been identified as essential for initiating and maintaining AF.

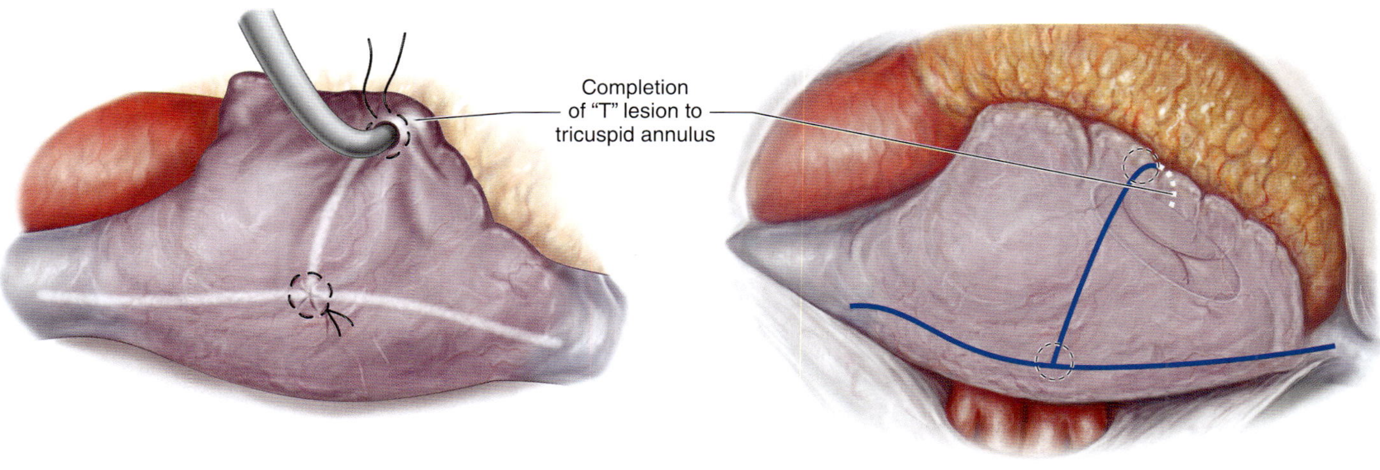

Fig. 17.2 *Left panel,* The second pursestring suture and stab incision near the atrioventricular groove at the end of the first right atrial free wall ablation line, followed by an endocardial cryolesion down to the tricuspid annulus at the 2 o'clock position. *Right panel,* Schematic illustration for clarification.

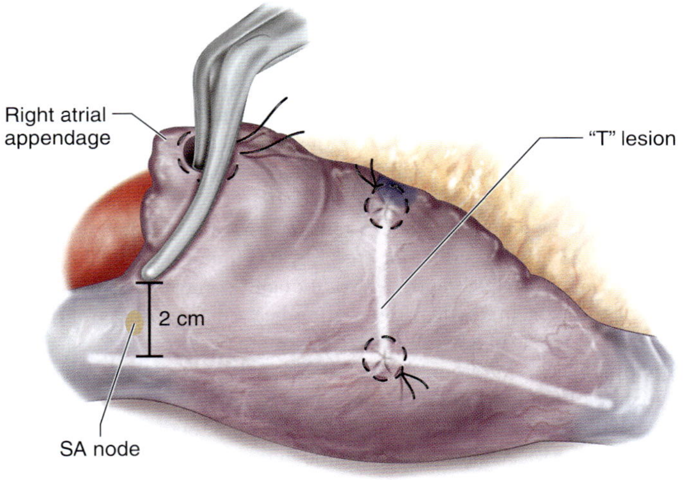

Fig. 17.3 The third pursestring suture at the base of the right atrial appendage and creation of a right atrial free wall lesion using a bipolar radiofrequency clamp. The end of this lesion should be at least 2 cm from the intercaval line. The position of the anatomic sinoatrial (SA) node varies.

Approximately 70% of ectopic atrial triggers in patients with concomitant PAF are located within this area (see Chapter 25).[25,26] Furthermore, our data have shown that even if the PVs are successfully isolated and all of the other left atrial and right atrial lesions are complete, failure to isolate the posterior wall of the LA results in only a 33% freedom from recurrent atrial tachyarrhythmias at 5 years.[24] Two randomized controlled studies showed that success rates for surgical PV isolation (PVI) are comparable to those of catheter PVI but with increased morbidity.[27,28] They also showed that PVI with either method that does not include exclusion of the posterior left atrial wall is an inadequate therapy for AF.

A linear lesion, known as the "left atrial isthmus line," or the "mitral line," connecting the box lesion to the posterior MV annulus is essential to prevent "atypical LA flutter," which is also called "perimitral flutter."[29] Moreover, studies dating as far back as the late 1970s during development of the left atrial isolation procedure have shown that the coronary sinus itself can conduct electrical impulses (see Chapter 9, Fig. 9.14). Therefore, to block conduction across the left atrial isthmus and prevent postoperative perimitral flutter, it is necessary to block conduction through both the coronary sinus with a cryolesion and conduction through the left atrial myocardium with the mitral line (see Chapter 48).[30]

Right PV isolation is typically performed on CPB before cross-clamping the aorta as part of the box lesion. After blunt dissection between the right pulmonary artery and the right superior PV and opening the oblique sinus posterior to the IVC, an umbilical tape is passed around the right PVs (Fig. 17.5), and pacing is performed before and after a bipolar RF clamp is applied to isolate the right PVs (Fig. 17.6). It is important to place the bipolar clamp well up onto the LA to isolate as large a cuff of atrial tissue as possible around the right PVs. When performing this ablation, three sets of two consecutive (double) ablations without unclamping are performed with slight adjustments in position between each set, effectively resulting in the creation of three closely positioned concentric circles in the LA around the orifices of the right PVs. We then document complete isolation of the PVs by testing for exit block (see Chapter 20).

Left-sided PV isolation is performed similarly to the right PVI if the Cox-Maze-IV procedure is performed through a standard median sternotomy. However, when the procedure is performed through a minimally invasive right mini-thoracotomy, left PV isolation is performed from the inside of the LA as it is done in the Cox-Maze-III procedure. After the placement of a left atrial retractor and lift system, the endocardial surfaces of the LA and MV are visualized (Fig. 17.7). Starting from the inferior aspect of the left atriotomy, the bipolar RF clamp is used to create an ablation line across the floor of the LA toward the left inferior PV orifice, commonly referred to as "inferior connecting lesion" or the "floor lesion" (Fig. 17.8). From the superior aspect of the left atriotomy, the bipolar RF clamp is used to create another ablation line across the roof of the LA toward the left superior PV, commonly referred to as the "superior connecting lesion" or the "roof lesion." The endpoints of the bipolar ablation lines are usually marked with methylene blue if they are challenging to visualize.

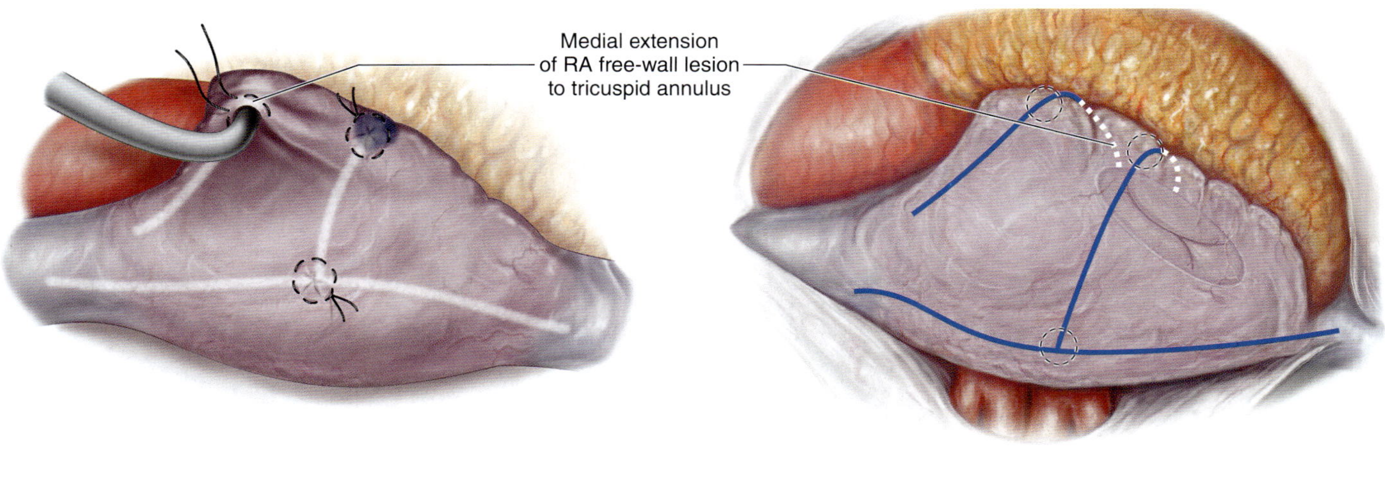

Fig. 17.4 *Left panel,* Completion of the right atrial (RA) lesion set by extending an endocardial cryolesion from the end of the RA free-wall lesion down to the 10 o'clock position on the tricuspid annulus. *Right panel,* Schematic illustration for clarification.

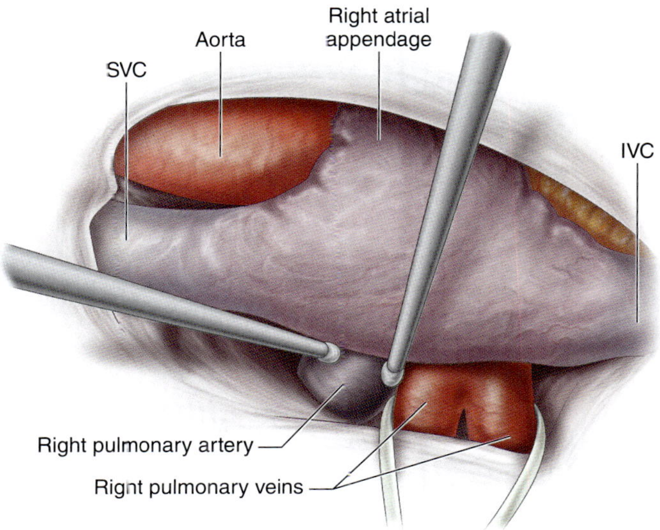

Fig. 17.5 Blunt dissection and mobilization of the space between the right superior pulmonary vein and the right pulmonary artery from underneath the superior vena cava (SVC). *IVC,* Inferior vena cava.

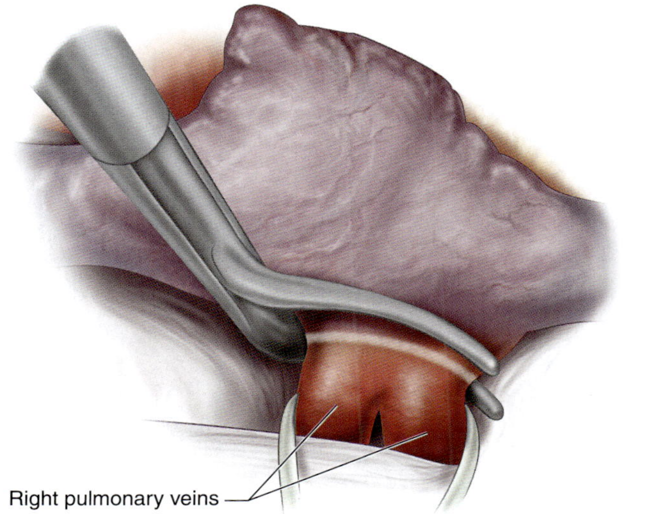

Fig. 17.6 Right-sided pulmonary vein isolation using a bipolar radiofrequency clamp.

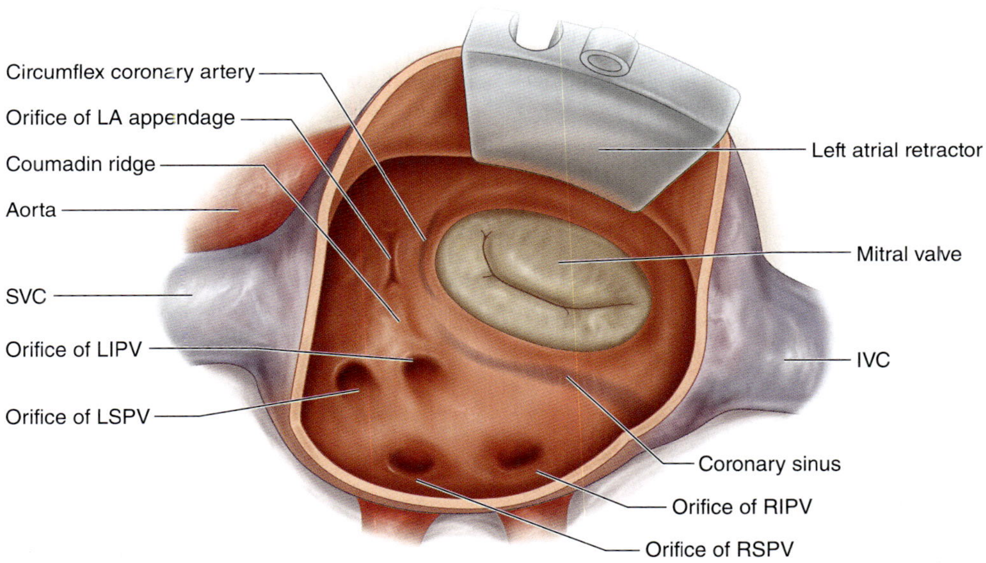

Fig. 17.7 Internal anatomy of the left atrium through a left atriotomy in Waterston's groove. *IVC,* Inferior vena cava; *LAA,* left atrial appendage; *LIPV,* left inferior pulmonary vein; *LSPV,* left superior pulmonary vein; *RIPV,* right inferior pulmonary vein; *RSPV,* right superior pulmonary vein; *SVC,* superior vena cava.

The mitral isthmus line is then created either with cryoablation alone or with a combination of bipolar RF and cryoablation depending on the anatomy of the mitral isthmus (Figs. 17.8 to 17.10). The presence of the AV groove fat pad and its contents in that area (see Chapter 3, Fig. 3.22) prevents the bipolar RF clamp from creating a transmural lesion all the way to the mitral annulus. The bipolar RF clamp is used, when needed, from the lower aspect of the left atriotomy to create an ablation line across the floor of the LA, heading toward the MV annulus and potentially across the coronary sinus (see Fig. 17.8). To bridge the gap of 1 to 2 cm and connect the bipolar ablation line to the annulus, an endocardial cryoablation is used toward the annulus (see Fig. 17.9). In many instances, a linear cryoprobe can complete this mitral isthmus lesion alone. Endocardial cryoablation is advantageous for preserving the heart's fibrous skeleton, making it well-suited for ablation on valvular tissue. If needed, placing a lap pad beneath the cryoprobe's shaft can reduce the risk of injury to the right phrenic nerve. To ensure complete conduction block across the LA isthmus, the coronary sinus cryolesion must be in line with the endocardial mitral line lesion (see Fig. 17.10).

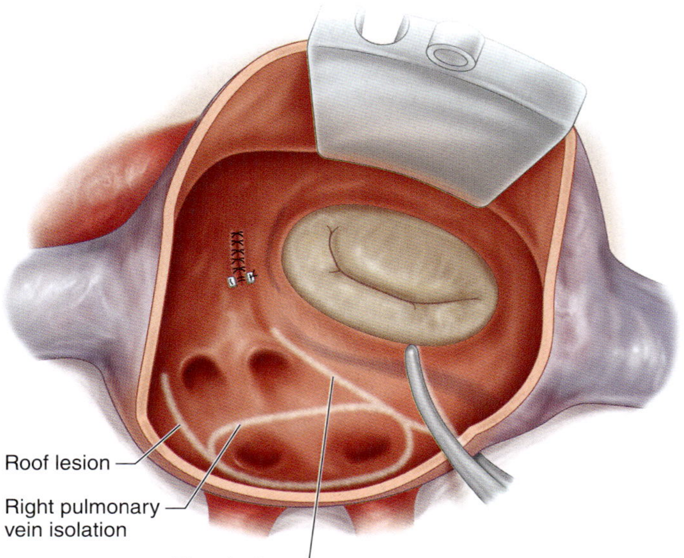

Fig. 17.8 Internal view of the right-sided pulmonary vein isolation with superior (roof) and inferior (floor) connecting lesions. Occasionally, the endocardial mitral line and the epicardial coronary sinus lesion can be created simultaneously with a bipolar radiofrequency clamp by the clamp from the lower end of the left atriotomy all the way to the mitral annulus. This should only be done in patients with dominant right coronary artery systems, and this lesion is placed between the last marginal branch of the distal circumflex coronary artery and the posterior descending branch of the right coronary artery in the so-called "watershed" area of the left atrioventricular groove. It should never be done in patients with either left-dominant or balanced coronary artery anatomy.

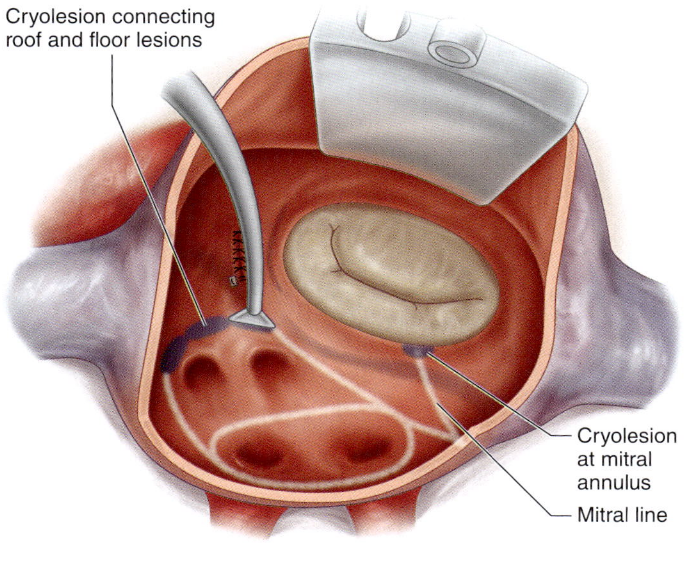

Fig. 17.9 In most instances, the proximal portion of the mitral line that is created with the bipolar radiofrequency clamp is confined to the atrial myocardium above the left atrioventricular groove. The remainder of the endocardial mitral line is completed with an endocardial linear cryolesion.

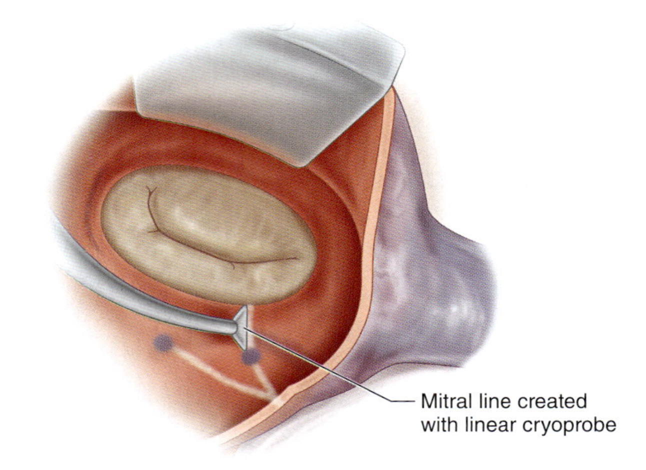

Fig. 17.10 Epicardial cryoablation of the coronary sinus using a linear cryoprobe overlying the coronary sinus.

This is accomplished using an epicardial application of cryoenergy. It is essential to highlight a potential risk to the circumflex artery when creating the left atrial isthmus lesion at the mitral annulus in patients with a left-dominant system. For patients with a right-dominant system, the isthmus line is typically directed toward the junction of the P2 and P3 scallops of the posterior leaflet. In patients with a left-dominant system, injury can be prevented by directing the ablation toward the posteromedial commissure.

Cryoablation is then performed around the left PVs and along the lateral ridge, connecting the roof and floor lesions to complete the box. This can be done using a linear cryoprobe as described in the Cox-CryoMaze-III procedure (Fig. 17.11).

The left atriotomy is then closed with a running polypropylene suture. The aorta is unclamped, and after rewarming, the heart is examined with TEE for retained air and ventricular and valvular function. The patient is subsequently weaned from CPB.

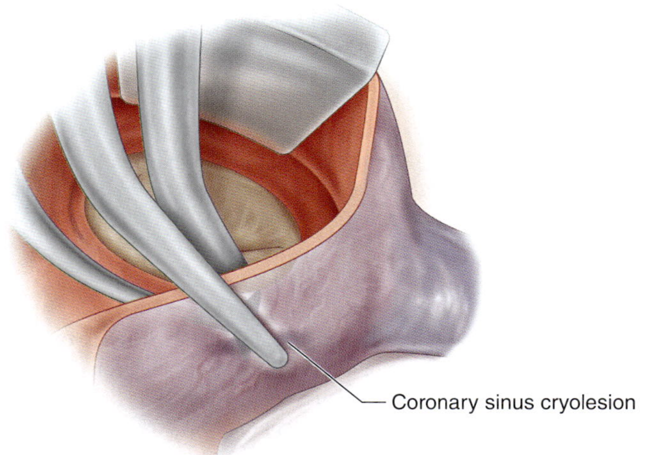

Fig. 17.11 Endocardial left-sided pulmonary vein isolation by cryoablation connecting the superior ("roof") and inferior ("floor") lesions with sequential cryolesions (depicted as *light blue lines*).

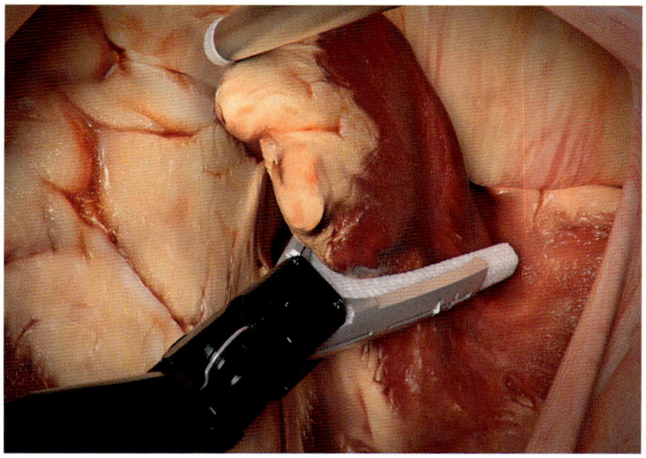

Fig. 17.12 Application of a left atrial appendage clip.

Left Atrial Appendage Management

Effective management of the LAA is crucial because the majority of thromboembolic strokes in patients with AF originate in the LAA. Thus removing or excluding the LAA significantly reduces the risk of stroke and systemic embolism.[31,32]

In our experience, we have found that either excising the LAA or using an epicardial exclusion device such as AtriClip (AtriCure, Inc.) is the most successful method for eliminating the LAA (Fig. 17.12). Unfortunately, stapler exclusion, oversewing, and ligation techniques have shown relatively high failure rates.[33,34] The appendage clip, specifically the AtriClip, has demonstrated excellent long-term success rates, accomplishing complete LAA occlusion with an excellent safety profile.[35,36] As a result, clipping the LAA is currently the most reasonable approach whether performed through minimally invasive or open surgical procedures. In a mini-thoracotomy approach, we usually clip the LAA through the transverse sinus prior to unclamping. This allows for possible endocardial oversewing of the LAA if placement of the clip is unsuccessful.

Regardless of whether the LAA is excised or clipped, it is imperative to avoid leaving a stump at the base of the occluded or excised appendage. Residual LAA tissue is thrombogenic when connected to the LA.[37] Thus even without a residual stump, if not properly anchored to electrically nonconductive tissue, the LAA exclusion line can still act as a potential source for a flutter circuit.[19] Therefore we also establish a lesion from the excluded LAA to the left PV lesion, connecting the LAA exclusion to the electrically excluded posterior LA, in a sternotomy approach. In the mini-thoracotomy approach, the cryoablation along the lateral ridge behind the left PVs connects the box to the base of the LAA (Video 17.1).

COMPLICATIONS AND PREVENTION STRATEGIES

The rate of major complications in our recently published series of 853 consecutive patients who underwent either stand-alone or concomitant Cox-Maze-IV procedures showed a 3.3% 30-day mortality rate, immediate or early postoperative atrial tachyarrhythmias rate of 56.9%, renal failure requiring dialysis rate of 5.6%, bleeding requiring reoperation rate of 2.5%, and cerebrovascular accident rate of 1.6%.[38] These adverse outcomes are reduced with the right mini-thoracotomy approach. In a large series of stand-alone Cox-Maze IV procedures recently published we have had no operative mortality.

Complications unique to the Cox-Maze procedure include rhythm disturbances such as immediate or early atrial tachyarrhythmias, sinus node dysfunction requiring pacemaker insertion (see Chapter 21), and late recurrence of atrial tachyarrhythmias. Early arrhythmias are common and typically managed with rate control and eventual cardioversion if persistent. These complications are described in more detail later.

The need for new permanent pacemakers after the Cox-Maze-IV procedure is reported to be 5% to 12%.[38,39] This can be attributed to various factors, including the unmasking of preexisting sick sinus, concomitant valve surgery, damage to autonomic nerve input as a result of excessive extracardiac dissection, premature implantation of a pacemaker after temporary junctional rhythm immediately postoperatively, surgical error, and patient selection.[40] See Chapter 21 for an in-depth discussion of this issue.

Potential Intraoperative Complications

Injury of the Large Vessels or Heart Structures

There is a risk of injuring large vessels and heart tissues during the external blunt dissection required to encircle the PVs to isolate them with a bipolar RF clamp in the Cox-Maze-IV procedure. Careful and gentle dissection should follow the plane between anatomic structures and should avoid forceful or direct impact on large vessels and heart structures. If slight bleeding is observed, the blunt dissection should be stopped immediately to identify the bleeding source. Patients with a history of multiple catheter ablations, prior cardiac surgery, or pericarditis may pose challenges during this external blunt dissection.

Tissue Injury Caused by Manipulation of the Cryoprobe While Freezing

Delicate cardiac tissues can be damaged by allowing slight manipulation of the cryoprobe during the freezing phase of surgical cryoablation. After the target tissue is frozen, if the cryoprobe is allowed to move, "cracks" can develop between the edge of the frozen tissue and the surrounding unfrozen tissue. When the area thaws, these "cracks" become lacerations, so it is extremely important for the surgeon to focus on keeping the cryoprobe absolutely stable during the freezing phase of cryoablation. This is especially true during creation of the mitral isthmus line, tricuspid annulus lesions, and coronary sinus lesions. These lesions should be completed before any valve repair or replacement procedure, and RF ablation should never be used near these delicate structures.

Injury of the Circumflex Coronary Artery

The circumflex coronary artery can theoretically be injured during the creation of a left atrial isthmus lesion ("mitral line") or during LAA clip placement. When creating the left atrial isthmus lesion, the line should be directed toward the P2 and P3 scallops of the MV in a right-dominant coronary system and toward the posteromedial commissure of the MV in a left-dominant system. The active administration of antegrade cardioplegia during cryoablation helps minimize the risk of coronary artery injury, though this is usually not necessary. During LAA clip placement, ensure that the entire clip and the appendage base are visualized. Position the clip parallel to the base of the appendage and then confirm visually that there is no residual stump.

Injury of the Phrenic Nerve

The most common nerve injury during the Cox-Maze-IV procedure is to the right phrenic nerve, which can occur when the pericardiotomy is performed with an electrocautery during a minimally invasive right mini-thoracotomy. The most common phrenic nerve injury during cryosurgery results from the handle of the cryoprobe inadvertently resting on the right phrenic nerve when performing the left atrial lesions through the right mini-thoracotomy. It is advisable to open the pericardium at least 2 cm anterior to the right phrenic nerve when using the minimally invasive right mini-thoracotomy approach. In addition, it is helpful to protect the nerve by placing a lap pad between it and the cryoprobe when the cryoprobe's shaft is near the phrenic nerve.

Potential Postoperative Complications

Acute Kidney Injury

Adding a concomitant Cox-Maze-IV procedure to CABG and valve surgery increases the risk of postoperative acute kidney injury but not the risk of permanent dialysis in some series.[41] Nephrotoxic drugs and imaging studies with nephrotoxic contrast (e.g., coronary angiography, CTA, contrast-enhanced CT/magnetic resonance imaging) should be avoided in the perioperative period if possible. Preferably, ablation surgery should be delayed for at least 1 to 2 weeks after these imaging studies to allow the kidneys to recover from potential contrast-induced injury.

Stenosis of the Pulmonary Vein Orifices

After RF ablation, tissue fibrosis and contraction occur during the healing process. Therefore, placing the bipolar RF clamp near the orifices of the PVs can result in scarring and PV stenosis. This has been a problem after RF catheter ablation but not so much for RF surgical ablation because of the direct vision by surgeons. Thus when isolating the PVs, the bipolar RF clamp should be positioned as far up onto the atrium as possible to create a large cuff of atrial tissue around the PVs to decrease the likelihood of causing later PV stenosis (see Fig. 17.6).

Special Consideration for Patients With Prior Cardiac Intervention

Patients with a history of failed catheter ablations require special attention because of the additional technical challenges they may present during surgery. In patients undergoing a stand-alone or concomitant Cox-Maze-IV procedure, 24% had experienced at least one prior failed catheter ablation,[38] with an incidence of 59% in the stand-alone group.[15]

Femoral Artery Access and Cannulation

Previous percutaneous femoral artery and vein catheterizations, especially after multiple or complicated procedures (e.g., hematoma formation), can result in scarring and fibrosis of the arterial wall and surrounding tissues. For this reason, imaging studies (e.g., CTA of the thoracic and abdominal aorta, iliac, and femoral vessels) should be conducted before surgery to evaluate the size, tortuosity, and wall thickness of the femoral arteries and surrounding tissues.

Pericardial Adhesions

Previous catheter ablations or transcatheter interventions may cause intrapericardial inflammation or bleeding, resulting in the development of intrapericardial adhesions. Dense pericardial adhesions between the right superior PV and right pulmonary artery can be a particular challenge. If dissection in this area to encircle the right PVs proves too difficult, one can create the left atrial box lesion from inside the LA under cardioplegic arrest as is done in the Cox-CryoMaze-III procedure (see Chapter 14).

Stiff and Scarred Atria

Multiple catheter ablations can lead to extensive damage and scarring of the left atrial endocardium. The success of cryoablations relies on close contact of the cryoprobe with the endocardium of the atrial wall, which is often challenging in nonpliable, stiff, and scarred atria. This challenge often results in interrupted ablation lines caused by "folding ablation gaps" or "gaps under the bridge" (see Chapter 20). When using a flexible cryoprobe, bend and adjust it to ensure close contact with the atrial wall throughout the length of the desired cryolesion. Moderate pressure should then be applied by the cryoprobe against the left atrial wall to flatten atrial folds and prevent gaps. If there is suspicion of a gap after the first cryoablation attempt, the cryolesion should be placed again.

Stiff and Scarred Pulmonary Veins and Restricted Left Atrium

Multiple catheter ablations can lead to extensive damage and scarring of the PVs and LA. This can cause differences in tissue compliance, leading to dissection and tearing between scarred and adjacent healthy tissue. The risk is significantly increased during concomitant CABG surgery such as circumflex coronary artery bypass grafting, which requires lifting or moving the heart. Thus care must be taken to minimize the risk of injury during heart manipulation, especially with lifting maneuvers.

Challenges With Occlusion of the Left Atrial Appendage

Scarring from multiple catheter ablations in the LAA and LA can occasionally impede mobilization and occlusion of the LAA. This can increase the risk of leaving an appendage stump. Therefore, caution should be exercised when performing LAA occlusion in patients with extensive scarring from multiple catheter ablations. In some situations, it is necessary to oversew the LAA from inside the LA, if the LAA can not be mobilized externally. This is usually done with a two-layer prolene closure. Late recannulization is higher with this approach compared to excision or clipping.

Iatrogenic Atrial Septal Defect

Transseptal access is necessary for LA catheter ablation procedures, and iatrogenic ASD is a known postprocedural complication.[42] In patients with a residual ASD after a previous catheter ablation, the right-sided lesions should be performed under cardioplegia arrest, and the ASD closed.

Severe Pulmonary Vein Stenosis or Occlusion

Catheter-based PV isolation may result in scarring and stenosis of the PV ostia. PV imaging should be performed in patients with previous catheter ablations to assess for PV stenosis or occlusion. If present and symptomatic, it can be addressed at the time of surgery.

POSTOPERATIVE MANAGEMENT

After a Cox-Maze-IV procedure, the primary objective in the immediate postoperative period is to optimize cardiac output. Continuous monitoring is vital for the early detection of potential complications such as bleeding, arrhythmias, and thromboembolic events. Adequate pain management is imperative to ensure patient comfort and promote timely mobilization. Optimal fluid management is essential for maintaining hemodynamic stability and preventing dehydration or fluid overload. However, rhythm management is the most unique postoperative consideration after a Cox-Maze-IV procedure. We routinely place temporary atrial and ventricular epicardial pacing wires in all patients undergoing an ablation procedure. These wires serve dual purposes: (1) to record unipolar and bipolar atrial electrograms to differentiate atrial and junctional rhythms and (2) to provide a means for atrial or AV sequential pacing postoperatively to optimize cardiac hemodynamics.

Regular interrogation of the underlying rhythm is conducted in the intensive care unit (ICU). A *junctional rhythm* is the most common arrhythmia after any iteration of the Cox-Maze procedure (see Chapter 21). A slow junctional escape rhythm (rate <60 beats/min) can be managed by A-pacing if AV conduction is normal or by AV sequential pacing if AV conduction is impaired. Drugs with a negative chronotropic effect, such as beta-blockers, amiodarone, and sotalol, should be discontinued in the presence of a postoperative junctional rhythm. *Nonparoxysmal AV junctional tachycardia* (rate 70–130 beats/min) results from enhanced automaticity in the bundle of His, suggested by a regular ventricular rate in patients with AF, which can be confirmed with an atrial electrogram. To establish AV synchrony, overriding pacing at a faster rate may suffice. Digoxin should be discontinued if the patient is taking this medication. If not, a beta-blocker or calcium channel blocker (diltiazem or verapamil) should be instituted to slow the junctional rhythm rate so that atrial or AV sequential pacing can then be used to establish AV synchrony.

Junctional rhythm typically resolves within several days after a Cox-Maze procedure. Antiarrhythmic drugs should not be initiated until sinus rhythm is restored, especially in patients with bradyarrhythmias. Patients with persistent bradycardia caused by a junctional rhythm are monitored for 5 to 7 days to allow the sinus node to recover, and antiarrhythmic drugs and beta-blockers are avoided. If symptomatic bradycardia persists, a dual-chamber pacemaker should be considered. In our practice, pacemaker insertion usually occurs after at least a 5-day observation period. In 5% to 12% of patients undergoing a Cox-Maze-IV procedure, a permanent pacemaker is required because of persistent heart block or sinus node dysfunction. This is more common in older adults and patients having concomitant valve surgery.[38,43]

Atrial tachyarrhythmias recur shortly after a Cox-Maze-IV procedure in approximately half of the patients. These arrhythmias are typically transient, resolving within the first month after surgery. Patients should be educated about the possibility of developing early arrhythmias and reassured that it is a normal part of the healing process related to atrial inflammation. The ability to record atrial electrograms can be of great help in diagnosing immediate postoperative atrial arrhythmias because the P wave may be small and difficult to see on a limb-lead tracing after a Cox-Maze procedure.

Patients with atrial arrhythmias are managed by pharmacologic rate control and Class I or Class III antiarrhythmic drugs. Elective cardioversion can be performed, ideally before hospital discharge. It can take 1 to 3 weeks after surgery for the inflammation to subside, so repeat cardioversion after hospital discharge is sometimes necessary. Antiarrhythmic drugs are typically continued for the first 2 months after surgery, with close monitoring of the QT interval.

Late atrial tachyarrhythmias that recur after the 3-month blanking period may require more aggressive treatment. Pharmacologic and nonpharmacologic treatments, along with lifestyle changes, are crucial. Collaboration among specialists, patient education, and follow-up visits are essential. Advanced therapies, including electrophysiologic studies and repeat catheter ablation, may be needed for difficult cases when the patient is symptomatic, although this has been unusual in our experience. A comprehensive, multidisciplinary approach is the key to optimal symptom control and rhythm stabilization after surgery.

Anticoagulation therapy is initiated in all Cox-Maze-IV patients without contraindications using either warfarin or a new class of direct anticoagulants such as apixaban or rivaroxaban for 3 to 6 months after surgery. Discontinuation of anticoagulation is considered after this period for patients free of both atrial tachyarrhythmias and antiarrhythmic drugs on prolonged monitoring and with no left atrial stasis or thrombus on echocardiography. This approach has proven effective in achieving a low stroke rate after the Cox-Maze-IV procedure, even in patients with high CHA_2DS_2-VASc scores.[24,44]

Regular follow-up visits and close monitoring of patients postoperatively are essential to assess surgical outcomes, detect complications, and adjust treatment as needed. In our clinic, patients are seen at 1,3, 6, and 12 months and then annually for life.

SURGICAL OUTCOMES

The Cox-Maze procedure is the most effective treatment for patients with AF and is widely recognized as the gold standard for the surgical treatment of AF. In its Cox-Maze-IV iteration, surgical incisions and linear cryolesions are supplanted by bipolar RF and linear cryolesions, which has resulted in significant shortening of the procedure while maintaining the exceptional success rate of the Cox-Maze-III procedure. A propensity score-matching analysis conducted by our group revealed no significant difference in freedom from AF at 3, 6, or 12 months between the Cox-Maze-III and the Cox-Maze-IV procedures.[6] However, the Cox-Maze-IV procedure demonstrated a significant reduction in operative time and lower complication rates than the original cut-and-sew Cox-Maze-III procedure while preserving the high success rate observed with the Cox-Maze-III procedure.[6,45] No direct comparison between the Cox-Maze-IV and the totally cryosurgical Cox-Maze-III (CryoMaze-III) procedure has been conducted.

The Cox-Maze-IV procedure has consistently demonstrated excellent long-term success rates in patients undergoing stand-alone and concomitant procedures, as evidenced by numerous studies including multiple centers shown in Table 17.1.[5,38,43,46–50,51] In our comprehensive series of 853 consecutive patients, the majority presented with non-PAF (60%), and 76% underwent prolonged monitoring during follow-up.

TABLE 17.1 Late Outcomes of the Cox-Maze Procedure

Reference	Study Type	Patients (*n*)	PAF (%)	Follow-up (years)	ATA Free or NSR	AAD Free or NSR	Stroke Free
Khiabani et al.[38]	Single center	853	40	10	92% at 1 year	84% at 1 year	NR
					84% at 5 years	71% at 5 years	
					77% at 10 years	61% at 10 years	
Gerdisch et al.[49]	Multicenter	807	33	3	88% at 1 year	81% at 1 year	
					85% at 3 years	73% at 3 years	94.8% at 3 years
Ad et al.[50]	Single Center	473	15	7	90% at 1 year	83% at 1 year	
					80% at 5 years	69% at 5 years	
					66% at 7 years	55% at 7 years	96.6% at 7 years
McCarthy et al.[43]	Multicenter	363	0	3	80% at 1 year	66% at 1 year	
					78% at 2 years	65% at 2 years	
					76% at 3 years	64% at 3 years	95.6% at 7 years

AAD, Antiarrhythmic drug; *ATA*, atrial tachyarrhythmia; *NR*, not reported; *NSR*, normal sinus rhythm; *TIA*, transient ischemic attack.

The freedom rates from atrial tachyarrhythmias were 92%, 84%, and 77% at 1, 5, and 10 years, respectively. Similarly, freedom from atrial tachyarrhythmias without the use of antiarrhythmic drugs was 84%, 71%, and 61% at 1, 5, and 10 years, respectively. Notably, no significant difference was found between stand-alone and concomitant Cox-Maze-IV patients with and without antiarrhythmic drugs across early, mid-term, and long-term follow-up periods. There was also no difference in late outcomes between patients with PAF and non-PAF. Perioperative morbidity remained low, with an overall 30-day mortality rate of 3.3%, a postoperative pacemaker insertion rate of 12.2%, and a cerebrovascular accident rate of 1.6%.[38]

Minimally invasive techniques represent the future of cardiac surgery. The Cox-Maze-IV procedure performed via a right mini-thoracotomy is equally effective as the same procedure performed through a median sternotomy with the added benefits of fewer complications, a reduced mortality rate, and shorter ICU and hospital stays.[17,38,52] We prefer a right mini-thoracotomy approach for the Cox-Maze-IV procedure rather than a median sternotomy for stand-alone procedures and for patients needing concomitant mitral and/or tricuspid valve surgery.[7,50] The Cox-Maze-IV procedure performed via a right mini-thoracotomy is equally effective for PAF and non-PAF with minimal morbidity and no deaths to date. Most patients in our series presented with non-PAF (75%). At 1, 5, and 10 years after a Cox-Maze-IV procedure, freedom from atrial tachyarrhythmias was 94%, 89%, and 77%, respectively. No significant difference was observed in freedom from arrhythmias between patients with PAF versus non-PAF or those undergoing sternotomy versus a minimally invasive approach. Factors such as increased left atrial size and the number of prior catheter ablations were associated with late AF recurrence, and only 6% of patients having a mini-thoracotomy approach experienced major complications with no 30-day deaths.[15]

Our most recent propensity score-matched study compared patients who underwent a concomitant Cox-Maze-IV and mitral surgery via a right mini-thoracotomy versus a median sternotomy. The mini-thoracotomy group showed superior 1- and 3-year freedom from atrial tachyarrhythmia recurrence compared with the median sternotomy group. Despite longer surgical durations, patients in the mini-thoracotomy group experienced shorter hospital stays, fewer postoperative transfusions, and a lower incidence of pacemaker implantation. Notably, freedom from atrial tachyarrhythmia recurrence at 1 year (99% versus 90%) and 3 years (94% versis 86%) was significantly higher in the mini-thoracotomy group. Pacemaker implantations occurred more frequently in the median sternotomy group (18% versus 4%), along with higher rates of postoperative transfusions (57% versus 41%). However, the groups had no significant differences in 30-day mortality or 8-year survival rates.

In conclusion, numerous studies have affirmed the efficacy of the Cox-Maze-IV for both stand-alone AF and concomitant AF. Performing the procedure using a minimally invasive approach offers comparable effectiveness to sternotomy with fewer complications, shorter hospital stays, and reduced mortality rates.

RECURRENCE OF ATRIAL TACHYARRHYTHMIAS

The recurrence of atrial tachyarrhythmias is defined as any episode lasting more than 30 seconds, including AF, atrial flutter, or atrial tachycardia, after a 3-month blanking period.[12,53] Although arrhythmia recurrence is common in the immediate and early postoperative period,[49,54] it is typically transient. It reflects the healing process rather than indicative of long-term failure. Therefore, assessing the success of the ablation procedure after a 90-day blanking period is standard practice.

In our previously mentioned series, Fine-Gray regression analysis identified age, left atrial size, and non-PAF as significant predictors of first arrhythmia recurrence over the 10-year follow-up period. Symptomatic recurrence after the Cox-Maze-IV procedure is rare, occurring in only 2% of cases at 5 years and 5% at 10 years.[38]

Early recurrences of arrhythmias (between 3 months and 1 year after the procedure) may result from technical challenges in creating ablation lines or complex cases with extensive atrial remodeling and fibrosis, thereby allowing AF to recur. In contrast, late recurrences of arrhythmias (>1 year after the procedure) may be attributed to progressive worsening of the substrate in the LA due to inadequate management of comorbidities, such as hypertension, diabetes, obesity, and sleep apnea. The importance of lifetime management of these risk factors can not be overemphasized. Our approach has been proactive in addressing these late failures by bringing patients back to the catheterization laboratory for an electrophysiologic study and potential ablation.

SUMMARY

Advancements in ablation technologies have had a significantly positive impact on the landscape of AF surgery. The shift from surgical incisions in the original Cox-Maze-I, -II, and -III procedures (1987–1992), to exclusively linear cryolesions in the CryoMaze-III procedure (1996), to the combination of RF and cryolesions in the Cox-Maze-IV procedure (2002), to the recent introduction of the modified cryosurgical Cox-CryoMaze-III procedure (2024) has shortened the time required to perform a Maze procedure and hopefully made it more accessible to a broader group of surgeons. Notably, these innovative ablation technologies have opened up possibilities for minimally invasive AF surgery, leading to ongoing efforts to devise more straightforward procedures.

Surgeons developing novel procedures or lesion sets must diligently monitor their outcomes and share their findings through peer-reviewed journals. Adherence to recently published guidelines for patient follow-up and determining procedure success or failure is imperative. Despite ongoing developments, the Cox-Maze-III cryosurgical procedure and the Cox-Maze-IV procedure, both boasting a 90% success rate across all types of AF, remain the benchmarks for alternative lesion sets and serve as a standard for newer, less invasive approaches currently in development.

REFERENCES

1. Cox JL. The first Maze procedure. *J Thorac Cardiovasc Surg*. 2011;141(5):1093–1097.
2. Cox JL, Schuessler RB, D'Agostino HJ, et al. The surgical treatment of atrial fibrillation: III. Development of a definitive surgical procedure. *J Thorac Cardiovasc Surg*. 1991;101(4):569–583.
3. Cox JL, Boineau JP, Schuessler RB, Jaquiss RDB, Lappas DG. Modification of the Maze procedure for atrial flutter and atrial fibrillation: I. Rationale and surgical results. *J Thorac Cardiovasc Surg*. 1995;110(2):473–484.
4. Prasad SM, Maniar HS, Camillo CJ, et al. The Cox Maze III procedure for atrial fibrillation: long-term efficacy in patients undergoing lone versus concomitant procedures. *J Thorac Cardiovasc Surg*. 2003;126(6):1822–1827.
5. Weimar T, Bailey MS, Watanabe Y, et al. The Cox-Maze IV procedure for lone atrial fibrillation: a single center experience in 100 consecutive patients. *J Intervention Cardiac Electrophysiol*. 2011;31(1):47–54.
6. Lall SC, Melby SJ, Voeller RK, et al. The effect of ablation technology on surgical outcomes after the Cox-Maze procedure: a propensity analysis. *J Thorac Cardiovasc Surg*. 2007;133(2):389–396.
7. Cox JL. The minimally invasive Maze-III procedure. *Op Tech Thorac Cardiovasc Surg*. 2000;5(1):79–92.

8. Cox JL. Cardiac surgery for arrhythmias. *PACE Pacing Clin Electrophysiol.* 2004;27(2):266–282.
9. Weimar T, Schena S, Bailey MS, et al. The Cox-Maze procedure for lone atrial fibrillation. *Circ Arrhythm Electrophysiol.* 2012;5(1): 8–14.
10. Ruaengsri C, Schill MR, Khiabani AJ, Schuessler RB, Melby SJ, Damiano Jr RJ. The Cox-Maze IV procedure in its second decade: still the gold standard? *Eur J Cardio-Thorac Surg.* 2018;53(suppl_1):i19–i25.
11. Mehaffey JH, Krebs E, Hawkins RB, et al. Variability and utilization of concomitant atrial fibrillation ablation during mitral valve surgery. *Ann Thorac Surg.* 2021;111(1):29–34.
12. Calkins H, Hindricks G, Cappato R, et al. 2017 HRS/EHRA/ECAS/APHRS/SOLAECE expert consensus statement on catheter and surgical ablation of atrial fibrillation. *Heart Rhythm.* 2017;14(10):e275–e444.
13. Badhwar V, Rankin JS, Damiano RJ, et al. The society of thoracic surgeons 2017 clinical practice guidelines for the surgical treatment of atrial fibrillation. *Ann Thor Surg.* 2017;103(1):329–341.
14. Wyler von Ballmoos MC, Hui DS, Mehaffey JH, et al. The society of thoracic surgeons 2023 clinical practice guidelines for the surgical treatment of atrial fibrillation. *Ann Thorac Surg.* 2024;118(2):291–310.
15. MacGregor RM, Bakir NH, Pedamallu H, et al. Late results after stand-alone surgical ablation for atrial fibrillation. *J Thorac Cardiovasc Surg.* 2022;164(5):1515–1528.e1518.
16. Melby SJ, Lee AM, Zierer A, et al. Atrial fibrillation propagates through gaps in ablation lines: implications for ablative treatment of atrial fibrillation. *Heart Rhythm.* 2008;5(9):1296–1301.
17. Yates T-A, McGilvray M, Schill MR, et al. Performance of an irrigated bipolar radiofrequency ablation clamp on explanted human hearts. *Ann Thor Surg.* 2023;116(2):307–313.
18. Khiabani AJ, MacGregor RM, Manghelli JL, et al. Bipolar radiofrequency ablation on explanted human hearts: how to ensure transmural lesions. *Ann Thorac Surg.* 2020;110(6):1933–1939.
19. Gillette PC, Kugler JD, Garson Jr A, Gutgesell HP, Duff DF, McNamara DG. Mechanisms of cardiac arrhythmias after the mustard operation for transposition of the great arteries. *Am J Cardiol.* 1980;45(6):1225–1230.
20. Robertson JO, Saint LL, Leidenfrost JE, Damiano Jr RJ. Illustrated techniques for performing the Cox-Maze IV procedure through a right mini-thoracotomy. *Ann Cardiothorac Surg.* 2014;3(1): 105–116.
21. Lancaster TS, Melby SJ, Damiano Jr RJ. Minimally invasive surgery for atrial fibrillation. *Trends Cardiovasc Med.* 2016;26(3): 268–277.
22. Shah DC, Jaïs P, Haïssaguerre M, et al. Three-dimensional mapping of the common atrial flutter circuit in the right atrium. *Circulation.* 1997;96(11):3904–3912.
23. Cuculich PS, Wang Y, Lindsay BD, et al. Noninvasive characterization of epicardial activation in humans with diverse atrial fibrillation patterns. *Circulation.* 2010;122(14) 1364–1372.
24. Henn MC, Lancaster TS, Miller JR, et al. Late outcomes after the Cox Maze IV procedure for atrial fibrillation. *J Thorac Cardiovasc Surg.* 2015;150(5):1168–1178.e1162.
25. Haïssaguerre M, Jaïs P, Shah DC, et al. Spontaneous initiation of atrial fibrillation by ectopic beats originating in the pulmonary veins. *N Engl J Med.* 1998;339(10):659–666.
26. Lin WS, Tai CT, Hsieh MH, et al. Catheter ablation of paroxysmal atrial fibrillation initiated by non-pulmonary vein ectopy. *Circulation.* 2003;107(25):3176–3183.
27. Castellá M, Kotecha D, van Laar C, et al. Thoracoscopic vs. catheter ablation for atrial fibrillation: long-term follow-up of the fast randomized trial. *Europace.* 2019;21(5):746–753.
28. Adiyaman A, Buist TJ, Beukema RJ, et al. Randomized controlled trial of surgical versus catheter ablation for paroxysmal and early persistent atrial fibrillation. *Circ Arrhythm Electrophysiol.* 2018;11(10):e006182.
29. Knecht S, Hocini M, Wright M, et al. Left atrial linear lesions are required for successful treatment of persistent atrial fibrillation. *Eur Heart J.* 2008;29(19):2359–2366.
30. Jimenez A, Shorofsky SR, Dickfeld TM, Anand R, Saliaris AP, Saba M. Left-sided atrial flutter originating in the coronary sinus after radiofrequency ablation of atrial fibrillation. *Pacing Clin Electrophysiol.* 2010;33(10):e96–e99.
31. Pet M, Robertson JO, Bailey M, et al. The impact of CHADS2 score on late stroke after the Cox Maze procedure. *J Thorac Cardiovasc Surg.* 2013;146(1):85–89.
32. Whitlock RP, Belley-Cote EP, Paparella D, et al. Left atrial appendage occlusion during cardiac surgery to prevent stroke. *N Engl J Med.* 2021;384(22):2081–2091.
33. Squiers JJ, Edgerton JR. Surgical closure of the left atrial appendage: the past, the present, the future. *J Atri Fibrill.* 2018;10(5):1642.
34. Lee R, Jivan A, Kruse J, et al. Late neurologic events after surgery for atrial fibrillation: rare but relevant. *Ann Thorac Surg.* 2013;95(1):126–131 discussion 131–122.
35. Emmert MY, Puippe G, Baumüller S, et al. Safe, effective and durable epicardial left atrial appendage clip occlusion in patients with atrial fibrillation undergoing cardiac surgery: first long-term results from a prospective device trial. *Eur J Cardiothorac Surg.* 2014;45(1):126–131.
36. Ailawadi G, Gerdisch MW, Harvey RL, et al. Exclusion of the left atrial appendage with a novel device: early results of a multicenter trial. *J Thorac Cardiovasc Surg.* 2011;142(5):1002–1009 1009 e1001.
37. Al-Saady NM, Obel OA, Camm AJ. Left atrial appendage: structure, function, and role in thromboembolism. *Heart.* 1999;82(5):547–554.
38. Khiabani AJ, MacGregor RM, Bakir NH, et al. The long-term outcomes and durability of the Cox-Maze IV procedure for atrial fibrillation. *J Thorac Cardiovasc Surg.* 2022;163(2):629–641.e627.
39. Robertson JO, Cuculich PS, Saint LL, et al. Predictors and risk of pacemaker implantation after the Cox-Maze IV procedure. *Ann Thor Surg.* 2013;95(6):2015–2021.
40. Cox JL, Ad N, Churyla A, et al. The Maze procedure and postoperative pacemakers. *Ann Thor Surg.* 2018;106(5):1561–1569.
41. Bakir NH, Khiabani AJ, MacGregor RM, et al. Concomitant surgical ablation for atrial fibrillation is associated with increased risk of acute kidney injury but improved late survival. *J Thorac Cardiovasc Surg.* 2022;164(6):1847–1857.e1843.
42. Lehrmann H, Schneider J, Jadidi AS, et al. Transseptal access for left atrial ablation: the catheter-probing techniques are not without risk. *J Cardiovasc Electrophysiol.* 2014;25(5):479–484.
43. McCarthy PM, Gerdisch M, Philpott J, et al. Three-year outcomes of the postapproval study of the atricure bipolar radiofrequency ablation of permanent atrial fibrillation trial. *J Thorac Cardiovasc Surg.* 2022;164(2):519–527.e514.
44. Ademir T, Khiabani AJ, Schill MR, et al. Surgical ablation of atrial fibrillation in patients with tachycardia-induced cardiomyopathy. *Ann Thorac Surg.* 2019;108(2):443–450.
45. Melby SJ, Zierer A, Bailey MS, et al. A new era in the surgical treatment of atrial fibrillation: the impact of ablation technology

and lesion set on procedural efficacy. *Ann Surg*. 2006;244(4): 583–592.
46. Damiano RJ, Bailey M. The Cox-Maze IV procedure for lone atrial fibrillation. *Multimed Man Cardiothorac Surg*. 2007;2007(723) mmcts.2007.002758.
47. Lawrance CP, Henn MC, Miller JR, Sinn LA, Schuessler RB, Damiano Jr RJ. Comparison of the stand-alone Cox-Maze IV procedure to the concomitant Cox-Maze IV and mitral valve procedure for atrial fibrillation. *Ann Cardiothorac Surg*. 2014;3(1):55–61.
48. McGilvray MMO, Bakir NH, Kelly MO, et al. Efficacy of the stand-alone Cox-Maze IV procedure in patients with long-standing persistent atrial fibrillation. *J Cardiovasc Electrophysiol*. 2021;32(10):2884–2894.
49. Gerdisch M, Lehr E, Dunnington G, et al. Mid-term outcomes of concomitant Cox-Maze IV: results from a multicenter prospective registry. *J Cardiol Surg*. 2022;37(10):3006–3013.
50. Ad N, Holmes SD, Massimiano PS, Rongione AJ, Fornaresio LM. Long-term outcome following concomitant mitral valve surgery and Cox Maze procedure for atrial fibrillation. *J Thorac Cardiovasc Surg*. 2018;155(3):983–994.
51. Lawrance CP, Henn MC, Miller JR, et al. A minimally invasive Cox Maze IV procedure is as effective as sternotomy while decreasing major morbidity and hospital stay. *J Thorac Cardiovasc Surg*. 2014;148(3):955–962.
52. Nitta T, Wai JWW, Lee SH, et al. 2023 APHRS expert consensus statements on surgery for AF. *J Arrhyth*. 2023;39(6):841–852.
53. Ishii Y, Gleva MJ, Gamache MC, et al. Atrial tachyarrhythmias after the Maze procedure. *Circulation*. 2004;110(11) II-164–II-168.
54. McCarthy PM, Cox JL, Kruse J, Elenbaas C, Andrei A-C. One hundred percent utilization of a modified CryoMaze III procedure for atrial fibrillation with mitral surgery. *J Thorac Cardiovasc Surg*. 2024;167(4):1278–1289.

18

Downsizing the Left Atrium and Right Atrium

Steven F. Bolling, Whitney W. Fu

CHAPTER OUTLINE

There is a pathophysiological association between left atrial enlargement and atrial fibrillation (AF), with left atrial enlargement being both an inciting factor and one of the sequelae of AF.[1–4] There are many components of left atrial remodeling and enlargement, and they are discussed in detail in Chapter 8. Left atrial enlargement is a well-established predictor of adverse events, including first-time AF, stroke, cardiovascular death, and all-cause mortality.[5–10] Given the strong relationship between left atrial enlargement and AF, downsizing of the left atrium (LA) can be an important component of the surgical treatment of patients with AF. This chapter focuses on the mechanisms of left atrial enlargement, the association between LA enlargement and the development and treatment of AF, and the indications and techniques for surgical downsizing of the LA. The chapter also briefly describes the surgical technique for downsizing the right atrium (RA) should it be necessary.

RELATIONSHIP OF LEFT ATRIAL ENLARGEMENT TO THE DEVELOPMENT OF ATRIAL FIBRILLATION

Left atrial enlargement and AF are commonly encountered together.[11] The literature suggests a 30% or higher risk for AF in the presence of left atrial enlargement than in a normal-sized atrium even after controlling for other AF risk factors. The risk of AF increases proportionally with the extent of left atrial enlargement.[12] This may be because left atrial enlargement and AF commonly occur together with valvular pathologies that create a pressure and/or volume overload of the LA. Increasing wall stress causes dilatation and subsequent myocardial fibrosis and associated functional impairment. The response of the LA to these pressure, volume, and pathological changes is explained by Laplace's law, $T = \frac{P \times R}{M}$, wherein T is wall tension, P is the pressure differential across the wall, R is the radius of the cylinder (i.e., the LA), and M is the wall thickness.[13] Kuppahally et al.[14] demonstrated an inverse relationship between fibrosis and wall strain (i.e., functional impairment) using echocardiography and delayed-enhancement magnetic resonance imaging (MRI).

Dilatation of the LA contributes to AF in two ways. First, fibrosis disrupts the electrical connections between left atrial muscle bundles.[11] In a normally functioning atrium, these connections are important for normal synchronized atrial contraction, and disruption of these connections can lead to heterogenous electrical and mechanical atrial activity.[15] Second, fibrosis effectively slows electrical conduction through the atrium, resulting in an increase in the cycle length of a potential reentrant circuit. The altered conduction characteristics caused by fibrosis results in an increased likelihood that multiple macro-reentrant circuits can be sustained and function as the drivers of persistent fibrillatory activity in AF.[4]

However, even in the absence of valvular or known structural heart disease, left atrial enlargement is still associated with an increase in AF. For example, paroxysmal AF can be encountered in young, tall, athletic males who have a large LA simply because of their body size and high exercise capacity.[1] Larger atrial size can accommodate macro-reentrant drivers that are too large to develop in a normal-sized atrium even with fibrotic pathology.[4]

Moreover, there is evidence that AF begets left atrial enlargement, and left atrial enlargement begets AF (see Chapter 8).[1] Because of the interdependence of these two factors, the modern surgeon must address both AF and left atrial enlargement for effective treatment of patients with AF. It is well known that successful treatment of AF can lead to "reverse remodeling" of the LA that can be measured by reduction of left atrial size and return of left atrial function after therapy.[16,17] Pharmacologic conversion, electrical cardioversion, and mitral valve repair have all been shown to decrease left atrial size, improve atrial function, and decrease AF over time.[2,18–20]

RELATIONSHIP OF LEFT ATRIAL SIZE TO THE FAILURE OF SURGICAL ABLATION FOR ATRIAL FIBRILLATION

It is well-documented that LA enlargement is a risk factor for failure of surgical ablation.[21–23] The landmark Atrial Fibrillation Follow-up Investigation of Rhythm Management (AFFIRM) trial found that an enlarged atrium was associated with recurrent AF after ablation in 46% of patients after 1 year and 84% of patients after 5 years.[21] Comparatively, in patients with a non-enlarged atrium, 1% of patients at 1 year and 5% of patients at 5 years had recurrent AF. Studies evaluating predictors of recurrent AF after surgical ablation consistently find that left atrial enlargement is associated with significantly higher odds of recurrent AF.[23–26] Traditionally, a left atrial diameter of 65 mm is considered to be the threshold size at which ablation becomes much less likely to be successful.[27–30]

As discussed in the preceding section, left atrial enlargement is largely the result of fibrosis, which disrupts the atrium's normal electrophysiology.[31] Some have suggested that surgical ablation of AF in an enlarged LA requires increased ablative energy, more extensive lesions, and longer aortic cross-clamp times to be successful.[22,32] Because surgical AF ablation is underused, the thought that more extensive lesion sets are needed in patients with an enlarged LA and the perceived difficulty of performing a complete Cox Maze-III/IV lesion set even in normal-sized left atria may serve as additional barriers to attaining a durable, successful ablation in the presence of left atrial enlargement.[33–35]

There are several possible explanations for the failure of surgical AF ablation in a large LA. First, the lesion sets that are used for surgical ablation may be inadequate to eradicate the macro-reentrant drivers of AF because the normal atrial and conduction architecture is disrupted.[36–38] Second, with atrial enlargement, there is a much greater surface area between the lesions of a Cox Maze-III/IV available to participate in the formation of macro-reentrant circuits that drive and sustain AF.[38,39] Together, these factors make successful ablation of AF in enlarged LA a challenging problem.

IMPORTANCE OF BIATRIAL ENLARGEMENT

In the Multi-Ethnic Study of Atherosclerosis (MESA), large right atrial size was found to be associated with a greater incidence of AF.[40] Some studies suggest that the adverse effects of right atrial enlargement are similar to those of the LA.[41] Emerging data support the concept that right atrial enlargement and biatrial enlargement are important predictors of suboptimal outcomes for AF ablation.[42,43] In a cohort of 519 patients with AF, Kong et al.[44] showed that biatrial enlargement was associated with an increased need for reablation independent of left atrial enlargement.

MEASUREMENTS THAT DEFINE LEFT ATRIAL ENLARGEMENT

The American Society of Echocardiography (ASE) recommends transthoracic echocardiography (TTE) for the evaluation of left atrial size. Several echocardiography metrics are used in the preoperative diagnosis of LA enlargement including left atrial diameter, left atrial volume, and left atrial volume index (LAVI).[45]

Left Atrial Diameter

Left atrial diameter is the length of the anteroposterior left atrial dimension in the parasternal long-axis view on standard TTE. According to the ASE guidelines, a normal LA is less than 41 mm in males and 39 mm in females. On the basis of left atrial diameter, left atrial enlargement can be classified as mild (41–46 mm in males, 39–42 mm in females), moderate (47–51 mm in males, 43–46 mm in females), or severe (≥52 mm in males, ≥47 mm in females). Left atrial diameter should not be used as the only determinant of left atrial size, particularly in the setting of a dilated LA, because it assumes that all dimensions enlarge uniformly.[45,46]

Left Atrial Volume and Left Atrial Volume Index

Although quantification of LA volume still requires several geometric assumptions, LA volume more accurately accounts for differences in LA dimensions in multiple directions. LA volume has been shown in a multitude of studies to be more closely correlated than LA diameter with outcomes in cardiac disease, including AF, congestive heart failure, ischemic stroke, heart transplant, long-term survival in degenerative mitral valve disease, and death.[45,47–50] Because there are normal physiologic differences in left atrial size between males and females, left atrial volume should be indexed to body surface area. The normal upper limit of LAVI is 34 mL/m^2 in both males and females.[45] These values are measured by two-dimensional echocardiography, but three-dimensional echocardiography, cardiac computed tomography, and MRI are being increasingly used in the evaluation of chamber size.[45]

Left Atrial Strain

Recently, left atrial strain calculation using speckle-tracking analysis has become perhaps the most common method for determining left atrial function (see Chapter 7). The most important left atrial strain measurements are longitudinal strain, fractional area change, reservoir strain, and strain rate, all of which have been used to improve prognostic and risk prediction models of cardiac disease.[50–52] Although large-volume clinical data are still lacking, many smaller studies have used these functional parameters successfully to quantify left atrial reverse remodeling in response to AF ablation and to predict long-term maintenance of sinus rhythm after ablation.[50,51]

INDICATIONS FOR DOWNSIZING THE LEFT ATRIUM

The most extreme indication for surgical downsizing of the LA is the presence of compressive symptoms on the enlarged LA from adjacent organs, commonly called "giant LA." Fortunately, this problem is rare in most current clinical practices. There is ample evidence that left atrial reduction in patients with an left atrial diameter of 65 mm or larger who are undergoing mitral valve surgery and/or AF ablation alone increases the success rate of surgical AF ablation. This approach is supported by evidence showing that an LA larger than 65 mm in diameter rarely return to normal size after mitral valve surgery.[13,53–55]

SURGICAL TECHNIQUES FOR DOWNSIZING THE LEFT ATRIUM

Our primary surgical technique for downsizing of the LA is an atrial reduction plasty performed in combination with the Cox Maze procedure. After the patient is placed on standard cardiopulmonary bypass with bicaval cannulation, a left atriotomy is performed in the interatrial groove ("Waterston's groove") and extended around the pulmonary veins. The left atrial appendage (LAA) is inverted, excised, and oversewn at the stump. A resection of the inferior portion of the posterior left atrial wall in the left atrial isthmus is then performed using two incisions (Fig. 18.1). One incision extends from the os of the right inferior pulmonary vein to the os of the left inferior pulmonary vein, and a second is placed parallel to the inferior pulmonary veins around the mitral annulus immediately above the atrioventricular (AV) groove fat pad. Finally, these two incisions are connected near the os of the left inferior pulmonary vein. Pulmonary vein isolation and LAA orifice isolation is then performed using radiofrequency ablation. The LA is closed, starting by sewing the pulmonary vein cuff to the remaining atrium above the mitral annulus.

Our standard technique also includes a right atrial reduction (Fig. 18.2). This is accomplished in a similar fashion to the left atrial

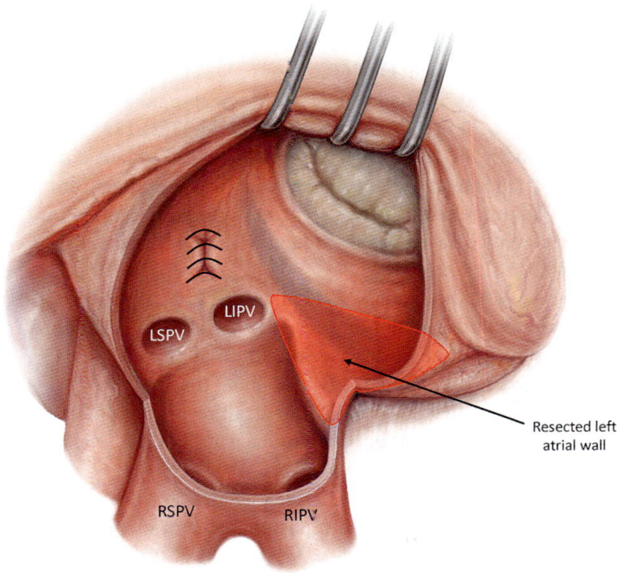

Fig. 18.1 Downsizing the left atrium (LA). Surgeons' view of the internal LA through a standard left atriotomy in Waterston's groove. After amputation of the left atrial appendage and closure of the resulting wall defect, the first lesion is created just beneath the two inferior pulmonary veins. A second lesion is then placed from the end of that incision near the left inferior pulmonary vein back toward the atrial septal side of the LA. These two lesions create a triangle of resected atrial wall in the left atrial isthmus between the inferior pulmonary veins and the left atrioventricular groove above the mitral annulus. *LIPV,* Left inferior pulmonary vein *LSPV,* left superior pulmonary vein; *RIPV,* right inferior pulmonary vein; *RSPV,* right superior pulmonary vein.

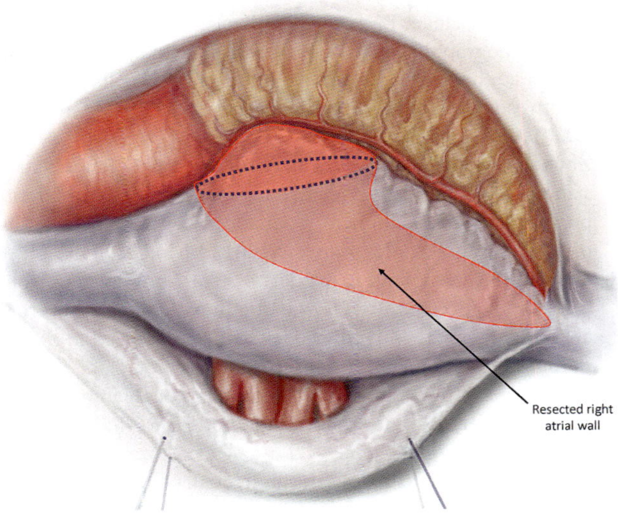

Fig. 18.2 Downsizing the right atrium. The right atrial appendage (RAA) is excised, and an incision is placed from the stump of the excised RAA parallel to the right atrioventricular groove down to the inferior vena cava (IVC). A separate incision is then placed from the IVC, back up to the RAA excision site near the superior vena cava, taking care to avoid the anatomic sinoatrial node.

reduction, starting with excision of the right atrial appendage (RAA). An incision made from the excised RAA stump toward the inferior vena cava (IVC) and parallel to the right AV groove is connected to a second more posterior longitudinal incision running from below the IVC orifice to above the superior vena cava orifice, with care taken to avoid the sinoatrial node. These two incisions accomplish excision of a sizeable portion of the lateral right atrial free wall, which is then followed by radiofrequency ablation lesions isolating the tricuspid annulus and across the atrial septum.[56]

Other described techniques include the following: (1) para-annular plication of the posteroinferior left atrial wall between the ostia of the inferior pulmonary veins and the posterior mitral annulus, superior plication between the right and left pulmonary veins, and then circumferentially around the left pulmonary veins toward the mitral annulus (Fig. 18.3)[57–59]; (2) resection of three triangular segments of the left posterior wall (Fig. 18.4)[60]; and (3) plication of both the posteroinferior wall and the superior wall of the LA through a combined superior and transeptal approach.[61]

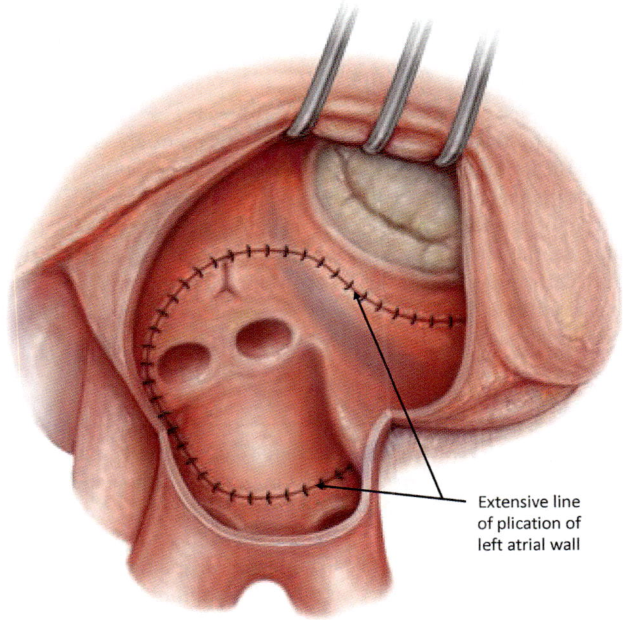

Fig. 18.3 Downsizing the left atrium. Extensive plication of the left atrial wall in the areas designated. See text for further discussion.

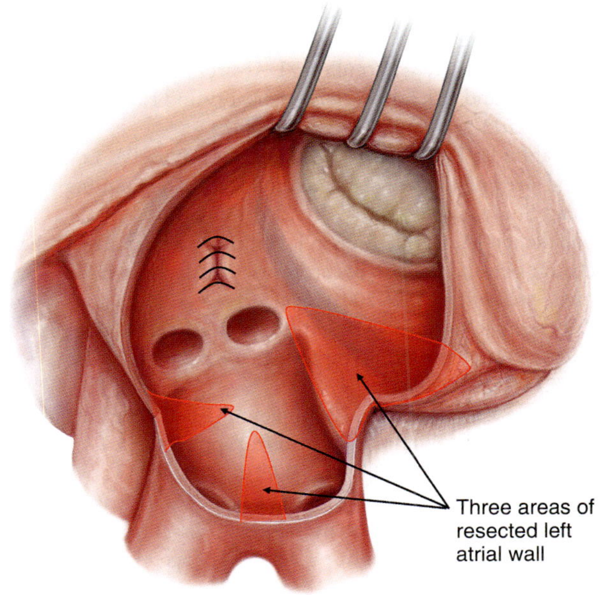

Fig. 18.4 Downsizing the left atrium. Resection of three areas of the left atrial wall. See text for further discussion.

RESULTS OF DOWNSIZING THE LEFT ATRIUM

A 2023 meta-analysis including 19 studies showed that left atrial reduction during the Cox Maze procedure was associated with higher restoration of sinus rhythm at discharge and fewer cases of perioperative stroke.[62] In addition, a recent 2021 randomized clinical trial of 140 patients compared 70 patients who had mitral valve surgery plus a Maze procedure only (MVR + Maze) and 70 who had mitral valve surgery plus a Maze procedure plus left atrial volume reduction (MVR + Maze + LAVR).[63] The left atrial volume reduction was accomplished by imbricating an extra portion of the LA lying just outside the roof and floor lesions of a Maze-IV procedure. Adding LA volume reduction to the Maze procedure had no impact on perioperative morbidity or mortality, but it improved the freedom from recurrent atrial arrhythmias, including AF, during a 24-month follow-up period.

SUMMARY

The pathophysiology of AF and atrial enlargement are closely interrelated. The literature increasingly supports the concept that AF begets atrial enlargement and atrial enlargement begets AF. Given the negative prognostic effect of atrial enlargement on the success of ablation, it is important to consider addressing the atrial enlargement directly. In this setting, downsizing of the LA with resection and/or plication and downsizing the RA when necessary can be a valuable adjunct in the surgical treatment of patients with AF.

REFERENCES

1. Sanfilippo AJ, Abascal VM, Sheehan M, et al. Atrial enlargement as a consequence of atrial fibrillation. A prospective echocardiographic study. *Circulation*. 1990;82(3):792–797.
2. Casaclang-Verzosa G, Gersh BJ, Tsang TS. Structural and functional remodeling of the left atrium: clinical and therapeutic implications for atrial fibrillation. *J Am Coll Cardiol*. 2008;51(1):1–11.
3. van de Vegte YJ, Siland JE, Rienstra M, van der Harst P. Atrial fibrillation and left atrial size and function: a Mendelian randomization study. *Sci Rep*. 2021;11(1):8431.
4. Nattel S, Burstein B, Dobrev D. Atrial remodeling and atrial fibrillation: mechanisms and implications. *Circ Arrhythm Electrophysiol*. 2008;1(1):62–73.
5. Bouzas-Mosquera A, Broullon FJ, Alvarez-Garcia N, et al. Left atrial size and risk for all-cause mortality and ischemic stroke. *CMAJ*. 2011;183(10):E657–E664.
6. Benjamin EJ, D'Agostino RB, Belanger AJ, Wolf PA, Levy D. Left atrial size and the risk of stroke and death. The Framingham Heart Study. *Circulation*. 1995;92(4):835–841.
7. Laukkanen JA, Kurl S, Eranen J, Huttunen M, Salonen JT. Left atrium size and the risk of cardiovascular death in middle-aged men. *Arch Intern Med*. 2005;165(15):1788–1793.
8. Zilberszac R, Gleiss A, Massetti M, et al. Left atrial size predicts outcome in severe but asymptomatic mitral regurgitation. *Sci Rep*. 2023;13(1):3892.
9. Abhayaratna WP, Seward JB, Appleton CP, et al. Left atrial size: physiologic determinants and clinical applications. *J Am Coll Cardiol*. 2006;47(12):2357–2363.
10. Abhayaratna WP, Fatema K, Barnes ME, et al. Left atrial reservoir function as a potent marker for first atrial fibrillation or flutter in persons >or = 65 years of age. *Am J Cardiol*. 2008;101(11):1626–1629.
11. Kirchhof P, Benussi S, Kotecha D, et al. 2016 ESC Guidelines for the management of atrial fibrillation developed in collaboration with EACTS. *Europace*. 2016;18(11):1609–1678.
12. Seko Y, Kato T, Haruna T, et al. Association between atrial fibrillation, atrial enlargement, and left ventricular geometric remodeling. *Sci Rep*. 2018;8(1):6366.
13. Apostolakis E, Shuhaiber JH. The surgical management of giant left atrium. *Eur J Cardiothorac Surg*. 2008;33(2):182–190.
14. Kuppahally SS, Akoum N, Burgon NS, et al. Left atrial strain and strain rate in patients with paroxysmal and persistent atrial fibrillation: relationship to left atrial structural remodeling detected by delayed-enhancement MRI. *Circ Cardiovasc Imaging*. 2010;3(3):231–239.
15. Allessie MA, de Groot NM, Houben RP, et al. Electropathological substrate of long-standing persistent atrial fibrillation in patients with structural heart disease: longitudinal dissociation. *Circ Arrhythm Electrophysiol*. 2010;3(6):606–615.
16. Thomas L, Abhayaratna WP. Left atrial reverse remodeling: mechanisms, evaluation, and clinical significance. *JACC Cardiovasc Imaging*. 2017;10(1):65–77.
17. Soulat-Dufour L, Lang S, Ederhy S, et al. Biatrial remodelling in atrial fibrillation: a three-dimensional and strain echocardiography insight. *Arch Cardiovasc Dis*. 2019;112(10):585–593.
18. Westenberg JJ, van der Geest RJ, Lamb HJ, et al. MRI to evaluate left atrial and ventricular reverse remodeling after restrictive mitral annuloplasty in dilated cardiomyopathy. *Circulation*. 2005;112(9 Suppl):I437–I442.
19. Reant P, Lafitte S, Jais P, et al. Reverse remodeling of the left cardiac chambers after catheter ablation after 1 year in a series of patients with isolated atrial fibrillation. *Circulation*. 2005;112(19):2896–2903.
20. Stassen J, van Wijngaarden AL, Butcher SC, et al. Prognostic value of left atrial reservoir function in patients with severe primary mitral regurgitation undergoing mitral valve repair. *Eur Heart J Cardiovasc Imaging*. 2022;24(1):142–151.
21. Olshansky B, Heller EN, Mitchell LB, et al. Are transthoracic echocardiographic parameters associated with atrial fibrillation recurrence or stroke? Results from the Atrial Fibrillation Follow-Up Investigation of Rhythm Management (AFFIRM) study. *J Am Coll Cardiol*. 2005;45(12):2026–2033.
22. Zhuang J, Wang Y, Tang K, et al. Association between left atrial size and atrial fibrillation recurrence after single circumferential pulmonary vein isolation: a systematic review and meta-analysis of observational studies. *Europace*. 2012;14(5):638–645.
23. Demarchi A, Neumann L, Rordorf R, et al. Long-term outcome of catheter ablation for atrial fibrillation in patients with severe left atrial enlargement and reduced left ventricular ejection fraction. *Europace*. 2021;23(11):1751–1756.
24. Amuthan R, Curtis AB. What clinical trials of ablation for atrial fibrillation tell us—and what they do not. *Heart Rhythm O2*. 2021;2(2):174–186.
25. Clarnette JA, Brooks AG, Mahajan R, et al. Outcomes of persistent and long-standing persistent atrial fibrillation ablation: a systematic review and meta-analysis. *Europace*. 2018;20(FI_3):f366–f376.
26. Gillinov AM, Sirak J, Blackstone EH, et al. The Cox Maze procedure in mitral valve disease: predictors of recurrent atrial fibrillation. *J Thorac Cardiovasc Surg*. 2005;130(6):1653–1660.
27. Kamata J, Kawazoe K, Izumoto H, et al. Predictors of sinus rhythm restoration after Cox Maze procedure concomitant with other cardiac operations. *Ann Thorac Surg*. 1997;64(2):394–398.
28. Kosakai Y, Kawaguchi AT, Isobe F, et al. Modified maze procedure for patients with atrial fibrillation undergoing simultaneous open heart surgery. *Circulation*. 1995;92(9 Suppl):II359–II364.
29. Sunderland N, Maruthappu M, Nagendran M. What size of left atrium significantly impairs the success of maze surgery for atrial fibrillation? *Interact Cardiovasc Thorac Surg*. 2011;13(3):332–338.

30. Damiano RJ Jr, Schwartz FH, Bailey MS, et al. The Cox Maze IV procedure: predictors of late recurrence. *J Thorac Cardiovasc Surg*. 2011;141(1):113–121.
31. Yue L, Xie J, Nattel S. Molecular determinants of cardiac fibroblast electrical function and therapeutic implications for atrial fibrillation. *Cardiovasc Res*. 2011;89(4):744–753.
32. McGilvray MMO, Bakir NH, Yates TE, et al. Surgical ablation for atrial fibrillation is efficacious in patients with giant left atria. *J Thorac Cardiovasc Surg*. 2024;167(2):680–691 e682.
33. Brancato SC, Wang M, Spinelli KJ, et al. Temporal trends and predictors of surgical ablation for atrial fibrillation across a multistate healthcare system. *Heart Rhythm O2*. 2022;3(1):32–39.
34. Badhwar V, Rankin JS, Ad N, et al. Surgical ablation of atrial fibrillation in the united states: trends and propensity matched outcomes. *Ann Thorac Surg*. 2017;104(2):493–500.
35. Ad N, Henry L, Hunt S, Holmes SD. Should surgical ablation for atrial fibrillation be performed in patients with a significantly enlarged left atrium? *J Thorac Cardiovasc Surg*. 2014;147(1):236–241.
36. Kirchhof P, Benussi S, Kotecha D, et al. 2016 ESC Guidelines for the management of atrial fibrillation developed in collaboration with EACTS. *Eur J Cardiothorac Surg*. 2016;50(5):e1–e88.
37. Oakes RS, Badger TJ, Kholmovski EG, et al. Detection and quantification of left atrial structural remodeling with delayed-enhancement magnetic resonance imaging in patients with atrial fibrillation. *Circulation*. 2009;119(13):1758–1767.
38. Verma A, Wazni OM, Marrouche NF, et al. Pre-existent left atrial scarring in patients undergoing pulmonary vein antrum isolation: an independent predictor of procedural failure. *J Am Coll Cardiol*. 2005;45(2):285–292.
39. Lin WS, Tai CT, Hsieh MH, et al. Catheter ablation of paroxysmal atrial fibrillation initiated by non-pulmonary vein ectopy. *Circulation*. 2003;107(25):3176–3183.
40. Xie E, Yu R, Ambale-Venkatesh B, et al. Association of right atrial structure with incident atrial fibrillation: a longitudinal cohort cardiovascular magnetic resonance study from the Multi-Ethnic Study of Atherosclerosis (MESA). *J Cardiovasc Magn Reson*. 2020;22(1):36.
41. Bax M, Ajmone Marsan N, Delgado V, Bax JJ, van der Bijl P. Effect of bi-atrial size and function in patients with paroxysmal or permanent atrial fibrillation. *Am J Cardiol*. 2022;183:33–39.
42. Wen S, Liu N, Bai R, et al. Right atrial diameter and outcome of catheter ablation of atrial fibrillation. *J Interv Card Electrophysiol*. 2017;49(2):157–164.
43. Ko KY, Jang JH, Choi SH, et al. Impact of right atrial enlargement on clinical outcome in patients with atrial fibrillation. *Front Cardiovasc Med*. 2022;9:989012.
44. Kong Q, Shi L, Yu R, et al. Biatrial enlargement as a predictor for reablation of atrial fibrillation. *Int J Med Sci*. 2020;17(18):3031–3038.
45. Lang RM, Badano LP, Mor-Avi V, et al. Recommendations for cardiac chamber quantification by echocardiography in adults: an update from the American Society of Echocardiography and the European Association of Cardiovascular Imaging. *Eur Heart J Cardiovasc Imaging*. 2015;16(3):233–270.
46. Lang RM, Bierig M, Devereux RB, et al. Recommendations for chamber quantification: a report from the American Society of Echocardiography's Guidelines and Standards Committee and the Chamber Quantification Writing Group, developed in conjunction with the European Association of Echocardiography, a branch of the European Society of Cardiology. *J Am Soc Echocardiogr*. 2005;18(12):1440–1463.
47. Pritchett AM, Jacobsen SJ, Mahoney DW, Rodeheffer RJ, Bailey KR, Redfield MM. Left atrial volume as an index of left atrial size: a population-based study. *J Am Coll Cardiol*. 2003;41(6):1036–1043.
48. Faustino A, Providencia R, Barra S, et al. Which method of left atrium size quantification is the most accurate to recognize thromboembolic risk in patients with non-valvular atrial fibrillation? *Cardiovasc Ultrasound*. 2014;12:28.
49. Essayagh B, Antoine C, Benfari G, et al. Prognostic implications of left atrial enlargement in degenerative mitral regurgitation. *J Am Coll Cardiol*. 2019;74(7):858–870.
50. Hoit BD. Left atrial size and function: role in prognosis. *J Am Coll Cardiol*. 2014;63(6):493–505.
51. Vieira MJ, Teixeira R, Goncalves L, Gersh BJ. Left atrial mechanics: echocardiographic assessment and clinical implications. *J Am Soc Echocardiogr*. 2014;27(5):463–478.
52. Stassen J, Namazi F, van der Bijl P, et al. Left atrial reservoir function and outcomes in secondary mitral regurgitation. *J Am Soc Echocardiogr*. 2022;35(5):477–485 e473.
53. Scherer M, Dzemali O, Aybek T, Wimmer-Greinecker G, Moritz A. Impact of left atrial size reduction on chronic atrial fibrillation in mitral valve surgery. *J Heart Valve Dis*. 2003;12(4):469–474.
54. Scherer M, Therapidis P, Miskovic A, Moritz A. Left atrial size reduction improves the sinus rhythm conversion rate after radiofrequency ablation for continuous atrial fibrillation in patients undergoing concomitant cardiac surgery. *Thorac Cardiovasc Surg*. 2006;54(1):34–38.
55. Choo SJ, Park NH, Lee SK, et al. Excellent results for atrial fibrillation surgery in the presence of giant left atrium and mitral valve disease. *Eur J Cardiothorac Surg*. 2004;26(2):336–341.
56. Romano MA, Bach DS, Pagani FD, Prager RL, Deeb GM, Bolling SF. Atrial reduction plasty Cox Maze procedure: extended indications for atrial fibrillation surgery. *Ann Thorac Surg*. 2004;77(4):1282–1287; discussion 1287.
57. Johnson J, Danielson GK, MacVaugh H 3rd, Joyner CR. Plication of the giant left atrium at operation for severe mitral regurgitation. *Surgery*. 1967;61(1):118–121.
58. Kawazoe K, Beppu S, Takahara Y, et al. Surgical treatment of giant left atrium combined with mitral valvular disease. Plication procedure for reduction of compression to the left ventricle, bronchus, and pulmonary parenchyma. *J Thorac Cardiovasc Surg*. 1983;85(6):885–892.
59. Fujita T, Kawazoe K, Beppu S, Manabe H. Surgical treatment on mitral valvular disease with giant left atrium-the effect of para-annular plication on left atrium. *Japanese Circ J*. 1982;46(4):420–426.
60. Sinatra R, Pulitani I, Antonazzo A, Melina G. A novel technique for giant left atrium reduction. *Eur J Cardiothorac Surg*. 2001;20(2):412–414.
61. Yuasa S, Soeda T, Masuyama S, Shimizu K, Matsuda M. Surgical treatment of giant left atrium using a combined superior-transseptal approach. *Ann Thorac Surg*. 2003;75(6):1985–1986.
62. Baudo M, Rosati F, Di Bacco L, D'Alonzo M, Benussi S, Muneretto C. Left atrium volume reduction procedure concomitant with Cox-Maze ablation in patients undergoing mitral valve surgery: a meta-analysis of clinical and rhythm outcomes. *Heart Lung Circ*. 2003;32(11):1386–1393.
63. Bogachev-Prokophiev AV, Ovcharov MA, Lavinykov SO, et al. Surgical atrial fibrillation ablation with and without left atrium reduction for patients scheduled for mitral valve surgery: a prospective randomised study. *Heart Lung Circ*. 2021;30(6):922–931.

19

When Is a Maze Procedure a Maze Procedure?

James L. Cox

CHAPTER OUTLINE

The Maze procedure was developed to preclude or interrupt the macro-reentrant drivers that sustain atrial fibrillation (AF). It was first performed clinically in 1987, some 11 years before Haïssaguerre showed that pulmonary vein (PV) triggers induced most episodes of AF.[1] Since that time, improvements have evolved in the lesion patterns and in the surgical tools to create them, but the basic concept of the Maze procedure has not changed. Radiofrequency (RF) energy was introduced for the catheter ablation of arrhythmias other than AF in the early 1990s, but attempts to reproduce the Maze procedure with RF catheters at that time proved to be futile. This was not because of an inadequate energy source but because of the limitations of the catheter technique in creating lesions in the essential areas of the atrium to interrupt the macro-reentrant drivers. The era of catheter ablation for AF began in 1998 when Haïssaguerre demonstrated that PV triggers induced AF and that the number of recurrent episodes of paroxysmal AF (PAF) could be dramatically reduced or completely abolished by isolating the PVs (PV isolation [PVI]) with RF catheters.[1] The use of PVI for more persistent forms of AF was not recommended by Haïssaguerre in that article, but despite this fact, PVI subsequently became widely applied for nonparoxysmal AF (non-PAF) as well. It soon became clear that although catheter PVI for PAF was quite successful, the results of PVI for more persistent forms of AF were dismal.[2–4]

After Haïssaguerre's seminal 1998 report, bipolar RF clamps and unipolar RF surgical devices were developed to provide surgeons with an alternative to surgical incisions and linear cryoprobes. The bipolar RF clamps have been quite successful for the treatment of AF when performing either PVI for PAF or in creating lesions of the Maze-III or Maze-IV procedure for more complex forms of AF.[5–7] There is no reason to expect that surgical PVI is any better than a well-performed catheter PVI for the treatment of non-PAF, but some surgeons were willing to accept the suboptimal results of PVI for non-PAF as long as the procedure could be performed off pump and through smaller chest incisions. This compromise represented a paradigm shift in the primary surgical objective of AF surgery from seeking the *best possible outcomes* to seeking the *least invasive procedures*. With rare exceptions, these "minimally invasive" procedures for AF eschewed the use of cardiopulmonary bypass (CPB) even though CPB has been the seminal tool that has allowed cardiac surgery to be performed safely for more than 70 years.

The desire to develop a surgical procedure less invasive than the Maze procedure for AF was, and remains, a laudable goal. However, there is concern that relatively uninformed patients are not always allowed to participate in the decision regarding which approach is to be used for their own surgery (i.e., the traditional "better outcomes" approach or the more recent "less invasive" approach). Nevertheless, the compromise between better outcomes and less invasion led to the development of the Wolf Mini-Maze procedure, the left atrial Maze procedure, the Dallas lesion set, the five-box Maze procedure, and many other unnamed and untested surgical interventions for the treatment of patients with all types of AF. In the process, the term "Maze procedure" became the generic designation for virtually any surgical procedure used to ablate AF.[8,9] This generic use of the term "Maze procedure" skews the perception of the success rates of an actual Maze procedure, leading to confusion not only among patients but also among surgeons and cardiologists.[10,11]

WOLF MINI-MAZE PROCEDURE

In 2005, Wolf and colleagues reported a series of 27 patients who underwent a minimally invasive surgical procedure for AF performed through bilateral mini-thoracotomies that included PVI with a bipolar RF clamp and occlusion of the left atrial appendage with a stapler (Fig. 19.1).[12] Two-thirds of the patients had PAF, and the patients were followed for an average of 6 months. Of the 25 patients followed for at least *3 months* (the usual blanking period), 91% (21 of 23) were free of AF. No mention was made of whether or not the patients were also free of atrial flutter and/or atrial tachycardia, both of which constitute procedural failure.[13,14] Nevertheless, this was an exciting initial report of a promising new minimally invasive approach for the treatment of patients with AF.

According to the current website (wolfminiMaze.com), Wolf has now performed "over 2,000 Wolf Mini-Maze procedures since the first one in 2003, and has demonstrated the procedure to over 800 heart surgeons worldwide."[15] Unfortunately, there is no evidence in the literature that this large personal series of Wolf mini-Maze procedures, or even a sizeable cohort of it, has ever been subjected to the peer-review process for publication of a scientific article. In a 2007 review article, the success rate for the procedure was again stated to be 91% with no other information on results provided.[16] A two-page update of

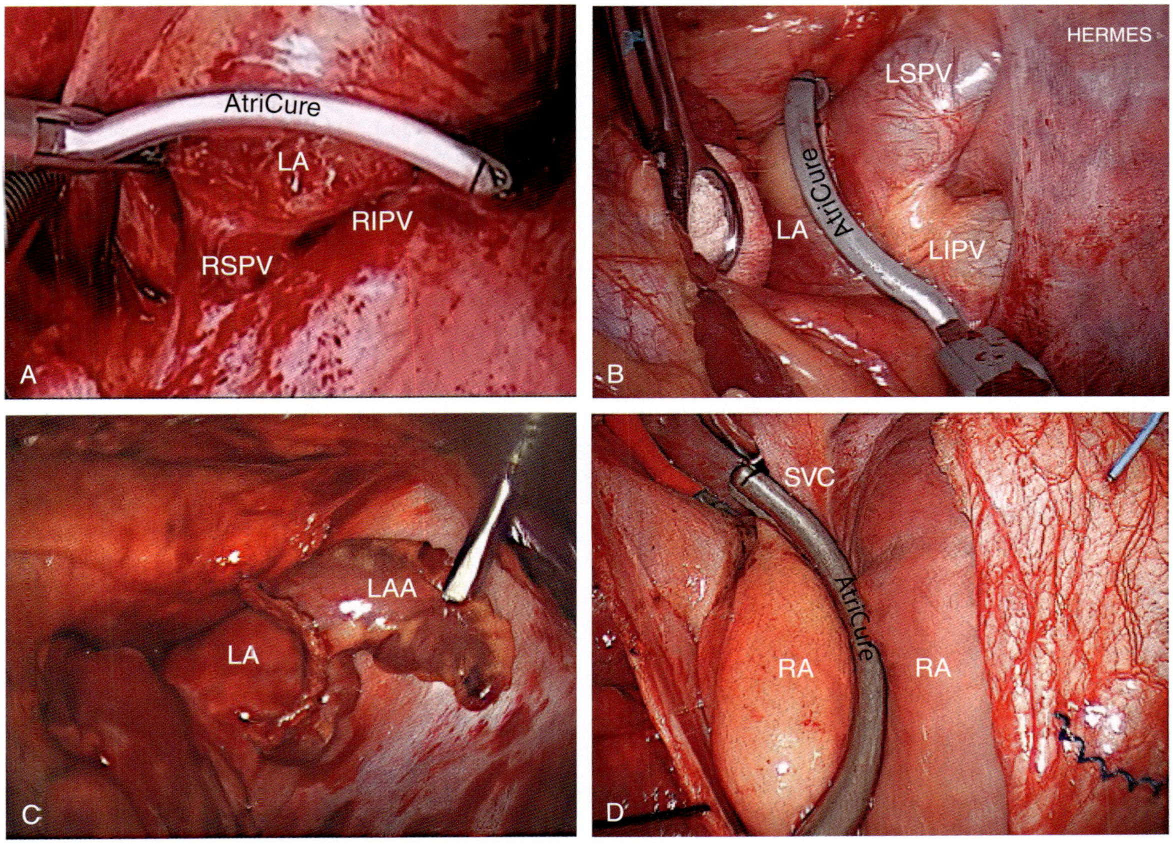

Fig. 19.1 The original Wolf mini-Maze procedure included isolation of the right pulmonary veins (A), isolation of the left pulmonary veins (B), and occlusion of the left atrial appendage (LAA) using a stapling device (C). In later iterations, the LAA was occluded with an AtriClip and ganglionic plexus ablation was added. Recently an SVC–inferior vena cava (IVC) intercaval lesion was included in which a bipolar radiofrequency clamp is placed on the posterior right atrial and left atrial walls as illustrated (D). *LA,* Left atrium; *LIPV,* left inferior pulmonary vein; *LSPV, left* superior pulmonary vein; *RA,* right atrium; *RIPV,* right inferior pulmonary vein; *RSPV,* right superior pulmonary vein.

the procedure published in 2014 contained no patient data but mentioned that ganglionic plexus ablation had been added to the procedure since its original description in 2005.[17] In a separate 2014 perspective article[18] it was stated:

> *"Recently we reviewed 157 patients who are now 1 to 9 years out from the Wolf procedure. The patients' ages ranged from 15 to 87 years old. The cure rate for paroxysmal AF was 92%, 85% for persistent AF, and 75% for long-standing persistent AF. The follow-up included 7-day continuous monitoring. There were no deaths (personal review)."*

No other information on freedom from recurrent arrhythmias, statistical analysis, or outcomes was provided and there was no reference for this data summary, leaving one to conclude that even this cohort of 157 patients had not been subjected to the peer-review process. A 2021 review titled "Surgical Treatment of Atrial Fibrillation" published in the *Methodist DeBakey Cardiovascular Journal*[19] again stated: *"The AF-free rate is 92% for paroxysmal AF, 85% for persistent AF, and 75% for long-standing persistent AF."* It was also mentioned that *"After more than 1,000 procedures using a stapler to close the LAA, we transitioned to clip closure of the LAA (Atriclip, Atricure, Inc.)."*

The only other outcomes mentioned in that 2021 review were those from the biatrial Maze procedure arm of the cardiothoracic surgical trials network (CTSN) Clinical Investigators prospective randomized trial.[11] As described in Chapter 13, the patients in that trial who had mitral valve (MV) or double valve surgery had persistent or long-standing persistent AF (LSpAF), and the results of concomitant surgical AF ablation are among the poorest in the literature (66% success at 1 year). Because the Wolf mini-Maze procedure is used in patients with stand-alone AF rather than concomitant AF in patients undergoing coronary artery bypass graft or valve surgery, perhaps it would have been appropriate to mention that in 2017, Ad and colleagues[20] reported their results with the minimal invasive CryoMaze-III procedure for stand-alone AF, 78% of which was LSpAF, as being successful in 73% of patients at 5 years. The year after the 2021 review, Damiano's group[21] reported their results for stand-alone AF, 75% of which was non-PAF, as being successful in 89% of patients at 5 years. It is unfortunate that after performing the Wolf mini-Maze procedure in more than 2000 patients, we still have only the original peer-reviewed report on 27 patients with an average of 6 months of follow-up to compare with the safety and efficacy of other minimally invasive surgical procedures for AF.

LEFT ATRIAL MAZE PROCEDURE

As mentioned in Chapter 13, there are several publications in the literature suggesting that the right atrial lesions are unnecessary or that they are only incidental to the success of the Maze procedure for the treatment of patients with AF.[22-24] Thus, it is understandable that surgeons might choose to delete the right atrial lesions and perform only the left atrial lesions of a Maze procedure, especially when ablating AF caused by left-heart problems such as coronary artery disease or left-sided valve abnormalities. Of course, if lesions are not placed in both atria, the procedure cannot rightfully be called a "Maze procedure" because a complete maze cannot be placed in only half of the contiguous atrial myocardial mass any more than a complete maze can be drawn in only half of a square. Thus the so-called "left atrial Maze" procedure is not a Maze procedure at all, even if every left atrial lesion of a Maze-III or Maze-IV procedure is created and placed perfectly.[10]

The major problem with the concept of performing a "left atrial Maze" procedure in patients with non-PAF is that up to 30% of the macro-reentrant drivers that sustain AF can be located in the *right* atrium (RA; Fig. 19.2).[25,26] As described in Chapter 13, if these potential right atrial drivers are not addressed, they can continue to sustain AF, and the left atrium (LA) will be a passive bystander in the fibrillation (Fig. 19.3).

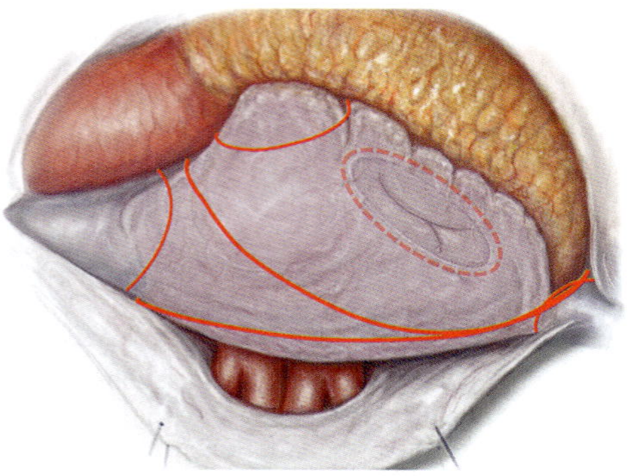

Fig. 19.2 Sites of documented right atrial macro-reentrant drivers of atrial fibrillation (AF). Up to 30% of all macro-reentrant drivers that can potentially sustain AF are located in the right atrium. See text for discussion.

In patients who have left-heart abnormalities such as coronary artery disease, aortic and/or MV disease, heart failure, or systemic hypertension causing AF, the location of the AF drivers may be confined to the LA early in the disease process because the RA is still normal and therefore incapable of harboring more than one macro-reentrant circuit at a time because of the long refractory periods in the RA (see Chapter 4, Figs. 4.14 and 4.15). Of course, both atria are fibrillating in these patients, but the RA is fibrillating *passively* in response to the multiple AF drivers in the LA that are sustaining the AF. Therefore, if a patient with MV regurgitation undergoes MV repair early in the course of the disease before the RA is actively involved in sustaining the AF, it would be expected that ablative lesions confined to the LA would be as effective as biatrial ablative lesions.[24] However, later in the course of the MV regurgitation when the RA is capable of actively sustaining AF drivers, deleting the RA lesions of the Maze procedure (Fig. 19.4) may result in failure of the surgical procedure (Fig. 19.5).

The problem faced by clinicians is that neither visual inspection nor preoperative imaging techniques are capable of determining if the RA is actively or passively involved in sustaining persistent AF in a given patient. Because electrocardiographic imaging mapping from the surface of the chest is non-invasive (see Chapter 6), this may be a viable way in the future to differentiate preoperatively which patients need biatrial ablative lesions and which patients might be just as well served by confining the ablative lesions to the LA.

As mentioned in Chapter 13, another reason that the results of AF ablation procedures confined to the LA might occasionally seem to be as successful as biatrial ablative lesions is that the biatrial lesions are either incomplete or are performed incorrectly. In this case, the results of the biatrial lesion set will be so poor that they may be no better than lesions confined to the LA. This was a major problem with the CTSN trial published in the *New England Journal of Medicine* in 2015.[11]

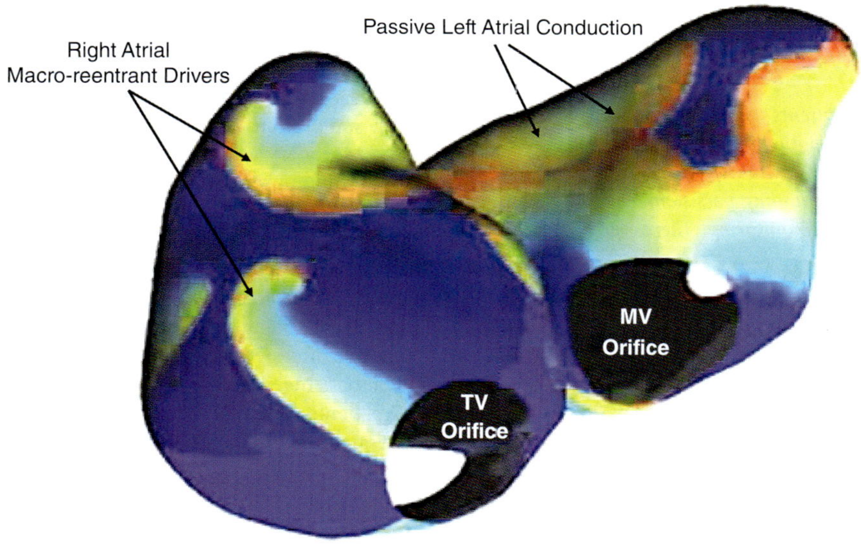

Fig. 19.3 Preoperative phase map of the atria a patient with non-paroxysmal atrial fibrillation (AF). In this single frame from a video of sustained AF, two active mac-o-reentrant drivers are clearly visible in the right atrium. Note that the entire left atrium is being passively activated in response to the two right atrial drivers. *MV,* Mitral valve; *TV,* tricuspid valve.

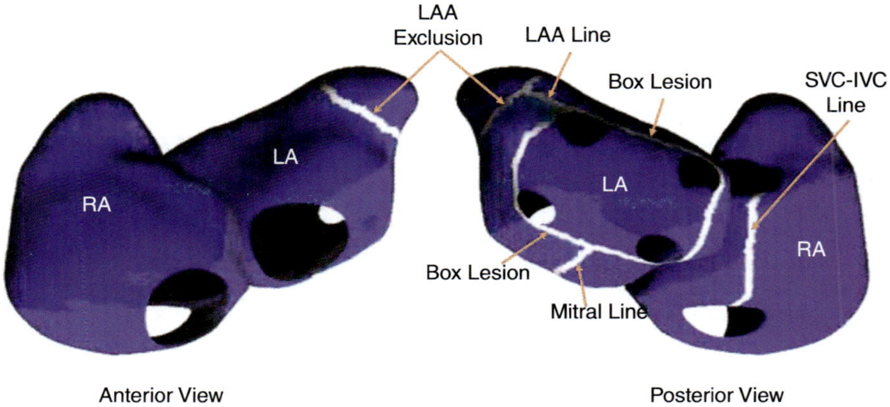

Fig. 19.4 Anterior and posterior views of the atria showing the locations of surgical lesions a "left atrial Maze" procedure for atrial fibrillation. In addition to the left atrial lesions, a right atrial intercaval lesion between the superior vena cava (SVC) and inferior vena cava (IVC) was added for unknown reasons in this particular patient. A coronary sinus lesion, not shown here, was also created in the plane of the mitral line to prevent postoperative peri-mitral flutter. Each of these left atrial lesions is placed in the perfect position, as is the intercaval line in the right atrium (RA). *LA,* Left atrium; *LAA,* left atrial appendage.

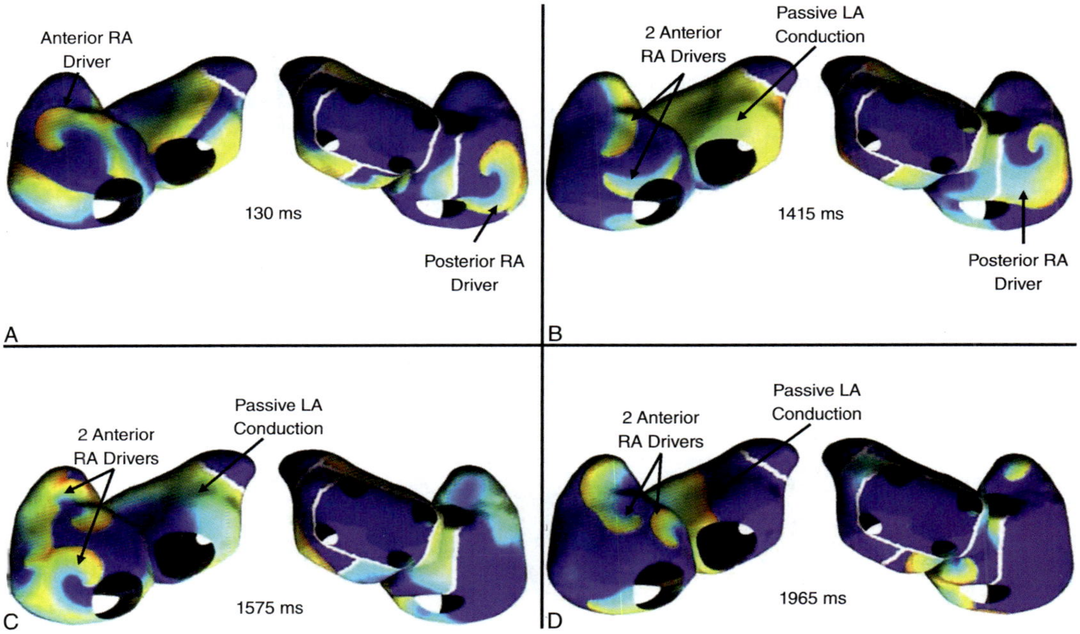

Fig. 19.5 Failed "left atrial Maze" procedure for non-paroxysmal atrial fibrillation (non-PAF).

- These are four frames from a postoperative video of recurrent AF after the left atrial Maze procedure shown in the Fig. 19.4 that demonstrate the importance of including the right atrial lesions in patients with non-PAF. They document that each of the left atrial lesions except the right atrial intercaval lesion is functioning perfectly as a line of bidirectional conduction block:
  - The four pulmonary veins and posterior left atrial wall are successfully isolated from the rest of the atrial myocardium by the box lesion (A–D).
  - The mitral line blocks conduction in both directions (A and B).
  - The LAA line blocks conduction in both directions (A and D).
- However, the right atrial intercaval line blocks conduction only from medial to lateral (C) but not from lateral to medial (B), so it has resulted in a unidirectional conduction block only. The drivers that are sustaining AF are clearly documented in all four frames of the video:
  - 130 ms after the beginning of the video, two macro-reentrant circuits are simultaneously driving AF, one located in the anterior right atrium (RA) and another in the posterior RA.
  - The 1415-ms frame shows three simultaneous AF drivers, two in the anterior RA and one in the posterior RA. Note the smooth, passive activation of the left atrium (LA) in response to the active AF drivers in the RA.
  - At 1575 ms, the two RA drivers are still apparent, and passive activation of the LA continues.
  - At 1965 ms, two drivers are still active in the RA, and a new passive wavefront generated by these two drivers is being conducted passively across the LA.

This series of snapshots from a video of sustained AF after a perfectly performed left atrial Maze procedure demonstrates the importance of performing the RA lesions when treating patients with non-PAF. They also show the futility of trying to use mapping to determine precisely where surgical or catheter lesions should be placed to ablate AF because these drivers change locations every few milliseconds. It is a graphic demonstration of why interventional therapy for AF cannot be map guided reliably even with the ready availability of such sophisticated mapping techniques.

DALLAS LESION SET

In 2009, Jimmy Edgerton and colleagues[27] introduced a modification of the left atrial Maze lesion pattern that adhered to the concept of a Maze procedure with the exception that the right atrial lesions were not included (Fig. 19.6). The combined posterior mitral line and coronary sinus lesions of the Maze procedure that prevent postoperative peri-mitral flutter (see Chapter 48) cannot be performed off pump epicardially, so these authors replaced the two lesions in the left atrial isthmus with a single epicardial "anterior trigone lesion" from the PVI roof line down to the left fibrous trigone. If this anterior trigone lesion is complete, it is as effective in preventing postoperative peri-mitral flutter as the posterior mitral line–coronary sinus lesion across the left atrial isthmus. In their initial report, the authors stated that all of the lesions were tested intraoperatively and successfully blocked conduction bidirectionally. Had they included the right atrial lesions with this pattern of left atrial lesions, the operation could rightly have deserved a new Roman numeral designation as another step in the series of Maze procedures, perhaps the "Maze-V" procedure. However, when one chooses to change a lesion from one location to another in the RA or LA lesion sets, one must be aware not only of the potential advantages of the new lesion but also of its potential negative consequences.

The problem with the anterior trigone lesion of the Dallas lesion set is twofold. First, it divides Bachmann's bundle and therefore forces sinus impulses to take a significantly longer route across the left atrial isthmus to reach the lateral LA (Fig. 19.7). The same problem was encountered in the Maze-I procedure and was one of the main reasons it had to be modified to the Maze-II procedure (see Chapter 12).

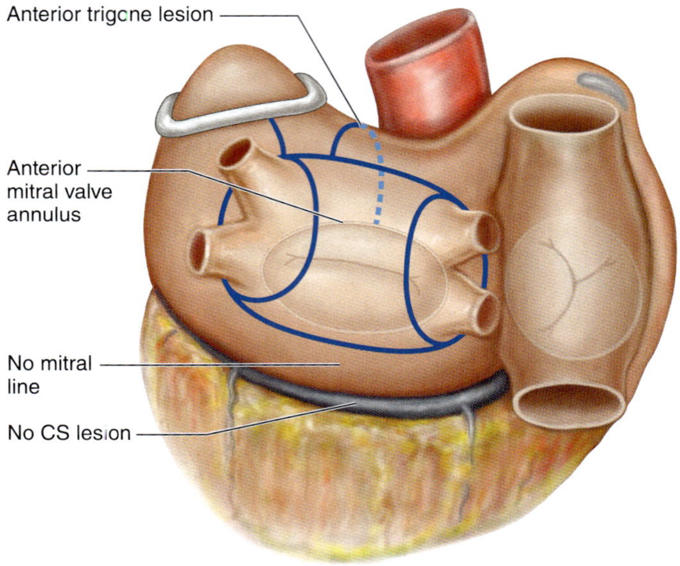

Fig. 19.6 Atrial lesions in the "Dallas lesion set." The mitral line and coronary sinus (CS) lesions that are designed to prevent postoperative perimitral flutter are eliminated and replaced by a single anterior trigone lesion from the roof of the box lesion, across Bachmann's bundle, down to the anterior mitral valve annulus. Because only one lesion is necessary to interrupt any reentrant circuit, the anterior trigone lesion was designed to interrupt the macro-reentrant circuit of peri-mitral flutter anteriorly rather than posteriorly where two lesions are required. (See text for further discussion.)

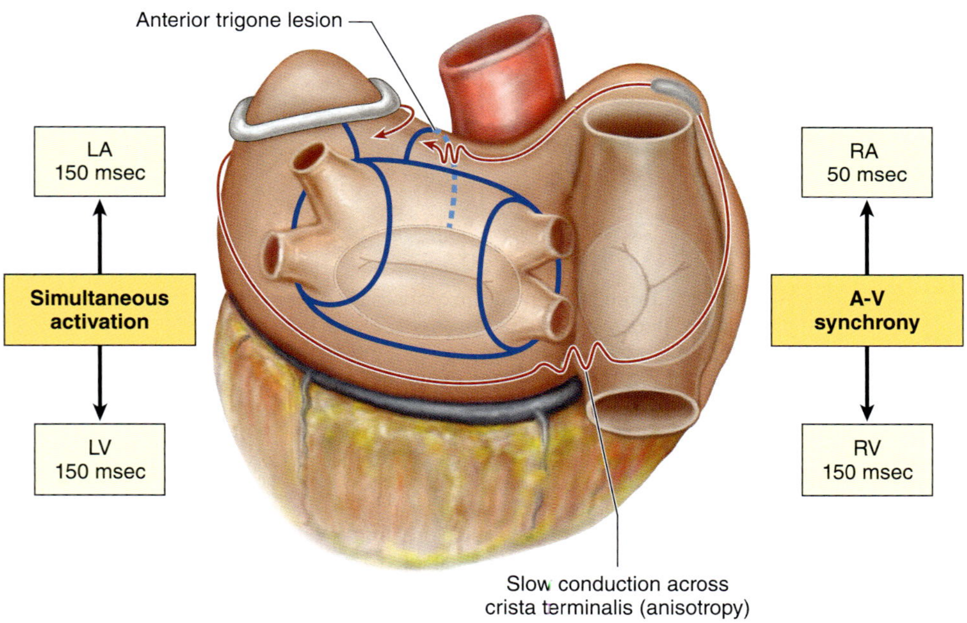

Fig. 19.7 It normally takes only about 40 ms for a sinus impulse in the right atrium (RA) to arrive in the left atrium (LA) because of the rapidity of impulse propagation across Bachmann's bundle. The anterior trigone lesion of the Dallas lesion set transects Bachmann's bundle and therefore delays the arrival of a sinus impulse in the left atrium by forcing it to reach the LA by propagating across the posteroinferior left atrial isthmus. In doing so, the impulse must traverse the crista terminalis in a direction that is perpendicular to its muscle fiber orientation, which slows the velocity of conduction in this area. If the delay is long enough (e.g., an extra 100–110 ms), the same sinus impulse will reach the LA at the same time it reaches the left ventricle (LV) through the atrioventricular node. This can result in the LA and LV being activated simultaneously and therefore, contracting simultaneously. In this situation, the LA will contract against a closed mitral valve and therefore, will lose its contribution to forward cardiac output. (See text for further discussion.) *RV,* Right ventricle.

Theoretically, the intraatrial conduction delay from the RA to the LA in the Dallas lesion set should not be as severe as it was in the Maze-I procedure because the forced posteroinferior conduction route across the left atrial isthmus is not completely blocked by the presence of the mitral line–coronary sinus lesions as it was in the Maze-I procedure. However, the sinus-generated impulse still must traverse the crista terminalis in a direction that is perpendicular to the orientation of its muscle fibers, which causes slowing of wavefront propagation in this area because of the phenomenon of anisotropy discussed in Chapter 3 (see Fig. 3.13). A severe interatrial conduction block can delay activation of the LA during sinus rhythm so much that the LA activates and contracts at the same time as the left ventricle, thereby abolishing effective LA transport function postoperatively. Unfortunately, neither the magnitude of the postoperative inter-atrial conduction delay nor the functional capacity of the LA has been evaluated after the Dallas lesion set.

The second problem with the anterior trigone lesion is that it is extremely difficult to create a permanent transmural lesion from the epicardium with a unipolar RF device in a normothermic beating, working heart (see Chapter 20) (Fig. 19.8). There are two problematic sites along the anterior trigone lesion, one at its distal end, where is it difficult to extend the lesion all the way to the left fibrous trigone, and another in subendocardium of Bachmann's bundle. This structure is a thick muscle bundle, and the "cooling sink" effect of intracavitary blood is often strong enough during epicardial RF ablation to prevent the atrial subendocardium of Bachmann's bundle from reaching a lethal temperature.

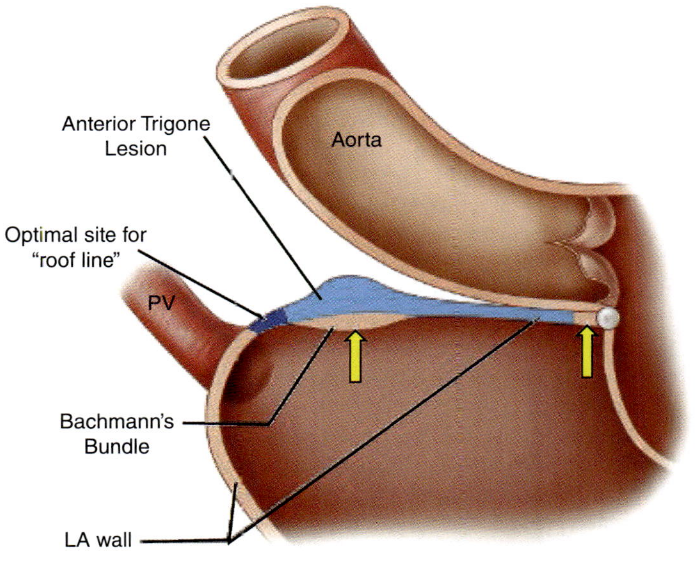

Fig. 19.8 Cross-section view of the relationship between the anterior left atrium (LA) and surrounding structures. The anterior trigone lesion *(light blue)* extends from the roof of a box lesion *(dark blue)* across Bachmann's bundle to the mitral valve annulus. Because this bundle is much thicker than the remainder of the anterior left atrial wall, it is difficult to create a transmural lesion through it using a unipolar radiofrequency (RF) ablation device placed on the epicardium, especially off-pump. Therefore, one common site of failure of the anterior trigone line is in the subendocardium of Bachmann's bundle *(left yellow arrow)*. Another vulnerable site for failure is near the level of the mitral annulus because it is difficult to reach all the way down to the annulus with an epicardial RF device *(right yellow arrow)*. *PV,* Pulmonary vein.

If the anterior trigone lesion fails at either of these sites, it establishes a potential macro-reentrant circuit in which electrical activity must travel in a larger circuit around the mitral annulus (i.e., it creates a potential macro-reentrant circuit just above the MV annulus with a *longer cycle length* than if the lesion had not been created at all). A longer cycle length dramatically increases the likelihood that a stable macro-reentrant circuit will develop (see Chapter 4). If it does, the result is postoperative peri-mitral flutter, the very problem that the anterior trigone lesion was designed to prevent. This means that a failed anterior trigone lesion is quite arrhythmogenic (i.e., it *promotes* the development of an arrhythmia). The difficulty of creating a permanent contiguous, uniformly transmural anterior trigone lesion from the epicardium off-pump and the pro-arrhythmic consequences of creating a failed lesion in this location have caused some authorities to abandon its use altogether.[28,29]

"FIVE-BOX MAZE" PROCEDURE

Another off-pump thoracoscopic surgical ablation procedure called the "five-box thoracoscopic Maze procedure" was proposed in 2012 (Fig. 19.9).[30] This approach includes isolation of the PVs in pairs (boxes 1 and 3) and roof and floor lesions to isolate the posterior left atrial wall (box 2). An anterior trigone lesion across Bachmann's bundle and a separate lesion across Bachmann's bundle from the roof line to the anterior trigone lesion isolates a portion of the anterosuperior left atrial wall designated as box 4. A circumferential lesion is also created in the RA to isolate the lower end of the superior vena cava (SVC; box 5). The problems associated with transecting Bachmann's bundle and those that arise from calling this a Maze procedure are the same as described for the three procedures discussed earlier. The needless addition of a right atrial lesion to isolate the lower end of the SVC from the RA is discussed in Chapter 13. Fortunately, this procedure has not received wide acceptance by arrhythmia surgeons.

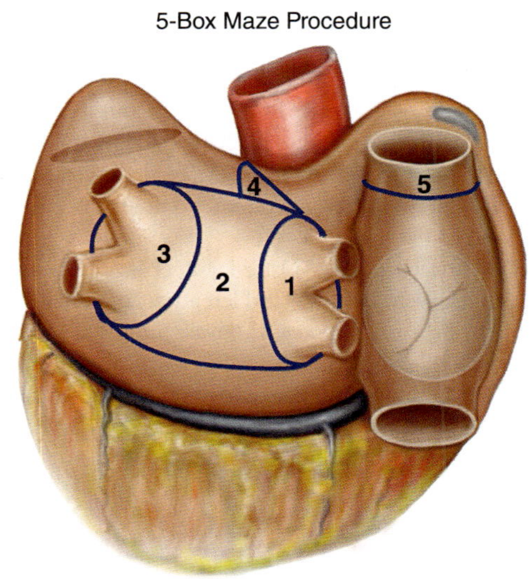

Fig. 19.9 The "five-box Maze" procedure. The title of this operation for atrial fibrillation takes its name from the five individual areas of the atrium that are isolated from the remainder of the atrial myocardium. They are shown in this illustration as numbers from *1* to *5*. (See text for further discussion.)

SUMMARY

The concept of a Maze procedure is to create atrial lesions in the pattern of a Maze to preclude or interrupt atrial macro-reentry and leave both atria capable of being activated during normal sinus rhythm. Thus the only Maze procedures are the historical Maze-I and Maze-II procedures and the contemporary Maze-III, Maze-IV, and Maze-V (Chapter 39) procedures because they are the only ones that adhere to the Maze concept for the treatment of AF. Procedures that do not adhere to this concept should not be called "Maze procedures."

REFERENCES

1. Haïssaguerre M, Jais P, Shah DC, et al. Spontaneous initiation of atrial fibrillation by ectopic beats originating the pulmonary veins. *N Engl J Med.* 1998;339:659–666.
2. Oral H, Knight BP, Tada H, et al. Pulmonary vein isolation for paroxysmal and persistent atrial fibrillation. *Circulation.* 2002;105(9):1077–1081 S.
3. Weerasooriya R, Khairy P, Litalien J, et al. Catheter ablation for atrial fibrillation: are results maintained at 5 years of follow-up? *J Am Coll Cardiol.* 2011;57(2):160–166.
4. Tilz RR, Rillig A, Thum AM, et al. Catheter ablation of long-standing persistent atrial fibrillation: 5-year outcomes of the Hamburg Sequential Ablation Strategy. *J Am Coll Cardiol.* 2012;60(19):1921–1929.
5. Gillinov AM, McCarthy PM. AtriCure bipolar radiofrequency clamp for intraoperative ablation of atrial fibrillation. *Ann Thorac Surg.* 2002;74(6):2165–2168.
6. McCarthy PM, Gerdisch M, Philpott J, et al. Three-year outcomes of the postapproval study of the atricure bipolar radiofrequency ablation of permanent atrial fibrillation trial. *J Thorac Cardiovasc Surg.* 2022;164(2):519–527.
7. Ruaengsri C, Schill MRR, Khiabani AJ, Schuessler RB, Melby SJ, Damiano Jr RJ. The Cox-Maze IV procedure in its second decade: still the gold standard? *Eur J Cardiothorac Surg.* 2018;53(1):i19–i25.
8. Ad N. How do we spell Maze? A dialogue concerning definitions and goals. *J Thorac Cardiovasc Surg.* 2006;132(6):1253–1255.
9. Ad N. How do we spell Maze (2.0)? A dialogue concerning definition and outcome. *J Thorac Cardiovasc Surg.* 2019;157(1):245–247.
10. Cox JL, Churyla A, Malaisrie SC, et al. When is a Maze procedure a Maze procedure? *Can J Cardiol.* 2018;34(11):1491–1492.
11. Gillinov Am, Gelijns AC, Parides MK, et al. Surgical ablation of atrial fibrillation during mitral-valve surgery. *N Eng J Med.* 2015;372(15):1399–1409.
12. Wolf RK, Schneeberger EW, Osterday R, et al. Video- assisted bilateral pulmonary vein isolation and left atrial appendage exclusion for atrial fibrillation. *J Thorac Cardiovasc Surg.* 2005;130:797–802.
13. Badhwar V, Rankin S, Damiano Jr RJ, et al. The society of thoracic surgeons 2017 clinical practice guidelines for the surgical treatment of atrial fibrillation. *Ann Thorac Surg.* 2017;103:329–341.
14. Ad N, Damiano Jr RJ, Badhwar V, et al. Expert consensus guidelines: examining surgical ablation for atrial fibrillation. *J Thor Cardiovasc Surg.* 2017;153(6):1330–1354.
15. WolfminiMaze.com.
16. Wolf RK. Minimally invasive surgical treatment of atrial fibrillation. *Semin Thorac Cardiovasc Surg.* 2007;19(4):311.
17. Wolf RK, Burgess S. Minimally invasive surgery for atrial fibrillation—wolf mini Maze procedure. *Ann Cardiothoracic Surg.* 2014;3(1):122–123.
18. Wolf RK. Treatment of lone atrial fibrillation: minimally invasive pulmonary vein isolation, partial cardiac denervation and excision of the left atrial appendage. *Ann Cardiothorac Surg.* 2014;3(1):98–104.
19. Wolf RK. Surgical treatment of atrial fibrillation. *Methodist DeBakey Cardiovasc J.* 2021;16(1):56–64.
20. Ad N, Holmes SD, Friehling T: Minimally invasive stand-alone Cox Maze procedure for persistent and long-standing persistent AF: perioperative safety and 5-year outcomes. Circ Arrhythm Electrophysiol, 10(11), p e005352.
21. MacGregor RM, Bakir NH, Pedamallu H, et al. Late results after stand-alone surgical ablation for atrial fibrillation. *J Thorac Cardiovasc Surg.* 2022;164(5):1515–1528.
22. Soni LK, Cedola SR, Cogan J, et al. Right atrial lesions do not improve the efficacy of a complete left atrial lesion set in the surgical treatment of atrial fibrillation but they do increase procedural morbidity. *J Thorac Cardiovasc Surg.* 2013;145(2):356–361.
23. Ad N, Holmes SD, Lamont D, Shuman DJ. Left-sided surgical ablation for patients with atrial fibrillation who are undergoing concomitant cardiac surgical procedures. *Ann Thorac Surg.* 2017;103:58–63.
24. Churyla A, Iddriss A, Andrei A-C, et al. Biatrial or left atrial lesion set for ablation during mitral surgery: risks and benefits. *Ann Thorac Surg.* 2017;103:1856–1865.
25. Lim HS, Hocini M, Dubois R, et al. Complexity and distribution of drivers in relation to duration of persistent atrial fibrillation. *J Am Coll Cardiol.* 2017;69(10):1257–1269.
26. Giorgios T, Antonio F, Limite LR, et al. Bi-atrial characterization of the electrical substrate in patients with atrial fibrillation. *Pacing Clin Electrophysiol.* 2022;45:752–760.
27. Edgerton JR, Jackman WM, Mack MJ. A new epicardial lesion set for minimal access left atrial Maze: the Dallas lesion set. *Ann Thorac Surg.* 2009;88:1655–1657.
28. Pison L, La Meir M, Crijns HJ. Left atrial flutter due to incomplete left fibrous trigone linear lesion. *J Thorac Cardiovasc Surg.* 2011;142(5):e149–e150.
29. Sawhney N, Anousheh R, Chen W, Feld GK. Circumferential pulmonary vein ablation with additional linear ablation results in an increased incidence of left atrial flutter compared with segmental pulmonary vein isolation as an initial approach to ablation of paroxysmal atrial fibrillation. *Circ Arrhythm Electrophysiol.* 2010;2:243–248.
30. Sirak J, Jones D, Schwartzman D. The five-box thoracoscopic Maze procedure. *Ann Thorac Surg.* 2012;95(3):986–989.

20

Lesion Integrity, Energy Sources, Ablation Devices, and Intraoperative Testing

James L. Cox, Ralph J. Damiano, Jr., Sydney L. Gaynor

CHAPTER OUTLINE

The two current types of energy sources available to create atrial lesions surgically in patients with arrhythmias are radiofrequency (RF) energy and cryothermia. Both are thermal energy sources, with RF ablation depending on tissue heating and cryoablation depending on freezing. RF and cryothermia operate on a temperature spectrum that ranges from 61°C, the critical lethal myocardial temperature of RF-generated heat,[1,2] to −30°C, the critical lethal temperature for cryothermia-generated cold (Fig. 20.1).[3–6]

Although there have been no randomized controlled trials (RCTs) to compare the efficacy of one ablation technology with another, these technologies have had proven clinical efficiency over the past two decades. To date, a prospective, multicenter, non-RCT, AtriCure Bipolar Radiofrequency Ablation of Permanent Atrial Fibrillation, has resulted in specific US Food and Drug Administration (FDA) approval for surgical treatment of patients with atrial fibrillation (AF).[7] This device was used on patients with nonparoxysmal AF undergoing concomitant coronary artery bypass graft and/or valve procedures and Maze-IV ablation and resulted in a 76% freedom from AF recurrence off antiarrhythmic drugs at 6 months.

Two factors determine the effectiveness of any surgical procedure for AF, and they are controlled by both the surgeon and the ablation technology: (1) the specific locations where the lesions are created in the atria and (2) the ability of the lesion to create conduction block, which has been shown to require transmural atrial necrosis throughout the entire lesion. It was not challenging to control both of these factors with the cut-and-sew Maze procedures because the same lesion pattern was used within each iteration of the Maze procedure, and surgical incisions precluded any concern about creating lesions with potential gaps or that were not transmural. When the cut-and-sew Maze-III procedure was converted to the minimally invasive CryoMaze procedure in the mid-1990s, the lesion pattern remained the same (see Chapter 14). By that time, N_2O-based cryosurgery had been used for more than 20 years to ablate cardiac arrhythmias clinically (see Chapter 9). Therefore each cryolesion in the CryoMaze procedure was believed to be complete, and it was not surprising that the outcomes of the two different surgical techniques for performing a Maze-III lesion pattern proved to be similar.

In 2004, Gaynor et al.[8] were the first to publish their findings on the use of a combination of bipolar RF and cryoablation in performing the Cox-Maze-IV procedure. This technique was introduced after rigorous experimental testing of the bipolar RF clamps, and after two decades, it is the most commonly performed surgical procedure for AF and the only surgical procedure to have an FDA indication to treat patients with AF. Experimental studies have suggested that the Cox-Maze-IV procedure can be performed on the beating heart.[9,10]

Soon after Haissaguerre and colleagues'[11] 1998 report showing that pulmonary vein isolation (PVI) with RF catheters was effective for the treatment of patients with paroxysmal AF, new atrial lesion patterns were proposed by both surgeons and interventional electrophysiologists, and industry adapted new energy sources for surgical ablation devices. Thus two variables were introduced that directly affected subsequent surgical outcomes, making it difficult to determine whether future failures were due to an inappropriate lesion pattern or to the inadequacy of the ablative energy source. This led a number of groups to go back to the research laboratory and investigate the efficacy of the new ablation technologies.[12] In the first decade after Haissaguerre et al.'s report, most interventional AF procedure failures were attributed

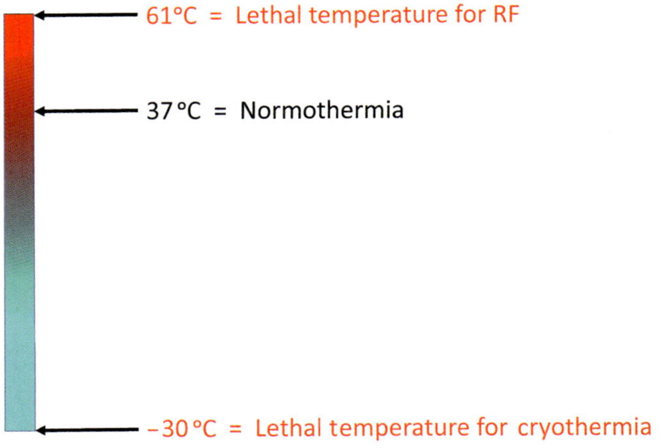

Fig. 20.1 Temperature scale from the critical lethal temperature using heat-based ablation devices such as radiofrequency (RF) catheters and surgical clamps (61°C) to the critical lethal temperature using cryothermia-based ablation devices such as cryoballoon catheters and surgical cryoprobes (−30°C).

to the ablative energy source rather than to the inappropriateness of the lesion pattern. For example, despite PVI alone being an inherently inadequate intervention for AF, its failure in treating persistent and long-standing persistent AF (LSpAF) was commonly attributed to the limitations of the ablative energy source. As a result, several ablative energy sources, such as microwave, laser, and high-intensity ultrasonography, were withdrawn from the market even though they had often been used to create lesion patterns that were likely inadequate for nonparoxysmal AF. However, experimental work did show that many of these energy sources were unable to create reliably transmural lesions.[13] During the past decade, more emphasis has been placed on the importance of creating an adequate lesion pattern for the various types of AF. This gradual change in emphasis was fueled by the dismal results of PVI alone for LSpAF (see Chapters 25 and 31) and led to the development of hybrid approaches using both thoracoscopic surgery and catheter ablation for the treatment of complex forms of AF (see Section IV).

LESION INTEGRITY

The efficacy of a specific lesion pattern depends on each of its individual lesions completely blocking electrical conduction. Because electrical wavefronts propagate through the full thickness of the atrial wall (Fig. 20.2), every lesion must be uniformly transmural and contiguous with no gaps (Fig. 20.3). For example, one of the most common technical errors during endocardial cryosurgery in an arrested heart is the creation of "folds" in the atrial wall that can occur across the line of intended ablation.[14] In this situation, the cryolesion will appear to be contiguous, but the folded portion of the atrial wall will not be ablated (Fig. 20.4, *upper panel*). When the lesion is allowed to thaw and the atrial wall resumes its normal shape, a gap will exist in the intended line of ablation (Fig. 20.4, *lower panel*), and the procedure will fail. This is why it is absolutely essential to smooth out all folds in the atrial wall and assure perfect apposition of the cryoprobe and the target atrial tissue without even the smallest of gaps before creating a linear cryolesion.

Similarly, several factors influence the ability of RF energy to create transmural lesions in myocardial tissue, including tissue thickness, overlying epicardial fat, char on the ablation device and tissue, and air pockets in folded tissue. The generators that supply RF energy operate on an impedance algorithm that acts as a surrogate for determining lesion transmurality. Any foreign body that increases impedance may impact the interpretation of lesion transmurality in a negative way. In a study by two of the authors (RJD and SLG), a single bipolar ablation did not result in consistent transmural ablation, with more than one-third of lesions being non-transmural. Performing two successive ablations without unclamping the device produced transmural lesions in 100% of histologic sections in *ex vivo* human hearts.[15] The technique reliably produced transmural lesions regardless of tissue characteristics (i.e., the presence of epicardial fat, atrial wall thickness) or ablation location. Based on these findings, surgeons performing AF ablation

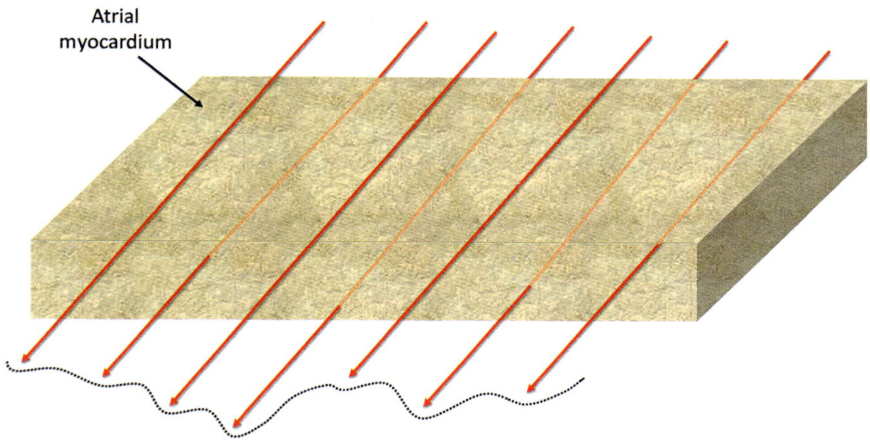

Fig. 20.2 Diagrammatic sketch of the atrial wall showing that electrical activation *(red arrows)* and wavefront propagation *(dotted black line)* occur in all layers of the atrial wall.

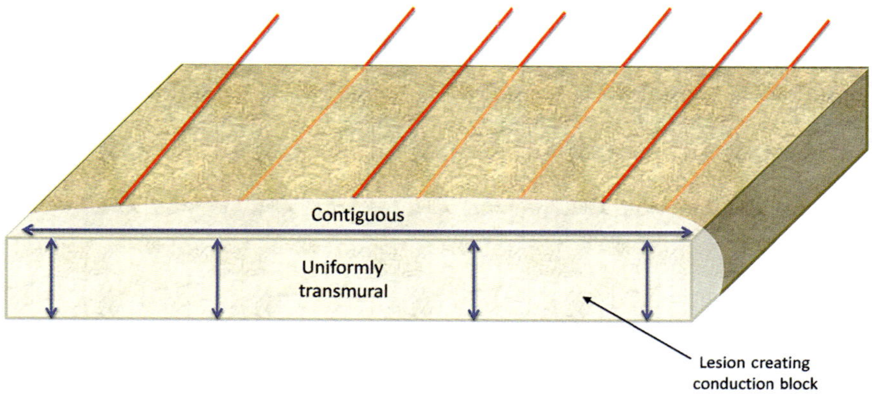

Fig. 20.3 The ideal lesion is contiguous (has no gaps) and uniformly transmural. Any lesion that meets these two simple criteria will block the conduction of electrical activity across it.

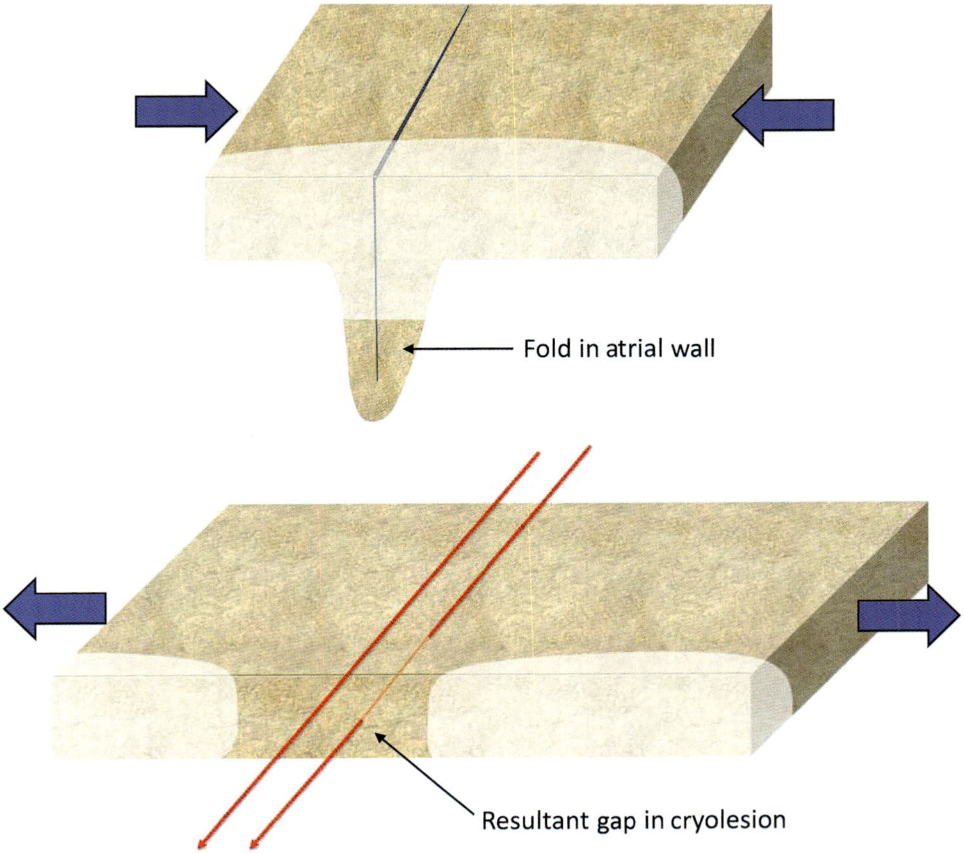

Fig. 20.4 *Upper panel,* A common cause of gaps in a lesion, especially cryolesions, occurs when the folds in the atrial wall are not smoothed out before application of the ablation energy. Thus the ablation does not penetrate to the distal portion of the folded wall. *Lower panel,* When the atrial wall is allowed to unfold, the nonablated portion will appear as a gap in the intended line of ablation.

with bipolar RF clamps should use a double-ablation technique to increase the likelihood of achieving conduction block.

Perhaps the most common reason that individual lesions fail is that they are not transmural. Immediately after the creation of an RF lesion or a cryolesion, there are a central area of irreversibly injured cells and a peripheral area around this dead zone where myocardial cells are still viable but temporarily incapable of conducting electrical activity. Immediate intraoperative testing may indicate that the newly created lesion is contiguous and uniformly transmural because it has blocked electrical conduction across the lesion (Fig. 20.5, *upper panel*). With time, however, the viable peripheral cells can recover from the acute injury and resume their ability to conduct electrical activity. In this case, the lesion that caused complete conduction block intraoperatively will no longer be transmural, and the procedure may fail (Fig. 20.5, *lower panel*). This highlights the necessity of careful experimental evaluation of each device to define efficacy, in which histologic assessment can be used to definitely define lesion transmurality. Unfortunately, ablation in experimental animals does not always reflect the clinical situation, requiring the development of more realistic models, such as human hearts turned down for transplantation.[15,16]

UNIPOLAR RADIOFREQUENCY ABLATION

The terminology describing RF devices has evolved, and because it can be confusing, it deserves clarification. RF energy can be delivered to myocardial tissue as either a unipolar or bipolar energy source. Unipolar RF devices are, by definition, unidirectional, meaning that the RF energy can be delivered from only one surface of the atrium at a time, either the epicardium or the endocardium. Unipolar RF devices are the so-called unipolar pens. Bipolar RF devices can be either uni directional or bidirectional. Bipolar unidirectional devices deliver RF via two adjacent electrodes that, like unipolar devices, can deliver ablative energy from either the endocardium or epicardium but not from both simultaneously: that is, they are technically bipolar devices but functionally are unidirectional devices that have to overcome the limitations of unipolar unidirectional devices. Examples of bipolar unidirectional devices are the Atricure Isolator RF pen and the AtriCure Coolrail device (Atricure, Inc., Mason, OH). Bipolar bidirectional devices have the electrodes embedded in the opposite jaws of a clamp, allowing the RF to be delivered from both sides of the target tissue simultaneously but requiring that it be encompassed in the jaws of a clamp. Both the Medtronic Cardioblate clamp and the Atricure Synergy clamp are bipolar bidirectional RF devices, even though the Cardioblate clamp has one electrode in each jaw of the clamp and the Synergy device has two electrodes in each jaw of the clamp. Although catheter techniques are restricted to the use of unipolar RF ablation, both unipolar RF and bipolar RF can be used for the surgical ablation. Unipolar RF devices can measure the electrode interface temperature with or without a suction stabilization device to enhance tissue contact. They can be either irrigated or non-irrigated. Despite

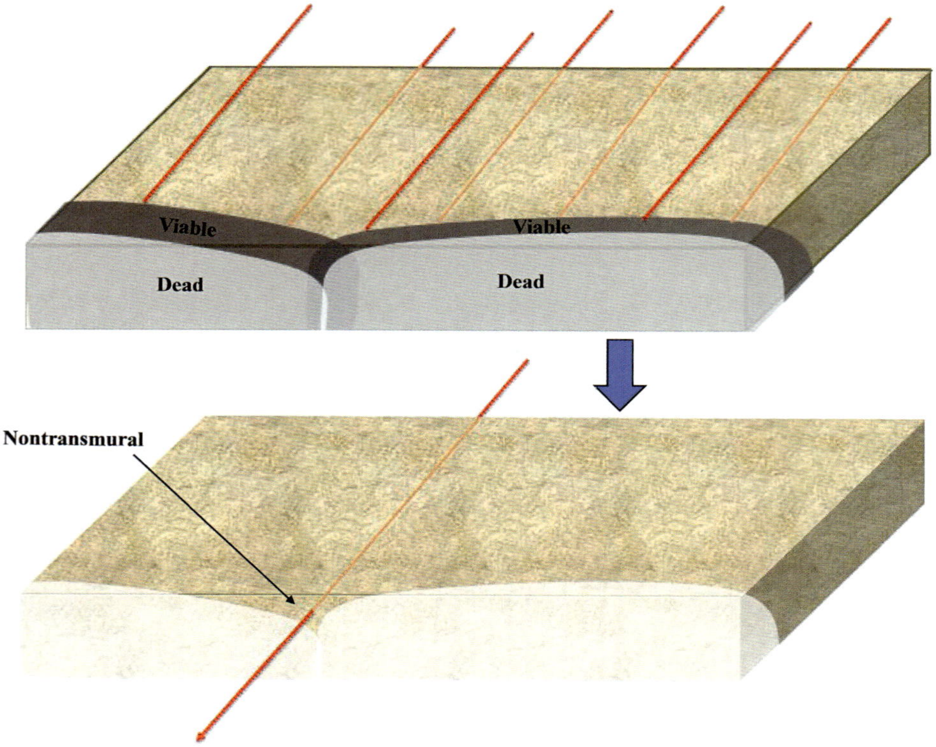

Fig. 20.5 *Upper panel,* A lesion created with any ablative energy source has a zone where the cells are killed acutely surrounded by a zone where the cells remain viable but are too damaged temporarily to conduct electrical activity. *Lower panel,* When enough time has passed for these viable cells to recover, they can resume their normal function and conduct electrical activity. Therefore, it is essential that the initial ablation procedure be sufficient to extend the "dead zone" all the way through the atrial wall.

the variety of unipolar devices, as mentioned earlier, they have had limited success in creating transmural lesions consistently.[12,17,18] None has been FDA approved for the surgical treatment of patients with AF. The only FDA-approved unipolar RF device is for hybrid therapy for persistent AF and LSpAF (EPi-Sense Guided Coagulation System with Visitrax, AtriCure) and is described below. The EPi-Sense device is a 3-cm-long, suction-assisted, irrigated unipolar RF device. The lesion transmurality of this device is variable,[12,19] but its clinical performance has been validated in the treatment of patients with persistent AF and LSpAF in the setting of the minimally invasive Convergent hybrid procedure (see Chapter 36).[20]

Unipolar RF ablation systems deliver RF energy between a single small electrode at the tip of a unipolar catheter or surgical pen and a large grounding patch typically placed on the skin of the abdomen or thigh. When the catheter or surgical pen is placed at the target site, alternating current (500–1000 kHz) is applied to the tip electrode, and RF current passes from the tip of the unipolar device to the grounding patch. Resistive heating occurs in the intervening tissue at a rate proportional to the square of current density, which is highest at the tissue-electrode interface at the tip of the unipolar device. As a result, significant resistive heating occurs only at this interface. Deeper unipolar RF lesions result from conductive heating of myocardium adjacent to the site of resistive heating.

The efficacy of unipolar RF ablation varies depending on the state of the heart and whether the unipolar RF is applied epicardially or endocardially. The use of unipolar RF can be problematic in totally thoracoscopic procedures and in hybrid procedures for AF because of the "cooling-sink" effect of circulating intracavitary blood. When the patient is off pump, the cavitary blood is not only normothermic but also flowing through the atrium at 4 to 5 L/min (Fig. 20.6, *upper panel*). Continuous cooling of the endocardial surface of the atrial wall by the intracavitary blood flow will prevent the subendocardium from reaching a critical lethal temperature, and the lesion will be non-transmural (Fig. 20.6, *lower panel*). Most transmural gaps that remain after the initial thoracoscopic step in hybrid procedures are located in the subendocardium, emphasizing the importance of performing the follow-up endocardial catheter ablation to close any remaining gaps. The problem of residual endocardial gaps also favors the theoretical advantage of delaying the follow-up catheter ablation long enough to allow the thoracoscopic lesions to heal. In extensive experimental evaluation, all unipolar RF devices have been shown to be incapable of creating reliable transmural lesions from the epicardial surface in the beating heart.[12] The same is true for cryoablation, which is also a unidirectional ablative energy source that relies on thermal cooling.

The ability to create transmural lesions with unipolar RF devices from the epicardium is enhanced by cardiopulmonary bypass (CPB) because the "cooling-sink" created by circulating cavitary blood is eliminated (Fig. 20.7).[13] However, both epicardial and endocardial unipolar RF is unpredictable even during normothermic CPB because there is no visual or quantitative feedback that confirms transmurality during the creation of a lesion. In a normothermic heart on or off CPB, RF ablative energy must increase the temperature of myocardial cells from 37°C to more than 61°C to ensure cell death. However, when unipolar RF ablation is performed endocardially during *cardioplegic arrest* when the targeted myocardial temperature is only 10° to 15°C, the magnitude of change in the myocardial temperature to ensure cell death is even

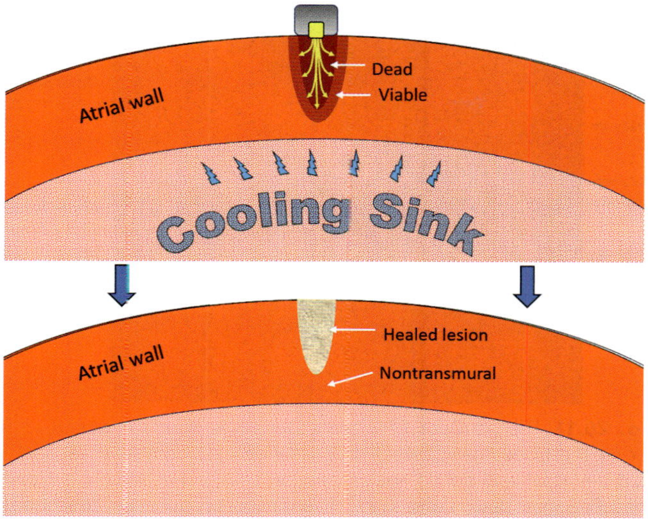

Fig. 20.6 **Unipolar radiofrequency (RF) ablation: epicardial, off pump.** *Upper panel,* When unipolar RF energy is applied epicardially to create a lesion in the atrial wall and the patient is not on cardiopulmonary bypass (CPB), the cavitary blood acts as a "cooling sink," making it difficult for the epicardial RF device to heat the subendocardium of the atrial wall to a lethal temperature. The "cooling-sink" effect results not only from the blood being normothermic but also because it is circulating through the atrium at 4 to 5 L/min, thereby enhancing its ability to keep the endocardium cool. *Lower panel,* If the epicardial unipolar RF device is unable to heat the subendocardium to a lethal temperature (61°C), the permanent lesion will not be transmural, and the lesion will fail to block electrical conduction.

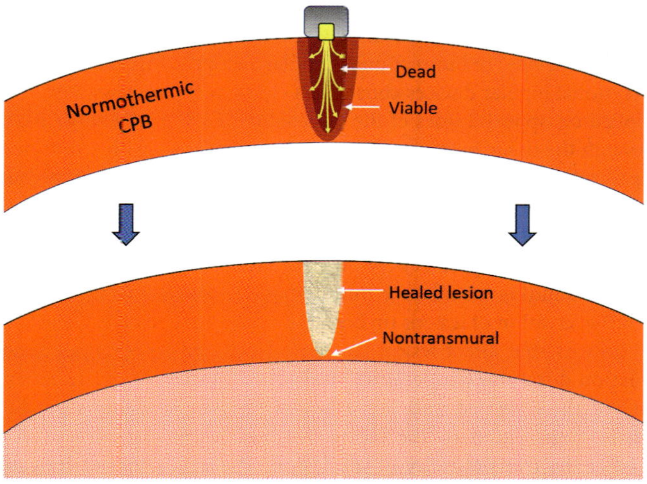

Fig. 20.7 **Unipolar radiofrequency (RF) ablation epicardial, on normothermic cardiopulmonary bypass.** *Upper panel,* Because there is no atrial cavitary blood on pump, unipolar RF applied to the epicardium is more likely to result in a transmural lesion than the same energy applied at the same site off pump. However, there is still no way to confirm in the operating room if the lesion is transmural or not. In this case, transmurality depends primarily on the thickness of the atrial wall in the target area. *Lower panel,* If the subendocardium does not reach the lethal temperature of 61°C, the permanent lesion will be non-transmural. It is not well established how large this remaining bridge of subendocardium has to be to conduct electrical activity and cause the lesion to fail. However, the accessory atrio-ventricular connections (which are residual strands of atrial muscle) responsible for bidirectional electrical conduction in the Wolfe-Parkinson-White syndrome are approximately the size of a human hair (see Chapter 1, Fig. 1.6).

greater (Fig. 20.8). Although unipolar RF can be capable of doing this in thin atrial tissue, its success depends on the persistence and patience of the surgeon to attain transmurality. Because unipolar linear lesions on the endocardium have to be created much like those with endocardial catheters (i.e., by creating a line of overlapping transmural "dots"), the use of endocardial unipolar RF in the arrested heart can be laborious and time consuming (Fig. 20.9). Using unipolar RF pens to simply

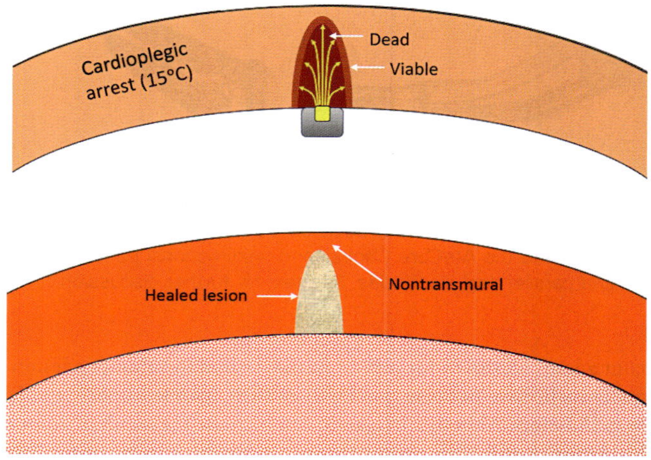

Fig. 20.8 **Unipolar radiofrequency (RF) ablation: endocardial, cardioplegic arrest.** *Upper panel,* The temperature of the atrial wall should be approximately 15°C during cardioplegic arrest, and there should be no warm blood circulating through the capillaries of the atrial wall. Therefore, either epicardial or endocardial RF ablation should be more successful under cardioplegic arrest than when the heart is normothermic on or off pump. *Lower panel,* The lesions are more likely to be transmural if they are performed under cardioplegic arrest, but they can still fail depending on the surgical technique and the thickness of the targeted atrial wall.

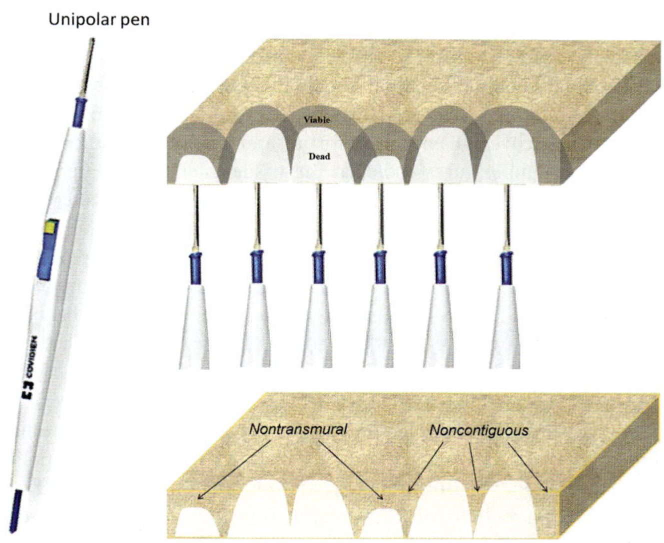

Fig. 20.9 **Unipolar radiofrequency (RF) ablation: endocardial, cardioplegic arrest.** *Upper panel,* To create a linear lesion using unipolar RF endocardially, multiple individual applications are required, and each of them must be transmural and contiguous with lesions on both sides. Each of these lesions has a zone of instant cell death and a surrounding zone of viable but nonconducting tissue. *Lower panel,* With time some of the viable but non-conducting tissue can heal and resume electrical conduction. Therefore, it is preferable to use bipolar RF clamps or cryoprobes to create the lesions when the heart is arrested.

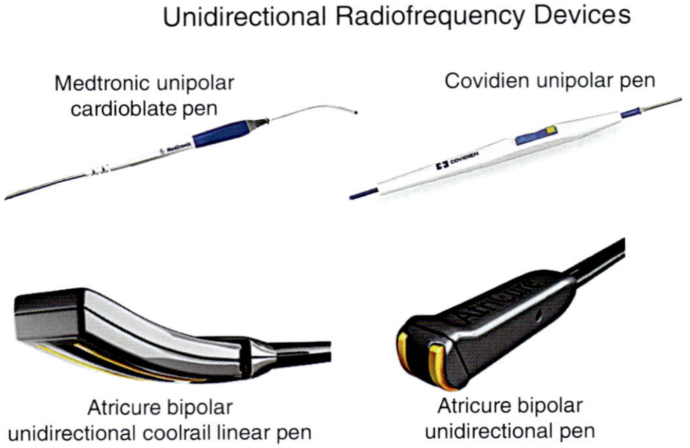

Fig. 20.10 The most commonly used unipolar and bipolar unidirectional devices. The Medtronic and Covidien unipolar pens both have single electrodes and the AtriCure Coolrail and unidirectional pens have adjacent and parallel dual electrodes. See text for further discussion.

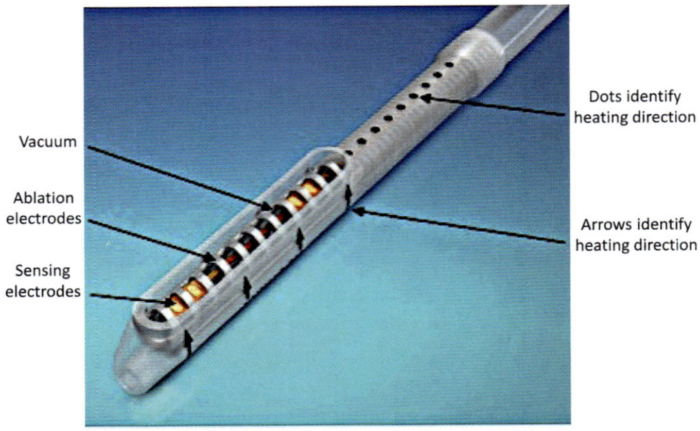

Fig. 20.11 The AtriCure EPi-Sense Device is specially designed for use in the Convergent hybrid procedure. It incorporates a vacuum to hold the atrial wall tightly against the sensing and ablation electrodes. The EPi-Sense device and the Convergent procedure are described in greater detail Chapter 36.

"paint a line" on the endocardium in the desired location of a lesion is usually ineffective because the depth of such "painted lines" is only a few millimeters. Although irrigation can increase the depth of unipolar RF ablation, it still does not reliably penetrate thick tissue or fat. Thus, these devices have been largely abandoned in clinical practice and have never received an indication to treat AF during concomitant surgery. It is preferable to avoid the use of unipolar RF surgical ablation devices in favor of bipolar RF clamps or cryosurgery whenever possible, as proposed in the Cox Maze-III and Cox Maze-IV procedures.

Currently, the most frequently used surgical ablation devices for the treatment of AF are manufactured by either AtriCure or Medtronic (Fig. 20.10). All of the AtriCure and Medtronic unipolar RF devices can be used to create epicardial and endocardial lesions in the atrium off-pump during normothermic CPB or under cardioplegic arrest. AtriCure bipolar unidirectional RF ablation devices include a pen and the Coolrail linear ablation pen as well as the EPi-Sense unidirectional device (see later). Medtronic unipolar RF ablation devices include a unipolar ablation pen.

RF energy can be delivered by either dry or irrigated electrodes. Irrigation helps deliver RF energy uniformly and to prevent char formation by keeping temperatures cooler at the tissue interface.[21] Unipolar RF ablation works by delivering RF energy from the probe directly to the tissue. The unipolar devices do not provide surgeons with transmurality indicators. In contrast, bidirectional bipolar RF (bipolar clamps) can be either directional or constrained, and transmurality can be implied by the manufacturer's dose-response algorithms. The unidirectional bipolar devices have two side-by-side electrodes that are applied to the target tissue surface, with the energy passing through the tissue between them.

Unlike bidirectional bipolar RF devices, unipolar and unidirectional bipolar devices have failed to consistently create transmural lesions and have a risk of forming endocardial char or thrombus when applied endocardially.[12,17,18,22] Both unipolar and unidirectional bipolar RF energy sources have had difficulty creating transmural lesions when used from the epicardial surface on the beating heart.[23] This difficulty is due to the circulating intracavitary blood flow, as stated earlier. To overcome this problem, devices have used suction to pull the atrial tissue into apposition, thus partially ameliorating the circulating heat sink.

The EPi-sense unipolar RF ablation device (Fig. 20.11) is specifically designed to be used in the Convergent hybrid procedure described in Chapter 36. It differs from other unipolar RF ablation devices by incorporating sensing electrodes and a vacuum system that holds the epicardium of the atrium in position against the ablating electrodes to enhance ablation efficacy. Because it is a unidirectional unipolar device, it does not always create transmural lesions when used off pump,[12] but because it is designed for use solely in the Convergent hybrid procedure, initial transmurality is less important. Since it is applied from the epicardial surface, virtually all remaining gaps are at the subendocardial level and can be easily closed during the obligatory endocardial catheter ablation portion of the hybrid procedure.

BIPOLAR RADIOFREQUENCY ABLATION

Bidirectional Bipolar Radiofrequency

As mentioned above, bipolar devices can be either unidirectional (Coolrail device) or bidirectional (bipolar clamps). The constrained bidirectional bipolar devices consist of a clamp with two jaws, which are applied on opposite sides of the targeted tissue. The RF energy passes through the tissue between the two jaws. RF ablation with constrained bipolar devices has provided faster and more efficient ablation because of direct contact with the tissue, with ablation time measured in seconds, as opposed to minutes. Because the tissue is ablated between the jaws of a clamp, the energy delivery is focused and isolated from the surrounding circulating intracavitary blood, allowing for more effective creation of lesions on both the beating and arrested heart.

Factors that affect lesion size and depth are power, impedance, ablation duration, temperature, and contact force.[15,24–26] The generators of the irrigated and nonirrigated bipolar RF clamps produce power transmitted to the electrodes, and these data are used to predict the transmurality of the lesion. The generators of irrigated clamps do this by measuring the impedance between electrodes, varying the power according to the impedance, and terminating power delivery once the feedback program detects a steady-state plateau.[21] On the other hand, the generators of nonirrigated clamps measure conductance and continue ablation until a stable low conductance is reached. Voltage is varied according to the conductance, resulting in a safe delivery of energy to the tissue.[15] Care should be taken to clean the electrodes after every two to three ablations with the nonirrigated clamps because char decreases conductance, which can result in nontransmural lesions.

Importantly, in a human heart ex vivo model, a double ablation without unclamping significantly improved lesion transmurality. Epicardial fat and muscle thickness can also decrease conductance and limit ablation depth.[15] The ablation duration affects the tissue temperature

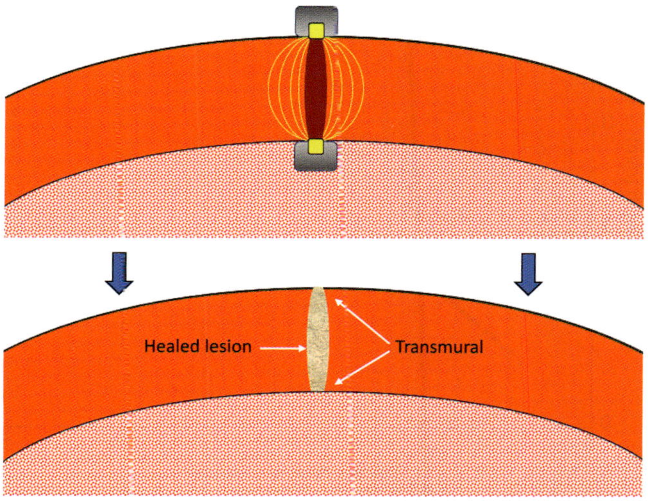

Fig. 20.12 **Bipolar radiofrequency (RF) ablation: off pump, on normothermic cardiopulmonary bypass, or cardioplegic arrest (one pair of electrodes).** *Upper panel,* Bipolar RF ablation can be performed safely and effectively off pump, on normothermic cardiopulmonary bypass, or under cardioplegic arrest. The arm of the bipolar RF clamp that is placed inside the atrium prevents cavitary blood from acting as a "cooling sink" in off-pump patients; therefore, bipolar RF ablation is far more effective than unipolar RF ablation when performing off-pump surgical ablation. *Lower panel,* RF energy is provided by both the epicardial and endocardial RF electrodes *(yellow lines)*, making the creation of a transmural lesion more reliable.

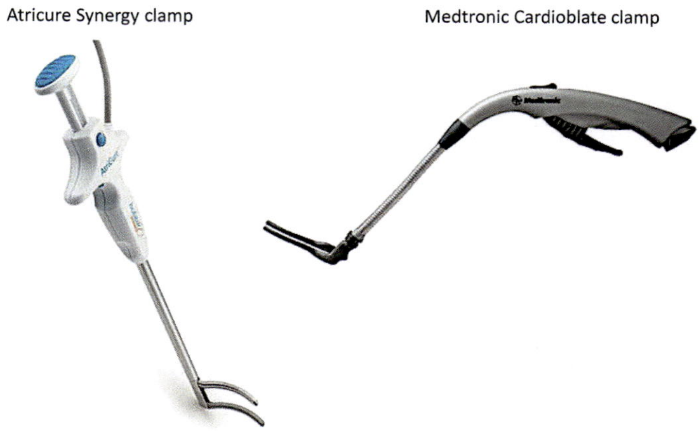

Fig. 20.13 The Medtronic Cardioblate bipolar atrial fibrillation (AF) clamp has a single pair of linear bipolar radiofrequency (RF) electrodes imbedded in each arm of the clamp as shown in Fig. 20.12. The AtriCure Synergy bipolar AF clamp has two pairs of linear bipolar RF electrodes imbedded in each arm of the bipolar clamp. See text for further discussion.

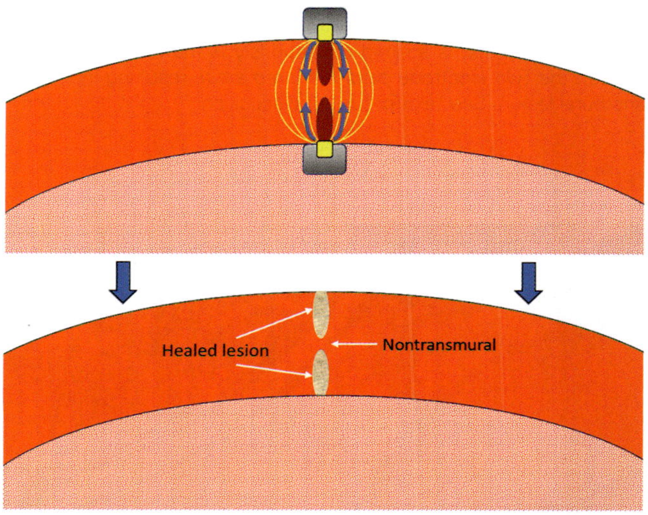

Fig. 20.14 **Bipolar radiofrequency (RF) ablation: off pump, no normothermic cardiopulmonary bypass, or cardioplegic arrest (one pair of electrodes).** *Upper panel,* One potential problem that can occur when using bipolar RF clamps with only a single ablation electrode on either side of the targeted atrial wall is that as the lesion forms, tissue impedance between the leading edges of the two ablation zones can increase enough to cause the RF energy to take the path of least resistance and circumvent the areas of higher impedance *(blue arrows)*. *Lower panel,* This can result in the mid-myocardium's failing to reach a lethal temperature, resulting in a nontransmural lesion.

profile. Cardiac muscle exposed to temperature of 50°C or higher for more than a few seconds will show irreversible coagulation necrosis.[27] Last, adequate but not excessive contact force is needed to achieve a reliable transmural lesion.[28,29]

Bipolar RF clamps can be used to treat patients with AF regardless of whether the heart is off pump, on normothermic CPB, or under cardioplegic arrest. A bipolar RF clamp can be used to create a lesion in the atrial free wall off pump by either completely surrounding a structure such as the pulmonary veins (PVs) or left atrial appendage or by placing one arm of the clamp inside and the other arm outside the atrium. The latter approach is not recommended in patients who are not on CPB because of bleeding and embolic risks. The endocardial arm of the clamp excludes the cavitary blood from the targeted tissue thus negating the "cooling-sink" effect that complicates epicardial unipolar RF (Fig. 20.12, *upper panel*). It also effectively prevents damage to collateral tissue. Bipolar RF ablation during surgery is commonly performed on CPB.

Currently, the most commonly used bipolar RF clamps for the treatment of AF are the AtriCure Isolator Synergy clamp and the Medtronic Cardioblate clamp (Fig. 20.13). One limitation of bipolar RF clamps that have only one electrode on each side of the target tissue is that as the lesion forms, tissue impedance between the leading edges of the two ablation zones can increase enough to cause the RF energy to take the path of least resistance and circumvent the areas of higher impedance (Fig. 20.14, *upper panel*). This can cause the lesions from each electrode to be shallow, resulting in a non-transmural lesion and procedural failure (Fig. 20.14, *lower panel*). The dual pairs of electrodes on the Synergy clamp deliver RF energy that alternates at 267 Hz with only one pair of opposing electrodes delivering RF energy at any one time (Fig. 20.15, *upper panel*). This creates a zone where RF energy is always being delivered where the alternating ablation fields overlap, resulting a wider and more reliable lesion (Fig. 20.15, *lower panel*). However, these clamps can still fail because of high tissue impedances.

Bipolar RF clamps are often used to create lesions in patients undergoing Maze procedures. They are commonly used for surgical isolation of the PVs (PVI). During isolation of the PVs in pairs, a bipolar clamp is placed on the posterior left atrium (LA) harboring the orifices of the right PVs and then on the posterior LA harboring the left PVs (Fig. 20.16). This results in the thickness of the target tissue being double that of bipolar ablation on the atrial free wall. The device can compensate for this with its algorithm and can vary power delivery up to 40-fold in thicker tissue. To overcome the problem of high impedance and thick tissue, most surgeons perform multiple ablations. The lack of consensus on the best method to ensure permanent transmurality of

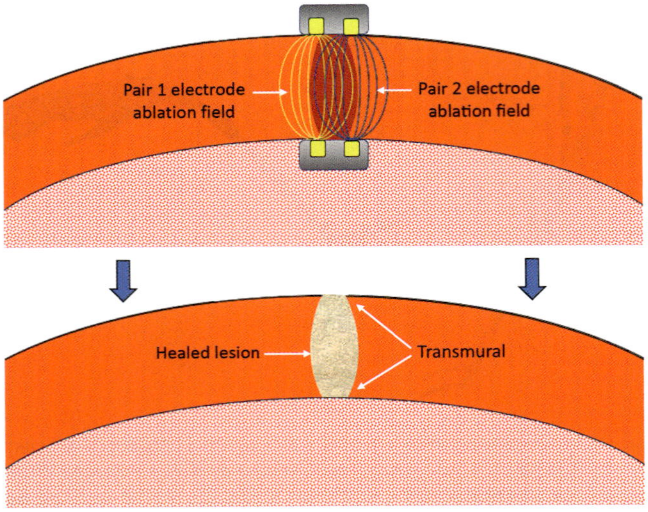

Fig. 20.15 **Bipolar radiofrequency (RF) ablation: off pump, no normothermic cardiopulmonary bypass, or cardioplegic arrest (two pairs of electrodes).** *Upper panel,* The two pairs of bipolar electrodes in the AtriCure Synergy bipolar RF clamp allow the ablative current to alternate between the two pairs at 267 Hz. *Lower panel,* The only portion of the atrial wall that is ablated continuously is the overlapping region between the two electrode pairs *(dark red area)*, resulting in a reliable transmural lesion. See text for further discussion.

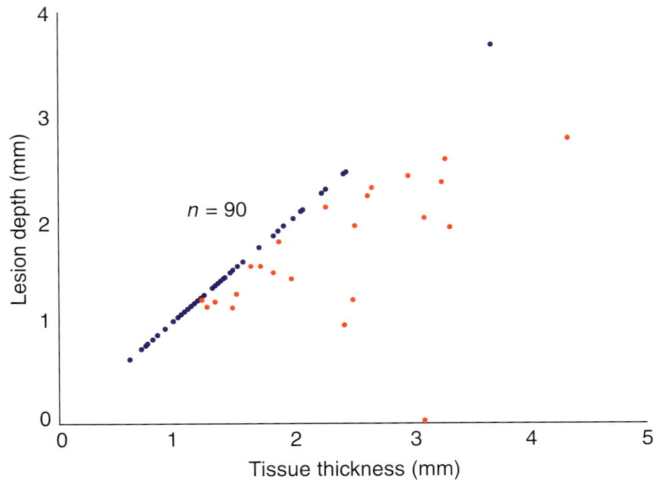

Fig. 20.17 Lesion depth plotted against tissue thickness following single-cycle bipolar radiofrequency (RF) ablation in seven human hearts that had been explanted during cardiac transplantation. Only 65% of the linear lesions were transmural throughout their entire length. See text for further discussion.

the lesions with bipolar RF devices was addressed by our group (Damiano and Gaynor) in 2020 when we used the Synergy bipolar RF clamp in nine human hearts that had been explanted after being turned down for cardiac transplantation.[15] In the first seven hearts, single bipolar ablation was transmural in 466 of 528 tissue sections (89%) (Fig. 20.17), but only 65% of the linear lesions were transmural throughout their entire length. This means that from a practical clinical standpoint, single bipolar RF clamp ablation would have failed 35% of the time. The nontransmural lesions were in areas where the atrial wall was thicker with more epicardial fat, and the lesions themselves were narrower than the transmural lesions (Fig. 20.18). In the last two hearts, bipolar RF lesions were performed twice in the same place without unclamping

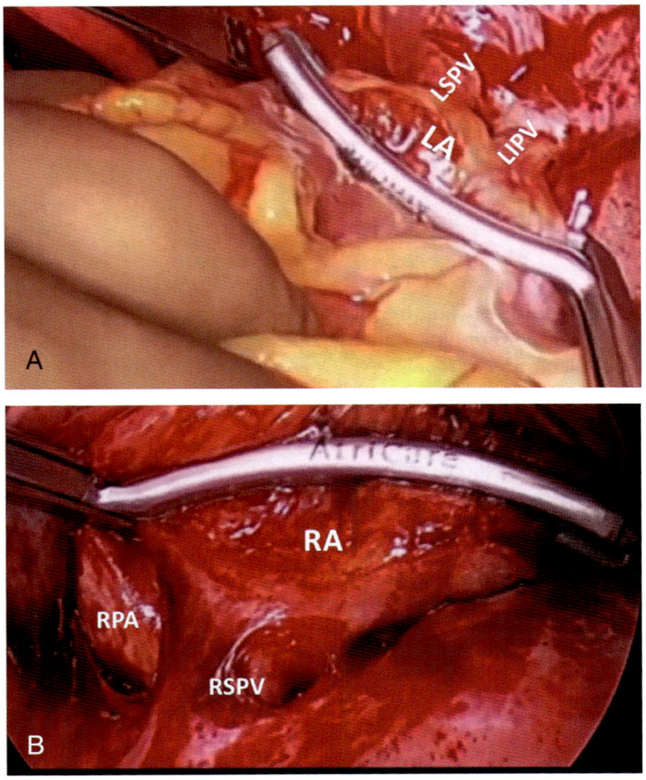

Fig. 20.16 Isolation of the left and right pulmonary veins with a bipolar radiofrequency clamp. Note that the clamp is placed well up onto the posterior atrial wall for the isolation of each pair of veins. *LA,* Left atrium; *LIPV,* left inferior pulmonary vein; *LSPV,* left superior pulmonary vein; *RA,* right atrium; *RPA,* right pulmonary artery; *RSPV,* right superior pulmonary vein.

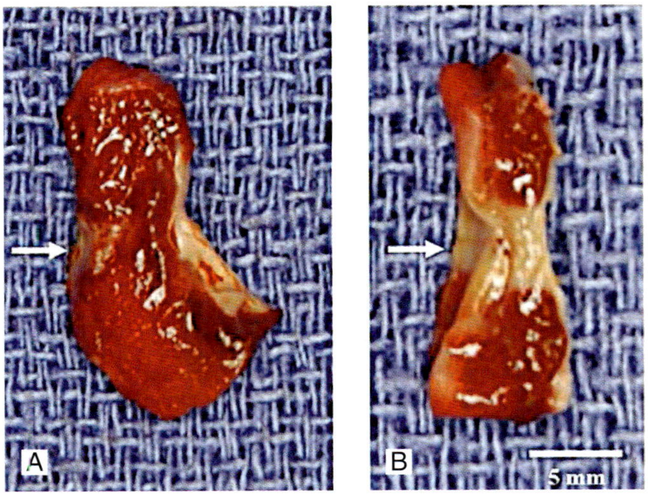

Fig. 20.18 Cross-section samples of nontransmural (A) and transmural (B) ablations after triphenyl tetrazolium chloride (TTC) staining. The ablation line is indicated by *arrows.* Devitalized tissue does not take up TTC, so the ablations appear white or pale. The non-transmural ablated tissue is indicated by a *red color.* The endocardial surface is on the right side of the tissue samples. (Reproduced from Vos LM, Bentala M, Geuzebroek GS, Molhoek SG, van Putte BP. Long-term outcome after totally thoracoscopic ablation for atrial fibrillation. *J Cardiovasc Electrophysiol.* 2020;31(1):40–45.)

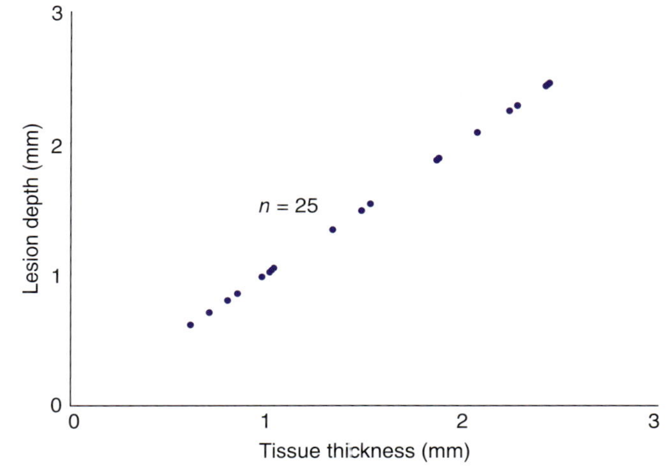

Fig. 20.19 Lesion depth plotted against tissue thickness after two cycles of bipolar radiofrequency (RF) ablation at the same target site in two human hearts that had been explanted during cardiac transplantation. See text for further discussion. All of the linear lesions were transmural throughout their entire length. (Reproduced from Vos LM, Bentala M, Geuzebroek GS, Molhoek SG, van Putte BP. Long-term outcome after totally thoracoscopic ablation for atrial fibrillation. *J Cardiovasc Electrophysiol.* 2020;31(1):40–45.)

between ablations. These lesions were transmural in 201 of 201 sections (100%), and 25 of 25 (100%) of the lesions were transmural throughout their entire length (Fig. 20.19). These observations demonstrated how bipolar RF ablation should be performed to ensure transmurality. It is recommended to perform a double ablation without unclamping. Most surgeons perform two or three sets of double ablations to ensure chronic lesion durability. The left atrial roof and floor lesions and most of the right atrial lesions of Maze procedures can be performed within minutes on pump with bipolar RF clamps.

Recently, the bipolar RF Encompass clamp was developed to create a box lesion around all four PVs and the intervening posterior left atrial wall (Fig. 20.20). In our experience, without a complete box isolation of the entire posterior LA and all four PVs, the rest of the Cox-Maze-IV lesion set has only a 33% success rate at 5 years.[30] Thus, the

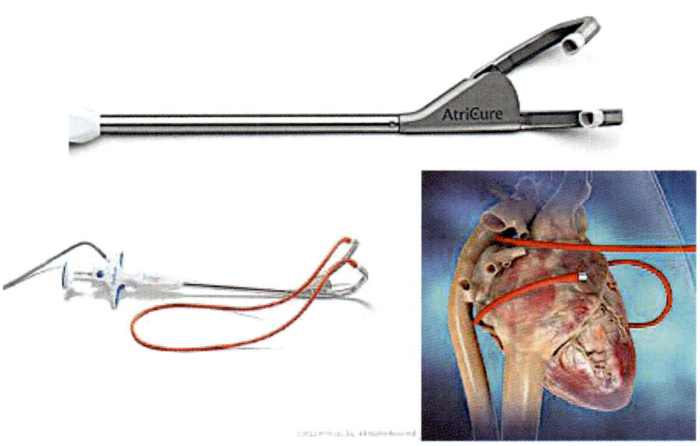

Fig. 20.20 Bipolar radiofrequency devices. *Upper panel,* The AtriCure Encompass Clamp was designed to encircle all four pulmonary veins and the intervening left atrial posterior wall to create a box lesion with one clamp. *Lower panels,* Special red rubber guides are passed around the posterior left atrium through the transverse sinus and the oblique sinus and attached to the two ends of the Encompass Clamp to guide it into place.

box is clearly the most important part of the procedure. Experimental studies have shown that the Encompass clamp is effective at creating a transmural box lesion.[31] This single clamp is a particular advantage to patients undergoing coronary artery bypass and/or aortic valve surgery who have concomitant paroxysmal AF because it does not require the surgeon to open the LA. However, there have been no long-term studies of efficacy of a box lesion alone during concomitant ablation, and these are desperately needed (see Chapter 25).

Unidirectional or Unconstrained Bipolar Devices

The Coolrail linear device is commonly used to create the roof and floor lines of a box lesion during thoracoscopic AF procedures and during the initial thoracoscopic stage of some hybrid AF procedures. This device delivers RF energy at a frequency of approximately 460 kHz, with a maximum output power range of 12 to 30 W. To counter the limitations of unidirectional ablation devices, it is recommended that when they are used, repeat ablation cycles should be applied at each targeted location to improve the likelihood of transmurality, especially when using them off pump. Although there is no universal algorithm for how unipolar RF should be applied, one effective technique when using the Coolrail device off pump is to apply multiple ablation cycles and use feedback from the ablation and sensing unit (ASU) monitor as an endpoint. The ASU monitor displays a graph of tissue conductance (current/voltage) versus time during each ablation cycle and no two ablations are the same. It usually takes several seconds for the tissue conductance of a given lesion to show a rapid decrease (Fig. 20.21,

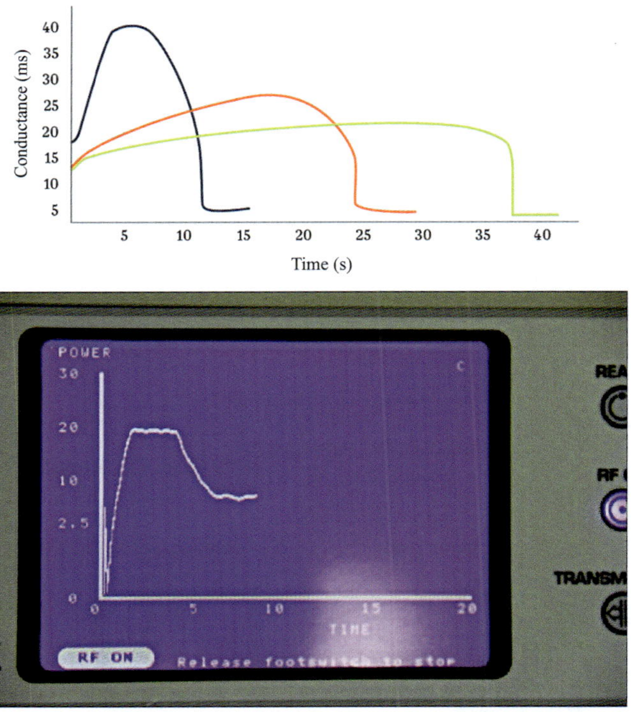

Fig. 20.21 *Upper panel,* The AtriCure Ablation and Sensing Unit (ASU) displays a graph of tissue conductance (current/voltage) versus time during each ablation cycle. Multiple ablation cycles are recommended when using unipolar ablation devices to create linear lesions. During the initial ablation cycle, it is typically several seconds before a rapid downward deflection in the tissue conductance occurs that indicates transmurality at the target site. With subsequent repeat ablation cycles, the rapid downward deflection occurs progressively earlier. *Lower panel,* Many experienced surgeons recommend repeat ablation cycles at the same site with a Coolrail device until the rapid downward deflection occurs within 5 seconds before moving to a new target site.

upper panel). Van Putte's group recommends repeat ablation cycles in the same location until the tissue conductance curve shows the rapid decrease within 5 seconds before considering the tissue to be permanently ablated transmurally (Fig. 20.21, *lower panel*).[32] However, there has been no experimental confirmation of this recommendation, and it makes little biophysical sense in that the energy delivered to the tissue is simply a product of voltage and tissue resistance. The devices only deliver energy within a relatively tight constant power zone. It has been shown that conductance below 15 ms was predictive of non-transmural lesions with bipolar devices. The heat sink of the circulating blood volume prevents the Coolrail and other unidirectional thermal devices from creating reliable conduction block. In at least one chronic experimental model, this device was ineffective in creating durable conduction block.[33]

The AtriCure Isolator RF Pen, is also classified as a unidirectional bipolar nonirrigated device. It uses similar bipolar technology as the Coolrail device.[12] In animal studies conducted at Washington University in St. Louis, it produced transmural lesions in all sections tested. However, the maximum tissue thickness tested was only 6 mm. The AtriCure Isolator RF Pen has shorter electrodes than the Coolrail device, and the ablation time for the AtriCure Isolator RF Pen was 15 seconds compared with 40 to 50 seconds for the Coolrail device. The device was shown to produce transmural lesions more consistently than the Coolrail device. One explanation for this may be that the Coolrail is often more difficult to hold in place on the beating atria.

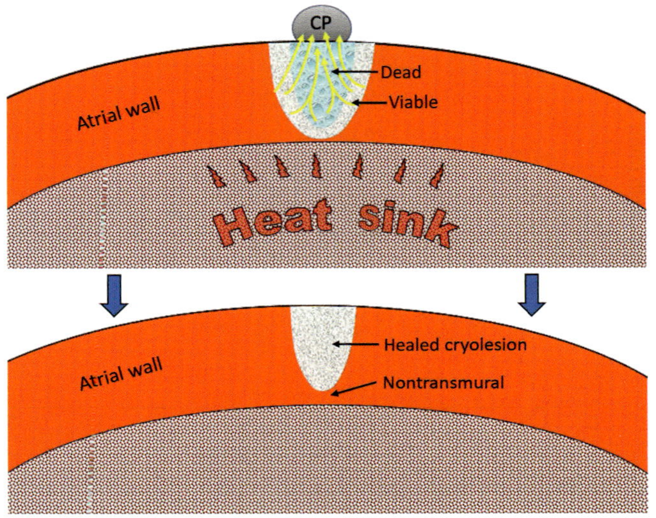

Fig. 20.23 Cryoablation: epicardial, off pump. Cryosurgery works by withdrawing heat from the target tissue so cavitary blood acts as a "heat sink" when cryoablation is performed from the epicardium off pump *(upper panel)*. It is extremely difficult for the extraction of heat from the epicardium to overcome the constant rewarming of the subendocardium by the cavitary blood, so epicardial cryosurgery usually is not able to create transmural lesions *(lower panel)*; and therefore is not recommended for off-pump atrial fibrillation ablation in thoracoscopic procedures.

CRYOSURGICAL ABLATION

Cryosurgery has been used to treat patients with cardiac arrhythmias for more than 50 years. Today, surgical cryoablation is performed with disposable, flexible cryoprobes with an internally circulating nitrous oxide (N_2O) cryogen (AtriCure) that cools the cryoprobe to −60°C or with an argon gas cryogen (Medtronic) that cools the cryoprobe to −160°C (Fig. 20.22). During the freezing phase of cryoablation, some cells die at tissue temperatures between 0°C and −10°C because of the slowing of enzyme function associated with hypothermia and cellular dehydration. The number of cells killed increases the longer these low temperatures are maintained. Intracellular ice crystals begin to form at a tissue temperature of −15°C, and all myocardial cells crystallize at −30°C, at which time they die. During the thawing phase, intracellular ice can form into larger crystals and damage or destroy cells that might have survived tissue temperatures between −15° and −30°C.

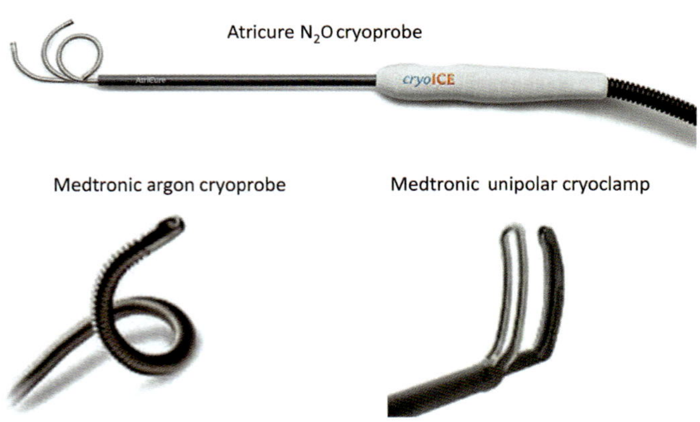

Fig. 20.22 Cryosurgical devices. The AtriCure nitrous oxide (N_2O) surgical cryoprobe *(upper panel)* and the Medtronic argon gas cryoprobe *(left lower panel)*, both of which are corrugated and flexible. Medtronic also has a cryoclamp *(right lower panel)* with one arm that freezes and the other arm that allows the transmurality of the cryolesion to be documented visually.

Cryothermic ablation creates atrial lesions by *withdrawing* heat from the myocardium rather than by creating heat like RF and other heat-based energy sources. Because cryoablation is performed from only one surface of the atrium at a time, it is functionally a unipolar energy source, so it has the same limitations as unipolar RF when used epicardially off pump. The ability of epicardial cryoablation to create transmural lesions is prevented by the "heat sink" of normothermic cavitary blood (Fig. 20.23). However, surgical cryoprobes can be used quite effectively off pump by placing them inside the atrium through a pursestring suture and freezing the atrial wall from the endocardial surface as described in Chapter 14 (see Figs. 14.9 to 14.13). The cryoprobe itself excludes cavitary blood from the blood-endocardial interface, so there is no "heat-sink" problem to prevent lesion transmurality (Fig. 20.24). Cryosurgery is used primarily during on-pump surgical procedures to treat concomitant AF associated with coronary artery or valvular heart disease. Information regarding the effectiveness of cryoablation during normothermic CPB is sparse because cryosurgery is usually performed in cardioplegically arrested hearts.

In summary, the two most effective ablation technologies both experimentally and clinically have been bipolar RF and cryoablation. The Cox-Maze-III and IV procedures depend on one or both of these ablation technologies, and they have proven to be as effective as the original cut-and-sew Maze-III procedure for the treatment of patients with AF.[34,35]

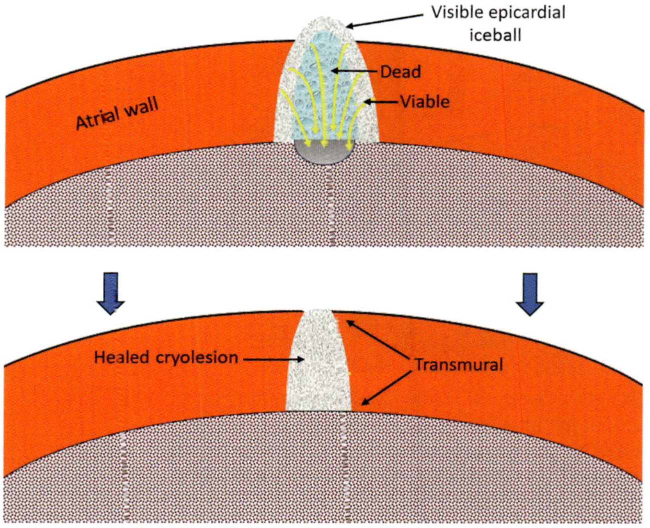

Fig. 20.24 Cryoablation: endocardial, off pump. *Upper panel,* Endocardial cryoablation can be performed safely and effectively off pump, on normothermic cardiopulmonary bypass, or under cardioplegic arrest. The cryoprobe that is placed inside the atrium prevents cavitary blood from acting as a "heat sink" in off-pump patients; therefore, endocardial cryoablation is far more effective than epicardial cryoablation when performing off-pump surgical ablation. See text for further discussion.

INTRAOPERATIVE TESTING

The impact of time on lesion transmurality is the reason that predicting long-term success based on immediate intraoperative testing is problematic. Intraoperative testing is invaluable if it shows that a given lesion is incomplete when electrical conduction persists across the ablation line. For example, if intraoperative testing shows that the PVs are not isolated after PVI, further ablation to complete the isolation is warranted. However, if intraoperative testing indicates that the PVI is complete, it does not ensure that the PVs will remain isolated in the future. Unfortunately, there is no way to determine the future integrity of an ablation lesion in the operating room or EP lab except to create the lesion by techniques that have proven to be effective experimentally or by past clinical experience. Furthermore, without the intraoperative availability of sophisticated multipoint computerized mapping systems, the only feasible intraoperative testing after surgery for AF is to determine if a specific area of the heart has been successfully isolated. This limits intraoperative testing to the PVs and the posterior wall of the LA.

Intraoperative Testing of Pulmonary Vein Isolation

Currently, the majority of surgical PVI procedures are performed using bipolar RF clamps to isolate the right and left PVs in pairs. After it is completed, the isolating lesion for each pair of PVs is tested for exit block to see if the heart can be paced from inside the isolated segments. (Fig. 20.25A). To demonstrate exit block, the heart has to be in sinus rhythm. If the patient is not in sinus rhythm, then the heart has to be electrically cardioverted to demonstrate exit block, thus confirming electrical isolation. Failure to conduct a pacing impulse from inside the isolated segment to the rest of the heart confirms exit block. Entrance block is tested by placing a *sensing* electrode inside the isolated segment of PVs and pacing the atrium from outside the isolated segment (Fig. 20.25B). If the sensing electrodes do not detect the outside paced or nonpaced electrical activity then entrance block is confirmed. Entrance block can be demonstrated without the heart being in sinus rhythm. However, this exercise can be challenging because interpretation can be confounded by far-field nonconducted electrical signals and electrical noise, which is not uncommon in the operating room environment. During surgical procedures, exit block is more commonly tested because it is simpler to demonstrate.

Intraoperative Testing of the Box Lesion of Cox-Maze Procedures

The box lesion of the Cox-Maze-IV procedure is created by first isolating the PVs with bipolar RF clamps and then isolating the intervening posterior left atrial wall with roof and floor lesions that connect the PVI lesions. In the Cox-Maze-III lesion pattern, the box lesion is created either by using an Encompass clamp or a flexible cryoprobe. It

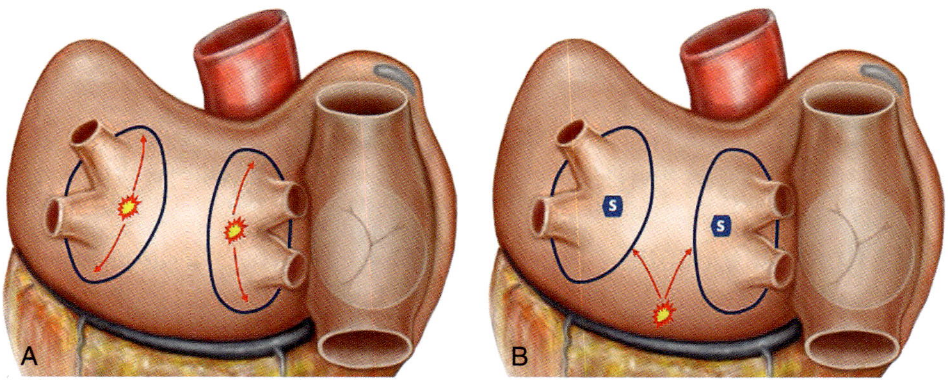

Fig. 20.25 Intraoperative testing after pulmonary vein isolation (PVI). After isolation of the pulmonary veins (PVI), the success or failure of the isolation procedure is tested by documenting exit block from the isolated areas and entrance block into the isolated areas. (A) Exit block is tested by pacing the tissue inside the isolated segments to see if the pacing captures the heartbeat. If it captures the heartbeat, the isolation procedure has failed, and more ablation is required. If it does not capture the heartbeat, exit block from the isolated segment is confirmed. (B) Entrance block is tested by pacing the atrium outside the isolated segment to see if the pacing impulse activates a sensing electrode inside the isolated segment. If an externally paced impulse conducts to the sensing electrode inside the isolated segment, the isolation procedure has failed, and more ablation is required. If it does not conduct to the sensing electrode inside the isolated segment, entrance block into the isolated segment is confirmed.

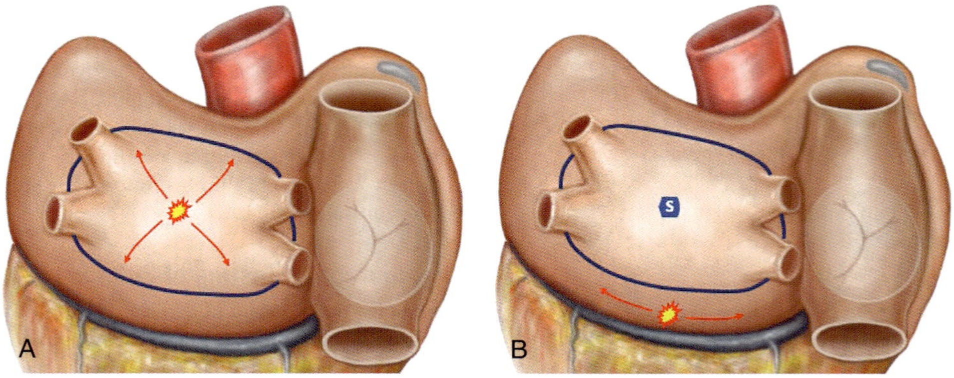

Fig. 20.26 Intraoperative testing after box lesion of the Maze-III procedure. In the Cox-Maze-III procedure, isolation of all four pulmonary veins and the intervening posterior left atrial wall is accomplished with a single lesion called the "box lesion." (A) Testing this box lesion for exit block requires pacing from anywhere within the box to see if it captures the heartbeat. (B) Entrance testing requires only a single sensing electrode inside the box lesion to determine if external pacing is conducted to the inside of the box.

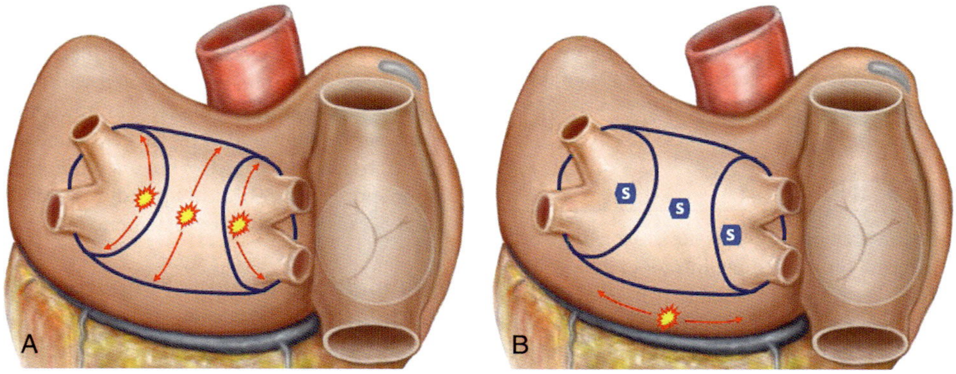

Fig. 20.27 Intraoperative testing after box lesion of the Maze-IV procedure. A box lesion is also a part of the Maze-IV procedure, but it is created by first isolating the pulmonary veins in pairs and then completing the box by adding roof and floor lines to isolate the posterior wall of the left atrium. Therefore there are three separate isolated compartments of atrium that should be tested for entrance and exit block in each compartment. (A) To test for exit block, each compartment must be paced individually to determine if the heartbeat is captured. (B) To test for entrance block, a sensing electrode must be placed in each individual compartment to determine if an external pacing stimulus can be conducted into that specific segment.

should be documented that all four PVs are isolated by confirming exit block (and entrance block when possible) before arresting the heart (Figs. 20.26 and 20.27).

POTENTIAL COMPLICATIONS OF VARIOUS ALTERNATIVE ENERGY SOURCES

The use of alternative energy sources to perform the Cox-Maze-III and IV procedures is not without potential risk, though proper surgical technique can mitigate against potential complications.

1. When isolating the PVs using bipolar clamps, it is important to place the clamp around the PVs with the clamp seated on the proximal cuff of atrial tissue and not on the PVs themselves to avoid PV stenosis. To our knowledge, there have been no reports of clamp-induced pulmonary stenosis using this technique. Double ablations without unclamping should be performed.
2. The RF or cryoablation devices should not be placed across coronary arteries to avoid the complication of late intimal hyperplasia and stenosis. The same is true when using an Encompass clamp to create the box lesion of a Cox Maze-III procedure.
3. RF devices, whether unidirectional or bidirectional, should never be placed across valvular tissue because RF ablation can damage valve tissue. On the other hand, cryothermia has been shown to be safe for ablating valvular tissue.
4. Cryoablation devices are contact-forgiving, and after the probe is frozen, it will adhere to neighboring tissue. Hence, caution should be observed, particularly in areas close to the phrenic nerve or sinoatrial nodal complex, to avoid permanent damage.

This chapter would not be complete without the mention of a newly introduced energy source, pulsed-field ablation (PFA), which is currently being evaluated when delivered by endocardial catheter devices.[36] PFA is discussed in detail in Chapter 52.

REFERENCES

1. Nath S, Lynch C 3rd, Whayne JG, Haines DE. Cellular electrophysiological effects of hyperthermia on isolated guinea pig papillary muscle. Implications for catheter ablation. *Circulation*. 1993;88:1826–1831.
2. Wood M, Goldberg S, Lau M, et al. Direct measurement of the lethal isotherm for radiofrequency ablation of myocardial tissue. *Circ Arrhythm Electrophysiol*. 2011;4:373–378.
3. Baust JG, Gage AA. The molecular basis of cryosurgery. *BJU Int*. 2005;95:1187–1191.
4. Cox JL, Malaisrie SC, Churyla A, et al. Cryosurgery for atrial fibrillation: physiologic basis for creating optimal cryolesions. *Ann Thorac Surg*. 2021;112:354–362.
5. Gage AA, Baust J. Mechanisms of tissue injury in cryosurgery. *Cryobiology*. 1998;37:171–186.
6. Gage AA, Baust JM, Baust JG. Experimental cryosurgery investigations in vivo. *Cryobiology*. 2009;59:229–243.
7. Philpott JM, Zemlin CW, Cox JL, et al. The ablate trial: safety and efficacy of cox maze-iv using a bipolar radiofrequency ablation system. *Ann Thorac Surg*. 2015;100:1541–1546 discussion 7-8.
8. Gaynor SL, Diodato MD, Prasad SM, et al. A prospective, single-center clinical trial of a modified Cox maze procedure with bipolar radiofrequency ablation. *J Thorac Cardiovasc Surg*. 2004;128:535–542.
9. Gaynor SL, Ishii Y, Diodato MD, et al. Successful performance of Cox-Maze procedure on beating heart using bipolar radiofrequency ablation: a feasibility study in animals. *Ann Thorac Surg*. 2004;78:1671–1677.
10. Voeller RK, Zierer A, Lall SC, Sakamoto S, Schuessler RB, Damiano RJ Jr. Efficacy of a novel bipolar radiofrequency ablation device on the beating heart for atrial fibrillation ablation: a long-term porcine study. *J Thorac Cardiovasc Surg*. 2010;140:203–208.
11. Haissaguerre M, Jais P, Shah DC, et al. Spontaneous initiation of atrial fibrillation by ectopic beats originating in the pulmonary veins. *N Engl J Med*. 1998;339:659–666.
12. Schuessler RB, Lee AM, Melby SJ, et al. Animal studies of epicardial atrial ablation. *Heart Rhythm*. 2009;6:S41–S45.
13. Melby SJ, Zierer A, Kaiser SP, Schuessler RB, Damiano RJ Jr. Epicardial microwave ablation on the beating heart for atrial fibrillation: the dependency of lesion depth on cardiac output. *J Thorac Cardiovasc Surg*. 2006;132:355–360.
14. Doll N, Kornherr P, Aupperle H, et al. Epicardial treatment of atrial fibrillation using cryoablation in an acute off-pump sheep model. *J Thorac Cardiovasc Surg*. 2003;51:267–273.
15. Khiabani AJ, MacGregor RM, Manghelli JL, et al. Bipolar radiofrequency ablation on explanted human hearts: how to ensure transmural lesions. *Ann Thorac Surg*. 2020;110:1933–1939.
16. Yates TA, McGilvray M, Schill MR, et al. Performance of an irrigated bipolar radiofrequency ablation clamp on explanted human hearts. *Ann Thorac Surg*. 2023;116:307–313.
17. Saint LL, Lawrance CP, Okada S, et al. Performance of a novel bipolar/monopolar radiofrequency ablation device on the beating heart in an acute porcine model. *Innovations (Phila)*. 2013;8:276–283.
18. Bugge E, Nicholson IA, Thomas SP. Comparison of bipolar and unipolar radiofrequency ablation in an in vivo experimental model. *Eur J Cardiothorac Surg*. 2005;28:76–80 discussion-2.
19. Kiser AC, Nifong LW, Raman J, Kasirajan V, Campbell N, Chitwood WR Jr. Evaluation of a novel epicardial atrial fibrillation treatment system. *Ann Thorac Surg*. 2008;85:300–303.
20. DeLurgio DB, Crossen KJ, Gill J, et al. Hybrid convergent procedure for the treatment of persistent and long-standing persistent atrial fibrillation: results of converge clinical trial. *Circ Arrhythm Electrophysiol*. 2020;13:e009288.
21. Hamner CE, Potter DD Jr, Cho KR, et al. Irrigated radiofrequency ablation with transmurality feedback reliably produces Cox Maze lesions in vivo. *Ann Thorac Surg*. 2005;80:2263–2270.
22. Thomas SP, Guy DJ, Boyd AC, Eipper VE, Ross DL. Chard RB: Comparison of epicardial and endocardial linear ablation using handheld probes. *Ann Thorac Surg*. 2003;75:543–548.
23. La Meir M. Surgical options for treatment of atrial fibrillation. *Ann Cardiothorac Surg*. 2014;3:30–37.
24. Jais P, Haissaguerre M, Shah DC, et al. Successful irrigated-tip catheter ablation of atrial flutter resistant to conventional radiofrequency ablation. *Circulation*. 1998;98:835–838.
25. Haines DE. The biophysics and pathophysiology of lesion formation during radiofrequency catheter ablation. In: Zipes D, Jalife J, Stevenson W, eds. *Cardiac Electrophysiology: From Cell to Bedside*. WB Saunders Co; 2005:1018–1027.
26. Melby SJ, Zierer A, Voeller RK, et al. Wide variations in energy delivery using an impedance-controlled algorithm in bipolar radiofrequency ablation: evidence against fixed time ablation. *Innovations (Phila)*. 2007;2:67–72.
27. Dewhirst MW, Viglianti BL, Lora-Michiels M, Hanson M, Hoopes PJ. Basic principles of thermal dosimetry and thermal thresholds for tissue damage from hyperthermia. *Int J Hyperthermia*. 2003;19:267–294.
28. Varzaly JA, Chapman D, Lau DH, et al. Contact force and ablation assessment of surgical bipolar radiofrequency clamps in the treatment of atrial fibrillation. *Interact Cardiovasc Thorac Surg*. 2019;28:85–93.
29. Reddy VY, Dukkipati SR, Neuzil P, et al. Randomized, controlled trial of the safety and effectiveness of a contact force-sensing irrigated catheter for ablation of paroxysmal atrial fibrillation: results of the TactiCath Contact Force Ablation Catheter Study for Atrial Fibrillation (TOCCASTAR) study. *Circulation*. 2015;132:907–915.
30. Henn MC, Lancaster TS, Miller JR, et al. Late outcomes after the Cox Maze IV procedure for atrial fibrillation. *J Thorac Cardiovasc Surg*. 2015;150:1168–1176 78 e1-2.
31. Yates TA, McGilvray M, Razo N, et al. Efficacy of a novel bipolar radiofrequency clamp: an acute porcine model. *Innovations (Phila)*. 2022;17:409–415.
32. Vos LM, Bentala M, Geuzebroek GS, Molhoek SG, van Putte BP. Long-term outcome after totally thoracoscopic ablation for atrial fibrillation. *J Cardiovasc Electrophysiol*. 2020;31:40–45.
33. Lee AM, Aziz A, Clark KL, Schuessler RB, Damiano RJ Jr. Chronic performance of a novel radiofrequency ablation device on the beating heart: limitations of conduction delay to assess transmurality. *J Thorac Cardiovasc Surg*. 2012;144:859–865.
34. Ad N, Holmes SD, Rongione AJ, et al. The long-term safety and efficacy of concomitant Cox Maze procedures for atrial fibrillation in patients without mitral valve disease. *J Thorac Cardiovasc Surg*. 2019;157:1505–1514.
35. MacGregor RM, Bakir NH, Pedamallu H, et al. Late results after stand-alone surgical ablation for atrial fibrillation. *J Thorac Cardiovasc Surg*. 2022;164:1515–1528.e8.
36. Verma A, Asivatham SJ, Deneke T, Castellvi Q, Neal RE 2nd. Primer on pulsed electrical field ablation: understanding the benefits and limitations. *Circ Arrhythm Electrophysiol*. 2021;14:e010086.

21

Maze Procedure and Postoperative Pacemakers

James L. Cox, Patrick M. McCarthy

CHAPTER OUTLINE

One of the persistent misconceptions in surgery for atrial fibrillation (AF) is that the right atrial (RA) lesions of the Maze procedure cause patients to need more permanent pacemakers (PPMs) postoperatively. There is no question that improperly placed RA lesions can damage the sinoatrial (SA) node and improperly placed atrial septal lesions can damage the atrioventricular (AV) node, both of which can result in the need for a postoperative pacemaker. However, if the Maze procedure is performed properly, its lesions will not damage either the SA node or the AV node, so it is misleading to characterize the need for a new PPM as a "complication" of the Maze procedure. More often, the need for a new pacemaker after a Maze procedure is actually a surrogate for having performed the procedure correctly. For example, dysfunction of the SA node with an abnormally slow sinus rhythm can result in AF, in which case the AF is simply an escape rhythm that occurs because of the slow heart rate. Thus the more successful a procedure is in ablating AF in patients with an underlying "sick sinus syndrome" (SSS), the more pacemakers will be required. On the other hand, if the AF is not successfully ablated, there will be no need for a pacemaker implantation. In other words, "*successful AF ablation begets more postoperative pacemakers.*"

If the Maze procedure itself were the culprit in requiring more postoperative pacemakers, the lesions of the procedure would have to do one of two things: (1) prevent the SA node's ability to generate an appropriate rate of spontaneously generated sinus impulses, or (2) impede the conduction of atrial impulses through the AV node–His bundle complex to the ventricles. Otherwise, the need for new pacemakers postoperatively would have to be attributed to causes other than the Maze procedure itself. There are two ways that any surgical procedure, including the Maze procedure, can injure the SA node or AV node–His bundle: traumatic injury or devascularization.

DAMAGE OF THE SINOATRIAL NODE

Traumatic Injury of the Sinoatrial Node

A group of surgical research fellows were once challenged to ablate normal sinus rhythm in a normal dog within 5 minutes using a 2-cm diameter cryoprobe. None could do it. This was an experiment to demonstrate how difficult it is to damage a normal SA node enough to require a PPM. This is largely because normal sinus rhythm can originate from anywhere within a large area of the right atrium (RA) (the atrial pacemaker complex) distant from the anatomic SA node. Thus, if a patient has an SA node that is entirely normal preoperatively, it is virtually impossible to traumatize it enough surgically to cause permanent dysfunction. Most cases of documented postoperative SA node dysfunction were in patients whose preoperative SA node function was never evaluated, and in addition, most dysfunction was also temporary. Nevertheless, it is prudent to avoid traumatic injury of the anatomic SA node by creating lesions as far away from it as possible and by avoiding excessive retraction during surgery.

The atrial pacemaker complex, including the SA node, can be traumatized temporarily by surgical retraction that is applied to gain exposure of the inside of the left atrium (LA), especially when a mitral valve procedure or a Maze procedure is performed through a median sternotomy. This can occur regardless of whether LA exposure is gained through Waterston's groove or by an anterior transseptal incision. Surgical approaches that require less traction for exposure, such as minimally invasive, thoracoscopic, and robotic Maze procedures, are associated with lower postoperative pacemaker requirements than are Maze procedures performed through a median sternotomy.[1–3] Another potential reason for fewer pacemakers being required after these minimally invasive approaches may be surgeon selection bias, as surgeons who perform the Maze procedure by these techniques usually have had more experience with the procedure.

Surgical traction injury of the SA node is manifest early as a slower postoperative sinus rate, but the effect is temporary.[4,5] Simultaneously, vagal innervation of the AV node is often suppressed by the LA lesions of the Maze procedure,[6,7] resulting in faster spontaneous AV node rates in the immediate postoperative period. The combination of a slower SA rate and a faster AV node rate immediately after a Maze procedure often results in a temporary junctional rhythm postoperatively. Because it can take several days for the SA node and AV node rates to return to normal with restoration of sinus rhythm, surgeons often

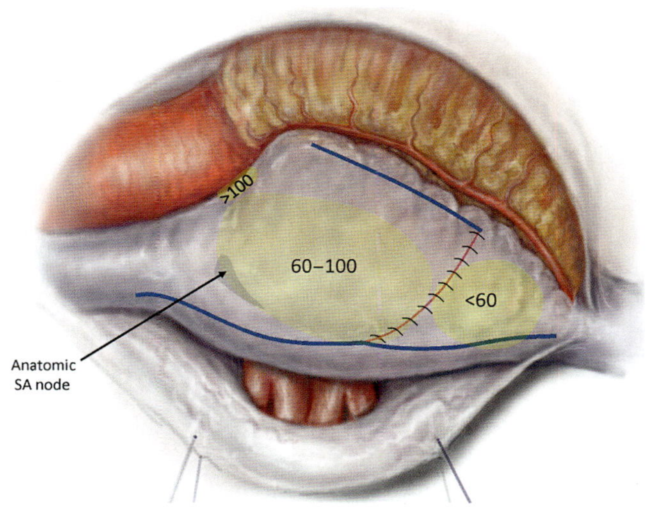

Fig. 21.1 Right atrial (RA) lesions and atrial pacemaker complex. The RA lesions of the Maze procedure are purposely positioned to create minimal damage to the atrial pacemaker complex. This includes the right atriotomy that creates the free-wall portion of the "T" lesion and provides exposure to the inside of the right atrium RA for the endocardial cryoablation extension of the lesion down to the tricuspid valve annulus.

implant PPMs for temporary junctional rhythm during this recovery phase to hasten hospital discharge. This scenario can also be seen after other LA procedures such as mitral valve surgery in patients who do not have a concomitant Maze procedure.

Some surgeons are reluctant to perform the superior vena cava (SVC) lesion of a Maze procedure because they are concerned that it is too close to the anatomic SA node and therefore may injure it. Although this concern is unwarranted, again, it is prudent to place all of the RA lesions in locations that are least likely to cause any damage to the SA node or the AV node. Thus, we always place the SVC lesion in the lateral portion of the SVC orifice, which keeps it well away from the anatomic SA node and avoids all other areas of the atrial pacemaker complex (Fig. 21.1). To our knowledge, there has never been a report documenting traumatic injury of the SA node caused by the SVC lesion, regardless of the energy source used and despite tens of thousands of Maze procedures having been performed.

In summary, it is virtually impossible to cause permanent SA node dysfunction by traumatic injury during surgery. Temporary SA node dysfunction caused by traction for surgical exposure invariably recovers if the SA node was normal preoperatively. However, one of the most common reasons that post-Maze patients receive a PPM is for the treatment of temporary postoperative junctional rhythm.

Devascularization of the Sinoatrial Node

There is a coronary artery branch that is designated the "SA node artery" because it passes directly through the anatomic SA node. Thus it is reasonable to assume that if this SA node artery were injured, it would result in SA node dysfunction, perhaps even severe enough to require a PPM implantation. However, the relationship between the SA node artery and the anatomic SA node is not that of an end-artery, so interruption of the SA node artery has little or no effect on SA node function or dysfunction.

I (JLC) was once honored to share a long train ride from Kiruna, Sweden, to Narvik, Norway, with the legendary cardiologist and pathologist Dr. Thomas N. James, who was universally regarded as one of medicine's greatest experts on coronary artery anatomy and the specialized conduction system. During that trip, Dr. James made a most enlightening comment regarding the blood supply of the SA node. He stated: *"The SA node artery reminds me of an interstate highway passing through a small town but with no off-ramps to that town because even though the SA node artery passes through the anatomic SA node, it has no identifiable branches to its specialized cells"* (see Chapter 3, Fig. 3.10). Dr. James' point was that yes, there is a coronary artery branch that passes through the anatomic SA node, and therefore we call it the "SA node artery," but there is no indication that it actually supplies blood to the SA node!

With this in mind, the fear that some clinicians have about interrupting the SA node artery with the SVC lesion of a Maze procedure is clearly unwarranted. Engle et al.[8] documented that no patients in their series with disease or total obstruction of the SA node artery had dysfunctional SA nodes. Therefore, the SA node artery does not serve as an end artery to the anatomic SA node and its occlusion does not cause SA node dysfunction. The clinical results of the Maze procedure further support the concept that the SA node is not dependent on a single end artery for its blood supply. Tens of thousands of patients have undergone properly performed Maze procedures in which the superior end of the intercaval lesion was placed into the orifice of the SVC. Undoubtedly, the SA node artery was either divided or frozen in many of these cases. However, no direct relationship has ever been demonstrated between the SVC lesion of a Maze procedure and the need for new postoperative pacemakers. SA node artery injury by the RA lesions of the Maze procedure is not a cause of increased postoperative pacemaker requirements.

DAMAGE OF THE ATRIOVENTRICULAR NODE–HIS BUNDLE COMPLEX

Traumatic Injury of the Atrioventricular Node–His Bundle Complex

The AV node and the proximal portion of the His bundle are located entirely within the atrial septum (see Chapter 3, Fig. 3.17). From the surgeon's view, they are located in the triangle of Koch (see Chapter 3, Fig. 3.18). This triangular anatomic space is bordered by the tendon of Todaro superiorly and the tricuspid valve annulus inferiorly with the os of the coronary sinus at its base and the membranous atrial septum at its apex. The AV node–His bundle complex is located near the apex of the triangle of Koch with the His bundle passing to the ventricles immediately posterior to the membranous septum. It is anatomically impossible for the lesions of the Maze procedure to injure the AV node–His bundle complex without crossing the tendon of Todaro and entering the triangle of Koch with an atrial septal lesion. The atrial septal lesions in the historical Maze-I and Maze-II procedures were surgical incisions that did not cross the tendon of Todaro and therefore were incapable of causing heart block. Likewise, the atrial septal lesion in the cut-and-sew Maze-III procedure, which is positioned more posteriorly in the atrial septum, also ends above the level of the tendon of Todaro. Neither the CryoMaze-III nor the Maze-IV procedure has an atrial septal lesion at all, so it is obviously impossible to injure the AV node–His bundle complex with either of these contemporary Maze procedures (Fig. 21.2).

One of the most frequently referenced surgical papers in the AF literature is the 2015 Cardiothoracic Surgery Network (CTSN) Clinical Trials article published in *The New England Journal of Medicine* documenting that patients with persistent AF who require mitral valve surgery have superior outcomes if the AF is ablated concomitantly during the mitral surgery than if the AF is ignored.[9] However, one of the major so-called "complications" in that trial was a dramatic increase in the need for postoperative pacemakers in patients who received biatrial Maze procedures

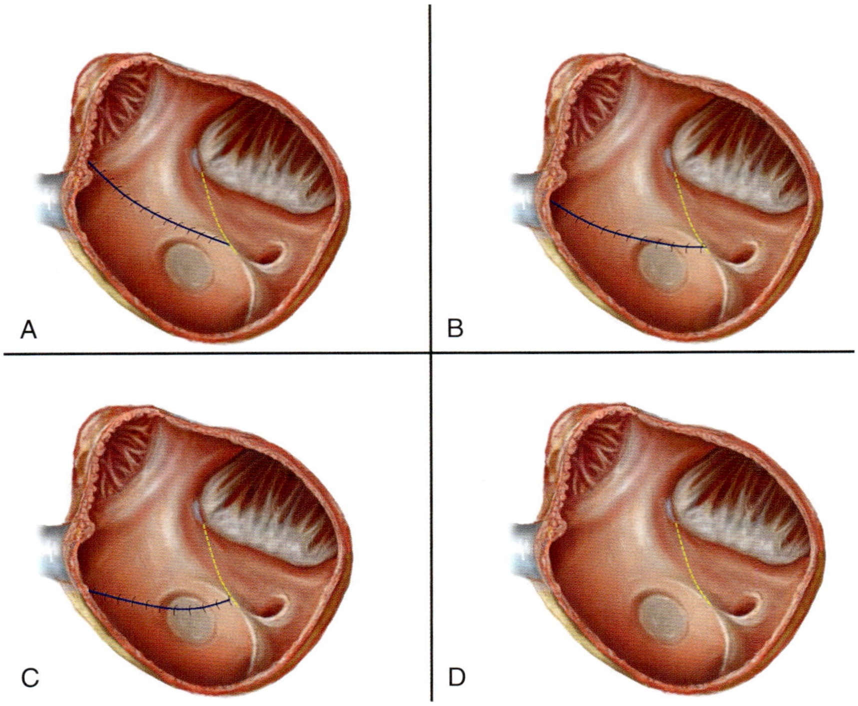

Fig. 21.2 The primary differences in the Maze-I, Maze-II, and cut-and-sew Maze-III lesion patterns was a progressive repositioning of the atrial lesion from anterior to posterior. (A) In the original Maze-I procedure, the superior end of the atrial septal lesion was anterior to the superior vena cava (SVC) orifice. (B) In the Maze-II procedure, the superior end of the septal lesion was in the medial portion of the SVC orifice. (C) In the cut-and-sew Maze-III procedure, the superior end of the septal lesion was posterior to the SVC orifice. (D) There is no atrial septal lesion in either the CryoMaze-III procedure or the Maze-IV procedure. Regardless of where the superior ends of the septal lesions were positioned in the first three iterations of the Maze procedure, the lower end of the septal lesion always terminated at the tendon of Todaro *(yellow dashed line)* just above the os of the coronary sinus and well away from the atrioventricular node–His bundle complex, which is located at the apex of the triangle of Koch.

rather than left-sided-only lesions. This observation was interpreted as confirmation that the RA lesions in the biatrial Maze group were responsible for the increased postoperative pacemaker requirements.

The problem with that interpretation is that according to their own data, the differences in postoperative pacemaker requirements were not due to SA node injury but to AV node–His bundle injury that caused postoperative heart block. Yet none of the biatrial Maze procedures in that study included an atrial septal lesion! The absence of an atrial septal lesion in these patients makes it anatomically impossible for the RA lesions to have created heart block necessitating a postoperative pacemaker. Other possible explanations for the increased need for pacemakers in the biatrial Maze group include the following: (1) more AF was successfully ablated with the biatrial Maze than with the LA-only lesions[10]; (2) more patients who received the biatrial Maze also underwent double valve replacement; (3) because of the more extensive valve surgery, the aortic cross-clamp times had to be longer in the biatrial Maze group; and (4) there was no documentation of preoperative SA node function in either group of patients. However, what can be stated with absolute certainty is that the RA lesions in the biatrial Maze group did not cause the increased incidence of heart block and subsequent pacemaker implantations because none of the RA lesions were anywhere near the AV node–His bundle complex.

Finally, it is worth recalling that for nearly 20 years before the first Maze procedure, *elective* His bundle ablation was a common surgical procedure to treat supraventricular tachyarrhythmias, including AF, that could not be controlled medically (see Chapter 11, Fig. 11.3). It seems that with the RA open on cardiopulmonary bypass and the ability to localize the site of the His bundle under direct vision using a handheld electrode, surgical division of the His bundle would be a simple operation. However, even after hours of blunt and sharp surgical dissection in the posterior septal space and triangle of Koch after map-guided localization of the His bundle, it was sometimes virtually impossible to create heart block on purpose. In fact, it was so difficult that in the mid-1970s, cryosurgery was introduced by our group at Duke University specifically to replace surgical dissection in the effort to create elective heart block more reliably.[11] This personal experience over 2 decades is why we are confident in stating that a single, carefully placed atrial septal lesion in the Maze procedure will not inadvertently create heart block, and it renders comical any suggestion that a surgical procedure that has no septal lesion at all can inadvertently create heart block. The RA lesions of the Maze procedure do not cause heart block.

Devascularization of the Atrioventricular Node

The AV node artery penetrates the posterior interventricular septum through the posterior septal space to reach the AV node located in the lower anterior interatrial septum (Fig. 21.3).[12] In the early years of Wolff-Parkinson-White syndrome surgery, patients with posterior–septal accessory pathways represented the greatest challenge to arrhythmia surgeons because of intense efforts to avoid surgical injury of the AV node artery.[13] At that time, the AV node artery was assumed

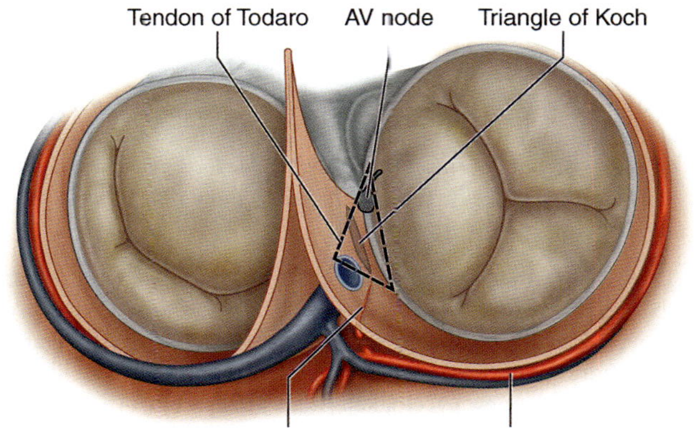

Fig. 21.3 The atrioventricular (AV) node artery typically penetrates the posterior ventricular septum to exit from the floor of the posterior septal space before entering the atrial septum to reach the AV node.

to be an end artery whose interruption would automatically lead to heart block. In the late 1970s, I (JLC) became suspicious that posterior–septal accessory pathways were intimately associated with the AV node artery and that its meticulous preservation was the primary reason why surgery for these accessory pathways failed so often. Therefore, a new surgical approach was developed in which the AV node artery was *purposely* divided in patients with posterior–septal accessory pathways.[14] During the ensuing 15 years, I purposely divided the AV node artery surgically in 115 consecutive patients with posterior–septal pathways, and not one patient developed heart block. This observation confirmed that like the SA node artery, the AV node artery is not an end artery, and its division will not cause heart block.

INCIDENCE AND IMPACT OF NEW PACEMAKER IMPLANTATION AFTER ATRIAL FIBRILLATION ABLATION PROCEDURES

The implantation rate for new pacemakers after cardiac surgery varies widely and it is not limited to the Maze or other AF ablation procedures. The Society of Thoracic Surgeons (STS) Adult Cardiac Surgery Database for the calendar year of 2019 showed that new pacemakers were required in approximately 2% of patients undergoing coronary artery bypass graft surgery, 11% having aortic valve surgery, 17% having mitral valve replacement, and 8% having mitral valve repair.[15] In one randomized clinical trial for combined mitral and tricuspid valve procedures, new pacemakers were implanted in 14% compared with 2.5% for mitral valve surgery alone.[16]

It is well established by STS database analyses,[17,18] randomized clinical trials,[19] and meta analyses[20,21] that in patients with concomitant AF, the need for new pacemakers is higher in patients undergoing surgical AF ablation than in patients whose AF is ignored. An STS Database analysis in 2008 showed that the need for new pacemakers was increased by approximately 25% in patients who had concomitant AF ablation versus those who did not undergo ablation.[17] The reported pacemaker implantation rates in mitral valve patients undergoing concomitant AF ablation range from highs of 17% to 24%[9,22] to lows of 5% to 8%.[23,24] At Northwestern University, our overall requirement for pacemakers after concomitant AF ablation in all cardiac surgery patients is 7.9%, but it varies considerably by operation and is less than 1% for patients undergoing AF ablation with isolated mitral valve repair.[24]

Finally, much is often made of the relationship between the implantation of a new pacemaker following AF ablation surgery and poorer long-term survival, but this is not a cause-and-effect relationship. The implantation of a pacemaker does not cause a patient to die sooner; otherwise it would not be implanted. Therefore, the observation that new pacemaker implantations after cardiac surgery are associated with an increase in the long-term mortality rate[21] is of no practical importance. Clearly, the need for a postoperative pacemaker is associated with poorer long-term survival time because patients who need pacemakers are generally in poorer health than patients who do not need pacemakers.

Pacemaker implantation is not always followed by pacemaker dependency. Our group recently showed that approximately 60% of all the new pacemakers that were implanted after biatrial Maze procedures and LA-only ablation procedures were no longer needed 3 months after implantation because by then, the patients were back in normal sinus rhythm.[25] This observation strongly suggests that postoperative pacemakers are being implanted too soon after surgery, though clinicians no longer have the freedom of routinely keeping patients hospitalized long enough for them to recover their sinus rhythm.

THE REASONS PACEMAKER REQUIREMENTS INCREASE AFTER MAZE PROCEDURES

Several of the reasons why patients may need PPMs after a successful Maze procedure have already been mentioned but generally, but they fall into four categories: (1) temporary postoperative junctional rhythm, (2) unmasking an underlying SSS, (3) improperly performed surgery, and (4) patient selection. Note that only one these categories is potentially related to the lesions of the Maze procedure and that is category 3 in which the procedure may be performed incorrectly.

Postoperative Junctional Rhythm

As previously mentioned, junctional rhythm is common immediately after a Maze procedure because of the combination of (1) a slower SA node rate caused by surgical traction on the upper part of the atrial pacemaker complex, and (2) a faster AV node rate caused by the release of vagal suppression of the AV node caused by the LA lesions.[6,6] Because of economic incentives to reduce hospital stay and a reluctance to discharge patients in junctional rhythm, many of these patients receive postoperative pacemakers prematurely. It is not always necessary to implant a PPM in patients with a postoperative junctional rhythm, and there are bedside methods of determining when pacemaker implantation is indicated and when it is safe to discharge patients with a postoperative junctional rhythm. Our criteria for the latter include (1) being able to capture the heartbeat by atrial pacing, confirming normal antegrade conduction through the AV node; (2) being able to document retrograde conduction through the AV node by pacing the ventricles and recording an atrial spike after each ventricular activation, and (3) having a baseline resting junctional rate of 50 beats/min or greater. Clearly, these bedside evaluations require the availability of temporary atrial and ventricular pacing wires, which we believe should be placed in all patients undergoing surgery for cardiac arrhythmias.

Unmasking a Sick Sinus Syndrome

The RA lesions of the Maze procedure are commonly blamed for the increase in postoperative pacemaker requirements.[7,9,21,26,27] However, if the preoperative functional status of the SA node is unknown, it is impossible to know after eliminating the AF whether any subsequent SA node dysfunction is due to the surgical procedure itself or to "unmasking" an underlying SSS. It is logical to assume that if the SVC lesion of the Maze procedure were responsible for postoperative SA node dysfunction, it would also cause damage to normal preoperative SA nodes at the same rate as abnormal preop SA nodes. However, in our original series of cut-and-sew Maze-I, Maze-II, and Maze-III procedures, the preoperative status of the SA node in patients with paroxysmal AF (PAF) was documented to be normal in 95% of patients and abnormal in the other 5%. Before surgery, we explained to the 5% with abnormal preoperative SA node function that they would need not only a Maze procedure but also a pacemaker implantation because of their SSS. However, in the 95% ($n = 114$) of patients[30] with PAF who had normal preop SA nodes, not one patient required a postoperative pacemaker after a Maze procedure.[28] This observation proved to us that the RA lesions of the Maze procedure, if complete and placed properly, do not cause postoperative SA node dysfunction and therefore are not the cause of increased postoperative pacemaker requirements following a Maze procedure.

On the other hand, the association of AF and SSS is well known, and several different causes of SA node dysfunction in patients with AF have been documented.[29,30] They include not only the most common intrinsic cause of SA node dysfunction, idiopathic atrial degenerative disease, but prolonged AF itself can also damage the SA node as a result of the remodeling of SA node ion channel expression and function.[28] In addition, beta-blockers, calcium channel blockers, digoxin, antihypertensive agents, and antiarrhythmic agents can cause SA node dysfunction, particularly in patients with non-PAF.

Approximately 20% of patients with non-PAF in our original cut-and-sew Maze series required PPMs postoperatively.[4,5,28] We did not determine the status of the SA node preoperatively in patients with persistent and long-standing persistent AF (non-PAF) because we were reluctant to cardiovert them for study during sinus rhythm because of the thromboembolic risks involved. Therefore, because of the known association between the SSS and AF and the lack of pacemaker requirements in patients with documented normal preoperative SA node function, we originally attributed the need for new pacemakers in this group solely to an "unmasking" of preoperative dysfunctional SA nodes rather than to the Maze procedure lesions. However, we later learned that unmasking a SSS in these non-PAF patients with unknown preoperative SA node functional status was not the only cause of postoperative pacemaker requirements.

From 1987 to 1997, all Maze procedures were performed through a median sternotomy and included extensive dissection of the pericardial reflections and associated connective tissues external to the right and left atria to gain better surgical exposure for the Maze-I, Maze-II, and Maze-III procedures. In 1997, we switched to performing the minimally invasive totally cryosurgical Maze-III procedure in which little or no extracardiac dissection was needed because of the superior exposure of the inside of the LA that was provided by the improved angle of vision through a right mini-thoracotomy. Using the same Maze-III lesion pattern in a similar cohort of patients with non-PAF, the pacemaker requirements dropped from 20% in the median sternotomy group to 6% in the minimally invasive patients.[28] This observation has now been confirmed by Ad et al.[23] in more than 700 patients undergoing the minimally invasive CryoMaze-III procedure. In addition, as mentioned earlier, McCarthy's group[24] reported a postoperative pacemaker rate of 7.9% after performing the CryoMaze-III procedure concomitantly via a median sternotomy but without extensive extracardiac dissection and fewer than 1% new pacemaker requirements in isolated mitral valve repair patients. As stated in the McCarthy group's report:

> *"It is clear that there is tremendous variability in the rate of a new PPM need when adding right atrial incisions to achieve a biatrial lesion pattern . . . and compounding the confusion, the majority of reports do not clearly identify whether the indication for a PPM was heart block, sick sinus syndrome, or some other conduction abnormality."*

Thus, it seems reasonable to conclude from the available literature that between 5% and 10% of patients with non-PAF and unknown preoperative SA node status will need a new pacemaker postoperatively, and the more often the AF ablation is successful, the more likely the patient will need a new pacemaker. Indeed, *"successful AF ablation begets postoperative pacemakers."*[28]

Improperly Performed Surgery

A properly performed Maze procedure includes creating the lesion pattern of either the Maze-III or Maze-IV procedure and being certain that each individual lesion in the pattern is uniformly transmural and contiguous as described in the Chapter 20. Unfortunately, strict adherence to these rigorous technical details was not designed into the CTSN investigators' randomized trial. For example, there was no mention in either the text of the article or in its supplemental materials of a coronary sinus lesion, and notoriously unreliable unipolar ablation devices were used to create 44% of the LA lesions and 100% of the RA lesions.[9] Thus, it is likely that the only consistently perfect lesions within the two surgical subgroups (LA lesions only and "biatrial Maze procedure") were those that isolated the pulmonary veins, which were created with bipolar radiofrequency clamps. This explains by there was no statistical difference between the results of a simple pulmonary vein isolation (PVI) and the so-called "biatrial Maze procedure" in these patients with non-PAF.

An even more puzzling observation in that multicenter clinical trial was that the only statistical difference in the surgically ablated group and the non-ablated group resulting in a need for new pacemakers was an increase in postoperative heart block in the surgical ablation group. There was no increase in SA node disfunction in the surgical ablation group (Fig. 21.4). However, as mentioned previously, it is anatomically impossible to create heart block with a surgical procedure that has no atrial septal lesion, as was the case in this study. Thus if faced with the question of "Which lesion of the biatrial Maze procedure caused the heart block and subsequent pacemaker implantation in these patients?" the answer is that none of them could possibly have damaged the AV node–His bundle complex because none of the lesions were anywhere near those atrial septal structures.

Improperly positioned RA lesions can permanently damage the atrial pacemaker complex and result in the need for new postoperative pacemakers, but this is a surgical error that results from the faulty design of "modified" RA lesions. Furthermore, if the *LA* lesions are performed improperly or incompletely, the addition of the RA lesions, however they are performed, will not have a significant impact on outcomes, and the success rate will be unacceptably low, as it was in the CTSN trial (66%). Again, that was a major problem in this trial that led the authors to suggest erroneously, that PVI was as effective as "biatrial Maze procedures" for the treatment of patients with concomitant non-PAF, a suggestion based on an admittedly inadequately powered analysis of the two surgical subgroups.[9,10]

Patient Selection

One of the most powerful determinants of whether or not a patient undergoing concomitant surgical AF ablation is the type of preoperative

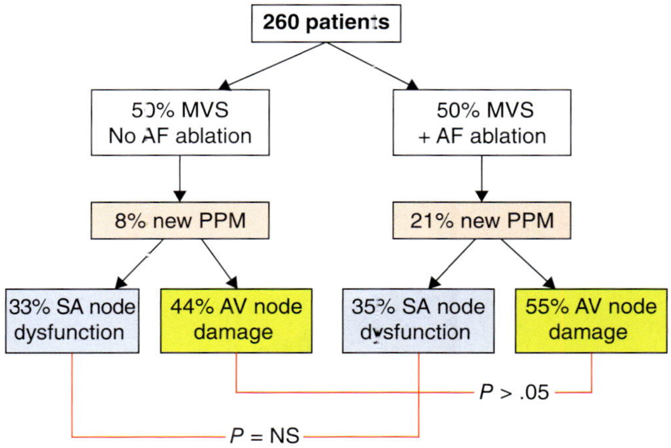

Fig. 21.4 Surgical ablation of nonparoxysmal atrial fibrillation (non-PAF) during mitral valve surgery (MVS). The highest incidence of new pacemaker requirements of any large clinical trial in cardiac surgery is the 21% reported for the surgical arm of the Cardiothoracic Surgery Network (CTSN) investigators controlled randomized trial.[9] The prevalence of postoperative sinoatrial (SA) node dysfunction was the same in the non-ablation group as in the atrial fibrillation (AF) ablation group, indicating that surgical AF ablation had no significant effect on SA node function postoperatively. However, atrioventricular (AV) node function was significantly worse in the AF ablation group than in the non-ablation group and led to the need for more permanent pacemaker (PPM) implantations postoperatively. The authors attributed this increased requirement for postoperative pacemakers to the right atrial (RA) lesions of the biatrial Maze procedure even though no atrial septal lesions were performed in the study, and the RA lesions were nowhere near the AV node or His bundle, which are located in the atrial septum. Because it is anatomically impossible for a surgical procedure that does not include an atrial septal lesion to injure the AV node–His bundle, some other explanation for the postoperative heart block has to exist. In this study, more patients who underwent AF ablation also had more double valve (mitral and tricuspid) procedures than in the non-ablated group, leading to more sutures being placed in the region of the AV node and His bundle, longer cardiopulmonary bypass times, and longer aortic cross-clamp times, all of which could have damaged the AV node–His bundle complex. *NS,* Not significant.

AF the patient has (Fig. 21.5).[28] If a patient has preoperative PAF, it is possible to determine the status of the SA node preoperatively during periods of sinus rhythm. In our original series of Maze patients, the preoperative status of the SA node was determined during periods of sinus rhythm in patients with PAF by performing "sinus node recovery times" and other tests of SA node function. As mentioned earlier, we found that 95% of patients with PAF had normal SA node function, and only 5% had sinus node dysfunction. Although all patients with documented SA node dysfunction preoperatively received new pacemakers postoperatively, not one of the patients with normal preoperative SA node function required a pacemaker after the Maze procedure.

If the preoperative status of the SA node is unknown, it is impossible to determine preoperatively whether the patient will the need a pacemaker postoperatively. This is the problem one faces in patients with non-PAF in whom it can be dangerous to cardiovert preoperatively simply to determine SA node function because of thromboembolic risks. Thus, when one is surgically ablating non-PAF, the preoperative functional status of the SA node is rarely known. Therefore, when the non-PAF is successfully ablated and the SA node is found to be abnormal postoperatively, it is impossible to know whether a SSS has been unmasked by the successful surgery or the actual ablation procedure itself damaged the SA node. Experience has taught us that approximately 10% of patients who have their AF ablated as a concomitant surgical procedure will require postoperative pacemakers because of unmasking an underlying SSS.

Fortunately, the presence of postoperative SSS does not always require a PPM. Thus, the range of expected postoperative pacemaker needs in patients with non-PAF is generally between 5% and 10%. Furthermore, several of the underlying SSS in patients with non-PAF have been induced by antiarrhythmic medications and/or continuous long-standing AF. Therefore, some of them will recover so that the patient becomes non–pacemaker dependent. Our group at Northwestern University recently reported a series of 6135 valve surgery patients that resulted in 282 patients (4.6%) who required a new predischarge PPM after concomitant surgical AF ablation.[31] PVI, LA-only, or a standard biatrial Maze procedure was used to ablate the AF concomitant with the mitral valve surgery. The new pacemakers were implanted for postoperative AV node dysfunction (75.3%), SSS (19.1%), both (5%),

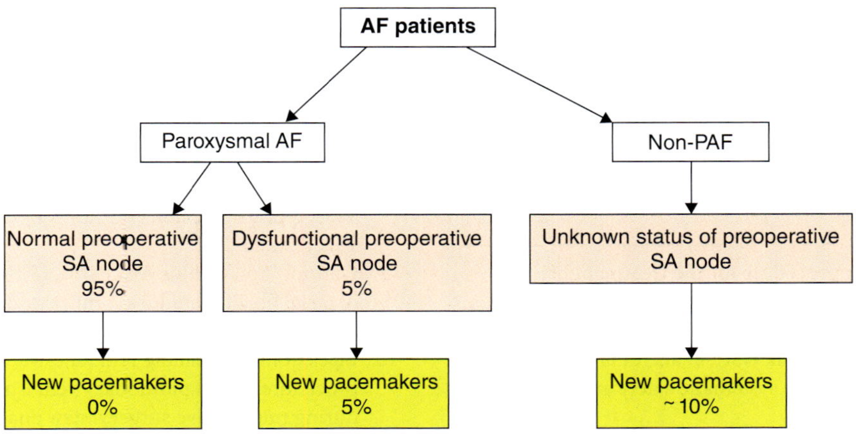

Fig. 21.5 The number of pacemakers required after surgical atrial fibrillation (AF) ablation largely depends on the distribution of paroxysmal (PAF) versus non-PAF within a given patient cohort. Using this chart, one can see that simply changing the distribution of patients from predominantly PAF to predominantly non-PAF will result in significantly more postoperative pacemakers and vice versa. See text for further discussion. *SA,* Sinoatrial.

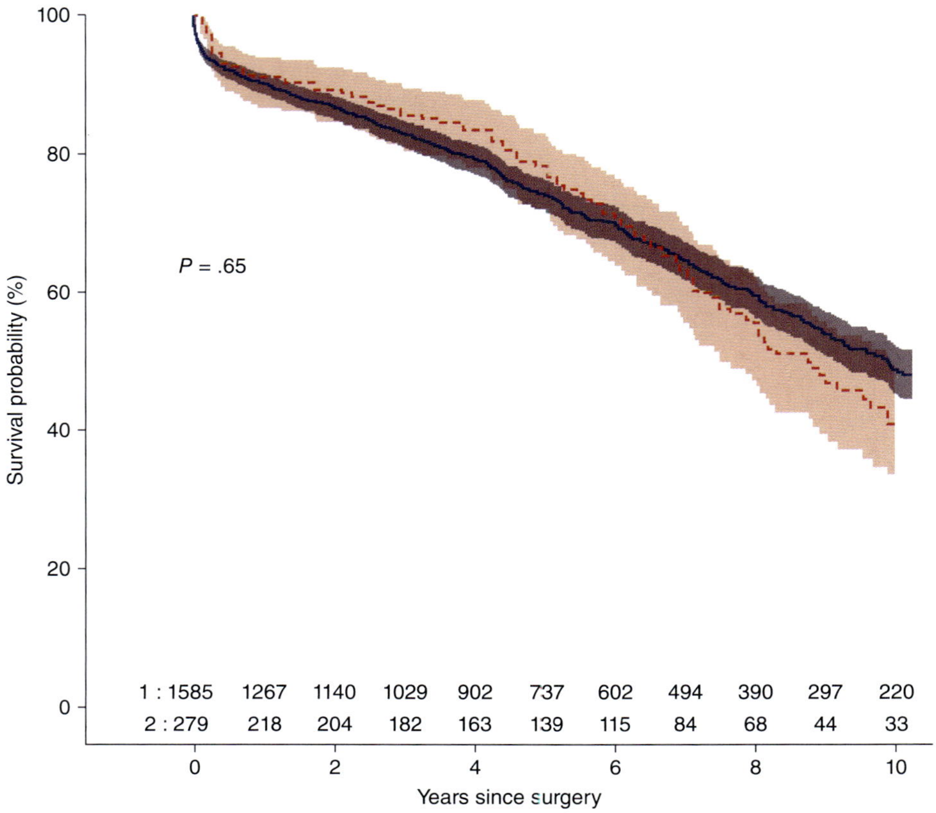

	Year 1	Year 2	Year 4	Year 6	Year 8	Year 10
No PreDC PPM	90.1%	86.7%	79.4%	69.9%	59.3%	48.7%
PreDC PPM	90.9%	89.2%	83.5%	70.7%	55.2%	40.9%

1 : No PreDC PPM ------ 2 : PreDC PPM

Fig. 21.6 Kaplan-Meier survival estimates of propensity score-matched patients with predischarge (PreDC) or without predischarge (no PreDC) permanent pacemaker (PPM) implantation. No statistically significant differences in 10-year survival rates were found between the two groups (*P* = .65).

and indeterminate (0.7%). The necessity for new pacemaker implantation was 3.0% after PVI, 6.1% after LA-only lesions, and 12.8% after a biatrial Maze procedure. By 3 months after concomitant surgical AF ablation, rhythm recovery was present in 56.5% of patients and did not differ by lesion set. Rhythm recovery rates were 44.7% in patients with postoperative AV node dysfunction and in 68.6% in patients with postoperative SSS. Propensity score matching showed that late survival was similar in patients who received new postoperative pacemakers and those who did not (Fig. 21.6).

REFERENCES

1. Ad N, Cox JL. The Maze procedure for the treatment of atrial fibrillation: a minimally invasive approach. *J Card Surg.* 2004;19:196–200.
2. Vos LM, Kotecha D, Geuzebroek GSC, et al. Totally thoracoscopic ablation for atrial fibrillation: a systematic safety analysis. *Europace.* 2018;20(11):1790–1797.
3. Cheema FJ, Weisberg JS, Khalid I, Roberts HG. Warm beating heart, robotic endoscopic Cox-cryomaze: an approach for treating atrial fibrillation. *Ann Thorac Surg.* 2009;87:966–968.
4. Cox JL, Boineau JP, Schuessler RB, Kater KM, Lappas DG. Five-year experience with the Maze procedure for atrial fibrillation. *Ann Thorac Surg.* 1994;56:814–824.
5. Cox JL, Schuessler RB, Lappas DG, Boineau JP. An 8 1/2 year clinical experience with surgery for atrial fibrillation. *Ann Surg.* 1996;224:267–275.
6. Takahashi N, Zipes DP. Vagal modulation of adrenergic effects on canine sinus and atrioventricular nodes. *Am J Physiol.* 1983;244:H775–H781.
7. Issa ZF, Miller JM, Zipes DP. Sinus node dysfunction. *Clinical Arrhythmology and Electrophysiology: A Companion to Braunwald's Heart Disease.* 2009:118–126.
8. Engel TR, Meister SG, Feltosa GS, Fischer HA, Frankl WS. Appraisal of sinus node artery disease. *Circulation.* 1975;52:286–291.
9. Gillinov Am, Gelijns AC, Parides MK, et al. Surgical ablation of atrial fibrillation during mitral-valve surgery. *N Eng J Med.* 2015;372(15):1399–1409.
10. Blackstone EH, Chang HL, Rajeswaran J, et al. Biatrial Maze procedure versus pulmonary vein isolation for atrial fibrillation during mitral valve surgery: new analytical approaches and end points. *J Thorac Cardiovasc Surg.* 2019;157(1):234–243.
11. Klein GJ, Sealy WC, Pritchett EL, et al. Cryosurgical ablation of the atrioventricular node-His bundle: long-term follow-up and properties of the junctional pacemaker. *Circulation.* 1980;61:8–15.
12. Cox JL. Anatomy of the "posterior septal space.". *Am J Cardiol.* 1991;68:675–677.

13. Sealy WC, Mikat EM. Anatomical problems with identification and interruption of posterior septal Kent bundles. *Ann Thorac Surg*. 1983;36:584–595.
14. Cox JL, Gallagher JJ, Cain ME. Experience with 118 consecutive patients undergoing surgery for the Wolff-Parkinson-White syndrome. *J Thorac Cardiovasc Surg*. 1985;90:490–501.
15. McCarthy PM, Churyla A, Kruse J, Cox JL. Reducing permanent pacemaker requirements following concomitant surgery for atrial fibrillation. *J Cardiovasc Electrophysiol*. 2022;33: 1978–1982.
16. Gammie JS, Chu MWA, Falk V, et al. Concomitant tricuspid repair in patients with degenerative mitral regurgitation. *N Engl J Med*. 2021;386:327–339.
17. Gammie JS, Haddad M, Milford-Beland S, et al. Atrial fibrillation correction surgery: lessons from the Society of Thoracic Surgeons National Cardiac Database. *Ann Thorac Surg*. 2008;85(3):909–914.
18. Badhwar V, Rankin JS, Ad N, et al. Surgical ablation of atrial fibrillation in the United States: trends and propensity matched outcomes. *Ann Thorac Surg*. 2017;104:493–500.
19. DeRose JJ Jr, Mancini DM, Chang HL, et al. Pacemaker implantation after mitral valve surgery with atrial fibrillation ablation. *J Am Coll Cardiol*. 2019;73:2427–2435.
20. Ma J, Wei P, Yan Q, et al. Safety and efficacy of concomitant ablation for atrial fibrillation in rheumatic mitral valve surgery: a meta-analysis. *J Cardiac Surg*. 2022;37:361–373.
21. Cappabianca G, Ferrarese S, Tutino C, et al. Safety and efficacy of biatrial vs left atrial surgical ablation during concomitant cardiac surgery: a meta-analysis of clinical studies with a focus on the causes of pacemaker implantation. *J Cardiovasc Electrophysiol*. 2019;30:2150–2163.
22. Henn MC, Lawrence CP, Sinn LA, et al. Effectiveness of surgical ablation in patients with atrial fibrillation and aortic valve disease. *Ann Thorac Surg*. 2015;100(4):1253–1259.
23. Ad N, Holmes SD, Ali R, Pritchard G, Lamont D. A single center's experience with pacemaker implantation after the Cox Maze procedure for atrial fibrillation. *J Thorac Cardiovasc Surg*. 2017;154(1):139–146.
24. Halas M, Kruse J, McCarthy PM. Concomitant treatment of atrial fibrillation during mitral valve surgery. *J Cardiovasc Electrophysiol*. 2021;32(10):2873–2878.
25. McCarthy PM, Churyla A, Kruse J, Cox JL. Reducing permanent pacemaker requirements following concomitant surgery for atrial fibrillation. *J Thorac Cardiovasc Surg*. 2022;33(8):1978–1982.
26. Soni LK, Cedola SR, Cogan J, et al. Right atrial lesions do not improve the efficacy of a complete left atrial lesion set in the surgical treatment of atrial fibrillation, but they do increase procedural morbidity. *J Thorac Cardiovasc Surg*. 2013;145:356–361.
27. Churyla A, Iddriss A, Andrei AC, et al. Biatrial or left atrial lesion set for ablation during mitral surgery: risks and benefits. *Ann Thorac Surg*. 2017;103:1858–1865.
28. Cox JL, Ad N, Churyla A, et al. The Maze procedure and postoperative pacemakers. *Ann Thorac Surg*. 2018;106:1561–1569.
29. Gomes JAC, Kang PS, Matheson M, Gough WB, El-Sheri. Coexistence of sick sinus rhythm and atrial flutter fibrillation. *Circulation*. 1981;63:80–86.
30. Van den Berg PM, van Gelder IC. Atrial fibrillation and sinus node dysfunction. *J Am Coll Cardiol*. 2001;38:1585–1586.
31. Churyla A, McCarthy PM, Kruse J, et al. Concomitant ablation of atrial fibrillation: new pacemakers and early rhythm recovery. *J Thorac Cardiovasc Surg*. 2023. S0022-5223(23)00987-X. https://doi.org/10.1016/j.jtcvs.2023.10.030.

22

Effect of the Maze Procedure on Left and Right Atrial Function

James L. Cox, Olga N. Kislitsina

CHAPTER OUTLINE

Atrial fibrillation (AF) can cause multiple adverse sequelae, including palpitations, decreased cardiac output, systemic thromboembolism, and tachycardia-induced ventricular cardiomyopathy. Typically, the first symptoms of *de novo* AF are palpitations and the consequences of decreased cardiac output such as fatigue, shortness of breath, and dyspnea on exertion. These symptoms are usually worse in patients with paroxysmal AF (PAF) than in patients who are in AF continuously. This paradox is likely because patients who have intermittent bouts of AF are simply more aware of their symptoms during AF because of the noticeable discrepancy between how they feel while in AF versus how they feel when they are not in AF. Although systemic thromboembolism occurs with equal frequency in patients with PAF and persistent AF,[1] tachycardia-induced ventricular cardiomyopathy occurs almost exclusively in patients with long-standing persistent AF (LSpAF) and poor rate control because of the time required for the ventricular cardiomyopathy to develop.

The primary objectives of catheter ablation for AF and surgical ablation for AF are fundamentally different; therefore, they can have different impacts on postprocedure atrial function. Catheter ablation is designed to *isolate* the triggers located primarily in and around the pulmonary vein orifices that are responsible for inducing AF episodes. The success of catheter ablation in restoring left atrial function depends largely on the extent of preexisting atrial fibrosis and the degree of additional scarring induced by the ablation procedure. Surgical ablation is designed to *ablate* the macro-reentrant circuits that sustain AF by creating a series of strategically placed linear lesions in the atria. Although the surgical Maze procedure has a higher success rate in achieving sinus rhythm, it is inherently more invasive than catheter ablation, raising concerns about its potential impact on postoperative atrial function. The degree of left atrial dysfunction after the Maze procedure has been associated with multiple factors such as the extent of preoperative atrial scarring, the number of surgical lesions created, and other preoperative conditions involving the left atrium (LA). Like patients having catheter ablation, surgical patients with preserved preoperative atrial function and minimal fibrosis are more likely to retain better atrial function postoperatively. Additionally, sinus rhythm restoration after the Maze procedure plays a pivotal role in promoting the functional recovery of both atria.

The ability to assess atrial function in an accurate and reproducible manner has evolved significantly with advancements in echocardiographic techniques.[2] Speckle-tracking echocardiography (STE) has become a key tool for quantifying atrial strain and identifying early functional impairment (see Chapter 7). Left atrial reservoir strain and pump strain have proven to be sensitive markers of atrial function, and they can be used as predictors of AF recurrence after both catheter ablation and the Maze procedure.

EXPERIMENTAL EVALUATION OF LEFT ATRIAL FUNCTION AFTER THE MAZE PROCEDURE

As mentioned in Chapter 1, there was initial concern that the multiple transmural atrial lesions of the Maze procedure might devascularize the atrial myocardium. Therefore, postmortem evaluation of the atria after experimental Maze procedures included injecting the right coronary artery with blue dye and the left main coronary artery with red dye to document that the coronary blood supply to the atria remained intact postoperatively (Fig. 22.1). In addition, histologic studies of both atria failed to show any ischemic injury in either atrium after the experimental Maze procedure. After the safety and efficacy of the Maze procedure was confirmed in animals, major efforts were expended to determine the effect of the procedure on both right and left atrial function.

In the first series of experiments, an electromagnetic flow probe was placed around the ascending aorta for continuous measurement of the cardiac output (minus coronary artery flow) in dogs that had undergone a Maze procedure. Atrioventricular (AV) sequential pacing was instituted at a constant rate and optimal A-V interval, and the cardiac output was allowed to stabilize for several minutes (Fig. 22.2). The atrial pacing wire was then suddenly disconnected from the pacemaker to convert from AV sequential pacing to ventricular pacing alone at the identical rate. The cardiac output immediately decreased by approximately 16% with the loss of synchronous atrial activation. After the cardiac output had stabilized with ventricular pacing, the atrial pacing wire was reattached to the pacemaker to restore AV sequential pacing, and the cardiac output returned to its previous level. This series of

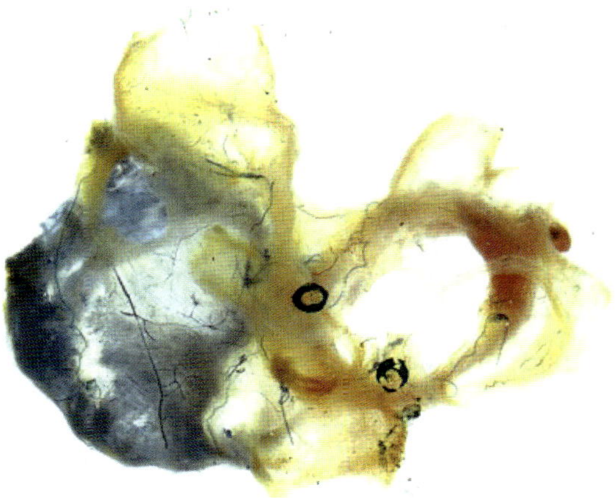

Fig. 22.1 Photo of the right and left atria after an experimental canine Maze procedure. The right coronary artery was injected with blue dye, and the left main coronary artery was injected with red dye to determine if the lesions of the Maze procedure interfered with the blood supply of the atria. The tests showed that the coronary artery blood supply of the atria was not affected by the Maze procedure. Histologic examination of random tissue samples from both atria also confirmed the absence of atrial myocardial ischemia after the Maze procedure.

experiments clearly demonstrated that the atria functioned well after a Maze procedure.

Although these experiments documented that the Maze procedure had no significantly adverse effect on *overall* atrial function, they did not exclude the possibility that the LA was adversely affected by the Maze procedure. Lessons learned from the left atrial isolation procedure years before were extremely important in the accurate assessment of the effects of the Maze procedure on atrial function. For example, we had documented that after isolation of the LA, the loss of all left atrial function had no impact on forward cardiac output in the presence of normal right atrial function, normal right atrial-right ventricular synchrony, and a normal left ventricle (LV) (Fig. 22.3). Thus we recognized that the experimental findings of preserved *overall* atrial function after the Maze procedure did not rule out the possibility that the procedure had injured the LA but not the RA. Therefore, we performed two-dimensional echocardiography and Doppler flow analysis after the Maze procedure specifically to evaluate postoperative function in the LA. Doppler flow across the mitral valve in the control group demonstrated excellent A-waves, indicating that the canine LA was functioning normally. Similar A-waves were consistently observed after the Maze procedure, indicating that the LA continued to function postoperatively (Fig. 22.4).

CLINICAL EVALUATION OF LEFT ATRIAL FUNCTION AFTER THE MAZE PROCEDURE

Beginning with the first patient who underwent the Maze procedure, we performed certain intraoperative tests to evaluate atrial function soon after discontinuing cardiopulmonary bypass. Repeated Swan-Ganz thermodilution cardiac outputs were recorded during atrioventricular (AV) sequential pacing versus ventricular pacing, and transesophageal echocardiography (TEE) was used to record evidence of right atrial and left atrial contractile activity. Perhaps more important than either test was to simply look at both the RA and LA and watch them contract. The LA was sometimes slow to recover its capacitance capabilities, but in virtually every patient, the left atrial myocardium could be seen to contract briefly just before ventricular systole. I made a habit of bringing my electrophysiology colleagues, who had been involved in the pre-Maze mapping process, back into the operating room specifically to confirm visually that the atria were contracting. All patients were in normal sinus rhythm or being A-paced or AV sequentially paced during these assessments, and all showed evidence of almost immediate return of atrial function. In view of the well-known delay in atrial function after successful electrical cardioversion of AF to sinus rhythm, we were quite surprised to see atrial function return so soon after being surgically converted from AF to sinus or A-paced rhythm. We still have no explanation for this unexpected phenomenon except that perhaps unlike surgical conversion, electrical cardioversion might "stun" the atrial myocardium, which then takes more time to recover.

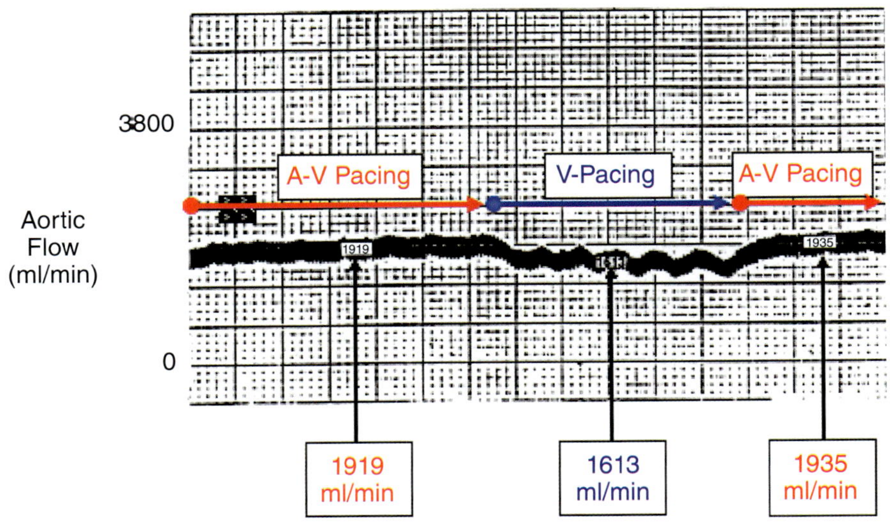

Fig. 22.2 Hemodynamic evaluation of atrial function after a canine Maze procedure. An electromagnetic flow probe was placed around the ascending aorta for the continuous measurement of cardiac output (minus coronary blood flow). The cardiac output was approximately 16% better in the presence of synchronous atrial contraction during atrioventricular sequential pacing than it was without synchronous atrial contraction during ventricular pacing at the same rate.

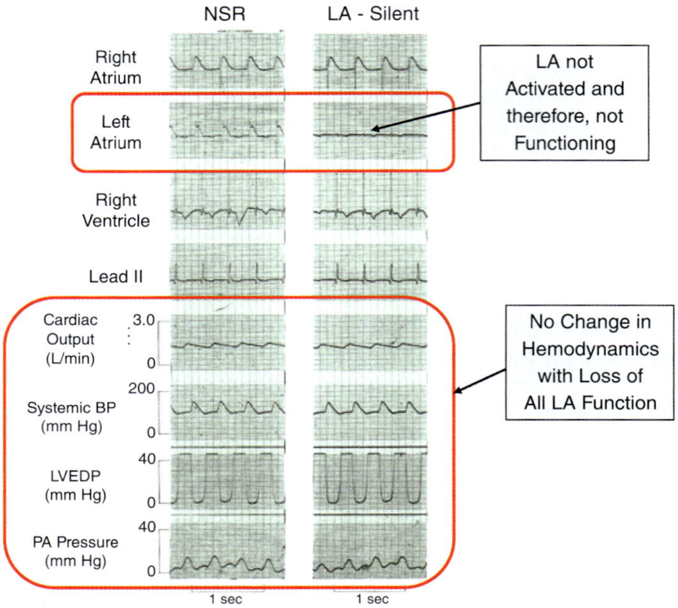

Fig. 22.3 Evaluation of the impact of left atrial contraction on multiple hemodynamic factors. The cardiac output (minus coronary blood flow) was continuously recorded with an electromagnetic flow probe around the ascending aorta. Systemic blood pressure (BP) was monitored continuously with an indwelling arterial cannula. Left ventricular end-diastolic pressure (LVEDP) was monitored continuously with a high-fidelity Millar catheter in the left ventricle. Continuous pulmonary artery (PA) pressure was monitored with a Swan-Ganz catheter located in the main PA. *Left panel,* After surgical electrical isolation of the left atrium (LA) from the rest of the heart, normal sinus rhythm (NSR) was reproduced by pacing the right atrium and LA with a 40-ms delay in pacing of the LA. Activation of the ventricles occurred normally through the AV node–His bundle complex. This precisely reproduced the electrical activation sequence of the heart during normal sinus rhythm in someone who had *not* undergone a left atrial isolation procedure. *Right panel,* The left atrial pacing wire was then suddenly disconnected, and the LA became electrically silent. Note that the complete loss of left atrial contraction did not affect the forward cardiac output, systemic BP, LVEDP, or PA pressure. (See text for further discussion.)

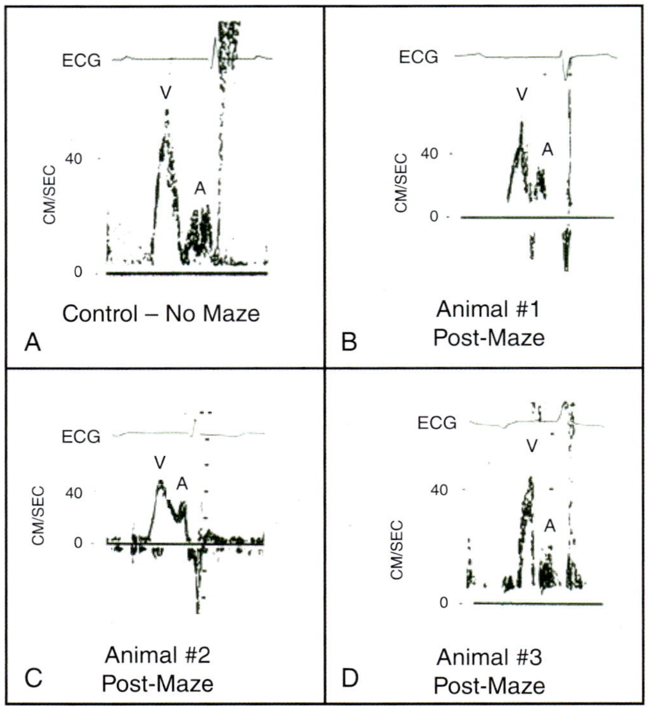

Fig. 22.4 Echocardiographic evaluation of left atrial function after a canine Maze procedure. (A) Transmitral Doppler flow in a normal dog. (B–D) Transmitral Doppler flow in three separate dogs after undergoing the Maze procedure. Persistence of the A-wave after the Maze procedure confirms the presence of post-Maze left atrial function. *ECG,* Electrocardiogram.

The first 69 patients undergoing the Maze-I ($n = 32$), Maze-II ($n = 14$), or Maze-III ($n = 23$) procedure had the following tests and evaluations performed 6 months after surgery:

1. Complete endocardial catheter electrophysiology study that included the identical programmed electrical stimulation protocol and burst-pacing protocol used preoperatively in an effort to induce AF. These stimulation protocols were performed both at rest and during isoproterenol infusion.
2. Swan-Ganz thermodilution cardiac output determinations during AV sequential pacing versus ventricular pacing. Cardiac output was recorded as the average of three separate thermodilution outputs performed during AV sequential pacing and during ventricular pacing
3. Standard 12-lead electrocardiography (ECG)
4. 24-hour Holter monitor
5. Dynamic magnetic resonance imaging (MRI) scans of the heart
6. Transthoracic echocardiography (TTE)
7. TEE if the TTE showed no apparent left atrial function

AF could not be induced in any of the 69 patients 6 months after having a Maze procedure. In a few patients, self-terminating atrial flutter was induced briefly during the infusion of isoproterenol, but it did not occur clinically either before or after the 6-month electrophysiology study. As observed in the experimental studies, cardiac output was consistently higher during AV sequential pacing than during ventricular pacing at the same rate, indicating the presence of atrial function. No AF was seen on either the 12-lead ECGs or on the 24-hour Holter monitors. Our electrophysiologists, Drs. Bruce Lindsay and Michael Cain, stopped performing the electrophysiology studies after the first 69 patients because they believed that the extensive efforts to induce AF in patients after a Maze procedure were "an unnecessary inconvenience to the patients and waste of our time and resources because the operation clearly works."

The results of the thermodilution cardiac outputs, dynamic MRI scans, and TTEs that were performed to evaluate postoperative atrial function did not always coincide. As a result, we took the position that if any one of these tests showed positive atrial function, then the results would be considered positive. Using this criterion, right atrial function was documented in 98% of patients, and left atrial function was documented in 93% of patients. Nine patients showed no apparent left atrial function in any of the tests, including the TTE. We proceeded with a TEE in these 9 patients, and definitive left atrial function was documented in 8 of them. This suggested that TEE was more sensitive than TTE in the assessment of left atrial function.

Over my (JLC) objection, our group published an article in 1994 describing only the Doppler echo results in 46 of the Maze patients and showed that using Doppler echocardiography only, right atrial function was present in 83%, and left atrial function was present in only 61%,[3] even though many of these same patients were shown to have biatrial function by one of the other tests, particularly the dynamic MRI scans. Thus this article resulted in a profound misconception that suggested that the LA "didn't work" in more than one-third of patients after the

Maze procedure, when in fact, left atrial function was documented by at least one test in 93% of them. Another 1997 study in 31 Maze patients, which was also confined to the evaluation of atrial function by Doppler echocardiography only, showed right atrial function in 81% and left atrial function in 71%.[4] This study noted that the mitral A-wave was "lower" after the Maze procedure, suggesting to the authors that the restored atrial function after a Maze procedure was "less than" that in control patients despite a significant decrease in both left atrial and right atrial sizes with no left atrial fractional area change postoperatively, though it remained below normal in both atria.

In 2008, Damiano and colleagues[5] reported a superb experimental study in pigs in which a group undergoing a Maze procedure via a median sternotomy and pericardiotomy was compared with a sham group undergoing only a median sternotomy and pericardiotomy. Postoperative left atrial function, including left atrial reservoir, conduit, and contraction parameters, was assessed by load-sensitive MRI and load-independent conductance catheter techniques. Their findings showed that "many of the previously-observed changes in LA function following the Cox Maze procedure are due to the median sternotomy and cardiotomy."

Several studies indicate that the restoration of atrial pump function after a Maze procedure is affected by comorbidities and the duration of AF.[6–8] In patients undergoing a Maze only or in conjunction with coronary artery bypass graft surgery, atrial function typically recovers quickly. However, patients with long-standing degenerative mitral regurgitation can have both global and regional atrial dysfunction that are exacerbated by preexisting conditions such as scar tissue, which can result in irreversible remodeling of the LA, resulting in an elevated risk of recurrent AF and stroke.

EVALUATION OF ATRIAL FUNCTION AFTER THE MAZE PROCEDURE USING CONVENTIONAL ECHOCARDIOGRAPHY AND SPECKLE-TRACKING ANALYSIS

Previously, left atrial function was assessed using invasive methods such as angiography, micro-manometry, and pulmonary artery pressure measurements.[9] However, advancements in noninvasive imaging techniques such as pulsed-wave Doppler echocardiography and speckle-tracking echocardiography (STE) analysis now provide more accurate and reproducible assessments of atrial mechanics, making it possible to diagnose early atrial dysfunction and guide therapeutic decisions (see Chapter 7). The three distinct phases of left atrial function as determined by STE, the reservoir, conduit, and booster phases, ensure efficient atrial contribution to left and right ventricular filling. A comprehensive evaluation of preoperative atrial strain and post-Maze atrial strain by STE analysis enables clinicians to predict AF recurrence, monitor atrial recovery, and optimize long-term management strategies. Atrial myocardial deformation (i.e., compliance) has emerged as a significant predictor of the maintenance of sinus rhythm, particularly after external cardioversion or surgical interventions such as the Maze procedure. Furthermore, understanding the status of both left atrial and right atrial function and their interplay before and after surgery is essential because atrial dysfunction in either atrium can have cascading effects on biventricular performance and overall cardiac output.

Traditional Echocardiographic Techniques

1. **Anteroposterior diameter and area measurements** (Fig. 22.5A and B): These conventional two-dimensional measurements are used to assess atrial enlargement and geometry. Left atrial size is often an indicator of chronic pressure or volume overload and is strongly associated with AF recurrence.
2. **Pulsed-wave Doppler** (Fig. 22.5C): Doppler echocardiography evaluates the transmitral and tricuspid inflow velocities, identifying atrial contribution to ventricular filling (A-wave) and distinguishing phases of diastolic dysfunction. Mitral inflow patterns, for instance, reflect conduit and booster-pump phases of left atrial function.
3. **Tissue Doppler imaging (TDI)** (Fig. 22.5D): TDI provides measurements of mitral annular velocities, particularly the A′-wave, which represents atrial contraction. These velocities help assess atrial mechanics and delays in atrial conduction.
4. **3D echocardiography** (Fig. 22.5E): Advances in three-dimensional imaging allow for accurate calculation of maximum left atrial volumes, minimizing geometric assumptions. It improves the assessment of global left atrial size and function and is increasingly used for preoperative evaluations.

Speckle-Tracking Echocardiography

STE (Figs. 22.5F and 22.6) has emerged as a superior method for assessing atrial strain and deformation, providing a deeper understanding of atrial mechanics beyond size and velocities. STE-derived longitudinal reservoir strain is particularly valuable in evaluating left atrial compliance and predicting atrial remodeling. Reduced left atrial reservoir strain has been shown to correlate with increased atrial pressures, AF recurrence, and impaired hemodynamics postintervention (see Chapter 7). The best measure of left atrial compliance is the peak left atrial reservoir strain, which is also referred to as the peak left atrial longitudinal strain.[10]

Similar to the LA, right atrial strain is evaluated using STE and is characterized by the same three functional phases: reservoir, conduit, and booster pump. Right atrial strain plays a pivotal role in assessing right ventricular filling pressure and has been shown to reflect early pathophysiological changes, offering a valuable tool for diagnosing and monitoring disease progression. For example, reduced right atrial strain correlates with elevated right ventricular afterload and impaired right ventricular diastolic function, which can result in poor clinical outcomes after a Maze procedure.[11] A detailed evaluation of right atrial strain and its clinical significance is provided in Chapter 7.

A-wave velocity—a critical indicator of left atrial contractile function—is significantly lower in patients post-Maze procedure compared with age-matched control subjects ($P < .001$). In contrast, right atrial function shows a more favorable recovery after a Maze procedure, as evidenced by tricuspid inflow velocities comparable to healthy control subjects. These findings underscore that although the Maze procedure effectively restores atrial function in most patients, the degree of recovery, particularly in the LA, remains less robust than in individuals without AF.[4]

Several studies have expanded on these findings. For example, in 2016, Nitta's group in Tokyo provided valuable insights into the comparative efficacy of two Maze procedure lesion sets: the U lesion and the box lesion in the LA.[12] Patients undergoing the U lesion demonstrated superior preservation of left atrial transport function, reflected by higher peak A/E ratios, a sensitive echocardiographic marker of left atrial contractility, underscoring improved left atrial mechanical recovery. Conversely, the box lesion set, although effective in maintaining sinus rhythm, resulted in greater impairment of left atrial transport function. Predictors of poorer outcomes, such as larger left atrial size and LSpAF, were identified in both groups, emphasizing the role of baseline atrial remodeling in postoperative recovery. Lönnerholm et al.[13] further evaluated patients undergoing the Cox Maze-III procedure and observed a significant reduction in left atrial fractional area change and transmitral A-wave velocity at 6 and 56 months of follow-up compared to baseline ($P < .001$). These findings suggest that postoperative reductions in atrial mechanical function could have

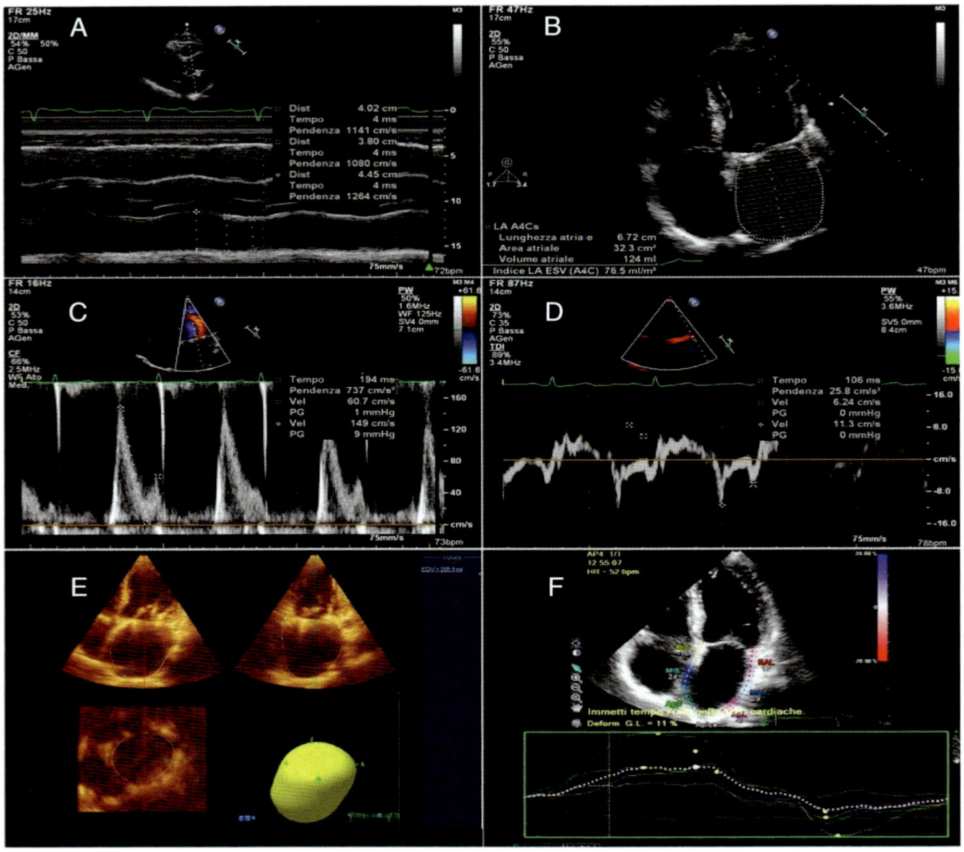

Fig. 22.5 Echocardiographic methods and measurements used to evaluation left atrial function. (A) Anteroposterior left atrial diameter. (B) Left atrial areas, volumes, and maximum superoinferior diameter. (C) Transmitral peak velocity of the late filling wave (A-wave). (D) Lateral mitral annulus peak velocity related to atrial contraction (a′ wave) and atrial conduction delay. (E) Maximum left atrial three-dimensional volume. (F) Left atrial global longitudinal strain. (Reproduced from Albirini A, Scalia GM, Murray RD, et al. Left and right atrial transport function after the Maze procedure for atrial fibrillation: an echocardiographic Doppler follow-up study. *J Am Soc Echocardiol.* 1997;10(9):937–945.)

clinical implications, including an elevated risk of thrombus formation.[13] Buber et al.[14] corroborated these findings, highlighting that approximately 31% of patients with sinus rhythm before and after surgery exhibited no evidence of left atrial mechanical contraction, resulting in a fivefold increased risk of thromboembolic stroke.

The Lonnerholm and Buber reports are at variance with most of the large clinical series that have been reported over the past 30 years as well as with the Society of Thoracic Surgeons guidelines for AF surgery (see Chapter 24). For example, why would Buber's results show a fivefold increase in thromboembolic stroke when other larger series, even those that included patients with previous preoperative strokes caused by AF, were more than 98% stroke free for up to 15 years after the Maze procedure?[15,16] There is no obvious explanation why some surgeons should get such dramatically different results from others, but these sporadic outlier reports underscore the need for continued monitoring of atrial transport function after AF surgery. Although postoperative left atrial mechanical function often improves over time, serial echocardiographic follow-up remains critical for identifying patients at risk for late thromboembolism caused by postoperative left atrial dysfunction.

Baalman et al.[17] demonstrated that TTE assessment of preoperative left atrial strain, particularly during the reservoir phase, serves as a reliable predictor of AF recurrence after thoracoscopic surgical ablation. The study found that reduced left atrial reservoir strain and increased mechanical dispersion of the conduit phase were associated with increased AF recurrence in patients with sinus rhythm or AF at baseline. These findings highlight the utility of left atrial strain as a valuable tool for improving preoperative risk stratification and guiding surgical strategies.[17]

Our group evaluated the predictive value of preoperative and postoperative four-chamber strain analysis, emphasizing the significance of both left atrial and right atrial function in determining outcomes after the Maze-IV procedure.[18] This study analyzed a cohort of 821 patients undergoing surgical AF ablation subdivided into those receiving biatrial lesions ($n = 290$) and left atrial–only lesions ($n = 531$). The study found that preoperative strain values for both the LA and RA were significant predictors of AF recurrence, with a 6% increased risk for recurrence per unit decrease in atrial reservoir strain. Interestingly, although preoperative left atrial reservoir strain was lower in the biatrial group compared with control subjects, its postoperative value emerged as a key predictor for cardiovascular events, including stroke. This highlights the prognostic value of left atrial strain, not just for rhythm control but also for assessing thromboembolic risk. Right atrial strain demonstrated similar predictive power for AF recurrence, underscoring the importance of preoperative and postoperative right atrial assessment. These findings suggest that preoperative evaluation of both left atrial and right atrial function is critical for surgical planning, particularly when deciding between biatrial and left atrial–only lesion sets. Our study suggests to us that integrating right atrial strain

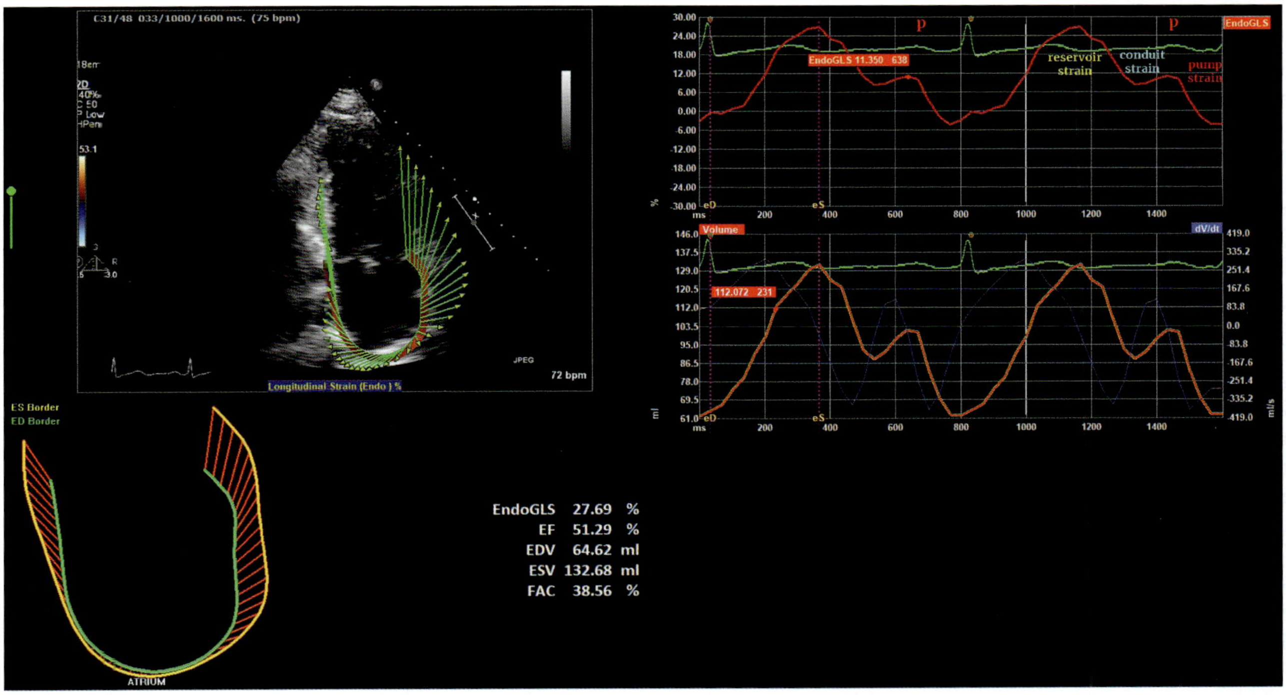

Fig. 22.6 Left atrial strain is calculated during the reservoir, conduit, and pump phases of the cardiac cycle using speckle-tracking echocardiographic analysis. (See text for further discussion.)

analysis into routine postoperative assessments might enhance patient-specific risk stratification, improving long-term outcomes and guiding the management of cardiovascular events after the Maze-IV procedure.

LEFT ATRIAL FRACTIONAL AREA CHANGE AS A MEASURE OF LEFT ATRIAL FUNCTION

Another useful parameter for assessing left atrial function is left atrial fractional area change (LA-FAC) (Fig. 22.7). This parameter can be calculated from standard echocardiograms or using speckle-tracking analysis. Unfortunately, LA-FAC is often misconstrued as being comparable to the left ventricular ejection fraction because it measures the change in the size of the LA during one cardiac cycle. In fact, it is often actually called the "left atrial ejection fraction."[19,20] However, this term is misleading because the area change that occurs in the LA is all *passive* deformation dependent on the compliance of the LA, not on its active contraction. Therefore it cannot be accurately called an "ejection fraction," which implies actively forcing blood out of the LA. However, active contraction of the LA does not occur at any time in the cardiac cycle except during the atrial twitch (brief pump phase) at left ventricular end-diastole. Thus the observed decrease in LA-FAC of approximately 8% after the Maze procedure likely reflects reduced left atrial compliance caused by procedural effects, including isolation of the pulmonary veins and posterior left atrial wall, as well as the inherent stiffness caused by the multiple ablation lesions. This postoperative reduction in compliance is expected, given the structural changes induced by the Maze procedure, which disrupt normal atrial tissue properties. LA-FAC remains a valuable parameter, particularly in clinical settings where advanced imaging technologies, such as STE, are not available. Despite their limitations, our studies have shown that LA-FAC can serve as a reliable surrogate for assessing left atrial reservoir function and compliance both before and after the Maze procedure.[10]

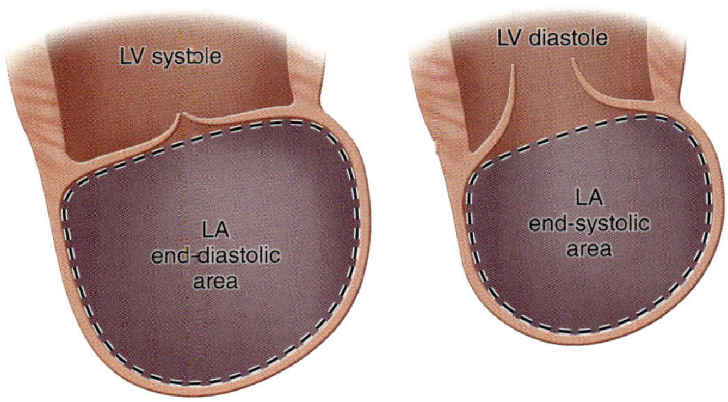

Fig. 22.7 The left atrial fractional area change is calculated using the formula $(A_{pre\text{-}a} - A_{min})/A_{pre\text{-}a}$, in which $A_{pre\text{-}a}$ is the left atrial area (cm^2) before atrial systole and A_{min} is the minimal left atrial area (cm^2) at the end of atrial systole. (See text for further discussion.) *LA*, Left atrium; *LV*, left ventricle.

In settings where only standard two-dimensional echocardiography is available, LA-FAC can provide critical insights into changes in atrial mechanics, aiding in the evaluation of left atrial function and the identification of patients at risk for adverse outcomes. Its availability and ease of use make it particularly relevant for hospitals without access to advanced echocardiographic technologies such as STE.

SUMMARY

The effects of the Maze procedure on postoperative atrial function can be summarized by the following observations:

- The Maze procedure rarely affects postoperative right atrial function. Right atrial recovery is often favorable, with post-Maze tricuspid inflow velocities comparable to healthy control subjects, highlighting the resilience of right atrial function postoperatively.

- Active left atrial contraction (pump phase) is somewhat diminished after the Maze procedure, particularly in patients with LSpAF. However, active left atrial contractile (pump) function is relatively unimportant as long as the RA is in synchrony with the right ventricle and the LV is normal (see Chapter 9). Left atrial pump function is more important in patients with reduced left ventricular ejection fraction or heart failure with preserved ejection fraction.
- Left atrial compliance (reservoir and conduit phases) may be slightly reduced after the Maze procedure but is vastly improved compared with the preoperative state during AF. This improvement underscores the value of restoring sinus rhythm because it normalizes atrial mechanics and enhances overall cardiac output despite minor reductions in compliance.
- Patients with no demonstrable left atrial reservoir function after a Maze procedure should be anticoagulated indefinitely even if the left atrial appendage has been successfully closed. The absence of left atrial mechanical contraction represents a significant thromboembolic risk, as demonstrated by studies linking reduced left atrial function and increased stroke risk.
- Evaluating right atrial strain, left atrial strain, and other echocardiographic parameters, such LA-FAC, provides insights into baseline atrial mechanics. These assessments are particularly relevant for patients with preexisting conditions such as pulmonary hypertension, hypertrophic cardiomyopathy, or valvular heart disease, in whom tailored lesion sets (e.g., left atrial versus biatrial) may optimize functional recovery and minimize recurrence of AF.

REFERENCES

1. Disertorei M, Franzosi MG, Barlera S, et al. Thromboembolic event rate in paroxysmal and persistent atrial fibrillation: data from the GISSI-AF trial. *BMC Cardiovasc Disord*. 2013;13:28.
2. Khan HR, Yakupoglu HY, Kralj-Hans I, et al. Left atrial function predicts atrial arrhythmia recurrence following ablation of long-standing persistent atrial fibrillation. *Circ Cardiovasc Imaging*. 2023;16(6):e015352.
3. Feinberg MS, Waggoner AD, Kater KM, Cox JL, Lindsay BD, Perez JE. Restoration of atrial function after the Maze procedure for patients with atrial fibrillation. Assessment by Doppler echocardiography. *Circulation*. 1994;90(5) II285-92.
4. Albirini A, Scalia GM, Murray RD, et al. Left and right atrial transport function after the Maze procedure for atrial fibrillation: an echocardiographic Doppler follow-up study. *J Am Soc Echocardiol*. 1997;10(9):937–945.
5. Voeller RK, Zierer A, Lall SC, et al. The effects off the Cox Maze procedure on atrial function. *J Thorac Cardiovasc Surg*. 2008;136(5):1257–1264.
6. Yamanaka K, Fujita M, Doi K, et al. Multislice computed tomography accurately quantifies left atrial size and function after the MAZE procedure. *Circulation*. 2006;114:15–19.
7. Buber J, Luria D, Sternik L, et al. Left atrial contractile function following a successful modified Maze procedure at surgery and the risk for subsequent thromboembolic stroke. *J Am Coll Cardiol*. 2011;58(15):1614–1621.
8. Kim JB, Yang DH, Kang J-W, et al. Left atrial function following surgical ablation of atrial fibrillation: prospective evaluation using dual-source cardiac computed tomography. *Yonsei Med J*. 2015;56(3):608–616.
9. Leischik R, Littwitz H, Dworrak B, et al. Echocardiographic evaluation of left atrial mechanics: function, history, novel techniques, advantages, and pitfalls. *Biomed Res Int*. 2015;2015:765921.
10. Kislitsina ON, Cox JL, Shah SJ, et al. Preoperative left atrial strain abnormalities are associated with the development of postoperative atrial fibrillation following isolated coronary artery bypass surgery. *J Thorac Cardiovasc Surg*. 2022;164(3):917–924.
11. Kislitsina O, Rigolin V, Thomas J, et al. Failure of the surgical ablation of paroxysmal atrial fibrillation: the importance of preoperative left atrial and right atrial function estimated by conventional and speckle-tracking echocardiography. *J Am Coll Cardiol*. 2022;79(9_Supplement)):74.
12. Nitta T, Ishii Y, Fujii M, et al. Restoration of sinus rhythm and atrial transport function after the Maze procedure: u lesion set versus box lesion set. *J Thorac Cardiovasc Surg*. 2016;151(4):1062–1069.
13. Lönnerholm S, Blomström P, Nilsson L, et al. Long-term effects of the Maze procedure on atrial size and mechanical function. *Ann Thorac Surg*. 2016;85:916–920.
14. Buber J, Luria D, Sternik L, et al. Left atrial contractile function following a successful modified Maze procedure at surgery and the risk for subsequent thromboembolic stroke. *J Am Coll Cardiol*. 2011;58:1614–1621.
15. Prasad SM, Maniar HS, Camillo CJ, et al. The cox Maze iii procedure for atrial fibrillation: long-term efficacy in patients undergoing lone versus concomitant procedures. *J Thorac Cardiovasc Surg*. 2003;126(6):1822–1827.
16. Weimar T, Schena S, Bailey MS, et al. The Cox-Maze procedure for lone atrial fibrillation: a single-center experience over 2 decades. *Circ Arrhythm Electrophysiol*. 2012;5(1):8–14.
17. Baalman SWE, van den Berg NWE, Neefs J, et al. Left atrial strain and recurrence of atrial fibrillation after thoracoscopic surgical ablation: a subanalysis of the AFACT study. *Int J Cardiovasc Imaging*. 2022;38(12):2615–2624.
18. Kislitsina ON, Jankowski M, Rigolin V H, et al. The impact of preoperative four-chamber strain on failure of the Maze IV procedure for atrial fibrillation: insights from conventional and speckle-tracking echocardiography. *Eur Heart J*. 2024;45(Supplement 1) ehae666.041.
19. Anselmino M, Rovera C, Marchetto G, et al. Left atrial function after atrial fibrillation cryoablation concomitant to minimally invasive mitral valve repair: a pilot study on long-term results and clinical implications. *Medicina*. 2019;55:709.
20. Kanagala P, Arnold JR, Cheng ASH, et al. Left atrial ejection fraction and outcomes in heart failure with preserved ejection fraction. *Int J Cardiovasc Imaging*. 2020;36(1):101–110.

23

Prevalence of Atrial Fibrillation Before Cardiac Surgery and the Benefits of Concomitant Ablation

Patrick M. McCarthy

CHAPTER OUTLINE

It is common for cardiac surgeons to encounter patients with a history of atrial fibrillation (AF) before undergoing other cardiac operations.[1–3] Originally, the Cox-Maze operations were performed on patients with stand-alone AF (i.e., patients with no known structural heart disease warranting cardiac surgery). After the procedure was established as safe and effective, we added it in patients with AF undergoing mitral valve (MV) repair.[4] AF predisposes patients to stroke, reduces survival and quality of life, and reduces the need for lifelong anticoagulation.[5] Adding a Maze operation to correct the arrhythmia, reduce AF-related complications and mortality, and reduce or eliminate the need for medications and anticoagulants was a logical next step when patients with AF needed cardiac surgery.

Small randomized clinical trials (RCTs) of the early efficacy of the Maze procedure were performed in the most common concomitant operation, MV surgery, to demonstrate the reduction of AF in treated patients versus untreated patients (Table 23.1). There were no randomized clinical trials performed to demonstrate the *late* effectiveness of adding a Maze procedure to other cardiac operations. They were not powered with enough patients or followed long enough to evaluate the important late clinical outcomes such as survival and freedom from stroke. Therefore, it took years and extensive database studies using propensity-matched studies to compile the evidence demonstrating the clinical benefit of adding a Maze procedure to other cardiac operations. This chapter reviews the current data of the combined operations

TABLE 23.1 Randomized Controlled Trials on the Early Efficacy of the Maze Procedure in Ablating Atrial Fibrillation

Reference (Year)	Patients (*n*)	Energy Source	Follow-up NSR in the No-Maze Group (%)	Follow-up NSR in the Maze Group (%)	*P* Value
Deneke et al.[50]	30	Unipolar cooled RF	26.7	80.0	<.01
Schuetz et al.[51]	43	Microwave	33.3	80.0	.036
Akpinar et al.[52]	67	Unipolar RF	9.4	93.6	.0001
Abreu Filho et al.[53]	70	Unipolar cooled RF	26.9	79.4	.001
Doukas et al.[54]	101	Unipolar RF	4.5	44.4	.001
Blomström-Lundqvist et al.[55]	69	Cryoablation	42.9	73.3	.013
Chevalier et al.[56]	43	Unipolar RF	4.0	57.0	.004
Gillinov et al.[26]	260	Unipolar RF, bipolar RF, cryoablation	29.0	63.2	.001

NSR, Normal sinus rhythm; *RF*, radiofrequency.

which serves as the basis for the Class I guideline recommendations from the Society of Thoracic Surgeons (STS) and European Association for Cardio-Thoracic Surgery (EACTS).[5-7]

PREVALENCE OF PREOPERATIVE ATRIAL FIBRILLATION IN CARDIAC SURGERY PATIENTS

Mitral Valve Procedures

Both mitral regurgitation and mitral stenosis are associated with left atrial pressure and volume overload, and both cause significant left atrial dilatation. Therefore, these patients are more prone to develop AF as the mitral valve disease progresses. For many years, if AF and mitral valve disease were clinically well tolerated, surgery was deferred until symptoms developed. In these patients, it was difficult to discern whether the dyspnea and fatigue were related to the AF or to the underlying mitral valve disease. Patients were often prescribed long-term diuretics and anticoagulants for AF until surgery was finally considered. In the interval, left ventricular dysfunction, pulmonary hypertension, and secondary (functional) tricuspid regurgitation associated with significant right atrial dilatation frequently developed. Preoperative sinus node dysfunction was not tested because the patient was in continuous AF but after surgery, sinus node dysfunction was often evident, requiring a permanent pacemaker implantation. MV surgery, with or without AF ablation, was considered high risk, and cardiac dysfunction may already have become irreversible. In a "Catch-22" mind-set, cardiologists were reluctant to refer patients for high-risk surgery, and the cycle continued with late referrals. Today, decades later, with more routine MV repair with concomitant AF surgery, the pattern has been broken, and asymptomatic patients with or without AF are commonly referred for surgery before left ventricular dysfunction and right heart changes occur.[8] Many patients now undergo surgery before they have developed AF,[9] but practices vary considerably across the world and depend on the patient's comorbidities and age.

In a study of Medicare-age patients, we found the prevalence of AF before cardiac surgery to be higher than previously reported.[2] In our study, up to 62% of patients in some subsets of MV surgery were found to have preoperative AF, and it varied by procedure between 45% and 62% of all MV operations (Fig. 23.1). This study may be the most accurate accounting of preoperative AF because it investigated Medicare records for 3 years in advance of surgery. The primary study evaluating this issue that was based on the STS database[10] showed a lower occurrence of preoperative AF in MV operations (34.4%; 30,011 of 87,214 patients). However, the STS database includes younger patients who are at a lower risk for AF, and it does not always capture paroxysmal AF (PAF) or AF that was not present on preoperative admission.[3] However, all database studies show that the prevalence of preoperative AF is higher in MV operations than in non-MV operations (Table 23.2).

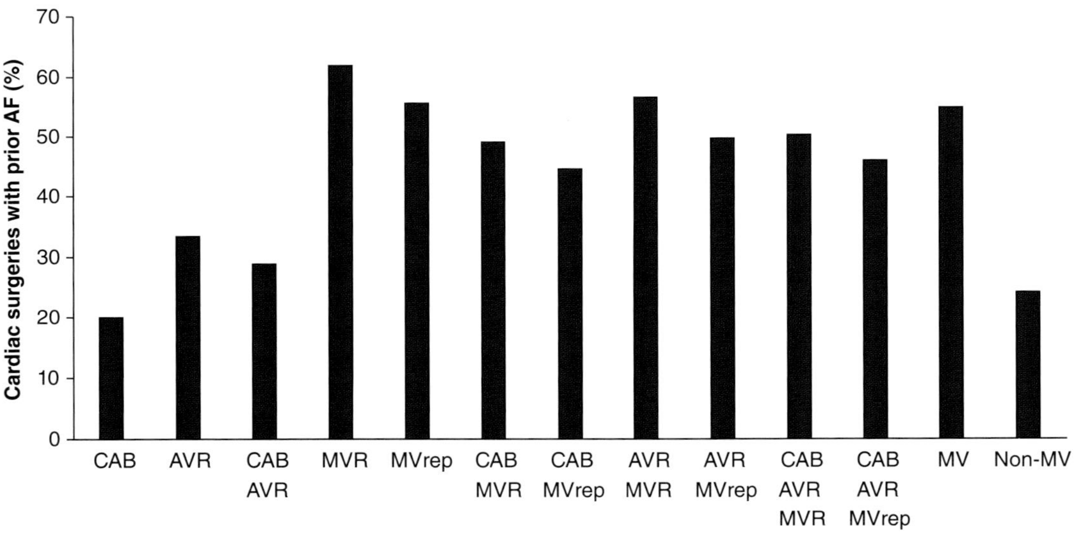

Fig. 23.1 Prevalence of preoperative atrial fibrillation (AF) in patients undergoing different cardiac procedures using a Medicare database. These numbers reflect an older population than Society of Thoracic Surgeons database reports and therefore, a higher prevalence of preoperative AF than previously reported. Preoperative AF was twice as common in mitral procedures as in non-mitral operations. *AVR,* Aortic valve replacement; *CAB,* coronary artery bypass; *MV,* mitral valve; *MVR,* mitral valve replacement; *MVrep,* mitral valve repair. (Reproduced from McCarthy PM, Davidson CJ, Kruse J, et al. Prevalence of atrial fibrillation before cardiac surgery and factors associated with concomitant ablation. *J Thorac Cardiovasc Surg.* 2020;159(6):2245–2253.)

TABLE 23.2 Prevalence of preoperative AF in Mitral Valve Operations Compared to Non-Mitral Valve Operations

Surgery Type	STS Prevalence (%)	Patients (*n*)	Medicare Prevalence (%)	Patients (*n*)
Mitral valve	34.4	87,214	61.8	5977
Aortic valve	17.8	87,426	33.4	8844
Coronary artery bypass	10.3	361,138	20.1	10,575

STS, Society of Thoracic Surgeons.

Non–Mitral Valve Procedures

Left atrial pressure, volume, and enlargement are generally much lower in patients undergoing coronary artery bypass grafting (CABG) and aortic valve replacement (AVR) than in mitral valve (MV) patients. The cause-and-effect relationship of AF to coronary artery disease or aortic valve disease may not be as apparent in non-MV structural heart disease except in patients with heart failure and reduced left ventricular function who often have a dilated left atrium (LA). Also, patients with coronary artery disease and aortic valve stenosis may be older, which is another risk factor for AF. In the Medicare study mentioned earlier, using 3 years of medical record searches before surgery, the prevalence of preoperative AF was almost twice as high as it was in the STS studies (Fig 23.1). CABG patients had a 20.1% prevalence of preoperative AF and AVR patients had a 33.4% prevalence in the Medicare study.[2] In the STS database, preoperative AF was recorded in 10.3% of 361,138 patients undergoing CABG[11] and in 17.8% of 87,426 patients undergoing AVR.[12] These reports showed the prevalence of preoperative AF recorded in the STS database to be approximately one-half of the prevalence recorded in the older Medicare patients.

Unfortunately, any type of concomitant surgical ablation for AF, including the least complex pulmonary vein isolation, was not common. In Medicare patients, surgical ablation was performed in only 22.2% overall and was highest for MV surgery patients (37.6%) compared with non-MV surgery patients (16.2%) (Fig. 23.2).[2] In comparison, MV surgery was performed in 25% of the STS population with AF (n = 86,941) and in these patients AF was ablated in 68.4%.[3] In 34,600 CABG patients with preoperative AF in the STS database, concomitant AF ablation was performed in 30.5%.[13] For AVR patients, concomitant ablation was performed in 33.1% of 15,596 patients.[12]

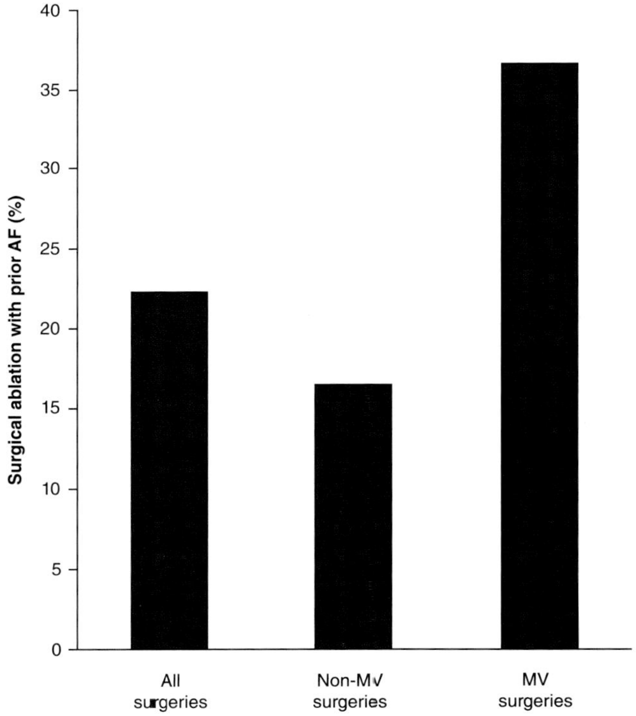

Fig. 23.2 Overall, concomitant surgical atrial fibrillation (AF) ablation was performed in 22.2% of patients with preoperative AF. Patients with mitral valve surgery had the highest AF treatment (37.6%) compared with nonmitral valve surgery (16.2%). *MV,* Mitral valve. (Reproduced from McCarthy PM, Davidson CJ, Kruse J, et al. Prevalence of atrial fibrillation before cardiac surgery and factors associated with concomitant ablation. *J Thorac Cardiovasc Surg.* 2020;159(6):2245–2253.)

The STS published guidelines supporting concomitant surgical AF ablation in 2017.[14] Following a study of concomitant surgical ablation in Florida and Maryland from 2016 to 2017, there was an increase in surgical ablation, but it was only from 2.1% to 17.4% (P <.001).[15] Concomitant surgical ablation for mitral surgery, and non-mitral surgery, now have Class I indications in the 2023 STS guidelines, and the benefits of surgical ablation are made clear.[16] Our hope is that with the new guidelines, wider education of surgeons and cardiologists regarding the data supporting safety and effectiveness, and publications such as this textbook, concomitant AF ablation will increase significantly.

BENEFITS OF THE CONCOMITANT ABLATION OF ATRIAL FIBRILLATION

Surgeons always need to balance the risks and benefits of surgery, and it is no different regarding the choice of performing concomitant AF ablation or ignoring the AF and allowing it to continue after surgery. Practically speaking, the decision depends on patient factors, the surgeon's experience, and the complexity of the ablation procedure to be used.[17] It was demonstrated years ago in large propensity-matched studies that patients with preoperative AF have significantly reduced survival times compared to patients with no preoperative AF (Fig. 23.3).[18–21] This was not surprising considering that in medical studies, we knew patients with AF have reduced survival and a significant risk for massive disabling or fatal strokes. The goal of concomitant AF surgical ablation should be to minimize any risk using an effective operation that has significant long-term benefits for the patient.

Thirty-Day Operative Mortality and Morbidity Rates

There have been multiple studies over the past several years demonstrating the safety of adding a Cox-Maze procedure to ablate AF concomitantly in patients undergoing coronary artery bypass graft (CABG) and/or valve surgery. Ad et al.[22] first showed in 2012 that adding a Cox-Maze-III procedure to isolated CABG or AVR procedures did not increase major morbidity or operative mortality rates. Al-Atassi et al.[23] confirmed in 2017 that "patients undergoing isolated CABG, AVR, or combined CABG and AVR with a history of AF can undergo concomitant AF ablation without increased surgical risk." These were particularly interesting studies because the LA had to be opened to perform the Cox-Maze-III procedure, which obviously is not normally required for either CABG or AVR. Damiano's group[24] in St. Louis first showed

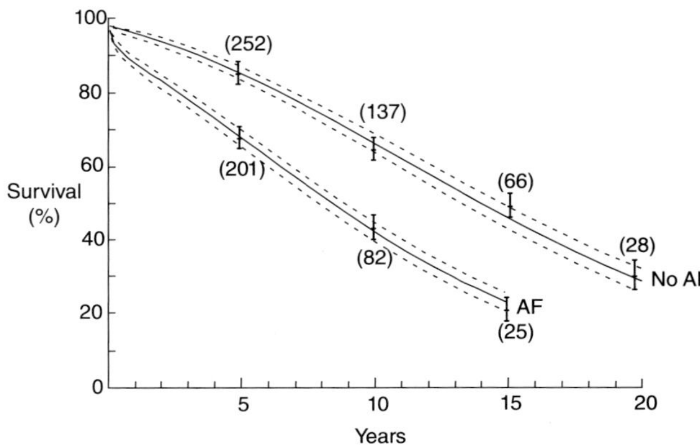

Fig. 23.3 Preoperative atrial fibrillation (AF) has long been shown to reduce survival compared with patients without preoperative AF over many years of follow-up. (Reproduced from Quader MA, McCarthy PM, Gillinov AM, et al. Does preoperative atrial fibrillation reduce survival after coronary artery bypass grafting? *Ann Thorac Surg.* 2004;77(5):1514–1522; discussion 1522–1524.)

in 2013 that adding a Cox-Maze-IV procedure to MV surgery "*did not* significantly affect the procedural mortality."

A propensity score-matched STS study by Badhwar et al.[3] in 2017 demonstrated that concomitant surgical ablation by a variety of ablation techniques resulted in an actual *reduction* in 30-day mortality rate (by 8%) and perioperative stroke rate (by 16%). In addition, a study by the Nationwide Inpatient Database also showed a reduction in operative mortality rate when concomitant AF was surgically ablated (3.6% treated vs 4.2% untreated; P <.001) and stroke (2.0% vs. 2.8%; P <.001).[25] Both of the latter were large studies of approximately 50,000 patients each. The STS CABG and AVR studies did not show any 30-day differences except for an increase in postoperative pacemaker requirements in the AF ablated AVR patients (6.8% vs 5.0; P <.001). Finally, these studies provided a major stimulus for the 2017 STS Guideline Committee to grant Class 1 recommendations for the concomitant surgical ablation of AF during MV surgery, CABG, AVR, and CABG plus AVR.[14]

Reduction in Atrial Fibrillation in Randomized Clinical Trials

The Cox-Maze procedure gradually evolved from "cut and sew" in the 1990s to the use of cryoablation, unipolar radiofrequency (RF) ablation, and eventually bipolar RF ablation beginning about 2000. With the advent of these new ablation tools, more surgeons adopted concomitant surgical ablation of AF, so more studies were performed to demonstrate the reduction in AF after surgical ablation (see Table 23.1). By current standards, the trials were not robust but nevertheless, using a variety of technologies and lesion sets and with variable types and duration of AF monitoring after the procedure, all of the initial RCTs demonstrated a higher freedom from AF in the surgical ablation groups. Also, there were no increased perioperative complications in these smaller series, until the cardiothoracic surgery network (CTS Net) trial published in 2015 showed a much higher requirement for new pacemakers in ablated patients than in nonablated patients (21.5% vs. 8.1% per 100 patient years; P = .01)[26] (see Chapter 21). It is well recognized and universally accepted that surgical ablation effectively treats patients with AF, but it took more time and larger studies with longer follow-up periods to demonstrate a clinical benefit. Also, there were various technologies, lesion sets, and patient populations used in the RCTs, which confounded the ability to judge clinical benefits.

Reduction in Long-Term Stroke

An issue of *Seminars in Thoracic and Cardiovascular Surgery* in 2000 convened a group of large-volume "cut-and-sew" Maze procedure patients reported from many centers, with a mix of concomitant and isolated Maze procedures.[27–29] The late stroke rate was very low, and for instance, at Washington University in St. Louis, the freedom from stroke after the concomitant ablation of AF with a Cox-Maze-III procedure was 99.6% at 11.5 years (Fig. 23.4).[30] Left atrial appendage occlusion (LAAO), or excision or exclusion, is an integral part of all iterations of the Maze procedure. Subsequent database studies showed a reduction in late stroke for patients with LAAO and a history of AF compared with those with no treatment.[31]

The definitive study proving that LAAO reduced the incidence of stroke in patients with preoperative AF was the LAAOS III trial. It showed that LAAO resulted in a 33% reduction in stroke over a mean follow-up period of 3.8 years in a study population of 2379 patients (Fig. 23.5).[32] More recently, a study by Mehaffey et al.[33] has shown that

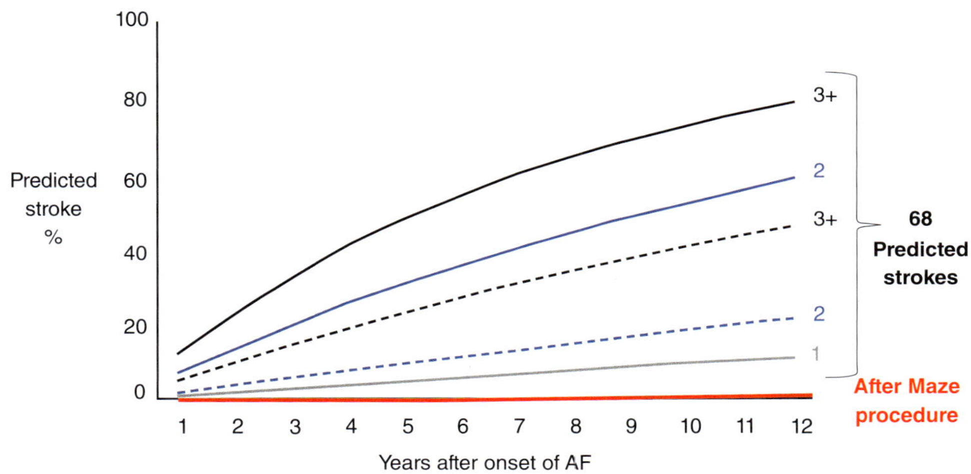

Fig. 23.4 Patients in atrial fibrillation (AF) needing surgical ablation who presented to Washington University in St. Louis had known risks for a future stroke based on what is now called the CHA_2DS_2-VASc scores. The *solid black line* represents the 12-year risk of a thromboembolic stroke in those patients with a score greater than 3 who were not anticoagulated, and the *dashed black line* shows the stroke risk after anticoagulating those patients with warfarin for 12 years. The *solid blue line* represents the 12-year risk of a thromboembolic stroke in patients with a score greater than 2 who were not anticoagulated, and the *dashed blue line* shows the stroke risk after anticoagulating those patients with warfarin for 12 years. The *solid gray line* represents the 12-year risk of a thromboembolic stroke in patients with a score greater than 1 who were not anticoagulated. This curve is essentially the same for anticoagulated patients if hemorrhagic strokes are included. By observing these known risks and calculating the number of strokes to be projected over 12 years, the entire group of patients would be projected to have a total of 68 thromboembolic strokes over the next 12 years if they were not treated with a Maze procedure. The *lower red line* is the actual number of thromboembolic strokes (one mild stroke) that occurred in this entire group of patients over the 12 years after a Cox-Maze-III procedure for AF. (Modified from Cox JL, Ad N, Palazzo T. Impact of the Maze procedure on the stroke rate in patients with atrial fibrillation. *J Thorac Cardiovasc Surg*. 1999;118(5):833–840.)

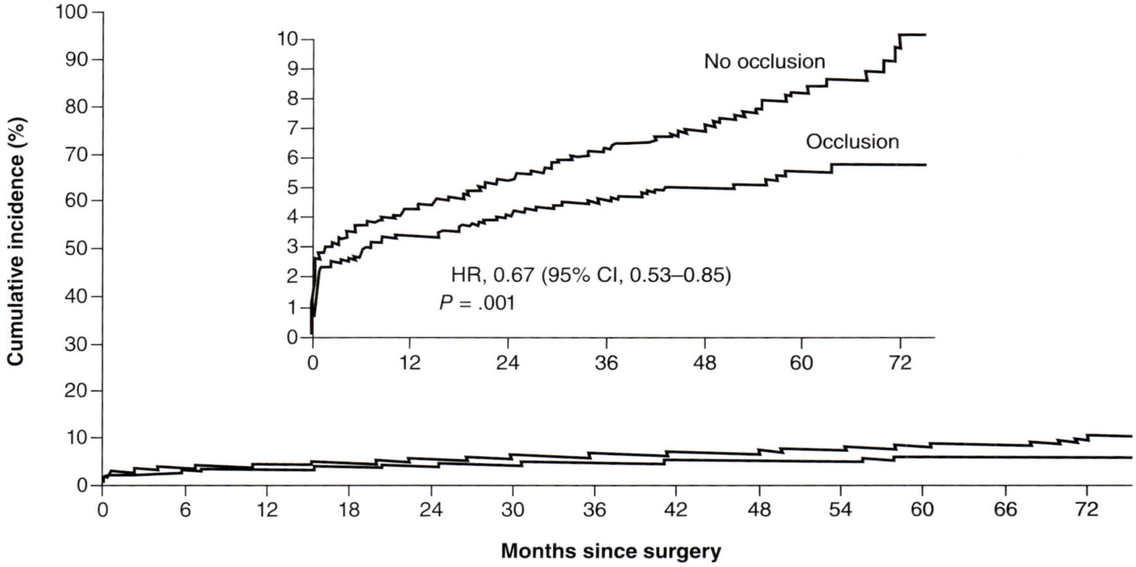

No. at risk													
No occlusion	2391	2134	2081	2030	1981	1897	1607	1291	1016	751	540	348	205
Occlusion	2379	2163	2105	2059	2020	1948	1642	1322	1046	781	550	349	199

Fig. 23.5 Results of the left atrial appendage occlusion study (LAAOS) III trial show a lower risk of stroke or systemic embolism in patients who had cardiac surgery treated with ongoing antithrombic therapy and left atrial appendage closure compared to those without it. *CI*, Confidence interval; *HR*, hazard ratio. (Reproduced from Whitlock RP, Belley-Cote EP, Paparella D, et al. Left atrial appendage occlusion during cardiac surgery to prevent stroke. *N Eng J Med.* 2021;384(22):2081–2091.)

ablation *and* LAAO are the ideal treatment for patients with concomitant AF in terms of stroke risk benefit with the highest survival rates identified in patients with both treatments (Fig. 23.6).

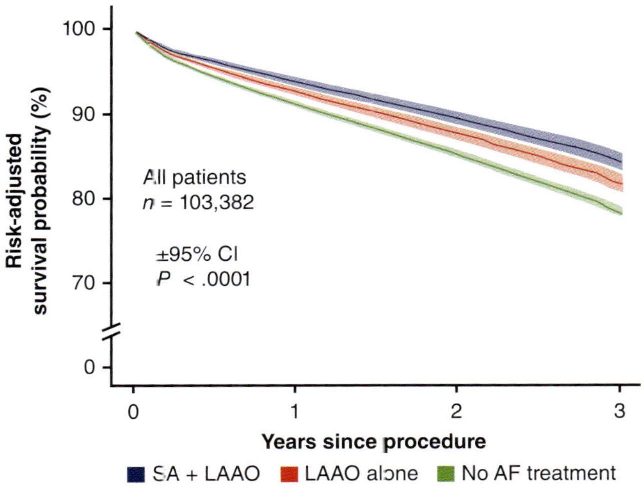

Fig. 23.6 Results of a study evaluating surgical ablation (SA) and left atrial appendage occlusion (LAAO) showed the highest survival compared with LAAO alone or no atrial fibrillation (AF) treatment. The curves steadily diverge over 3 years of follow-up. *CI*, Confidence interval. (Reproduced from Mehaffey JH, Hayanga JWA, Wei L, Mascio C, Rankin JS, Badhwar V. Surgical ablation of atrial fibrillation is associated with improved survival compared with appendage obliteration alone: an analysis of 100,000 Medicare beneficiaries. *J Thorac Cardiovasc Surg.* 2024;168(1):104–116.)

Improved Late Survival

The recent surgical society guidelines from STS and EACTS[7,14] review the literature extensively regarding the most critical issue: does concomitant surgical ablation of AF reduce the long-term mortality rate after cardiac surgery? An entire review of these data is beyond the scope of this chapter. The most convincing data come from large database studies that use propensity score matching to balance the comorbidities, age, and other demographic parameters of concomitant AF patients and those with no history of AF.

The benefits of surgical ablation and LAAO become more evident over time. An STS database study compared the outcomes of three groups: (1) patients with AF with no treatment, (2) patients with AF who received LAAO alone, (3) patients with AF who received both surgical ablation and LAAO. These curves steadily diverge over time (see Fig. 23.6).[33] The same was true for CABG patients in the study by Malaisrie et al.[13] that included a landmark analysis at 2 years (Fig. 23.7). Also, this difference was significant for patients with PAF (Fig. 23.8).[34] Although the STS propensity-matched studies are the largest and most influential, there have been other important studies from outside the United States using large databases, including from South Korea (Fig. 23.9)[35] and Poland, reporting data from the KROK (Polish National Registry of Cardiac Surgery Procedures) Registry (Fig. 23.10).[36] The KROK registry found that the greatest mortality reduction was associated with surgical ablation with LAAO, followed by surgical ablation alone and LAAO alone (log-rank $P < .001$).

Single-center and multi-center studies showed similar findings, including the first papers in 2012 and 2013 from our group demonstrating improved survival after concomitant AF ablation (Fig. 23.11).[37] Patients with PAF who were treated surgically had the same survival rates as

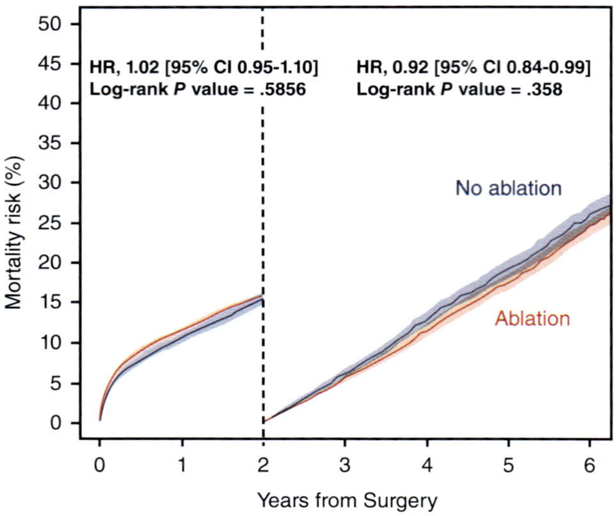

Numbers at risk: matched

No ablation	9771	7754	6452	5088	3722	2516	1529
Ablation	9771	7565	6240	5040	3822	2678	1606

Fig. 23.7 Data from a Medicare-linked Society of Thoracic Surgeons database study examining outcomes in coronary arty bypass patients with preoperative atrial fibrillation (AF). Landmark analysis in matched patients found a lower mortality rate from 2 to 5 years in those who had AF ablation compared with those who did not. *CI,* Confidence interval; *HR,* hazard ratio. (Reproduced from Malaisrie SC, McCarthy PM, Kruse J, et al. Ablation of atrial fibrillation during coronary artery bypass grafting: late outcomes in a Medicare population. *J Thorac Cardiovasc Surg.* 2021;161(4):1251–1261.)

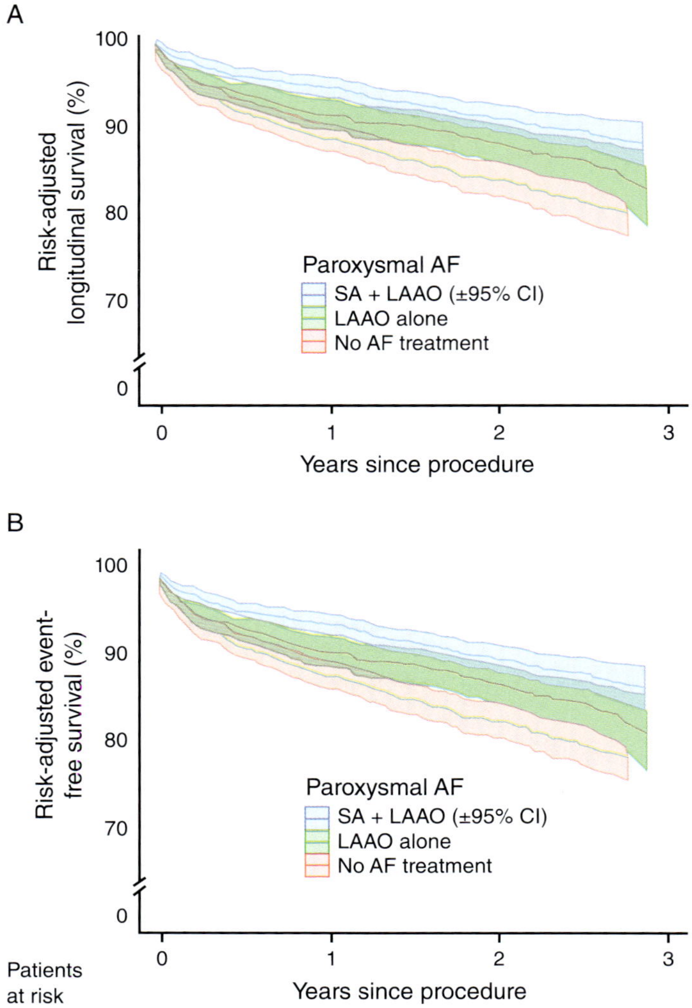

Patients at risk	0	1	2	3
SA + LAAO	2243	1522	789	232
LAAO alone	1342	897	476	87
No AF Tx	2055	1493	873	200

Fig. 23.8 In a study of Medicare beneficiaries with paroxysmal atrial fibrillation (AF) undergoing mitral valve surgery, the 3-year survival rate (A) and freedom from stroke or death (B) were significantly lower in those with no treatment compared with those with surgery plus left atrial appendage occlusion (LAAO). *CI,* Confidence interval; *SA,* surgical ablation; *Tx,* treatment. (Reproduced from Darehzereshki A, Mehaffey JH, Hayanga JWA, et al. Concomitant surgical ablation in paroxysmal vs persistent atrial fibrillation during mitral surgery. *Ann Thorac Surg.* 2025;119(2):389–397.)

patients who had no AF, including in patients with PAF (Fig. 23.12).[38] Improved survival rates for AF ablated patients was also reported from Washington University (Fig. 23.13A)[39] and from the multicenter Northern New England Cardiovascular Disease Study Group (Fig. 23.13B).[40] These findings influenced us such that all Northwestern patients with AF are considered for concomitant ablation (see Chapter 15).[17,41] Interestingly, the Northwestern University study showed more benefit for patients with successful ablation ($P = .03$) than for patients who failed to return to sinus rhythm (Fig. 23.14).[37] These granular-level data highlight a limitation of registry data because late freedom from AF cannot be ascertained from registry studies. It points out the importance of achieving a high efficacy of ablation and not just doing a minimal ablation or using a non-transmural technology or technique.

Other Benefits of Surgical Atrial Fibrillation Ablation

Like catheter ablation studies, surgical ablation has been associated with improved left ventricular ejection (LVEF) fraction in patients with preoperative left ventricular dysfunction and tachycardia-mediated cardiomyopathy. Restoration of sinus rhythm and normalization of LVEF were demonstrated after stand-alone AF surgery in patients who had failed other therapies to control AF.[42,43] We believe some of these "tachycardia-mediated" cardiomyopathy patients may have an unrecognized underlying genetic cardiomyopathy.[44]

Quality-of-life (QoL) studies are difficult to interpret for patients undergoing concomitant AF surgery because QoL typically improves from the underlying cardiac operation itself in AF treated groups.[45] A pilot study in 2000 from the Netherlands showed marked improvement in QoL after surgery for lone PAF.[46] However, this group reported an early randomized trial in 2003 studying patients with AF undergoing MV surgery with and without AF surgery. Improved QoL did not differ between groups.[47] A meta-analysis reviewing outcomes of both concomitant and stand-alone surgery for AF found significant improvement in QoL for those who were in sinus rhythm at 1 year.[48] A Swedish study for lone patients with AF undergoing the Cox-Maze-III procedure showed postoperative QoL scores improved to the level of the general population and were sustained through 35 months of follow-up.[49]

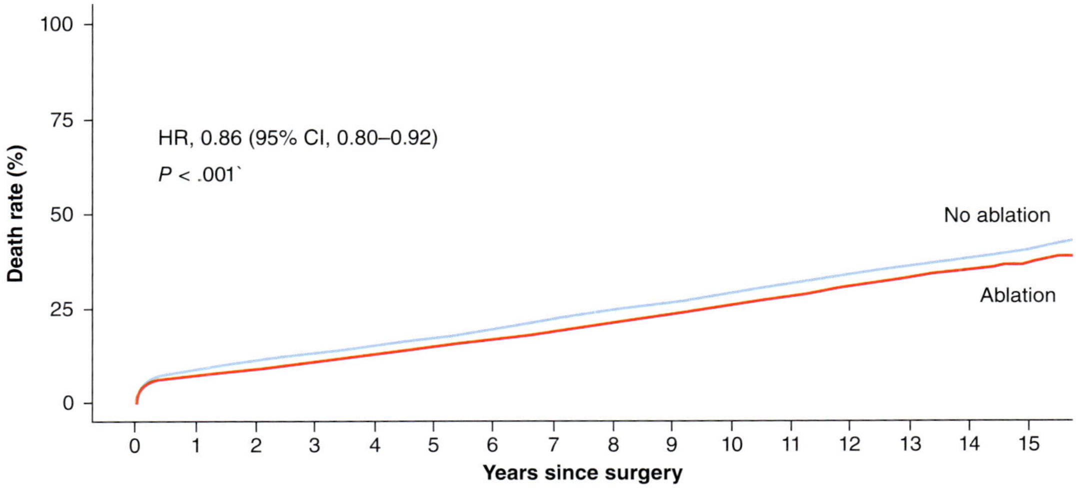

Fig. 23.9 This study from South Korea shows only a small difference in the 15-year survival rates for patients undergoing concomitant atrial fibrillation ablation at the time of cardiac surgery. *CI,* Confidence interval; *HR,* hazard ratio. (Reproduced from Kim HJ, Kim YJ, Kim M, et al. Surgical ablation for atrial fibrillation during aortic and mitral valve surgery: a nationwide population-based cohort study. *J Thorac Cardiovasc Surg.* 2024;167(3):981–993.)

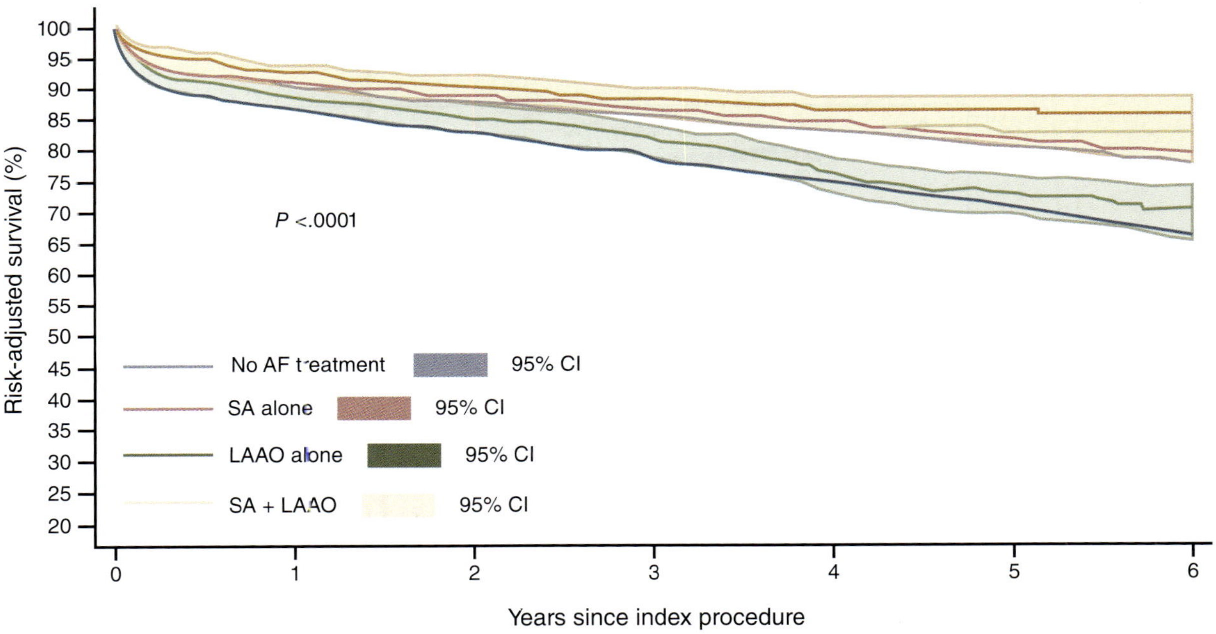

Fig. 23.10 This study from the Poland KROK (Polish National Registry of Cardiac Surgery Procedures) registry shows improved survival in patients treated with concomitant surgical ablation (SA). *AF,* Atrial fibrillation; *CI,* confidence interval; *LAAO,* left atrial appendage occlusion. (Reproduced from Pasierski M, Batko J, Kuzma L, et al. Surgical ablation, left atrial appendage occlusion or both? Nationwide registry analysis of cardiac surgery patients with underlying atrial fibrillation. *Eur J Cardiothorac Surg.* 2024;65(3):ezae014.)

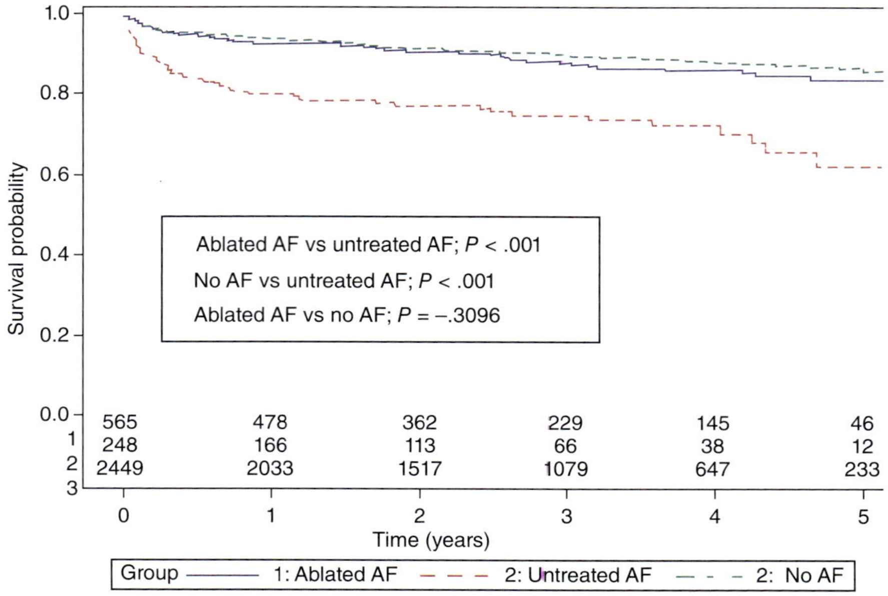

Fig. 23.11 Matched comparison of survival in patient receiving concomitant ablation for atrial fibrillation (AF) in patients without AF, in those surgically treated, and in those with AF who were untreated. The AF surgically treated patients' 5-year survival rate was the same as in patients who had never had AF, and both were markedly better than the untreated AF patient survival rates. (Reproduced from Lee R, McCarthy PM, Wang EC, et al. Midterm survival in patients treated for atrial fibrillation: a propensity-matched comparison to patients without a history of atrial fibrillation. *J Thorac Cardiovasc Surg.* 2012;143(6):1341–1351; discussion 1350.)

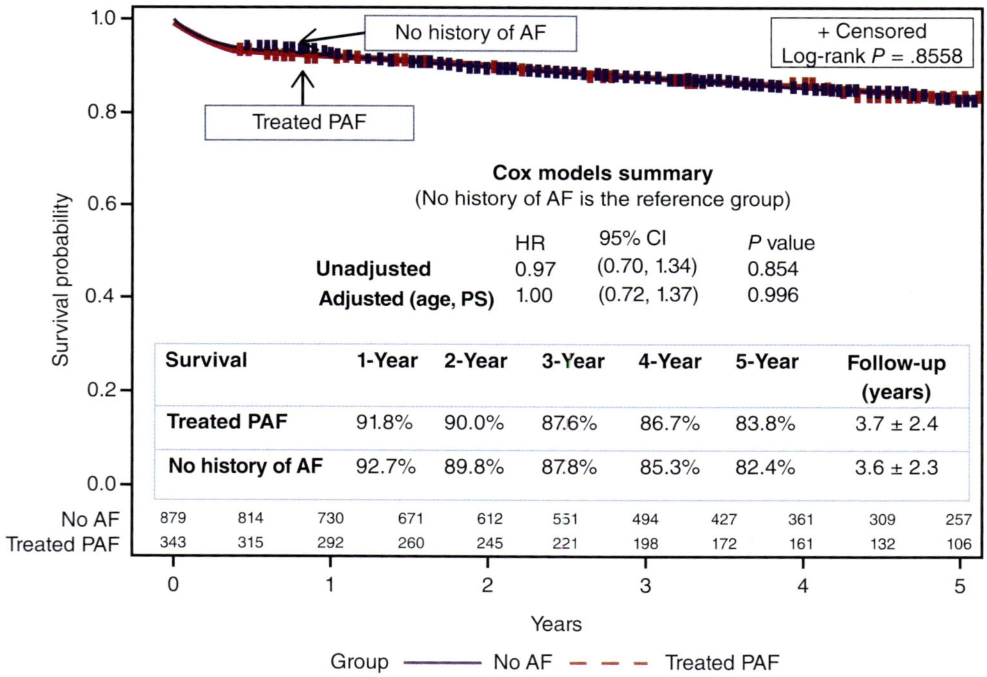

Fig. 23.12 Matched comparison of patients with treated paroxysmal atrial fibrillation (AF) and those with no history of AF showing similar survival rates. *CI,* Confidence interval; *HR,* hazard ratio; *PAF,* paroxysmal atrial fibrillation. (Reproduced from McCarthy PM, Manjunath A, Kruse J, et al. Should paroxysmal atrial fibrillation be treated during cardiac surgery? *J Thorac Cardiovasc Surg.* 2013;146(4):810–823.)

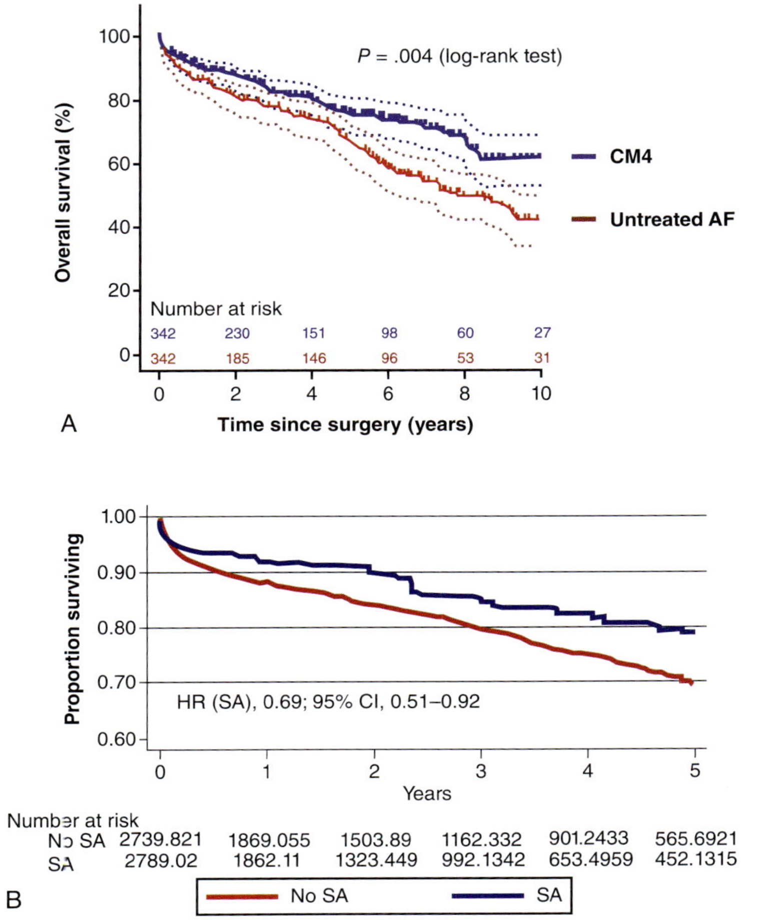

Fig. 23.13 (A) Washington University data reporting improved survival in patients with atrial fibrillation (AF) undergoing the Cox-Maze-IV procedure compared with no AF treatment. (B) Data from the Northern New England Cardiovascular Disease Study Group showing similar findings. *CI,* Confidence interval; *HR,* hazard ratio; *SA,* surgical ablation. (A reproduced from Musharbash FN, Schill MR, Sinn LA, et al. Performance of the Cox-Maze IV procedure is associated with improved long-term survival in patients with atrial fibrillation undergoing cardiac surgery. *J Thorac Cardiovasc Surg.* 2018;155(1):159–170. B reproduced from Iribarne A, DiScipio AW, McCullough JN, et al. Surgical atrial fibrillation ablation improves long-term survival: a multicenter analysis. *Ann Thorac Surg.* 2019;107(1):135–142.)

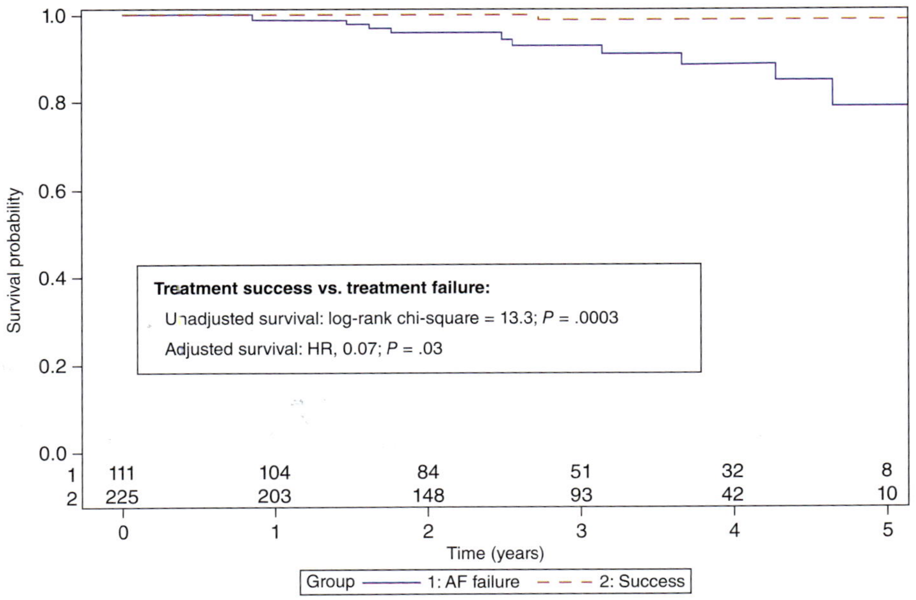

Fig. 23.14 A Northwestern study showed improved survival benefit in those with successful ablation compared with those who did not return to sinus rhythm. *AF,* Atrial fibrillation; *HR,* hazard ratio. (Reproduced from Lee R, McCarthy PM, Wang EC, et al. Midterm survival in patients treated for atrial fibrillation: a propensity-matched comparison to patients without a history of atrial fibrillation. *J Thorac Cardiovasc Surg.* 2012;143(6):1341–1351; discussion 1350.)

SUMMARY

There is now a large body of evidence from many sources across the globe documenting early and late benefits of combining surgical AF ablation with LAAO. The perioperative risks are low and predominantly reflect pacemaker use, which we believe can be minimized by avoiding the atrial pacemaker complex and performing the operation correctly (see Chapters 15 and 21). The data clearly support the Class I recommendations for both LAAO and concomitant AF ablation in most patients (see Chapter 24).

REFERENCES

1. Gammie JS, Haddad M, Milford-Beland S, et al. Atrial fibrillation correction surgery: lessons from the society of thoracic surgeons national cardiac database. *Ann Thorac Surg*. 2008;85(3):909–914.
2. McCarthy PM, Davidson CJ, Kruse J, et al. Prevalence of atrial fibrillation before cardiac surgery and factors associated with concomitant ablation. *J Thorac Cardiovasc Surg*. 2020;159(6):2245–2253.
3. Badhwar V, Rankin JS, Ad N, et al. Surgical ablation of atrial fibrillation in the United States: trends and propensity matched outcomes. *Ann Thorac Surg*. 2017;104(2):493–500.
4. McCarthy PM, Cosgrove 3rd DM, Castle LW, White RD, Klein AL. Combined treatment of mitral regurgitation and atrial fibrillation with valvuloplasty and the Maze procedure. *Am J Cardiol*. 1993;71(5):483–486.
5. Tanaka Y, Shah NS, Passman R, Greenland P, Lloyd-Jones DM, Khan SS. Trends in cardiovascular mortality related to atrial fibrillation in the United States, 2011 to 2018. *J Am Heart Assoc*. 2021;10(15):e020163.
6. Wyler von Ballmoos MC, Hui DS, Mehaffey JH, et al. The society of thoracic surgeons 2023 clinical practice guidelines for the surgical treatment of atrial fibrillation. *Ann Thorac Surg*. 2024. https://doi.org/10.1016/j.athoracsur.2024.01.007.
7. Van Gelder IC, Rienstra M, Bunting KV, et al. 2024 ESC guidelines for the management of atrial fibrillation developed in collaboration with the European Association for Cardio-Thoracic Surgery (EACTS). *Eur Heart J*. 2024;45(36):3314–3414.
8. Otto CM, Nishimura RA, Bonow RO, et al. 2020 ACC/AHA guideline for the management of patients with valvular heart disease: a report of the American College of Cardiology/American Heart Association Joint Committee on clinical practice guidelines. *Circulation*. 2021;143(5):e72–e227.
9. Desai A, Thomas JD, Bonow RO, et al. Asymptomatic degenerative mitral regurgitation repair: validating guidelines for early intervention. *J Thorac Cardiovasc Surg*. 2021;161(3):981–994.
10. Gammie JS, Chikwe J, Badhwar V, et al. Isolated mitral valve surgery: the Society of Thoracic Surgeons Adult Cardiac Surgery Database analysis. *Ann Thorac Surg*. 2018;106(3):716–727.
11. Malaisrie SC, McCarthy PM, Kruse J, et al. Burden of preoperative atrial fibrillation in patients undergoing coronary artery bypass grafting. *J Thorac Cardiovasc Surg*. 2018;155(6):2358–2367.
12. Churyla A, Andrei AC, Kruse J, et al. Safety of atrial fibrillation ablation with isolated surgical aortic valve replacement. *Ann Thorac Surg*. 2021;111(3):809–817.
13. Malaisrie SC, McCarthy PM, Kruse J, et al. Ablation of atrial fibrillation during coronary artery bypass grafting: late outcomes in a Medicare population. *J Thorac Cardiovasc Surg*. 2021;161(4):1251–1261.
14. Badhwar V, Rankin JS, Damiano RJ Jr, et al. The Society of Thoracic Surgeons 2017 clinical practice guidelines for the surgical treatment of atrial fibrillation. *Ann Thorac Surg*. 2017;103(1):329–341.
15. Jenkins HN, Weiss AJ, Maigrot JA, et al. Trends in surgical ablation at the time of cardiac surgery among patients with atrial fibrillation. *JTCVS Open*. 2023;16:333–341.
16. Joglar JA, Chung MK, Armbruster AL, et al. 2023 ACC/AHA/ACCP/HRS guideline for the diagnosis and management of atrial fibrillation: a report of the American College of Cardiology/American Heart Association Joint Committee on clinical practice guidelines. *Circulation*. 2024;149(1):e1–e156.
17. McCarthy PM, Cox JL. Practical approaches to concomitant surgical ablation of atrial fibrillation: matching the ablation to the patient. *J Thorac Cardiovasc Surg*. 2024. https://doi.org/10.1016/j.jtcvs.2024.03.023.
18. Ngaage DL, Schaff HV, Mullany CJ, et al. Does preoperative atrial fibrillation influence early and late outcomes of coronary artery bypass grafting? *J Thorac Cardiovasc Surg*. 2007;133(1):182–189.
19. Quader MA, McCarthy PM, Gillinov AM, et al. Does preoperative atrial fibrillation reduce survival after coronary artery bypass grafting? *Ann Thorac Surg*. 2004;77(5):1514–1522; discussion 1522-1524.
20. Ngaage DL, Schaff HV, Mullany CJ, et al. Influence of preoperative atrial fibrillation on late results of mitral repair: is concomitant ablation justified? *Ann Thorac Surg*. 2007;84(2):434–442; discussion 442-443.
21. Ngaage DL, Schaff HV, Barnes SA, et al. Prognostic implications of preoperative atrial fibrillation in patients undergoing aortic valve replacement: is there an argument for concomitant arrhythmia surgery? *Ann Thorac Surg*. 2006;82(4):1392–1399.
22. Ad N, Henry L, Hunt S, Holmes SD. Do we increase the operative risk by adding the Cox Maze III procedure to aortic valve replacement and coronary artery bypass surgery? *J Thorac Cardiovasc Surg*. 2012;143(4):936–944.
23. Al-Atassi T, Kimmaliardjuk D-M, Dagenais C, Bourke M, Lam B-K, Rubens FD. Should we ablate atrial fibrillation during coronary artery bypass grafting and aortic valve replacement? *Ann Thorac Surg*. 2017;104:515–522.
24. Saint LL, Damiano RJ Jr, Cuculich PS, et al. Incremental risk of the Cox-Maze IV procedure for patients with atrial fibrillation undergoing mitral valve surgery. *J Thorac Cardiovasc Surg*. 2013;146(5):1072–1077.
25. Elbadawi A, Elgendy IY, Mahmoud AH, et al. Outcomes of surgical ablation in patients with atrial fibrillation undergoing cardiac surgeries. *Ann Thorac Surg*. 2019;107(5):1395–1400.
26. Gillinov AM, Gelijns AC, Parides MK, et al. Surgical ablation of atrial fibrillation during mitral-valve surgery. *N Eng J Med*. 2015;372(15):1399–1409.
27. McCarthy PM, Gillinov AM, Castle L, Chung M, Cosgrove D 3rd. The Cox-Maze procedure: the Cleveland Clinic experience. *Sem Thorac Cardiovasc Surg*. 2000;12(1):25–29.
28. Schaff HV, Dearani JA, Daly RC, Orszulak TA, Danielson GK. Cox-Maze procedure for atrial fibrillation: mayo clinic experience. *Sem Thorac Cardiovasc Surg*. 2000;12(1):30–37.
29. Arcidi 3rd Jr, Doty DB, Millar RC. The Maze procedure: the LDS Hospital experience. *Sem Thorac Cardiovasc Surg*. 2000;12(1):38–43.
30. Cox JL, Ad N, Palazzo T. Impact of the Maze procedure on the stroke rate in patients with atrial fibrillation. *J Thorac Cardiovasc Surg*. 1999;118(5):833–840.

31. Friedman DJ, Piccini JP, Wang T, et al. Association between left atrial appendage occlusion and readmission for thromboembolism among patients with atrial fibrillation undergoing concomitant cardiac surgery. *J Am Med Assoc*. 2018;319(4):365–374.
32. Whitlock RP, Belley-Cote EP, Paparella D, et al. Left atrial appendage occlusion during cardiac surgery to prevent stroke. *N Eng J Med*. 2021;384(22):2081–2091.
33. Mehaffey JH, Hayanga JWA, Wei L, Mascio C, Rankin JS. Badhwar V: Surgical ablation of atrial fibrillation is associated with improved survival compared with appendage obliteration alone: an analysis of 100,000 Medicare beneficiaries. *J Thorac Cardiovasc Surg*. 2024;168(1):104–116.
34. Darehzereshki A, Mehaffey JH, Hayanga JWA, et al. Concomitant surgical ablation in paroxysmal vs persistent atrial fibrillation during mitral surgery. *Ann Thorac Surg*. 2024. https://doi.org/10.1016/j.athoracsur.2024.06.020.
35. Kim HJ, Kim YJ, Kim M, et al. Surgical ablation for atrial fibrillation during aortic and mitral valve surgery: a nationwide population-based cohort study. *J Thorac Cardiovasc Surg*. 2024;167(3):981–993.
36. Pasierski M, Batko J, Kuzma L, et al. Surgical ablation, left atrial appendage occlusion or both? Nationwide registry analysis of cardiac surgery patients with underlying atrial fibrillation. *Eur J Cardiothorac Surg*. 2024;65(3). https://doi.org/10.1093/ejcts/ezae014.
37. Lee R, McCarthy PM, Wang EC, et al. Midterm survival in patients treated for atrial fibrillation: a propensity-matched comparison to patients without a history of atrial fibrillation. *J Thorac Cardiovasc Surg*. 2012;143(6):1341–1351; discussion 1350.
38. McCarthy PM, Manjunath A, Kruse J, et al. Should paroxysmal atrial fibrillation be treated during cardiac surgery? *J Thorac Cardiovasc Surg*. 2013;146(4):810–823.
39. Musharbash FN, Schill MR, Sinn LA, et al. Performance of the Cox-Maze IV procedure is associated with improved long-term survival in patients with atrial fibrillation undergoing cardiac surgery. *J Thorac Cardiovasc Surg*. 2018;155(1):159–170.
40. Iribarne A, DiScipio AW, McCullough JN, et al. Surgical atrial fibrillation ablation improves long-term survival: a multicenter analysis. *Ann Thorac Surg*. 2019;107(1):135–142.
41. McCarthy PM, Cox JL, Kruse J, Elenbaas C, Andrei AC. One hundred percent utilization of a modified CryoMaze III procedure for atrial fibrillation with mitral surgery. *J Thorac Cardiovasc Surg*. 2024;167(4):1278–1289.
42. Pozzoli A, Taramasso M, Coppola G, et al. Maze surgery normalizes left ventricular function in patients with persistent lone atrial fibrillation. *Eur J Cardiothorac Surg*. 2014;46(5):871–876.
43. Adademir T, Khiabani AJ, Schill MR, et al. Surgical ablation of atrial fibrillation in patients with tachycardia-induced cardiomyopathy. *Ann Thorac Surg*. 2019;108(2):443–450.
44. Baman JR, Cox JL, McCarthy PM, et al. Atrial fibrillation and atrial cardiomyopathies. *J Cardiovas Electrophysiol*. 2021;32(10):2845–2853.
45. Chernyavskiy A, Kareva Y, Pak I, Rakhmonov S, Pokushalov E, Romanov A. Quality of life after surgical ablation of persistent atrial fibrillation: a prospective evaluation. *Heart, Lung Cir*. 2016;25(4):378–383.
46. Jessurun ER, van Hemel NM, Defauw JA, et al. Results of Maze surgery for lone paroxysmal atrial fibrillation. *Circulation*. 2000;101(13):1559–1567.
47. Jessurun ER, van Hemel NM, Defauw JJ, et al. A randomized study of combining Maze surgery for atrial fibrillation with mitral valve surgery. *J Cardiovasc Surg (Torino)*. 2003;44(1):9–18.
48. Maesen B, van der Heijden CAJ, Bidar E, Vos R, Athanasiou T, Maessen JG. Patient-reported quality of life after stand-alone and concomitant arrhythmia surgery: a systematic review and meta-analysis. *Interact Cardiovasc Thorac Surg*. 2022;34(3):339–348.
49. Lundberg C, Albage A, Carnlof C, Kenneback G. Long-term health-related quality of life after Maze surgery for atrial fibrillation. *Ann Thorac Surg*. 2008;86(6):1878–1882.
50. Deneke T, Khargi K, Grewe PH, et al. Efficacy of an additional MAZE procedure using cooled-tip radiofrequency ablation in patients with chronic atrial fibrillation and mitral valve disease. A randomized, prospective trial. *Eur Heart J*. 2002;23(7):558–566.
51. Schuetz A, Schulze CJ, Sarvanakis KK, et al. Surgical treatment of permanent atrial fibrillation using microwave energy ablation: a prospective randomized clinical trial. *Eur J Cardiothorac Surg*. 2003;24(4):475–480.
52. Akpinar B, Guden M, Sagbas E, et al. Combined radiofrequency modified maze and mitral valve procedure through a port access approach: early and mid-term results. *Eur J Cardiothorac Surg*. 2003;24(2):223–230.
53. Abreu Filho CA, Lisboa LA, Dallan LA, et al. Effectiveness of the maze procedure using cooled-tip radiofrequency ablation in patients with permanent atrial fibrillation and rheumatic mitral valve disease. *Circulation*. 2005;112(9 Suppl):I20–I25.
54. Carteaux Doukas G, Samani NJ, Alexiou C, et al. Left atrial radiofrequency ablation during mitral valve surgery for continuous atrial fibrillation: a randomized controlled trial. *JAMA*. 2005;294(18):2323–2329.
55. Blomström-Lundqvist C, Johansson B, Berglin E, et al. A randomized double-blind study of epicardial left atrial cryoablation for permanent atrial fibrillation in patients undergoing mitral valve surgery: the SWEDish Multicentre Atrial Fibrillation study (SWEDMAF). *Eur Heart J*. 2007;28(23):2902–2908.
56. Chevalier JP, Corbineau H, Caus T, et al. Left atrial radiofrequency ablation during mitral valve surgery: a prospective randomized multicentre study (SAFIR). *Arch Cardiovasc Dis*. 2009102(11):769–775.

24

Current American and European Guidelines for Atrial Fibrillation Surgery

Patrick M. McCarthy, Piotr Suwalski

CHAPTER OUTLINE

Society clinical practice guidelines have significant potential to change clinical practice (Fig. 24.1).[1] They are authored by experts in the field and undergo a rigorous development and review process to reach consensus, ideally reflecting the best and most recent information used to shape clinical practice.[2] Guidelines are summarized in a concise format, with extensive supporting references, and are presented in a way that makes them easily accessible for busy clinicians. They focus on the latest information on a variety of issues facing clinicians, some of which are common and others that are rare and are updated periodically as clinical care evolves. Guidelines must be interpreted considering each patient's clinical situation because they cover generalities, and individual patients may have comorbidities or other reasons that the guidelines may not be the "best" therapy for a particular patient.

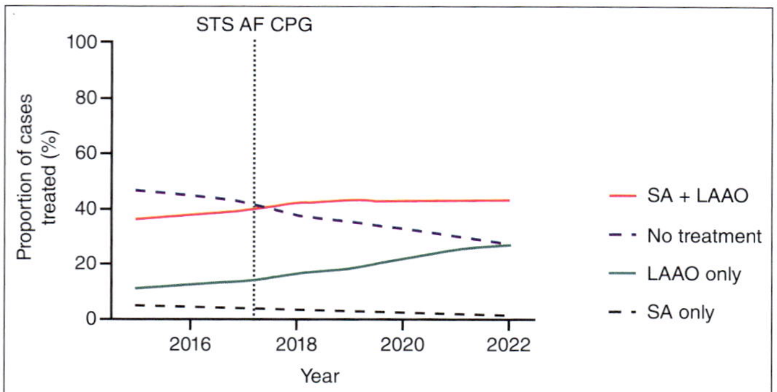

Fig. 24.1 Percentage of treatment of documented atrial fibrillation (AF) undergoing first-time, non-emergent cardiac surgery being treated with surgical ablation (SA) only, left atrial appendage occlusion (LAAO) alone, no treatment or surgical ablation plus LAAO. *CPG,* The Society of Thoracic Surgeons 2017 Clinical Practice Guidelines on the Surgical Treatment of Atrial Fibrillation; *STS,* Society of Thoracic Surgeons. (Reproduced from Wyler von Ballmoos MC, Hui DS, Mehaffey JH, et al. The Society of Thoracic Surgeons 2023 clinical practice guidelines for the surgical treatment of atrial fibrillation. *Ann Thor Surg.* 2024;118(2):291–310.)

Many societies have guidelines that cover various aspects of atrial fibrillation (AF) diagnosis, medical therapy, and interventional treatment, but not all are applicable to surgical patients.[1,3,4] There are also various types of clinical practice documents (Table 24.1).[2] The most relevant of these to the surgical treatment of AF are the 2024 Society of Thoracic Surgeons (STS) Guidelines and the European Society of CardioThoracic Surgery Guidelines.[1,4] This chapter focuses on these two sets of guidelines and builds off Chapter 23 on the benefits of concomitant AF ablation. There are a few caveats. The guidelines in general are not specific to which technology, approach, or lesion set should be used. Randomized trials are typically the most definitive data, but often they are not available, so surgical guideline recommendations are often based on systematic reviews, meta-analyses, large database studies, multicenter trials, and single-center reports with a generous helping of expert opinion. There are more data available for concomitant mitral valve (MV) surgery than for concomitant aortic valve replacement (AVR) or coronary artery bypass graft (CABG) operations, and the Level of Evidence (LOE) behind these latter recommendations is more limited. There is even less information about many other important areas of care, including the various types of stand-alone and "hybrid" operations, best practices for postoperative care such as anticoagulation, and the 'best" treatment for patients with aortic stenosis and AF, surgical AVR with concomitant ablation versus transcatheter AVR.

SHARED DECISION MAKING AND HEART TEAM ASSESSMENT

One principle common to all clinical practice guidelines is that the patient should be informed of options and have a role in decision making. As surgeons, we balance the risks and benefits of any procedure. Part of the informed consent of concomitant left atrial appendage occlusion (LAAO) and surgical ablation should include discussions of the potential near-term risks of adding LAAO and surgical ablation to what is almost always some other reason for undergoing cardiac surgery. The decision making for most patients is not complex because most patients are happy to have the AF and left atrial appendage (LAA) treated at the same time as the primary surgery. For "stand-alone" procedures, these discussions are more complex. The alternative treatments include continued medical therapy, or perhaps more catheter ablation. In the case of surgical AVR (SAVR) with LAAO and surgical ablation compared with transcatheter AVR (TAVR), the discussions can be quite extensive. These discussions typically center around improvement in symptoms and quality of life and reduction in stroke (Table 24.2).

Heart transplantation always functioned as a team of surgeons, cardiologists, and associated specialists. Complex decision making and care are best addressed with the combined skills of a variety of subspecialists. The "heart team" concept entered the everyday lexicon of practice with the launch of the placement of aortic transcatheter valves (PARTNER) Trials and eventually expanded to include MV therapies, coronary artery disease, and the treatment of AF and other arrhythmias. The STS Guidelines recommend (Class 1; LOE C) using a multidisciplinary heart team approach to the patients covered in the Guidelines. The European Association for Cardio-Thoracic Surgery (EACTS) multidisciplinary team recommendation is Class IIA.

GUIDELINES FOR THE CONCOMITANT ABLATION OF ATRIAL FIBRILLATION

Mitral Valve Surgery

The STS and EACTS recommend concomitant AF ablation for patients undergoing first-time nonemergency MV surgery (Table 24.3).[1,4] Reflecting the many randomized clinical trials, the recommendations are based on the success of restoring sinus rhythm compared with untreated patients with AF (see Table 23.1). Also, and importantly, they based this upon new information documenting improved long-term outcomes regarding survival and freedom from stroke (Fig. 24.2).[1] The data behind these recommendations are summarized in Chapter 23. This recommendation has the highest rating from both STS and EACTS: Class I; LOE A. The EACTS document also gives its highest recommendation to concomitant surgical ablation with MV surgery. The EACTS guideline committee relied primarily on meta-analyses to support their recommendations.[5–8]

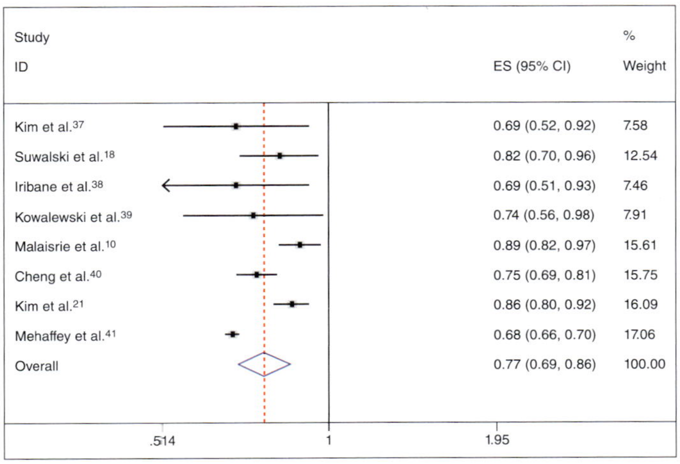

Fig. 24.2 Studies with a follow-up of 2 years or more (median follow-up range, 2.6–6.7 years; $n = 8$ studies) and the pooled effect estimates for all-cause mortality associated with surgical ablation of atrial fibrillation (hazard ratio, 0.77; 95% confidence interval [CI], 0.69–0.86). *ES*, estimate. (Reproduced from Reproduced from Wyler von Ballmoos MC, Hui DS, Mehaffey JH, et al. The Society of Thoracic Surgeons 2023 clinical practice guidelines for the surgical treatment of atrial fibrillation. *Ann Thor Surg.* 2024;118(2):291–310.)

Non–Mitral Valve Surgery

The data for concomitant non-MV surgery in which the left atrium is normally not opened are not as robust as they are for MV surgery in which the left atrium is always open because concomitant surgery is performed far less often in non-MV surgery. As discussed in Chapter 23, there are multiple STS database studies[9,10] and meta-analyses[8,11–15] focused on how to treat concomitant AF in patients undergoing CABG or AVR. The STS gave a Class 1 recommendation for concomitant AF surgical ablation in any first-time none-mergent non-mitral operation but an LOE B because the data supporting this recommendation are non-randomized (Table 24.4). Surgical ablation for AF is recommended for any first-time non-emergent concomitant non-mitral operation to restore sinus rhythm and improve long-term outcomes. EACTS gave a more reserved recommendation of IIa in these patients and suggested that concomitant ablation "should be considered". This conservative recommendation is LOE B because there are fewer studies of this combination. This recommendation is primarily based upon meta-analyses.[8,11–27] The STS apparently places more emphasis on the STS database studies of CABG patients that show reduced stroke and mortality rates in the treated group. More well-designed studies of AF ablation in patients undergoing CABG and AVR will be helpful for the formulation of the next guidelines.

Left Atrial Appendage Management

Multiple studies supporting concomitant LAA closure for patients with preoperative AF to reduce the risk of stroke have created some of the most impressive datasets in cardiac surgery (see Chapter 23).[28–31] Therefore, it was no surprise that both the STS and EACTS support this as a Class I recommendation. The American Heart Association gives this a Class 1 recommendation with LOE A on the strength of the LAAOS III randomized clinical trial (Table 24.5).[1,3,4] LAAO treatment should be considered the minimum treatment for any patient with AF undergoing cardiac surgery because of the high safety and late reduction in stroke.[30,32]

Patients Being Considered for Transcatheter Valve Therapies

Patients with AF and aortic stenosis who can be treated with transcatheter valve replacement (TAVR) deserve a thorough and careful discussion about TAVR versus SAVR with surgical AF ablation and LAAO. The prognosis for patients with AF undergoing TAVR is significantly worse than for TAVR patients without AF.[33,34] Large, matched database trials demonstrated better late survival for patients treated with SAVR and surgical AF ablation compared with those undergoing TAVR alone,[35,36] which is not surprising. It is important that the patient receive SAVR with surgical AF ablation and LAAO to receive this benefit, and because this is untreated in the United States, there is a significant opportunity to improve our results and provide these patients with the best late outcomes (Table 24.6).[1] The EACTS has no comparable recommendation. This STS recommendation also applies to MV surgery patients who could be treated with either transcatheter therapy or MV surgery and AF surgical ablation with LAAO. Because adoption of concomitant surgical AF ablation is more common in MV patients, it seems that should be a more preferred choice, especially in low-risk and moderate-risk patients.

Stand-Alone Atrial Fibrillation and Hybrid Surgery

Stand-alone (non-concomitant) AF surgery is covered extensively in this book in other chapters. There are successful programs that typically have a strong heart team approach to difficult cases of AF, such as patients who have failed prior catheter ablation attempts. However, there are a variety of approaches, lesion sets, and technologies available but only a handful of surgeons and programs with much experience. This led to only one recommendation being given a level A rating based on the randomized "Converge trial" showing rhythm superiority of a hybrid procedure to catheter ablation alone.[4,42,43] Nevertheless, uniform Class IIa recommendations from all three societies (Tables 24.7 and 24.8) represents progress compared with years ago and reflects more data availability.[1,3,4]

TABLE 24.1 Types of Clinical Practice Documents

	Clinical Practice Guidelines	Expert Consensus Statements	Clinical Statements or White Papers
Definition	Evidence-based documents containing systematically developed recommendations with an explicit clinical scope and explicit consideration of benefits, harms, values, and preferences	Expert position on a controversial or specific clinical topic, formulated as a statement of facts based on available evidence and expert consensus in situations where high-level evidence is unavailable	Extensive reports outlining positions on critical clinical issues while highlighting areas of ongoing uncertainty or concern for patient safety
Source of evidence	Randomized controlled trials (RCTs) are available and serve as the primary source of information; observational data are used if considered robust.	Robust observational data are available and serve as the primary source of information in conjunction with a limited number of RCTs.	Any research and health care regulations
Number of writing committee members	≤20	≤20	≤10
Review	After the writing committee's established composition principles, a lead reviewer and up to five anonymous reviewers from each participating entity in collaboration with the governing bodies	After the writing committee's established composition principles, a lead reviewer and up to five anonymous reviewers from each participating entity in collaboration with the governing bodies	After the writing committee's established composition principles, up to three anonymous reviewers from each participating entity
Length	≤30,000 words and a total of 500 references	≤15,000 words and a total of 300 references	≤5000 words and a total of 50 references
Time frame (months)	24	12	6

Reproduced from Milojevic M, Freemantle N, Hayanga JWA, et al. Harmonizing guidelines and other clinical practice documents: a joint comprehensive methodology manual by the American Association for Thoracic Surgery (AATS), European Association for Cardio-Thoracic Surgery (EACTS), European Society of Thoracic Surgeons (ESTS), and Society of Thoracic Surgeons (STS). *J Thorac Cardiovasc Surg.* 2025;169(1):170–185.

TABLE 24.2 Guideline Recommendations for a Team Approach to Treatment Decision Making

Guideline	Recommendation: Team Approach	Class of Recommendation	Level of Recommendation
Wyler von Ballmoos et al., STS[1]	Multidisciplinary heart team assessment and treatment planning and long-term follow-up with periodic continuous rhythm monitoring	I	C
Van Gelder et al.,[4] EACTS	Education directed to patients, family members, caregivers, and health care professionals is recommended to optimize shared decision-making, facilitating open discussion of both the benefits and risks associated with each treatment option	I	C
Van Gelder et al.,[4] EACTS	Access to patient-centered management according to the AF-CARE principles is recommended in all patients with AF, regardless of gender, ethnicity, and socioeconomic status, to ensure equality in health care provision and improve outcomes	I	C
Van Gelder et al.,[4] EACTS	Patient-centered AF management with a multidisciplinary approach should be considered in all patients with AF to optimize management and improve outcomes.	IIa	B

AF, Atrial fibrillation; *AF-CARE,* Atrial fibrillation—[C] Comorbidity and risk factor management, [A] Avoid stroke and thromboembolism, [R] Reduce symptoms by rate and rhythm control, [E] Evaluation and dynamic reassessment; *EACTS,* European Association for Cardio-Thoracic Surgery; *STS,* Society of Thoracic Surgeons.

TABLE 24.3 Society of Thoracic Surgeons, European Society of Cardiology, and European Association for Cardio-Thoracic Surgery Recommendations for Surgical Atrial Fibrillation Ablation During Mitral Operations

Guideline: STS	Recommendations: Mitral Operations	Class of Recommendation	Level of Recommendation
Wyler von Ballmoos et al.[1]	Surgical ablation for AF is recommended for first-time nonemergent concomitant mitral operations to restore sinus rhythm and improve long-term outcomes.	I	A
Guideline: ESC/EACTS	**Recommendations: Mitral Operations**	**Class of Recommendation**	**Level of Recommendation**
Van Gelder et al.,[4] EACTS	Concomitant surgical ablation is recommended in patients undergoing MV surgery and AF suitable for a rhythm control strategy to prevent symptoms and recurrence of AF, with shared decision making supported by an experienced team of electrophysiologists and arrhythmia surgeons.	I	A

AF, Atrial fibrillation; *EACTS,* European Association for Cardio-Thoracic Surgery; *ESC,* European Society of Cardiology; *MV,* mitral valve; *STS,* Society of Thoracic Surgeons.

TABLE 24.4 Society of Thoracic Surgeons, European Society of Cardiology, and European Association for Cardio-Thoracic Surgery Recommendations for Surgical Atrial Fibrillation Ablation During Nonmitral Operations

Guideline: STS	Recommendations: Nonmitral Operations	Class of Recommendation	Level of Recommendation
Wyler von Ballmoos et al.[1]	Surgical ablation for AF is recommended for any first-time nonemergent concomitant nonmitral operation to restore sinus rhythm and improve long-term outcomes.	I	B-NR
Guideline: ESC/EACTS	**Recommendations: Nonmitral Operations**	**Class of Recommendation**	**Level of Recommendation**
Van Gelder et al.,[4] EACTS	Concomitant surgical ablation should be considered in patients undergoing non–MV cardiac surgery and AF suitable for a rhythm control strategy to prevent symptoms and recurrence of AF, with shared decision making supported by an experienced team of electrophysiologists and arrhythmia surgeons.	IIa	B

AF, Atrial fibrillation; *EACTS,* European Association for Cardio-Thoracic Surgery; *ESC,* European Society of Cardiology; *MV,* mitral valve; *STS,* Society of Thoracic Surgeons.

TABLE 24.5 Guideline Recommendations for Left Atrial Appendage Management During Cardiac Surgery

Guideline	Recommendations: Left Atrial Appendage	Class of Recommendation	Level of Recommendation
Wyler von Ballmoos et al.[1]	LAAO for AF is recommended for all first-time nonemergent cardiac surgery procedures, with or without concomitant surgical ablation, to reduce morbidity from thromboembolic complications.	I	B-NR
Van Gelder et al.,[4] EACTS	Surgical closure of the LAA is recommended as an adjust to oral anticoagulation in patients with AF undergoing cardiac surgery to prevent ischemic stroke and thromboembolism	I	B
Joglar et al.[3]	In patients with AF undergoing cardiac surgery with a CHA2DS2-VASc score of ≥2 or equivalent stroke risk, surgical LAA exclusion, in addition to continued anticoagulation, is indicated to reduce the risk of stroke and systemic embolism.	I	A

ACC, American College of Cardiology; *AHA,* American Heart Association; *ACCP,* American College of Clinical Pharmacy; *AF,* atrial fibrillation; *EACTS,* European Association for Cardio-Thoracic Surgery; *HRS,* Heart Rhythm Society; *LAAO,* left atrial appendage obliteration; *STS,* Society of Thoracic Surgeons.

TABLE 24.6 Society of Thoracic Surgeon Recommendations for Patients With Atrial Fibrillation Considering Transcatheter Valve Therapies

Guideline: STS	Recommendations: Patients Considering Transcatheter Valve Therapies	Class of Recommendation	Level of Recommendation
Wyler von Ballmoos et al.[1]	For patients with symptomatic valve disease and AF, who are deemed of low to intermediate surgical risk, surgical valve repair or replacement with concomitant surgical ablation and LAAO is reasonable over isolated transcatheter valve repair or replacement alone to restore sinus rhythm and improve long-term outcomes	IIa	B-NR

AF, Atrial fibrillation; *LAAO,* left atrial appendage obliteration; *STS,* Society of Thoracic Surgeons.

TABLE 24.7 Society of Thoracic Surgeon Recommendations for Stand-Alone Surgical Ablations

Guideline: STS	Recommendations: Stand-Alone Surgical Ablations	Class of Recommendation	Level of Recommendation
Wyler von Ballmoos et al.[1]	Surgical ablation for symptomatic AF in the absence of structural heart disease refractory to class I/III antiarrhythmic drugs, catheter-based therapy, or both is reasonable as a primary stand-alone procedure to restore sinus rhythm.	IIa	B-NR
	Surgical ablation for symptomatic persistent or long-standing persistent AF in the absence of structural heart disease is reasonable as a stand-alone procedure using the Cox-Maze-III or -IV lesion set as the preferred procedure.	IIa	B-NR
	Surgical ablation for symptomatic AF in the setting of left atrial enlargement (≥4.5 cm) or more than moderate mitral regurgitation by PVI alone is not recommended.	III	C

AF, Atrial fibrillation; *PVI,* pulmonary vein isolation; *STS,* Society of Thoracic Surgeons.

TABLE 24.8 European Society of Cardiology, European Association for Cardio-Thoracic Surgery, American College of Cardiology, American Heart Association, American College of Chest Physicians, and Heart Rhythm Society Recommendations for Stand-Alone Atrial Fibrillation Surgical Ablation

Guideline: ESC/EACTS	Recommendations: Endoscopic and Hybrid AF Ablation	Class of Recommendation	Level of Recommendation
Van Gelder et al.,[4] EACTS	Endoscopic and hybrid ablation procedures should be considered in patients with symptomatic persistent AF refractory to antiarrhythmic drug therapy to prevent symptoms, recurrence, and progression of AF, within a shared decision-making rhythm control team of electrophysiologists and surgeons.	IIa	A
Guideline: ACC/AHA/ACCP/HRS	**Recommendations: Hybrid epicardial and endocardial AF Ablation[44–46]**	**Class of Recommendation**	**Level of Recommendation**
Joglar et al.[3]	For patients with symptomatic, persistent AF refractory to antiarrhythmic drug therapy, a hybrid epicardial and endocardial ablation might be reasonable to reduce the risk of recurrent atrial arrhythmia.	IIa	B-R

ACC, American College of Cardiology; *AHA,* American Heart Association; *ACCP,* American College of Clinical Pharmacy; *AF,* atrial fibrillation; *EACTS,* European Association for Cardio-Thoracic Surgery; *ESC,* European Society of Cardiology; *HRS,* Heart Rhythm Society.

REFERENCES

1. Wyler von Ballmoos MC, Hui DS, Mehaffey JH, et al. The Society of Thoracic Surgeons 2023 clinical practice guidelines for the surgical treatment of atrial fibrillation. *Ann Thor Surg*. 2024;118(2):291–310.
2. Milojevic M, Freemantle N, Hayanga JWA, et al. Harmonizing guidelines and other clinical practice documents: a joint comprehensive methodology manual by the American Association for Thoracic Surgery (AATS), European Association for Cardio-Thoracic Surgery (EACTS), European Society of Thoracic Surgeons (ESTS), and Society of Thoracic Surgeons (STS). *J Thorac Cardiovasc Surg*. 2025;169(1):170–185.
3. Joglar JA, Chung MK, Armbruster AL, et al. 2023 ACC/AHA/ACCP/HRS guideline for the diagnosis and management of atrial fibrillation: a report of the American College of Cardiology/American Heart Association Joint Committee on clinical practice guidelines. *Circulation*. 2024;149(1):e1–e156.
4. Van Gelder IC, Rienstra M, Bunting KV, et al. 2024 ESC Guidelines for the management of atrial fibrillation developed in collaboration with the European Association for Cardio-Thoracic Surgery (EACTS). *Eur Heart J*. 2024;45(36):3314–3414.
5. Cheng DC, Ad N, Martin J, et al. Surgical ablation for atrial fibrillation in cardiac surgery: a meta-analysis and systematic review. *Innovations*. 2010;5(2):84–96. https://doi.org/10.1097/IMI.0b013e3181c9199b.
6. McClure GR, Belley-Cote EP, Jaffer IH, et al. Surgical ablation of atrial fibrillation: a systematic review and meta-analysis of randomized controlled trials. *Europace*. 2018;20(9):1442–1450.
7. Phan K, Xie A, Tian DH, Shaikhrezai K, Yan TD. Systematic review and meta-analysis of surgical ablation for atrial fibrillation during mitral valve surgery. *Ann Cardiothorac Surg*. 2014;3(1):3–14.
8. Huffman MD, Karmali KN, Berendsen MA, et al. Concomitant atrial fibrillation surgery for people undergoing cardiac surgery. *Cochrane Database Syst Rev*. 2016;2016(8):CD011814.
9. Churyla A, Andrei AC, Kruse J, et al. Safety of atrial fibrillation ablation with isolated surgical aortic valve replacement. *Ann Thor Surg*. Mar 2021;111(3):809–817.
10. Malaisrie SC, McCarthy PM, Kruse J, et al. Ablation of atrial fibrillation during coronary artery bypass grafting: late outcomes in a Medicare population. *J Thorac Cardiovasc Surg*. 2021;161(4):1251–1261.
11. Pokushalov E, Romanov A, Corbucci G, Cherniavsky A, Karaskov A. Benefit of ablation of first diagnosed paroxysmal atrial fibrillation during coronary artery bypass grafting: a pilot study. *Eur J Cardiothorac Surg*. 2012;41(3):556–560.
12. Yoo JS, Kim JB, Ro SK, et al. Impact of concomitant surgical atrial fibrillation ablation in patients undergoing aortic valve replacement. *Circ J*. 2014;78(6):1364–1371.
13. Malaisrie SC, Lee R, Kruse J, et al. Atrial fibrillation ablation in patients undergoing aortic valve replacement. *J Heart Valve Dis*. 2012;21(3):350–357.
14. Rankin JS, Lerner DJ, Braid-Forbes MJ, Ferguson MA, Badhwar V. One-year mortality and costs associated with surgical ablation for atrial fibrillation concomitant to coronary artery bypass grafting. *Eur J Cardiothorac Surg*. 2017;52(3):471–477.
15. Schill MR, Musharbash FN, Hansalia V, et al. Late results of the Cox-Maze IV procedure in patients undergoing coronary artery bypass grafting. *J Thorac Cardiovasc Surg*. 2017;153(5):1087–1094.
16. Musharbash FN, Schill MR, Sinn LA, et al. Performance of the Cox-Maze IV procedure is associated with improved long-term survival in patients with atrial fibrillation undergoing cardiac surgery. *J Thorac Cardiovasc Surg*. 2018;155(1):159–170.
17. Rankin JS, Lerner DJ, Braid-Forbes MJ, McCrea MM, Badhwar V. Surgical ablation of atrial fibrillation concomitant to coronary-artery bypass grafting provides cost-effective mortality reduction. *J Thorac Cardiovasc Surg*. 2020;160(3):675–686.
18. Suwalski P, Kowalewski M, Jasinski M, et al. Survival after surgical ablation for atrial fibrillation in mitral valve surgery: analysis from the Polish National Registry of Cardiac Surgery Procedures (KROK). *J Thorac Cardiovasc Surg*. 2019;157(3):1007–1018.
19. Suwalski P, Kowalewski M, Jasinski M, et al. Surgical ablation for atrial fibrillation during isolated coronary artery bypass surgery. *Eur J Cardiothorac Surg*. 2020;57(4):691–700.
20. Wehbe M, Albert M, Lewalter T, et al. The German cardiosurgery atrial fibrillation registry: 1-year follow-up outcomes. *Thorac Cardiovasc Surg*. 2023;71(4):255–263.
21. Kim HJ, Kim YJ, Kim M, et al. Surgical ablation for atrial fibrillation during aortic and mitral valve surgery: a nationwide population-based cohort study. *J Thorac Cardiovasc Surg*. 2024;167(3):981–993.
22. Ad N, Henry L, Hunt S, Holmes SD. Do we increase the operative risk by adding the Cox Maze III procedure to aortic valve replacement and coronary artery bypass surgery? *J Thorac Cardiovasc Surg*. 2012;143(4):936–944.
23. Maesen B, van der Heijden CAJ, Bidar E, Vos R, Athanasiou T, Maessen JG. Patient-reported quality of life after stand-alone and concomitant arrhythmia surgery: a systematic review and meta-analysis. *Interact Cardiovasc Thorac Surg*. 2022;34(3):339–348.
24. Osmancik P, Budera P, Talavera D, et al. Five-year outcomes in cardiac surgery patients with atrial fibrillation undergoing concomitant surgical ablation versus no ablation. The long-term follow-up of the PRAGUE-12 Study. *Heart Rhythm*. 2019;16(9):1334–1340.
25. Lee R, Jivan A, Kruse J, et al. Late neurologic events after surgery for atrial fibrillation: rare but relevant. *Ann Thor Surg*. 2013;95(1):126–131; discussion 131-2.
26. Kowalewski M, Pasierski M, Kolodziejczak M, et al. Atrial fibrillation ablation improves late survival after concomitant cardiac surgery. *J Thorac Cardiovasc Surg*. 2023;166(6):1656–1668.
27. Cox JL, Ad N, Palazzo T. Impact of the Maze procedure on the stroke rate in patients with atrial fibrillation. *J Thorac Cardiovasc Surg*. 1999;118(5):833–840.
28. Whitlock RP, Belley-Cote EP, Paparella D, et al. Left atrial appendage occlusion during cardiac surgery to prevent stroke. *N Eng J Med*. 2021;384(22):2081–2091.
29. Baudo M, Sicouri S, Yamashita Y, et al. Stroke prevention with prophylactic left atrial appendage occlusion in cardiac surgery patients without atrial fibrillation: a meta-analysis of randomized and propensity-score studies. *Circ Cardiovasc Interv*. 2024;17(10):e014296.
30. Pasierski M, Batko J, Kuzma L, et al. Surgical ablation, left atrial appendage occlusion or both? Nationwide registry analysis of cardiac surgery patients with underlying atrial fibrillation. *Eur J Cardiothorac Surg*. 2024;65(3). https://doi.org/10.1093/ejcts/ezae014.
31. Brescia AA, Groskurth JD, Murphy ET, et al. Increasing adoption of left atrial appendage occlusion in isolated coronary artery bypass grafting. *Ann Thor Surg*. 2024;118(4):854–862.
32. McCarthy PM, Cox JL. Practical approaches to concomitant surgical ablation of atrial fibrillation: matching the ablation to the patient. *J Thorac Cardiovasc Surg*. 2024. https://doi.org/10.1016/j.jtcvs.2024.03.023.

33. Shahim B, Malaisrie SC, George I, et al. Atrial fibrillation and outcomes after transcatheter or surgical aortic valve replacement (from the PARTNER 3 trial). *Am J Cardiol.* 2021;148:116–123.
34. Mengi S, Cepas-Guillen PL, Ternacle J, et al. Clinical outcomes in atrial fibrillation patients undergoing transcatheter aortic valve replacement with contemporary devices. *Can J Cardiol.* 2024. https://doi.org/10.1016/j.cjca.2024.12.007.
35. Patrick WL, Chen Z, Han JJ, et al. Patients with atrial fibrillation benefit from SAVR with surgical ablation compared to TAVR Alone. *Cardiol Ther.* 2022;11(2):283–296.
36. Mehaffey JH, Kawsara M, Jagadeesan V, et al. Atrial fibrillation management during surgical vs transcatheter aortic valve replacement. *Ann Thor Surg.* 2024. https://doi.org/10.1016/j.athoracsur.2024.03.020.
37. Kim WK, Kim HJ, Kim JB, et al. Concomitant ablation of atrial fibrillation in rheumatic mitral valve surgery. *J Thorac Cardiovasc Surg.* 2019;157:1519–1528.e5.
38. Iribarne A, DiScipio AW, McCullough JN, et al. Surgical atrial fibrillation ablation improves long-term survival: a multicenter analysis. *Ann Thorac Surg.* 2019;107:135–142.
39. Kowalewski M, Wanha W, Litwinowicz R, et al. Stand-Alone Left Atrial appendage occlusion for throMboembolism prevention in nonvalvular Atrial fibrillatioN DiseasE Registry (SALAMANDER): protocol for a prospective observational nationwide study. *BMJ Open.* 2022;12:e063990.
40. Cheng Y-T, Huang Y-T, Tu H-T, et al. Long-term outcomes of concomitant surgical ablation for atrial fibrillation. *Ann Thorac Surg.* 2023;116:297–305.
41. Mehaffey JH, Hayanga JWA, Wei L, Mascio C, Rankin JS, Badhwar V. Surgical ablation of atrial fibrillation is associated with improved survival compared with appendage obliteration alone: an analysis of 100,000 Medicare beneficiaries. *J Thorac Cardiovasc Surg.* 2024;168(1):104–116.
42. Cox JL, Churyla A, Malaisrie SC, et al. When is a Maze procedure a Maze procedure? *Can J Cardiol.* 2018;34(11):1482–1491.
43. DeLurgio DB, Crossen KJ, Gill J, et al. Hybrid convergent procedure for the treatment of persistent and long-standing persistent atrial fibrillation: results of CONVERGE clinical trial. *Circ Arrhythm Electrophysiol.* 2020;13(12):e009288.
44. Kress DC, Erickson L, Choudhuri I, et al. Comparative effectiveness of hybrid ablation versus endocardial catheter ablation alone in patients with persistent atrial fibrillation. *JACC Clin Electrophysiol.* 2017;3(4):341–349.
45. Mannakkara NN, Porter B, Child N, et al. Convergent ablation for persistent atrial fibrillation: outcomes from a single-centre real-world experience. *Eur J Cardiothorac Surg.* 2022;63(1). https://doi.org/10.1093/ejcts/ezac515.
46. Gersak B, Zembala MO, Muller D, et al. European experience of the convergent atrial fibrillation procedure: multicenter outcomes in consecutive patients. *J Thorac Cardiovasc Surg.* 2014;147(4):1411–1416.

25

Surgical Options for the Treatment of Concomitant Atrial Fibrillation

James L. Cox

CHAPTER OUTLINE

Most of what is known about atrial fibrillation (AF) has come from basic electrophysiologists and clinical electrophysiologists, and this knowledge has accrued primarily from the study of what we clinically call *stand-alone AF*. This refers to AF that is not associated with other heart problems that are severe enough to warrant cardiac surgery. AF that develops as a result of left-heart problems that are severe enough to warrant surgery (e.g., coronary artery disease, mitral or aortic valve disease, or other left-heart abnormalities) is called *concomitant AF* and is in the domain of surgeons.

There are several differences between stand-alone AF and concomitant AF. For example, patients with concomitant AF tend to have more atrial scarring and larger, thicker left atria. Early in the stage of left-heart disease, only the left atrium (LA) may be affected, and the right atrium (RA) can be entirely normal. The longer left-heart disease remains untreated, the greater the likelihood of the RA's becoming involved in the adaptive response, especially in mitral and aortic valve disease. When both atria are adversely affected by the left-heart problem, the patient is more likely to develop AF. Thus, if the primary left-heart structural problem is not surgically corrected early in the course of coronary artery or valve disease, the RA is more likely to be involved in sustaining the AF, and the patient is more likely to need a biatrial AF ablation procedure.

Another difference between stand-alone AF and concomitant AF is that approximately 90% of the atrial triggers that induce stand-alone AF are located in and around the pulmonary veins.[1] However, only approximately 70% of the atrial triggers are located in the pulmonary vein area in patients with concomitant paroxysmal AF (PAF)[2–4] (Fig. 25.1). These differences in both the anatomy and the electrophysiology of stand-alone AF and concomitant AF dictate that the outcomes for the same interventional procedure will be different in the two groups. Thus, a perfect box lesion that isolates all four pulmonary veins and the posterior left atrial wall can reach a maximum success rate of 90% for stand-alone AF but a maximum success rate of only 70% for concomitant AF.

Because surgeons rarely treat stand-alone AF, the most important decisions we have to make regarding the treatment of AF in patients undergoing coronary artery or valve surgery relate to concomitant AF only. The first, and by far the most important, thing that surgeons must determine in these patients is whether they have PAF (repeatedly induced by atrial triggers) or non-paroxysmal AF (non-PAF sustained by atrial macro-reentrant drivers).

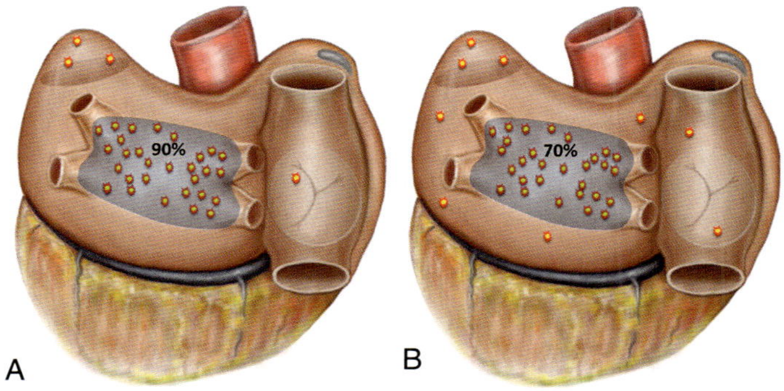

Fig. 25.1 (A) In stand-alone atrial fibrillation (AF), approximately 90% of AF triggers are located in and around the pulmonary veins. (B) In concomitant AF, approximately 70% of atrial triggers are located in and around the pulmonary veins.

PAROXYSMAL ATRIAL FIBRILLATION

Patients with PAF usually spend most of their time in normal sinus rhythm (NSR). They then have the spontaneous discharge of an automatic or micro-reentrant focus (trigger), usually located in or around the pulmonary veins, that induces macro-reentrant drivers in the atria resulting in AF (see Chapter 5, Fig. 5.34). In patients with PAF, the resultant episode of AF may last from several minutes up to 7 days before it self-terminates or is terminated with drugs, and NSR resumes (Fig. 25.2). For another episode of AF to occur, it must again be induced by an atrial trigger, which may or may not be the same one that induced the previous AF episode. This is the repetitive cycle of NSR–PAF–NSR that patients with PAF experience.

The goal of AF surgery in patients with PAF is to isolate as many of the AF triggers as possible from the rest of the heart. Because we know that roughly 70% of these triggers are located in and around the pulmonary veins, it is logical to isolate this area of the heart with a box lesion around the pulmonary veins and intervening posterior left atrial wall (the "pulmonary vein cuff"), which should result in a 70% success rate. Over the years, we have learned the approximate distribution of the other non-pulmonary vein atrial triggers (Fig. 25.3), so we can

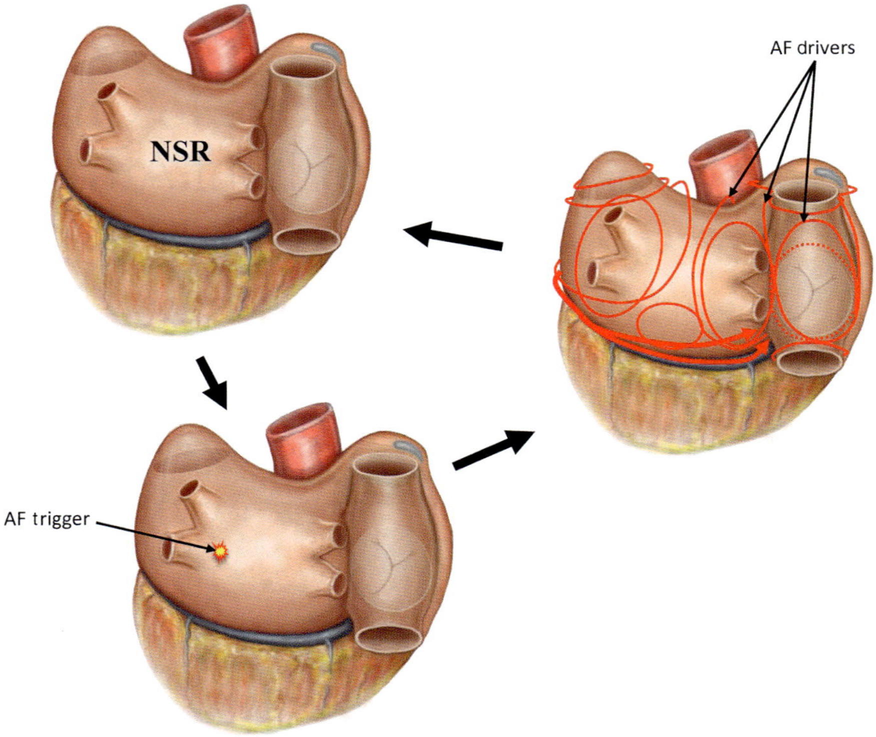

Fig. 25.2 Paroxysmal atrial fibrillation (PAF): self-limiting episode of AF. Patients with PAF are usually in normal sinus rhythm (NSR). When an AF trigger suddenly fires *(lower panel)*, it induces an episode of AF *(right panel)* that is either self-limited or can be terminated by antiarrhythmic drugs or electrical cardioversion in less than 1 week from its onset. The objective of interventional therapy (catheter ablation or surgical ablation) for PAF is to isolate as many triggers in and around the pulmonary veins and intervening posterior left atrial wall as possible to decrease the likelihood of the induction of an episode of AF.

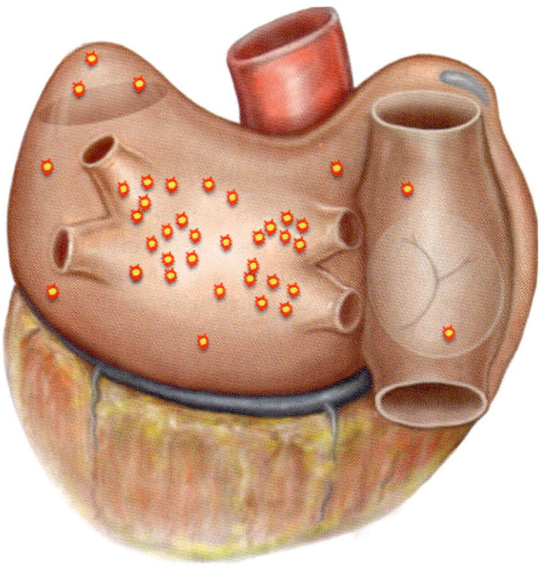

Fig. 25.3 Distribution of atrial triggers in concomitant paroxysmal atrial fibrillation (PAF). AF triggers can be located anywhere in either atrium, but approximately 70% of them are located in and around the pulmonary veins and in the posterior left atrial wall between the two pairs of pulmonary veins. We refer to this area encompassing all four pulmonary veins and the intervening posterior left atrial wall as the "pulmonary vein cuff."

now predict the success of any AF isolation or ablation procedure that one might use for concomitant PAF. Of the triggers within the pulmonary vein cuff, 20% or more are located in the posterior left atrial wall (Fig. 25.4). The remaining 50% within the pulmonary vein cuff are in the right and left pulmonary veins, and we assume that they are equally distributed between the two pairs of veins. Thus, simple isolation of the pulmonary veins in pairs with a bipolar clamp can be expected to produce a success rate of approximately 50% in patients with concomitant PAF (Fig. 25.5). Adding a roof and floor lesion to the pulmonary vein isolation (PVI) to isolate the additional 20% of triggers in the posterior left atrial wall creates a box lesion around the entire pulmonary vein cuff and therefore increases the expected success rate in PAF to 70% (Fig. 25.6). At least 10% of the atrial triggers in patients with PAF reside in the left atrial appendage (LAA). Thus, if LAA occlusion (LAAO), which includes LAA electrical isolation or LAA amputation, is added to a box lesion in patients with PAF, the success rate can be expected to reach approximately 80% (Fig. 25.7). It is important to understand that catheter-based devices that are used to close the LAA endocardially do not *electrically* isolate the LAA from the LA even though the LAA may be successfully occluded. Likewise, neither endocardial nor epicardial suture closure of the LAA electrically isolates the LAA; therefore, neither of them improves the success rate of adding LAAO to a box lesion for patients with PAF. The only currently available LAA occluding devices that electrically isolate the LAA are epicardial devices that devascularize the musculature of the LAA itself, such as the surgical AtriClip and the catheter-based LARIAT device. Of course, surgical amputation of the LAA serves the same purpose.

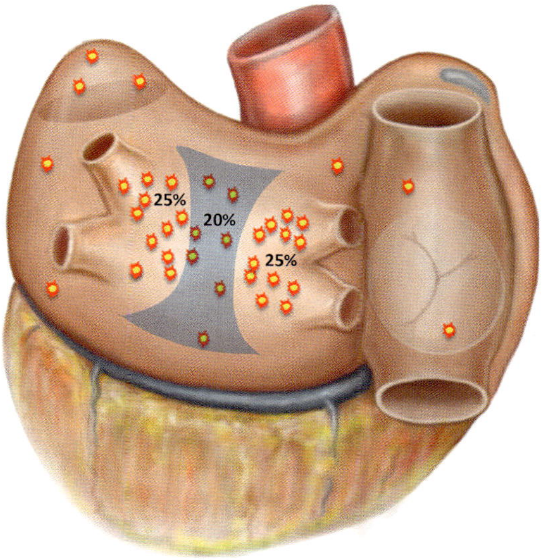

Fig. 25.4 Proportional distribution of "pulmonary vein cuff" triggers in concomitant paroxysmal atrial fibrillation (PAF). Approximately 20% of the atrial triggers are located in the posterior left atrial wall between the two pairs of pulmonary veins *(shadowed area)*. This means that the remaining 50% of triggers within the pulmonary vein cuff are located within or in the immediate vicinity of the pulmonary veins. If they are distributed evenly between the two pairs of pulmonary veins, then each pair of pulmonary veins harbors approximately 25% of the atrial triggers present in patients with concomitant PAF.

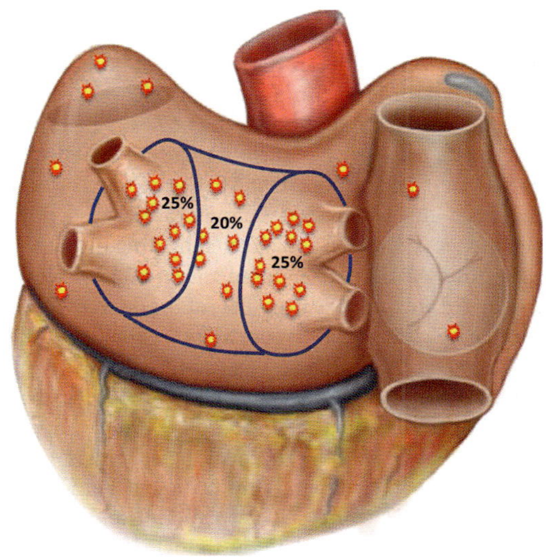

Fig. 25.6 Box lesion for concomitant paroxysmal atrial fibrillation (PAF). A box lesion encompassing all four pulmonary veins and the posterior left atrial wall would be expected to have a success rate of approximately 70% in patients with concomitant PAF.

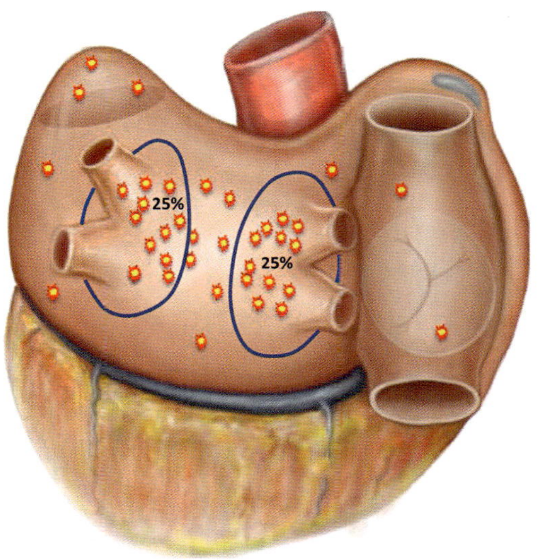

Fig. 25.5 Pulmonary vein isolation (PVI) for concomitant paroxysmal atrial fibrillation (PAF). On the basis of the distribution of potential atrial triggers, PVI alone would be expected to have a success rate of approximately 50% in patients with concomitant PAF.

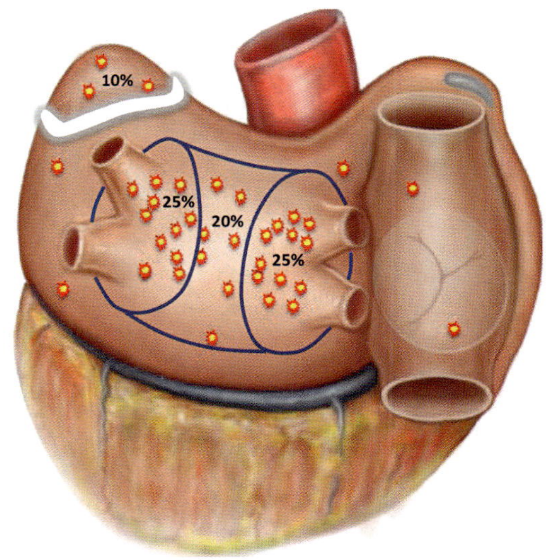

Fig. 25.7 Box lesion plus left atrial appendage occlusion (LAAO) for concomitant paroxysmal atrial fibrillation (PAF). The combination of a box lesion with LAAO would be expected to have a success rate of approximately 80% in patients with concomitant PAF. Because this combination of lesions can be performed without opening the left atrium, it is a reasonable alternative to the Maze procedure in patients undergoing coronary bypass graft (CABG), aortic valve replacement (AVR), or CABG plus AVR by surgeons less experienced in arrhythmia surgery.

One disadvantage of performing only a box lesion plus LAAO for concomitant PAF in patients undergoing coronary artery bypass graft (CABG) and/or aortic valve replacement (AVR) is that these lesions do not render the atria incapable of fibrillating. It only decreases the likelihood of having recurrent episodes of AF by isolating most of the potential triggers that induce each episode. Thus, nonpulmonary vein triggers, arrhythmia triggers, and nonarrhythmia triggers can still induce AF (see Chapter 5). The only way the atria can become incapable of fibrillating is by performing a Maze procedure, but this requires opening the atrium. Most experienced arrhythmia surgeons perform Maze procedures routinely in patients with any type of AF who require cardiac surgery. However, a box lesion plus LAAO is a reasonable alternative for the treatment of concomitant PAF, especially for surgeons who are less experienced in arrhythmia surgery.

NON-PAROXYSMAL ATRIAL FIBRILLATION

The current classification of AF is not always helpful in deciding which interventional approach is best in a given patient with AF because it is based solely on the duration of the episodes of AF (see Chapter 52). PAF episodes last less than 1 week, persistent AF episodes last between 1 week and 1 year, and long-standing persistent AF (LSpAF) lasts more than 1 year. After AF has been initiated, macro-reentrant drivers sustain the AF until it spontaneously terminates or is terminated by drug therapy or electrical cardioversion. After AF has been induced, the electrophysiologic events in the atria during AF are the same regardless of the duration of the episode. Thus, the primary physiologic difference in PAF, persistent AF, and LSpAF is the electrical stability of the macro-reentrant AF drivers (Fig. 25.8).

Because atrial triggers are responsible for inducing the recurrent individual episodes of PAF, their isolation is the primary interventional goal in patients with PAF. On the opposite end of the spectrum, persistent and long-standing persistent AF occur because the macro-reentrant drivers of AF become self-perpetuating and the triggers have little or nothing to do with sustaining the AF (Fig. 25.9). Therefore, while the goal of AF ablation surgery in patients with PAF is to isolate as many focal triggers as possible, the goal of ablation in patients with non-PAF is to interrupt, or preclude the development of, as many potential macro-reentrant circuits that can sustain AF as possible.

The cumulative experience of approaching the different types of AF based on this concept suggests that the classification of AF should probably be further subdivided. For example, if the episodes of persistent AF (more than 1 week) are relatively shorter in duration, say,

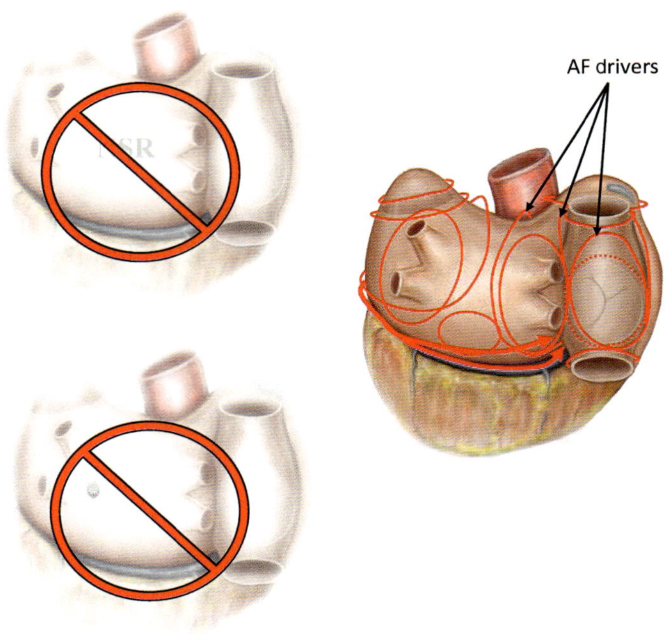

Fig. 25.8 Non-paroxysmal atrial fibrillation (non-PAF; persistent AF and long-standing persistent AF) is sustained by self-perpetuating macro-reentrant circuits (drivers). The focal atrial triggers that likely induced the AF originally have little or nothing to do with sustaining AF.

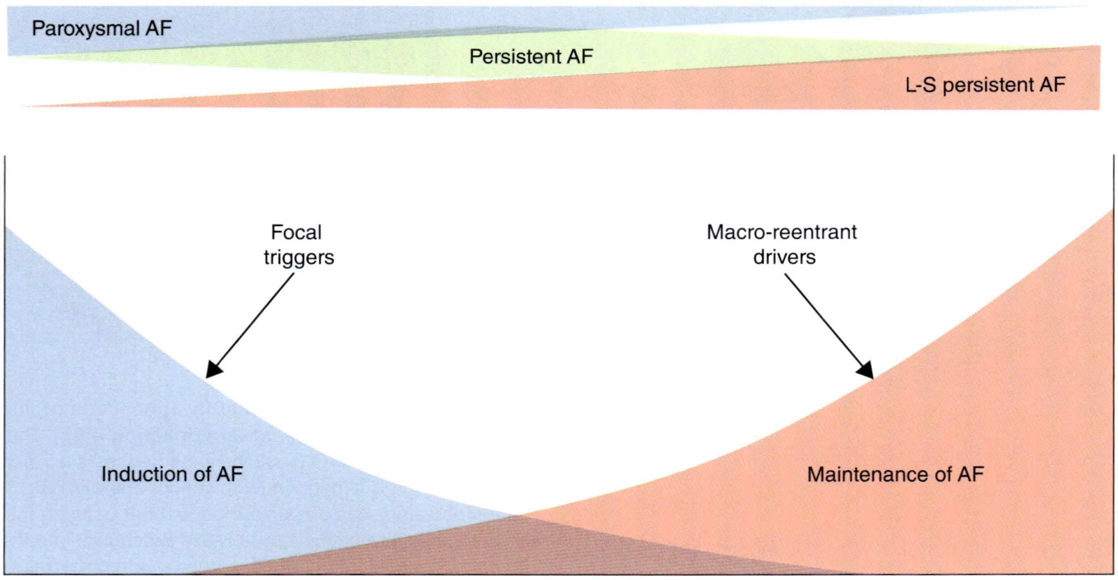

Fig. 25.9 The classification of atrial fibrillation (AF) into the categories of paroxysmal AF (PAF), persistent AF, and long-standing persistent AF (LSpAF) is based solely on the duration of AF episodes, but the underlying electrophysiology in each category is the same. However, focal atrial triggers are more important in PAF because they are necessary to induce each of the recurring self-limiting episodes of AF. As the individual episodes of AF become longer in persistent AF, the focal triggers become less important, and the drivers that sustain AF become more important. Therefore, simple isolation of the focal triggers in patients with persistent AF is less successful for persistent AF than it is for PAF. As the drivers become even more self-perpetuating in LSpAF, the focal drivers lose their importance entirely, and interventional treatment (catheter ablation or surgery) must be focused on interrupting the macro-reentrant drivers that are sustaining the AF. Thus as one moves from PAF to persistent AF to LSpAF, the focal triggers become less important, and the stability of the macro-reentrant drivers becomes more important. In addition, the objective of interventional therapy must also evolve across this spectrum to attain optimal interventional results.

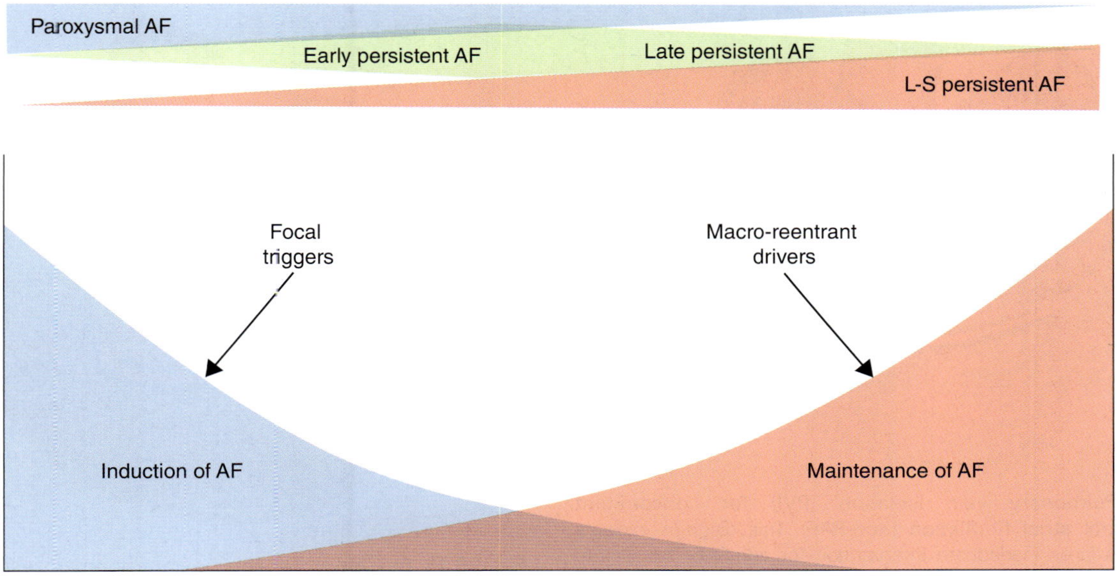

Fig. 25.10 Interventional electrophysiologists typically treat both paroxysmal atrial fibrillation (PAF) and persistent AF with pulmonary vein isolation (PVI). However, because of their mixed results in persistent AF, many now subdivide persistent AF into "early persistent AF" and "late persistent AF." There is no specific cutoff between these two subcategories, but it is clear that as AF episodes increase in duration, PVI alone becomes less effective. Therefore current practice is to treat patients with PAF and early persistent AF with PVI alone and to treat those with late persistent AF and long-standing persistent AF by PVI plus some type of "substrate modification." From a surgical standpoint, it is best to classify AF into only two categories, PAF and everything else (i.e., "non-PAF"). Patients with PAF can be treated satisfactorily by PVI alone, and those with non-PAF are best treated with a Maze procedure.

less than 5 or 6 months, the persistent AF can be treated relatively successfully by isolating the pulmonary vein triggers (PVI), which is the standard intervention for patients with PAF. Electrophysiologists now refer to this as "early persistent AF" (Fig. 25.10). However, if the persistent AF is longer, say, 6 to 12 months in duration ("late persistent AF"), it does not respond as well to PVI alone; rather, it should be treated more as if it were LSpAF, that is, by interrupting the macro-reentrant drivers.

Much like the known trigger locations in PAF already mentioned, we originally predicted the potential locations of atrial macro-reentrant drivers that sustain non-PAF. In fact, the *predicted* locations of potential large macro-reentrant circuits was, and remains, the basis of the Maze procedure. Subsequent mapping confirmed that the macro-reentrant drivers were, in fact, found to be in the predicted locations. Understanding the characteristics of atrial macro-reentry, including where macro-reentrant drivers can potentially form, explains the success rates of different ablative procedures for non-PAF. The most vulnerable atrial locations where individual macro-reentrant drivers are likely to form have now been documented many times both experimentally and clinically (Fig. 25.11). If any two or more of these macro-reentrant circuits form simultaneously in the atria, the atria will fibrillate. The *anatomic* locations of the drivers may change from one region to another within a few milliseconds (see Chapter 19, Fig. 19.5), but they are capable of remaining *electrically* stable for indefinite periods of time while moving from one anatomic location to another. Therefore, the best way to prevent these electrically stable but anatomically changing macro-reentrant drivers is to create lesions of conduction block in strategic areas of the atrium so that they simply cannot form anywhere in either atrium. That can be accomplished with a Maze procedure. This is an anatomically based procedure that does not depend on atrial mapping to guide placement of the atrial lesions because they are created in the same anatomic locations in all patients with AF. There are five ways a Maze procedure can fail:

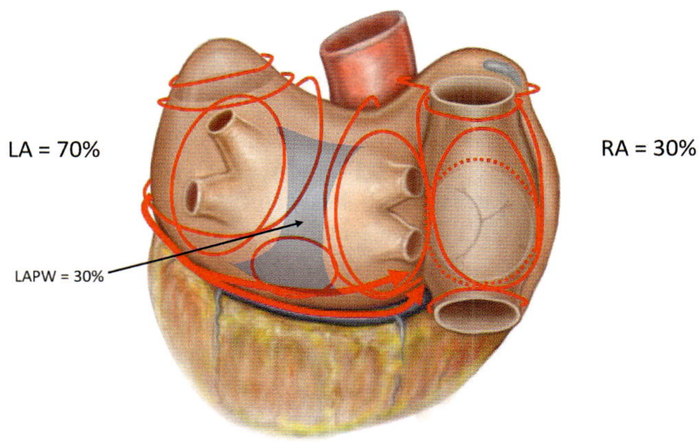

Fig. 25.11 Potential locations of atrial drivers in concomitant non-paroxysmal atrial fibrillation (non-PAF). These are the most common locations for the macro-reentrant drivers of AF in the two atria. Approximately 70% of them reside in the left atrium and 30% in the right atrium. Approximately 30% use the posterior left atrial wall between the two pairs of pulmonary veins as a critical part of their macro-reentrant circuit *(shadowed area)*. *LA,* Left atrium; *LAPW,* left atrial posterior wall; *RA,* right atrium.

1. The lesions are placed in the wrong places.
2. All lesions of the procedure are not performed.
3. One or more of the lesions is either non-contiguous or non-transmural.
4. The lesions end up being too far apart because of atrial enlargement.
5. The macro-reentrant drivers are small-diameter rotors that are located between the lesions.

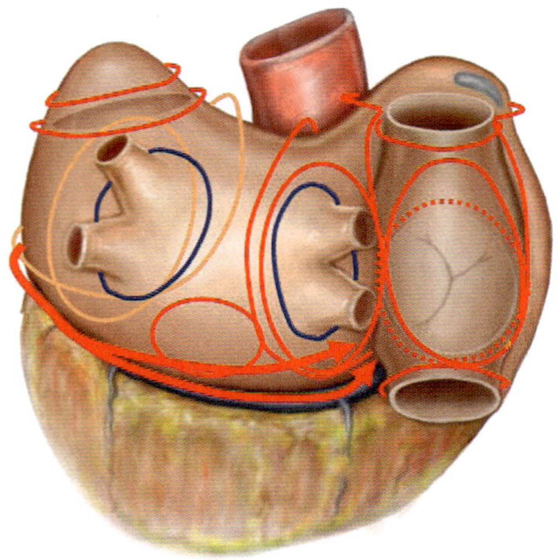

Fig. 25.12 Pulmonary vein isolation (PVI) for concomitant non-paroxysmal atrial fibrillation (non-PAF). This diagram explains why PVI alone is an inadequate intervention for non-PAF. This is true whether it is being performed for stand-alone non-PAF or concomitant non-PAF. The *red circles* represent potentially active macro-reentrant drivers of non-PAF that remain after completing PVI alone for non-PAF. The *tan circles* represent potential macro-reentrant drivers of non-PAF that are interrupted by performing PVI alone. The maximum long-term success rate after PVI alone for non-PAF is approximately 20%.

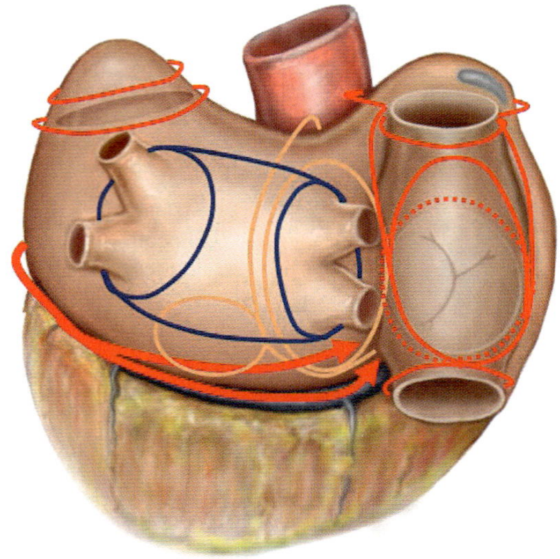

Fig. 25.13 Box lesion for concomitant non-paroxysmal atrial fibrillation (non-PAF). A box lesion is successful in approximately 30% of patients with non-PAF, primarily because it interrupts the macro-reentrant drivers that use the posterior left atrial wall as a part of their reentrant circuit. A box lesion created by isolation of the individual pairs of pulmonary veins in the Maze-IV procedure plus roof and floor lesions (as shown here) or as a single circumferential lesion that encompasses all four pulmonary veins and the posterior left atrial wall (as in the Maze-III procedure) are equally effective. The *red circles* represent potentially active macro-reentrant drivers of non-PAF that remain after completing a box lesion for non-PAF. The *tan circles* represent the additional potential macro-reentrant drivers of non-PAF that are precluded by performing a box lesion. The expected success rate after a box lesion for non-PAF is approximately 30%.

Except for the Maze procedure, the same surgical procedures have markedly different results in PAF and non-PAF. For example, simple isolation of the pulmonary veins (PVI) is successful in roughly 50% of patients with PAF but in very few patients with non-PAF unless the PVI, by chance, inadvertently interrupts a few of the macro-reentrant drivers that use the posterior LA wall as a part of their reentrant circuit (Fig. 25.12). Thus, it is no mystery why a single catheter ablation procedure has a 60% 5-year success rate for stand-alone PAF[5] but only a 20% 5-year success rate for stand-alone LSpAF.[6] Although adding roof and floor lesions to PVI to create a box lesion around the pulmonary vein cuff results in a success rate of 70% for PAF, a box lesion is only approximately 30% successful for non-PAF (Fig. 25.13).[4] Although the combination of a box lesion and LAAO can be successful in up to 80% of patients with PAF, the LAAO adds little or nothing in patients with non-PAF because macro-reentrant drivers rarely use the LAA as part of their circuit (Fig. 25.14). In addition, LAAO does not eliminate the reentrant circuit that uses the coumadin ridge between the LAA orifice and the left superior pulmonary vein, a very common site of macro-reentrant circuits.

It has been shown repeatedly that approximately 30% of the drivers of non-PAF are located in the RA, leaving approximately 70% in the LA.[7,8] Therefore, some surgeons perform a so-called "LA Maze" procedure for concomitant non-PAF (Fig. 25.15). Therefore, they can expect a 70% success rate with this approach and that is acceptable to many surgeons. One reason these surgeons do not include the right atrial lesions is the fear of increasing the requirements for postoperative pacemakers without significantly improving the AF ablation success rate. However, both of these concerns are unwarranted (see Chapters 13 and 21).

Adding the right atrial lesions to complete a Maze-III or Maze-IV procedure precludes the 30% of potential macro-reentrant drivers in the RA from developing and therefore, improves the expected success rate of a Maze procedure to greater than 90% (Fig. 25.16).

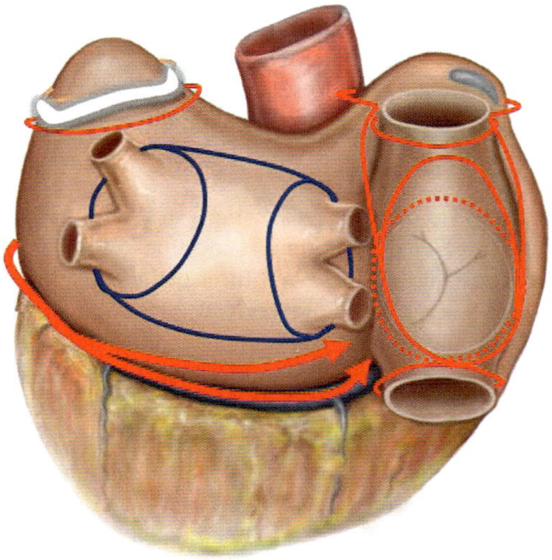

Fig. 25.14 Box lesion plus left atrial appendage occlusion (LAAO) for concomitant non-paroxysmal atrial fibrillation (non-PAF). Excluding the LAA in addition to performing a box lesion has little effect on the overall success of a box lesion in patients with non-PAF. (See text for further discussion.) Note that although this combination of lesions is up to 80% successful in patients with PAF, it is far less successful in patients with non-PAF. The *red circles* represent potentially active macro-reentrant drivers of non-PAF that remain after completing a box lesion plus LAAO for non-PAF. The *tan circles* represent the additional potential macro-reentrant drivers of non-PAF that are precluded by performing a box lesion plus LAAO. The maximum success rate after a box lesion and LAAO for non-PAF is approximately 30%.

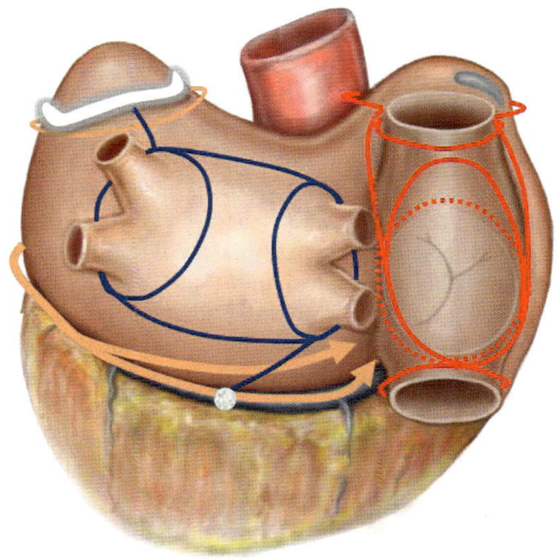

Fig. 25.15 **"LA (left atrial) Maze"-IV procedure for concomitant non-paroxysmal atrial fibrillation (non-PAF).** Completing the left atrial lesions but not the right atrial lesions of a Maze procedure is roughly 70% successful for the treatment of patients with non-PAF. The *red circles* represent potentially active macro-reentrant drivers of non-PAF that remain after completing an "LA Maze" procedure for non-PAF, and they are all in the right atrium. The *tan circles* represent the additional potential macro-reentrant drivers of non-PAF that are precluded by performing an "LA Maze" procedure.

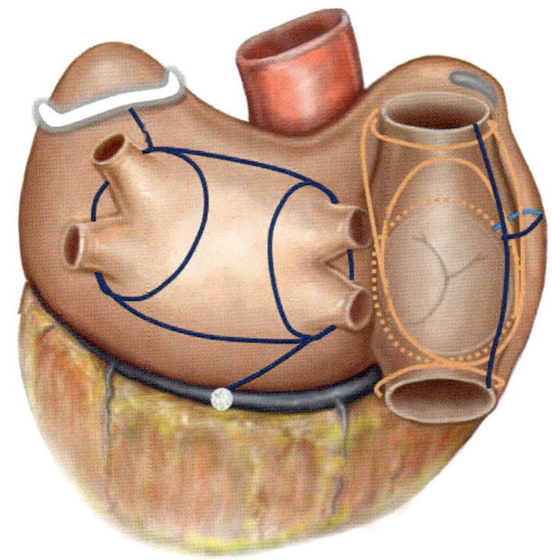

Fig. 25.16 **Maze-IV procedure for concomitant non-paroxysmal atrial fibrillation (non-PAF).** The Maze procedure is typically more than 90% successful for the treatment of patients with non-PAF because it interrupts all of the potential macro-reentrant drivers that sustain atrial fibrillation. The *tan circles* represent the additional potential macro-reentrant drivers of non-PAF that are precluded by performing a Maze-III or Maze-IV procedure (shown here). The expected success rate after a Maze procedure for non-PAF is more than 90%.

SUMMARY

The maximum success rates that can be expected in concomitant PAF and concomitant non-PAF with each type of surgical ablation procedure are summarized in Table 25.1. Several items should be of particular interest. PVI alone is successful in approximately 50% of patients with concomitant PAF but in only approximately 20% with concomitant persistent or LSpAF. The box lesion combined with LAAO is successful in 80% of patients with concomitant PAF but in only 30% with concomitant persistent or LSpAF. Thus if a surgeon's standard approach to AF in a CABG patient is to use a box lesion plus LAAO, the surgeon can expect to relieve the patient of AF 80% of the time if the patient has PAF but only 30% of the time if the patient has non-PAF. This fact emphasizes the importance of distinguishing between patients with PAF and those with non-PAF *preoperatively* because they should be approached surgically in entirely different ways.

The recommended type of AF ablation procedure that should be applied concomitantly also depends on the type of primary surgery that is required (Table 25.2). Concomitant AF, whether PAF or non-PAF, is handled the same in patients undergoing CABG, AVR or CABG plus AVR because neither CABG nor AVR requires opening the LA. The results of a concomitant Maze-III or Maze-IV procedure is always superior to the results any other AF ablation procedure but requires that the LA be opened. The addition of a Maze procedure to CABG, AVR, or CABG plus AVR procedure has been shown many times to be just as safe and even more effective than any other concomitant AF ablation approach. For this reason, most experienced AF surgeons routinely add a Maze procedure in any patient who has any type of concomitant AF and who is undergoing any type of primary cardiac surgical procedure.

TABLE 25.1 Maximum Success Rates[a]

Procedure	Maximum Success Rate for PAF (%)	Maximum Success Rate for Non-PAF (%)
Ignore the AF	0	0
LAAO	10	<5
PVI	50	<10
Box lesion	70	30
Box lesion + LAAO	80	30
LA Maze	80	70
Maze III/IV	>90	>90

[a]The approximate success rates that surgeons can expect from different procedures for concomitant atrial fibrillation (AF) ablation during cardiac surgery are listed. See text for further discussion.
LA, Left atrial; *LAAO,* left atrial appendage occlusion; *non-PAF,* nonparoxysmal atrial fibrillation; *PAF,* paroxysmal atrial fibrillation; *PVI,* pulmonary vein isolation.

TABLE 25.2 Recommended Atrial Fibrillation Ablation Procedures[a]

Primary Surgery	PAF	Non-PAF
CABG	Box lesion[b] + LAAO	Maze-III/IV
AVR	Box lesion[b] + LAAO	Maze-III/IV
CABG + AVR	Box lesion[b] + LAAO	Maze-III/IV
MVR	Maze-III/IV	Maze-III/IV

[a]A summary of the current recommendations for the type of concomitant AF ablation procedure that should be added when the primary cardiac procedure is coronary artery bypass grafting (CABG), aortic valve replacement or repair (AVR), CABG + AVR, or mitral valve repair or replacement (MVR).
[b]A box lesion encompasses all four pulmonary veins and the intervening posterior wall of the left atrium.
LAAO, Left atrial appendage occlusion; *non-PAF,* nonparoxysmal atrial fibrillation; *PAF,* paroxysmal atrial fibrillation.

However, if less experienced surgeons wish to avoid opening the LA for AF ablation during CABG and/or AVR surgery, it is reasonable to perform a box lesion plus LAAO because this approach is successful in 80% of patients with PAF *but not in patients with non-PAF.*

It is recommended that all patients with any type of AF associated with mitral valve surgery undergo a concomitant Maze-III or Maze-IV procedure because the LA already has to be opened for the mitral surgery. However, if the patient's concomitant AF is asymptomatic or the patient has prohibitive comorbidities, it may be wise to ignore the AF entirely rather than perform a non-Maze procedure with a poor chance of helping the patient. At the very least, though, all such patients should have their LAA occluded.

REFERENCES

1. Haïssaguerre M, Jaïs P, Shah DC, et al. Spontaneous initiation of atrial fibrillation by ectopic beats originating in the pulmonary veins. *N Eng J Med.* 1998;339(10):659–666.
2. Stulak JM, Suri RM, Burkhart HM, et al. Surgical ablation for atrial fibrillation for two decades: are the results of new techniques equivalent to the Cox Maze III procedure? *J Thorac Cardiovasc Surg.* 2014;147(5):1478–1486.
3. Onorati F, Mariscalco G, Rubino AS, et al. Impact of lesion sets on mid-term results of surgical ablation procedure for atrial fibrillation. *J Am Coll Cardiol.* 2011;57(8):931–940.
4. Sef D, Trkulja V, Raja SG, Hooper J, Turina MI. Comparing mid-term outcomes of Cox-Maze procedure and pulmonary vein isolation for atrial fibrillation after concomitant mitral valve surgery: a systematic review. *J Card Surg.* 2022;37:3801–3810.
5. Takagawa M, Takahashi A, Kuwahara T, et al. Long-term outcome after catheter ablation of paroxysmal atrial fibrillation: impact of different atrial fibrillation foci. *Int J Cardiol.* 2017;227:407–412.
6. Tilz RR, Rillig A, Thum AM, et al. Catheter ablation of long-standing persistent atrial fibrillation: 5-year outcomes of the Hamburg sequential ablation strategy. *J Am Coll Cardiol.* 2012;60(19):1921–1929.
7. Lim HS, Hocini M, Dubois R, et al. Complexity and distribution of drivers in relation to duration of persistent atrial fibrillation. *J Am Coll Cardiol.* 2017;69(10):1257–1269.
8. Osorio-Jaramillo E, Cox JL, Klenk S, et al. Dynamic electrophysiological mechanism in patients with long-standing persistent atrial fibrillation. *Front Cardiovasc Med.* 2022;9:953622. Published 2022 Sep 29. doi:10.3389/fcvm.2022.953622.

26

How I Do It: Atrial Fibrillation Ablation Plus Coronary Artery Bypass Grafting

S. Chris Malaisrie

CHAPTER OUTLINE

Preoperative atrial fibrillation (AF) is present in 10% to 20% of patients undergoing coronary artery bypass grafting (CABG).[1,2] Although the prevalence of AF is much higher in those with valvular heart disease,[2] far more CABG procedures than valve procedures are performed, so the absolute number of patients with concomitant AF requiring cardiac surgery is highest in patients undergoing CABG. In 2017, both the Society of Thoracic Surgeons (STS) guidelines and the Association for Thoracic Surgery Expert Consensus statement on AF treatment recommended that all patients with AF undergoing CABG should have concomitant AF ablation unless specific contraindications exist (see Chapter 24).[3,4] This recommendation was further strengthened in the 2024 STS guidelines.[5] Because concomitant AF ablation is a Class 1A guideline recommendation, failure to treat AF in patients undergoing CABG falls below the contemporary standard of care. Absent specific contraindications, simply ignoring the concomitant AF is not a justifiable option.

Surgeons have several options to treat patients with concomitant AF, including left atrial appendage occlusion (LAAO), pulmonary vein isolation (PVI) alone, PVI plus LAAO, a box lesion, a box lesion plus LAAO, and the Maze procedure. As described in Chapter 25, the expected results of each of these approaches varies widely depending on whether the patient has paroxysmal AF (PAF) or nonparoxysmal AF (non-PAF, persistent AF or long-standing persistent AF [LSpAF]). The choice of surgical approach must also consider that of these options, only the Maze procedure requires opening the left atrium (LA).

ATRIAL FIBRILLATION ABLATION PROCEDURE OPTIONS

The choice of AF ablation procedure for concomitant AF during CABG surgery hinges on the type of concomitant AF being treated. The importance of distinguishing between PAF and non-PAF and the rationale for different lesions sets has been discussed in detail in Chapter 25. In patients with PAF, the best options are either a box lesion plus LAAO without opening the LA with an expected 80% success rate or a Maze procedure, which requires opening the LA with an expected success rate of more than 90%. We recommend performing a Maze procedure in all patients with non-PAF because it is highly successful compared with the other procedures, which have remarkably low success rates for non-PAF (see Chapter 25).

When comparing the results of these various lesion sets for PAF and non-PAF, the assumption is that every individual lesion in a particular lesion set is contiguous (no gaps) and uniformly transmural. If this assumption is incorrect and one or more of the individual lesions is less than perfect, it is meaningless to compare one lesion set with another. The integrity of individual lesions is independent of the lesion pattern; rather, it depends on the choice of ablation device, the energy source, and the surgeon. Unipolar radiofrequency (RF) ablation devices are notoriously unreliable for the creation of transmural lesions off pump because of the cooling-sink of the cavitary blood. When possible, bipolar RF clamps should be used to create off-pump lesions, and either bipolar RF clamps or cryosurgery should be used under cardioplegic arrest. Because CABG does not require opening the LA but performance of a Maze procedure does, we tend to reserve the use of the Maze procedure for patients undergoing CABG with LSpAF or permanent AF.

Clinical assessment is also important in deciding the appropriate lesion set for patients with concomitant AF in CABG. A careful history should be taken to distinguish between the symptoms related to the AF and those related to the coronary artery disease. AF-related symptomatology can include complications such as stroke, systemic embolization, heart failure, anticoagulation-related problems, and aggravated angina pectoris. We recommend a Maze procedure for patients who have had multiple catheter ablation failures before presenting for CABG surgery. On the other hand, some patients are asymptomatic from their AF and are at elevated operative risk for CABG from comorbidities. In such patients, it may be prudent to perform LAAO alone to lessen their long-term risk of stroke while expediting the CABG procedure.

In non-PAF, the available options for AF ablation procedures are the same as those for PAF, but the expected results for a given lesion set can be profoundly different in non-PAF. For example, in non-PAF, a box lesion plus LAAO achieves only 30% efficacy compared with 80% efficacy in PAF (see Chapter 25). Thus we do not recommend performing either PVI alone or a box lesion alone for concomitant non-PAF. The optimal choices for AF intervention during CABG for non-PAF with better than a 30% success rate are a left-sided Maze procedure (70%) and a biatrial Maze procedure (>90%), both of which require opening the LA. The decision to open the LA should be based on clinical factors and surgical risk in the opinion of the operating surgeon. Several studies have demonstrated that adding a Maze procedure to CABG does not impact the operative mortality or operative morbidity rates of the procedure.[6,7] However, in cases of emergency CABG with shock, an LAAO alone is reasonable.

CANNULATION TECHNIQUES FOR CORONARY ARTERY BYPASS GRAFTING AND ATRIAL FIBRILLATION ABLATION

Typical cannulation for CABG surgery performed on cardiopulmonary bypass (CPB) is to place the arterial cannula in the distal ascending aorta and a single dual-stage venous return cannula in the right atrial appendage. Antegrade cardioplegia is administered through a line in the ascending aorta and retrograde cardioplegia through a cannula positioned into the coronary sinus through the right atrial wall. Cannulation for CPB in a CABG patient who requires concomitant AF ablation is modified depending on the concomitant AF ablation procedure to be performed. We recommend bicaval venous cannulation in patients undergoing AF ablation and CABG if a Maze procedure is to be performed (Fig. 26.1) because it does not interfere with the right atrial lesions, offers better exposure for the left atrial lesions, and keeps the atria colder (see Chapter 47, Figs. 47.8 and 47.9). Ideally, a right-angle venous return cannula is placed in the intrapericardial segment of the SVC approximately 2 cm cephalad to the SVC–right atrium (RA) junction, and a right-angle venous cannula is placed low and anterior in the RA near the level of the inferior vena cava (IVC)–RA junction. The retrograde cardioplegia cannula should be placed in the lower third of the RA where the diagonal atriotomy will be placed as a part of the right atrial T-lesion. If the planned AF ablation procedure does not require opening of either atrium, a single dual-stage venous return cannula is satisfactory.

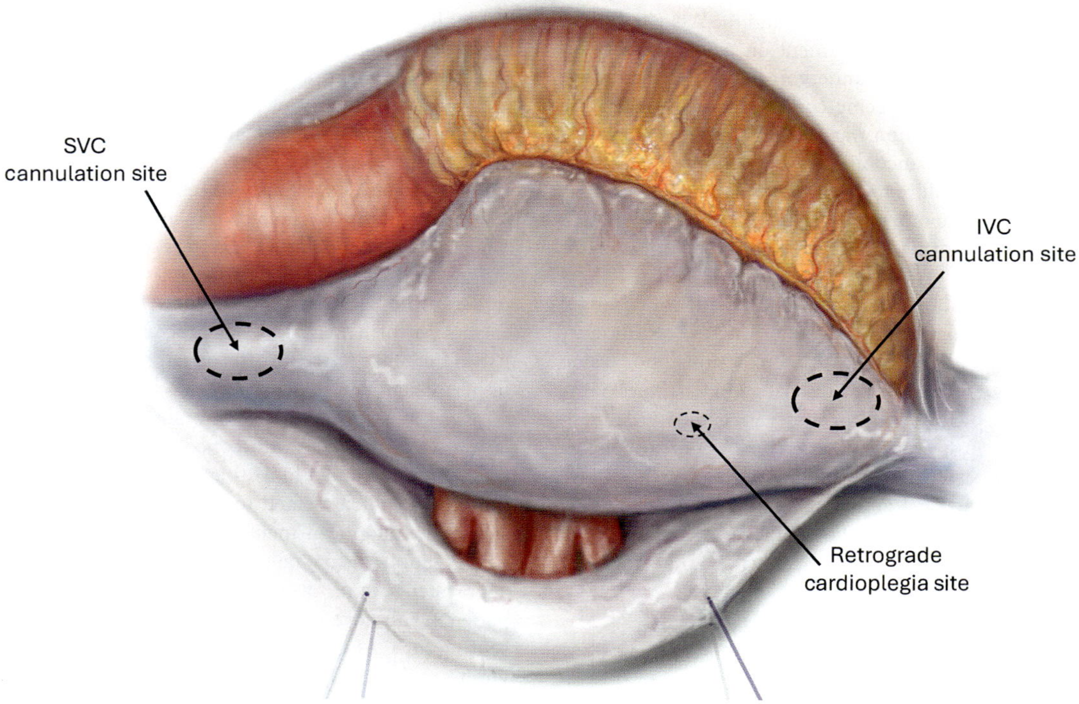

Fig. 26.1 Cannulation sites for cardiopulmonary bypass (CPB) in patients undergoing coronary artery bypass grafting (CABG) and atrial fibrillation (AF) ablation. Optimal venous cannulation sites for CPB and retrograde cardioplegia in CABG patients undergoing the concomitant ablation of AF using a Maze procedure. The superior vena cava (SVC) is cannulated anteriorly 2 cm above the SVC–right atrium (RA) junction. The inferior vena cava (IVC) is cannulated as low and anterior as possible. Bicaval cannulation at these two sites results in less interference with performance of the right atrial lesions and better exposure of the internal left atrium. The retrograde cardioplegia cannula is placed through a stab wound in the lateral RA in a position that will be included in the right atriotomy used to create the right atrial lesions.

CONDUCT OF THE COMBINED SURGICAL PROCEDURE

In LAAO alone with CABG, we recommend placing an epicardial LAAO device on the left atrial appendage (LAA) immediately after arresting the heart to enhance the ability to position it at the true base of the LAA to avoid leaving a stump. It is preferable to construct bypass grafts to the left circumflex artery, which avoid direct contact with the external LAAO device.

For concomitant AF ablation procedures that do not require opening the atria, we recommend performing the AF ablation procedure before constructing the coronary artery bypass grafts. After institution of CPB, Waterston's groove is developed to expose the LA wall. The oblique sinus is opened underneath the IVC, and a plane of dissection is established between the right superior pulmonary vein (PV) and the right pulmonary artery to allow complete encirclement of the right PVs. A bipolar RF clamp can then be applied well up onto the posteromedial LA to avoid RF injury of the orifices of the right PVs (Fig. 26.2). Next, the heart is arrested with antegrade and retrograde cardioplegia. The heart is then retracted to the right to expose the left PVs and LAA. (Fig. 26.3). The retraction of the heart in this manner stretches the

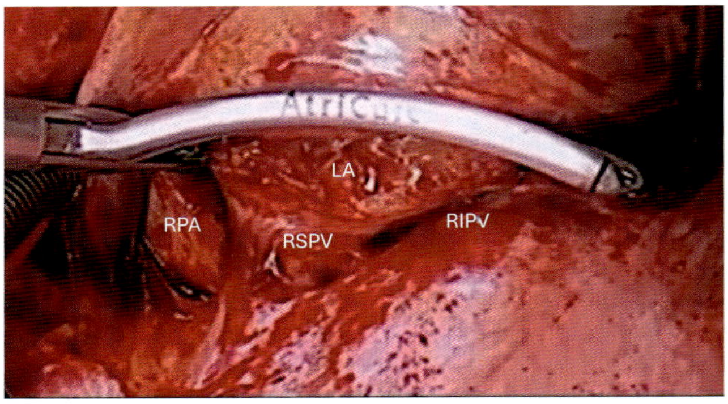

Fig. 26.2 Isolation of the right pulmonary veins (PVs). Waterston's groove separating the posterior right atrium (RA) and left atrium (LA) is first developed, and then a plane of dissection is established between the right superior pulmonary vein (RSPV) and the right pulmonary artery (RPA). A bipolar radiofrequency ablation clamp is then placed well up onto the LA as far as possible away from the PV orifices, and the right PVs are isolated. *RIPV,* Right inferior pulmonary vein.

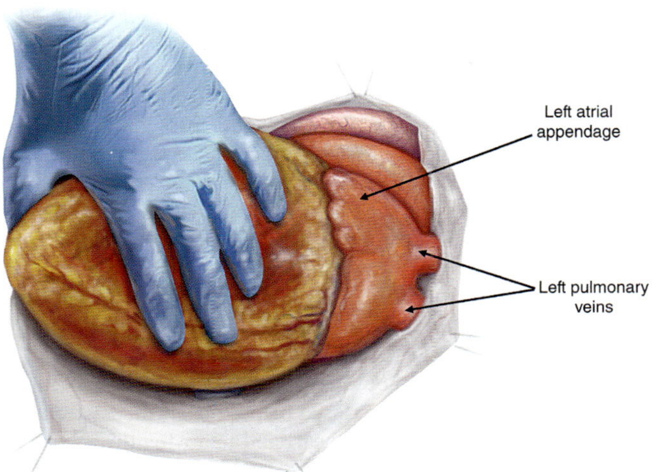

Fig. 26.3 Exposure of the left pulmonary veins (PVs) and the left atrial appendage (LAA). The heart is retracted to the patient's right to expose the left PVs and the LAA

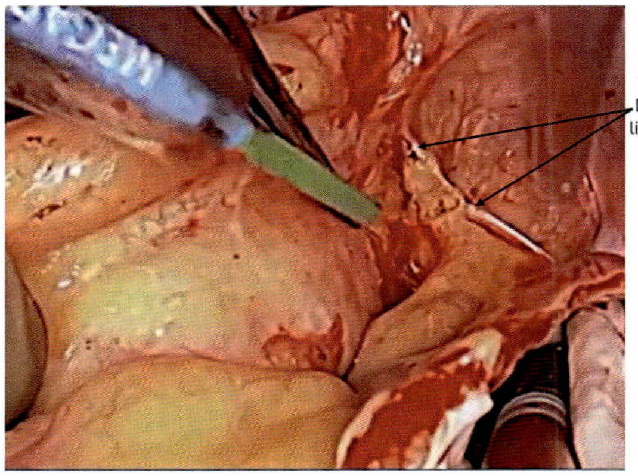

Fig. 26.4 Transection of the ligament of Marshall. The ligament of Marshall is exposed in its position just above the left superior pulmonary vein and is divided using an electrocautery.

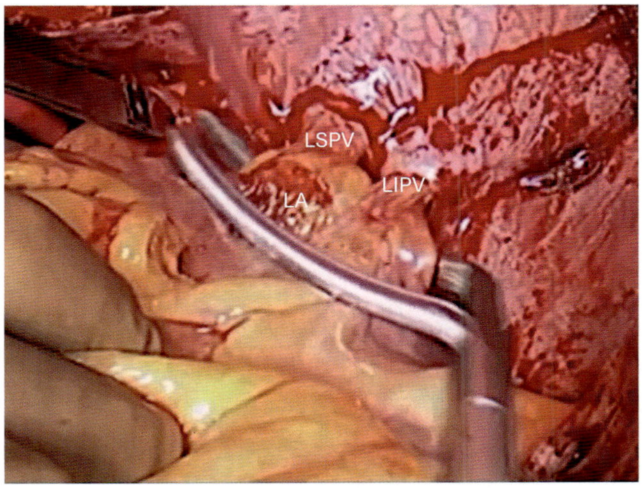

Fig. 26.5 Isolation of the left pulmonary veins (PVs). After transecting the Ligament of Marshall, dissection is continued just above the left superior pulmonary vein (LSPV) to divide the pericardial reflection and allow encirclement of the two left PVs. A bipolar radiofrequency ablation clamp is placed well up onto the left atrium (L)A as far away as possible from the PV orifices. *LIPV,* Left inferior pulmonary vein.

ligament of Marshall, making it easier to identify and divide with electrocautery (Fig. 26.4). The potential space between the left pulmonary artery and left upper PV is developed, and the left PVs are encircled. A bipolar RF clamp is then applied as high on the LA and away from the left PV orifices as possible (Fig. 26.5). An epicardial LAAO device is then applied to the base of the LAA to exclude it and to complete the ablation lesion set (Fig. 26.6). The advantage of performing the AF ablation before the CABG procedure is to avoid injury to the bypass grafts or coronary anastomoses during AF ablation.

The preceding paragraph describes how to do a PVI plus LAAO procedure for PAF during a CABG procedure (Fig. 26.7). This ablation procedure results in a maximum success rate of approximately 60% for concomitant PAF. It is preferable to convert the PVI lesions into a box lesion by adding roof and floor lines that connect the two pairs of PVs and isolates not only the PVs but also the posterior wall of the LA (Fig. 26.8). Because approximately 20% of the AF triggers in PAF reside in the posterior left atrial wall (see Chapter 25), the results of this box

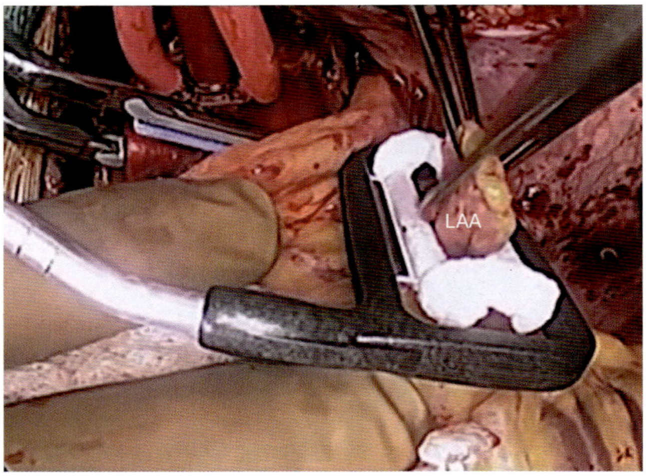

Fig. 26.6 Left atrial appendage occlusion (LAAO). The left atrial appendage (LAA) is closed epicardially with an epicardial LAAO device placed at its base.

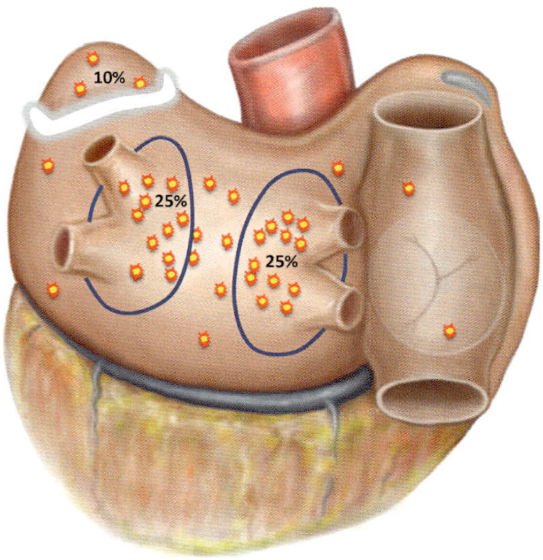

Fig. 26.7 Pulmonary vein isolation (PVI) plus left atrial appendage occlusion (LAAO) for concomitant paroxysmal atrial fibrillation (PAF). PVI results in the isolation of approximately 50% of the atrial triggers responsible for inducing individual episodes of PAF. It is assumed that the right and left pulmonary veins harbor approximately equal numbers of atrial triggers. LAAO with an epicardial LAAO device excludes another 10% of the atrial triggers that induce PAF. Thus the expectation is that a PVI plus LAAO procedure will reduce the episodes of PAF by approximately 60%.

lesion plus LAAO approach are in the range of 80% because the combined techniques isolate 80% of the known triggers of PAF. However as mentioned, the combined box lesion and LAAO interrupts only approximately 30% of the macro-reentrant drivers of non-PAF, so it not recommended in CABG patients with non-PAF.

Traditionally, the only way to create the roof and floor lines off-pump has been with a unipolar RF device such as the dual-electrode, unipolar Coolrail device (see Chapter 20, Fig. 20.10). Another

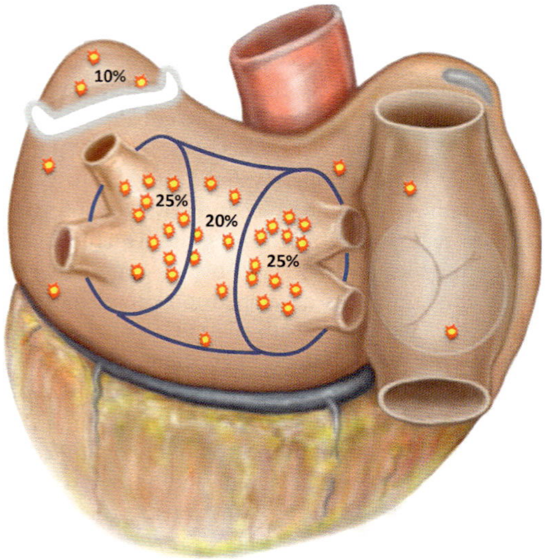

Fig. 26.8 Box lesion plus atrial appendage occlusion (LAAO) for concomitant paroxysmal atrial fibrillation (PAF). Adding roof and floor lesions to a pulmonary vein isolation (PVI) procedure results in the creation of a "box" that isolates another 20% of the atrial triggers that induce PAF. Thus the expectation is that a box lesion plus left LAAO procedure will reduce the episodes of PAF by approximately 80%.

method for creating the roof and floor lines using a bipolar RF clamp is described in Chapter 39 as the "Maze V" procedure. Recently, the bipolar RF "EnCompass" clamp (Atricure, Inc.) was introduced specifically for creating a box lesion without opening the LA, taking advantage of the superiority of bipolar RF ablation over unipolar RF ablation. Preclinical studies using the EnCompass clamp suggest that it is highly successful in creating a box lesion without opening the LA.[8] If this new clamp is as successful clinically as it is experimentally, it will represent a major step in improving the surgical treatment of concomitant PAF in patients undergoing CABG and aortic valve replacement.

As mentioned earlier, we recommend a Maze procedure in CABG patients with non-PAF. The specific technique that we use is the CryoMaze-III procedure described in Chapter 14 with the recent modification described in Chapter 15. An intraoperative transesophageal echocardiogram is used to check for the presence of a patent foramen ovale or LAA thrombus. The bicaval venous cannulae and the retrograde cardioplegia cannula are placed as described earlier. After arresting the heart, a saphenous vein bypass graft to the right coronary artery is often constructed (if one is necessary in the CABG procedure) to deliver additional antegrade cardioplegia. The heart is retracted to the right, and the external LAAO device is positioned in place. The LA is opened through Waterston's groove. The retrograde coronary sinus cannula is withdrawn to the ostium of the coronary sinus to allow creation of the coronary lesion externally. After closing the LA, the retrograde cardioplegia cannula is checked for positioning in the coronary sinus. The remaining bypass grafts are then completed and warm retrograde cardioplegia is given. If a PFO is present, the RA is opened and the PFO is closed before the aortic cross clamp is released. After de-airing the left heart and removing the aortic cross clamp, the right atrial cryolesions are created (see Chapter 13) during the rewarming and reperfusion period. Performing the right atrial lesions during the reperfusion and rewarming period adds no additional cross-clamp time and therefore has no detrimental effect on postpump cardiac or renal function.

RESULTS OF ATRIAL FIBRILLATION ABLATION IN PATIENTS UNDERGOING CORONARY ARTERY BYPASS GRAFTING

Concomitant AF ablation during CABG procedures has no impact on operative mortality or operative morbidity rates,[3–7] is effective in restoring sinus rhythm,[9,10] and reduces the risk of long-term death and stroke.[3,4] Two randomized controlled trials in CABG patients with preoperative AF have demonstrated the benefits of concomitant AF ablation. Pokushalov et al [11] randomized 35 patients with PAF undergoing CABG in which 18 patients received PVI using RF and 17 patients underwent CABG alone. At 18 months, 89% of patients in the CABG plus PVI group were free from AF compared with 47% in the CABG=only group (log-rank test, $P = .007$). Cherniavsky et al.[12] randomized 95 patients with persistent AF undergoing CABG, in which 61 patients received CABG with either PVI or left atrial RF ablation and 34 patients underwent CABG alone. Patients with concomitant AF ablation had greater than 80% freedom from AF compared with 44.1% in the CABG-only patients.

Three population-based studies have analyzed the long-term results of concomitant AF ablation in CABG patients. Rankin et al.[13] using the Medicare Standard Analytic File, showed an improved 2-year survival rate after AF ablation during CABG (hazard ratio [HR], 0.71; 95% confidence interval [CI], 0.52–0.97).[13] The authors also documented higher associated costs of concomitant AF ablation at 1 year but no difference in costs at 2 years.[14] In 2021, we reported the results of a propensity score-matched 2-year landmark analysis of an STS database, Medicare-linked study showing that survival was better with the addition of AF ablation in CABG patients (HR, 0.89; 95% CI, 0.82–0.97; $P = .0358$).[15] The study also showed a 13% reduction in stroke and systemic embolization at 5 years. In 2023, Cheng et al.[16] reported the results of the Taiwan registry study showing that concomitant AF ablation was associated with reduced risk of death in the entire cardiac surgery group (HR, 0.75; 95% CI, 0.69–0.81) and in a subset analysis of CABG only patients ($P = .0176$).[16]

SUMMARY

AF is common in patients undergoing CABG. Randomized clinical trials and population-based studies in CABG patients with AF have clearly demonstrated the benefit of concomitant AF ablation. The Maze procedure is the most effective surgical procedure for concomitant AF ablation, but it requires that the LA be opened, which is not a part of a CABG procedure. Therefore, a box lesion plus LAAO that isolates up to 80% of the atrial triggers without opening the LA is reasonable in patients with PAF but not in patients with non-PAF. At a minimum, patients with AF who undergo CABG should receive an epicardial LAAO device to reduce the risk of stroke even if AF ablation is omitted because of concerns of surgical risk.

REFERENCES

1. Malaisrie SC, McCarthy PM, Kruse J, et al. Burden of preoperative atrial fibrillation in patients undergoing coronary artery bypass grafting. *J Thor Cardiovasc Surg*. 2018;155(6):2358–2367.
2. McCarthy PM, Davidson CJ, Kruse J, et al. Prevalence of atrial fibrillation before cardiac surgery and factors associated with concomitant ablation. *J Thor Cardiovasc Surg*. 2020;159(6):2245–2253.
3. Badhwar V, Rankin JS, Damiano RJ Jr, et al. The society of thoracic surgeons 2017 clinical practice guidelines for the surgical treatment of atrial fibrillation. *Ann Thorac Surg*. 2017;103(1):329–341.
4. Ad N, Damiano RJ Jr, Badhwar V, et al. Expert consensus guidelines: examining surgical ablation for atrial fibrillation. *J Thorac Cardiovasc Surg*. 2017;153(6):1330–1354.
5. Wyler von Ballmoos MC, Hui DS, Mehaffey JH, et al. The society of thoracic surgeons 2023 clinical practice guidelines for the surgical treatment of atrial fibrillation. *Ann Thorac Surg*. 2024. S0003-497(24)00057-2. https://doi.org/10.1016/j.athoracsur.2024.01.007.
6. Ad N, Henry L, Hunt S, Holmes SD. Do we increase the operative risk by adding the Cox Maze III procedure to aortic valve replacement and coronary artery bypass surgery? *J Thor Cardiovasc Surg*. 2012;143(4):936–944.
7. Al-Amassi T, Kimmaliardjuk D-M, Dagenais C, Bourke M, Lam B-K, Rubens FD. Should we ablate atrial fibrillation during coronary artery bypass grafting and aortic valve replacement? *Ann Thorac Surg*. 2017;104:515–522.
8. Yates T-A, McGilvvray M, Razo N, et al. Efficacy of a novel bipolar radiofrequency clamp: an acute porcine model. *Innovations*. 2022;17(5):409–415.
9. Louagi Y, Buche M, Eucher P, et al. Improved patient survival with concomitant Cox Maze III procedure compared with heart surgery alone. *Ann Thorac Surg*. 2009;87(2):440–446.
10. Forlani S, De Paulis R, Guerrieri WL, et al. Conversion to sinus rhythm by ablation improves quality of life in patients submitted to mitral valve surgery. *Ann Thorac Surg*. 2006;81(3):863–867.
11. Pokushalov E, Romanov A, Corbucci G, Cherniavsky A, Karasdov A. Benefit of ablation of first diagnosed paroxysmal atrial fibrillation during coronary artery bypass grafting: a pilot study. *Eur J Cardiothorac Surg*. 2012;41(3):556–560.
12. Cherniavsky A, Kareva Y, Pak I, et al. Assessment of results of surgical treatment for persistent atrial fibrillation during coronary artery bypass grafting using implantable loop recorders. *Interact Cardiovasc Thorac Surg*. 2014;18(6):727–731.
13. Rankin JS, Lerner DJ, Braid-Forbes MJ, McCrea MM, Badhwar V. Surgical ablation of atrial fibrillation concomitant to coronary artery bypass grafting provides cost-effective mortality reduction. *J Thor Cardiovasc Surgery*. 2020;160(3):675–686.
14. Rankin JS, Lerner DJ, Braid-Forbes MJ, Ferguson MA, Badhwar V. One-year mortality and costs associated with surgical ablation for atrial fibrillation concomitant to coronary artery bypass grafting. *Eur J Cardiothorac Surg*. 2017;52(3):471–477.
15. Malaisrie SC, McCarthy PM, Kruse J, et al. Ablation of atrial fibrillation during coronary artery bypass grafting: late outcomes in a Medicare population. *J Thorac Cardiovasc Surg*. 2021;161(4):1251–1261.
16. Cheng Y-T, Huang Y-T, Tu H-T, et al. Long-term outcomes of concomitant surgical ablation for atrial fibrillation. *Ann Thorac Surg*. 2023;116(2):297–305.

27

How I do it: Atrial Fibrillation Ablation with Mitral Valve Surgery plus/minus Tricuspid Valve Surgery and Coronary Artery Bypass Grafting

Patrick M. McCarthy

CHAPTER OUTLINE

INTRODUCTION

The goals of concomitant treatment of atrial fibrillation (AF) are to achieve high efficacy as measured by late freedom from AF and stroke, to minimize morbidity, and to be efficient so as not to prolong the operative time.[1] When we achieve these goals, we can extend treatment to as many patients as possible. If the procedure is safe, effective, and efficient, then it should be uniformly adopted as recommended by the Society of Thoracic Surgeons Guidelines.[2] Concomitant left atrial appendage occlusion (LAAO) has become the standard of care and should be considered the most basic addition to the primary cardiac operation.[1–3] Surgical ablation of AF is equally important and adds a late survival advantage to LAAO alone in all types of AF, including paroxysmal AF.[4–6] It is easier to perform LAAO and concomitant ablation in operations with an open left atrium (LA), generally mitral valve (MV) surgery, than in those in which the LA is not opened (LA closed) such as coronary artery bypass (CAB), aortic valve replacement, and aortic aneurysms. The operations with the LA closed are covered in other chapters (see Chapters 26 and 29). This chapter focuses on the details of MV operations with surgical ablation and LAAO. It is common for MV operations to include tricuspid valve operations and CAB. We discuss these additional procedures as well. We report the technique of the modified CryoMaze-III procedure,[7,8] which includes epicardial clip closure of the left atrial appendage (LAA).[9,10]

SETUP AND EXPOSURE

The operation is generally performed through a small incision median sternotomy and can be done through a lower or upper hemisternotomy. It also can be performed through a right thoracotomy, with or without use of a robotic assistance, although placement of the LAA clip can be more challenging through a thoracotomy. This chapter is written as if through a sternotomy approach, and surgeons can adapt the technique to another approach if desired. The technique has been described before.[10]

Prepping and draping the patient are routine. Transesophageal echocardiography (TEE) is standard, and routine measurements are made for the MV repair (length of A2; distance between the septum and coaptation point of the mitral leaflets in systole).[11] Routine examination of all valves, ventricular function, and left ventricular dimensions are performed. The preoperative examination in patients with AF includes LAA thrombus and "smoke" and left atrial and right atrial dimensions with close attention to tricuspid diameter and grade of tricuspid regurgitation. A Swan-Ganz catheter is optional in patients with normal biventricular function and normal preoperative pulmonary artery pressures. A percutaneous wire is placed in the femoral vein (typically on the right) and advanced into the right atrium (RA). If needed for CAB, the saphenous vein is harvested using an endoscopic approach. After sternotomy, the left internal mammary artery (LIMA) is prepared for bypass grafting if desired. The patient is given therapeutic doses of heparin, and the pericardium is opened. The ascending aorta is cannulated in the standard fashion in the distal ascending aorta. A 28-Fr percutaneous multihole venous cannula is advanced from the femoral vein. It is positioned both with the guidance of TEE and by palpation of the RA–inferior vena cava (RA-IVC) junction. The tip of the cannula should be 1 or 2 cm caudal to the junction. Cardiopulmonary bypass with vacuum assistance is initiated, and a 26-Fr right-angle superior vena cava (SVC) cannula is placed. Retrograde cardioplegia is not used; therefore, for an "LA-only" ablation, there are no incision, no perforation, no suturing, and no significant manipulation of the RA. A caval tape is placed around the RA-IVC junction, pulled up, and attached to the drapes inferiorly. This is a standard procedure to optimize MV exposure at the medial commissure. No epicardial dissection is required for a modified CryoMaze-III operation.

The cross-clamp is applied, and 1500 cc of Del Nido cardioplegia is given antegrade (200 cc more if there is mild aortic insufficiency). Cold saline (no ice) is poured on the right ventricle. The LA is opened in the interatrial groove as cardioplegia is infusing. The incision is extended below the SVC and below the IVC as is standard for mitral surgery. No dissection along the left atrial dome is needed to perform the modified CryoMaze-III procedure.

LEFT ATRIAL APPENDAGE OCCLUSION AND LEFT ATRIAL ABLATION

When cardioplegia is complete, the heart is lifted out of the pericardium toward the right chest and held by the surgeon's left hand with a sponge (Fig. 27.1). The LAA is readily visible and collapsed because the LA is open. In the right hand, the surgeon takes a 35-mm AtriClip ACH2

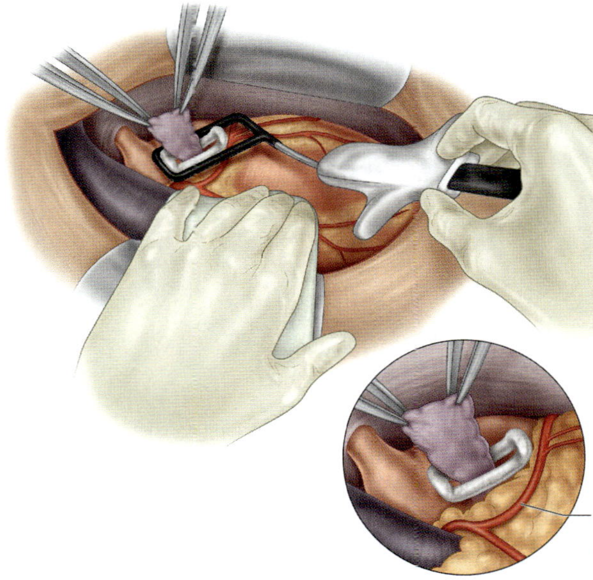

Fig. 27.1 When cardioplegia is complete and the left atrium (LA) is open, the left ventricle is elevated and tipped to the patient's right to expose the left atrial appendage (LAA). The LAA is empty, like a deflated balloon, because the LA is open. The surgeon takes a 35-mm AtriClip and squeezes to open the clip for positioning over the LAA while an assistant uses forceps to pull the LAA into the clip and align at the base. After releasing tension on the clip handle, visual confirmation and repositioning are performed to achieve symmetrical placement at least 2 mm from the circumflex artery, and the clip is at the LAA base. The sutures are cut, and the handle is removed to release the clip. The clip will cause tissue necrosis and electrical isolation of the LAA.

(AtriCure, Inc.) and opens the clip by squeezing the handle. Because the LAA is deflated, there is no need to measure the base of the appendage. It is like a deflated balloon, and the 35-mm clip can accommodate even a large LAA when it is empty. The clip is opened (the surgeon squeezes the handle) and positioned so the assistant can pull the LAA into the clip using two forceps as the surgeon lowers the clip to the base of the LAA. The surgeon releases tension on the handle to close the clip and inspects the base of the clip. Visually, the surgeon confirms it is at least 2 mm away from the circumflex coronary artery, which is typically visible near the base of the appendage (Fig. 27.1, *inset*). The surgeon and assistant also inspect the clip placement to look for symmetry. One side or the other may not be as low as desired on the LAA. If so, the clip is reopened and repositioned with traction from the assistant. Most often repositioning is not necessary because placement is very straightforward. When both are satisfied with the clip position, the assistant cuts the sutures, and the surgeon removes the handle to release the clip. The heart is placed back in the pericardium. On average, this whole process from the time of lifting the heart, positioning and releasing the clip, removing the handle, and replacing the heart in the pericardium takes less than 2 minutes.

If CAB is to be performed with saphenous vein grafts, then the distal anastomoses are performed at this time. This allows for redosing of cardioplegia down the vein graft if desired. The LIMA to left anterior descending (LAD) anastomosis can be performed at this point, or more often, just before removing the cross-clamp. After placing the clip (and CAB distals), attention is returned to the LA. Two self-retaining retractor blades are placed in the same position for the modified CryoMaze-III procedure as for mitral exposure.

Our modification of the minimally invasive CryoMaze-III procedure recreates all of the lesions of the original minimally invasive CryoMaze-III lesion set (see Chapter 14), which in turn recreated the lesion pattern of the original cut-and-sew Maze-III procedure (see Chapter 12) (Fig. 27.2).[10] However, all of these lesions are created in our

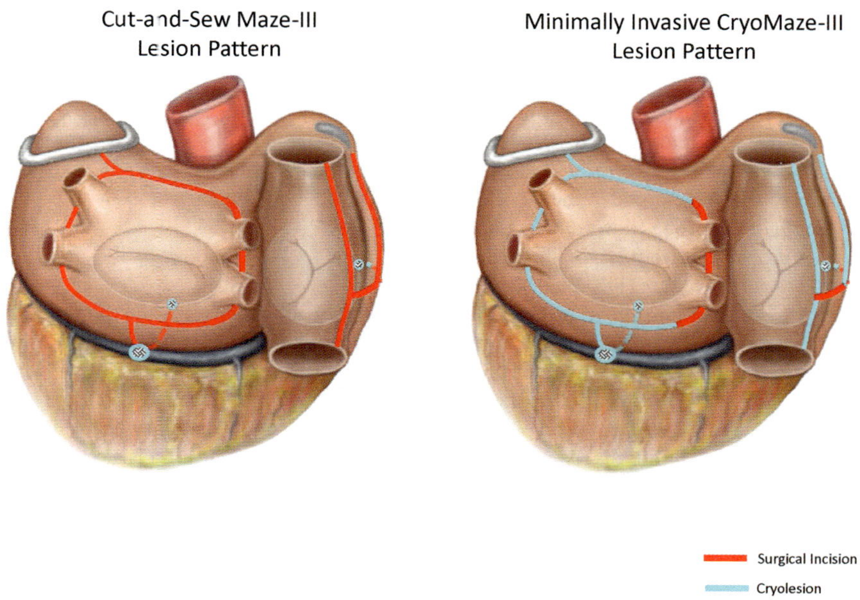

Fig. 27.2 (A) Cut-and-sew Maze-III lesion pattern. Virtually all of the lesions of the original cut-and-sew Maze-III procedure were performed using a knife and/or scissors *(red lines)*. However, there were several specific places in the lesion pattern where cryosurgery was used, those being at the mitral and tricuspid annuli and across the coronary sinus. (B) Minimally invasive CryoMaze-III lesion pattern. In the mid-1990s, the minimally invasive CryoMaze-III procedure replaced the original cut-and-sew Maze-III procedure, but the lesion patterns remained identical. However, with the exception of the two atriotromies performed for exposure purposes, all of the lesions in the CryoMaze-III procedure were performed using nondisposable linear cryoprobes *(pale cyan lines)*. When the modern disposable, flexible, linear cryoprobes became available, they became the tools used to perform the minimally invasive CryoMaze-III procedure.

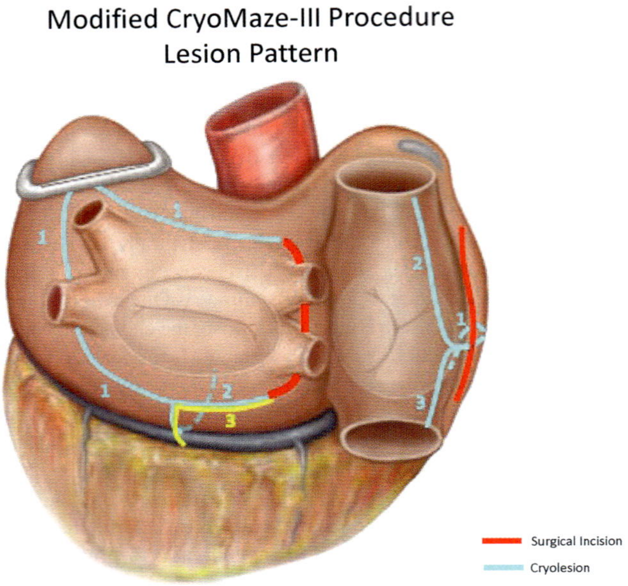

Fig. 27.3 Modified CryoMaze-III procedure lesion pattern. The modified CryoMaze-III procedure was developed to make the CryoMaze-III procedure quicker and easier to perform. The modern long, flexible, linear cryoprobes can be formed into virtually any desirable shape, which allowed us to use them to create all of the Maze-III lesion pattern with only three cryoablation applications in the left atrium and three cryoablation applications in the right atrium. Comparing this figure with Fig. 27.2 confirms that all of the biatrial Maze-III lesions can be created with these six cryoablation applications.

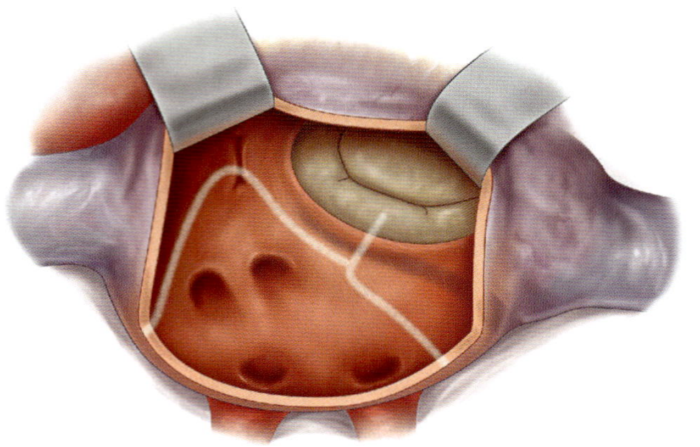

Fig. 27.4 The modified CryoMaze III procedure consists of three left atrial ablations that reproduce the Cox Maze III lesion set. The cryoablation lines must be transmural, contiguous, and anchored to tissue that cannot conduct an electrical wavefront such as the valve annulus. The lesion set, as drawn, reproduces the box lesion, mitral isthmus line, and coronary sinus ablation (not pictured). The left atrial appendage (LAA) has been closed with an epicardial AtriClip, which induces left atrial necrosis; therefore, the LAA is electrically silent. The ablation line across the dome of the left atrium also crosses the base of the LAA, so there is no need for a separate ablation line to the LAA.

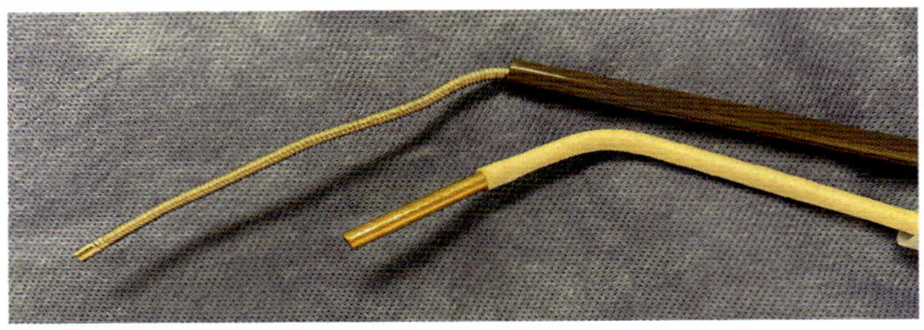

Fig. 27.5 The disposable 10-cm flexible cryoprobes *(top)* have several advantages over the older, shorter, reusable cryoprobes *(bottom)*. The disposable cryoprobe can easily and rapidly be bent into the proper form for each ablation. It can also be manipulated into a variety of shapes. Pressure on the probe or outside the atrium, pushing atrial tissue onto the probe, allows long, continuous ablation lines with no gaps. The longer length of the probe allows for the creation of long ablation lines with fewer applications than the reusable probes can provide.

modification with only three cryoablation applications in the LA and three cryoablation applications in the RA (Fig. 27.3). This modification simplifies the procedure and shortens the time needed to create the entire biatrial Maze-III lesion pattern. As in all previous iterations of the Maze procedure, the ablation lines should be uniformly transmural, contiguous (no gaps), and anchored to an area that cannot conduct an electrical wavefront (mitral or tricuspid annulus, or SVC/IVC in the RA) (Fig. 27.4). The 10-cm flexible cryoprobe (AtriCure Cryo Flex) can achieve these goals, and the ability to shape the probe to the atrial wall makes it easy to use. The long length of the probe allows a longer ablation line than the shorter reusable probes that were originally used for arrhythmia surgery, including the Maze procedure (Fig. 27.5).

The first ablation line outlines the superior portion of the box lesion around the pulmonary veins (PVs) and the LAA (Fig. 27.6). It covers the dome of the LAA and the base of the LAA, and the tip of the probe is usually (depending on LA size) about at the level of P2. For the first line, the probe is bent into a C shape. The base of the probe is positioned at the superior extent of the atriotomy under the SVC. The gentle curve of the probe covers the dome of the LA and, importantly, the LAA. The portion of the probe near the distal end extends along the left side of the LA, midway between the PVs and the mitral annulus. With a small LA, the tip of the probe may extend to P3. The probe may be quickly reshaped and repositioned at the distal end so that it is in good atrial contact and in the correct position between the PVs and mitral annulus. The surgeon pushes the probe into contact with the atrial wall with gentle pressure. Forceps or a sucker tip may help maintain contact and eliminate a small tissue fold. When the probe is in good position, a 3-minute freeze is begun. The probe quickly adheres to the tissue. The surgeon may release the forceps holding the probe in place because the probe sticks to the tissue rapidly and will not move. The assistant can hold the probe in place while the surgeon begins to inspect the MV, so no cross-clamp time is wasted. At 3 minutes the probe is thawed and removed from the tissue. It is important to confirm visually that there were no small folds that could leave a gap in the cryolesion. If so, a "spot" freeze on the gap may be needed, although this is unusual.

The second application is also 3 minutes and completes the box lesion and the line to the MV annulus (Fig. 27.7). The atrial wall is more prone to have a fold in this location, especially if the LA is very dilated. Avoiding a tissue fold and subsequent gap may be more difficult than the first ablation line across the dome. There are a variety of ways to reduce the amount of folding. Applying firm pressure when the probe is in contact with the atrium may remove the fold. Using a sucker tip or forceps and pushing the tissue against the probe from the epicardial side of the tissue may work. A sponge on the epicardial side may also help. Sometimes releasing the inferior retractor blade may provide enough tissue flexibility so there is uniformly good contact. The surgeon may have to be creative to avoid a fold. Again, if one is seen after the probe has been removed, then a spot freeze at the gap should

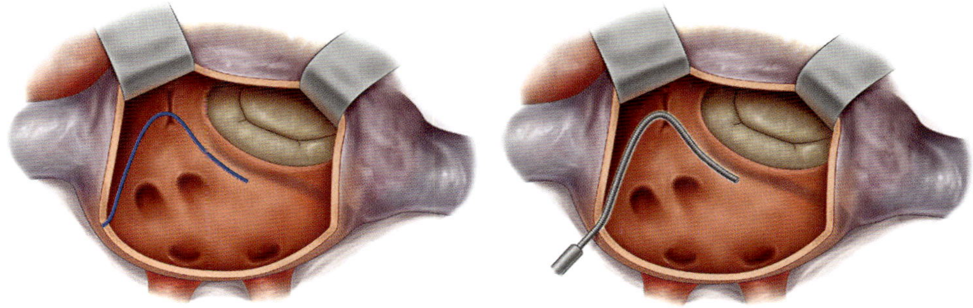

A B

Fig. 27.6 (A) The proper placement of the first lesion *(blue line)* is shown with the probe on the endocardial surface crossing the base of the clipped atrial appendage, which prevents a macro-reentrant circuit from using the bridge (Coumadin ridge) between the left atrial appendage and box lesion. (B) The probe is bent into a C shape to allow ablation across the dome of the left atrium (LA), base of the appendage, and to the mid-P2 (with a small LA, it may extend to P3). The proximal part of the probe is placed adjacent to the superior portion of the atriotomy. The probe can be reshaped as needed to get proper placement (no tissue folds), and contact is enhanced by applying pressure on the probe, such as with pickups or a sucker tip. When satisfied there are no gaps, a 3-minute freeze is performed. The cryolesion is then inspected for any gaps that might require further ablation.

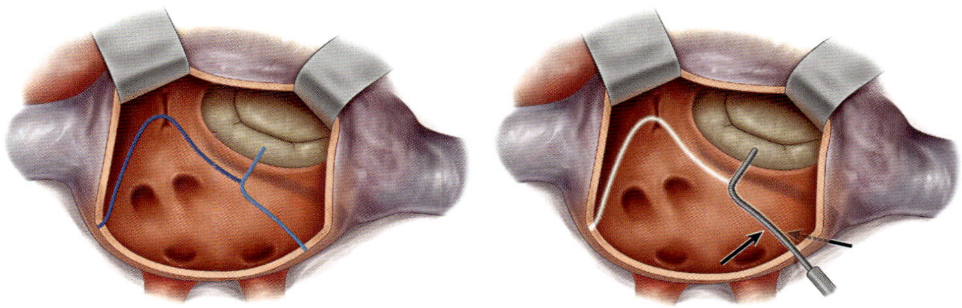

A B

Fig. 27.7 The second line completes the box lesion on the endocardial surface with the distal 2 cm of the probe bent to connect to the mitral annulus (A). It is important that this lesion overlap the end of the prior lesion (typically at P2); otherwise, there could be a gap. The lesion must be placed before a mitral ring or valve is placed. If it is a reoperation, the ring or valve must be removed before the mitral isthmus lesion is applied. Tissue folds are reduced by using firm pressure on the probe using forceps or sucker tip to push the probe against the endocardial surface (B, *arrows*). Alternatively, atrial tissue can be pushed against the probe with pressure from the epicardial surface. The probe can be held by an assistant as it sticks to the tissue. This allows the surgeon to inspect the valve to reduce cross clamp time during the 3-minute lesion. Again, any gaps should be treated with a spot freeze.

be placed. The probe is typically straight across the inferior LA, but at the distal end it is bent for about 2 cm so that it crosses the mitral isthmus onto the base of the MV leaflet (see Fig. 27.7B). The resulting ablation line completes the box lesion and extends across the annulus onto the leaflet.

The timing of ablation is important and must be done before mitral repair or replacement. If there is a prosthesis on the annulus, then the surgeon will not be able to ablate all the way to the annulus, which can lead to atrial flutter. Similarly, if this is a reoperation with a mitral prosthesis, then the ring or valve must be removed before the mitral isthmus lesion.

The third lesion is a spot lesion on the coronary sinus (CS) and is placed on the epicardium through the oblique sinus that was opened to place the IVC tape (Fig. 27.8). The freeze from the second lesion leaves ice on the epicardial surface of the LA and may already be full thickness across the CS. Because atrial flutter across the CS is potentially very symptomatic and difficult to treat later with catheter ablation, we add a 2-minute ablation just below the second lesion.

The three left atrial modified CryoMaze III lesions have recreated the Cox Maze-III lesion set; therefore, the pattern of the original cut-and-sew Cox Maze-III lesion pattern as well (see Figs. 27.2 and 27.3). The box lesion is the same and electrically isolates the four PVs and the intervening posterior wall of the LA. The LAA was originally excised in the cut-and-sew operation and an ablation line placed from the box lesion to the base of the LAA.[12] At the Cleveland Clinic, we excised the entire LAA as part of the box lesion so there was no additional line needed. When the LAA has been treated with an AtriClip, it is electrically isolated.[13] Therefore, in the CryoMaze-III procedure and in our modification of it, the clip across the base of the LAA combined with lesion number 1 replaces the old line to the LAA. CS and mitral annular lines done with cryoablation are in the same locations as the classic Cox Maze-III lesion set.

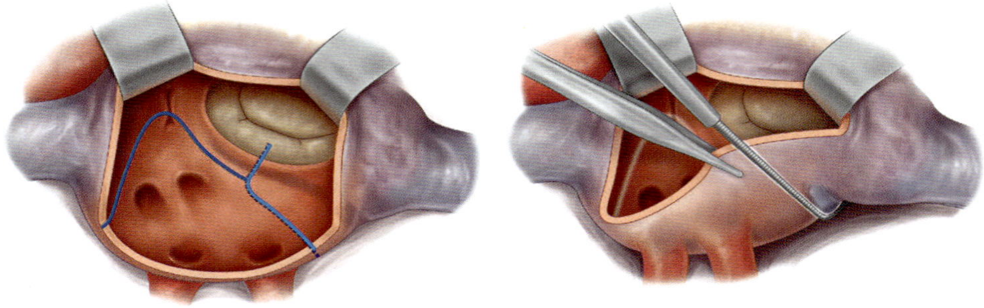

A B

Fig. 27.8 (A) The third and final left atrial lesion is placed epicardially through the oblique sinus (which was opened to place the inferior vena cava tape). The probe does not need to be reshaped, as the intention is to align this lesion directly under the second endocardial lesion and across the coronary sinus (CS). It is important to overlap lesions 2 and 3 to prevent gaps, which could allow the formation of re-entry conduction circuits. (B) If a retrograde cardioplegia catheter is used, it can be partially withdrawn to allow proper lesion placement. Because the CS was partially frozen with the second lesion (an epicardial iceball may be visible), the overlapping epicardial lesion is ablated for only 2 minutes. After this freeze, attention turns to the mitral valve, away from the frozen area until the treated areas are completely thawed.

RIGHT ATRIAL ABLATION

Right atrial ablation can be performed with the cross-clamp on or off pump. We prefer to do the initial ablation from the right atriotomy to the tricuspid annulus with the cross-clamp on because blood return from the CS may obscure the field and warm the cryoprobe. However, when the cross-clamp is off, it is not difficult to control the CS return with a basket and pump sucker when the IVC and SVC lines are placed.

The proper locations of the right atriotomy and the ablation lines are important to reduce sinus node dysfunction (Fig. 27.9). No ablation lines are near the atrioventricular node, so heart block is not caused by properly placed Maze lesions (see Chapter 21). Sinus node function is dependent on more than the anatomic sinoatrial (SA) node at the lateral junction of the RA and SVC. The surrounding lateral right atrial wall is the location of the atrial pacemaker complex (APC),[14,15] which is not clearly delineated by anatomic structures. For tricuspid valve surgery, we prefer a near-horizontal incision so the self-retaining retractor blades have enough tissue to stay in position. However, a vertical right atriotomy is also acceptable, but it should be inferior to the APC.

The first right atrial ablation line (see Fig. 27.9) is from the right atriotomy to the tricuspid annulus at the posterior leaflet. We prefer to ablate along the tricuspid annulus for 1 to 2 cm. The probe is roughly straight at this point, and pulling the RA tissue easily removes any folds. The right atrial tissue is thinner than the left atrial tissue, so a 2-minute freeze is acceptable in the RA. After the ablation to the tricuspid annulus, the probe is directed from the atriotomy into the IVC (Fig. 27.10). The final lesion is placed from the right atriotomy to the SVC (Fig. 27.11). The probe should pass below the SA node and far posterior in the RA. The probe is placed on the endocardial side of the crista terminalis, which may be as much as 1 cm thick. Often it will not freeze full thickness with only an endocardial freeze, even after 3 minutes (Fig. 27.12A). Rather than applying the probe longer, it is

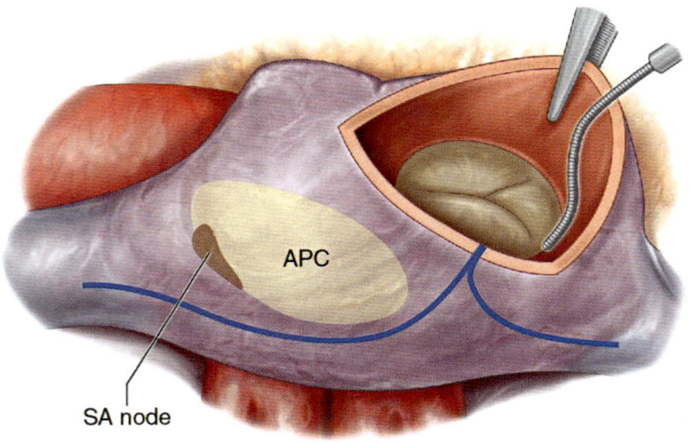

Fig. 27.9 Most often right-side ablation is performed along with tricuspid valve repair through a nearly horizontal right atriotomy. For all right atrial ablations, it is important to be aware of the atrial pacemaker complex (APC) which extends inferiorly from the sinoatrial (SA) node (see Chapter 1, Fig. 1.9). Incisions, trauma, and ablation in this area can lead to sinus node dysfunction. The first ablation is typically performed while the cross-clamp is on for convenience to avoid warm coronary sinus blood to contact the cryoablation lesion. This first ablation extends from the right atriotomy to the tricuspid annulus and along the posterior leaflet for approximately 1 cm. There is no need for a second tricuspid annular lesion because the potential macro-reentrant circuit needs to be prevented by only one lesion to the tricuspid valve.

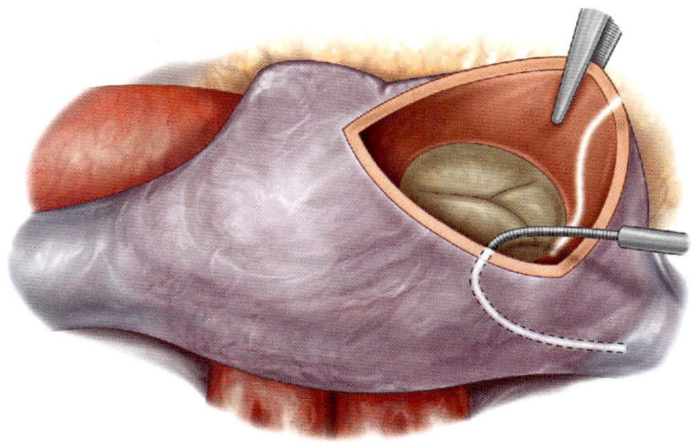

Fig. 27.10 The next lesion is simple and is placed from the right atriotomy to the inferior vena cava (IVC). It should be extended to the posterior part of the right atrium before curving down into the IVC orifice. This is thin tissue that rapidly freezes.

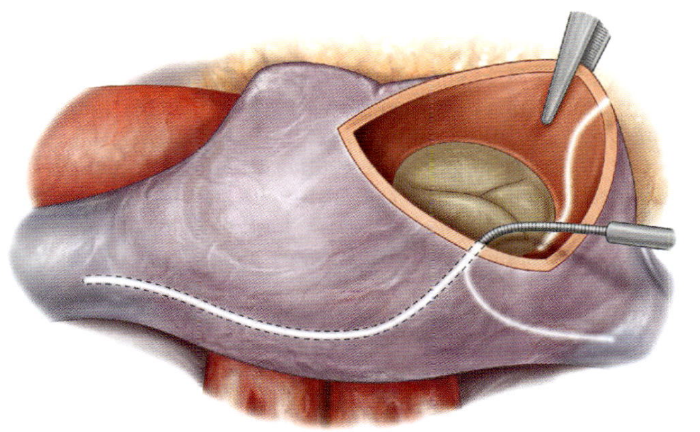

Fig. 27.11 The third and final right atrial cryolesion extends from the right atriotomy, posteriorly to avoid the atrial pacemaker complex, and then cephalad into the superior vena cava as diagrammed.

easy to place the probe on the epicardium over the crista terminalis for another 1 or 2 minutes (Fig. 27.12B). When freezing the IVC and SVC, ablation lines take care to assure the probe is not in contact with the pericardium because the right phrenic nerve is at that level. It is helpful to have an assistant hold a sucker or forceps to keep the pericardium and phrenic nerve away from the probe. After the right atrial ablation, the tricuspid valve is repaired in the usual fashion. Before weaning from bypass, TEE is used to measure the LAA stump and confirm it is less than 10 mm and that there is no flow across the base of the AtriClip into the LAA (Fig. 27.13). In personal experience with approximately 200 clip applications, this has not happened.

REOPERATIONS

Patients with prior cardiac surgery need a different approach for the LAA closure.[1] The left and right atrial ablation is performed the same way. However, pericardial adhesions make LAA clip placement much more difficult, and in an operation with a patent LIMA-LAD it is too dangerous to dissect out the LAA. The LAA can be closed from within the LA before ablation. We use suture closure for this. The technique described by Badhwar and coworkers[16] using a double-layer internal closure seems to be a good option, although we have not yet seen late clinical results with this technique.

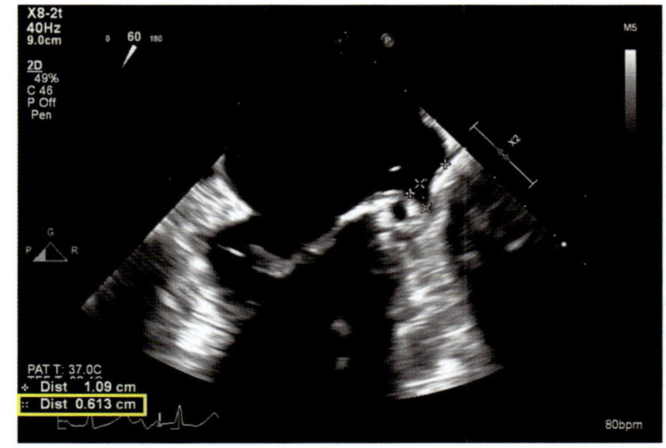

Fig. 27.13 Measurement of the residual left atrial appendage (LAA) stump after LAA clip closure. After weaning from cardiopulmonary bypass, transesophageal echocardiography should be used to confirm appropriate placement of the LAA occlusion clip. The depth of the "stump" can be measured and should be less than 10 mm. This is easily achieved when applying the clip to a completely empty LAA while the left atrium is open for mitral surgery. The horizontal reference line is drawn from the level of the left circumflex artery to the Coumadin ridge, marking the ostium of the appendage. The measurement of the greatest depth *(yellow)* between the ostium and the clip shows a stump of 6 mm. (Courtesy Dr. Kiran Belani, MD.)

RESULTS

Northwestern University data from 2012 indicated improved late survival with concomitant AF ablation in all types of AF.[17] Therefore, we routinely treated concomitant AF in all mitral patients starting in 2013. The patient characteristics, brief review of the procedure, and early and midterm results have been published.[9] All mitral patients with preoperative AF ($n = 277$) were treated with concomitant ablation with no exceptions for AF duration or type, LA size, or type of mitral surgery. These patients were propensity matched to mitral patients who underwent surgery by the same surgeon (PMM) with 161 patients in each group. The MV surgery with AF ablation group had only 10.5-minute longer cross-clamp time and 13.4-minute longer bypass time, confirming the efficiency of the procedure. There were no differences in 30-day mortality or morbidity rates, including pacemaker use and renal dysfunction, confirming there was no added morbidity from adding the modified CryoMaze-III procedure. Postoperative strokes were lower in

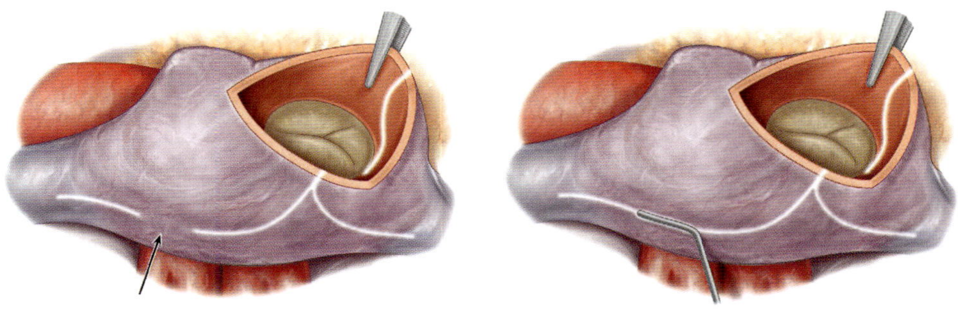

A B

Fig. 27.12 The third right atrial lesion crosses the crista terminalis, which in some cases is quite thick (1 cm) and will not be entirely frozen with a transmural lesion. (A) In this case, after the 2-minute freeze, a gap may be evident *(arrow)* on the epicardium inferior to the sinoatrial node. (B) If so, a spot lesion should be applied that connects the incomplete line. The spot lesion must overlap the ablation lines on either side of the gap.

the modified CryoMaze-III group at 30 days (5% versus 0.6%; $P = .018$). Five-year freedom from stroke was similar in both groups (98.3% CryoMaze-III versus 97.4% control). Late survival was no different between groups, as in prior reports, showing survival returned to normal for AF treated patients.[17] In a unique new analysis, the modified CryoMaze-III group had the same late survival rate as a control age- and sex-matched patient population from the Centers for Disease Control and Prevention database. The rate of late freedom from AF off antiarrhythmics was 77% for the entire group. However, when patients with only a 3-minute freeze for the box lesion were included (our standard approach since 2018), the rate of 12-month freedom from AF off antiarrhythmics was 90%. In subsequent publications for the 3-minute freeze group, the rates of 2- and 3-year freedom from AF off antiarrhythmics were 89% and 82%, respectively.[1]

SUMMARY

Surgeons have been reluctant to routinely add concomitant AF ablation and LAA occlusion despite a Class I indication. We are optimistic that a straightforward procedure for LAA clipping with ablation, such as our modified CryoMaze-III procedure, will encourage them that the operation poses no increased perioperative risk, can be performed without clinically significant increases in operative times, has excellent late survival and freedom from stroke and AF, and is easy to learn. We hope this significantly increases the adoption of this procedure.

REFERENCES

1. McCarthy PM, Cox JL. Practical approaches to concomitant surgical ablation of atrial fibrillation: matching the ablation to the patient. *J Thorac Cardiovasc Surg*. 2025;169(3):907–915.
2. Wyler von Ballmoos MC, Hui DS, Mehaffey JH, et al. The Society of Thoracic Surgeons 2023 clinical practice guidelines for the surgical treatment of atrial fibrillation. *Ann Thorac Surg*. 2024;118(2):291–310.
3. Whitlock RP, Belley-Cote EP, Paparella D, et al. Left atrial appendage occlusion during cardiac surgery to prevent stroke. *N Engl J Med*. 2021;384(22):2081–2091.
4. Mehaffey JH, Hayanga JWA, Wei L, Mascio C, Rankin JS, Badhwar V. Surgical ablation of atrial fibrillation is associated with improved survival compared with appendage obliteration alone: an analysis of 100,000 Medicare beneficiaries. *J Thorac Cardiovas Surg*. 2024;168(1):104–116.e7.
5. Mehaffey JH, Rankin JS, Wei LM, Badhwar V. Outcome benefits of surgical ablation and left atrial appendage obliteration for atrial fibrillation during adult cardiac surgery. *J Thorac Cardiovasc Surg*. 2025;169(5):1491–1498.
6. McCarthy PM, Manjunath A, Kruse J, et al. Should paroxysmal atrial fibrillation be treated during cardiac surgery? *J Thorac Cardiovasc Surg*. 2013;146(4):810–823.
7. Cox JL. The minimally invasive Maze-III procedure. *Oper Tech Thorac Cardiovasc Surg*. 2000;5(1):79–92.
8. Ad N, Cox JL. The Maze procedure for the treatment of atrial fibrillation: a minimally invasive approach. *J Card Surg*. 2004;19(3):196–200.
9. McCarthy PM, Cox JL, Kruse J, Elenbaas C, Andrei AC. One hundred percent utilization of a modified CryoMaze III procedure for atrial fibrillation with mitral surgery. *J Thorac Cardiovasc Surg*. 2024;167(4):1278–1289 e3.
10. McCarthy PM. Simple but effective modifications to the Cox Maze procedure using only cryoablation. *Oper Tech Thorac Cardiovasc Surg*. 2024;29(2):134–148. https://doi.org/10.1053/j.optechstcvs.2023.05.006.
11. McCarthy PM, Herborn J, Kruse J, Liu M, Andrei AC, Thomas JD. A multiparameter algorithm to guide repair of degenerative mitral regurgitation. *J Thorac Cardiovasc Surg*. 2022;164(3):867–876 e5.
12. Cox JL, Schuessler RB, D'Agostino HJ, Jr., et al. The surgical treatment of atrial fibrillation. III. Development of a definitive surgical procedure. *J Thorac Cardiovasc Surg*. 1991;101(4):569–583.
13. Ali Hassan SM, Paleczny S, Yanagawar B, Glover B, Bileri G. Electrical isolation following thoracoscopic left atrial appendage exclusion during hybrid ablation for longstanding persistent atrial fibrillation. *J Atr Fibrillation Electrophysiol*. 2022. http://www.jafib.com/PMC/XML/Inprogress/FullIssue/2022-01-31.pdf#page=51.
14. Boineau JP, Canavan TE, Schuessler RB, Cain ME, Corr PB, Cox JL. Demonstration of a widely distributed atrial pacemaker complex in the human heart. *Circulation*. 1988;77(6):1221–1237.
15. Efimov IR, Schuessler R. Architecture of the atrial pacemaker complex coming into focus. *JACC Clin Electrophysiol*. 2021;7(6):703–704.
16. Badhwar V, Scott Rankin J, Lee R, McCarthy PM, Wei LM. Contemporary left atrial appendage management during adult cardiac surgery. *J Thorac Cardiovasc Surg*. 2023;165(4):1398–1404.
17. Lee R, McCarthy PM, Wang EC, et al. Midterm survival in patients treated for atrial fibrillation: a propensity-matched comparison to patients without a history of atrial fibrillation. *J Thorac Cardiovasc Surg*. 2012;143(6):1341–1351; discussion 1350-1.

28

How I Do It: Minimally Invasive Atrial Fibrillation Ablation During Mitral Valve Surgery With or Without Tricuspid Valve Surgery

Niv Ad, Stephen D. Waterford

CHAPTER OUTLINE

Only approximately 60% of patients undergoing mitral valve (MV) surgery who have preoperative atrial fibrillation (AF) undergo concomitant ablation of their AF in addition to their MV surgery.[1] This chapter describes the technical aspects of AF surgical ablation at the time of minimally invasive MV surgery, focusing exclusively on the biatrial Maze-III procedure. The chapter also discusses how to incorporate the Maze procedure into minimally invasive MV operations that include tricuspid valve (TV) repair or replacement.

RATIONALE AND INDICATIONS

Surgical ablation of AF at the time of MV surgery is recommended by multiple different professional society guidelines.[2–5] It is clear that there are several early and late clinical benefits associated with concomitant AF ablation such as a reduction in cerebrovascular events, preservation or improved left ventricular function, improvement in quality of life, and better long-term survival. Most patients undergoing MV surgery with or without TV surgery are good candidates for a concomitant Cox Maze procedure whether the valve surgery is to be performed through a median sternotomy or by a minimally invasive technique.

The addition of concomitant AF ablation to MV surgery is both safe and effective.[6,7] Because the left atrium (LA) has to be opened for the index MV surgery, performance of the LA lesions of the Maze procedure adds little time to the MV procedure. The right atrial lesions can be created through a small right atriotomy or through multiple right atrial purse-string sutures while the patient is being rewarmed and reperfused after cardioplegic arrest (see Chapter 14). Performing the right atrial lesions during this period avoids extra aortic cross-clamp time or prolongation of cardiopulmonary bypass time. The right atrial lesion pattern has been designed to minimize the need for new postoperative pacemakers by avoiding the atrial pacemaker complex as much as possible (see Chapter 13) and in addition, no properly performed Cox Maze procedure should ever cause heart block (see Chapter 21). However, because the biatrial surgical approach is more successful in ablating AF than a unilateral LA-only approach, more preexisting sick sinus syndrome is exposed with the biatrial approach and therefore may require a new pacemaker after surgery unless the sick sinus node recovers within a few days. When TV surgery is performed, the right atriotomy necessary for the index procedure makes the right atrial lesions even easier to perform.

SCREENING OF PATIENTS

Preoperative evaluation is especially important before any minimally invasive cardiac surgical procedure is performed. We recommend computed tomography angiography (CTA) of the chest, abdomen, and femoral vessels to determine if retrograde perfusion can be performed safely. The ascending aorta can also be assessed to ensure that it is of suitable caliber and to detect any aortic calcification that might preclude aortic cross-clamping for cardioplegic arrest. Prohibitive ascending aortic calcification can be overcome using fibrillatory arrest provided there is no significant aortic insufficiency.

In the case of significant CTA findings that are prohibitive of retrograde arterial perfusion, axillary cannulation can be performed, and in the presence of a normal-appearing ascending aorta, direct cannulation of the aorta is also possible. Axillary cannulation is also recommended in patients with significant iliofemoral disease. We accomplish this by direct femoral artery cannulation rather than with a side-arm technique. As mentioned, direct aortic cannulation is also possible. Finally, it is important to exclude significant aortoiliac calcification when performing femoral perfusion to minimize the incidence of stroke. This is a matter of individual judgment, but significant calcific burden, or the presence of soft plaque in the descending aorta and iliac arteries, should be approached with caution when considering femoral arterial perfusion.

FEMORAL CANNULATION TECHNIQUE

We advise minimal dissection of the femoral vessels before cannulation to minimize the risk of postoperative lymphatic leaks. To further reduce the risk of postoperative lymphatic problems, we recommend placing the percutaneous arterial cannula on one side and the venous cannula on the opposite side. Ultrasound is used to guide the incision and the arterial cutdown such that it is very limited in size. Another option for femoral cannulation that is gaining popularity is percutaneous cannulation using either x-ray or ultrasound guidance and using specific closure devices to secure the vessels upon decannulation.[8] Cannulation of the superior vena cava (SVC) is not necessary in the majority of patients, including those having tricuspid operations, so we use a single femoral venous cannula, being certain that it is advanced into the SVC. For operations in which bicaval venous cannulation is preferred, percutaneous low jugular vein cannulation at the base of the neck with a 6- to 8-Fr catheter can be performed by the anesthesiologist. This access can be upsized as needed, thus avoiding the need for insertion of a percutaneous large-bore jugular vein cannula.

MINIMALLY INVASIVE THORACOTOMY ACCESS

After peripheral cannulation, a 6-cm or smaller right mini-thoracotomy or a totally endoscopic approach (robotic or a single endoscope) is used. This can be done laterally or anterolaterally depending on surgeon preference. The more lateral the approach, the narrower the intercostal space. Thus, retraction pain may be worse with more lateral mini-thoracotomies. Therefore, we prefer a more medial (anterolateral) access around the nipple area. In addition, when TV operations are involved, a more anterolateral incision is often advantageous for exposure.

To facilitate visibility of the atria, we recommend placing an endoscope in the same interspace as the mini-thoracotomy (usually the fourth interspace) just posterior to the incision. Alternate sites include a second interspace camera port or a port placed one interspace below the mini-thoracotomy incision. We secure the cardioplegia site in the ascending aorta with a pledgeted suture and use antegrade del Nido cardioplegia. This can then be secured with a titanium fastener after weaning off bypass and de-airing of the heart.[9] For antegrade cardioplegia, IntraClude can be used as well.[10] The retrograde cardioplegia cannula can be placed directly into the right atrium (RA) and coronary sinus or by the anesthesiologist, but it may interfere with the application of the epicardial coronary sinus lesion as part of the ablation. The most common technique that we use currently is fibrillatory arrest via a single bipolar pacing wire placed on the surface of the right ventricle (RV) that is connected to a fibrillatory or a standard external pacemaker using the rapid pacing mode. During fibrillatory arrest, the perfusion pressure is kept slightly higher than normal, preferably around 70 mm Hg, and the systemic perfusion temperature is kept between 28° and 32°C.

LEFT ATRIAL LESIONS OF THE CRYOMAZE-III PROCEDURE

After initiation of cardiopulmonary bypass, the oblique sinus is exposed to facilitate access to the posterior pericardium. The LA is then opened in Waterston's groove, and the first lesion performed is the epicardial coronary sinus lesion that creates an iceball that can be seen inside the LA. While the iceball is still visible on the LA endocardium, we mark it with methylene blue to be certain exactly where the coronary sinus lesion has been created after the iceball has thawed and disappeared (Fig. 28.1). We then place the endocardial "mitral line" from the lower end of the left atriotomy, across the site of the previous iceball (methylene blue mark), down to the MV isthmus (Fig. 28.2). If no iceball forms on the endocardium of the LA during the application of the epicardial coronary sinus lesion, it should serve a warning sign, and reapplication of the coronary sinus cryolesion is warranted to achieve visual confirmation that the coronary sinus cryolesion is circumferential. It is crucial that the mitral line and coronary sinus lesions overlap in exactly the same plane because a residual gap between them can

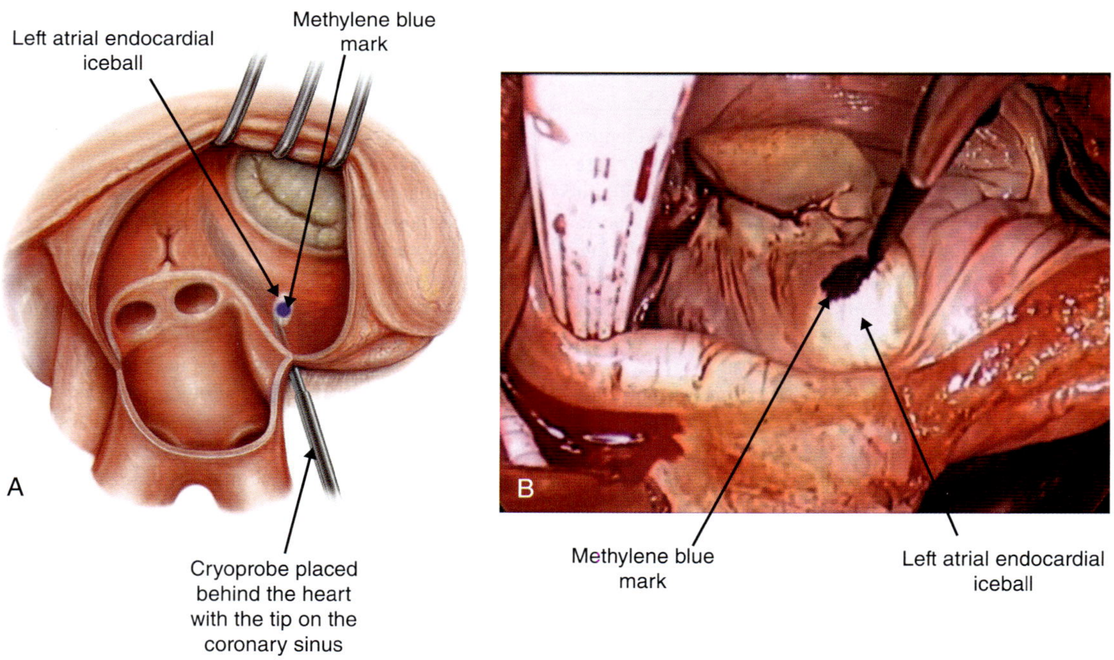

Fig. 28.1 (A) Diagram of a cryoprobe passed behind the heart with its tip pressing upward (toward the viewer) against the coronary sinus that collapses the coronary sinus and results in an iceball *(white spot)* forming on the inside (endocardium) of the left atrium during epicardial freezing of the coronary sinus. The site of the endocardial left atrial iceball is marked with methylene blue dye *(blue mark)* so that when the coronary sinus freezing is discontinued and the iceball disappears, the exact site where the coronary sinus lesion was created will be marked. (B) Operative photo of left atrial endocardial iceball being marked with methylene blue during freezing of the coronary sinus from the epicardium to serve as guidance for the proper placement of the left atrial mitral line.

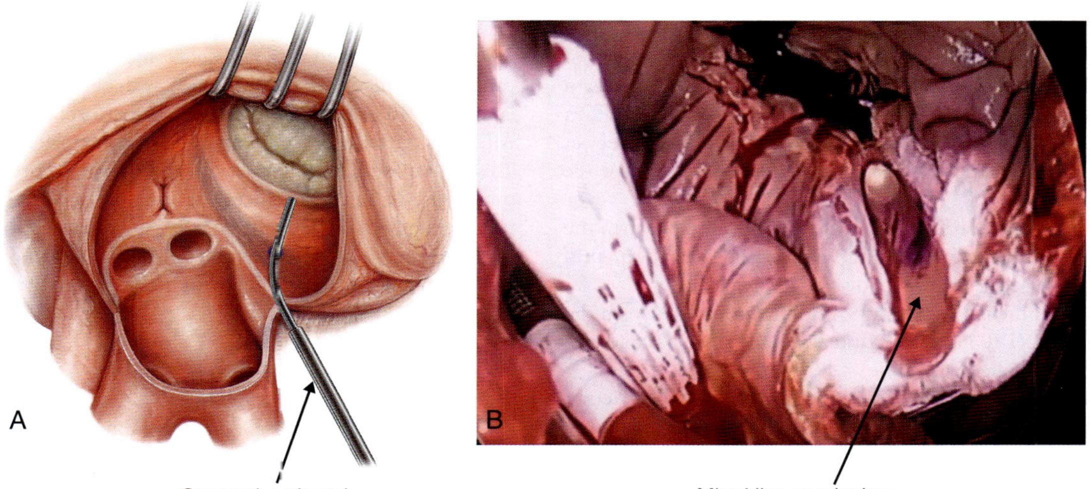

Fig 28.2 (A) Diagram showing the left atrial endocardial methylene blue mark being used to guide the placement of the linear cryoprobe used to create the mitral line in the let atrium so that it will line up precisely with the coronary sinus cryolesion. (B) Operative photo of the left atrial mitral line created in precisely the correct location extending from the lower end of the left atriotomy, across the methylene blue mark, to the mitral annulus.

result in postoperative peri-mitral flutter (see Chapter 48, Fig. 48.6). Experimental and clinical models have shown that neither the endocardial mitral line alone nor the epicardial coronary sinus cryolesion alone will ensure conduction block across the left atrial isthmus, a critical arm of the peri-mitral flutter wave.[11] In patients with a right-dominant coronary circulation (90% of patients), these lesions are usually placed between at the level of the P2 or P3 leaflets of the MV. In patients with a left-dominant coronary circulation (10% of patients), these lesions are placed closer to the posteromedial commissure in the direction of the P3 leaflet. Visual verification of the location of the circumflex coronary artery is always preferred before ablation regardless of coronary artery dominance. Following these two lesions, one can place a suture near P3 and exteriorize it through the back wall of the LA to expose the LA for the MV operation. This suture is placed after the mitral line and coronary sinus lesions have been completed across the left atrial isthmus to avoid obstructing placement of these lesions.

With the LA retracted open by the left atrial lift and posterior left atrial wall suture, a box lesion encompassing all four pulmonary veins (PVs) and the intervening posterior left atrial wall can be completed using either cryoablation alone or a combination of cryoablation and radiofrequency (RF) ablation. For cryoablation alone, we preshape the cryoprobe into a U and use it to complete the roof lesion from the upper end of the left atriotomy above the right superior PV over to a point above the left superior PV and then around the left PVs ending underneath the left inferior PV. The probe is then straightened, and a lesion is created from the inferior aspect of the left atriotomy to the spot where the prior lesion ended underneath the left inferior PV. If the os of the left atrial appendage (LAA) is not incorporated in one of these lesions, it is important to add another lesion to connect the left PVs with the LAA (see Chapter 14, Fig. 14.24). Most commonly, the LAA is closed with an epicardial clip applied through the transverse sinus or by endocardial suture closure in two layers, although the latter is less effective.[12] We usually apply the LAA clip before closure of the left atriotomy to assure that the clip is placed close to the base of the LAA. However, in 5% to 10% of patients, after applying the LAA clip, additional endocardial suturing is required to ensure that there is no residual LAA stump. If the appendage is closed endocardially without a clip, it should be done at this stage of the operation.

If the roof and floor lesions of the box lesion are created using bipolar RF clamps, it is still necessary to use cryoablation to completely encircle the left PVs and the LAA because an RF clamp is difficult to place in this location through a right mini-thoracotomy whether performed under direct vision or endoscopically.[13]

After the LA lesions of the Maze procedure have been completed, we complete the MV operation. The left atrial lesions of the Maze procedure are created first because this allows for the endocardial mitral line across the left atrial isthmus to be extended across the MV annulus before an annuloplasty ring or valve replacement is implanted.

With respect to the duration of cryolesion application, we apply a 2-minute cryolesion when using an argon gas source and a 3-minute cryolesion when using a nitrous oxide gas source. We also use 3-minute ablations for the left-sided lesions except for the epicardial coronary sinus lesion (2 minutes). All right-sided lesions are created by applying the cryoprobe for 2 minutes.

RIGHT ATRIAL LESIONS OF THE MAZE PROCEDURE WHEN NO TRICUSPID VALVE OPERATION IS PERFORMED

After completion of the LA lesions of the Cox Cryo Maze-III procedure and completion of the MV operation, the right atrial lesions can be performed either in the arrested heart, or the aortic cross-clamp can be released and the right atrial lesions performed in the empty beating heart. We prefer the latter because the heart has to be rewarmed and reperfused for a certain period of time, and the right atrial lesions can be completed during that time. With this technique, the right atrial lesions do not add any cross-clamp time or bypass time to the operation.

If no atriotomy is needed to address the TV, two or three purse-string sutures are used to perform the right-sided lesions of the Maze procedure depending on whether the original right atrial lesion pattern of the Cox-Maze-III procedure is performed with two separate lesions to the TV annulus (see Chapter 13, Fig. 13.13) or its recent modification is used in which a lesion is placed across the anterior lateral aspect of the right atrial wall to the tip of the right atrial appendage (RAA; see Chapter 13, Fig. 13.14).

If no TV surgery is needed and the surgeon prefers to perform the right atrial lesions on an empty, beating, reperfusing heart, our preferred purse-string placement is as follows:

1. The lateral part of the RA, right in the middle distance between the inferior vena cava (IVC) and SVC and anterior to the crista terminalis (along the so called white line)
2. Right atrial lateral wall about 1 to 2 cm from the atrioventricular (AV) groove. Enough distance from the AV groove itself is allowed so that if repair sutures are required, the right coronary artery is not endangered.
3. The tip of the RAA[14,15]

Through purse-string 1, the SVC and IVC lesions are then performed. With regards to the SVC lesion, when looking up the SVC, this is placed at the 7 o'clock position to avoid the anatomical sinoatrial node that is located more medially and on the anterior wall of the RA. It is important when performing the SVC and IVC lesions to separate the probe from the pericardium because these lesions can otherwise result in right phrenic nerve injury when performed with cryoablation because nerves are sensitive to cryoablation.

Through purse-string 2, the cryoprobe is placed across the TV into the RV to perform the 2 o'clock lesion. A second lesion is then performed with the cryoprobe down to purse-string 1. This represents the free-wall lesion.

Through purse-string 3, the cryoprobe is placed across the TV from this position, completing the 10 o'clock lesion. An alternate to this is to place the probe through the AV groove purse-string and direct it to the tip of the RAA. As described in Chapter 14, Dr. Cox prefers a slightly different placement of the right atrial purse-string sutures.

The right-sided lesions can also be performed through the purse-string sutures with a combination of RF ablation and cryoablation. The AV groove purse-string is used to complete a right atrial free-wall lesion down to the lower purse-string. This can also be down from the lower purse-string up to the AV groove purse-string if orientation of the RF clamp is easier. The lower purse-string is then used to complete the SVC and IVC lesions. The 2 o'clock and 10 o'clock lesions are then performed with cryoablation across the tricuspid annulus.

Some tips for the right-sided lesions include the following. If the heart is full of blood, this will be an impediment to cryoablation because the probe only starts timing down when the temperature reaches a threshold temperature, and tissue ablation also requires a lower temperature. A pump sucker can be placed through the purse-string that is not being used to empty the heart. This will collect blood from the coronary sinus. Although low flow can be used intermittently to empty the heart, if vacuum assisted drainage is being used, this can also result in an air lock in the cannula and worse venous drainage.

RIGHT ATRIAL LESIONS OF THE MAZE PROCEDURE WITH TRICUSPID VALVE SURGERY

When a TV operation is required, the right atrial lesions of the Maze procedure are easier to perform. The right atriotomy should be oriented diagonally to connect the areas where purse-strings 1 and 2 would be placed avoiding the atrial pacemaker complex.[16] This is the opposite of the incision orientation many surgeons use for tricuspid annuloplasty and is theoretically important to minimize the incidence of pacemaker placement. After the atriotomy, the 2 o'clock lesion across the tricuspid annulus is performed with cryoablation. Next the SVC and IVC lesions can be performed as described earlier, with either RF ablation or cryoablation. The 10 o'clock lesion can then be performed as described earlier. After this the tricuspid annuloplasty or valve replacement is performed. This allows for the annular lesions to be done before placement of the prosthesis. In summary, there are multiple acceptable techniques for performing both the left and right atrial lesions of a minimally invasive Maze procedure, but optimal outcomes still depend on creating perfect individual lesions and placing them in the pattern of a maze.

REFERENCES

1. Mehaffey JH, Charles EJ, Berens M, Clark MJ, Fonner CE, Kron I, et al. Barriers to atrial fibrillation during mitral valve surgery. *J Thorac Cardiovasc Surg*. 2023;165:650–658.
2. Ad N, Damiano RJ, Badhwar V, Calkins H, La Meir M, Nitta T, et al. Expert consensus guidelines: examining surgical ablation for atrial fibrillation. *J Thorac Cardiovasc Surg*. 2017;153:1330–1354.
3. Von Ballmoos M, Hui DS, Mehaffey JH, Malaisrie SC, Vardas PN, Gillinov AM, et al. The Society of Thoracic Surgeons 2023 Clinical Practice Guidelines for the Surgical Treatment of Atrial Fibrillation. *Ann Thorac Surg*. 2024;118:291–310.
4. Tzeis S, Gerstenfeld EP, Kalman J, Saad EB, Shamloo AS, Andrade JG, et al. 2024 European Heart Rhythm Association/Heart Rhythm Society/Asia Pacific Heart Rhythm Society/Latin American Heart Rhythm Society expert consensus statement on catheter and surgical ablation of atrial fibrillation. *Europace*. 2024;26:euae043.
5. Van Gelder IC, Rienstra M, Bunting KV, Casado-Arroyo R, Caso V, Crijns H, et al. 2024 ESC guidelines for the management of atrial fibrillation developed in collaboration with the European Association for Cardiothoracic Surgery. *Eur Heart J*. 2024;45:3314–3414.
6. Yanagawa B, Holmes SD, Henry L, Hunt S, Ad N. Outcome of concomitant Cox Maze III procedure using an argon-based cryosurgical system: a single-center experience with 250 patients. *Ann Thorac Surg*. 2013;95:1633–1639.
7. Ad N, Holmes SD, Massimiano PS, Rongione AJ, Fornaresio LM. Long-term outcome following concomitant mitral valve surgery and Cox Maze procedure for atrial fibrillation. *J Thorac Cardiovasc Surg*. 2018;155:983–994.
8. Cheema T, Venero C, Champaneria S, Younas S, Khan M, Anjum I, et al. Systematic review and meta-analysis comparing Manta device and Perclose device for closure of large bore arterial access. *J Vasc Access*. 2024;8:11297298231222314.
9. Nasif A, Masroor S. Using automated suture fastening system for securing aortic cannulation sites in minimally invasive mitral valve surgery: *Authorea* Feb 11, 2022.
10. Balkhy HH, Grossi EA, Kiaii B, Murphy D, Geirsson A, Guy S, et al. A retrospective evaluation of endo-aortic balloon occlusion compared to external clamping in minimally invasive mitral valve surgery. *Semin Thorac Cardiovasc Surg*. 2024;36:27–36.
11. Cox JL, Ad N, Palazzo T, Fitzpatrick S, Suyderhoud JP, DeGroot KW, et al. Current status of the Maze procedure for the treatment of atrial fibrillation. *Semin Thorac Cardiovasc Surg*. 2000;12:15–19.
12. Ad N, Massimiano PS, Shuman DJ, Pritchard G, Holmes SD. New approach to exclude the left atrial appendage during minimally invasive cryothermic surgical ablation. *Innovations*. 2015;10:323–327.

13. Robertson JO, Saint LL, Leidenfrost JE, Damiano RJ. Illustrated techniques for performing the Cox Maze IV procedure through a right mini-thoracotomy. *Ann Cardiothorac Surg*. 2014;3:105–116.
14. Ad N. The multi-purse string Maze procedure: a new surgical technique to perform the full Maze procedure without atriotomies. *J Thorac Cardiovasc Surg*. 2007;134:717–722.
15. Ad N: Cox IV cryoablation on bypass. *CTSnet.org* October 6, 2016.
16. Cox JL, Malaisrie SC, Kislitsina ON, McCarthy PM. The electrophysiologic basis for lesions of the contemporary Maze operation. *J Thorac Cardiovasc Surg*. 2019;157:584–590.

29

How I Do It: Atrial Fibrillation Ablation With Aortic Valve Surgery and Ascending Aortic Aneurysm Repair

Christopher K. Mehta, Stephen F. Chiu

CHAPTER OUTLINE

PATHOPHYSIOLOGY AND IMPACT OF ATRIAL FIBRILLATION

Atrial fibrillation (AF) is common in patients requiring aortic valve surgery. Although age is a risk factor for both AF and aortic valve disease,[1,2] there is a direct relationship between the severity of aortic stenosis (AS) and the presence of AF, with up to one-third of AS patients having concomitant AF.[3,4] It is thought that the increased incidence of AF in patients with AS is due to increased left ventricular pressure overload that can result in a cascade of left ventricular diastolic dysfunction leading to left atrial enlargement that in turn promotes the development of AF. Laenens et al.[5] reported in a prospective multicenter registry that patients with both AS and AF had a worse 10-year survival rate than AS patients in sinus rhythm. However, in patients with no echocardiography markers of left ventricular diastolic dysfunction, AF was not an independent predictor of death.[5] Kubala and colleagues[6] reported the results of a retrospective single-center study of 1838 patients who underwent aortic valve replacement for severe AS. In those who underwent surgical or transcatheter aortic valve replacement, the 5-year survival rate was 86% in patients who were in sinus rhythm compared with only 77% in patients who were in AF.[6] Furthermore, the 2023 Society of Thoracic Surgeons guidelines gave a Class I recommendation for concomitant surgical AF ablation in patients undergoing non–mitral valve surgery.[7] Therefore, all cardiac surgeons should be facile in concomitant surgical AF ablation and left atrial appendage occlusion (LAAO) and excision.

Several studies have demonstrated that there is a relationship between AF and thoracic aortic aneurysms, though the pathologic relationship is unclear. A 2020 study of 1000 consecutive patients with AF showed by cross-section chest computed tomography scanning that 20% had previously undetected thoracic aortic dilatation.[8] The authors suggested that a surveillance strategy for thoracic aortic disease should be considered in all patients with AF, particularly in those with other risk factors for aortic disease. A 2021 Danish study of 14,989 patients identified AF as an independent risk factor for ascending and descending thoracic aortic aneurysms, and the presence of these two localized aneurysms increased the incidence of aortic arch aneurysms by a factor of 6–8.[9]

CHOICE OF ATRIAL FIBRILLATION ABLATION PROCEDURE IN PATIENTS UNDERGOING AORTIC VALVE SURGERY AND/OR THORACIC ANEURYSM SURGERY

In patients undergoing surgery for aortic valve disease and/or thoracic aortic aneurysms who have concomitant AF, the specific AF ablation technique of choice depends primarily on whether the patient has paroxysmal AF (PAF) or nonparoxysmal AF (non-PAF). The choice of surgical ablation technique in these patients is further affected by the fact that the Maze procedure requires opening the left atrium (LA), which is not necessary in either aortic valve or thoracic aneurysm surgery. Fortunately, other surgical ablation approaches can yield satisfactory results without opening the LA, though they are not as successful as Maze procedures. The optimal treatment objectives in concomitant PAF and non-PAF are discussed in detail in Chapter 25.

Paroxysmal Atrial Fibrillation and Aortic Valve Surgery

The objective of treating PAF in patients requiring aortic valve surgery is to isolate as many atrial triggers as possible to decrease the likelihood of AF episodes being induced. Because 70% of the triggers in patients with concomitant PAF are located in, around, and between the pulmonary veins (PVs) (Fig. 29.1), a box lesion around all four PVs and the intervening left atrial posterior wall will isolate these atrial triggers, thereby reducing the likelihood of future AF episodes by 70%. In addition, approximately 10% of concomitant PAF triggers are located in the left atrial appendage (LAA), so if it is either amputated or electrically isolated with an epicardial LAA clip, the overall result will be isolation of 80% of the atrial triggers. Thus in patients with AS and/or thoracic aneurysm with concomitant PAF, the surgical options are as follows: (1) ignore the concomitant AF, resulting in the same level of AF as the patient experienced preoperatively; (2) amputate or clip the LAA, resulting in 10% less AF postoperatively; (3) perform a box lesion and apply an LAA clip, resulting in 80% less AF postoperatively; or (4) open the LA and perform a Maze procedure, resulting in over 90% less AF postoperatively.

The creation of a box lesion without opening the LA has traditionally been performed by external isolation of the PVs with a bipolar radiofrequency (RF) clamp and then creating roof and floor lesions with a dual-electrode unipolar Coolrail device (Fig. 29.2). However, the creation of a box lesion has recently become much easier and promises to be more effective using an Encompass clamp (Atricure, Inc.) (Fig. 29.3). The Encompass clamp is a bipolar RF clamp designed so that one arm can be placed above the superior PVs and one arm below the inferior PVs to create a complete box

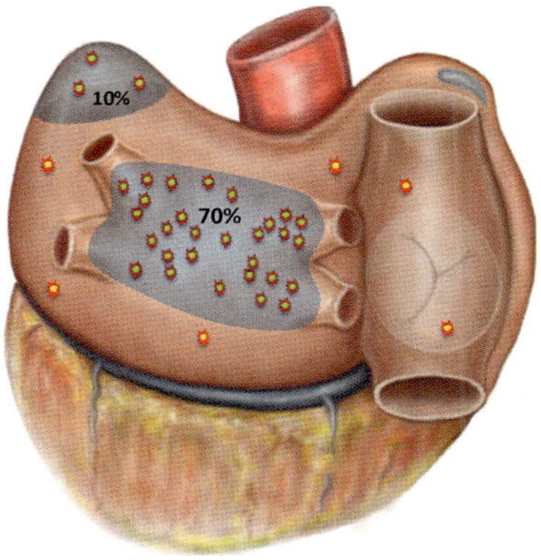

Fig. 29.1 Locations of atrial triggers in concomitant paroxysmal atrial fibrillation (PAF). Atrial triggers are responsible for the induction of atrial fibrillation (AF) and therefore for each of the individual recurrent AF episodes in patients with PAF. The objective of surgical intervention for PAF in patients with aortic valve disease and/or thoracic aortic aneurysms is the isolation of as many of these AF triggers as possible in hopes of decreasing the likelihood of another AF episode occurring. Seventy percent of these AF triggers reside in or near the pulmonary veins (PVs) and the posterior left atrial wall between the two pairs of PVs. Approximately 10% of them are in the left atrial appendage (LAA), and the other 20% are widely scattered throughout the two atria.

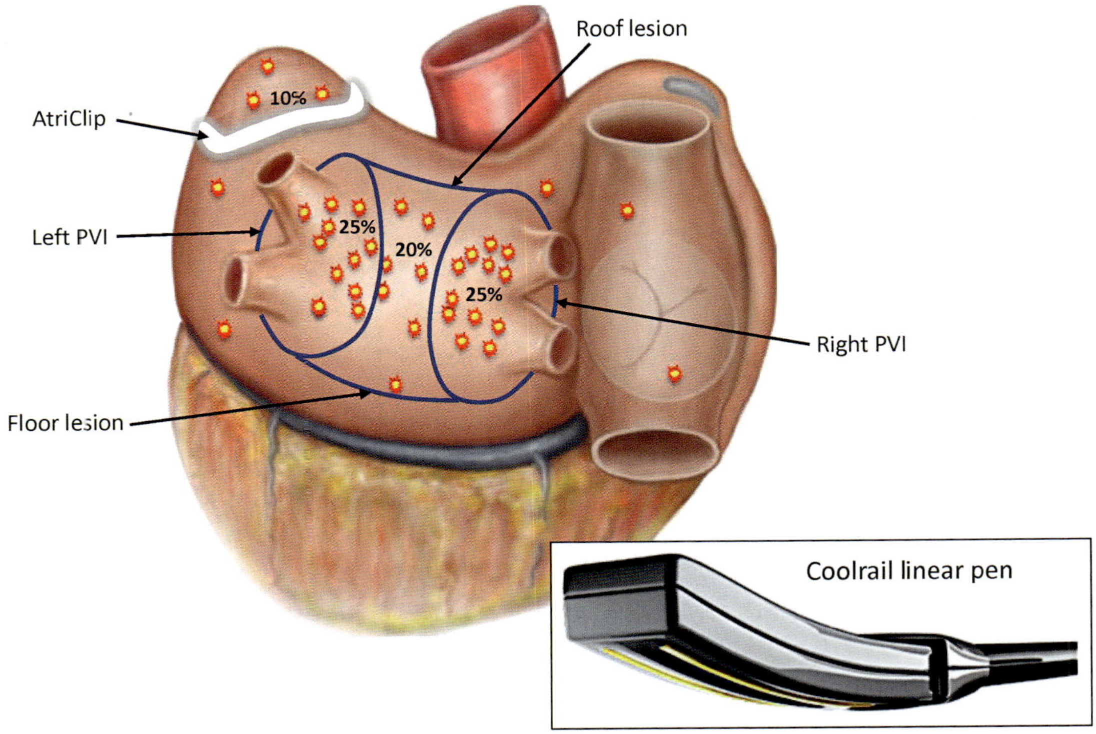

Fig. 29.2 Box lesion plus left atrial appendage occlusion for concomitant paroxysmal atrial fibrillation (PAF). A box lesion encompassing all four pulmonary veins (PVs) and the intervening posterior left atrial wall isolates 70% of the atrial fibrillation (AF) triggers, and an epicardial left atrial appendage (LAA) clip isolates another 10%. Therefore, the creation of a box lesion plus clipping the LAA results in 80% less PAF afterward. One way that a box lesion can be created is by isolating the PVs in pairs and then creating roof and floor lines with a Coolrail device *(inset)* to complete the box lesion as is done in the Maze-IV procedure. The PVs are isolated using bipolar radiofreqency (RF) clamps while the roof and floor lesions are created using less reliable unipolar RF devices. If successful, this technique isolates the 20% of AF triggers in the posterior left atrial wall plus the 50% of AF triggers in and around the PVs themselves. It is assumed that this latter 50% of PV triggers are distributed roughly equally between the left and right pairs of PVs.

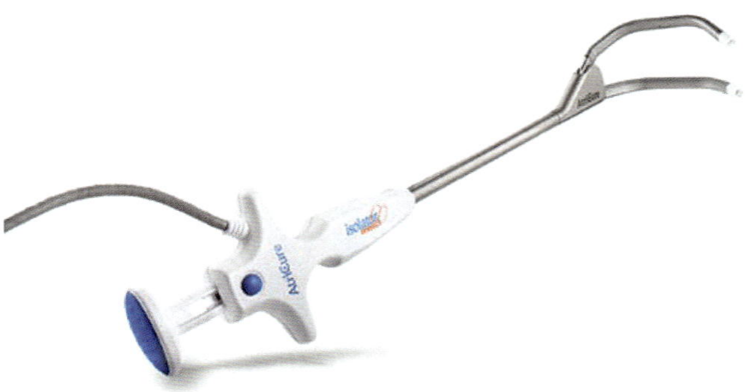

Fig. 29.3 Bipolar radiofrequency (RF) Encompass clamp. This clamp is designed to encompass the entire "box" in the left atrium (LA) that includes all four pulmonary veins and the intervening posterior wall of the LA. Therefore, in patients with concomitant atrial fibrillation (AF), this clamp should isolate 70% of all the AF triggers in the LA. Because this is a bipolar RF clamp, it eliminates the problem of having to create the roof and floor lines of the box lesion with unipolar RF devices that are known to be less reliable than bipolar RF devices.

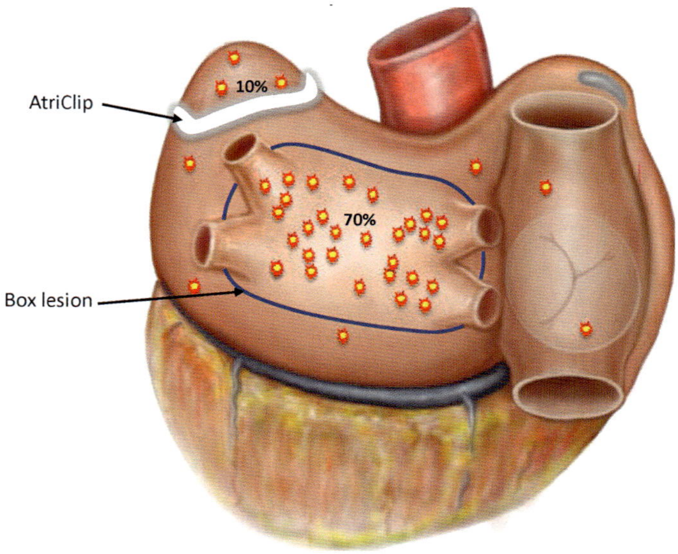

Fig. 29.4 Box lesion with Encompass clamp plus left atrial appendage occlusion for concomitant paroxysmal atrial fibrillation (PAF). Nonparoxysmal atrial fibrillation (non-PAF; persistent and long-standing persistent atrial fibrillation [AF]) depends on larger macro-reentrant circuits (drivers) for sustaining episodes of AF after the triggers have induced the AF. The maintenance of AF after it has been induced has little or nothing further to do with AF triggers, so the objective of surgery for non-PAF should have nothing to do with isolating them. Rather, the objective of surgery for non-PAF is to interrupt as many of the macro-reentrant drivers as possible.

lesion in one step (Fig. 29.4). In patients with PAF who require aortic valve and/or thoracic aneurysm surgery, we prefer to open the LA and perform a CryoMaze-III procedure when possible, but we consider performing a box lesion plus LAAO to be a satisfactory alternative.

Nonparoxysmal Atrial Fibrillation and Aortic Valve Surgery

Non-PAF includes persistent AF and long-standing persistent AF, neither of which depend on atrial triggers for its maintenance but rather on large macro-reentrant drivers that maintain and sustain the AF (see Chapters 5 and 25). Thus the objective of treating patients with non-PAF is not to isolate atrial triggers but to interrupt as many of the macro-reentrant drivers as possible. Unfortunately, only about 30% of the macro-reentrant AF drivers use the posterior wall of the LA between the PVs as a part of their reentrant circuit (Fig. 29.5), and virtually none of the AF drivers use the LAA or the PVs. Therefore, a box lesion plus epicardial clip LAAO in patients with non-PAF is far less successful than in patients with PAF, and neither LAA occlusion nor simple PV isolation has much effect on the elimination of non-PAF (Fig. 29.6).[10]

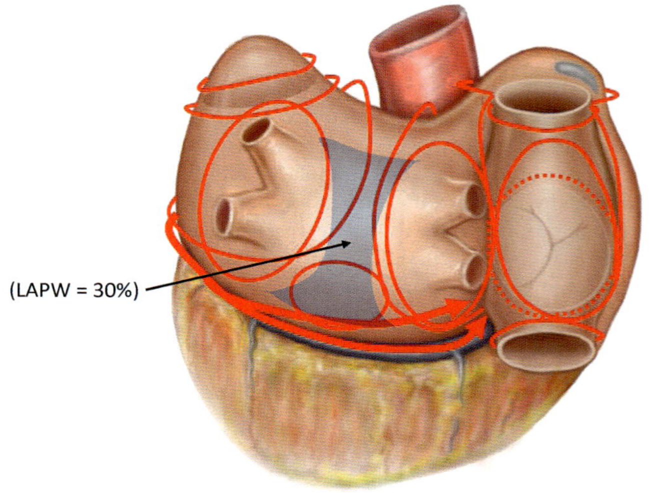

Fig. 29.5 Potential locations of atrial drivers in concomitant nonparoxysmal atrial fibrillation (non-PAF). Only about 30% of the macro-reentrant drivers that sustain non-PAF use the posterior left atrial wall between the right and left pulmonary veins (PVs) as a part of their reentrant circuits, and virtually none of them use the orifices of the PVs or the left atrial appendage. *LAPW*, Left atrial posterior wall.

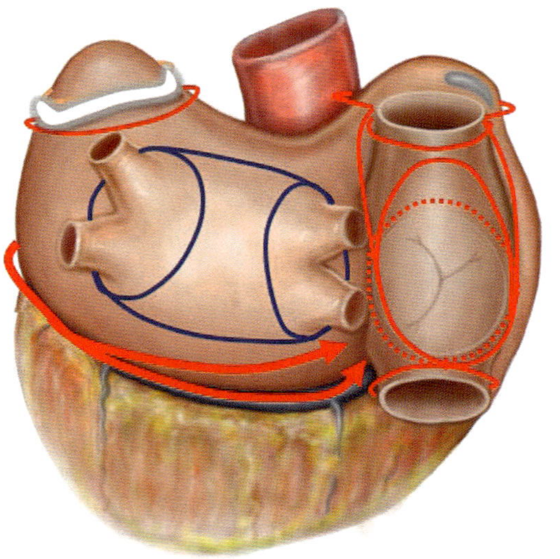

Fig. 29.6 Box lesion plus left atrial appendage occlusion (LAAO) for concomitant nonparoxysmal atrial fibrillation (non-PAF). Unlike patients with paroxysmal atrial fibrillation, combining a box lesion with LAAO results in terminating the atrial fibrillation (AF) in only around 30% of patients with non-AF because some 70% of the macro-reentrant AF drivers do not use the pulmonary veins, the posterior left atrial wall, or the left atrial appendage as a part of their reentrant circuits.

As in patients with PAF, in patients with non-PAF who require aortic valve and/or thoracic aneurysm surgery, we prefer to open the LA and perform a CryoMaze-III procedure because we do not consider performing a box lesion plus LAAO to be a satisfactory alternative in patients with non-PAF. However, if the surgeon decides that an open Maze procedure is not feasible, a box lesion with an EnCompass clamp plus LAAO with an AtriClip would be the next alternative, though it must be recognized that the success rate will be far less in patients with non-PAF than in patients with PAF (see Chapter 25, Table 25.1). The last resort for patients with concomitant non-PAF is to simply clip the LAA, which will not affect the presence of AF but will offer some protection against thromboembolic stroke. We will describe our approach for a CryoMaze III procedure performed concomitantly with aortic valve surgery as well as with thoracic aortic aneurysm repair.

SURGICAL SETUP AND CANNULATION

After median sternotomy, aortic cannulation strategy should always be dictated by the operation to be performed. For aortic valve replacement, the distal ascending aorta is cannulated, but for type A ascending aortic aneurysms, the aortic cannula should be placed in the aortic arch to facilitate cross-clamp placement as high as possible in the ascending aorta. For ascending aorta replacement with circulatory arrest, the aortic cannula is placed proximal to the innominate artery to exclude the cannulation site once a hemi-arch anastomosis is performed.

Bicaval venous cannulation is typically used to facilitate the CryoMaze III procedure. A right-angle superior vena cava (SVC) cannula is placed in the upper right atrium, with care taken to ensure that the purse-string sutures are not too close to the anatomic sinoatrial node. Alternatively, the SVC can be cannulated directly. Inferior vena cava (IVC) cannulation can be performed using a dual-lumen venous return cannula placed through the right atrial appendage, a right-angle single-stage cannula placed near the IVC, or a femoral venous cannulation advanced up the IVC to near the IVC–RA junction. Importantly, venous cannulation should avoid the atrial pacemaker complex as much as possible (see Chapter 3, Fig. 3.9). An umbilical tape is placed around the IVC and is eventually snared before the right atriotomy. Some surgeons prefer to place an umbilical tape around the SVC as well.

SEQUENCE OF ATRIAL FIBRILLATION ABLATION AND AORTIC VALVE REPLACEMENT AND/OR THORACIC ANEURYSM REPAIR

Left Atrial Appendage Closure

Cardiopulmonary bypass is initiated, and the aorta is cross-clamped. Cardioplegia is administered antegrade into the aortic root and/or retrograde via coronary sinus catheter depending on surgeon preference. During antegrade cardioplegia infusion, the LA is opened in the interatrial groove to vent the left side of the heart. After the delivery of cardioplegia has been completed, the heart is lifted and retracted to the right, and the LAA is occluded with an epicardial clip.

Left Atrial Lesions of the CryoMaze-III Procedure

The left atriotomy is then extended at both ends, and a self-retaining mitral valve retractor is positioned to enhance surgical exposure of the internal LA. The modified CryoMaze-III procedure is performed entirely with a cryoprobe starting in the LA.[11,12] The total time required for creation of the LA cryolesions should be no more than 8 to 10 minutes, with freezing for 3 minutes to create each of the first two cryolesions and 2 minutes for the third cryolesion. Our technique for performing the LA cryolesions is described in detail in Chapter 15. After completion of the LA cryolesions, a left ventricular vent may be placed within the suture line and snared in place to facilitate the impending aortic valve and/or aortic root surgery.

Aortic Valve Replacement and/or Thoracic Aortic Aneurysm Repair

After the LAA has been occluded and the LA lesions of the CryoMaze-III procedure have been completed, patients needing an aortic valve replacement undergo aortic valve replacement (AVR) at this stage of the operation. In patients with thoracic aortic aneurysms, the heart is arrested in the aforementioned manner, and the patient is cooled to a target temperature of moderate or deep hypothermia while the left atrial cryolesion set is being performed. If exposure to the LA is limited, the aneurysmal aorta can be transected to improve exposure. During these few minutes, the aneurysmal mid-ascending aorta and aortic root can be resected if exposure permits.

After the patient is cooled systemically to the target temperature, the aortic cross-clamp is removed, and an open distal hemi-arch anastomosis is performed. The patient is then rewarmed, and the focus turns toward the aortic root and/or aortic valve. Aortic valve or root replacement is performed at this time, and the proximal anastomosis of the aneurysm repair is completed at the native sinotubular junction for concomitant AVR or to the graft of an aortic root replacement.

Right Atrial Lesions of the CryoMaze-III Procedure

With the aortic cross-clamp still in place, the IVC is snared using the previously placed umbilical tape, and the SVC is clamped using a Cooley vena caval occlusion clamp to complete the right atrial cryolesion set. Total cryoablation time for the right atrial lesions is 6 minutes (three lesions for 2 minutes each), so performing the right atrial lesions should add less than 10 minutes to the aortic cross-clamp time. Our technique for performing the right atrial cryolesions is described in detail in Chapter 15. In contrast to the Cox Maze III procedure, we omit a cryolesion to the right atrial appendage because we have never seen a failure of the CryoMaze-III procedure caused by postoperative reentry around the RA appendage.

Some surgeons prefer to perform the right atrial lesions after releasing the aortic cross-clamp during the rewarming phase to save both pump time and aortic cross-clamp time in these combined procedures. Regardless of whether the right atrial lesions are performed under cardioplegic arrest or during the rewarming phase of the procedure, the right atriotomy is closed with a double layer of 4-0 polypropylene suture, temporary ventricular pacing wires are placed on the right ventricle, and the patient is weaned off cardiopulmonary bypass. Transesophageal echocardiography is used to assess the aortic valve prosthesis and/or the thoracic aneurysm repair and the LAA for residual connection with the LA and for a residual pouch of 10 mm or larger.

REFERENCES

1. Heeringa J, van der Kuip DA, Hofman A, et al. Prevalence, incidence and lifetime risk of atrial fibrillation: the Rotterdam study. *Eur Heart J*. 2006;27(8):949–953.
2. Miyasaka Y, Barnes ME, Gersh BJ, et al. Secular trends in incidence of atrial fibrillation in Olmsted County, Minnesota, 1980 to 2000, and implications on the projections for future prevalence. *Circulation*. 2006;114(2):119–125.

3. Greve AM, Gerdts E, Boman K, et al. Prognostic importance of atrial fibrillation in asymptomatic aortic stenosis: the Simvastatin and Ezetimibe in Aortic Stenosis study. *Int J Cardiol.* 2013;166(1):72–76.
4. Stortecky S, Buellesfeld L, Wenaweser P, et al. Atrial fibrillation and aortic stenosis: impact on clinical outcomes among patients undergoing transcatheter aortic valve implantation. *Circ Cardiovasc Interv*. 2013;6(1):77–84.
5. Laenens D, Stassen J, Galloo X, et al. The impact of atrial fibrillation on prognosis in aortic stenosis. *Eur Heart J Qual Care Clin Outcomes*. 2023;9(8):778–784.
6. Kubala M, Bohbot Y, Rusinaru D, Marechaux S, Diouf M, Tribouilloy C. Atrial fibrillation in severe aortic stenosis: prognostic value and results of aortic valve replacement. *J Thorac Cardiovasc Surg*. 2023;166(3):771–779.
7. Wyler von Ballmoos MC, Hui DS, Mehaffey JH, et al. The society of thoracic surgeons 2023 clinical practice guidelines for the surgical treatment of atrial fibrillation. *Ann Thorac Surg*. 2024.
8. Ramchand J, Bansal A, Seedazn MB, et al. Incidental thoracic aortic dilatation on chest computed tomography in patients with atrial fibrillation. *Am J Cardiol*. 2020;140:78–82.
9. Obel LM, Diederrichsen AC, Steffensen FH, et al. Population-based factors for ascending, arch, descending, and abdominal aortic dilatations for 60-74-year-old individuals. *J Am Coll Cardiol*. 2021;78(3):201–211.
10. Cox JL, Malaisrie SC, Kislitsina ON, McCarthy PM. The electrophysiologic basis for lesions of the contemporary Maze operation. *J Thorac Cardiovasc Surg*. 2019;157(2):584–590.
11. McCarthy PM, Cox JL, Kruse J, Elenbaas C, Andrei AC. One hundred percent utilization of a modified CryoMaze III procedure for atrial fibrillation with mitral surgery. *J Thorac Cardiovasc Surg*. 2022;167(4):1278–1289. https://doi.org/10.1016/j.jtcvs.2022.08.028.
12. Cox JL, Malaisrie SC, Churyla A, et al. Cryosurgery for atrial fibrillation: physiologic basis for creating optimal cryolesions. *Ann Thorac Surg*. 2021;112(2):354–362.

30

Ganglionic Plexus Ablation

Marc W. Gerdisch, Taras Lysyy, Ralph J. Damiano, Jr.

CHAPTER OUTLINE

Ganglionic plexi (GP) ablation can be used to treat patients with various cardiac arrhythmias by selectively disrupting clusters of autonomic nerve cells, known as ganglia, on the epicardial surface of the heart. GP influence cardiac physiology through complex neural connections that can play a role in the etiology of various cardiac arrhythmias including atrial fibrillation (AF).[1–3] GP are the targets of various catheter-based and surgical ablation techniques to treat arrhythmias as either standalone procedures or adjunctive procedures in patients undergoing cardiac surgery.[4,5] This chapter discusses the rationale for GP ablation, the techniques for the identification and ablation of the GP, and the efficacy of GP ablation in the management of arrhythmias.

NEUROANATOMY OF THE HEART

The cardiac autonomic nervous system (ANS) consists of *extrinsic* (central) and *intrinsic* (peripheral) components (Fig. 30.1).[6,7] The intrinsic cardiac ANS is a complex network of epicardial GP, interconnected neurons, and axons.[6,8] These GP are extensions of mediastinal nerves that terminate in the epicardium around the ascending aorta, pulmonary artery trunk, pulmonary veins (PVs), and venae cavae.[6,9] Multiple anatomic studies have consistently identified seven discrete areas on the epicardium where densely concentrated clusters of these ganglionic cells form.[4,6,8] Two plexi innervate the right atrium (RA) and three innervate the left atrium (LA). One GP innervates the right ventricle (RV) and three innervate the left ventricle (LV).[8]

Epicardial ganglia are most densely concentrated on the posterior and posterolateral surfaces of the LA near the junctions of the PVs and LA, where about 50% of all cardiac ganglia are located.[8,10] Individual GP are located near the four PV ostia and innervate the myocardial sleeves of the PVs.[6,8] To ensure accurate description during ablation procedures, these GP near the PVs have been assigned names that reflect their association with a specific adjacent PV.[9] The superior left ganglionic plexus (SLGP) is located on the LA roof just medial to the left superior PV (Fig. 30.2). The inferior left ganglionic plexus (ILGP) is located just below the left inferior PV, extending toward the inferior

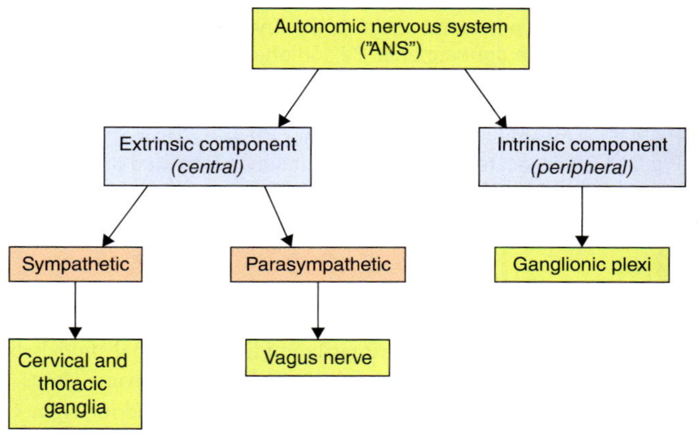

Fig. 30.1 Flow diagram of the cardiac autonomic nervous system. The anatomic structures responsible for all facets of the autonomic nervous system are the cervical and thoracic sympathetic ganglia, the vagus nerve parasympathetic fibers, and the ganglionic plexi on the surface of the atria and the proximal great vessels.

aspect of the left atrial posterior wall. It is connected to the atrioventricular (AV) node and is pivotal in ventricular slowing.[5] The anterior right ganglionic plexus (ARGP) is situated anterior to the right superior and right inferior PVs and is the only GP immediately adjacent to a PV. It delivers signals to the sinoatrial (SA) node, including integrating signals from the extrinsic ANS.[5] The inferior right ganglionic plexus (IRGP) is located just below the right inferior PV and extends toward the inferior aspect of the left atrial posterior wall. It delivers signals to the AV node. The IRGP and ILGP are known as the "oblique sinus GP."[5] The ligament of Marshall ganglionic plexus (LOM GP) is positioned between the left superior PV and the left atrial appendage (LAA) and is the only GP not embedded in epicardial fat. The LOM is a vestigial remnant of the embryonic left superior vena cava (SVC) that harbors predominately parasympathetic fibers of the left vagus nerve

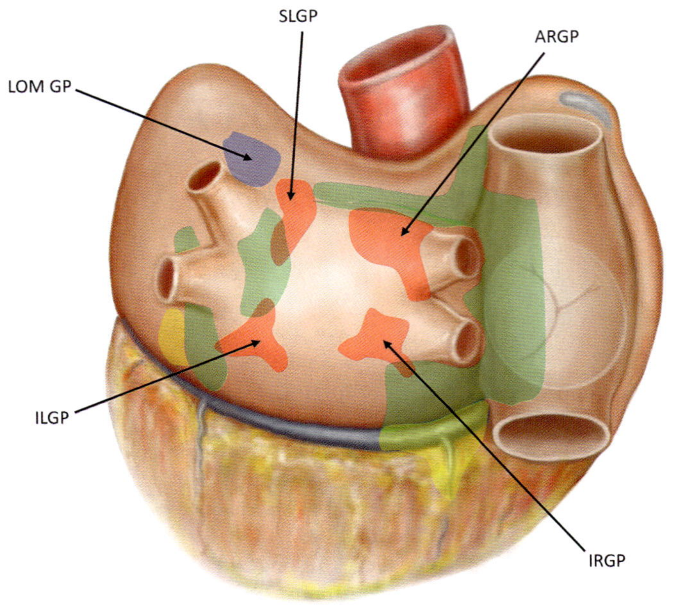

Fig. 30.2 Approximate locations of the ganglionic plexi (GP) in the posterior left atrium (LA). The GP near each pulmonary vein (PV) orifice have been given names to reflect their association with the corresponding PV. These GP innervate the sleeves of left atrial endocardium that extend up into the PVs. The superior left GP (SLGP) is located on the roof of the LA near the left superior PV and often extending to the medial aspect of left atrial appendage (LAA). The anterior right GP (ARGP) is located near the right superior PV and often extends inferiorly to the area near the right inferior PV. The inferior left GP (ILGP) is located just below the junction of the left inferior PV and the LA. The inferior right GP (IRGP) is located near the right inferior PV. The ligament of Marshall GP (LOM GP) is located between the left superior PV and the LAA. It is the only GP in the atrium that is not embedded in an epicardial fat pad.

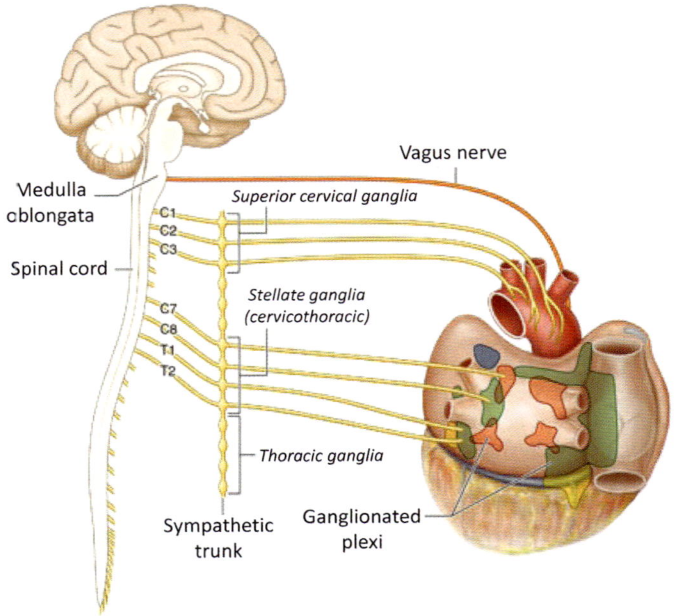

Fig. 30.3 The autonomic nervous system (ANS) of the heart. See text for further discussion.

that innervate parts of the LA.[11] It transforms into the vein of Marshall as it connects to the coronary sinus.

Less accessible atrial GP, primarily studied in animal models because of limited endocardial access, include the transverse sinus or great artery GP and the SVC–aortic (SVC-Ao) or superior right GP (SRGP).[5] Experimental canine models have identified the SVC-Ao GP as the "head station" connecting the extrinsic and intrinsic ANS. This characterization is due to the finding that the majority of vagosympathetic fibers carrying signals from the CNS to heart innervation pass through the SVC-Ao GP. There are numerous interconnections between the GP, and there is a final common pathway to the sinus node via the ARGP and to the AV node via the IRGP.[7,12] GP embedded within epicardial fat pads and in the LOM form a complex neural network that modulates autonomic innervation.[13–15] They also facilitate communication between intrinsic and extrinsic components of the ANS.[16–18]

The extrinsic component of the ANS is divided into two parts: *sympathetic* and *parasympathetic* (Fig. 30.3). The sympathetic component originates from major autonomic ganglia located along the cervical and thoracic spinal cord, including the superior cervical ganglia (connected with C1–C3), the stellate ganglia (connected with C7–C8 to T1–T2), and the thoracic ganglia (extending down to the seventh thoracic ganglion).[18] Most postganglionic sympathetic neurons have cell bodies in these ganglia. Their axons form the superior, middle, and inferior cardiac nerves, connecting with GP neurons.[19] The parasympathetic component derives primarily from the nucleus ambiguus and the dorsal motor nucleus of the medulla oblongata, which houses preganglionic neurons. These neurons send their axons primarily through the vagus nerve to reach postganglionic neurons located in the GP.[17,20]

NEUROPHYSIOLOGY OF THE HEART

The ANS maintains cardiovascular homeostasis by balancing sympathetic and parasympathetic inputs to regulate heart rate, contractility, and conduction. Sympathetic stimulation, via norepinephrine release, exerts positive chronotropic, inotropic, and dromotropic effects on the heart. Activation of β-adrenergic receptors enhances SA node automaticity, increases myocardial contractility, and facilitates AV conduction, thereby augmenting cardiac output to meet increased metabolic demands during stress or exercise. Conversely, the parasympathetic activation, predominantly mediated by acetylcholine, exerts negative chronotropic, inotropic, and dromotropic effects. Stimulation of vagal nerve fibers decreases heart rate by slowing SA node depolarization, reduces AV conduction velocity, and diminishes myocardial contractility. Thus vagal input has an important role during rest and recovery.

GP are recognized as "integration centers" between the intrinsic and extrinsic ANS and therefore can play a role in the induction of AF.[12] Evidence suggests that the extrinsic component of the ANS suppresses the intrinsic component, and loss of this inhibition may lead to the induction of AF.[4,21] Animal studies have also indicated that a hyperactive intrinsic ANS may create an environment conducive to the induction of AF.[22–24]

GANGLIONIC PLEXUS MAPPING AND ABLATION

Localization and mapping of the GP can be performed using high-frequency stimulation (HFS).[9,12] The primary goal of GP ablation for AF is to ablate the five major GP in the LA, the four associated with specific PVs and one in the LOM.[4,9,21,25] These GP have been targeted in both endocardial and epicardial ablation procedures because of their proximity to the PVs and left atrial posterior wall. Although electrophysiological mapping provides a general estimate of the GP locations, precise localization of the plexi remains challenging.

Epicardial electrophysiologic mapping of GP was first reported during thoracoscopic surgical ablation in 2007 by Mehall et al.[26] Subsequent mapping and ablation were also demonstrated in both limited thoracotomy and open chest surgical approaches.[27,28] Identification of an active GP involves low-voltage, HFS while monitoring for a vagal response. An active GP is identified when HFS of the atrial epicardial surface elicits a bradycardic response, with a greater than 50% increase in the R-to-R interval, resulting in a more than 50% heart rate reduction (Fig. 30.4). An example of HFS parameters for GP identification is an 18-V impulse with a 1.5-ms pulse width at 1000 pulses per minute.[29,30] In the surgical setting, HFS is performed by using a transpolar pen that can pace, sense, and ablate.

As previously discussed, GP have both sympathetic and parasympathetic innervation. Because the sympathetic response is delayed until after the immediate parasympathetic response, HFS is delivered for 2 to 5 seconds to elicit the initial parasympathetic response and avoid interference from the later sympathetic response.[9] The same transpolar pen used to identify the GP can then be used to ablate it. HFS that fails to illicit a vagal response at the same site after ablation confirms GP denervation (Fig. 30.5).

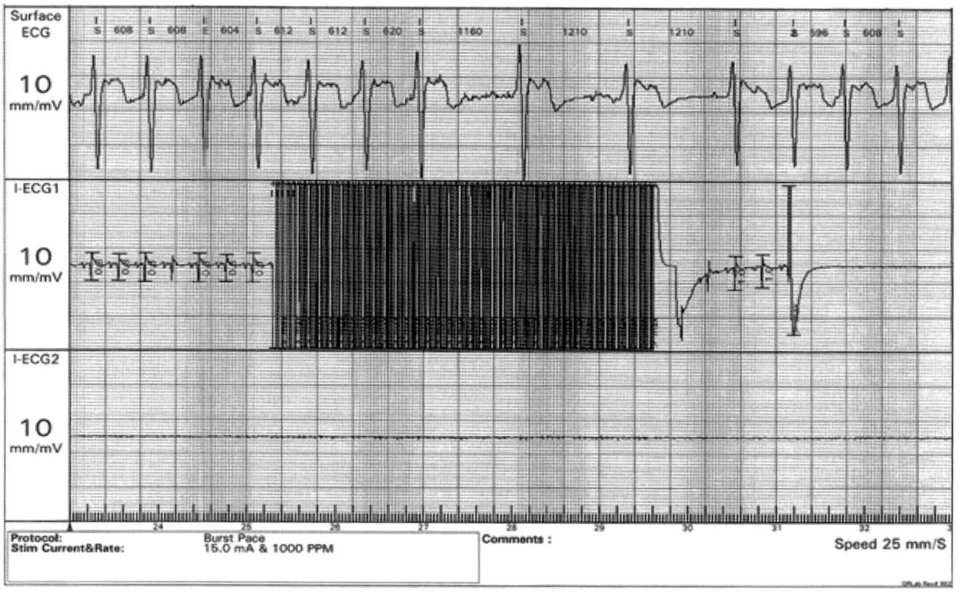

Fig. 30.4 Identification of a ganglionic plexus. The surface electrocardiogram documents that high-frequency stimulation yields a vagal response with slowing of the intrinsic heart rate.

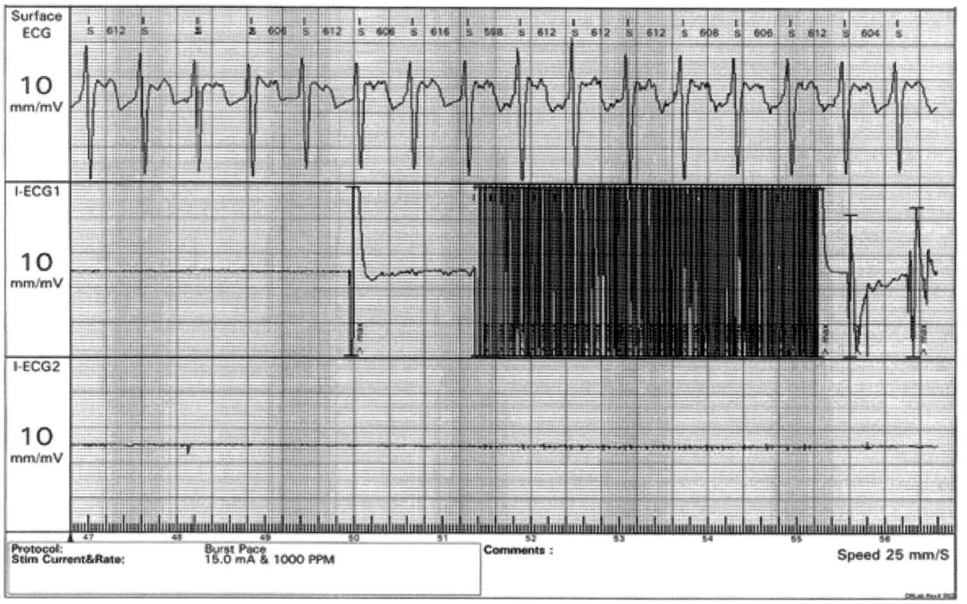

Fig. 30.5 Documentation of successful ganglionic plexus ablation. The surface electrocardiogram documents that high-frequency stimulation at the same site after ablation fails to elicit the vagal response of a slowing of the intrinsic heart rate.

EXPERIMENTAL STUDIES ON GANGLIONIC PLEXUS ABLATION FOR ATRIAL FIBRILLATION

Numerous animal studies have examined the long-term effects of autonomic denervation after RF GP ablation. Permanently damaging nerve cells requires destruction of the bodies of the cells within the GP. However, GP consist not only of cell bodies but also of interconnecting axons. Because of neuroplasticity, they can regenerate and even increase innervation through nerve sprouting in response to axonal injury.[31] Thus neuroplasticity suggests the possibility of GP reinnervation after ablation, with heterogeneous reinnervation and proarrhythmic potential. Damiano et al.[32] examined the acute and chronic effects of surgical GP ablation alone or with additional surgical ablation (pulmonary vein isolation [PVI], PVI plus box lesion) in canines. To ensure lesion transmurality, they dissected epicardial fat pads. Postoperatively, vagosympathetic trunk stimulation elicited significantly reduced responses from the atrial conduction system and myocardium, confirming initial atrial denervation. However, evidence of parasympathetic reinnervation was observed 4 weeks after surgery, revealing transient and nonuniform denervation, potentially increasing vulnerability to the development of a new arrhythmogenic substrate.

Mao et al.[33] observed similar findings when they studied the electrophysiologic outcomes of GP ablation in dogs. They divided the dogs into three groups: group 1, pre- and postablation of four major GP and LOM GP; group 2, 8 weeks after ablation of four major GP and LOM GP; and group 3, sham-operated controls at 8 weeks. Immediately after GP ablation, group 1 exhibited significantly prolonged atrial refractory periods compared with preablation levels. However, at 8 weeks, group 2 showed a significantly shortened atrial refractory periods compared with the group 3 control subjects and the preablation levels in group 1. Moreover, the refractory periods were significantly shorter in the LA compared with the RA in group 2, which was not observed in group 3 control subjects. In group 1, atrial tachyarrhythmia (ATA) inducibility decreased immediately after GP ablation compared with before the ablation. However, after 8 weeks, dogs in group 2 showed significantly higher ATA inducibility. In group 2, ATA inducibility was higher in the LA than in the RA, unlike in the group 3 control subjects. Furthermore, immunohistochemical staining showed a significantly higher nerve density in GP-ablated dogs at 8 weeks (group 2) than controls (group 3). The authors suggested that incomplete denervation, along with factors such as axonal regeneration, nerve sprouting in response to RF energy nerve injury, and repeated HFS of GP, could have contributed to the observed changes in atrial refractory periods and ATA inducibility at 8 weeks after ablation.

Wang et al.[34] evaluated the longer-term effectiveness of GP ablation in dogs at 6 and 12 months after ablation. Similar to Mao et al.,[33] they focused solely on ablating the RIGP and ARGP without performing PV or posterior wall isolation. Although there was an initial refractory period prolongation 1 month after GP ablation, refractory periods returned to preablation values at 6 and 12 months. AF was not inducible immediately before or after GP ablation. However, the ability to induce AF improved 1 month after the procedure and remained elevated compared with control subjects at 6 and 12 months. Immunohistochemical staining revealed reduced nerve density 1 month after GP ablation, but nerve density was similar to control subjects by 6 and 12 months.

As previously mentioned, the GP at the junction of the SVC, right pulmonary artery, and aorta is the primary relay between the extrinsic and intrinsic ANS. Po et al.[23] ablated this "headway station" GP in five dogs and assessed atrial refractory periods acutely and after 10 weeks. A control group of five dogs underwent refractory period measurements without GP ablation. Although the refractory periods were prolonged initially after GP ablation, they were significantly shortened after 10 weeks, which contrasted with no change in the refractory periods in the control group. Furthermore, significant AF and ATA burden increased in the ablated group but not in the control group.

CLINICAL OUTCOMES OF GANGLIONIC PLEXUS ABLATION FOR ATRIAL FIBRILLATION

Surgical GP ablation has the advantage of direct access to the GP embedded in fat. In contrast, endocardial ablation requires penetrating through the myocardium to reach the GP, leading to difficulty in achieving complete GP ablation.[25] During surgical access to the LAA, management often includes dissecting or ablating the LOM GP. Avazzadeh et al.[5] provided a comprehensive review of surgical and catheter-based GP ablation studies in 2020. The following sections discuss selected observational and randomized studies.

Nonrandomized Studies of Surgical Ganglionic Plexus Ablation for Atrial Fibrillation

Nonrandomized studies of GP ablation during surgical ablation procedures have yielded mixed results regarding efficacy when added to traditional lesion sets.

Doll et al.[30] conducted a small prospective study involving GP testing and ablation in 12 patients with paroxysmal AF (PAF) or persistent AF (4.5 ± 1.5 years' duration) undergoing concomitant left atrial surgical ablation. They reported a sinus rhythm rate of 83% after 12 months of follow-up, concluding that GP ablation was feasible.

Onorati et al.[35] performed a prospective study on 75 patients undergoing mitral valve surgery, in whom biatrial ablation procedures were conducted with or without additional GP ablation. The "mini-Maze" procedure, conducted using bipolar and monopolar RF ablation, involved PVI, mitral isthmus, and left superior PV to LAA ablation on the left side and SVC, IVC, cavotricuspid isthmus, right atrial appendage, and terminal crest ablation on the right side. Septal isthmus ablation was also performed if a patient had a large RA. They observed improved sinus rhythm rates with the addition of GP ablation. They also extended resection of the epicardial fat pads along Waterston's groove, the LOM, and the left PVs for histological evaluation of GP post-operatively.[35] Ware et al.[27] compared 20 patients who received biatrial or left atrial surgical ablation with GP mapping and ablation during different valve replacement procedures to case-matched control subjects who had concomitant surgical ablation without GP ablation. They reported higher sinus rhythm rates at 12 months of follow-up with the addition of GP ablation.[27] In a much larger retrospective study of 519 patients with nonparoxysmal AF (PAF) who underwent Cox Maze-IV ablation, the incorporation of GP ablation did not improve the maintenance of sinus rhythm or reduce AF recurrence.[36]

Randomized Clinical Trials of Surgical Ganglionic Plexus Ablation for Atrial Fibrillation

The two randomized clinical trials that have evaluated GP ablation for AF were performed during open chest and minimally invasive thoracoscopic procedures, but the results did not favor GP ablation. The Japan Ganglionated Plexi Ablation Trial (JGPAT) was a multicenter randomized trial comparing 69 patients who underwent surgical Maze procedures with and without GP ablation during concomitant open chest structural heart procedures.[37] Approximately 80% of patients had persistent or long-standing persistent AF (LSpAF). In the Maze plus GP ablation arm, ablation was performed at known anatomic GP sites and at 28 additional sites identified by HFS stimulation. The mean number of active GPs identified was 4.5. Postoperative pacemaker implantation rates and complications were similar with and without GP ablation. With a mean follow-up period of 16.3 months, there was no significant difference in freedom from AF or ATA between the two arms, with rates of 86.8% after Maze plus GP ablation and 91.4% after the Maze without GP ablation. The investigators speculated that in the control arm (Maze without GP ablation), the Maze procedure itself may have disrupted the GP by cardiac dissection and epicardial fat ablation, leading to denervation despite the lack of targeted GP testing and ablation.

The Atrial Fibrillation Ablation and Autonomic Modulation via Thoracoscopic Surgery (AFACT) trial was a single-center, randomized trial of 240 patients with advanced PAF and persistent AF who underwent thoracoscopic RF ablation and LAA exclusion with and without GP ablation.[25] Thoracoscopic RF ablation involved PVI with a bipolar RF clamp for all patients and additional superior connecting and trigone lines for those with persistent AF. In the GP ablation arm, the GP were identified using either HFS or an anatomic approach, resulting in the ablation of all four major GP and the LOM GP. After the procedure, vagal responses were present in 0% of the GP ablation arm and 87% of the no GP ablation arm. Major adverse events were significantly higher in the GP ablation arm compared with the no GP ablation arm (19% versus 8%; $P = .022$), mainly because of bleeding, SA node dysfunction, and pacemaker implantation. At 1-year follow-up, freedom from ATA was comparable between the GP ablation arm and no GP ablation arm (70.9% versus 68.4%; $P = .696$), as were freedom from AF rates when analyzed by AF type. However, ATA recurrences were significantly more frequent in the GP ablation arm than the no GP ablation arm (78.1% versus 51%; $P = .026$). At 2-year follow-up, no additional procedure-related complications occurred, and rates of freedom from ATA remained similar between arms (55.6% in the GP ablation arm and 56.1% in the no GP ablation arm).[38] As a result of these findings, the investigators advised against thoracoscopic GP ablation in this patient population. As a result of both trials, adjunctive GP ablation has largely been abandoned in most centers during either stand-alone, hybrid, or concomitant surgical ablation.

Randomized Clinical Trials of Catheter Electrophysiology Ablation for Atrial Fibrillation

The efficacy of GP ablation via endocardial catheter ablation approach has yielded mixed results in randomized studies. After showing that extensive anatomically guided endocardial catheter GP ablation was more effective than HFS-guided ablation,[39] Katritsis et al. demonstrated in a randomized trial that anatomically guided GP ablation added to PVI improved freedom from arrhythmia recurrence in patients with PAF.[40] Similarly, a two-center randomized trial involving 242 patients with PAF showed that combining PVI with GP ablation achieved a higher rate of sinus rhythm (74%) after 2 years compared with GP ablation alone (48%) and PVI alone (56%) without any reported complications related to GP ablation.[41] However, it remains unclear whether the improved outcomes after extensive anatomically guided ablation were due to true GP denervation, more extensive ablation targeting other AF drivers, reduced critical mass, or a combination of these factors.

In the ectopy triggering ganglionated plexus ablation to prevent atrial fibrillation (GANGLIA-AF) trial involving 102 patients with PAF across three centers, GP ablation alone was compared with PVI alone. GP were mapped using HFS and ablated until nonfunctional. At 12-month follow-up, freedom from atrial arrhythmias was 50% with GP ablation compared with 64% with PVI, showing a trend but not reaching statistical significance (log-rank, $P = .09$). However, more than half of the patients who underwent GP ablation were able to discontinue antiarrhythmic drugs compared with approximately one-third of patients who had PVI.[42]

In another randomized trial, 264 patients with persistent or LSpAF were compared using endocardial catheter PVI with additional linear lesions (PVI plus LL) versus PVI with GP ablation. At 12 months, sinus rhythm (SR) was achieved in 47% of PVI plus LL patients and 54% of PVI plus GP ablation patients, with no significant difference. However, at 3 years, SR maintenance rates were 34% for PVI plus LL and 49% for PVI plus GP ($P = .035$). Atrial flutter was more common in PVI plus LL (18% versus 6%; $P = .002$). After the second procedure, the long-term success rates were 52% for PVI plus LL and 68% for PVI plus GP ($P = .006$), suggesting superior outcomes with PVI plus GP ablation.[43]

In some cases, AF is primarily driven by heightened parasympathetic activity, known as "vagal AF." These are typically younger patients without structural heart disease who may experience episodes of AF that are triggered by eating, drinking, or alcohol consumption or during periods of resting or sleep. In a cohort of patients with suspected vagal AF, Danik et al.[44] found that solely targeting endocardial GP ablation did not reliably eliminate vagal AF.

Surgical Ablation of the Ligament of Marshall

The LOM is located between the LAA and the left superior PV. It harbors axonal extensions of both sympathetic and parasympathetic fibers of the ANS as well as a GP that connects atrial myocardium and coronary sinus muscle sleeves.[45] The LOM may serve as a source of triggers and drivers for AF, contributing to both paroxysmal and persistent forms of arrhythmia.[46] Mapping and ablating the LOM can be clinically beneficial for managing atrial arrhythmias, whether performed during catheter procedures or surgical AF ablation.

Animal studies have demonstrated that ablating the LOM attenuates AF inducibility and prolongs atrial refractory periods.[47,48] LOM ablation combined with other procedures has improved success rates in treating AF in humans. Endocardial ablation techniques and alternative methods such as ethanol infusion can potentially eliminate parasympathetic responses and reduce AF induction.[49] In the randomized vein of marshall ethanol for untreated persistent AF (VENUS) trial, ethanol infusion into the vein of Marshall during endocardial catheter ablation for persistent and LSpAF showed promising results.[50] At 6 and 12 months, there was a statistically significant improvement of 11% in freedom from AF and atrial tachycardia without antiarrhythmic drugs compared with catheter ablation alone. However, despite adjunctive ethanol infusion, the recurrence rate remained high at 51%, highlighting the challenges of managing advanced AF solely with endocardial catheter ablation.

CHALLENGES AND FUTURE DIRECTIONS

Limitations of Ganglionic Plexus Testing and Ablation

Because GP are not exclusively innervated by parasympathetic nerves, accurate detection of the entire GP region can be challenging because the expected parasympathetic response (bradycardia or hypotension) may not always occur.[41] High-voltage endocardial HFS, usually performed under general anesthesia, may generate a parasympathetic response; it is unclear if GP that are unresponsive to HFS are truly inactive. Suwalski et al.[51] found that 15% of patients undergoing concomitant surgical ablation had no detectable GP despite the use of HFS for identification and ablation. Only a lower heart rate was significantly associated with positive GP detection.[51] They speculated that a patient's higher baseline parasympathetic activity might increase the likelihood of an HFS response during GP testing. Because of the challenges of accurate GP testing, some authors, such as Katritsis and colleagues,[40] preferred an anatomic approach to GP ablation.

Current Guideline Recommendations

Contemporary societal guidelines and consensus statements emphasize the significant role of both intrinsic and extrinsic cardiac ANS in initiating and perpetuating AF. However, they acknowledge the lack of evidence supporting GP ablation as a beneficial adjunct to catheter or surgical ablation strategies. The 2023 Society of Thoracic Surgeons guidelines classify ganglionic ablation as "minimally efficacious" and "no longer considered as an additive application to surgical ablation."[52] Similarly, the Korea Surgical Ablation Network and Heart Rhythm Society also acknowledge GP ablation's limited evidence and uncertain utility.[53,54]

Future Directions in Ganglionic Plexus Ablation

As AF management continues to evolve, promising avenues are being explored to improve the safety and efficacy of GP ablation. Advancements in imaging (e.g., high-resolution cardiac magnetic resonance imaging) and mapping technologies (e.g., three-dimensional electroanatomic mapping systems) could enhance *GP localization precision*, leading to optimized procedures and reduced procedural times. Developing technologies for precisely *targeted energy delivery to GP* sites, such as laser ablation, pulsed-field ablation, and focused ultrasonography, could improve efficacy with minimal collateral tissue damage and fewer side effects. *Tailoring ablation strategies* based on individual patient characteristics and ANS function may optimize treatment outcomes. Continued research into the mechanisms of neural regeneration is essential for refining strategies and developing more targeted and effective treatment approaches.

SUMMARY

Although the ANS, including GP, plays a role in the initiation and perhaps the maintenance of AF, the aggregation of experimental and clinical evidence, including randomized clinical trials, does not support GP ablation as an addition to conventional surgical AF ablation procedures. Transient effects of GP ablation may be observed during and after various surgical ablation approaches. The creation of the left atrial posterior wall box and PV isolation may provide transient GP inhibition. However, as documented experimentally, neural connections appear to regenerate within a few weeks. Furthermore, heterogenous hyper-reinnervation may initiate AF by contributing to an arrhythmogenic substrate. Considering the lack of a durable effect and the risk of promoting arrhythmogenicity, GP ablation does not play a role in modern surgical AF ablation strategies. Nonetheless, the role of GP in chronotropic and dromotropic cardiac performance and their influence on arrhythmogenic substrate perpetuate interest in creating a means to manipulate them for arrhythmia management. As precision mapping and perhaps durable neuronal interruption evolve, GP therapies may eventually be tailored to modulate patient-specific rhythm disorders.

REFERENCES

1. Nishida K, Datino T, Macle L, et al. Atrial fibrillation ablation: translating basic mechanistic insights to the patient. *J Am Coll Cardiol*. 2014;64(8):823–831.
2. Shen MJ, Choi E-K, Tan AY. Neural mechanisms of atrial arrhythmias. *Nat Rev Cardiol*. 2011;9(1):30–39.
3. Schauerte P, Scherlag BJ, Patterson E. Focal atrial fibrillation: experimental evidence for a pathophysiologic role of the autonomic nervous system. *J Cardiovasc Electrophysiol*. 2001;12(5):592–599.
4. Stavrakis S, Po S. Ganglionated plexi ablation: physiology and clinical applications. *Arrhythm Electrophysiol Rev*. 2017;6(4):186–190.
5. Avazzadeh S, McBride S, O'Brien B, et al. Ganglionated plexi ablation for the treatment of atrial fibrillation. *J Clin Med*. 2020;9(10):3081.
6. Armour JA. Functional anatomy of intrathoracic neurons innervating the atria and ventricles. *Heart Rhythm*. 2010;7(7):994–996.
7. Armour JA. Cardiac neuronal hierarchy in health and disease. *Am J Physiol-Reg Integ Compar Physiol*. 2004;287(2):R262–R271.
8. Pauza DH, Skripka V, Pauziene N, Stropus R. Morphology, distribution, and variability of the epicardiac neural ganglionated subplexuses in the human heart. *Anat Rec*. 2000;259(4):353–382.
9. Po SS, Nakagawa H, Jackman WM. Localization of left atrial ganglionated plexi in patients with atrial fibrillation. *J Cardiovasc Electrophysiol*. 2009;20(10):1186–1189.
10. Tan AY, Li H, Wachsmann-Hogiu S, Chen LS, Chen P-S, Fishbein MC. Autonomic innervation and segmental muscular disconnections at the human pulmonary vein-atrial junction: implications for catheter ablation of atrial-pulmonary vein junction. *J Am Coll Cardiol*. 2006;48(1):132–143.
11. Pappone C, Santinelli V, Mangusa F, et al. Pulmonary vein denervation enhances long-term benefit after circumferential ablation for paroxysmal atrial fibrillation. *Circulation*. 2004;109(3):327–334.
12. Hou Y, Scherlag BJ, Lin J, et al. Ganglionated plexi modulate extrinsic cardiac autonomic nerve input: effects on sinus rate, atrioventricular conduction, refractoriness, and inducibility of atrial fibrillation. *J Am Coll Cardiol*. 2007;50(1):61–68.
13. Shivkumar K, Ajijola OA, Anand I, et al. Clinical neurocardiology defining the value of neuroscience-based cardiovascular therapeutics. *J Physiol*. 2016;594(14):3911–3954.
14. Lemery R, Birnie D, Tang ASL, Green M, Gollob M. Feasibility study of endocardial mapping of ganglionated plexuses during catheter ablation of atrial fibrillation. *Heart Rhythm*. 2006;3(4):387–396.
15. Rysevaite K, Saburkina I, Pauziene N, et al. Immunohistochemical characterization of the intrinsic cardiac neural plexus in whole-mount mouse heart preparations. *Heart Rhythm*. 2011;8(5):731–738.
16. Armour JA, et al. Gross and microscopic anatomy of the human intrinsic cardiac nervous system. *Anat Rec*. 1997;247(2):289–298.
17. Scridon A, Şerban RC, Chevalier P. Atrial fibrillation: neurogenic or myogenic? *Arc Cardiovasc Dis*. 2018;111(1):59–69.
18. Armour JA, Murphy DA, Yuan BX, Macdonald S, Hopkins DA. Potential clinical relevance of the "little brain" on the mammalian heart. *Experim Physiol*. 2008;93(2):165–176.
19. Kawashima T. The autonomic nervous system of the human heart with special reference to its origin, course, and peripheral distribution. *Anat Embryol*. 2005;209(6):425–438.
20. Chiou CW, Eble JN, Zipes DP. Efferent vagal innervation of the canine atria and sinus and atrioventricular nodes: the third fat pad. *Circulation*. 1997;95(11):2573–2584.
21. Stavrakis S, Nakagawa H, Po SS, Scherlag BJ, Lazzara R, Jackman WM. The role of the autonomic ganglia in atrial fibrillation. *JACC Clin Electrophysiol*. 2015;1(1):1–13.
22. Choi E-K, Shen MJ, Han S, et al. Intrinsic cardiac nerve activity and paroxysmal atrial tachyarrhythmia in ambulatory dogs. *Circulation*. 2010;121(24):2615–2623.
23. Lo LW, Scherlag BJ, Chang H-Y, Lin Y-J, Chen S-A, Po SS. Paradoxical long-term pro-arrhythmic effects after ablating the "head station" ganglionated plexi of the vagal innervation to the heart. *Heart Rhythm*. 2013;10(5):751–757.
24. Chugh A. Ganglionated plexus ablation in patients undergoing pulmonary vein isolation for paroxysmal atrial fibrillation: here we go again. *J Am Coll Cardiol*. 2013;62(24):2326–2328.
25. Driessen AHG, Berger WR, Krul SPJ, et al. Ganglion plexus ablation in advanced atrial fibrillation: the AFACT study. *J Am Coll Cardiol*. 2016;68(11):1155–1165.

26. Mehall JR, Kohut Jr RM, Schneeberger EW, Taketani T, Merrill WH, Wolf RK. Intraoperative epicardial electrophysiologic mapping and isolation of autonomic ganglionic plexi. *Ann Thorac Surg*. 2007;83(2):538–541.
27. Ware AL, Suri RM, Stulak JM, Sundt 3rd TM, Schaff HV. Left atrial ganglion ablation as an adjunct to atrial fibrillation surgery in valvular heart disease. *Ann Thorac Surg*. 2011;91(1):97–102.
28. McClelland J, Duke D, Reddy R. Preliminary results of a limited thoracotomy: new approach to treat atrial fibrillation. *J Cardiovasc Electrophysiol*. 2007;18(12):1289–1295.
29. Han FT, Kasirajan V, Kowalski M, et al. Results of a minimally invasive surgical pulmonary vein isolation and ganglionic plexi ablation for atrial fibrillation: single-center experience with 12-month follow-up. *Circ Arrhythm Electrophysiol*. 2009;2(4):370–377.
30. Doll N, Pritzwald-Stegmann P, Czesla M, et al. Ablation of ganglionic plexi during combined surgery for atrial fibrillation. *Ann Thorac Surg*. 2008;86(5):1659–1663.
31. Scherlag BJ, Jackman WM. Unravelling the paradoxical effects of ganglia ablation. *Circ Arrhythm Electrophysiol*. 2014;7(4):570–572.
32. Sakamoto S, Schuessler RB, Lee AM, Aziz A, Lall SC, Damiano RJ. Vagal denervation and reinnervation after ablation of ganglionated plexi. *J Thorac Cardiovasc Surg*. 2010;139(2):444–452.
33. Mao J, Yin X, Zhang Y, et al. Ablation of epicardial ganglionated plexi increases atrial vulnerability to arrhythmias in dogs. *Circ Arrhythm Electrophysiol*. 2014;7(4):711–717.
34. Wang X, Zhang M, Zhang Y, et al. Long-term effects of ganglionated plexi ablation on electrophysiological characteristics and neuron remodeling in target atrial tissues in a canine model. *Circ Arrhythm Electrophysiol*. 2015;8(5):1276–1283.
35. Onorati F, Curcio A, Santarpino G, et al. Routine ganglionic plexi ablation during Maze procedure improves hospital and early follow-up results of mitral surgery. *J Thorac Cardiovasc Surg*. 2008;136(2):408–418.
36. Gelsomino S, Lozekoot P, La Meir M, et al. Is ganglionated plexi ablation during Maze IV procedure beneficial for postoperative long-term stable sinus rhythm? *Int J Cardiol*. 2015;192:40–48.
37. Sakamoto SI, Ishii Y, Otsuka T, et al. Multicenter randomized study evaluating the outcome of ganglionated plexi ablation in maze procedure. *Gen Thorac Cardiovasc Surg*. 2022;70(10):908–915.
38. Berger WR, Neefs J, van den Berg NWE, et al. Additional ganglion plexus ablation during thoracoscopic surgical ablation of advanced atrial fibrillation: intermediate follow-up of the AFACT Study. *JACC Clin Electrophysiol*. 2019;5(3):343–353.
39. Pokushalov E, Romanov A, Shugayev P, et al. Selective ganglionated plexi ablation for paroxysmal atrial fibrillation. *Heart Rhythm*. 2009;6(9):1257–1264.
40. Katritsis DG, Giazitzoglou E, Zografos T, Pokushalov E, Po SS, Camm JA. Rapid pulmonary vein isolation combined with autonomic ganglia modification: a randomized study. *Heart Rhythm*. 2011;8(5):672–678.
41. Katritsis DG, Pokushalov E, Romanov A, et al. Autonomic denervation added to pulmonary vein isolation for paroxysmal atrial fibrillation: a randomized clinical trial. *J Am Coll Cardiol*. 2013;62(24):2318–2325.
42. Kim MY, Coyle C, Tomlinson DR, et al. Ectopy-triggering ganglionated plexuses ablation to prevent atrial fibrillation: GANGLIA-AF study. *Heart Rhythm*. 2022;19(4):516–524.
43. Pokushalov E, Romanov A, Katritsis DG, et al. Ganglionated plexus ablation vs linear ablation in patients undergoing pulmonary vein isolation for persistent/longstanding persistent atrial fibrillation: a randomized comparison. *Heart Rhythm*. 2013;10(9):1280–1286.
44. Danik S, Neuzil P, d'Avila A, et al. Evaluation of catheter ablation of periatrial ganglionic plexi in patients with atrial fibrillation. *Am J Cardiol*. 2008;102(5):578–583.
45. Kim DT, Lai A.C., Hwang C, et al. The ligament of Marshall: a structural analysis in human hearts with implications for atrial arrhythmias. *J Am Coll Cardiol*. 2000;36(4):1324–1327.
46. Hwang C, Chen PS. Ligament of Marshall: why it is important for atrial fibrillation ablation. *Heart Rhythm*. 2009;6(12):S35–S40.
47. Liu X, Yan Q, Hui L, et al. Ablation of ligament of Marshall attenuates atrial vulnerability to fibrillation induced by inferior left atrial fat pad stimulation in dogs. *J Cardiovasc Electrophysiol*. 2010;21(9):1024–1030.
48. Ulphani JS, Arora R, Cain JH, et al. The ligament of Marshall as a parasympathetic conduit. *Am J Physiol-Heart Circ Physiol*. 2007;293(3):H1629–H1635.
49. Baez-Escudero JL, Keida T, Dave AS, Okishige K, Valderrabano M. Ethanol infusion in the vein of Marshall leads to parasympathetic denervation of the human left atrium: implications for atrial fibrillation. *J Am Coll Cardiol*. 2014;63(18):1892–1901.
50. Valderrabano M, Peterson LE, Swarup V, et al. Effect of catheter ablation with vein of Marshall ethanol infusion vs catheter ablation alone on persistent atrial fibrillation: the VENUS randomized clinical Trial. *J Am Med Assoc*. 2020;324(16):1620–1628.
51. Suwalski G, Marczewska MM, Kaczejko K, et al. Left atrial ganglionated plexi detection is related to heart rate and early recurrence of atrial fibrillation after surgical ablation. *Braz J Cardiovasc Surg*. 2017;32(2):118–124.
52. Wyler von Ballmoos MC, Hui DS, Mehaffey JH, et al. The society of thoracic surgeons 2023 clinical practice guidelines for the surgical treatment of atrial fibrillation. *Ann Thorac Surg*. 2024;118(2):291–310.
53. Je HG, Choi JW, Hwang HY, et al. 2023 KASNet Guidelines on atrial fibrillation surgery. *J Chest Surg*. 2024;57(1):1–24.
54. Calkins H, Hindricks G, Cappato R, et al. 2017 HRS/EHRA/ECAS/APHRS/SOLAECE Expert consensus statement on catheter and surgical ablation of atrial fibrillation. *Heart Rhythm*. 2017;14(10):e275–e444.

31

Results of Catheter Ablation for Stand-Alone Atrial Fibrillation

James L. Cox

CHAPTER OUTLINE

The development of catheter ablation for the treatment of patients with cardiac arrhythmias represents one of the seminal achievements in the history of heart disease therapy. The first catheter-based approach for interventional arrhythmia treatment was described in 1982 when Mel Scheinman and Fred Morady of the University of California San Francisco reported a method called "catheter fulguration" for creating heart block with an endocardial catheter.[1] The precise location of the His bundle was first determined by endocardial mapping of the atrial septum just above the tricuspid valve annulus. After it was located, an electrical shock was delivered through the catheter to create permanent heart block, and a permanent ventricular pacemaker was then implanted.

Elective heart block by the catheter fulguration technique was used to treat patients with various intractable supraventricular tachyarrhythmias throughout the 1980s.[2–4] The objective of elective His bundle ablation was not to ablate the atrial fibrillation (AF) but rather to confine it to the atria and protect the ventricles from the irregularly irregular rhythm associated with AF (see Chapter 11). Sealy and Gallagher[5] had been performing elective His bundle ablation that required open-heart surgery for almost 10 years before Scheinman's catheter fulguration technique was introduced. However, the far less invasive catheter technique proved to be as successful in creating heart block as the surgical approach had been, so the latter receded into history. After radiofrequency (RF) catheters became available[6] in the late 1980s, the catheter fulguration technique was abandoned.[7]

Before the availability of RF catheters, successful surgical procedures had been developed for the treatment of Wolff-Parkinson-White syndrome (1968),[8] ischemic ventricular tachycardia (1978),[9,10] nonischemic ventricular tachycardia (1979),[11] automatic atrial tachycardias (1980),[12] atrioventricular node reentry tachycardia (1982),[13] and AF (1987).[14] However, the ability to perform RF catheter ablation in the early 1990s quickly replaced all of these surgical approaches except the Maze procedure for the treatment of patients with AF.[15–18]

Multiple attempts at creating a Maze-like pattern of atrial lesions with an endocardial RF catheter were unsuccessful, but in 1998, Michel Haissaguerre and Pierre Jais reported that most episodes of AF were induced by pulmonary vein (PV) triggers and that the frequency of paroxysmal AF (PAF) episodes could be decreased, or even abolished, by isolating the triggers to the PVs.[19] This seminal article initiated the era of catheter ablation for AF that has dominated its interventional treatment to the present day.

IMPACT OF ATRIAL FIBRILLATION TYPE ON THE RESULTS OF CATHETER ABLATION

After Haissaguerre and coworkers' 1998 article, pulmonary vein isolation (PVI) with RF catheters proved to be quite successful for the treatment of patients with PAF. In their original article, Haissaguerre et al.[19] reported a success rate with PVI for PAF of 62%.Thousands of publications on the results of catheter ablation for AF have appeared in the literature since that time. In 2023, Roger Winkle and his associates[20] in Redwood City and Palo Alto, California, published a remarkable and unique article reporting their personal series of 5200 patients who underwent 7145 catheter ablation procedures over a period of two decades (2003–2023).[20] To include the most contemporary ablation devices and techniques, they divided the years into three treatment eras. Catheter ablation was performed in 101 patients using solid big-tip catheters from 2003 to 2005. From 2005 to 2016, 2143 patients had ablation with open irrigated-tip catheters, and from 2016 to 2021, 2956 patients were ablated using contact force catheters. There was some overlap in the types of catheters used in the last two eras. Winkle et al. also reported the patient results at 5, 10, and 16 years according to whether the patient had PAF, persistent AF, or long-standing persistent AF (LSpAF). Their report demonstrated a significant difference in the results of catheter ablation depending primarily on the type of AF being treated (Fig. 31.1).

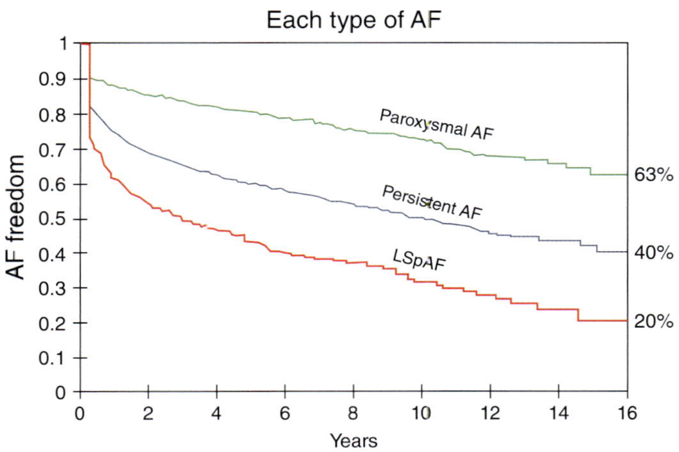

Fig. 31.1 Sixteen-year success rates of catheter ablation for paroxysmal atrial fibrillation (AF), persistent AF, and long-standing persistent AF (LSpAF) in 5200 patients. At 16 years, the success rates were 63% for paroxysmal AF, 40% for persistent AF, and 20% for LSpAF. (Modified and reproduced from Winkle RA, Mead RH, Engel G, et al. Very long term outcomes of atrial fibrillation ablation. *Heart Rhythm.* 2023;20:680–688.)

CATHETER ABLATION FOR PAROXYSMAL ATRIAL FIBRILLATION

Winkle et al.'s article documented that the AF-freedom rates after their final catheter ablation for PAF at 5, 10, and 16 years were 80%, 73%, and 63%, respectively. In 2014, Takigawa and colleagues[21] reported a success rate of 75% at 9 years in 1220 patients with PAF who had catheter PVI in addition to "focal ablation for nonpulmonary vein foci." It is interesting that Winkle and colleagues' 9-year success rate of 75% for patients with PAF was identical to that of Takigawa and colleagues (Fig. 31.2).

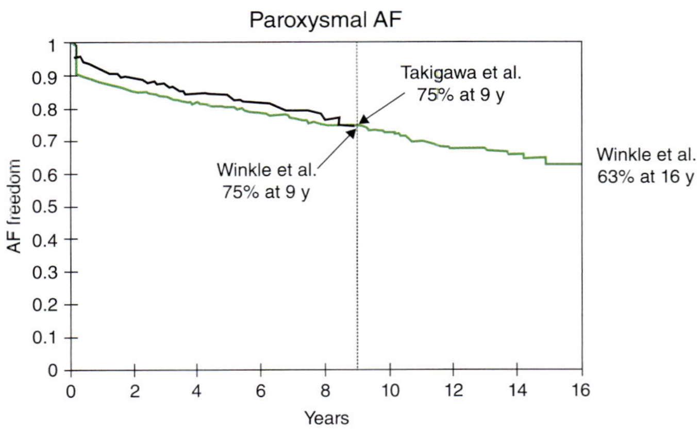

Fig. 31.2 Winkle et al.[20] and Takigawa et al.'s[21] catheter ablation success rates at 9 years for paroxysmal atrial fibrillation (AF) were identical (75%). Winkle et al.'s patients went on to have a 63% success rate at 16 years. (Modified and reproduced from Winkle RA, Mead RH, Engel G, et al. Very long term outcomes of atrial fibrillation ablation. *Heart Rhythm.* 2023;20:680–688 and Takigawa M, Takahashi A, Kuwahara T, et al. Long-term follow-up after catheter ablation of paroxysmal atrial fibrillation. *Circ Arrhythm Elecctrophysiol.* 2014;7:267–273).

The fact that these two large studies, one with 5200 patients and another with 1220 patients, had identical 9-year success rates supports the validity of the subsequent 16-year results reported by Winkle and coworkers.

CATHETER ABLATION FOR PERSISTENT ATRIAL FIBRILLATION

Because of the rather arbitrary nature of the classification of AF (see Chapter 52), reports on the treatment of persistent AF often include LSpAF, making it difficult to determine the results of catheter ablation specifically for patients with persistent AF. Thus there is a paucity of information on the results of catheter ablation specifically for those with persistent AF, especially at 5 years. Fortunately, in 2015, a group of three centers in Germany reported a 56% success rate at 5 years for multiple catheter ablations performed solely for persistent AF in 549 patients.[22] In Winkle and colleagues' report, the 5-year success rate for the catheter ablation of persistent AF was 60%, only 4% different from the German centers' results (Fig. 31.3).

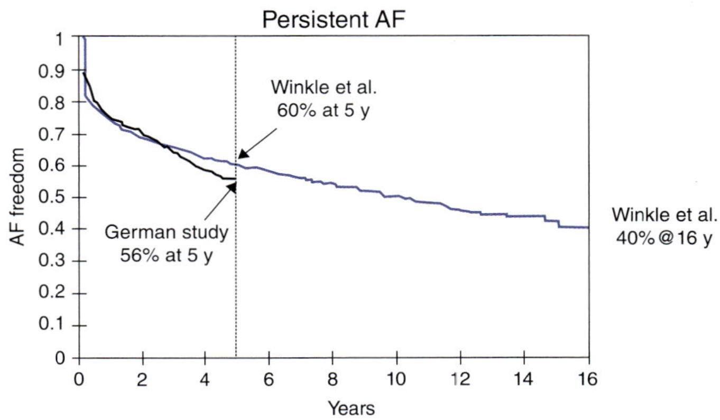

Fig. 31.3 Winkle et al.[20] and Takigawa et al.'s[21] catheter ablation success rates at 5 years for persistent atrial fibrillation (AF) were 60% and 56%, respectively. Winkle's patients went on to have a 40% success rate at 16 years. (Modified and reproduced from Winkle RA, Mead RH, Engel G, et al. Very long term outcomes of atrial fibrillation ablation. *Heart Rhythm.* 2023;20:680–688 and Schreiber D, Rostock TR, Frolich M, et al. Five-year follow-up after catheter ablation of persistent atrial fibrillation using the stepwise approach and prognostic factors for success. *Circ Arrhythm Elecctrophysiol.* 2015;8:308–317).

CATHETER ABLATION FOR LONG-STANDING PERSISTENT ATRIAL FIBRILLATION

The most important previous study evaluating the effectiveness of catheter ablation for LSpAF was the 2012 Hamburg Study.[23] That landmark study showed that the 5-year success rate after a single catheter ablation for LSpAF was only 20%, but that it increased to 45% after multiple catheter ablations. Winkle et al.'s study showed an identical 45% 5-year success rate for the catheter ablation of LSpAF (Fig. 31.4), again validating the data reported by Winkle et al. at 10 and 16 years after the last catheter ablation.

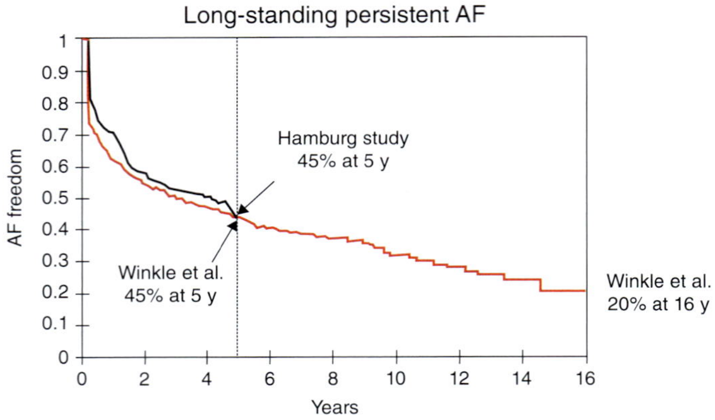

Fig. 31.4 Winkle et al.[20] and the Hamburg Study's[23] catheter ablation success rates at 5 years for long-standing persistent atrial fibrillation (AF) were identical (45%). Winkle et al.'s patients went on to have a 20% success rate at 16 years. (Modified and from Winkle RA, Mead RH, Engel G, et al. Very long term outcomes of atrial fibrillation ablation. *Heart Rhythm.* 2023;20:680–688 and Tilz RR, Rillig A, Thum et al. Catheter ablation of long-standing persistent atrial fibrillation: 5-year outcomes of the Hamburg Sequential Ablation Strategy. *J Am Coll Cardiol.* 2012;60(19):1921–1929.)

CATHETER ABLATION FOR ALL PATIENTS WITH ATRIAL FIBRILLATION

Winkle et al. reported that success rates for catheter ablation improved over the entire study period in the patient groups with PAF and persistent AF, but they did not improve in patients with LSpAF. The overall success rates for catheter ablation in all patients in the study (combined PAF, persistent AF, and LSpAF) at 5 years, 10 years, and 16 years were 65%, 58%, and 47%, respectively. The 5-year success rate of 65% was the same as the 5-year overall success rate reported in the 2020 randomized CABANA trial (64%)[24] (Fig. 31.5). Again, this documents that

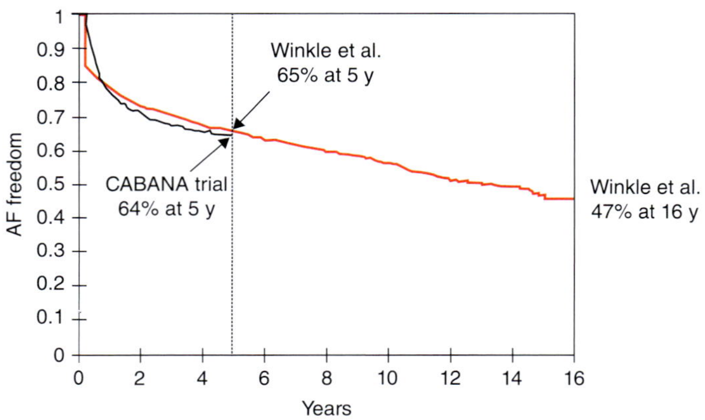

Fig. 31.5 Winkle et al.[20] and the CABANA trial's[24] catheter ablation success rates at 5 years for all patients with atrial fibrillation (AF) were 65% and 64%, respectively. Winkle et al.'s patients went on to have a 47% overall success rate at 16 years. (Modified and reproduced from Winkle RA, Mead RH, Engel G, et al. Very long term outcomes of atrial fibrillation ablation. *Heart Rhythm.* 2023;20:680–688 and Poole JE, Bahnson TD, Monahan KH, et al. Recurrence of atrial fibrillation after catheter ablation or antiarrhythmic drug therapy in the CABANA trial. *J Am Coll Cardiol.* 2020;75(25):3105–3118).

Winkle et al.'s data were consistent with previously reported trials and that their 10-year and 16-year data are reliable indicators of the overall long-term effectiveness of catheter ablation for AF.

CATHETER ABLATION COMPARED WITH OTHER TREATMENT MODALITIES

The satisfactory results of catheter ablation for patients with PAF have resulted in PVI being a first-line therapy for those with PAF in many centers. Several meta-analyses have suggested that catheter ablation is superior to medical therapy and might even be considered as a first-line therapy in patients with persistent AF.[25,26] Two separate meta-analyses of randomized controlled trials also suggested that catheter ablation is superior to medical therapy in persistent patients with AF, especially those with heart failure.[27,28] However, the randomized AMICA trial failed to show any benefit of catheter ablation over medical therapy in patients with persistent AF and advanced heart failure.[29]

CATHETER ABLATION VERSUS SURGICAL THERAPY FOR LONG-STANDING PERSISTENT ATRIAL FIBRILLATION

The suboptimal results of catheter ablation for LSpAF raised the issue of whether or not these patients should be treated surgically rather than by catheter ablation. The 2011 randomized controlled FAST trial demonstrated that minimally invasive surgery (combined PVI, ganglionic plexus ablation, and left atrial appendage occlusion [LAAO]) was superior to catheter ablation for persistent AF.[30] However, that same year, the randomized controlled CASA-AF trial showed that a thoracoscopic surgical ablation (combined box lesion, ganglionic plexus ablation, and LAAO) was no better than catheter ablation for the treatment of patients with LSpAF.[31] These equivocal results from two well-controlled trials supported the idea that a hybrid procedure combining thoracoscopic surgical ablation and catheter ablation might be a better choice. Thus the poor catheter results for more persistent forms of AF and the introduction of thoracoscopic surgical techniques led to the development of the hybrid procedures that are presented in the following chapters in this section.

REFERENCES

1. Scheinman MM, Morady F, Hess DS, Gonzalez R. Catheter- induced ablation of the atrioventricular junction to control refractory supraventricular arrhythmias. *J Am Med Assoc.* 1982;248:851–855.
2. Gallagher J, Svenson RH, Kasell JH, et al. Catheter technique for closed- chest ablation of the atrioventricular conduction system: a therapeutic alternative for the treatment of refractory supraventricular tachycardia. *N Engl J Med.* 1982;306:194–200.
3. Gallagher J, Trantham JL. Observations during catheter ablation of the atrioventricular conduction system in humans. In: Fontaine G, Scheinman MM, eds. *Ablation in Cardiac Arrhythmias.* Futura Publishing Co; 1987:117–137.
4. Rosenqvist M, Lee MA, Moulinier L, et al. Long-term follow-up of patients after transcatheter direct current ablation of the atrioventricular junction. *J Am Coll Cardiol.* 1990;16:1467–1474.
5. Sealy WC, Gallagher J, Kasell J. His bundle interruption for control of inappropriate ventricular responses to atrial arrhythmias. *Ann Thorac Surg.* 1981;32:429–438.
6. Rowland E, Cunningham D, Rickards AF. Transvenous ablation of AV conduction using a new energy source (abstract). *Circulation.* 1986;74(supplI) I-386.

7. Langberg J, Chin MC, Rosenqvist M, et al. Catheter ablation of the atrioventricular junction with radiofrequency energy. *Circulation*. 1989;80:1527–1535.
8. Cobb FR, Blumenschein SD, Sealy WC, Boineau JP, Wagner GS, Wallace AG. Successful surgical interruption of the bundle of Kent in a patient with Wolff-Parkinson-White syndrome. *Circulation*. 1968;38:1018.
9. Guiraudon G, Fontaine G, Frank R, Escande G, Etievent P, Cabrol C. Encircling endocardial ventriculotomy: a new surgical treatment for life-threatening ventricular tachycardias resistant to medical treatment following myocardial infarction. *Ann Thor Surg*. 1978;26(5):438–444.
10. Harken AH, Horowitz LN, Josephson ME. The surgical treatment of ventricular tachycardia. *Ann Thor Surg*. 1980;30(5):499–508.
11. Cox JL, Bardy GH, Damiano RJ, et al. Right ventricular isolation procedures for nonischemic ventricular tachycardia. *J Thorac Cardiovasc Surg*. 1985;90:212.
12. Williams JM, Ungerleider RM, Lofland GK, Cox JL. Left atrial isolation: new technique for the treatment of supraventricular arrhythmias. *J Thorac Cardiovasc Surg*. 1980;80:373.
13. Cox JL, Holman WL, Cain ME. Cryosurgical treatment of atrioventricular node reentry tachycardia. *Circulation*. 1987;76:13291336.
14. Cox JL. The surgical treatment of atrial fibrillation: IV. Surgical technique. *J Thorac Cardiovasc Surg*. 1991;101:584–592.
15. Jackman WM, Wang XZ, Friday KJ, et al., Catheter ablation of accessory atrioventricular pathways (Wolff-Parkinson-White syndrome by radiofrequency current. N Engl J Med, 324(23):1605-1611.
16. Haissaguerre M, Warin JF, Lematayer P, Saoudi N, Guillem JP, Blanchot P. Closed-chest ablation of retrograde conduction in patients with atrioventricular nodal reentrant tachycardia. *N Engl J Med*. 1989;320:426–433.
17. Fisher JD. Stimulation as a key to tachycardia localization and ablation. *J Am Coll Cardiol*. 1988;11:889–893.
18. Fitzgerald DM, Friday KJ, Yeung Lai Wah JA, Lazzara R, Jackman WM. Electrogram patterns predicting successful catheter ablation of ventricular tachycardia. *Circulation*. 1988;77:806–814.
19. Haissaguerre M, Jais P, Shah DC, et al. Spontaneous initiation of atrial fibrillation by ectopic beats originating in the pulmonary veins. *N Eng J Med*. 1998;339(10):659–665.
20. Winkle RA, Mead RH, Engel G, et al. Very long term outcomes of atrial fibrillation ablation. *Heart Rhythm*. 2023;20:680–688.
21. Takigawa M, Takahashi A, Kuwahara T, et al. Long-term follow-up after catheter ablation of paroxysmal atrial fibrillation. *Circ Arrhythm Elecctrophysiol*. 2014;7:267–273.
22. Schreiber D, Rostock TR, Frolich M, et al. Five-year follow-up after catheter ablation of persistent atrial fibrillation using the stepwise approach and prognostic factors for success. *Circ Arrhythm Elecctrophysiol*. 2015;8:308–317.
23. Tilz RR, Rillig A, Thum AM, et al. Catheter ablation of long-standing persistent atrial fibrillation: 5-year outcomes of the Hamburg Sequential Ablation Strategy. *J Am Coll Card*. 2012;60(19):1921–1929.
24. Poole JE, Bahnson TD, Monahan KH, et al. Recurrence of atrial fibrillation after catheter ablation or antiarrhythmic drug therapy in the CABANA Trial. *J Am Coll Card*. 2020;75(25): 3105–3118.
25. Khan AR, Khan S, Sheikh MA, Khuder S, Grubb B, Moukarbel GV. Catheter ablation and antiarrhythmic drug therapy as first-or second-line therapy in the management of atrial fibrillation: systematic review and meta-analysis. *Circ Arrhythm Electrophysiol*. 2014;7(5):853–860.
26. Shi LZ, Heng R, Liu SM, Leng FY. Effect of catheter ablation versus antiarrhythmic drugs on atrial fibrillation: a meta-analysis of randomized controlled trials. *Therap Med*. 2015;10(2): 816–822.
27. Chen C, Zhou X, Zhu M, et al. Catheter ablation versus medical therapy for patients with persistent atrial fibrillation: a systematic review and meta-analysis of evidence from randomized controlled trials. *J Interv Card Electrophysiol*. 2018;52:9–18.
28. Zhu M, Zhou X, Cai H, et al. Catheter ablation versus medical rate control or persistent atrial fibrillation in patients with heart failure. *Medicine*. 2016;95:30.
29. Kuch K-H, Merkely B, Zahn R, et al. Catheter ablation versus best medical therapy in patients with persistent atrial fibrillation and congestive heart failure: the randomized AMICA Trial. *Circ Arrhythm Electrophysiol*. 2019;12(12):e007731.
30. Boersma LVA, Castella M, van Boven W, et al. Atrial fibrillation catheter ablation versus surgical ablation treatment (FAST) a 2-center randomized clinical trial. *Circulation*. 2012;125:23–30.
31. Haldar S, Khan JR, Boyalla V, et al. Catheter ablation vs. thoracoscopic surgical ablation in long-standing persistent atrial fibrillation: CASA-AF randomized controlled trial. *Eur Heart J*. 2020;41(47):4471–4480.

32

Totally Thoracoscopic Left Atrial Modified Maze Procedure

Bart P. van Putte

CHAPTER OUTLINE

The Cox Maze procedure has been performed routinely since its first description in 1991.[1–4] However, the degree of invasiveness precluded the widespread adoption of the Cox Maze procedure, limiting its use to only the most recalcitrant stand-alone AF cases and to concomitant AF ablation during cardiac surgery. Less invasive catheter ablation procedures for AF were introduced by Haissaguerre et al. in 1998,[5] and although they have since become the procedure of choice for the interventional treatment of patients with paroxysmal AF (PAF), they have yielded less favorable results for persistent AF and long-standing persistent AF[6] (see Chapter 31). Several "minimally invasive" surgical procedures were proposed to address this dilemma,[7–9] but they proved to be little better than catheter ablation for PAF. In addition, while they were somewhat better than catheter ablation for non-PAF[10] and were less invasive than a Cox Maze procedure, they were still far more invasive than catheter ablation. The dilemma of the success of interventional AF procedures being inversely related to their degree of invasiveness ultimately led to the development of thoracoscopic surgery for AF.

DEVELOPMENT OF THORACOSCOPIC SURGERY FOR ATRIAL FIBRILLATION

In 2003, thoracoscopic surgery using a microwave energy source was described as a less invasive procedure than open surgery for performing pulmonary vein isolation (PVI).[11] Unfortunately, this limited lesion set is adequate only for the isolation of AF triggers in the pulmonary veins (PVs). Nevertheless, the disappointing results of microwave PVIs for the overall treatment of patients with AF (i.e., all types of AF) were attributed to the use of microwave energy rather than to the fact that PVI is an inadequate operation for non-PAF. Thus, after this initial publication, microwave energy was abandoned and replaced by radiofrequency (RF) as the preferred new energy source for surgical AF ablation. Different minimally invasive and thoracoscopic surgical techniques were proposed for the surgical treatment of patients with AF, including bilateral video-assisted RF ablation and bilateral closed-chest RF ablation.[7,12] These attempts at AF ablation using only thoracoscopic surgical approaches were disappointing and as a result, the concept of a "hybrid procedure" was introduced in which thoracoscopic surgeons and interventional electrophysiologists joined forces to treat patients with AF.[13] The incentive for such a procedure is to combine the best of the two worlds, epicardial RF surgical ablation and endocardial RF catheter ablation. Although the hybrid ablation procedures were promising and have proven to be useful, they were never directly compared with epicardial thoracoscopic ablation alone without follow-up endocardial catheter ablation. Our group observed early on that thoracoscopic epicardial RF ablation had similar success rates as hybrid procedures, so we persisted in this thoracoscopic-only approach for the treatment of stand-alone AF.

The FAST trial, which compared endocardial catheter ablation with closed-chest surgical RF isolation of the PVs, ganglionic plexus ablation, and left atrial appendage (LAA) closure in patients with persistent AF and PAF demonstrated that epicardial surgical ablation was superior to endocardial catheter ablation for rhythm control (66% vs 37%, respectively; $P = .0022$), although the procedural adverse event rate (mainly pneumothorax) was significantly higher for surgical ablation.[10]

A multicenter cohort registry in 475 patients confirmed results for the thoracoscopic ablation of AF and showed an overall freedom from arrhythmia of 69% after a mean follow-up of almost 2 years.[14] A systematic safety analysis in 558 patients confirmed the safety of thoracoscopic AF ablation and emphasized an interaction between the incidence of complications, age and gender, resulting in older female patients being more prone to complications than others.[15] Another study in 222 patients showed a stroke rate of only 0.5% per 100 patient-years after LAA occlusion with postoperative oral anticoagulation in 43% of patients.[16]

In 2016, the European Association for Cardio-Thoracic Surgery (EACTS)/European Society of Cardiology (ESC) guidelines for the management of AF awarded a Class 2A recommendation for the thoracoscopic ablation of AF.[17] Despite this important validation, there remains some concern among patients and cardiologists regarding postoperative pain, which can lead to prolonged recovery. However, despite the natural increase in the number of patients with AF and demonstration of the safety and efficacy of thoracoscopic AF ablation, we did not experience the expected increase in the number of referrals for this therapy. This encouraged surgeons to find even less invasive ways to treat patients with AF. In 2020 and 2021, surgeons from the Netherlands introduced the unilateral right-chest and unilateral left-chest approaches for thoracoscopic ablation that limited the postoperative pain to one side.[18,19] This experience emphasizes the importance of reducing postoperative pain as much as possible and the lowest possible level of pain seems to have been reached with these unilateral approaches. In our current technique, only two 5-mm and one 1-mm incisions are required to do the entire operation. However, no matter how minimally invasive we can make surgery, it will always be more invasive than catheter ablation, which requires only the puncture of a vein in the groin. On the contrary, catheter ablation must compete with the efficacy of surgical ablation, which remains the gold standard for the interventional treatment of patients with AF. Although catheter-based technology has evolved significantly over the years, any energy delivered through a catheter will always be from a single unipolar device that targets the tissue from only one side while being guided by fluoroscopy rather than direct vision. Therefore, achieving reliably contiguous and uniformly transmural lesions will remain a major challenge for the catheter ablation of AF.

CURRENT SURGICAL TECHNIQUE

The 2020 ESC/EACTS guidelines for the management of AF state that there is no supporting evidence for the use of catheters, which are unipolar, to create atrial lines other than those around the PVs.[20] Currently, bipolar RF clamps are used to isolate the PVs, and unipolar radiofrequency (RF) pens are the only devices available to create additional atrial lesions from the epicardium. However, as in catheter ablation, it is difficult to create reliably transmural and contiguous linear lesions with unipolar RF pen devices. In 2022, we described a unilateral right-chest approach in which the entire left atrial box lesion was created with bipolar RF clamps only, thereby ameliorating the need for unipolar devices and substantially reducing the risk for incomplete lesions and treatment failure.[21] The major challenge to overcome during the development of this off-pump approach was to make sure that cardiac output and adequate blood pressure are maintained throughout the ablation. This means that all four PVs cannot be clamped simultaneously. The left PVs are first isolated as described in the right sided unilateral approach (Fig. 32.1). Next, the roof and floor lesions are created in two stages. First, the two right PVs and the left inferior PV are clamped simultaneously and ablated, leaving the left superior PV open (Fig. 32.2). Then the two right PVs and the left superior PV are clamped and ablated, leaving the left inferior PV open (Fig. 32.3). This completes

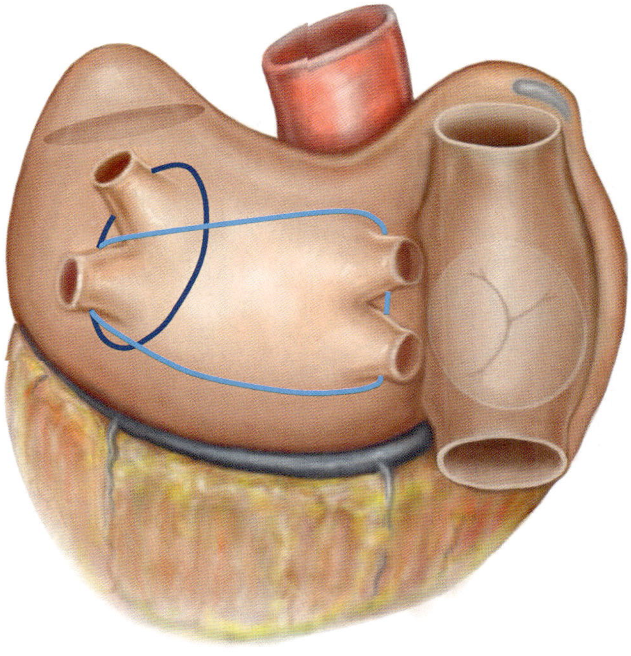

Fig. 32.2 The right pulmonary veins (PVs) and the left inferior PV are clamped simultaneously with a bipolar radiofrequency clamp, leaving the left superior PV open *(light blue circle)*.

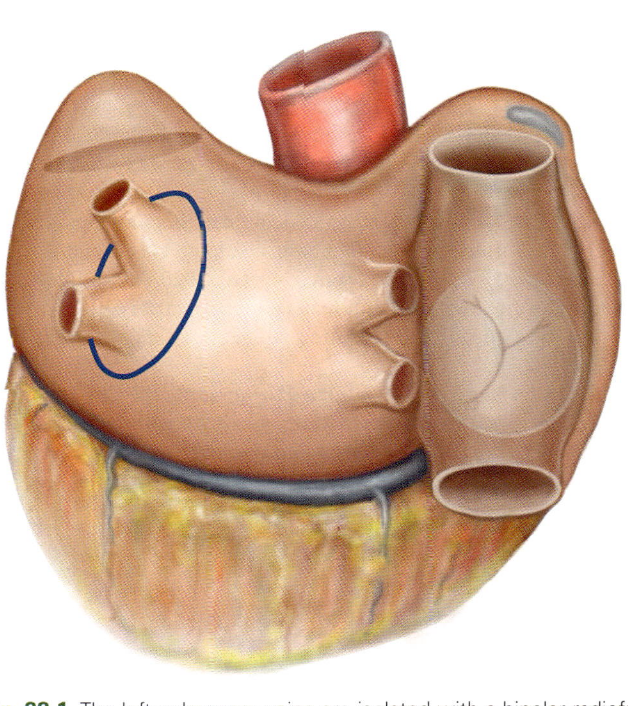

Fig. 32.1 The left pulmonary veins are isolated with a bipolar radiofrequency clamp *(dark blue circle)*.

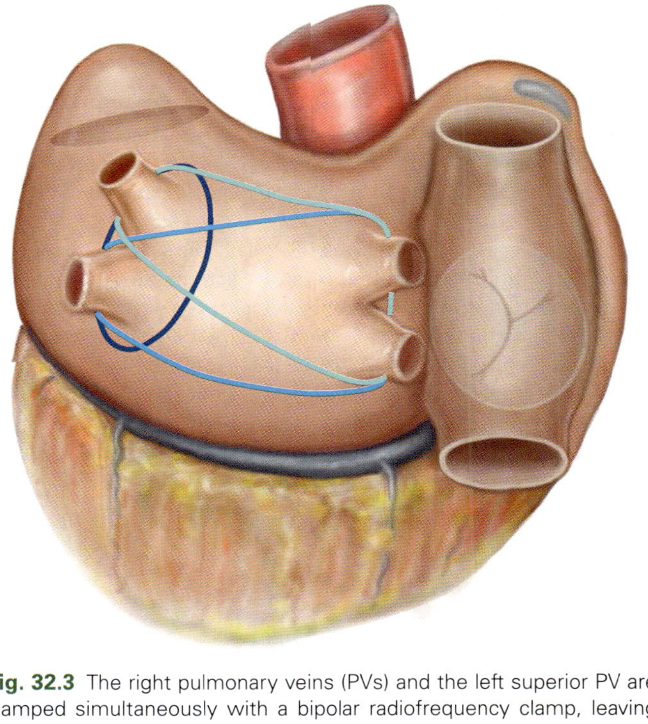

Fig. 32.3 The right pulmonary veins (PVs) and the left superior PV are clamped simultaneously with a bipolar radiofrequency clamp, leaving the left inferior PV open *(cyan circle)*.

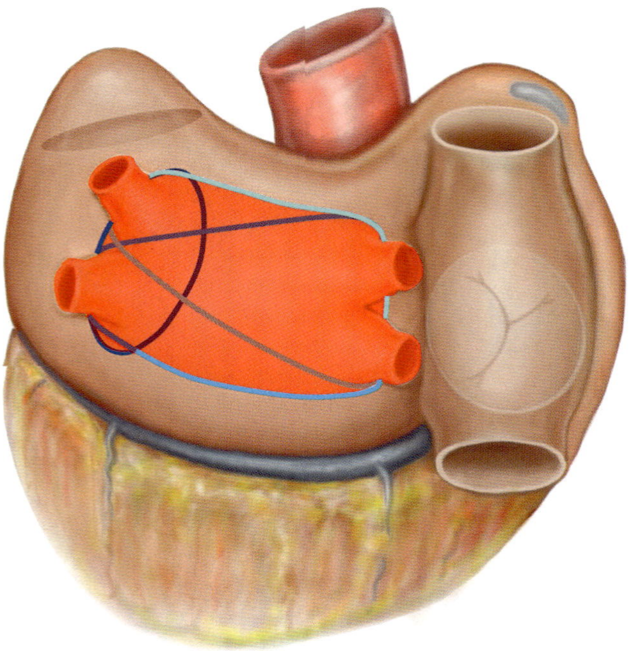

Fig. 32.4 The three separate lesions created with a bipolar radiofrequency clamp complete the box lesion isolating all four pulmonary veins and the intervening posterior left atrial wall *(red-shaded area)*.

the box lesion isolating all four PVs and the intervening posterior left atrial wall (Fig. 32.4).

Creating the box lesion using only bipolar RF clamps overcomes the need to use unipolar pens to create the roof and floor lesions. This improves the efficacy of the box lesion, and it can be performed much more quickly than a box lesion in which the two pairs of PVs are isolated with bipolar RF clamps and the roof and floor lesions are created with unipolar RF devices.

REFERENCES

1. Cox JL, Schuessler RB, Boineau JP. The surgical treatment of atrial fibrillation: I. Summary of the current concepts of the mechanisms of atrial flutter and atrial fibrillation. *J Thorac Cardiovasc Surg*. 1991;101:402–405.
2. Cox JL, Canavan TE, Schuessler RB, et al. The surgical treatment of atrial fibrillation: II. Intraoperative electrophysiologic mapping and description of the electrophysiologic basis of atrial flutter and atrial fibrillation. *J Thorac Cardiovasc Surg*. 1991;101:406–426.
3. Cox JL, Schuessler RB, D'Agostino Jr HJ, et al. The surgical treatment of atrial fibrillation: III. Development of a definitive surgical procedure. *J Thorac Cardiovasc Surg*. 1991;101:569–583.
4. Cox JL. The SURGICAL treatment of atrial fibrillation: IV. Surgical technique. *J Thorac Cardiovasc Surg*. 1991;101:584–592.
5. Haissaguerre M, Jais P, Shah DC, et al. Spontaneous initiation of atrial fibrillation by ectopic beats originating in the pulmonary veins. *N Eng J Med*. 1998;339(10):659–666.
6. Winkle RA, Mead RH, Engel G, et al. Very long term outcomes of atrial fibrillation ablation. *Heart Rhythm*. 2023;20:680–688.
7. Wolf RK, Schneeberger EW, Osterday R, et al. Video-assisted bilateral pulmonary vein isolation and left atrial appendage exclusion for atrial fibrillation. *J Thorac Cardiovasc Surg*. 2005;130:797–802.
8. Edgerton JR, Jackman WM, Mack MJ. A new epicardial lesion set for minimal access left atrial Maze: the Dallas lesion set. *Ann Thorac Surg*. 2009;88:1655–1657.
9. Sirak J, Jones D, Schwartzman D. The five-box thoracoscopic Maze procedure. *Ann Thorac Surg*. 2012;95(3):986–989.
10. Boersma LVA, Castella M, van Boven W, et al. Atrial fibrillation catheter ablation versus surgical ablation treatment (FAST): a 2-center randomized clinical trial. *Circulation*. 2012;125(1):23–30.
11. Saltman AE, Rosenthal LS, Francalancia NA, Lahey S. A completely endoscopic approach to microwave ablation for atrial fibrillation. *Heart Surg Forum*. 2003;6(3):E38–E41.
12. Hu QM, Li Y, Han J, Zhang HB, Meng X. Analysis of risk factors for recurrence after video-assisted pulmonary vein isolation of lone atrial fibrillation – results of 5 years of follow-up. *J Thorac Cardiovasc Surg*. 2014;148(5):2174–2180.
13. Pison L, La Meir M, van Opstal J, Maessen J, Crijns HJ. Hybrid thoracoscopic surgical and transvenous catheter ablation of atrial fibrillation. *J Am Coll Cardiol*. 2012;60(1):54–61.
14. Van Laar C, Bentala M, Weimar T, et al. Thoracoscopic ablation for the treatment of atrial fibrillation: a systematic outcome analysis of a multicentre cohort. *Europace*. 2019;21(6):893–899.
15. Vos LM, Kotecha D, Geuzebroek GSC, et al. Totally thoracoscopic ablation for atrial fibrillation: a systematic safety analysis. *Europace*. 2018;20(11):1790–1797.
16. Van Laar C, Verberkmoes NJ, van Es HW, et al. Thoracoscopic left atrial appendage clipping: a multicenter cohort analysis. *JACC Clin Electerophysiol*. 2018;4(7):893–901.
17. Kirchof P, Benussi S, Kotecha D, et al. 2016 ESC guidelines for the management of atrial fibrillation developed in collaboration with EACTS. *Eur Heart J*. 2016;37(38):2893–2962.
18. Fleerakkers J, Hofman FN, van Putte BP. Totally thoracoscopic ablation: a unilateral right sided approach. *Eur J Cardiothorac Surg*. 2020;58(5):1088–1090.
19. Maesen B, La Meir M. Unilateral left-sided thoracoscopic ablation of atrial fibrillation. *Ann Thor Surg*. 2020;110(1):e63–e66.
20. Hindricks G, Potpara T, Dagres N, et al. 2020 ESC Guidelines for the diagnosis and management of atrial fibrillation developed in collaboration with EACTS. *Eur Heart J*. 2021;42(5):373–498.
21. Vos LM, Fleerakkers J, Hofman FN, van Putte BP. Closed-chest unilateral thoracoscopic ablation: box lesion with radiofrequency clamps only. *Eur J Cardiothorac Surg*. 2022;62(1):ezac316. doi:10.1093/ejcts/ezac316.

33

An Overview of Hybrid Procedures for the Treatment of Atrial Fibrillation

Gianluigi Bisleri

CHAPTER OUTLINE

The concept of hybrid ablation—combining a surgical and catheter-based approach—for the treatment of patients with atrial fibrillation (AF) was first proposed nearly 20 years ago.[1] Over the past decade, several technologies and techniques have been introduced in an attempt to overcome the limitations of both catheter and surgical AF ablation by combining them. Although catheter ablation has remained the first-line interventional treatment for stand-alone AF, the success rates have consistently been suboptimal for the treatment of persistent and long-standing persistent AF (LSpAF) (see Chapter 31).

Although the Cox-Maze procedure has remained the most effective interventional treatment for stand-alone AF, its level of invasiveness as a major cardiac surgical procedure requiring cardiopulmonary bypass has prevented its adoption as a first-line therapy for AF. Instead, off-pump minimally invasive and totally thoracoscopic epicardial surgical ablation procedures have become preferable even though they usually limit the atrial lesions that can be applied with the expected, and accepted, decrease in efficacy.[2]

RATIONALE FOR THE HYBRID ABLATION OF ATRIAL FIBRILLATION

Several modifications of AF catheter ablation techniques have been proposed in an effort to improve outcomes, ranging from pulmonary vein isolation (PVI), to wider inclusion of the antrum of the pulmonary veins (PVs), to including the posterior wall of the left atrium (LA) in a box lesion, to substrate modification by ablating complex atrial fractionated electrograms and trying to create linear lesions in the atrium.[2–4] Unfortunately, only the inclusion of the posterior LA wall in a box lesion has clearly proven to be superior to PVI alone. However, the potential risk of esophageal injury associated with isolation of the posterior LA wall using an endocardial radiofrequency (RF) catheter has resulted in simple PVI remaining as the primary technique for the catheter ablation of AF. Unfortunately, success rates below 50%, even after multiple catheter ablation procedures for LSpAF, have dampened the enthusiasm of the electrophysiology community for treating such a complex subset of patients at all.[5] Furthermore, recent studies have shown that in LSpAF, the macroreentrant drivers that sustain AF are more complex than originally thought and may exhibit epicardial–endocardial dissociation on electroanatomic mapping.[6,7]

PATIENT SELECTION

Most patients referred for the surgical ablation of AF have undergone multiple prior catheter ablations. Endocardial catheter PVI is associated with high success rates in patients with paroxysmal AF (PAF); therefore, hybrid procedures are rarely required in those patients. However, some patients with recurrent AF after PVI who are thought to have complete isolation of the PVs on the basis of endocardial maps can have epicardial breakthroughs that go undetected by endocardial mapping. This phenomenon can result in failure of an endocardial catheter PVI that requires thoracoscopic epicardial ablation.[8] However, most catheter ablation failures occur in patients with persistent AF or LSpAF. Hybrid procedures offer these patients a complementary solution to address problems with a prior PVI as well as incomplete isolation of the posterior wall of the LA. Only recently has a complete Cox-Maze lesion set has been accomplished with a hybrid approach[9]; the hybrid Maze procedure is described in Chapter 37.

Left atrial dimensions as determined by echocardiography and the duration of AF are also considered in the selection of patients to undergo hybrid procedures. Prior failed catheter ablation is a risk factor for AF recurrence following thoracoscopic epicardial surgical ablation. This is likely due to the presence of a complex substrate in the atrium with significant atrial remodeling and endocardial scar formation.[10] Previous cardiac surgery is considered to be a contraindication for hybrid procedures because of pericardial adhesions.

SURGICAL TECHNIQUES

Different minimally invasive surgical approaches have been described for performing the initial epicardial surgical ablation in a hybrid procedure, including mini-thoracotomies, thoracoscopy, and a subxiphoid approach. In addition, several different ablative lesion sets have been used in hybrid procedures, but the common goal has been to create an off-pump, epicardial-only surgical approach performed in conjunction with endocardial catheter ablation. Hybrid procedures can be performed as a "joint" procedure at the time of the initial thoracoscopic surgery or as a "staged" procedure in which the endocardial catheter ablation portion of the procedure is delayed several weeks to allow time for the epicardial lesions to mature.

The ablative energy source that is currently used for the initial epicardial ablation is either unipolar or bipolar RF. Although bipolar RF clamps were used most commonly in the early experience with minimally invasive approaches, different linear devices have since been developed that augment lesion sets and minimize surgical manipulation. Cryoablation is not effective for off-pump epicardial ablation because of the "heat sink" caused by the circulating normothermic cavitary blood (see Chapter 20). This is also a challenge for off-pump unipolar RF epicardial ablation in which the cavitary blood acts as a "cooling sink." Other energy sources, such as microwave and high-intensity focused ultrasound, have been proposed in the past but are no longer in use.

The primary objective of the initial thoracoscopic epicardial ablation of a hybrid procedure is to create a box in the LA that isolates all four PVs and the intervening posterior left atrial wall. The most common technique for creating the box in hybrid procedures is to isolate the right and left PVs in pairs using bipolar RF clamps passed through bilateral mini-thoracotomies or thoracoscopic ports. Floor and roof lesions are then created to isolate the posterior left atrial wall and complete the posterior box. These lesions have traditionally been created using a dual-electrode, unipolar Coolrail linear pen (Atricure Inc.).[11,12] Other techniques and devices to create the box lesion included a linear RF ablation device that could be wrapped around all four PVs and the posterior left atrial wall to create a complete box lesion, but it is no longer in use. More recently, a novel approach, the Convergent procedure, was introduced in which the posterior left atrial wall is ablated rather than isolated and the PVs are then isolated by endocardial catheter ablation (see Chapter 36). One advantage of the Convergent procedure is that it mitigates the risk of esophageal injury during isolation of the posterior left atrial wall that can occur with extensive endocardial catheter ablation. Another advantage is that it is performed through a small subxiphoid incision, though if the left atrial appendage is to be closed, it requires a separate left chest incision.

Hybrid procedures allow for the intraoperative validation of both epicardial and endocardial entrance and exit block as well as for advanced high-density mapping to confirm the acute results of the epicardial ablation. The role of the electrophysiologist is to detect and address any endocardial gaps in the surgical ablation lines or, during the convergent procedure, to complete the isolation of the PVs.

CLINICAL OUTCOMES OF HYBRID PROCEDURES

The clinical results of different hybrid procedures vary significantly due to a variety of factors that affect outcomes. These factors include the type of being treated (PAF versus nonparoxysmal AF [non-PAF]), the duration of (<5 years versus >5 years), the selected surgical approach (thoracotomy versus thoracoscopy versus subxiphoid), the choice of ablation device (bipolar RF versus unipolar RF), and the preferred ablation lesion set (PVI versus box lesion versus posterior wall ablation). Most published data are based on single-center experiences with limited cohorts of patients. The overall aggregate success rate of hybrid procedures in terms of freedom from AF ranges from approximately 60% to approximately 80%, and complication rates vary between 2% and 6%.[2,3,13]

Recently, three prospective randomized trials of hybrid procedures (CONVERGE, HARTCAP, CEASE-AF) that used different surgical techniques and technologies demonstrated a superiority of hybrid procedures over catheter ablation with an absolute increase in sinus rhythm restoration, especially in patients with LSpAF, ranging between 20% and 40%.[14–16] Most of the published series report only 1- to 3-year follow-up data, so there is a paucity of information regarding the long-term results of hybrid procedures.[17–19] Therefore, additional clinical evidence from either institutional experiences or prospective randomized trials is needed to assess the impact of hybrid procedures on long-term outcomes such as quality of life, stroke, heart failure, and mortality.

GUIDELINE RECOMMENDATIONS

There have been a few different guideline recommendations regarding hybrid procedures, including the 2020 European Association for Cardio-Thoracic Surgery/European Society of Cardiology guidelines, that recommended hybrid procedures in patients who have symptomatic PAF or persistent AF that is refractory to medical therapy (Class IIa, B) and in patients with persistent AF with risk factors for recurrences (Class IIb, C).[20] The 2023 American College of Cardiology/American Heart Association/American College of Clinical Pharmacy/Heart Rhythm Society guidelines also recommended hybrid procedures for patients with symptomatic persistent AF refractory to medical therapy (Class IIb).[21] The most recent 2024 Society of Thoracic Surgeons guidelines did not provide specific recommendations for hybrid procedures, but they confirmed a Class IIa recommendation for the use of surgical ablation for stand-alone AF with a preference for the use of the cryosurgical Maze procedure for patients with LspAF.[22] The US and European guidelines are discussed in greater detail in Chapter 24.

SUMMARY

Hybrid ablation has evolved and expanded over the past decade thanks to the development of multidisciplinary teams that integrate newly described minimally invasive and thoracoscopic surgical techniques with the most advanced mapping and catheter ablation techniques. The group of patients who are being offered hybrid ablation is rapidly evolving, especially among those with LSpAF. It is clear that hybrid procedures are superior to catheter ablation for non-PAF, but longer follow-up data are needed to establish the proper position of hybrid procedures in the spectrum of AF ablation procedures.

REFERENCES

1. Bisleri G, Curnis A, Bottio T, Mascioli G, Muneretto C. The need of a hybrid approach for the treatment of atrial fibrillation. *Heart Surg Forum*. 2005;8(5):E326–E330.
2. Bisleri G, Pandey AK, Verma S, et al. Combined minimally invasive surgical and percutaneous catheter ablation of atrial fibrillation. *J Am Coll Cardiol*. 2023;81(6):606–619.
3. Varzaly JA, Lau DH, Chapman D, Edwards J, Worthington M, Sanders P. Hybrid ablation for atrial fibrillation: a systematic review and meta-analysis. *J Thorac Cardiovasc Surg Open*. 2021;7:141–154.
4. Bisleri G, Glover B. Hybrid ablation for atrial fibrillation: current approaches and future directions. *Curr Opin Cardiol*. 2017;32(1):17–21.
5. van der Heijden CAJ, Vroomen M, Luermans JG, et al. Hybrid versus catheter ablation in patients with persistent and longstanding persistent atrial fibrillation: a systematic review and meta-analysis. *Eur J Cardiothorac Surg*. 2019;56(3):433–443.
6. Parameswaran R, Kalman JM, Royse A, et al. Endocardial-epicardial phase mapping of prolonged persistent atrial fibrillation recordings: high prevalence of dissociated activation patterns. *Circ Arrhythm Electrophysiol*. 2020;13(8):e008512.
7. Verheule S, Eckstein J, Linz D, et al. Role of endo-epicardial dissociation of electrical activity and transmural conduction in the development of persistent atrial fibrillation. *Prog Biophys Mol Biol*. 2014;115(2-3):173–185.
8. Ariss RW, Khan Minhas AM, Patel NJ, et al. Contemporary trends and in-hospital outcomes of catheter and stand-alone surgical ablation of atrial fibrillation. *EP Europace*. 2022;24:218–225.

9. Cox JL, Churyla A, Malaisrie SC, et al. A hybrid Maze procedure for long-standing persistent atrial fibrillation. *Ann Thorac Surg.* 2019;107:610–618.
10. Wesselink R, Vroomen M, Overeinder I, et al. A failed catheter ablation of atrial fibrillation is associated with more advanced remodeling and reduced efficacy of further thoracoscopic ablation. *Revista Española de Cardiología.* 2023;76:417–426.
11. Gelsomino S, Van Breugel HN, Pison L, et al. Hybrid thoracoscopic and transvenous catheter ablation of atrial fibrillation. *Eur J Cardiothorac Surg.* 2014;45:401–407.
12. Hassan SM, Hong K, Rosati F, et al. Hybrid ablation for atrial fibrillation: the importance of achieving transmurality and lesion validation. *Minerva Cardioangiol.* 2019;67(2):115–120.
13. Jiang YQ, Tian Y, Zeng LJ, et al. The safety and efficacy of hybrid ablation for the treatment of atrial fibrillation: a meta-analysis. *PLoS One.* 2018;13(1):e0190170.
14. DeLurgio DB, Crossen KJ, Gill J, et al. Hybrid convergent procedure for the treatment of persistent and long-standing persistent atrial fibrillation: results of CONVERGE clinical trial. *Circ Arrhythm Electrophysiol.* 2020;13(12):e009288.
15. van der Heijden CAJ, Weberndörfer V, Vroomen M, et al. Hybrid ablation versus repeated catheter ablation in persistent atrial fibrillation: a randomized controlled trial. *JACC Clin Electrophysiol.* 2023;9(7 Pt 2):1013–1023.
16. Doll N, Weimar T, Kosior DA, et al. Efficacy and safety of hybrid epicardial and endocardial ablation versus endocardial ablation in patients with persistent and longstanding persistent atrial fibrillation: a randomized, controlled trial. *E Clinical Medicine.* 2023;61:102052.
17. Mahapatra S, LaPar DJ, Kamath S, et al. Initial experience of sequential surgical epicardial-catheter endocardial ablation for persistent and long-standing persistent atrial fibrillation with long-term follow-up. *Ann Thorac Surg.* 2011;91(6):1890–1898.
18. Pannone L, Mouram S, Della Rocca DG, et al. Hybrid atrial fibrillation ablation: long- term outcomes from a single-centre 10-year experience. *Europace.* 2023;25(5):euad114.
19. Muneretto C, Baudo M, Rosati F, et al. Thoracoscopic surgical ablation of lone atrial fibrillation: long-term outcomes at 7 years. *Ann Thorac Surg.* 2023;116(6):1292–1299.
20. Hindricks G, Potpara T, Dagres N, et al. 2020 ESC guidelines for the diagnosis and management of atrial fibrillation developed in collaboration with the European Association for Cardio-Thoracic Surgery (EACTS). *Eur Heart J.* 2021;42:373–498.
21. Joglar JA, Chung MK, Armbruster AL, et al. 2023 ACC/AHA/ACCP/HRS guideline for the diagnosis and management of atrial fibrillation: a report of the American College of Cardiology/American Heart Association Joint committee on clinical practice guidelines. *Circulation.* 2024;149(1):e1–e156.
22. Wyler von Ballmoos MC, Hui DS, et al. The society of thoracic surgeons 2023 clinical practice guidelines for the surgical treatment of atrial fibrillation. *Ann Thorac Surg.* 2024 S0003-4975(24)00057-2.

34

Thoracoscopic Left-Chest Only Hybrid Procedure for Stand-Alone Atrial Fibrillation

Mark La Meir

CHAPTER OUTLINE

Rhythm control of atrial fibrillation (AF) by interventional ablation is historically based on two major developments. First, the surgical Maze procedure (and its modifications) was introduced by Cox and included both left and right atrial lesions designed to extinguish the multiple macro-reentrant drivers that sustain AF while maintaining atrioventricular synchrony. The second was learning that pulmonary veins (PVs) are an important source of ectopic atrial beats that serve as triggers that induce frequent paroxysms of AF, by Haïssaguerre and coworkers.[1,2] During the past several decades, a significant number of alternative procedures that may or may not respect these fundamental concepts were developed. The latest surgical evolution in concomitant ablation is addressed in a recent invited expert opinion by McCarthy, stating, "The maze IV operation is not always the best choice: Matching the procedure to the patient."[3] This was an attempt to identify which patients needed a biatrial procedure versus a left-sided Maze pattern of lesions versus a simple pulmonary vein isolation (PVI). Although this type of procedural approach can be "tailored" for certain patients, McCarthy's article did not suggest that the individual lesions of the chosen procedures could be guided by intraoperative mapping. The "procedure tailoring" for individual patients was confined to three different well-established anatomic lesion sets: a biatrial Cox-Maze procedure, a left-atrial-only Maze lesion set, or a PVI. "Procedure tailoring," which uses the lesions of three different well-established anatomy-based surgical procedures, does not require intraoperative mapping. However, map-guided "lesion tailoring" involves placing individual ablative lesions in specific locations based on the electrophysiologic characteristics of AF at the particular moment of mapping. Our hybrid approach differs from others in that it is based on intraoperative mapping with "lesion tailoring" and has no predetermined lesion set that is used for all hybrid procedures.

Hybrid AF procedures were defined in the 2012 Heart Rhythm Society/European Heart Rhythm Association/European Cardiac Arrhythmia Society in an expert consensus statement on catheter and surgical ablation of AF as a joint AF ablation procedure that is a part of a single combined thoracoscopic/catheter procedure or performed as two preplanned staged ablation procedures separated by no more than 6 months.[4] Since this introduction, hybrid treatment of AF has been included in all major society consensus statements and guidelines on AF.

DEVELOPMENT OF A NOVEL HYBRID PROCEDURE

Starting with the Cox-Maze procedure, nonconcomitant AF ablation has evolved toward a minimally invasive video-assisted procedure with dedicated ablation tools using cryothermia and/or radiofrequency (RF) energy to isolate the PVs and create linear lesions without opening the heart. These ablation tools that replaced the cut-and-sew technique cannot always guarantee durable transmural lesions. Furthermore, linear lesions such as the isthmus lines cannot be made solely from the epicardium, and proving epicardial bidirectional block can be challenging. Therefore, our Maastricht group introduced a novel hybrid procedure for patients with paroxysmal AF (PAF) and persistent AF based on a combined simultaneous thoracoscopic surgical and transvenous catheter procedure.[5] These two complementary techniques performed in combination bear the potential of treating AF on a long-term basis with a single off-pump procedure. The workflow of the stepwise approach was designed to overcome the limitations of both thoracoscopy and catheter ablation, the absence of mapping in surgery, and the difficulty of consistently achieving transmural lesions with catheter ablation. During a stepwise ablation, structures contributing to the initiation and maintenance of AF (PVs, left atrial roof, left atrial posterior wall, mitral isthmus and cavotricuspid isthmus [CVI]) are sequentially targeted as needed.

Our hybrid procedure was originally performed using bilateral thoracoscopy and consisted of a minimal lesion set of bilateral PVI made with a bipolar RF clamp. The end point for the PVI was entrance and exit block. In the case of sinus rhythm after PVI, reinduction of AF was attempted by pacing, and if AF was not inducible, isoproterenol was infused. If AF had not been terminated or was still inducible, linear lesions were added. First, a roof line was performed followed by a floor line, left atrial isthmus line, right atrial intercaval line, superior caval vein isolation, and/or a CVI line if needed. In 23% of the patients, the epicardial lesions were not transmural, and an endocardial touch-up was necessary, proving the importance of simultaneous endocardial mapping and ablation. A single-procedure success rate (sinus rhythm without antiarrhythmic drugs and/or redo procedure) of 79% at 1 year for PAF (11 of 14 patients) and 90% for persistent AF (9 of 10 patients), and an overall single-procedure success rate of 83% at 1 year was obtained. Our results were published in 2012 along with an editorial by Calkins[6] discussing the potential limitations of this novel approach. In essence, Calkins discussed the need for expertise of both teams in the same center and the challenging logistics of organizing a simultaneous joint procedure.[5] The need for expertise is still a challenge, but the logistics have been solved with the creation of dedicated hybrid rooms used for the percutaneous treatment of patients with structural heart disease.

Based on this need for surgical expertise and the better understanding of the potentials of the hybrid procedure, it seemed important to minimize the surgical technique further by limiting the approach to one side of the chest. This made the procedure more teachable and increased our patient referrals. Therefore, we developed a left-side-only thoracoscopic approach to facilitate surgery, to avoid right-sided complications and reduce postoperative pain.[7] We had previous experience with a right-side-only approach, but many cardiac surgeons do not like to close the left atrial appendage (LAA) through the transverse sinus, and LAA occlusion is a bit more difficult to control with that approach.

LEFT-CHEST-ONLY HYBRID PROCEDURE: SURGICAL TECHNIQUE

When approaching the heart through the left chest, the camera has to be positioned inside the transverse and oblique sinuses to dissect the pericardial folds between the superior vena cava and the right superior PV (RSPV), between the inferior vena cava and the right inferior PV (RIPV), and the roof and posterior wall of the left atrium. Although this results in a reduced working space compared to the right-sided approach, the dissection is more straightforward because important cardiac structures are easily visualized, and the surgeon works toward the pericardium (safe space) instead of toward the heart. After this dissection, the connecting roof and inferior lines are created with the Coolrail device (Atricure, Inc.) as well as a line medial to the right PVs inside the oblique sinus. Performing these lines also melts the fat on the pericardial reflection between the transverse and oblique sinus and therefore facilitates the passage of the light dissector around the left PVs. When creating these linear ablations, it is mandatory to follow three steps to avoid the potential for an atrioesophageal fistula. The first step is to identify the anatomic position of the esophagus by looking for the tip of the transesophageal echocardiograpy (TEE) scope bulging through the pericardium. The second step is to push the ablated tissue away from the posterior pericardium. The third step is to flush the pericardial space with saline for at least 30 seconds after the ablation and before removing the ablation device.[8] Bipolar RF clamp ablation of the left PVs is performed medial to the ligament of Marshall and includes the coumadin ridge to exclude these structures. The remaining ganglionic plexi are then ablated. Next, we carefully position the clamp in the oblique sinus and guide it toward the opened reflection at the base of the RIPV and over the right PVs, and the ablation is performed. Finally, LAA occlusion (LAAO) is performed under echocardiographic guidance.

The most difficult part of this left-side-only approach is completely isolating the RIPV. Although we perform this surgically with a bipolar RF clamp, we do not recommend that this step be performed unless the surgeon is very experienced. Rather, we advise that the lateral part of the RIPV be isolated by the electrophysiologist (EP) with the endocardial catheter. This is a safe and straightforward alternative because the surgeon has already created a linear lesion on the inferior border of the RIPV, the superior border of the RSPV, and the medial side of the PVs in the oblique sinus. Thus only a lesion around the lateral side of the right PVs remains to be created by the EP for completion of the PV isolation. The left lung is insufflated, and the EP continues with endocardial confirmation of transmurality of the epicardial lesion set and, if needed, an endocardial touch-up. Then areas involved in the maintenance of AF, left-sided atrial tachycardias, and flutter are mapped and ablated.

WHY CHOOSE A HYBRID PROCEDURE?

The challenge of any epicardial ablation tool on the beating heart is the creation of reliable, safe, and long-lasting transmural lesions. The quality of each lesion can be impacted by the presence of epicardial fat, thickness of the tissues, histologic variations, and cardiac output. During surgery, if no intraoperative testing is performed to confirm lesion integrity and the efficacy of the lesion set, it is likely that the procedure will be less successful for the long term (see Chapter 20). Performing endocardial mapping after an epicardial ablation immediately provides valuable information regarding the efficacy of the ablation tool used and whether the number of applications (amount of energy delivered) was sufficient. Apart from the bipolar RF clamping devices and properly used cryoprobes, none of the other tools have proven to provide consistent, reliable transmural lesions.[9] This problem was emphasized in the **C**atheter **A**blation vs. Thoracoscopic **S**urgical **A**blation in Long-standing Persistent **A**trial **F**ibrillation (CASA-AF) randomized controlled trial (RCT).[10] The single-center CASA-AF pilot study in patients with long-standing persistent AF (LSpAF; 26 surgical ablations, 25 catheter ablations) showed a clear superiority of the thoracoscopic approach compared to the percutaneous approach. To ensure robust assessment of conduction block for surgical ablation lesions, block was confirmed by EP-guided testing. Of the 22 patients who had both surgical and EP catheter testing, 3 patients were found to have remaining PV connections, and 2 patients had conduction into the box lesion, all of which were deemed isolated after surgical pen testing. Therefore, EP catheter testing prompted further ablation to achieve conduction block in 23% (5 of 22) of patients. Haldar et al.[11] concluded, "In LSPAF, meticulous EP guided thoracoscopic SA [surgical ablation] as a first line strategy can provide excellent single procedure success rates as compared to catheter ablation (CA), but there is an increased upfront risk of non-fatal complications." The follow-up randomized controlled trial (RCT) did not achieve similar outcomes for the surgical group, and this time the authors concluded that "Single procedure thoracoscopic SA [surgical ablation] is not superior to CA in treating LSPAF." So, what changed? Analyzing the article, apart from the multicenter RCT, the only major difference between the two studies was the surgical device used for the creation of the connecting lesions (roof and floor line), which was the Atricure Coolrail device for the first study[10] and the Atricure Multi-Polar Pen (MLP) for the second.[11] In addition, the results of the EP-guided testing of surgical ablation conduction block and the need for further ablation to achieve conduction block were not published. Our group has studied both devices in our hybrid procedures. Whereas the Coolrail device resulted in more than 90% acute isolation, the MLP device always needed an endocardial touch-up to complete the lesion. The nontransmurality of the surgical lesion set easily explains the difference in outcome of the two studies. A hybrid procedure would have overcome this problem and proven the superiority of the combined procedure as demonstrated in the (**H**ybrid Thoracoscopic Surgical and Transvenous Catheter **A**blation Versus **T**ransvenous **C**atheter **A**blation in **P**ersistent and Longstanding Persistent **A**trial **F**ibrillation (HART-CAP AF) randomized controlled trial.[12]

ARE COMPLICATION RATES INCREASED WITH HYBRID PROCEDURES?

When discussing the potential for improved clinical outcomes of a surgical AF program with the EP, cardiologist, and patient, the sinus rate outcome is not always the primary concern. It is essentially the perceived potential increase of complication rates because of the invasiveness of the surgical procedure that most often limits referrals. A first step was to address this concern by eliminating the use of extracorporeal circulation (although it has not been demonstrated to increase complications) and to perform the ablation on the beating heart. The second step was to minimize surgical access first by bilateral thoracotomy, followed by bilateral thoracoscopy, then using a single-side thoracoscopy approach, and finally performing the ablation through a subxiphoid nonthoracic approach. This stepwise evolution required the development and honing of thoracoscopic skills, the availability of nonclamping ablation devices to create many of the lesions, and addressing the inability to create the left atrial isthmus and CTI lines from the epicardium alone. The hybrid approach can overcome these issues because the EP can help the surgeon reach areas deemed unsafe to approach surgically. For example, a difficult passage of the light dissector around the PVs for positioning of the bipolar clamp can be eliminated and the right PVI can be performed by the EP without taking the risk of surgical perforation. Je et al.[13] performed a systematic analysis of AF ablation techniques and compared the safety and efficacy of the minimally invasive Cox CryoMaze-III procedure, beating-heart epicardial ablation, and hybrid procedures. They showed that the incidence of conversion to a median sternotomy was 0%, 2.4%, and 2.5%, respectively, and the incidence of reoperation for bleeding was 1.0%, 1.5%, and 2.2%, respectively. However, the main limitation of this analysis was the lack of studies directly comparing these treatment strategies. Data do exist for hybrid versus EP only ablation, including RCTs. Van der Heijden et al.[14] conducted a systematic literature review and meta-analysis of hybrid versus catheter ablation in patients with persistent AF or LSpAF. Hybrid ablation resulted in higher freedom of atrial arrhythmias in patients with persistent and LSpAF than catheter ablation (70.7–49.9%). Another limitation of Je and coworkers'[13] report is that most published hybrid series are performed sequentially (not as a joint procedure), which could theoretically increase the risk for complications. Because the EP tests the integrity of the lesions in a hybrid procedure and can expose incomplete lesions, the likelihood of leaving acutely incomplete lesions is markedly decreased. In our experience, we never had a conversion because of perforation, even with the left-side-only technique. This can be explained not only by our large volume of cases but also by the fact that the surgeon does not have to take risks because the EP is present and can immediately close any gap in the epicardial surgical lesions. In "Hybrid ablation of atrial fibrillation: A unilateral left-sided thoracoscopic approach," van der Heijden et al.[15] evaluated the efficacy and safety of our unilateral left-sided thoracoscopic approach. A total of 119 patients were analyzed (LSpAF, 71%; previous catheter ablation, 44%). In all patients, a unilateral left-sided hybrid approach consisting of PV isolation, posterior left atrial wall isolation, and LAAO was done. Epicardial (n = 59) and/or endocardial validation (n = 81) was performed, and endocardial touch-up was performed in 33 patients. Major perioperative complications occurred in 5% of all patients (no incidences of stroke, conversion to sternotomy, or death). After 12 months, the probability of being free from supraventricular tachyarrhythmia recurrence was 80% (73–87%), and at 24 months it was 67% (58–76%), when including patients who required antiarrhythmic drugs after the procedure.

FUTURE OF HYBRID PROCEDURES FOR ATRIAL FIBRILLATION

Further improvement of mapping tools by the development of new multielectrode mapping catheters and the increased efficacy of catheter ablative energy sources, such as pulsed-field ablation (PFA)[16] and ultra-low cryoablation[17] with or without PFA (so-called PFCA), could be seen as a challenge to the hybrid program as well as to all stand-alone surgical AF treatment. Because hybrid procedures combine both surgery and catheter ablation, they are capable of taking advantage of improvements in both fields. Recurrence of AF after percutaneous ablation may be caused by PV reconnection but can also manifest in the presence of antral PV isolation. Even with improvement of ablation technology, PV reconnection rates are high. For example, during repeat endocardial ablations after cryoballoon ablation, reconnection rates still vary between 18% and 31%,[18] and it is similar after RF PVI. Approximately one-third of reconnections occur at the coumadin ridge between the LSPV and LAA, and approximately one-fourth occur at the level of the carina of the right PVs. These areas are more easily isolated with epicardial clamping technology than with endocardial catheters. After PV isolation is confirmed, the sinus rate outcome can be improved by isolation of the posterior wall ("box lesion"), by LAAO if we perform a non-hybrid procedure and, some believe, by ganglionic plexus ablation. However, without any intraoperative mapping, we cannot target remaining AF triggers, atrial tachycardias, or atrial flutters.

CONCLUSION

An arrhythmia surgeon without partnership with EPs will always have limited referrals and a small number of difficult to treat patients with AF, which results in overall suboptimal surgical outcomes. By working simultaneously within a hybrid program, both the surgeon and the EP engage in a collaboration based on mutual respect aiming for a safe and optimal approach with long-term sinus rate and improvement of quality of life. All patients with a history of symptomatic PAF, persistent AF, or LSpAF, refractory to or intolerant to at least one class I or III antiarrhythmic drugs, with or without a previous catheter ablation, are candidates for this ever-evolving state-of-the-art team approach.[19,20]

REFERENCES

1. Cox JL. The surgical treatment of atrial fibrillation. IV. Surgical technique. *J Thorac Cardiovasc Surg*. 1991;101(4):584–592.
2. Haïssaguerre M, Jaïs P, Shah DC, et al. Spontaneous initiation of atrial fibrillation by ectopic beats originating in the pulmonary veins. *N Engl J Med*. 1998;339(10):659–666.
3. McCarthy PM. The Maze IV operation is not always the best choice: matching the procedure to the patient. *J Thorac Cardiovasc Surg Techniques*. 2023;17:79–83.
4. Calkins H, Kuck KH, Cappato R, et al. 2012 HRS/EHRA/ECAS expert consensus statement on catheter and surgical ablation of atrial fibrillation: recommendations for patient selection, procedural techniques, patient management and follow-up, definitions, endpoints, and research trial design: a report of the Heart Rhythm Society (HRS) Task Force on Catheter and Surgical Ablation of Atrial Fibrillation. Developed in partnership with the European Heart Rhythm Association (EHRA), a registered branch of the European Society of Cardiology (ESC) and the European Cardiac Arrhythmia Society (ECAS); and in collaboration with the American College of Cardiology (ACC), American Heart Association (AHA), the Asia Pacific Heart Rhythm Society (APHRS), and the Society of Thoracic Surgeons (STS). Endorsed by the governing bodies of the American College of Cardiology Foundation, the American Heart Association, the European Cardiac Arrhythmia Society, the European Heart Rhythm Association, the Society of Thoracic Surgeons, the Asia Pacific Heart Rhythm Society, and the Heart Rhythm Society. *Heart Rhythm*. 2012;9(4):632–696.

5. Pison L, La Meir M, van Opstal J, Blaauw Y, Maessen J, Crijns HJ. Hybrid thoracoscopic surgical and transvenous catheter ablation of atrial fibrillation. *J Am Coll Cardiol*. 2012;60(1):54–61.
6. Calkins H. Hybrid thoracoscopic and transvenous catheter ablation of atrial fibrillation. Is this the answer we are searching for? *J Am Coll Cardiol*. 2012;60(1):62–63.
7. Maesen B, La Meir M. Unilateral left-sided thoracoscopic ablation of atrial fibrillation. *Ann Thorac Surg*. 2020;110(1):e63–e66.
8. Kronenberger R, Van Loo I, de Asmundis C, et al. Esophageal findings in the setting of a novel preventive strategy to avoid thermal lesions during hybrid thoracoscopic radiofrequency ablation for atrial fibrillation. *J Clin Med*. 2021;10(21):4981.
9. MacGregor RM, Melby SJ, Schuessler RB, Damiano RJ. Energy sources for the surgical treatment of atrial fibrillation. *Innovations*. 2019;14(6):503–508.
10. Haldar SK, Jones DG, Bahrami T, et al. Catheter ablation vs electrophysiologically guided thoracoscopic surgical ablation in long-standing persistent atrial fibrillation: the CASA-AF Study. *Heart Rhythm*. 2017;14(11):1596–1603.
11. Haldar S, Khan HR, Boyalla V, et al. Catheter ablation vs. thoracoscopic surgical ablation in long-standing persistent atrial fibrillation: CASA-AF randomized controlled trial. *Eur Heart J*. 2020;41(47):4471–4480.
12. van der Heijden CAJ, Weberndörfer V, Vroomen M, et al. Hybrid ablation versus repeated catheter ablation in persistent atrial fibrillation: a randomized controlled trial. *JACC Clin Electrophysiol*. 2023;7(2):1013–1023.
13. Je HG, Shuman DJ, Ad N. A systematic review of minimally invasive surgical treatment for atrial fibrillation: a comparison of the Cox-Maze procedure, beating-heart epicardial ablation, and the hybrid procedure on safety and efficacy. *Eur J Cardiothorac Surg*. 2015;48(4):531–540 discussion 540-1.
14. van der Heijden CAJ, Vroomen M, Luermans JG, et al. Hybrid versus catheter ablation in patients with persistent and longstanding persistent atrial fibrillation: a systematic review and meta-analysis. *Eur J Cardiothorac Surg*. 2019;56(3):433–443.
15. van der Heijden CAJ, Weberndörfer V, Luermans JGLM, et al. Hybrid ablation of atrial fibrillation: a unilateral left-sided thoracoscopic approach. *J Card Surg*. 2022;37(12):4630–4638.
16. Duytschaevver M, De Potter T, Grimaldi M, et al. Paroxysmal atrial fibrillation ablation using a novel variable-loop biphasic pulsed field ablation catheter integrated with a 3-dimensional mapping system: 1-year outcomes of the multicenter inspire study. *Circ Arrhythm Electrophysiol*. 2023;16(3):e011780.
17. De Potter T, Klaver M, Babkin A, et al. Ultra-low temperature cryoablation for atrial fibrillation: primary outcomes for efficacy and safety: the Cryocure-2 Study. *JACC: Clin Electrophysiol*. 2022;8(8):1034–1039.
18. Mugnai G, Cecchini F, Stroker E, et al. Durability of pulmonary vein isolation following cryoballoon ablation: lessons from a large series of repeat ablation procedures. *Int J Cardiol Heart Vasc*. 2022;40:101040.
19. Maesen B, Luermans JGLM, Bidar E, et al. A hybrid approach to complex arrhythmias. *Europace*. 2021;23:ii28–ii33.
20. Van Loo I, de Asmundis C, La Meir M. The 7 pillars of a successful hybrid atrial fibrillation program. *Innovations*. 2019;14(6):493–497.

35

Thoracoscopic Non-Maze Hybrid Procedure for Stand-Alone Atrial Fibrillation

Armin Kiankhooy, Gansevoort Dunnington

CHAPTER OUTLINE

The number of off-pump surgical ablation approaches to treat patients with atrial fibrillation (AF) has increased in the past several years. In the most recent Society of Thoracic Surgeons (STS) analysis, Ad et al.[1] reported that 3252 patients with stand-alone AF underwent off-pump surgical techniques, with an annual average growth per site of 8% per year. The two most common approaches are the subxiphoid Convergent procedure (see Chapter 36) and the totally thoracoscopic (TT) techniques (see Chapter 34). In both approaches, epicardial surgical ablation is combined with endocardial catheter ablation as a hybrid procedure to treat patients with stand-alone AF. The 2023 American College of Cardiology/American Heart Association/American College of Clinical Pharmacy/Heart Rhythm Society (HRS) Guidelines for the Diagnosis and Management of Atrial Fibrillation provided a Class IIB recommendation for hybrid procedures for the treatment of patients with symptomatic persistent AF refractory to antiarrhythmic drug therapy.[2] In addition, left atrial appendage occlusion (LAAO) with an epicardial occlusion device is a key component of the TT hybrid procedure described in this chapter.

RATIONALE FOR PERFORMING TOTALLY THORACOSCOPIC HYBRID PROCEDURES

TT hybrid procedures (Fig. 35.1) attempt to replicate as many of the left atrial lesions of the on-pump surgical Cox-Maze-III or -IV procedures as possible.[3] However, off-pump TT surgical lesions in hybrid procedures are inherently limited to epicardial lesions only. The left atrial lesions that we perform epicardially are bilateral pulmonary vein isolation (PVI), left atrial posterior wall isolation, lesions across the Coumadin ridge from the left superior pulmonary vein (PV) to the left atrial appendage (LAA), selected ganglionic plexus ablation, and LAA occlusion. Additional endocardial lesions are performed either jointly or after a delay to create more of the Cox-Maze-III or -IV lesions and to "touch up" any incomplete epicardial lesions. Thus the TT approach depends on a partnership between surgeons and electrophysiologists who perform endocardial lesions including the mitral isthmus line, the coronary sinus lesion, and the right atrial cavotricuspid isthmus (CTI) lesion, none of which can be performed epicardially. TT hybrid procedures are less invasive than the Cox-Maze-III and -IV procedures, but they also have fewer final ablative lesions and therefore an expected higher failure rate than the more invasive on-pump surgical procedures.

PATIENT SELECTION FOR TOTALLY THORACOSCOPIC HYBRID PROCEDURES

Patients referred for a hybrid procedure have usually failed medical therapy and multiple catheter ablations. However, the success of a hybrid procedure depends primarily on whether the patient has paroxysmal AF (PAF) or nonparoxysmal AF (non-PAF; persistent AF or long-standing persistent AF [LSpAF]), on the size of the left atrium (LA), and on the duration of the AF.[4,5] Surgeons should explain the possibility of needing a new pacemaker, especially if the procedure is successful in ablating the AF.[6] If the clinical history cannot identify the patient's AF type, continuous ambulatory monitoring (e.g., Holter, iRhythm ZioPatch, Philips BioTel) for at least 7 days should be performed. Continuous ambulatory monitoring also detects the presence or absence of sick sinus syndrome, which is a major reason for needing a new postoperative pacemaker (see Chapter 21). left atrial size is determined by transesophageal echocardiography or contrast-enhanced cardiac computed tomography.[7] A left atrial size greater than 5.5 cm is a known risk factor for decreased procedural success[4] as is an AF duration of more than 5 years.[5]

The clinical presentation of stand-alone AF may vary considerably. Paradoxically, those patients with longer-duration AF may express a lack of symptoms because of their gradual insidious deterioration, but more recently diagnosed patients can present with the typical findings of palpitations, dyspnea on exertion, chest pain, anxiety, and lightheadedness.[8] Seemingly asymptomatic patients should also be made aware that AF is associated with heart failure,[9] cognitive decline, and dementia, especially in the younger patient (younger than 70 years old) population.[10,11]

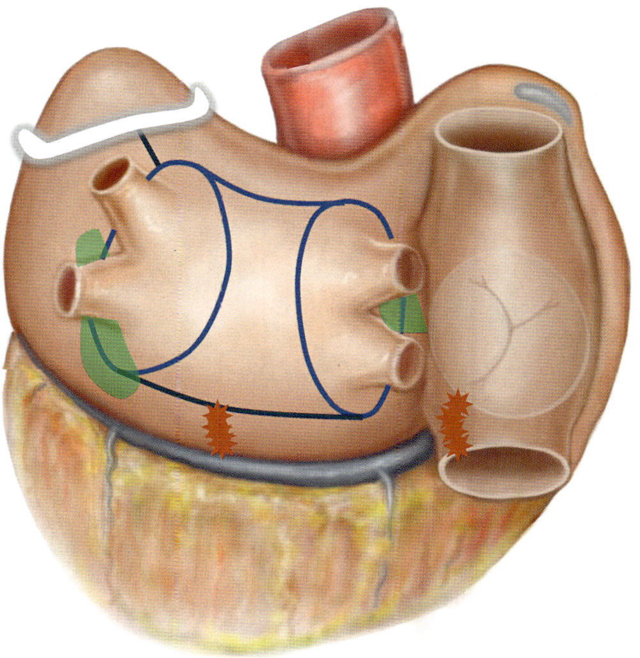

Fig. 35.1 Combined epicardial and endocardial catheter lesions in a totally thoracoscopic (TT) hybrid procedure. *Blue lines*, thoracoscopic epicardial ablation; *rust lines*, endocardial catheter ablation; *green areas*, ganglionic plexus ablation. An AtriClip is shown in place occluding the left atrial appendage

INDICATIONS FOR PERFORMING TOTALLY THORACOSCOPIC HYBRID PROCEDURES

The 2017 HRS/European Heart Rhythm Association/European Cardiac Arrhythmia Society/Asia Pacific Heart Rhythm Society/Latin American Society of Cardiac Stimulation and Electrophysiology guidelines recommended isolated catheter ablation of PAF (Class I, Level A), persistent AF (Class IIa, Level B-NR), and LSpAF (Class IIb, C-LD).[12] The most recent National Cardiovascular Data Registry AF Ablation Registry analysis (2016–2020) reflects the real-world implementation of these guidelines, demonstrating that catheter ablations were performed for 76,219 patients and were divided between PAF (55.8%), persistent (41.6%) and LSpAF (2.3%).[13] These recommendations are based on the high success rate of PVI with catheter ablation and excellent safety profile. Metaanalysis of randomized controlled trials (RCTs) evaluating radiofrequency (RF) catheter ablation versus medical management of PAF reveal 65% to 71% freedom from recurrent AF at 1 year,[14] and the recent STOP-AF trial[15] revealed nearly 75% freedom from AF recurrence at 1 year when comparing balloon cryotherapy versus a rhythm control medical management approach in a PAF population. Therefore, surgeons who are referred patients with stand-alone PAF should first refer these patients to an electrophysiology colleague for evaluation of an isolated endocardial catheter ablation before considering a TT hybrid approach.

Patients with stand-alone persistent AF, however, pose a challenge to an isolated catheter ablation approach (see Chapter 31). As mentioned, patients with persistent AF develop atrial substrate abnormalities beyond the PVs and necessitate an ablation strategy targeted at reentrant circuits (drivers) that sustain AF.[16] Linear ablation lesions based on the Cox-Maze-III or -IV lesion sets are required to interrupt these macro-reentrant drivers of AF. The crux of any ablation procedure, including catheter ablation, is lesion transmurality and continuity of the linear ablations without an increase in complications such as atrial perforation and atrial-esophageal fistulas. Several studies have now shown that epicardial-endocardial gaps exist in nearly one-third of patients undergoing catheter ablation,[17] and often an adipose layer is present between these layers, which can act as a barrier to effective transmural ablation. This nontransmurality problem is not an issue with open surgical ablation using the cut-and-sew technique, cryosurgery, or bipolar RF clamps, but it is a major problem when using unipolar RF ablative approaches such as endocardial catheter ablation or off-pump epicardial surgical approaches. However, a bidirectional hybrid ablation approach can overcome the technical difficulty of creating transmural lesions.[18] Several trials have now demonstrated that isolated catheter ablation that includes additional lesions beyond the PVI do not yield significantly improved freedom from AF when compared with isolated PVI alone.[19,20] The reason the additional lesions had no impact on the catheter ablation outcomes is because of the extreme difficulty in creating contiguous transmural linear lesions anywhere in the atrium with the tip of a long, moving catheter. It is also problematic for the surgeon to create the floor and roof lesions of the box lesion around all four PVs with a unipolar RF device whether it is a single or dual electrode device. The recent CAPLA study reported a disappointing 52.4% freedom from AF with a first-time catheter ablation of PVI and posterior wall isolation, which was not significantly improved over PVI alone (53.6%).[19] Thus in patients with persistent AF and LSpAF, a TT hybrid procedure should be considered.

Patients with LSpAF are so difficult to treat with catheter ablation that patients with this type of AF often go untreated,[13] but this is where hybrid procedures offer their greatest potential value. The CONVERGE trial was the first RCT to evaluate the efficacy and safety of a hybrid procedure to treat patients with these complex forms of non-PAF[21] and it is discussed extensively in Chapter 36. The recent gHARTCAP-AF trial was also an RCT that compared a hybrid procedure versus catheter ablation in patients with LSpAF.[22] Patients undergoing the hybrid approach showed superior 12-month rhythm success compared with those undergoing catheter ablation (89% vs 41%, respectively; relative risk [RR], 1.78; $P = .002$). The more recent CEASE-AF RCT in patients with LSpAF (19.5%) again showed the superiority of hybrid procedures over catheter ablation at 12 months (71.6% vs 39.2%, respectively; RR, 1.83; $P < .001$).[23]

On the basis of these RCTs and other prior nonrandomized comparisons, we believe that the indications for performing a hybrid procedure include (1) recurrent PAF despite multiple prior catheter ablations; (2) persistent AF with an enlarged or heavily scarred LA, left atrial fibrosis, or multiple prior failed catheter ablations; and (3) the presence of LSpAF.

CONTRAINDICATIONS TO PERFORMING TOTALLY THORACOSCOPIC HYBRID PROCEDURES

Only patients with stand-alone AF are considered to be candidates for a hybrid procedure. Patients with significant concomitant cardiac disease requiring coronary artery bypass grafting (CABG) or valve surgery should not be offered a hybrid procedure, and their AF should be addressed according to the STS guidelines.[24] Contraindications to a hybrid procedure include anatomic and physiologic considerations to both the off-pump epicardial surgical component and the ability to complete a subsequent endocardial catheter ablation. Strict contraindications to any combined hybrid approach include (1) the presence of left atrial thrombus, (2) an inability to tolerate anticoagulation, and (3) severe esophageal disease that would prohibit safe TEE.[25] Other secondary contraindications include (1) prior atrial septal defect closure device., (2) an incomplete inferior vena cava (IVC), (3) prior cardiac surgery or mediastinal radiation, (4) previous pericarditis, (5) advanced liver disease, and (6) advanced pulmonary disease requiring home oxygen therapy.[8] Increased body mass index (>45 kg/m^2), depressed left ventricular ejection fraction (LVEF) (<25%), chronic kidney disease (stage >3), and a history of prior thoracic surgery can increase the technical difficulty of the epicardial surgical component but can be overcome safely with increasing surgeons experience.

PREOPERATIVE PLANNING

Preoperative patient evaluation for a TT hybrid procedure includes (1) carotid duplex ultrasonography to evaluate for flow-limiting carotid stenosis leading to an increased risk of periprocedural stroke; (2) echocardiography and left heart catheterization to evaluate for concomitant structural heart disease warranting open cardiac surgery; (3) noncontrast computed topography to evaluate for left atrial, PV(s), and LAA anatomy; (4) pulmonary function tests to ascertain suitability for single lung ventilation; and (5) standard blood work to assess for other potential contraindications like end-stage liver disease or significant thrombocytopenia.

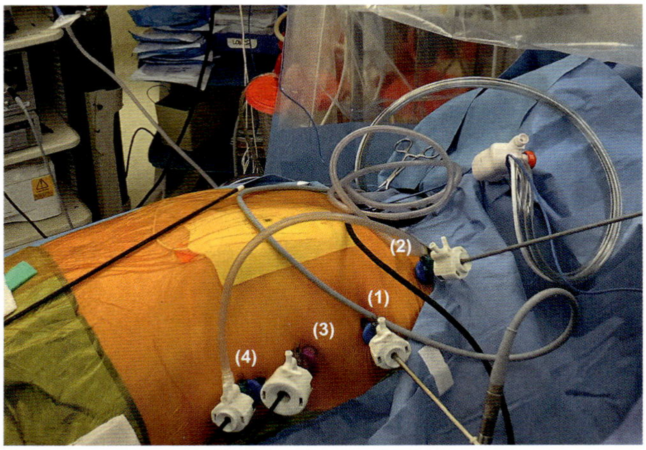

Fig. 35.2 Left chest port placement for thoracoscopic non-Maze hybrid ablation. Port placement: *(1)* 5-mm port at the fourth intercostal space along the anterior axillary line, *(2)* 12-mm port at the second intercostal space at the midclavicular line, *(3)* 12-mm port at the sixth intercostal space along the midaxillary line, and *(4)* 5-mm port at the eighth intercostal space along the midaxillary line.

SURGICAL TECHNIQUE

The non-Maze TT hybrid procedure is performed under general anesthesia, and double-lumen endotracheal intubation is performed in the operating room. The patient is positioned supine with inflatable bags aligned under each scapula to allow for differential inflation of each hemithorax during the procedure. Monitoring lines should include central venous access, an arterial line for blood pressure monitoring, and a Foley catheter. Transesophageal echocardiography is required to rule out the presence of LAA thrombus. Esophageal temperature monitoring is not routinely performed in our TT hybrid procedure. Defibrillator pads should be positioned to allow for appropriate port access and permit emergent conversion to sternotomy if needed. We prefer the use of sterile defibrillator pads. Intravenous (IV) unfractionated heparin is not routinely administered during a TT hybrid procedure. The patient is prepped with insufflation of both inflatable bags to maximize posterior-lateral exposure and optimize the area of skin prep from the neck to the posterior axillary lines and inferiorly to the groins bilaterally.

There are several iterations of TT hybrid procedures, and we will describe our institutional preference. We begin with a left-chest approach. Single right lung ventilation is initiated, and the left hemithorax is elevated with an inflatable Roho or 500-cc IV solution bag to aid with positioning of the left mediastinum. The patient is rotated a few degrees to the right to shift the mediastinal structures slightly rightward. The first port is 5 mm and inserted into the fourth intercostal space at the anterior axillary line to will act as the main camera port. The port should be inserted perpendicular to the chest wall and aimed at the pulmonary hilum. The ideal port placement is just anterior to the pulmonary hilum and in line with the PV carina. A 30-degree 5-mm camera is inserted to confirm appropriate placement. Carbon dioxide insufflation is initiated at 8 cm H_2O with a flow rate greater than 15 L/min. Deflation of the left lung results in excellent visualization of the left pulmonary hilum, pericardium, left phrenic nerve, and left hemidiaphragm.

A second 12-mm port is then placed at the second intercostal space at the lateral third of the clavicle and aimed toward the pulmonary hilum. This port is for insertion of the primary surgeon's right-hand instrument. A third 12-mm port is placed at the sixth intercostal space at the midaxillary line and again directed at the pulmonary hilum. This port is for insertion of the primary surgeon's left-hand instrument. A fourth and final 5-mm port is placed through the eighth intercostal space at the posterior axillary line to will serve as the assistant surgeon's left-hand instrument. The overall configuration of the four-port placement should mimic a "hockey stick" with orientation around the pulmonary hilum and just posterior to the phrenic nerve (Fig. 35.2). The typical instrument placement includes:

- Port 1: a 5-mm 30-degree camera
- Port 2: an Endo Kittner, a 32-cm laparoscopic monopolar hook Bovie cautery (set at 30-W coagulation), an Epicardial AtriCure MLP1 ablation device, and a 48-inch Endo Stitch (Medtronic)
- Port 3: a suction irrigator and an Epicardial AtriCure MLP1 ablation device
- Port 4: an Endo Kittner

A longitudinal pericardiotomy is then created with an electrocautery 2 to 3 cm posterior to the left phrenic nerve to expose the heart from the level of the pulmonary hilum to the level of the coronary sinus. If the patient has undergone prior catheter ablation, the PVs are tested for entrance and exit block (see Chapter 20). The ligament of Marshall is then divided with an electrocautery.

Encircling the PVs (left or right) is the most technically challenging component of the TT approach. A lighted-tip dissector passed via the third port site is helpful in developing the proper planes of dissection around the PVs. After the clamp has encircled the PVs beyond the anterior pericardial reflection, it should be moved as medial as possible near the base of the LAA to maximize left atrial antral ablation and minimize the risk of PV stenosis. The ablation clamp is then applied, and three "doublet" ablations are performed to ensure completion of a transmural ablation.[26] When the final ablation has been completed, the PVs are tested for entrance and exit block to confirm their isolation.

The roof and floor of the LA are created next. The roof lesion is started just above the left superior PV and extended as far medially across the transverse sinus as possible. The floor lesion is started similarly just below the left inferior PV and extended across the posterior LA to the right inferior PV (Fig. 35.3). We prefer to apply a constant 10-minute total ablation time to complete these simultaneous lesions.[3] Other centers have used the 3-cm internally cooled linear ablation device (MCR1, AtriCure) with similar success.[27] Before occlusion of the LAA, a lesion is placed from the left superior PV across the "Coumadin ridge" to the LAA. This ablation is performed for a total of 5 minutes.

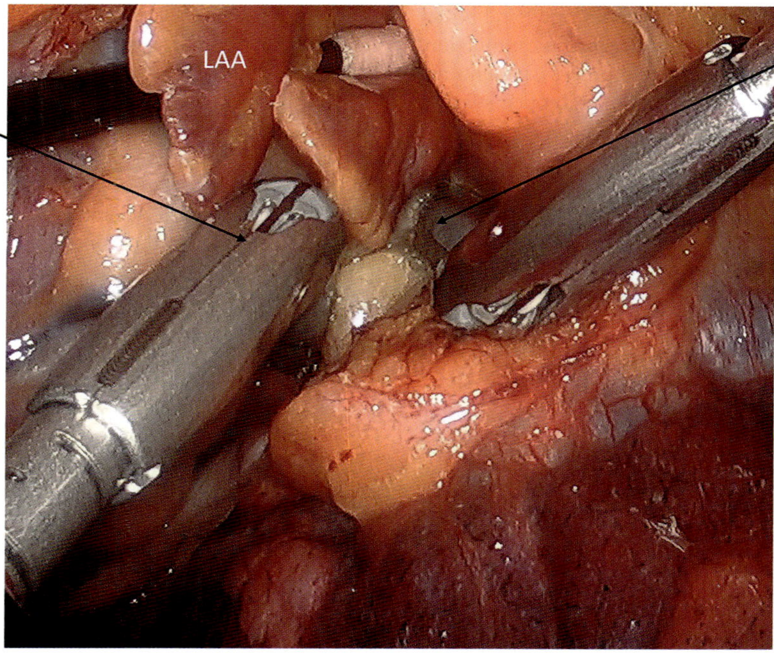

Fig. 35.3 Intraoperative depiction of left-sided "roof" and "floor" ablation creation with simultaneous ablation with unidirectional linear ablation devices. Interconnecting lesions from the left superior pulmonary vein (PV) and left inferior PV are created and anchored to the left PV isolation. These partial "roof" and "floor" lesions are then completed in an identical fashion from the right side to complete the left atrial "box." *LAA,* Left atrial appendage.

The final step of the left-sided thoracoscopic approach is LAAO with an epicardial clip, which is discussed in detail in other chapters of this book.

The right-sided ports are placed slightly more anterior than the left because the right-sided structures lie more anterior in the mediastinum than the left-sided structures, allowing the pericardium to be opened *anterior* to the phrenic nerve. To connect with the partial roof and floor lesions created earlier through the left-chest ports, both the oblique sinus and the transverse sinus are opened. In some instances, the partial floor lesion from the left side can be seen through the oblique sinus; therefore, completion of the floor lesion from the right side is usually easy to accomplish. To expose the partial roof lesion and to isolate the right PVs, a plane of dissection is established behind the superior vena cava between the right pulmonary artery and the right superior PV using blunt dissection. The right PVs and the isolated posterior left atrial wall should then be tested separately for entrance and exit block (see Chapter 20). We have found that in cases in which block is not confirmed, the most likely area for incomplete ablation is at the junction of the right superior PV and the interconnecting roof line. Unlike a left pericardiotomy, an open right pericardiotomy allows for herniation of the right atrium that can cause significant hemodynamic consequence. Therefore, we use a single Endo Stitch to close the right pericardiotomy. Double-lung ventilation is then resumed, and the patient is typically extubated in the operating room before to transfer to the postanesthesia care unit and subsequently to the monitored telemetry floor.

POSTOPERATIVE CARE

Patients who exhibit a ventricular rate greater than 80 beats/min are routinely started on IV continuous amiodarone (0.5 mg/min). Patients are also started on a proton pump inhibitor (pantoprazole 40 mg/day by mouth [PO]), a loop diuretic (furosemide 40 mg IV twice a day [BID]), and colchicine (0.6 mg/day PO). Standard postoperative analgesia medications and deep venous thrombosis prophylaxis (heparin 5000 units three times a day or enoxaparin 40 mg BID) are also initiated. On postoperative day 1, most patients are transitioned to oral amiodarone (200 mg PO BID), chest drains are removed, and oral anticoagulation is resumed (novel oral anticoagulant [NOAC] or warfarin, depending on the patient's preoperative routine). On postoperative day 2, most patients are discharged home with a 2-week course of amiodarone (200 mg po BID), preoperative NOAC or warfarin, colchicine 0.6 mg/day PO, pantoprazole 40 mg/day PO, and furosemide 40 mg PO BID. Patients are instructed to follow up in our clinic in 2 to 3 weeks and to schedule their second-stage endocardial mapping and ablation in 6 weeks with their electrophysiologist. It is important for the surgeon and patient to have a clear understanding that upon discharge, nearly 10% of patients will experience AF, atrial flutter, or tachyarrhythmias after the TT surgical stage of the hybrid procedure before the catheter ablation stage is performed.[3]

COMPLICATIONS OF INITIAL THORACOSCOPIC EPICARDIAL ABLATION

Early technical complications of the TT non-Maze hybrid procedure include perforation of the posterior LA during encircling of the PVs, perforation of the right atrium during right pericardiotomy creation, perforation of the LAA or left pulmonary artery during left pericardiotomy creation, perforation of the dome of the LA during transverse sinus mobilization, and perforation of the IVC during oblique sinus mobilization. In our opinion, the best ways to mitigate these complications are with direct mentorship and repeated case observations with experienced TT surgeons. In general, most perforations of the LA (roof or dome) can be resolved with thoracoscopic gauze packing and hemostatic agents without the need for suture placement or conversion to sternotomy or thoracotomy. In cases when uncontrollable bleeding occurs and the patient requires conversion to sternotomy, gauze packing still allows for safe mediastinal entry (sternotomy) and initiation of cardiopulmonary bypass via central or peripheral cannulation. We recommend that during the surgical consent process, patients are informed of this potential risk and consent to undergo open surgical ablation in these rare circumstances.

FOLLOW-UP ENDOCARDIAL CATHETER ABLATION

We allow at least 6 weeks between the first-stage epicardial surgical ablation and the second-stage endocardial catheter ablation. Initial endocardial mapping of the surgical ablation often reveals complete isolation of bilateral PVs and often complete left atrial posterior wall ablation (Fig. 35.4). However, in approximately one-third of cases, the electrophysiologist will need to perform additional "touch-up" endocardial ablation to achieve complete left atrial posterior wall isolation. The addition of a mitral line across the left atrial isthmus and/or the addition of a right atrial lesion across the CTI is left to the discretion of the electrophysiologist.

OUTCOMES

We have published our single-center retrospective series of 455 patients who underwent our TT non-Maze hybrid approach and observed a 12-month HRS-defined success freedom from AF, atrial flutter, and atrial tachycardia and off-antiarrhythmic drugs rate of 81%.[3] Our major complication rate included 1.1% conversion to sternotomy rate and a 1.1% mortality rate. Conversion is associated with poor patient outcomes,[1] and we highly recommend that surgeons interested in the TT approach participate in direct mentorship programs with highly experienced surgeons with both in-person and virtual proctoring to mitigate the potential higher complication rates of this approach. In addition, we have reported our technique in patients with tachycardia-mediated cardiomyopathy (TCM)[28] and with prior CABG.[29] Stand-alone AF patients who underwent our TT hybrid ablation approach with TCM experienced (at 12-month follow-up) on average a 12% increase in LVEF% (34.5% before hybrid ablation vs 46.5% after hybrid ablation; $P < .0001$) and a decrease in left atrial dilation (5.25 cm before hybrid ablation vs 4.82 cm after hybrid ablation; $P = .0078$). Patients with prior CABG were also effectively treated, with an 82.3% (14 of 17) 12-month rhythm success rate and safe exclusion of the LAA with an epicardial clip in all cases.

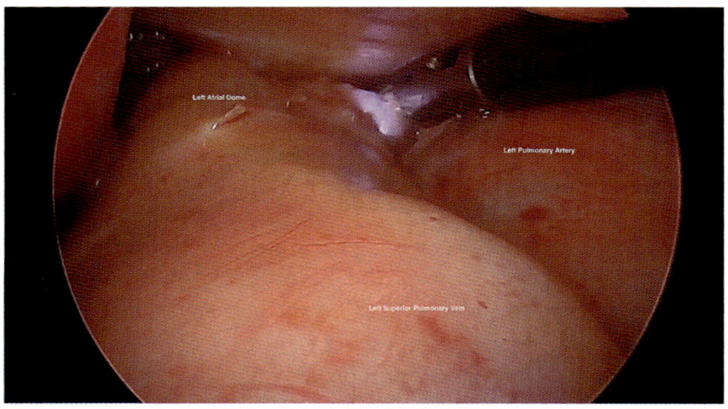

Fig. 35.4 Endocardial voltage map of thoracoscopic non-Maze hybrid ablation 6 weeks after epicardial off-pump creation of left atrial box lesion and left atrial appendage exclusion with an AtriClip. The first-stage epicardial ablation results in complete isolation of the left atrium and pulmonary veins with at times only scant *(red)* areas of voltage remaining completely outside the box lesion. *LIPV,* Left inferior pulmonary vein; *LSPV,* left superior pulmonary vein; *RIPV,* right inferior pulmonary vein; *RSPV,* right superior pulmonary vein.

SUMMARY

A heart team hybrid off-pump surgical epicardial ablation TT combined with an endocardial catheter ablation can provide patients with stand-alone persistent AF and LSpAF an improved freedom from AF compared with isolated catheter ablation.

REFERENCES

1. Ad N, Holmes SD, Roberts HG, Rankin JS, Badhwar V. Surgical treatment for stand-alone atrial fibrillation in North America. *Ann Thorac Surg.* 2020;109(3):745–752.
2. Joglar JA, Chung MK, Armbruster AL, et al. 2023 ACC/AHA/ACCP/HRS guideline for the diagnosis and management of atrial fibrillation: a report of the American College of Cardiology/American Heart Association Joint Committee on Clinical Practice Guidelines. *Circulation.* 2024;149(1):e1–156.
3. Dunnington GH, Pierce CL, Eisenberg S, et al. A heart-team hybrid approach for atrial fibrillation: a single-centre long-term clinical outcome cohort study. *Eur J Cardiothorac Surg.* 2021;60(6):1343–1350.
4. Ad N, Henry L, Hunt S, Holmes SD. Should surgical ablation for atrial fibrillation be performed in patients with a significantly enlarged left atrium? *J Thorac Cardiovasc Surg.* 2014;147(1):236–241.
5. Ad N, Holmes SD, Shuman DJ, Pritchard G. Impact of atrial fibrillation duration on the success of first-time concomitant Cox Maze procedures. *Ann Thorac Surg.* 2015;100(5):1613–1619.
6. Cox JL, Ad N, Churyla A, et al. The Maze procedure and postoperative pacemakers. *Ann Thorac Surg.* 2018;106(5):1561–1569.
7. Kiankhooy A. Talk like a duck, walk like a duck: a cardiac surgeon's understanding of complex imaging in the management of atrial fibrillation. *J Card Surg.* 2022;37(12):4178–4185.
8. Atrial Fibrillation | cdc.gov. 2020. https://www.cdc.gov/heartdisease/atrial_fibrillation.htm, 2020
9. Ambrosio G, Bassand JP, Corbalan R, et al. Characteristics, treatment, and outcomes of newly diagnosed atrial fibrillation patients with heart failure: GARFIELD-AF. *ESC Heart Fail.* 2021;8(2):1139–1149.
10. Bunch TJ. Atrial fibrillation and dementia. *Circulation.* 2020;142(7):618–620.
11. Bunch TJ, Weiss JP, Crandall BG, et al. Atrial fibrillation is independently associated with senile, vascular, and Alzheimer's dementia. *Heart Rhythm.* 2010;7(4):433–437.
12. Calkins H, Hindricks G, Cappato R, et al. 2017 HRS/EHRA/ECAS/APHRS/SOLAECE expert consensus statement on catheter and surgical ablation of atrial fibrillation: executive summary. *J Arrhyth.* 2017;33(5):369–409.
13. Hsu JC, Darden D, Du C, et al. Initial findings from the National Cardiovascular Data Registry of Atrial Fibrillation Ablation Procedures. *J Am Coll Cardiol.* 2023;81(9):867–878.
14. Nair GM, Nery PB, Diwakaramenon S, Healey JS, Connolly SJ, Morillo CA. A systematic review of randomized trials comparing radiofrequency ablation with antiarrhythmic medications in patients with atrial fibrillation. *J Cardiovasc Electrophysiol.* 2009;20(2):138–144.
15. Wazni OM, Dandamudi G, Sood N, et al. Cryoballoon ablation as initial therapy for atrial fibrillation. *N Engl J Med.* 2021;28(4):316–324 384.

16. Calkins H, Kuck KH, Cappato R, et al. 2012 HRS/EHRA/ECAS expert consensus statement on catheter and surgical ablation of atrial fibrillation: recommendations for patient selection, procedural techniques, patient management and follow-up, definitions, endpoints, and research trial design: a report of the Heart Rhythm Society (HRS) Task Force on Catheter and Surgical Ablation of Atrial Fibrillation. Developed in partnership with the European Heart Rhythm Association (EHRA), a registered branch of the European Society of Cardiology (ESC) and the European Cardiac Arrhythmia Society (ECAS); and in collaboration with the American College of Cardiology (ACC), American Heart Association (AHA), the Asia Pacific Heart Rhythm Society (APHRS), and the Society of Thoracic Surgeons (STS). Endorsed by the governing bodies of the American College of Cardiology Foundation, the American Heart Association, the European Cardiac Arrhythmia Society, the European Heart Rhythm Association, the Society of Thoracic Surgeons, the Asia Pacific Heart Rhythm Society, and the Heart Rhythm Society. *EP Europace*. 2012;1(4):528–606 14.
17. Ishikura M, Kobori A, Sasaki Y, et al. Importance of the relative epicardial connection locations and right-sided pulmonary vein isolation line for successful pulmonary vein isolation. *J Cardiovasc Electrophysiol*. 2023;34(4):841–848.
18. Vroomen M, Olsthoorn JR, Maesen B, et al. Quantification of epicardial adipose tissue in patients undergoing hybrid ablation for atrial fibrillation. *Eur J Cardio-Thorac Surg*. 2019;56(1):79–86.
19. Kistler PM, Chieng D, Sugumar H, et al. Effect of catheter ablation using pulmonary vein isolation with vs without posterior left atrial wall isolation on atrial arrhythmia recurrence in patients with persistent atrial fibrillation: the CAPLA randomized clinical trial. *J Am Med Assoc*. 2023;329(2):127–135.
20. Verma A, Jiang CY, Betts TR, et al. Approaches to catheter ablation for persistent atrial fibrillation. *N Eng J Med*. 2015;372(19):1812–1822.
21. DeLurgio DB, Crossen KJ, Gill J, et al. Hybrid convergent procedure for the treatment of persistent and long standing persistent atrial fibrillation: results of CONVERGE clinical trial. *Circ Arrhythm Electrophysiol*. 2020;13(12):e009288.
22. van der HCAJ, Weberndörfer V, Vroomen M, et al. Hybrid ablation versus repeated catheter ablation in persistent atrial fibrillation. *JACC Clin Electrophysiol*. 2023;9(72):1013–1023.
23. Doll N, Weimar T, Kosior DA, et al. Efficacy and safety of hybrid epicardial and endocardial ablation versus endocardial ablation in patients with persistent and longstanding persistent atrial fibrillation: a randomised, controlled trial. *eClinicalMedicine*. 2023;61:102052.
24. von Ballmoos MCW, Hui DS, Mehaffey JH, Gillinov AM, Sundt TM, Badhwar V. The Society of Thoracic Surgeons 2023 clinical practice guidelines for the surgical treatment of atrial fibrillation. *Ann Thor Surg*. 2024;118(2):291–310.
25. Makati KJ, Sood N, Lee LS, et al. Combined epicardial and endocardial ablation for atrial fibrillation: best practices and guide to hybrid convergent procedures. *Heart Rhythm*. 2021;18(2): 303–312.
26. Khiabani AJ, MacGregor RM, Manghelli JL, et al. Bipolar radiofrequency ablation on explanted human hearts: how to ensure transmural lesions. *Ann Thor Surg*. 2020;1(6):1933–1939 110.
27. Maesen B, Pison L, Vroomen M, et al. Three-year follow-up of hybrid ablation for atrial fibrillation. *Eur J Cardiothorac Surg*. 2018;1(1):i26–i32 53.
28. Kiankhooy A, Pierce C, Burk S, Phillips A, Eisenberg S, Dunnington G. Hybrid ablation of persistent and long-standing persistent atrial fibrillation with depressed ejection fraction: a single-center observational study. *J Thorac Cardiovasc Surg Open*. 2022;1(12):137–146.
29. Kiankhooy A, Pierce CL, Eisenberg S, et al. Hybrid ablation of atrial fibrillation in patients with prior coronary artery bypass grafting: a single center retrospective cohort study. *Video-Assisted Thoracic Surgery*. 2023;8. https://vats.amegroups.org/article/view/7679.

36

The Convergent Hybrid Procedure for Stand-Alone Atrial Fibrillation

Kevin J. Makati, Andrew J. Sherman

CHAPTER OUTLINE

Several off-pump, minimally invasive surgical procedures were developed in the early 2000s for the treatment of patients with stand-alone atrial fibrillation (AF) in an effort to make AF surgery less invasive and more accessible to a larger number of cardiac surgeons.[1–3] The minimally invasive, off-pump procedures incorporated epicardial lesions only and were performed either via bilateral mini-thoracotomies[2] or totally thoracoscopically with or without video assistance.[1,3] In 2007, Dr. Andy Kiser described a novel approach to surgical AF ablation called the "Ex-Maze" (extra-cardiac Maze) procedure[4] in which a small midline incision was made in the upper abdomen and a specially designed pericardioscope was inserted into the abdominal cavity. The abdomen was then insufflated to separate the liver from the diaphragm, and the posterior pericardial space was entered through the dome of the diaphragm to expose the posterior left atrium (LA) and pulmonary veins (PVs). He then created multiple epicardial lesions in the left and right atria using radiofrequency (RF) (Fig. 36.1).

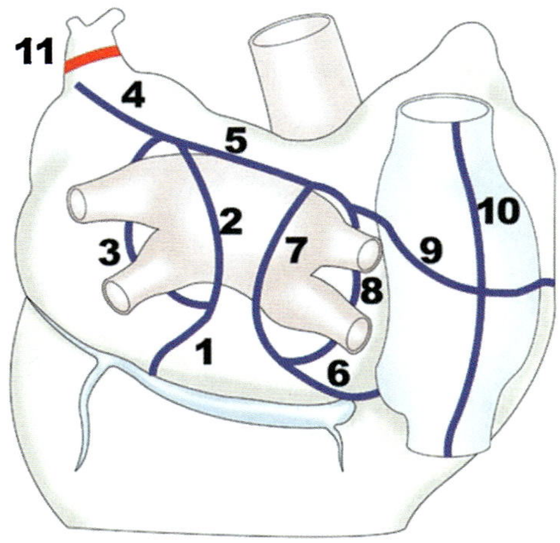

Fig. 36.1 Lesions of the original extracardiac Maze ("Ex-Maze") procedure performed on a beating heart. The back of the heart was accessed by a minimally invasive, trans-abdominal, trans-diaphragmatic route, and all lesions were performed epicardially using a vacuum-assisted unipolar radiofrequency ablation device. (Reproduced from Kiser AC, Wimmer-Greinecker G, Chitwood WR. Totally extracardiac Maze procedure performed on the beating heart. *Ann Thorac Surg*. 2007;84:1783–1785.)

This original trans-abdominal, trans-diaphragmatic surgical approach was eventually replaced by a subxiphoid approach as the Ex-Maze procedure evolved into the contemporary Convergent hybrid procedure.[5–7]

Although left atrial appendage occlusion (LAAO) was not a part of the original Convergent procedure, thoracoscopic LAAO through the left chest has become a common part of the procedure since 2017.[8] Other means of addressing the left atrial appendage (LAA) have also included percutaneous endocardial devices and external suture ligation.[9]

The initial version of Convergent ablation was conducted as a "joint" or same-day procedure, but the addition of LAAO and practical workflow considerations necessitated a "staged" approach in which endocardial catheter ablation is delayed until recovery of the thoracoscopic epicardial lesions. Follow-up catheter ablation in a staged Convergent hybrid procedure can be performed within the same hospitalization or several weeks after the initial thoracoscopic stage.

ROLE OF POSTERIOR LEFT ATRIAL WALL ISOLATION OR ABLATION IN SURGERY FOR ATRIAL FIBRILLATION

Although PV isolation remains the cornerstone of all catheter and surgical AF ablation procedures, the posterior left atrial wall between the right and left PVs is also important in the genesis and perpetuation of AF.[10] This area is complex in structure, sharing similar origins developmentally with the PVs and presumably maintaining their propensity to induce episodes of AF. Indeed, failure to isolate this area effectively was the only predictor of poor outcomes in an analysis of the late clinical results of one version of the Cox Maze-IV procedure.[11] The presence of varying myocardial fiber orientation and discrete septo-pulmonary and septo-atrial bands[12] creates anisotropy of conduction, leading to slow conduction[13] (see Chapter 3, Fig. 3.13). The posterior wall of the LA between the right and left PVs is believed to harbor approximately 20% of the atrial triggers responsible for inducing concomitant AF and some 30% of the macro-reentrant drivers responsible for sustaining persistent and long-standing persistent AF (LSpAF) use this area as a part of their reentrant circuit. Therefore, if this area is neither isolated nor ablated, it will result in an obligatory failure rate of at least 20% in patients with paroxysmal AF and at least 30% in patients with non-paroxysmal AF undergoing catheter or surgical ablation of AF (see Chapter 25).

CONVERGENT PROCEDURE TECHNIQUE

Whereas the box lesions of the on-pump surgical Maze-III and Maze-IV procedures are created to *isolate* the posterior left atrial (LA) wall along with the four PVs, the off-pump hybrid Convergent procedure is designed to *ablate* the posterior LA wall and isolate the PVs by combining thoracoscopic epicardial ablation and catheter-based endocardial ablation.

Thoracoscopic Closure of the Left Atrial Appendage

The patient is positioned supine with a bump placed under the left thorax toward the spine. Standard anesthetic monitoring includes an arterial line, central venous access, large-bore peripheral intravenous lines, and an oropharyngeal temperature probe positioned under fluoroscopic guidance to monitor esophageal temperature during the epicardial ablation. A bronchial blocker or double-lumen endotracheal tube is commonly used for intubation to allow for single right lung ventilation and left lung decompression during the initial thoracoscopic closure of the LAA. If the LAA is not closed thoracoscopically, a single lumen endotracheal tube can be used. We perform a transesophageal echocardiography (TEE) at the outset of the operation to ensure that there is no thrombus in the LA or atrial appendage and to assess left ventricular function and valvular competency. TEE is also used during the thoracoscopic LAAO to confirm complete LAA exclusion using multiple views, including three-dimensional reconstruction. Although the stages of the surgical procedure can be performed in different orders, our current practice is to perform the thoracoscopic LAAO before the subxiphoid epicardial ablation.

In addition to elevating the left chest, the operating table can be positioned in the reverse Trendelenburg position and tilted to the right to improve visualization. A 5-mm 30-degree scope is inserted in the sixth intercostal space (ICS) along the mid-axillary line, the pleural space is insufflated with carbon dioxide, and all pleural adhesions are divided. A second 5-mm port is inserted in the fourth ICS at the mid-axillary line, and a final 12-mm port in the eighth ICS at the posterior axillary line for delivery of the LAA clip. The phrenic nerve is identified, and the pericardium is incised 1 to 2 cm posterior to it. The pericardiotomy is extended caudally to the mid-ventricular level and cephalad to the main pulmonary artery trunk level. An endo-Kittner is used to expose the LAA through the pericardiotomy, and the Ligament of Marshall is identified and divided with an electrocautery (Fig. 36.2). The LAA is then closed with an AtriClip (AtriCure, Inc.) while proper clip application is confirmed by TEE.

In our current practice, we create a partial anterior lesion from the base of the LAA toward the mitral valve epicardially that is completed later endocardially by catheter. This combination of epicardial and endocardial lesions is created to prevent conduction across the so-called "mitral vestibule" (see Chapter 41, Figs. 41.2 through 41.4), also called the "LAA–MV isthmus" (see Chapter 48, Figs. 48.8, 48.9, and Fig. 48.11 through 48.13). As demonstrated anatomically in Chapter 41 and described functionally in Chapter 48, this isthmus of atrial myocardium between the LAA and the mitral valve annulus can potentially participate in postoperative peri-mitral atrial flutter if neither an anterior trigone lesion nor the combined posterior mitral line–coronary sinus lesions are used to prevent postoperative peri-mitral flutter. However, if either of those more traditional measures to prevent postoperative peri-mitral flutter is used, this LAA–MV isthmus lesion is unnecessary.

Subxiphoid Posterior Left Atrial Wall Ablation

A 3- to 4-cm incision is placed over the xiphoid process to expose the pericardium and a 4- to 6-cm transverse pericardiotomy is created to expose the posterior surface of the heart. A SUBTLE cannula (AtriCure, Inc., Mason, OH) is inserted into the pericardial space for suction and irrigation (Fig. 36.3), a 5- to 7-mm 0-degree scope is then inserted through the cannula, and both are positioned behind the heart. The cleft of the cannula is pointed toward the heart, and the beveled tip of the cannula is oriented toward the middle aspect of the posterior pericardial space. Gentle clockwise and counterclockwise twisting of the cannula helps maneuver it within the pericardial space to expose the posterior wall of the LA (Fig. 36.4). The superior PVs are rarely visible given the cephalad extent of

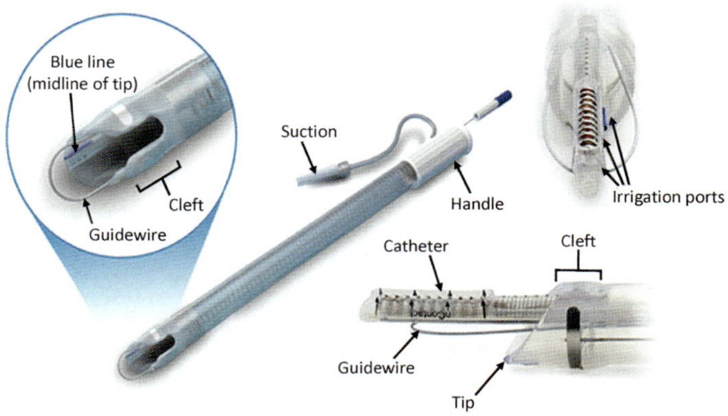

Fig. 36.3 The SUBTLE cannula and the EPi-Sense monopolar, vacuum-assisted, saline-irrigated radiofrequency ablation system. (See text for further discussion.)

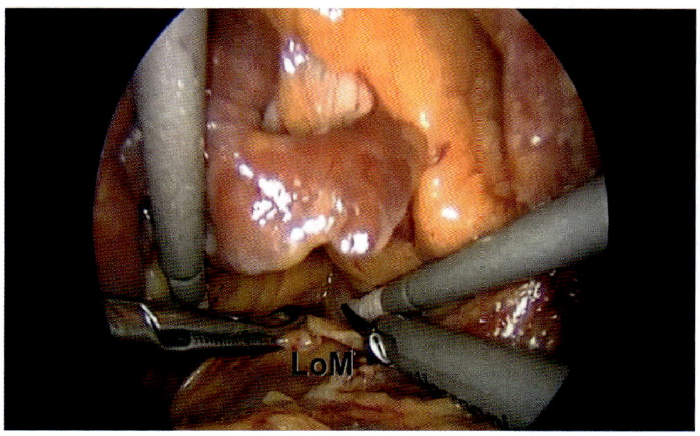

Fig. 36.2 Thoracoscopic exposure and division of the ligament of Marshall (LoM).

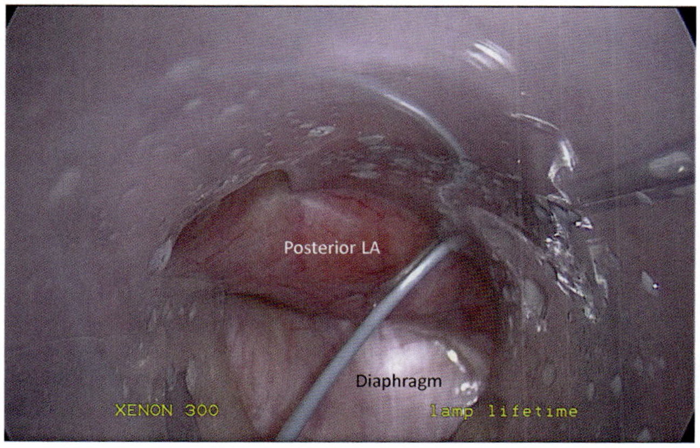

Fig. 36.4 Surgeon's initial view of the back of the heart through a pericardioscopy placed via the subxiphoid approach. *LA,* Left atrium.

the pericardial reflections. After the scope is inserted into the cannula, the first structure that is usually visible is the coronary sinus. With advancement of the cannula to the patient's right side from the coronary sinus, the LA will then come into view. If the right atrium is identified initially, advancing the cannula to the patient's left side will successfully guide the surgeon to the posterior left atrial space. Cephalad movement of the cannula will expose the left inferior PV. Sweeping the cannula and focusing on the patient's right will bring the right inferior PV into view. Ablation can begin after these three landmark structures above have been clearly identified. The EPi-Sense Coagulation Device (AtriCure, Inc., Mason, OH) is then inserted through the cannula (Fig. 36.5).

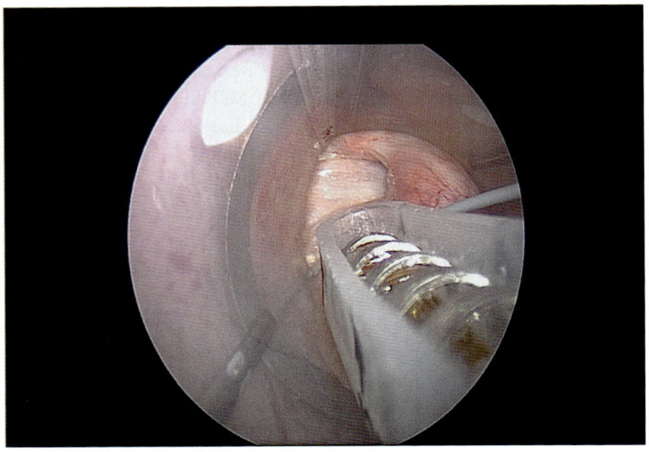

Fig. 36.5 The EPi-Sense ablation device being positioned on the posterior wall of the left atrium between the right and left pulmonary veins.

Ablation lines are initially created adjacent to the posterior aspect of the right PVs, advancing the cannula as far superior as the pericardial reflections will allow to achieve ablation of a portion of the posterior right superior PV and carina between the right PVs. The ablation catheter is moved in the cephalad direction until resistance is met by pericardial reflections, indicating that the catheter has been placed as far superiorly as possible. Vacuum suction is initiated through the Epi-Sense ablation device to create optimal contact with the posterior left atrial wall. Baseline esophageal temperature is recorded, and saline is infused into the field before ablation is initiated. The ablation catheter coil must always face the heart to avoid inadvertent energy delivery through the posterior pericardium in the oblique sinus where the esophagus resides. For this reason, endoscopic visualization of the guiding markers located along the open ablation face of the catheter is used as an additional visual reference. RF energy is applied at 30 watts for 90 seconds to create each lesion. Sequential ablation lines are created by moving from a cephalad to a caudal direction, ensuring each ablation lesion slightly overlaps the previous lesion. Ablated myocardium has a blanched appearance that assists in the placement of the next lesion (Fig. 36.6A). The availability of sensing electrodes on the ablation device is also extremely helpful in identifying residual electrical activity characteristic of incompletely ablated tissue (Fig. 36.6B. In addition, a "sawtooth" pattern on the sensing electrodes sometimes occurs as a consequence of epicardial fat, further indicating incomplete ablation (Fig. 36.6C).

It is sometimes difficult to ablate the antrum of the right PVs epicardially because of the angle of the PV-posterior wall junction, but fortunately, these areas can be easily ablated later with the endocardial catheter. Sequential epicardial ablation lesions are continued until the posterior aspect of the left PVs is identified and ablated. The area between the inferior PVs and the coronary sinus should remain

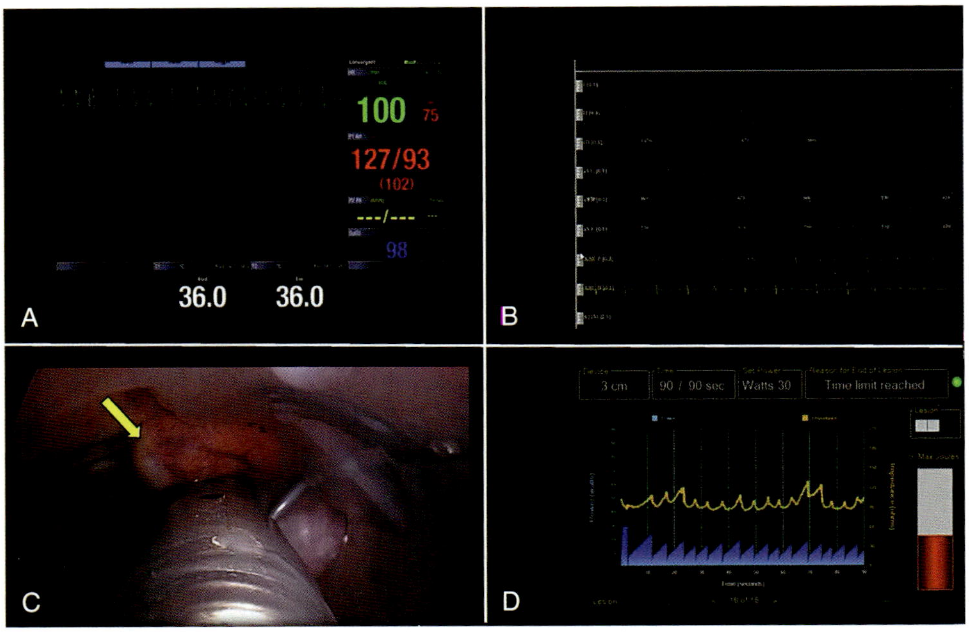

Fig. 36.6 Real-time monitoring of atrial ablation. (A) Display of standard hemodynamic parameters and esophageal temperature. (B) Sensing electrodes on the EPi-Sense ablation device reveals residual slow electrical activity in the ablated area, indicating that additional ablation is needed at this point. (C) The previous lesion *(yellow arrow)* is blanched in appearance compared with the surrounding nonablated tissue. (D) "Sawtooth" pattern on sensing electrode indicating incompletely ablated tissue that can be caused by epicardial fat.

unablated because incomplete ablation in this region can be proarrhythmic. The epicardial ablation endpoint is a homogenous area of ablation extending from the right PVs to the left PVs limited superiorly by the pericardial reflection and inferiorly by several centimeters of atrial myocardium above the coronary sinus. The anterior portions of the PVs on either side can also be ablated, although complete PV isolation is not possible because of pericardial reflections.

Endocardial Catheter Ablation

The purposes of the catheter ablation stage of the Convergent procedure are to audit the epicardial ablation and to complete a comprehensive epicardial–endocardial hybrid AF ablation lesion set. Patients who have been previously ablated may still derive benefit from endocardial mapping to ensure that all ablation targets have been addressed. The timing of the catheter ablation stage is a matter of practicality because the optimal timing to assess ablated tissue remains unclear. For programs that are early in the experience of hybrid AF ablation, we recommend performing the endocardial catheter procedure soon after the epicardial ablation stage to help the surgeon develop an understanding of how their ablation lesions translate on endocardial mapping.

Mapping software now provides high-resolution and ultrasensitive detection of viable myocardium as well as wavefront propagation, which may be a more sensitive measure of nonviable tissue than voltage measurements might provide.[14]

Scar or ablated tissue that is no longer viable is typically denoted by a gray color. An example of an endocardial map after epicardial ablation of the posterior wall demonstrates a large scar along the posterior wall and a portion of the left atrial isthmus (Fig. 36.7). Another map from the same patient shows the final result of both epicardial and endocardial ablation hallmarked by scar (gray color) along the PVs and left atrial posterior wall (Fig. 36.8). Variability within pericardial reflections alters the extent of endocardial ablation.

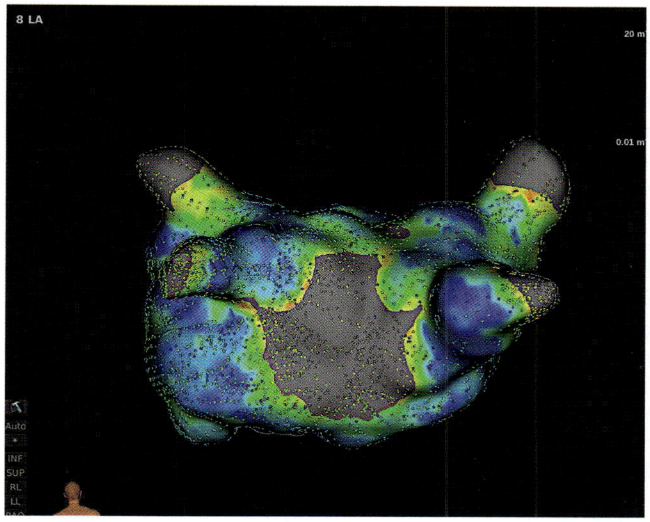

Fig. 36.8 An endocardial electroanatomic map of the left atrial posterior wall in the same patients as shown in Fig. 36.7 after both epicardial ablation with the EPi-Sense device and endocardial catheter ablation. The large *gray area* in the left atrial posterior wall indicates transmurality and successful ablation.

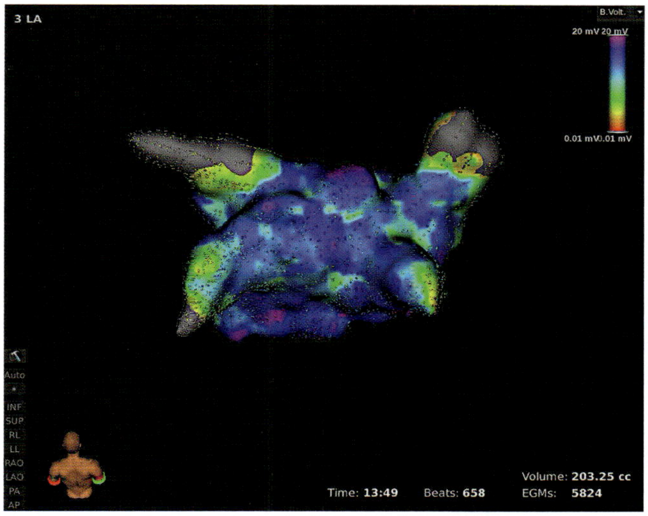

Fig. 36.7 An *endocardial* electroanatomic map of the left atrial posterior wall after *epicardial* ablation only, demonstrating a large scar along the posterior wall including a portion of the left atrial isthmus.

RESULTS OF THE CONVERGENT PROCEDURE

Convergent ablation has been studied extensively, and although worldwide experience has established its role as an effective treatment strategy, applying outcome data to clinical practice has been complex given the rapidly evolving landscape of endocardial ablation technologies. Furthermore, modifications made in the content and conduct of the Convergent procedure have influenced the safety and outcome data as well. At the current time, data supporting catheter-based posterior wall isolation remains mixed in part because of heterogenous endocardial energies used in studies, varied ablation strategies, and modes of endpoint analysis.[15–18] Outcome data using the original transabdominal entry without appendage management has been summarized in a meta-analyses of Convergent ablation confirming effectiveness in maintaining sinus rhythm as high as 84.3% at 12 months at the expense of adverse events as high as 9%. The great majority of complications involved pericardial effusion, bleeding related to surgery, tamponade, and cerebrovascular events with a small but relevant rate of mortality,[19,20] prompting the creation of best practice guidelines to mitigate common complications associated with the procedure in 2020.[21] The subxiphoid approach to the pericardial space has largely replaced the original trans-abdominal approach and has resulted in a significant reduction in complications from 23% to 3.8%.[22] The first observational studies using a subxiphoid approach reported no mortalities with complication rates ranging from 0% to 1.6%.[23,24]

A significant advance in understanding the true outcomes of the Convergent procedure occurred with completion of the first prospective, multicenter, randomized clinical trial, Convergence of Epicardial and Endocardial RF Ablation of the Treatment of Symptomatic Persistent AF (CONVERGE; NCT01984346).[25,26] The CONVERGE trial randomized 153 patients with persistent AF or LSpAF in a 2:1 ratio to either

Convergent ablation or endocardial catheter ablation. The control arm mandated PV isolation using RF with a connecting roof lesion and ablation of complex fractionated electrograms, which was popular when the trial was designed in 2013. The investigation arm included patients treated with the Convergent procedure first via the trans-diaphragmatic approach and then using the subxiphoid approach, and all were performed as joint procedures on the same day. A substantial proportion of the enrolled patients (42%) had LSpAF with a duration of more than 4 years. The CONVERGE trial showed that 67.7% of patients achieved the primary endpoint of no AF, no atrial flutter, and no atrial tachycardia off new drugs or without increased doses of previously failed antiarrhythmic drugs through 12 months compared with 50.0% in the catheter ablation group (relative risk, 1.35; $p = .036$). A subgroup analysis of patients with LSpAF only showed a greater absolute difference of 28.8% ($p = .022$) that was sustained through 18 months and a reduction in AF burden of at least 90% in 74% of Convergent ablation patients, as opposed to 55% in the control arm ($p = .0395$).[27]

Complementing the results of the CONVERGE trial was the emergence of real-world data using alternative forms of endocardial energy (cryothermy) and procedural staging validating the effectiveness of Convergent ablation in non-paroxysmal AF and as an effective method to reduce AF burden. We followed more than 200 patients in a prospective registry using Convergent epicardial ablation and endocardial cryoballoon ablation without appendage management and demonstrated an impressive freedom from AF, atrial flutter, and atrial tachycardia off amiodarone in 70%, with residual AF burden of 1% or less by implantable monitors in 80%.[28] Finally, the addition of surgical appendage management to Convergent ablation showed freedom from AF in 73.8% of patients using cardiac implantable electronic devices.[29] Although electrical isolation of the PVs and posterior left atrial wall can be performed endocardially, the surgical approach for the epicardial ablation of the posterior left atrial wall allows for easy access and division of the ligament of Marshall, now recognized to support AF arrhythmogenesis.[30]

SUMMARY

The off-pump hybrid Convergent procedure is a safe and effective treatment for patients with advanced forms of AF. When LAA management is added to hybrid AF ablation, the salutary benefits are additive. Potential improvements in the ability to expand the lesion set of all hybrid procedures, including the Convergent procedure, will likely improve freedom from AF in the future. These include the addition of lesions to prevent post-procedure peri-mitral atrial flutter and creating lesions in the right atrium.

REFERENCES

1. Manasse E, Infante M, Ghiselli S, et al. A video-assisted thoracoscopic technique to encircle the four pulmonary veins: a new surgical intervention for atrial fibrillation ablation. *Heart Surg Forum*. 2002;5:337–339.
2. Wolf RK, Schneeberger EW, Osterday R, et al. Video-assisted bilateral pulmonary vein isolation and left atrial appendage exclusion for atrial fibrillation. *J Thorac Cardiovasc Surg*. 2005;130:797–802.
3. Yilmaz A, Van Putte BP, Van Boven WJ. Completely thoracoscopic bilateral pulmonary vein isolation and left atrial appendage exclusion for atrial fibrillation. *J Thorac Cardiovasc Surg*. 2008;136:521–522.
4. Kiser AC, Wimmer-Greinecker G, Chitwood WR. Totally extracardiac Maze procedure performed on the beating heart. *Ann Thorac Surg*. 2007;84:1783–1785.
5. Makati K, Sherman A. Long term outcome in persistent atrial fibrillation patients undergoing concurrent epicardial radiofrequency/endocardial cryoballoon hybrid ablation. *Heart Rhythm*. 2017;14(5).
6. Gegechkori N, Yang F, Miller A, et al. Comparison of hybrid ablation for persistent atrial fibrillation with and without left atrial appendage closure. Report of 1 year follow up (abstract). *J Interv Card Electrophysiol*. 2020;57:164.
7. Tonks R, Lantz G, Mahlow J, et al. Short and intermediate term outcomes of the convergent procedure: initial experience in a tertiary referral center. *Ann Thorac Cardiovasc Surg*. 2019;20:13–21.
8. Lee LS. Subxiphoid minimally invasive epicardial ablation (convergent procedure) with left thoracoscopic closure of the left atrial appendage. *Op Tech Thorac Cardiovasc Surg*. 2018;23:152–165.
9. Ellis C, Badhwar N, Tschopp D, et al. Subxiphoid hybrid epicardial-endocardial atrial fibrillation ablation and LAA ligation: initial sub-X hybrid MAZE registry results. *J Am Coll Cardiol EP*. 2020;6(13):1603–1615.
10. Suenari K, Chen YC, Kao YH, et al. Discrepant electrophysiological characteristics and calcium homeostasis of left atrial anterior and posterior myocytes. *Basic Res Cardiol*. 2011;106:65–74.
11. Saint LL, Bailey MS, Prasad S, et al. Cox-Maze IV results for patients with lone atrial fibrillation versus concomitant mitral disease. *Ann Thor Surg*. 2012;93(3):789–795.
12. Ho SY, Anderson RH, Sanchez-Quintana D. Atrial structure and fibres: morphologic bases of atrial conduction. *Cardiovasc Res*. 2002;54:325–336.
13. Roberts-Thomson Kurt C, Stevenson I, Kistler PM, et al. The role of chronic atrial stretch and atrial fibrillation on posterior left atrial wall conduction. *Heart Rhythm*. 2009;6(8):1109–1117.
14. Frontera A, Pagani S, Limite LR, et al. Slow conduction corridors and pivot sites characterize the electrical remodeling in atrial fibrillation. *JACC Clin Electrophysiol*. 2022;8(5):561–577.
15. Ibrahim AA, Elaraby A, Almaadawy O, et al. Adjunctive left atrial posterior wall isolation for atrial fibrillation: an updated systematic review and meta-analysis. *Pacing Clin Electrophysiol*. 2024;47:1108–1123.
16. Jiang X, Liao J, Zhiyu L, et al. Adjunctive left atrial posterior wall isolation in treating atrial fibrillation: insight from a large secondary analysis. *JACC Clin Electrophysiol*. 2022;8(5):605–618.
17. Salih M, Darrat Y, Ibrahim AM, et al. Clinical outcomes of adjunctive posterior wall isolation in persistent atrial fibrillation: a meta-analysis. *J Cardiovasc Electrophysiol*. 2020;31:1394–1402.
18. Kozlov AV, Durmanov SS, Bazylev VV. Left atrial posterior wall isolation in persistent atrial fibrillation does not influence the efficacy of catheter ablation: a pilot study. *Vestnik Aritmologii*. 2022;29(3):5–12.
19. Luo X, Li B, Zhang D, et al. Efficacy and safety of the convergent atrial fibrillation procedure: a meta-analysis of observational studies. *Interact Cardiovasc Thorac Surg*. 2019;28:169–176.
20. Khan Z, Hamandi M, Khan H, DiMaio JM, Evans M. Convergent epicardial-endocardial ablation for treatment of long-standing persistent atrial fibrillation: a review of literature. *J Card Surg*. 2020;35(6):1306–1313.
21. Makati KJ, Sood N, Lee LS, et al. Combined epicardial and endocardial ablation for atrial fibrillation: best practices and guide to hybrid convergent procedures. *Heart Rhythm*. 2021;18(2):303–312.

22. Larson J, Merchant FM, Patel A, et al. Outcomes of convergent atrial fibrillation ablation with continuous rhythm monitoring. *J Cardiovasc Electrophysiol.* 2020;31(6):1270–1276.
23. Gegechkori N, Yang F, Miller A, et al., Comparison of hybrid ablation for persistent atrial fibrillation with and without left atrial appendage closure. Report of 1 year follow up (abstract). Presented at Venice Arrythmias 2019, 2019.
24. Sabzwari SRA, Garg L, Mehta N, et al. Convergent Ablation for the Treatment of Long-Standing Persistent Atrial Fibrillation—A Single Center Experience. Presented at American Heart Association Scientific Sessions, 2019.
25. DeLurgio DB, Ferguson E, Gill J, et al. Convergence of epicardial and endocardial RF ablation for the treatment of symptomatic persistent AF (CONVERGE Trial): rationale and design. *Am Heart J.* 2020;224:182–191.
26. DeLurgio DB, Crossen KJ, Gill J, et al. Hybrid convergent procedure for the treatment of persistent and long-standing persistent atrial fibrillation: results of CONVERGE clinical trial. *Circ Arrhythm Electrophysiol.* 2020;13:e009288. https://doi.org/10.1161/CIRCEP.120.009288.
27. DeLurgio DB, Blauth C, Halkos ME, et al. Hybrid epicardial-endocardial ablation for long-standing persistent atrial fibrillation: a subanalysis of the CONVERGE trial. *Heart Rhythm.* 2023;4(2):111–118.
28. Makati KJ, Sherman AJ, Gerogiannis I, Sood N. Safety and efficacy of convergent hybrid procedure using cryo as endocardial energy source for the treatment of atrial fibrillation. *Circ Arrhythm Electrophysiol.* 2020;13(11):e008556.
29. Ahmed A, Ghazal R, Bawa D, et al. Outcomes of hybrid surgical ablation and concomitant left atrial appendage exclusion in long-standing persistent atrial fibrillation. *J Cardiovasc Electrophysiol.* 2024. https://doi.org/10.1111/jce.16405.
30. Jiang R-H, Jiang CY, Sheng X, et al. Marked suppression of pulmonary vein firing after circumferential pulmonary vein isolation in patients with paroxysmal atrial fibrillation: is pulmonary vein firing an epiphenomenon? Is pulmonary vein firing an epiphenomenon? *J Cardiovasc Electrophysiol.* 2014;25(2):111–118.

37

A Complete Hybrid Maze Procedure for Stand-Alone Atrial Fibrillation

James L. Cox, Andrei Churyla

CHAPTER OUTLINE

Past experience with both the catheter and surgical ablation of atrial fibrillation (AF) has provided several observations that should be considered when designing an off-pump hybrid procedure:

1. The Maze procedure is the most effective intervention for AF.
2. The Maze procedure is too invasive to be feasible as first-line therapy for AF.
3. A Maze procedure cannot be performed by thoracoscopic surgery alone.
4. A Maze procedure cannot be performed by catheter ablation alone.
5. Interventional electrophysiologists (EPs) are excellent at closing the "gaps" of failed surgical lesions.
6. Interventional EPs are excellent at ablating focal areas of the atrium.

These observations suggest that if the ultimate goal of a hybrid procedure is to attain the best possible outcomes by the least invasive technique, the ideal hybrid procedure would be one that combines surgical lesions and catheter lesions to create a complete biatrial Maze procedure. Thus, although current hybrid procedures are more successful for long-standing persistent AF (LSpAF) than catheter ablation,[1,2] they cannot attain the success of the open-heart Maze procedures because none of current hybrid procedures reproduce all of the lesions of a complete biatrial Maze procedure.

The success rates of hybrid procedures for the treatment of AF fall between those for the open surgical Maze-III and Maze-IV procedures and those for catheter ablation (see Chapter 39, Fig. 39.1). The major advantage of hybrid procedures is that virtually all of the gaps in lesions that remain after the initial epicardial thoracoscopic lesions occur at the subendocardial level. This is because of the difficulty in creating complete and permanent transmural lesions with unipolar devices applied only to the epicardium in off-pump patients (see Chapter 20, Fig. 20.6). Fortunately, the residual lesion gaps in the subendocardium can be closed with a high degree of success during the follow-up endocardial catheter ablation portion of most hybrid procedures. Therefore, the primary reason that hybrid procedures are less successful than open on-pump surgical Maze procedures is that several critical lesions of the on-pump Maze procedures are routinely not included as a part of off-pump hybrid procedures. Thus, even when the thoracoscopic epicardial lesions are combined with the endocardial catheter lesions, they still do not create the complete pattern of a biatrial Maze procedure.

Following the growing popularity and acceptance of off-pump hybrid procedures, it occurred to us that it should be possible to create *all* of the lesions of a biatrial Maze procedure with the combination of epicardial thoracoscopic surgery and endocardial catheter ablation in which case the results of such an off-pump "hybrid Maze procedure" would be identical to those of an on-pump surgical biatrial Maze procedure. The conduct and technique of such an off-pump complete hybrid Maze procedure is described in this chapter.

TECHNICAL OBJECTIVES IN CURRENT NON-MAZE HYBRID PROCEDURES

Initial Thoracoscopic Surgery

There is a fundamental difference in the goal of a surgical procedure when it is performed as sole therapy for AF and a surgical procedure when it is performed as the first step in a hybrid procedure for AF. When surgery is used as sole therapy for AF and performed on cardiopulmonary bypass, it is essential to create *all* of the lesions of a Maze procedure because it is the only chance the surgeon will have to cure the arrhythmia. However, when thoracoscopic surgery is performed as the initial step in a hybrid procedure, it is not only impossible but also unnecessary to create a complete maze pattern because it will always be followed by an obligatory catheter ablation. The objective of the initial thoracoscopic surgery in a hybrid Maze procedure is to create as many of the linear lesions of the Maze procedure as possible to limit the complexity of the subsequent catheter lesions required to ablate the AF.

Follow-Up Catheter Ablation

A primary objective of the catheter ablation in all hybrid procedures is to "touch up" any gaps in the thoracoscopic lesions. Because the follow-up catheter ablation is performed endocardially, it is usually simple to close any gaps in the thoracoscopic lesions as mentioned earlier. It seems more logical to us to perform staged hybrid procedures rather than joint procedures because the former allow the thoracoscopic lesions to heal and the gaps to declare themselves before the follow-up catheter ablation. However, experienced teams who have performed both staged and joint hybrid procedures have found no significant differences in the results.[3,4] This observation speaks well for the ability to create permanent transmural lesions by combining epicardial surgical and endocardial catheter lesions in one setting. However, as currently practiced, neither staged nor joint hybrid procedures overcome the problem of misplaced and/or arbitrarily deleted lesions in critical areas of the atria.

After the initial thoracoscopic lesions have been created, three options remain for the catheter ablation portion of a hybrid procedure. The first option is to perform catheter mapping to localize and ablate extrapulmonary vein sites such as complex fragmented atrial electrogram spots, focal "rotors," and so on or to map-guide the placement of additional linear lesions in the atrium. An example of this approach is described in Chapter 34. This effort to "tailor" the treatment of each individual patient results in variations of the final lesion pattern of the hybrid procedure from one patient to another.[5] The desire to tailor AF therapy based on the patient's specific intraprocedure maps is a laudable goal, but it disregards the futility of previous efforts to map-guide both surgical and catheter procedures for AF.[6–8] Optimal long-term results are difficult to attain with map-guided interventional procedures primarily because of the changing nature of AF drivers with time as discussed in Chapter 6 (see Fig. 6.12) and Chapter 12. The second option for the catheter ablation portion of a hybrid procedure is to create the same predetermined hybrid lesion pattern in all patients. Examples of this approach are described in Chapters 35 and 36.[9,10] The third option is to create additional lesions during the catheter ablation that result in the final combined lesion set to be that of a Maze procedure. However, the ability to complete a biatrial Maze procedure during the follow-up catheter ablation depends on the lesion pattern that was created during the initial thoracoscopic surgery.

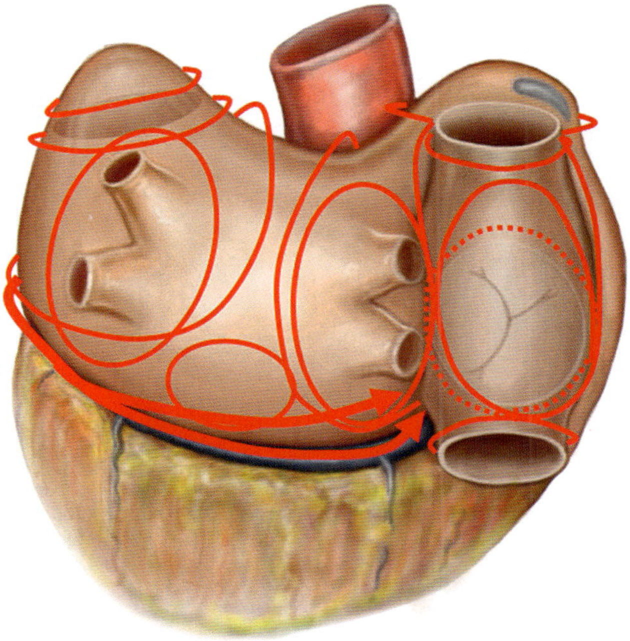

Fig. 37.1 Potential locations of atrial drivers in non-paroxysmal atrial fibrillation (AF). The *red circles* represent the actual macro-reentrant circuits that have been documented during AF. Note that they can and do occur in both the right atrium (RA) and left atrium. The long reentrant circuit in the RA, which may travel either anterior or posterior to the superior vena cava orifice, and the reentrant circuit around the tricuspid valve are the ones responsible for typical atrial flutter. The long circuits crossing the inferior left atrial isthmus between the inferior pulmonary veins and the mitral annulus, one of which is passing through the coronary sinus, are the pathways of postintervention atypical left atrial flutter, also known as perimitral flutter.

HYBRID MAZE PROCEDURE

As discussed in Chapter 19, use of the term "Maze procedure" as a generic term for anything done surgically to the atrium to treat AF can be misleading. Unfortunately, this practice has been especially common during the development of hybrid procedures over the past decade. The catchy phrase "totally thoracoscopic Maze procedure" has made it even easier to be misled into thinking that actual Maze procedures are being performed when that is not the case. For example, articles specifically including the term "Maze procedure" in their titles[11,12] lead one to believe that a technique for performing a complete Maze procedure had already been described. However, none of the patients reported in these articles received a Maze procedure. In fact, most of them had no right atrial lesions at all, and a significant number had no left atrial appendage (LAA) closure, both of which are critical elements of a Maze procedure.

The Maze procedure was designed to interrupt *all* of the potential macro-reentrant drivers that sustain AF while leaving the atria capable of being activated by a sinus-generated impulse after surgery. Although the macro-reentrant drivers may be stable or fleeting in nature, the regions in both atria that are capable of sustaining them have been well-defined (Fig. 37.1). This has allowed the concept of the Maze procedure to remain the same for the Maze-I, Maze-II, Maze-III (both the cut-and-sew and cryosurgical techniques), and Maze-IV iterations as well as for the off-pump hybrid Maze procedure described later.[13]

Thoracoscopic Surgery via the Right Chest

Right Atrial Lesions

As discussed in Chapter 13, the possible locations of macro-reentrant drivers in the right atrium (RA) have been identified, and they are present in up to 30% of patients with AF (Fig. 37.2).[14–16] Therefore, the RA should not be ignored in any surgical procedure designed to ablate AF.

The first right atrial lesion to perform is the superior vena cava (SVC) lesion, which precludes the development of macro-reentry around the orifice of the SVC and interrupts one of the three macro-reentrant circuits that can cause classic atrial flutter (Fig. 37.3). As opposed to when the on-pump Maze-III or Maze-IV procedure is performed, *the SVC lesion is specifically not extended into the inferior vena cava (IVC) in the off-pump hybrid Maze procedure.* The IVC lesion is unnecessary because a CTI lesion will be performed later during the follow-up catheter ablation procedure. However, following the creation of the SVC lesion, there are still several potential right atrial sites where macro-reentrant drivers can form (Fig. 37.4).

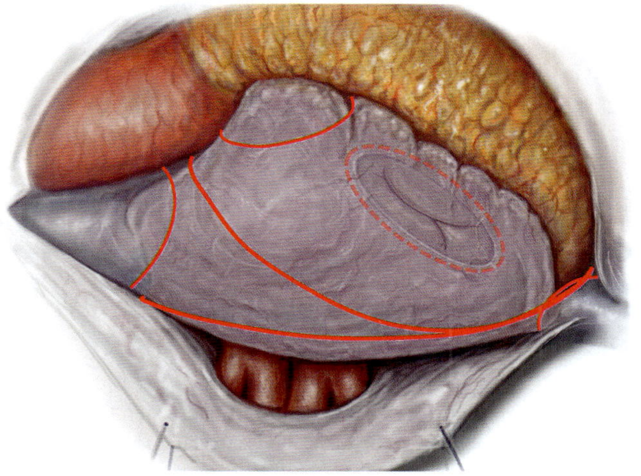

Fig. 37.2 Right atrial drivers of atrial fibrillation (AF). The *red circles* represent the locations of the macro-reentrant circuits that can occur in the right atrium and serve as drivers of AF.

In an off-pump complete surgical Maze procedure, the distal end of the "T" lesion terminates at the tricuspid valve annulus (see Chapter 13, Figs. 13.8 and 13.13). However, the "T" lesion cannot be extended to

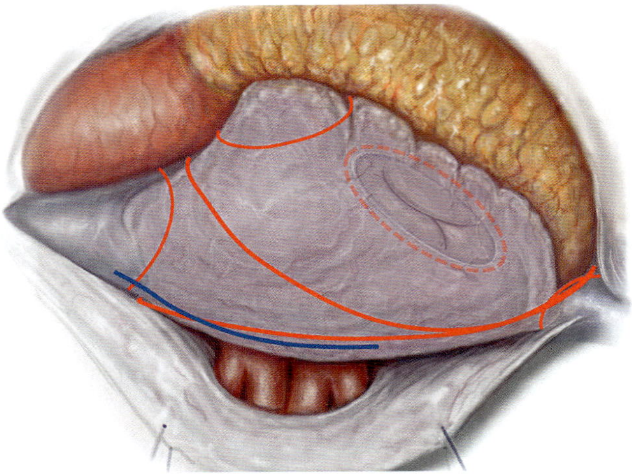

Fig. 37.3 Superior vena cava (SVC) lesion. The SVC lesion *(blue line)* extends from the SVC two-thirds of the way down to the inferior vena cava (IVC), *but it is not extended into the IVC.* It is positioned parallel and immediately anterior to the edge of the crista terminalis, where the right atrial wall is thin.

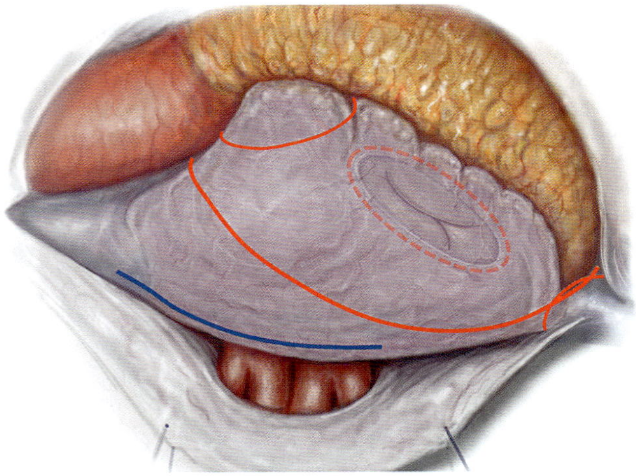

Fig. 37.4 Potential right atrial drivers after the superior vena cava (SVC) lesion completed. The SVC lesion prevents macro-reentry around the orifice of the SVC, and it also interrupts the macro-reentrant circuit passing posterior to the SVC orifice that is one of the three right atrial circuits than can drive atrial flutter.

the tricuspid annulus thoracoscopically. Instead, when the right atrioventricular groove is reached, the lesion is curved up along the anterior edge of the RA and extended to the tip of the right atrial appendage (RAA; Fig. 37.5). This lesion is a combination of the proximal free-wall portion of the "T" lesion and the RAA lesion described in Chapter 13, and it interrupts another of the three potential drivers of atrial flutter and prevents macro-reentry around the base of the RAA.

After these RA lesions have been created, the only sites in the RA where macro-reentry can occur are around the tricuspid valve annulus and around the orifice of the IVC (Fig. 37.6). Fortunately, both of these potential RA drivers use the cavotricuspid isthmus (CTI) and can easily be blocked by the creation of a CTI lesion during the follow-up catheter ablation (see later).

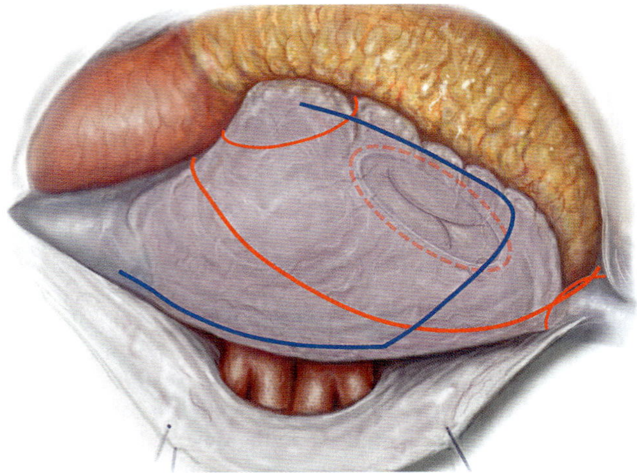

Fig. 37.5 Modified "T" lesion combined with right atrial appendage (RAA) lesion. The "T" lesion of an open on-pump Maze procedure is modified in the off-pump hybrid Maze procedure in which it purposely is not extended to the tricuspid valve annulus. Instead, when it reaches the anterior edge of the right atrium, the lesion is curved upward and is extended to the tip of the RAA. The IVC lesion in the open Maze procedure is created to prevent reentry around the orifice of the IVC. However, a CTI lesion performed during the follow-up catheter ablation in a hybrid procedure prevents reentry around the IVC orifice, so the surgical IVC lesion is unnecessary.

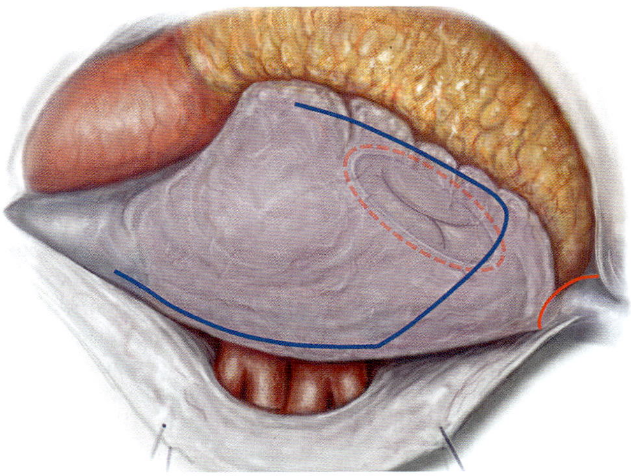

Fig. 37.6 Potential right atrial drivers after completion of all thoracoscopic right atrial lesions. After completion of the thoracoscopic right atrial lesions, the only remaining potential right atrial reentrant drivers are one around the tricuspid annulus and one around the inferior vena cava orifice. Both of these potential drivers use the cavotricuspid isthmus (CTI) and can be easily interrupted during the follow-up catheter ablation by performing a CTI lesion.

All of the thoracoscopic right atrial lesions in the hybrid Maze procedure are created using a dual-electrode, unipolar Coolrail device (AtriCure, Inc.) (Fig. 37.7, *right inset*). As mentioned, because these lesions are created epicardially, they are most likely to fail endocardially, so any gaps are quite amenable to being closed during the follow-up endocardial catheter ablation.

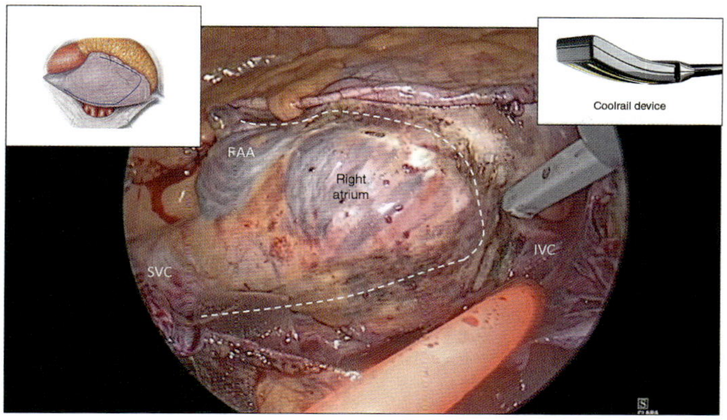

Fig. 37.7 Complete right atrial thoracoscopic lesion set. Operative photo of the thoracoscopic right atrial lesions of the hybrid Maze procedure *(dashed white lines). Left inset,* Diagrammatic sketch of the corresponding right atrial lesions. *Right inset,* Photo of the dual-electrode, unipolar Coolrail device used to create the right atrial lesions epicardially. *IVC,* Inferior vena cava; *RAA,* right Atrial appendage; *SVC,* superior vena cava.

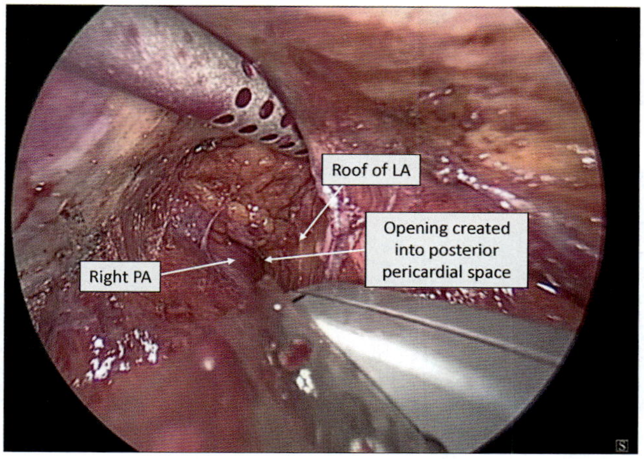

Fig. 37.9 Exposure of transverse sinus. Right chest thoracoscopic view of exposure of the transverse sinus. The dissection plane is between the right pulmonary artery (PA) and the top of the left atrium (LA) at the upper end of Waterston's groove. Blunt dissection is continued toward the left until an opening is created into the free space of the posterior pericardium.

Left Atrial Lesions

Waterston's groove is developed to expose the medial portion of the posterior left atrial septum (Fig. 37.8). At the upper end of Waterston's groove, dissection is continued between the top of the left atrium (LA) and the right pulmonary artery to open the transverse sinus that extends to the posterior pericardial space (Fig. 37.9). At the lower end of Waterston's groove, the thin pericardial reflection off the posterior wall of the IVC is divided to expose the oblique sinus (Fig. 37.10). Opening both the transverse sinus above and the oblique sinus below allows a guiding device to be passed around the posterior LA medial to the orifices of the right pulmonary veins (PVs; Fig. 37.11). One arm of a bipolar radiofrequency (RF) clamp is then placed around the posterior LA using a rubber drain guide, and the right PVs are isolated (Fig. 37.12).

Through the newly created entrance into the transverse sinus, a partial roof lesion is created with a Coolrail device as far over toward the LAA as possible (Fig. 37.13). Through the oblique sinus, a partial floor lesion is created in the same manner as far toward the left inferior PV as possible (Fig. 37.14).

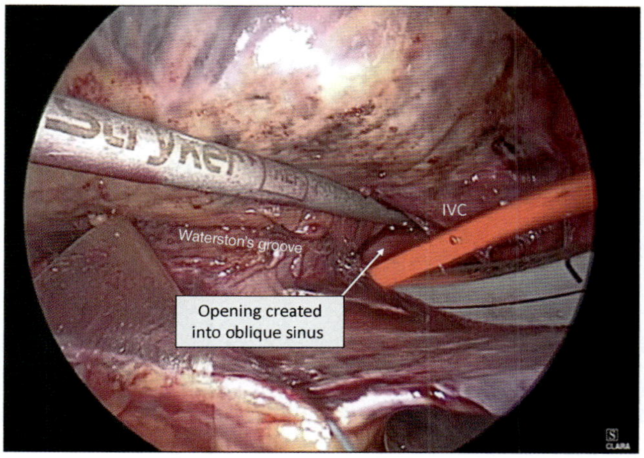

Fig. 37.10 Exposure of Oblique Sinus. Right chest thoracoscopic view of the opening in the pericardial reflection beneath the inferior vena cava to expose the oblique sinus.

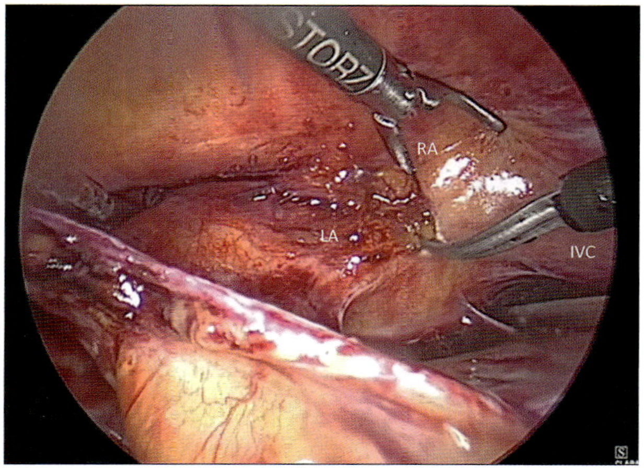

Fig. 37.8 Dissection of Waterston's Groove. Right chest thoracoscopic view of dissection of Waterston's groove to expose the left atrium (LA). *IVC,* Inferior vena cava; *RA,* right atrium.

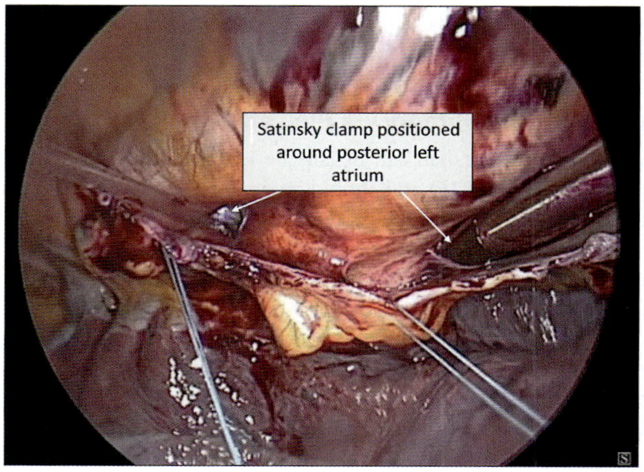

Fig. 37.11 Encirclement of the right pulmonary veins (PVs). Right chest thoracoscopic view of a Satinsky clamp passed around the posterior left atrium in preparation for isolating the right PVs.

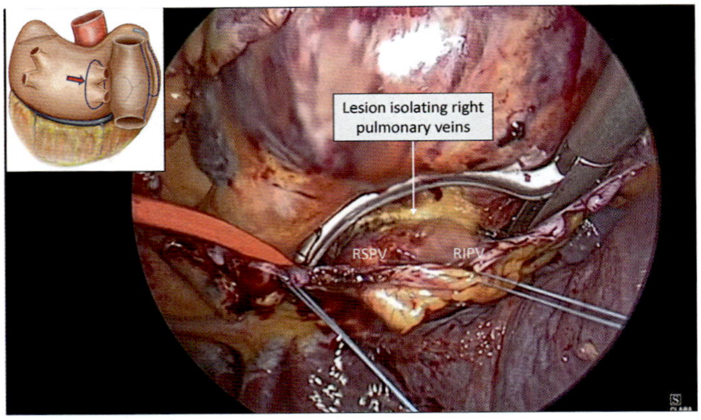

Fig. 37.12 Isolation of right pulmonary veins. Right chest thoracoscopic view of isolation of the right pulmonary veins with a bipolar radiofrequency clamp. The rubber drain was used to pass the posterior arm of the clamp around the pulmonary veins safely. The isolating lesion is placed on the left atrium well away from the orifices of the right pulmonary veins to prevent postoperative pulmonary vein stenosis. *Inset,* Diagrammatic sketch showing the location of the circumferential lesion that isolates the right pulmonary veins *(red arrow). RSPV,* Right superior pulmonary vein.

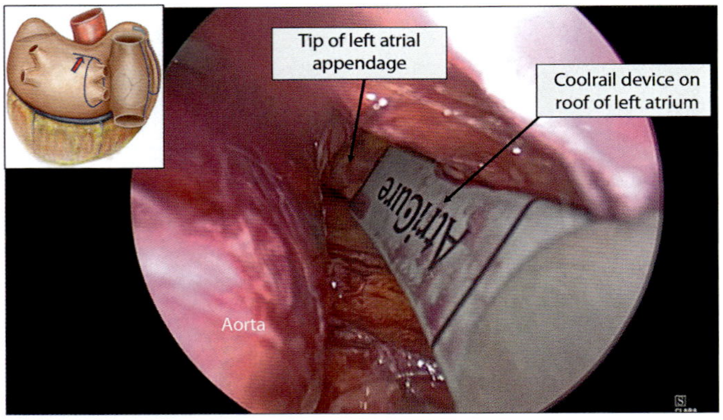

Fig. 37.13 Partial roof lesion via transverse sinus. Right chest thoracoscopic view of the creation of a partial roof line across the upper left atrium (LA) through the transverse sinus. The lesion is created from the right pulmonary vein isolation lesion to approximately halfway across the roof of the LA toward the left superior pulmonary vein. It is often possible to see the left atrial appendage during the creation of this lesion. *Inset,* Diagrammatic sketch showing the location of the partial roof lesion *(red arrow).*

Thoracoscopic Surgery via the Left Chest

The ligament of Marshall can usually be identified just above the left superior PV (Fig. 37.15) and should be divided by electrocautery. The left PVs are dissected free and isolated using a bipolar RF clamp placed across the posterolateral portion of the LA wall encompassing the orifices of the left superior and left inferior PVs (Fig. 37.16). The partial roof and floor lesions created through the right chest are easily identified and completed through the left chest (Fig. 37.17). This completes the box lesion in the LA (Fig. 37.18) A lesion is then created across the coumadin ridge from the left superior PV to the base of the LAA, and the LAA is closed with an AtriClip (Fig. 37.19).

To simplify the creation of the mitral line and coronary sinus lesions by catheter ablation in case they are needed later in 10–15% of patients vulnerable to the development of postoperative peri-mitral flutter, a cryolesion should be placed on the coronary sinus directly below

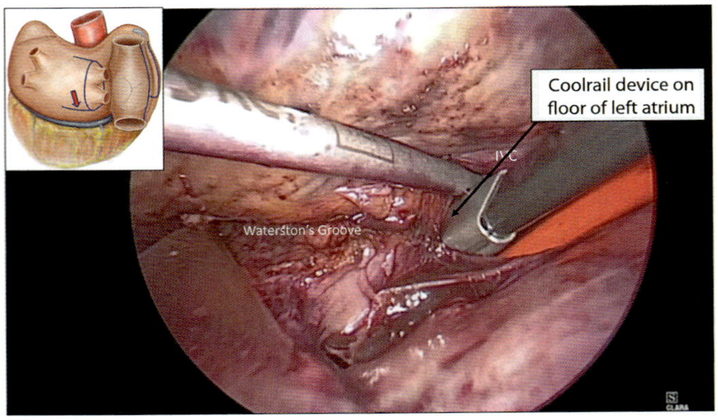

Fig. 37.14 Partial floor lesion via oblique sinus. Right chest thoracoscopic view of the creation of a partial floor line through the oblique sinus. The lesion is created from the right pulmonary vein isolation lesion to approximately halfway across the floor of the left atrium toward the left inferior pulmonary vein. *Inset,* Diagrammatic sketch showing the location of the partial floor lesion *(red arrow). IVC,* Inferior vena cava.

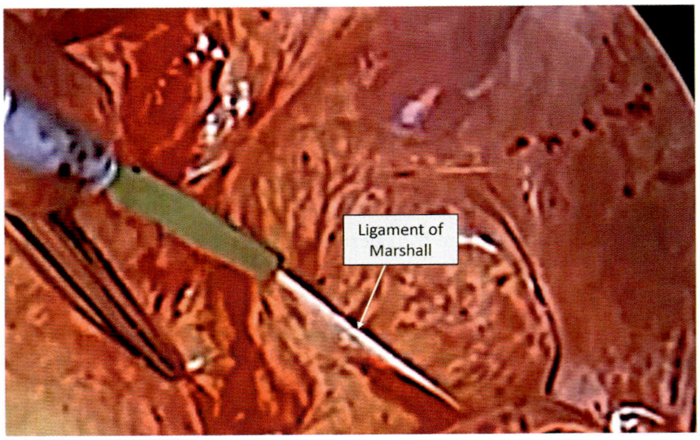

Fig. 37.15 Division of the ligament of Marshall. Left chest thoracoscopic view of the ligament of Marshall, which is located just above the left superior pulmonary vein. It is not absolutely essential to divide this structure, though it should be divided if it can be done expeditiously.

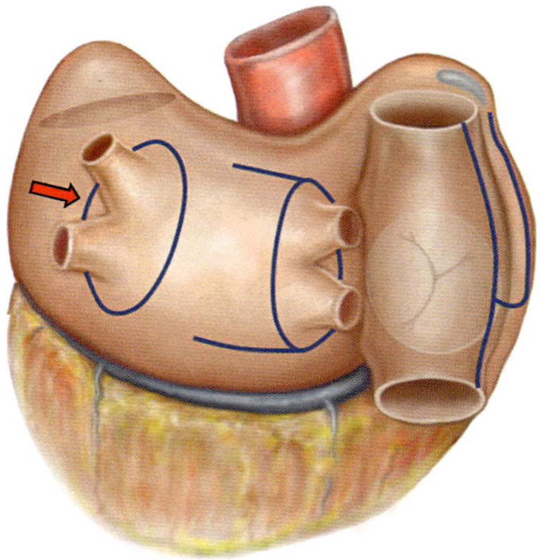

Fig. 37.16 Isolation of left pulmonary veins through left chest. Diagrammatic sketch showing the anatomic relationship of the left pulmonary vein (PV) isolation lesion to the previous lesions that have been created to this point in the thoracoscopic procedure.

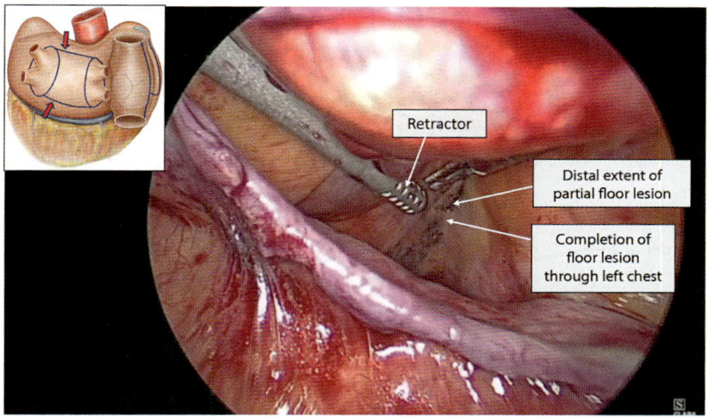

Fig. 37.17 Completion of floor lesion through left chest. The end of the partial floor lesion that was created from the right chest is easily identified through the left chest and a lesion is then placed from the left pulmonary vein isolation lesion to the end of the previously created partial floor lesion. The partial roof lesion is completed from the left chest in the same manner.

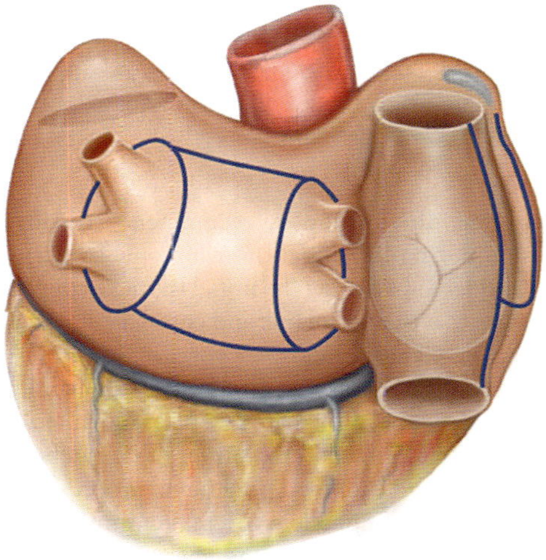

Fig. 37.18 Complete box lesion in left atrium. Diagrammatic sketch showing completion of the box lesion in the left atrium and the previously created lesions in the right atrium.

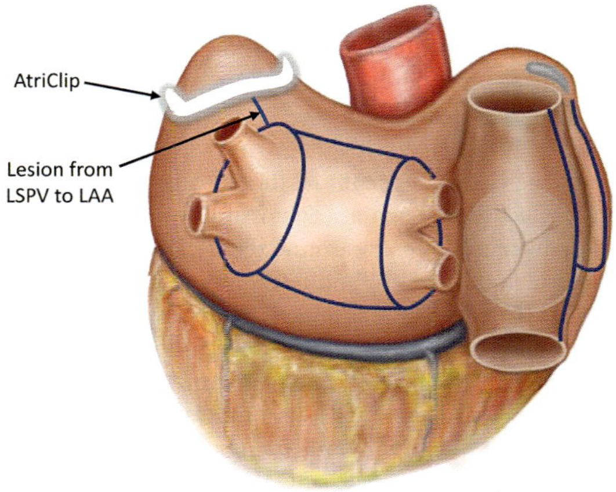

Fig. 37.19 Closure of the left atrial appendage. Diagrammatic sketch showing the location of the left superior pulmonary vein to left atrial appendage (LSPV-LAA) lesion across the coumadin ridge and application of an AtriClip device to occlude the LAA. The AtriClip not only occludes the LAA but also electrically isolates the myocardium of the LAA to prevent it from participating in atrial fibrillation.

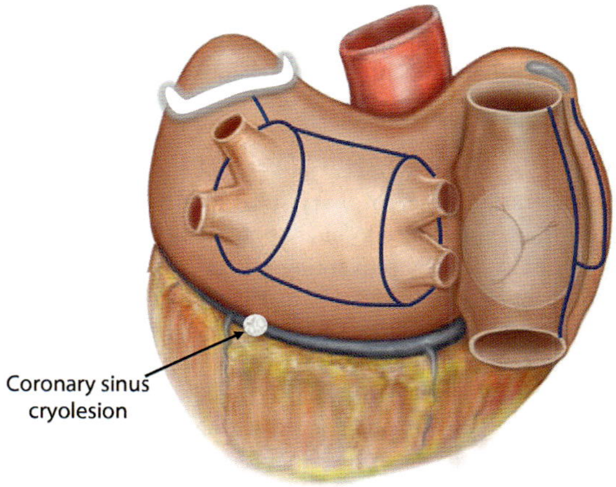

Fig. 37.20 Cryolesion on the coronary sinus. A cryolesion is placed on the coronary sinus below the left inferior pulmonary vein to preclude having to do it during the follow-up catheter ablation. If the patient has post-thoracoscopy peri-mitral atrial flutter and needs to have conduction blocked across the left atrial isthmus at the time of the follow-up catheter ablation, the only lesion that needs to be created is the mitral line. Cryolesions on the coronary sinus have no effect on its function, so it is of no consequence if it is not needed later.

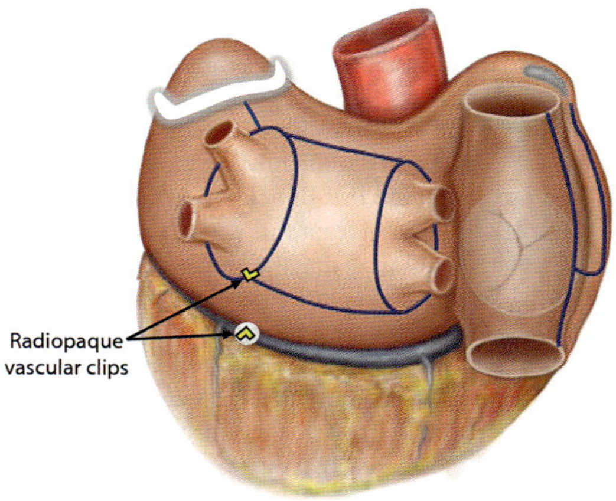

Fig. 37.21 Marking for catheter-based mitral line. Radiopaque vascular clips *(yellow)* are placed directly over the coronary sinus cryolesion and immediately below the left inferior pulmonary vein to make it easier for the interventional electrophysiologist to perform the mitral line (if needed) during the follow-up catheter ablation procedure.

the left inferior PV during the thoracoscopic procedure (Fig. 37.20). Radiopaque vascular clips should then be placed on the coronary sinus cryolesion and just beneath the left inferior PV within the confines of the box lesion (Fig. 37.21). The clips identify exactly where the mitral line should be created endocardially if needed during the follow-up catheter ablation procedure.

This completes all of the thoracoscopic lesions of the hybrid Maze procedure. The only lesions that need to be performed later are the mitral line in the LA to prevent the development of atypical peri-mitral atrial flutter and the CTI lesion in the RA to prevent classic right atrial flutter.

Follow-Up Catheter Ablation

"Touch-Up" of Surgical Lesions

During the follow-up catheter ablation procedure, the integrity of the previously placed thoracoscopic lesions is evaluated, and any detected gaps in the lesions are ablated. The roof and floor lesions and the lesion from the left superior PV to the LAA are more likely to need an endocardial "touch-up" than the pulmonary vein isolation (PVI) lesions during the follow-up catheter ablation because they are created with a unipolar RF device, and the PVI lesions are created with a bipolar RF clamp.

Ablation of Post-thoracoscopic Peri-Mitral Atrial Flutter

Combined mitral line and coronary sinus lesions are included in every surgical Maze procedure to block potential conduction across the left atrial isthmus, thereby preventing postoperative peri-mitral atrial flutter. However, because only 10% to 15% of patients will eventually develop perimitral flutter after a Maze procedure, 85% to 90% of the patients do not actually benefit from the mitral line or coronary sinus lesions during the Maze procedure. The dilemma is that we do not know which 10% to 15% of patients will develop postoperative perimitral flutter and need the lesions, so they should be performed in every patient undergoing an on-pump Maze procedure to avoid surgical failure in the 10% to 15% of patients who will develop peri-mitral fluter without them.

We can expect the same incidence of perimitral flutter after the initial thoracoscopic surgery of a hybrid procedure so that means that only 10% to 15% of patients will need to have catheter ablation for peri-mitral flutter as a second step of the procedure. If the patient has experienced atypical peri-mitral flutter during the blanking period, or if it can be induced during the follow-up catheter procedure, the interventional EP should create an endocardial mitral line between the two radiopaque vascular clips that can be seen easily on fluoroscopy (Fig. 37.22).

Although interventional EPs routinely create CTI lesions in a matter of minutes, they often have difficulty creating an endocardial mitral line. They usually blame this difficulty on the atrial wall's being thicker in the left atrial isthmus, but this is rarely, if ever, the problem. The reason EPs have trouble creating the endocardial mitral line is that they routinely try to create it before first blocking conduction across the coronary sinus lesion because creating an endocardial coronary sinus cryolesion requires a different ablation catheter (see Chapter 48). However, it is absolutely essential that a coronary sinus lesion be created *before* the mitral line because if the mitral line is attempted first, conduction through the coronary sinus can mask what is actually a perfect mitral line. This is why we recommend creating a coronary sinus cryolesion during the initial thoracoscopic surgery. Adding the radiopaque vascular clips during the initial thoracoscopy simply makes it easier to ensure that the mitral line and coronary sinus cryolesion are created in the same plane (see Chapter 48).

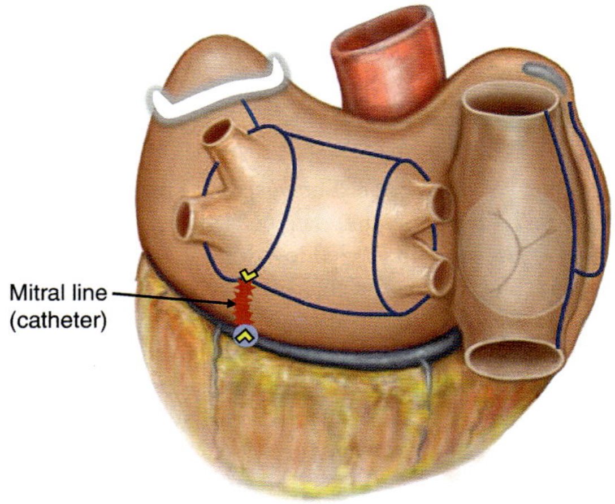

Fig. 37.22 Mitral line created by catheter ablation. If peri-mitral atrial flutter is present or can be induced during the follow-up catheter ablation, a mitral line is created between the radiopaque vascular clips. The presence of the vascular clips ensures that the mitral line and the coronary sinus lesion will be in proper alignment (seeChapter 48). The *blue lines* indicate epicardial thoracoscopic lesions, and the *rust line* indicates the endocardial catheter lesion.

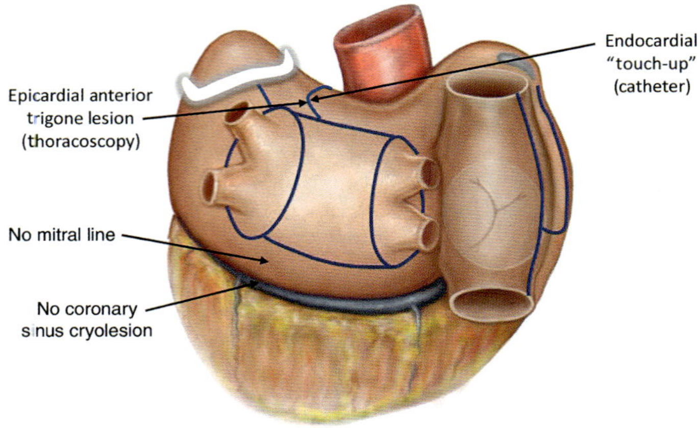

Fig. 37.23 Anterior trigone lesion created during initial thoracoscopy. A transmural anterior trigone lesion is as effective as the mitral line/coronary sinus lesion in preventing postoperative perimitral atrial flutter. The problem is that it is difficult to attain transmurality reliably because of the thickness of Bachmann's bundle in this area. However, that problem can be overcome in a hybrid procedure during the endocardial catheter ablation. This is why a totally epicardial thoracoscopic so-called "totally thoracoscopic Maze" procedure alone will have a 10% to 15% failure rate because of postoperative peri-mitral flutter and will therefore, require an obligatory follow-up catheter ablation.

Another option for preventing postoperative perimitral flutter in a hybrid Maze procedure is to create an epicardial anterior trigone lesion during the initial thoracoscopic surgery that can be "touched up" endocardially during the follow-up catheter procedure (Fig. 37.23). Although it is virtually impossible to create a uniformly transmural anterior trigone lesion solely from the epicardial surface of the atrium because of the thickness of Bachmann's bundle (see Chapter 19, Fig. 19.8), it can be reliably "touched up" endocardially during the follow-up catheter ablation (Fig. 37.24). Therefore, it is quite reasonable to create the anterior trigone lesion during the initial thoracoscopic portion of a hybrid Maze procedure rather to create the coronary sinus cryolesion during initial thoracoscopy and the mitral line during the follow-up catheter procedure.

Completion of Right Atrial Lesions

As mentioned earlier, after the initial thoracoscopic right atrial lesions have been created, there remains the possibility of having classic atrial flutter caused by macro-reentry around the tricuspid valve annulus and around the orifice of the IVC, and both potential drivers use the CTI (see Fig. 37.6). Thus the final lesion of the hybrid Maze procedure is a CTI lesion that is created during the second-stage catheter ablation (Fig. 37.25). A CTI lesion should be performed during the follow-up catheter ablation regardless of whether or not the patient has had classic atrial flutter after the initial thoracoscopic surgery. Although the resulting RA lesion pattern is not exactly the same as that of an on-pump Maze-III or Maze-IV procedure, it is equally effective in preventing the development of right atrial macro-reentry. The final combination of biatrial lesions in either of these hybrid Maze procedures (Fig. 37.26) can be expected to yield the same results as those of an on-pump Maze-III or Maze-IV procedure.

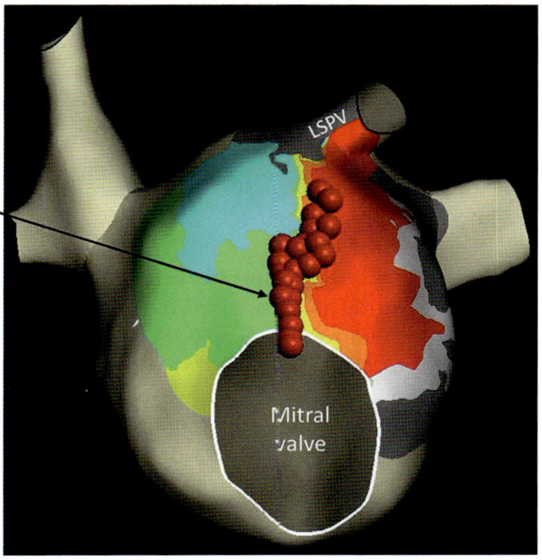

Fig. 37.24 Post–hybrid Maze procedure: map after anterior trigone lesion. If an anterior trigone lesion fails after the initial thoracoscopy, it can usually be completed by catheter ablation later as shown in this atrial activation map. The *red dots* represent the sites of endocardial catheter ablation that were necessary at follow-up to stop the patient's post-thorascopic peri-mitral flutter. Wavefront propagation from the earliest activation of atrium in this region *(red area)* is blocked by the anterior trigone lesion that was initially non-transmural but was rendered transmural by a combination of the initial epicardial thoracoscopic ablation and the endocardial catheter ablation several weeks later. *LSPV,* Left superior pulmonary vein.

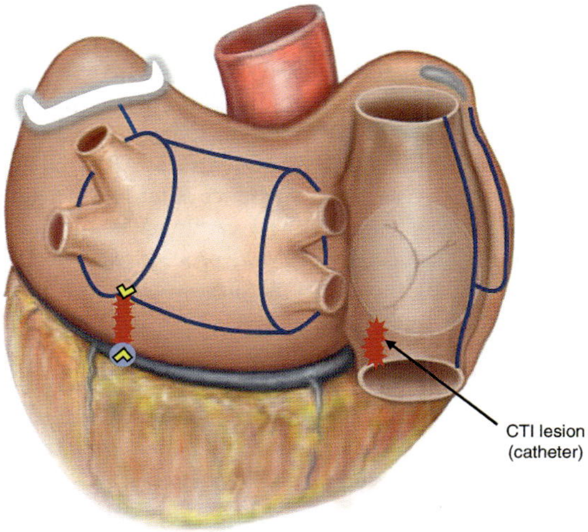

Fig. 37.25 Cavotricuspid isthmus (CTI) lesion created by catheter ablation. The right atrial lesions of the initial thoracoscopic procedure did not preclude the possibility of macro-reentry around the tricuspid valve annulus or the inferior vena cava orifice. Therefore, a CTI lesion is created during the follow-up catheter ablation to complete the right atrial lesions of the Maze procedure. The *blue lines* indicate epicardial thoracoscopic lesions, and the *rust lines* indicate endocardial catheter lesions.

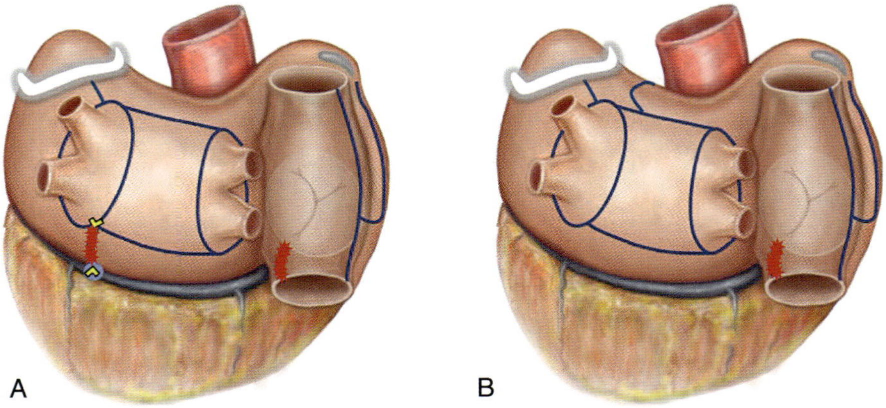

Fig. 37.26 A critical component of any Maze procedure is creating a lesion or lesions that will preclude the development of postoperative peri-mitral flutter. The hybrid Maze procedure can accomplish this goal in one of two ways: (1) by blocking conduction across the left atrial isthmus with the combination of a mitral line and a coronary sinus (CS) lesion (A), or (2) by blocking conduction in the anterior left atrium with an anterior trigone lesion (B). As long as all of the lesions are contiguous and uniformly transmural in either of these approaches, the off-pump hybrid Maze procedure can be expected to be as successful as the on-pump Maze-III and Maze-IV procedures for the treatment of atrial fibrillation. The *blue lines* indicate epicardial thoracoscopic lesions, and the *rust lines* indicate endocardial catheter lesions.

PRELIMINARY CLINICAL RESULTS OF THE HYBRID MAZE PROCEDURE

To our knowledge, the only clinical experience with the hybrid Maze procedure has been at our institution, and our experience has been very limited. A hybrid Maze procedure is more time-consuming to perform than some of the other non-Maze hybrid procedures, so at our institution, the Convergent procedure is currently preferred. However, Drs. Andrei Churyla (surgeon) and Rod Passman (interventional EP) have now performed the hybrid Maze procedure in 20 patients, but not all of them have agreed to have a follow-up catheter ablation, so they are not technically hybrid procedures, and they did not receive a complete Maze procedure. The types of AF treated in these 20 patients were 15% paroxysmal AF, 20% persistent AF, and 65% LSpAF. A total of 19 of the 20 patients (95%) were free of AF or atrial flutter at 1 year, and there were no major adverse events. Of the 14 patients who had both thoracoscopic surgery and a follow-up catheter ablation performed 6 to 12 weeks later, 100% were free of AF, atrial flutter, and atrial tachycardia at 1 year. This experience is far too meager to draw any meaningful conclusions, but these early results are encouraging, and they document that a complete Maze procedure can be performed off-pump by combining thoracoscopic surgery and catheter ablation.

REFERENCES

1. Van der Heijden CAJ, Weberndorfer Vroomen M, Luemans JG, et al. Hybrid versus catheter ablation in patients with persistent and longstanding persistent atrial fibrillation: a systematic review and meta-analysis. *Eur J Cardio-Thorac Surg*. 2019;56:433–443.
2. Van der Heijden CAJ, Weberndorfer V, Vroomen M, et al. Hybrid ablation versus repeated catheter ablation in persistent atrial fibrillation. *JACC Clin Electrophysiol*. 2023;9(7):1013–1023.
3. Umbrain V, Verborgh C, Chierchia G-B, de Asmundis C, Brugada P, La Meir M. One-stage approach for hybrid atrial fibrillation treatment. *Arrhythm Electrophysiol Rev*. 2017;6(4):210–216.
4. Bisleri G, Glover B. Hybrid ablation for persistent atrial fibrillation: how to merge the best from both worlds. *J Thorac Dis*. 2017;9(12):4837–4839.
5. Maesen G, Luermans JGLM, Bidar E, et al. A hybrid approach to complex arrhythmias. *Europace*. 2021;23:ii28–ii33.
6. Cox JL, Schuessler RB, D'Agostino HJ Jr, et al. The surgical treatment of atrial fibrillation: III. Development of a definitive surgical procedure. *J Thorac and Cardiovasc Surg*. 1991;101:569–583.
7. Haissaguerre M, Jais P, Shah DC, et al. Spontaneous initiation of atrial fibrillation by ectopic beats originating the pulmonary veins. *N Engl J Med*. 1998;339:659–666.
8. Baykaner T, Lalani GG, Schricker A, Krummen DE, Narayan SM. Mapping and ablating stable sources for atrial fibrillation: summary of the literature on Focal Impulse and Rotor Modulation (FIRM). *J Interv Card Electrophysiol*. 2014;40(3):237–244.
9. Dunnington GH, Pierce CL, Eisenberg S, et al. A heart-team hybrid approach for atrial fibrillation: a single-centre long-term clinical outcome cohort study. *Eur J Cardiothorac Surg*. 2021. https://doi.org/10.1093/ejcts/ezab197.
10. Delurgio DB, Crossen KJ, Gill J, et al. Hybrid convergent procedure for the treatment of persistent and long-standing persistent atrial fibrillation: results of the CONVERGE clinical trial. *Circ Arrhythm Electrophysiol*. 2020;13(12):e009288. doi:10.1161/CIRCEP.120.009288. Epub 2020 Nov 13.
11. Sirak JH, Schwartzman D. Interim results of the 5-box thoracoscopic Maze procedure. *Ann Thor Surg*. 2012;94(6):1880–1884.
12. Van Laar C, Johannes K, van Putte BP. The totally thoracoscopic Maze procedure for the treatment of atrial fibrillation. *Int Cardiovasc Thorac Surg*. 2017;24(1):102–111.
13. Cox JL, Churyla A, Malaisrie SC, et al. A hybrid Maze procedure for long-standing persistent atrial fibrillation. *Ann Thorac Surg*. 2019;107:610–618.
14. Santucci PA, Varma N, Cytron J, et al. Electroanatomic mapping of postpacing intervals clarifies the complete active circuit and variants in atrial flutter. *Heart Rhythm*. 2009;6(11):1586–1595.
15. Lim HS, Hocini M, Dubois R, et al. Complexity and distribution of drivers in relation to duration of persistent atrial fibrillation. *J Am Coll Cardiol*. 2017;69(10):1257–1269.
16. Osorio-Jaramillo E, Cox JL, Klenk S, et al. Dynamic electrophysiological mechanism in patients with long-standing persistent atrial fibrillation. *Front Cardiovasc Med*. 2022;9:953622. eCollection 2022. https://doi.org/10.3389/fcvm.2022.953622.

38

Minimally Invasive CryoMaze-III Procedure for Stand-Alone Atrial Fibrillation

Niv Ad, Stephen D. Waterford

CHAPTER OUTLINE

Over the past two decades, many different surgical ablation procedures have been proposed to replace the Maze procedure, but the stand-alone Maze procedure for lone atrial fibrillation (AF) remains the best single procedure for rhythm control for all types of AF. The cut-and-sew Maze procedure was originally introduced in 1987 after extensive research and rigid follow-up assessment that included complete electrophysiological studies 6 months postoperatively in the first 69 patients in the original series. In 1997, the minimally invasive CryoMaze-III procedure emerged as the preferred surgical approach for patients with stand-alone AF. When the minimally invasive approach was first developed, cryoablation was the only alternative to the cut-and-sew technique for creating atrial lesions. Even today, the minimally invasive CryoMaze-III procedure under direct vision or endoscopically guided[2,3] remains one of the most frequently used surgical techniques for the treatment of patients with stand-alone AF, although the group at Washington University uses a combination of bipolar radiofrequency and cryothermal energy for minimally invasive stand-alone Maze procedures.[4]

RATIONALE AND SURGICAL INDICATIONS

Although catheter ablation is associated with acceptable outcomes for paroxysmal AF with short duration and small left atria,[5] the success rates are much lower for persistent AF and long-standing persistent AF (LSpAF; see Chapter 31).[6–8] Surgical ablation in general, and the Maze procedure in particular, continues to offer the best long-term freedom from AF and atrial flutter in these patients and remains underused.[9–11] In addition, the Cox-Maze procedure provides the largest reduction in stroke rates. The literature also shows that on-pump procedures such as the Maze procedure are not associated with higher periprocedural morbidity compared with off-pump surgical ablation options.

The hybrid Convergent procedure has demonstrated an absolute increase in freedom from AF and previously failed class I and III antiarrhythmic drugs of 17% when compared with catheter ablation alone for persistent AF and LSpAF.[11] Like all hybrid procedures, the Convergent procedure includes both the initial epicardial ablation and an obligatory follow-up catheter ablation. Totally thoracoscopic (TT) left atrial ablation with or without follow-up catheter ablation is another option for stand-alone AF surgery, although it is suboptimal for persistent and LSpAF because it does not provide consistent transmural lesions because some of the critical left atrial lesions are performed with unipolar radiofrequency. Therefore, the success of off-pump procedures remains limited even after follow-up catheter ablation is performed as part of a planned hybrid procedure. When confronted with patients with a large left atrium (LA) and a long duration of persistent AF or LSpAF,[12] a Cox Maze procedure offers the best single procedure rhythm outcomes with no added perioperative morbidity. Patients who undergo the minimally invasive CryoMaze-III procedure and have a documented recurrence of atrial arrhythmia should be referred for an electrophysiologic study and a touch-up ablation, which has been reported to be extremely successful.[13]

In summary, there are currently several surgical options for patients who have persistent AF or LSpAF, including a traditional open surgical Maze procedure, a minimally invasive or robotic CryoMaze-III procedure, TT left atrial ablation without an obligatory follow-up catheter ablation, thoracoscopic–catheter hybrid procedures, and the Convergent procedure.[14] In our opinion, the minimally invasive CryoMaze-III procedure offers a more comprehensive ablation scheme for the treatment for AF and atrial flutter, and despite requiring 60 to 90 minutes of cardiopulmonary bypass (CPB), morbidity rates are often lower than they are for off-pump hybrid or TT procedures.[9,15] Nevertheless, approximately 80% of surgical ablation for AF in the United States is performed off pump, and there is no left atrial appendage (LAA) management in 50% of those patients. By contrast, a full Maze procedure can be performed through a small incision or through a port, with no added morbidity compared with off-pump modalities.[16] Patients should be particularly encouraged to pursue a full Maze procedure for late persistent AF and LSpAF, long duration of AF, and an enlarged LA, the most important predictors of failure after interventional AF therapy.

SCREENING OF PATIENTS

When evaluating a patient for a minimally invasive CryoMaze-III procedure, it is important to document any prior failed catheter ablations or prior off-pump surgical ablations. Echocardiography is important to rule out valvular disease and cardiac catheterization is helpful not only to rule out coronary artery disease but also to identify coronary artery anatomy in the left atrioventricular (AV) groove near the mitral isthmus and LAA and to note whether the patient has a left- or right-dominant circulation. Importantly, 22% of our referred patients had a diagnosis of significant valvular or coronary artery disease that led to a concomitant surgical procedure.

Preoperative evaluation should also include computed tomography angiography (CTA) of the chest, abdomen, and femoral vessels to ensure that femoral access vessels are usable and to determine whether retrograde arterial perfusion during CPB is possible. Patients who are not eligible for retrograde perfusion during CPB because of diseased femoral arteries or aortoiliac disease can be considered for axillary cannulation or direct aortic cannulation through the thoracotomy incision. The diameter of the ascending aorta should also be less than 45 mm and free of significant calcific disease. Rhythm monitors and electrocardiograms are reviewed to determine the type of atrial arrhythmia, although similar to the open surgical Maze-III and Maze-IV procedures, the CryoMaze-III procedure is equally successful in all forms of AF and atrial flutter. Finally, body mass index (BMI) is a factor for consideration. When first initiating a program, it is recommended to limit patient selection to those with a BMI under 30 kg/m^2, but with more experience, larger BMIs can also be undertaken. Recently, we added an option of implanting a loop recorder preoperatively, which enhances our ability to establish baseline arrhythmia burden and improve our follow-up decision making, especially regarding anticoagulation management.

THORACOTOMY UNDER DIRECT VISION OR ENDOSCOPICALLY GUIDED

A 3- to 5-cm mini-thoracotomy is placed along the right breast anterolateral fold. This affords a reduction in pain compared to more lateral thoracotomies, and it facilitates performance of the right atrial lesions of the Maze procedure, which are more anteriorly located. We use a special retractor and perform the operation under fibrillatory arrest if the patient has no significant aortic insufficiency, but we provide a description of the operation with use of an aortic cross-clamp and antegrade cardioplegia. If the aorta is cross-clamped, a standard Chitwood clamp or similar clamp (detachable or not) may be used. The advantages of a detachable clamp that can be placed through the incision are that it avoids a separate incision and sometimes offers a lower profile in the chest. Finally, an endo-balloon can also be used to provide aortic occlusion and deliver antegrade cardioplegia.

PRINCIPLES OF CRYOABLATION

There are two commercially available cryoablation devices that utilize either nitrous oxide or argon gas as the cryogen.[16] Nitrous oxide devices cool the cryoprobe to approximately minus 60°C and argon-based devices usually cool the cryoprobe to approximately minus 160°C. The cryoprobe itself has a hollow shaft and records the probe temperature at its distal tip for the argon-based device and at the proximal end for the nitrous oxide device. The liquid cryogen is stored in a tank and is released through a valve into the shaft of the probe, at which point it converts into a gas. This results in cooling of the probe by the Joule-Thomson effect. Tissue cells are destroyed by direct formation of ice crystals and early and late apoptosis, disrupting the cell membrane as well as cell organelles (see Chapter 14).[17] Of note, cryoablation, unlike RF, does not result in destruction of tissue architecture and does not destroy collagen. This is why cryothermia is the only ablative energy that can be safely used to ablate myocardial tissue anywhere in the heart without fear of structural injury. This includes the annulus, leaflets, chordae tendineae, and papillary muscles of cardiac valves and the coronary sinus while performing a Maze procedure. The optimal length of time one should apply a cryoprobe to myocardial tissue varies depending on multiple factors, including the temperature of the cryoprobe as well as the temperature and perfusion status of the target tissue. This topic is discussed in Chapters 14 and 20 and has been described in detail in a 2021 report by Cox and colleagues.[18]

LEFT ATRIAL LESIONS OF THE CRYOMAZE-III PROCEDURE

After CPB is established, the oblique sinus is opened to allow for later creation of the epicardial coronary sinus lesion. After arresting the heart, the LAA can be closed with an epicardial device either at the beginning of the procedure or immediately after the LA lesions are completed and before closure of the LA. The LAA can be closed with endocardial sutures or preferably with an AtriClip (AtriCure, Inc.) passed behind the ascending aorta through the transverse sinus with the aid of a 3-0 pledgeted Prolene suture to help guide the clip to the true base of the LAA.[19] Regardless of the stage when the LAA epicardial AtriClip is placed, the LAA orifice should be examined afterward from inside the LA to ensure that the device has been positioned all the way to the base of the LAA and has left no residual pouch.

Next, the LA is opened and the left atrial lift system is positioned to expose the mitral valve (MV) as the ablation begins with the "mitral line" across the LA isthmus and the accompanying coronary sinus lesion. These lesions must be created in the same plane, so the coronary sinus lesion is performed first, and the resultant left atrial endocardial iceball is marked with methylene blue dye to ensure overlap (see Chapters 14 and 48). The mitral line across the left atrial isthmus is then performed, taking care to cross the MV annulus onto the leaflets to ensure that there are no gaps at the annular level that could result in atypical left atrial flutter (Fig. 38.1).[20] There is significant morbidity associated with left atrial peri-mitral flutter as an iatrogenic rhythm because rates can be faster than AF, the rhythm less chemically sensitive to antiarrhythmic medications, and the patient more symptomatic than with AF.

In the 90% of patients with a right-dominant coronary circulation, the mitral line–coronary sinus lesions should be placed in the so-called "watershed area" between the last marginal branch of the circumflex coronary artery and the posterior descending branch of the right coronary artery where there is no coronary artery in the AV groove. Endocardially, the lesions end up being between the P2 and P3 leaflets of the MV. With a left-dominant coronary circulation, they are placed around P3 near the posteromedial commissure. Although cryoablation does not appear to damage coronary arteries, there is some evidence for late intimal hyperplasia,[21] so it is prudent to avoid placing the cryoprobe in direct contact with the coronary artery if possible. However, one

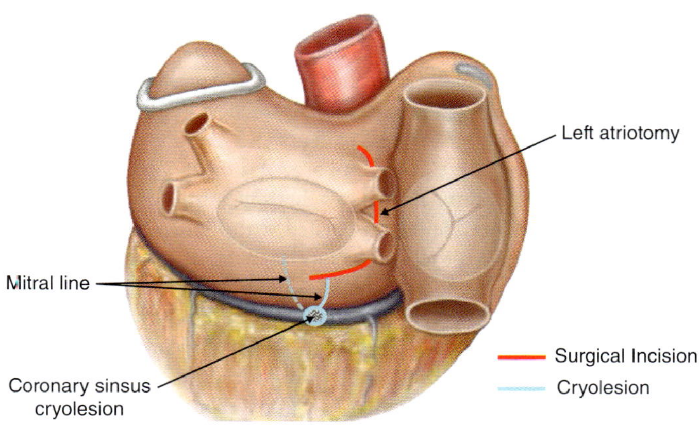

Fig. 38.1 Minimally invasive CryoMaze-III lesions: mitral line–coronary sinus. The surgical left atriotomy is illustrated in *red*, and the endocardial mitral line cryolesion and epicardial coronary sinus cryolesion are illustrated in *cyan*. Note that the mitral line and coronary sinus lesions are in the same plane. These two lesions prevent postoperative peri-mitral atrial flutter.

clinical study using CTA after the CryoMaze-III procedure revealed no late coronary artery damage resulting from cryoablation near the coronary arteries.[22]

After completion of these lesions, a box lesion that encompasses all four pulmonary veins (PVs) and the intervening posterior left atrial wall is created. We can usually create a complete box lesion with only two applications of the cryoprobe, although massive enlargement of the LA can necessitate a third application. With the first application, the cryoprobe is shaped into a U, and the linear cryolesion is created from the top of the atriotomy, around the left PVs, ending just below the left inferior PV (Fig. 38.2). With the second application, the cryoprobe is shaped more linearly, and the lesion is placed from the atriotomy to just below the left inferior PV, where it overlaps with the first linear cryolesion (Fig 38.3). After the completion of the box lesion set, the atriotomy is closed, and the LA is de-aired. After de-airing of the heart, the aortic cross-clamp is removed.

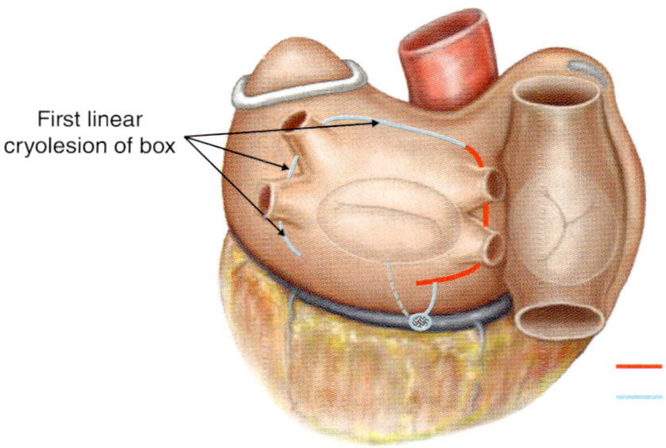

Fig. 38.2 Minimally invasive CryoMaze-III lesions: first endocardial cryolesion of the box around the pulmonary veins (PVs). The first linear cryolesion of the left atrial box lesion extends from the upper end of the left atriotomy, across the roof of the left atrium, around the left PVs, and ends below the left inferior pulmonary vein.

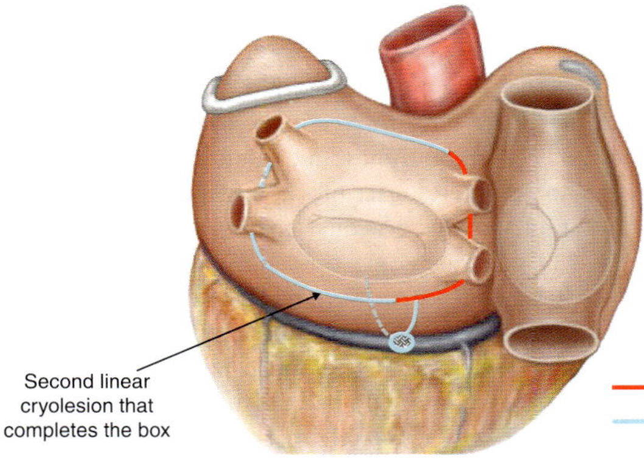

Fig. 38.3 Minimally invasive CryoMaze-III lesions: completion of the box around the pulmonary veins (PVs). The second linear endocardial cryolesion that completes the box lesion around all four PVs and the intervening posterior left atrial wall extends from the lower end of the left atriotomy to the end of the first linear cryo esion.

RIGHT ATRIAL LESIONS OF THE CRYOMAZE-III PROCEDURE

The right atrial (lesions can be performed with aorta still cross-clamped to minimize flooding the surgical field with blood from the coronary sinus. However, the right atrial lesions are usually performed during the reperfusion period immediately after release of the aortic cross-clamp to decrease ischemic time and avoid extending CPB time. Vacuum-assisted venous drainage is helpful during this phase of the procedure.

A diagonal right atriotomy is placed in the lower third of the right atrial to avoid injury to the atrial pacemaker complex in hopes of decreasing the need for postoperative pacemakers (Fig. 38.4). After the atriotomy, a cryolesion is created from its distal end down to tricuspid valve annulus where it intersects at the 2 o'clock position (Fig. 38.5). It is

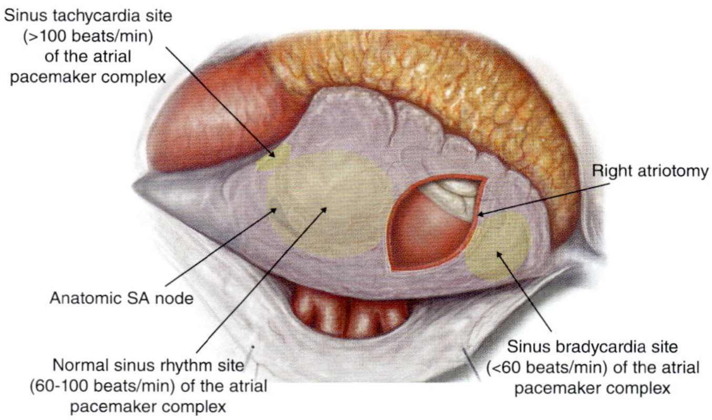

Fig. 38.4 Diagonal right atriotomy that makes the remainder of the right atrial lesions easier to perform, and it also exposes the tricuspid valve if concomitant tricuspid valve repair or replacement is required. The atriotomy is placed near the transition zone between the part of the atrial pacemaker complex *(yellow shaded areas)* that generates normal sinus rhythm at rates between 60 and 100 beats/min and the sinus bradycardia portion responsible for normal sinus bradycardia (<60 bpm) during rest or sleep (see Chapter 3, Fig. 3.9). *SA,* Sinoatrial.

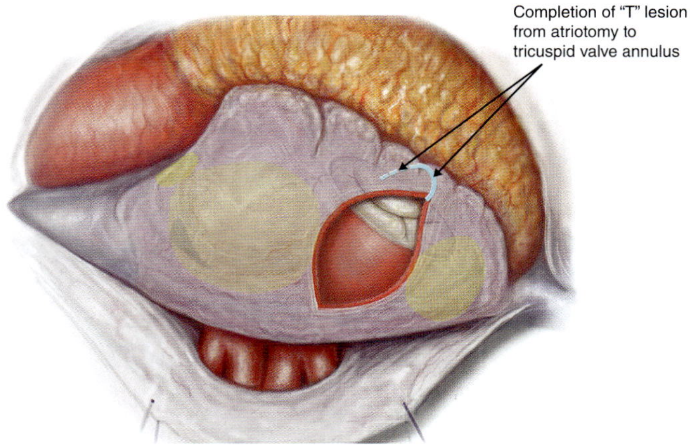

Fig. 38.5 Extension of the conduction block caused by the right atriotomy down to the level of the tricuspid valve annulus with a linear cryolesion from the distal end of the atriotomy to the tricuspid annulus (cyan line). In the Maze procedure, this is traditionally called the "T" lesion, and it intersects with the tricuspid annulus in the 2 o'clock position.

important that this lesion extend across the tricuspid valve annulus to avoid postoperative right atrial flutter caused by macro-reentry around the tricuspid annulus. Next, the inferior vena cava (IVC) lesion is placed from the proximal end of the right atriotomy down into the orifice of the IVC, and the superior vena cava (SVC) lesion is placed from the proximal end of the atriotomy up into the SVC orifice (Fig. 38.6). The SVC lesion should be placed as far lateral and posterior as possible to decrease the likelihood of injury of the anatomic sinoatrial node. During the creation of both the SVC and IVC lesions, it is important that the probe be kept well away from the pericardium because the right phrenic nerve runs parallel to the caval veins and if inadvertently frozen, it can result in paralysis of the right hemidiaphragm. Finally, a small opening can be made in the tip of the right atrial appendage (RAA) to allow for the so-called "counterlesion" to be created from the tip of the RAA to the medial tricuspid valve annulus where it intersects an the 10 o'clock position on the annulus (Fig. 38.7). The purpose of the "counterlesion" is to prevent reentry around the base of the RAA, but it has to be anchored on the tricuspid annulus to be effective. Because two ablation lines across the annulus are not required to prevent

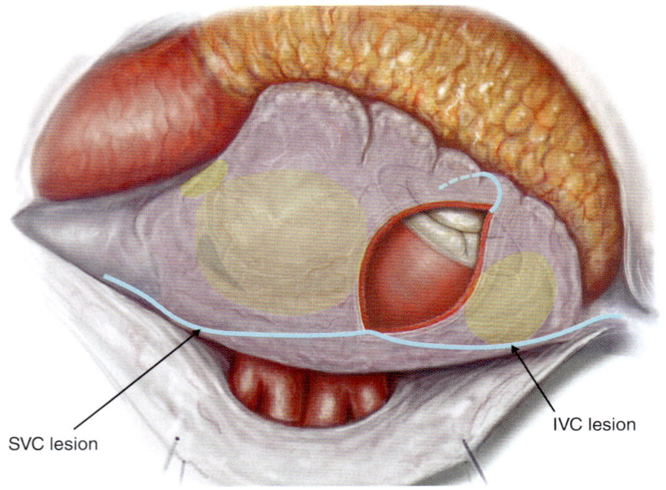

Fig. 38.6 The intercaval linear cryolesion from the superior vena cava (SVC) to the inferior vena cava (IVC).

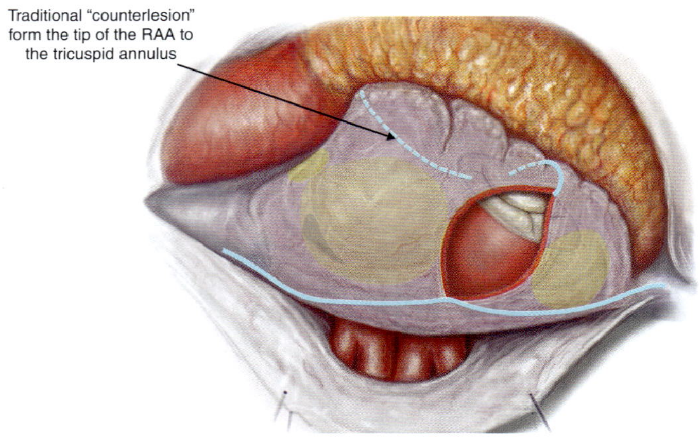

Fig. 38.7 Traditional so-called "counterlesion" from the tip of the right atrial appendage (RAA) to the medial tricuspid valve annulus at the 10 o'clock position. This lesion is included to prevent reentry around the base of the RAA and by necessity has to be anchored on the valve annulus.

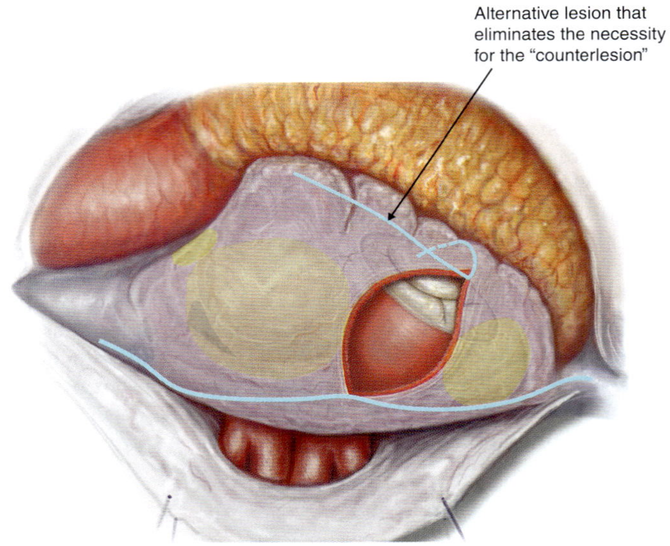

Fig. 38.8 Recent modification of the lesion to prevent reentry around the base of the right atrial appendage (RAA). The traditional "counterlesion" is replaced by a linear lesion from the distal end of the right atriotomy to the tip of the RAA.

postoperative reentry around the tricuspid annulus, a recent proposed modification of the right atrial lesions has been to replace "counterlesion" with a linear cryolesion from the distal right atriotomy to the tip of the right atrial appendage to prevent reentry around the base of the RAA (Fig. 38.8).[23] In addition, we prefer to extend the right atriotomy posteriorly across the crista terminalis, though no advantage or disadvantage of this extension has been confirmed.

Creation of the right atrial lesions during the rewarming and reperfusion period can occasionally result in blood from the coronary sinus flooding the operative field and interfering with the integrity of the cryolesions. This can be avoided by placing a drop sucker in the coronary sinus. The major points of emphasis regarding creation of the right atrial lesions is to place the atriotomy in the least vulnerable location of the atrial pacemaker complex as described, keeping the SVC lesion as far posterior and lateral as possible and being certain that the newly recommended lesion from the atriotomy to the tip of the RAA is placed as far anterior as possible along the edge of the right atrium.

RESULTS OF THE CRYOMAZE-III PROCEDURE

With the techniques described, pacemaker implantation can be limited to 7% or less, as reported in our series of 739 patients undergoing the Cox-CryoMaze-III procedure. Interestingly, 67% of these pacemakers were required because of unmasking an underlying sick sinus syndrome, 23% due to complete heart block, and 10% due to sinus bradycardia.[24] All patients received a dual-chamber, rate-responsive pacemaker. Of the 739 patients, some operations were stand-alone CryoMaze-III procedures, but others were performed concomitantly with valve operations. Patients who had two or more concomitant valve operations had the highest incidence of pacemaker implantation (14%). Finally, the group of patients who had a stand-alone CryoMaze-III procedure were significantly less likely to require a postoperative pacemaker (10%) than patients who underwent a CryoMaze-III procedure concomitantly with valve surgery (22%). In addition, patients who underwent stand-alone CryoMaze-III procedures had 80% lower odds for pacemaker implantation than patients who had the procedure in combination with valve surgery.

In terms of rhythm control after the technique described in a series of 133 patients, 90% of the patients had a sinus rhythm 5 years after a single surgical procedure regardless of the use of class I or III antiarrhythmic drug or cardioversion, and sinus rhythm off antiarrhythmic drugs at 5 years was 79%. Using the Heart Rhythm Society Guidelines definition of sinus rhythm off antiarrhythmic drugs and with no follow-up catheter ablations, success after a single surgical intervention was 73% 5 years after surgery. There were no operative or late deaths, strokes, or renal failure in this series of patients. In addition, 5-day Holter monitors were provided to all asymptomatic patients with no evidence of atrial arrhythmia at 2 years after surgery. Seven of the 105 patients who participated in this follow-up evaluation had AF recurrence, and of these, 2 had episodes less than 5 minutes. Only one of them had continuous AF. Although 86% of the patients were discharged on anticoagulation after the CryoMaze-III procedure, 73% of patients had oral anticoagulation discontinued at 4-year follow-up, and 69% of patients had discontinued both antiarrhythmic drugs and anticoagulation. Moreover, the patients included were those with risk factors for failure: 78% had LSpAF, and 22% had persistent AF (0% had paroxysmal AF). The mean left atrial diameter was 4.9 cm with 25% having a left atrial diameter larger than 5.5 cm. These data demonstrate that proper performance of the minimally invasive CryoMaze-III procedure can provide excellent rhythm outcomes in patients with LSpAF even in the presence of enlarged left atria.

SUMMARY

We describe the technical aspects of performing a minimally invasive CryoMaze-III procedure using cryoablation alone rather than a combination of radiofrequency ablation and cryoablation. Using this procedure routinely in patients with persistent and LSpAF will result in minimal operative morbidity, improved operative times, and superior long-term rhythm outcomes compared with alternative procedures such as hybrid procedures and TT left atrial ablation procedures.

REFERENCES

1. Cox JL. Introduction. *Op Techs Thorac Cardiovasc Surg.* 1999;4:97.
2. Ad N, Holmes SD, Friehling T. Minimally invasive stand-alone Cox Maze procedure for persistent and long-standing persistent atrial fibrillation: perioperative safety and 5-year outcomes. *Circ Arrhythm Electrophysiol.* 2017;10:e005352.
3. Moten S, Rodriguez E, Cook RC, Nifong W, Chitwood WR. New ablation techniques for atrial fibrillation and the minimally invasive Cryo-Maze procedure in patients with lone atrial fibrillation. *Heart Lung Circ.* 2007;16(Suppl 3):S88–S93.
4. Khiabani AJ, Schuessler RB, Damiano RJ. Surgical ablation of atrial fibrillation in patients with heart failure. *J Thorac Cardiovasc Surg.* 2021;162:1100–1105.
5. Imberti JF, Ding WY, Kotalczyk A, Zhang J, Boriani G, Lip G, Andrade J, Gupta D. Catheter ablation as first-line treatment for paroxysmal atrial fibrillation: a systematic review and meta-analysis. *Heart.* 2021;107:1630–1636.
6. Weerasooriya R, Khairy P, Litalien J, Macle L, Hocini M, Sacher F, et al. Catheter ablation for atrial fibrillation: are results maintained at 5 years of follow-up? *J Am Coll Cardiol.* 2011;57:160–166.
7. Kirchhof P, Calkins H. Catheter ablation in patients with persistent atrial fibrillation. *Eur Heart J.* 2017;38:20–26.
8. Koch-Buettner K, Kottmaier M, Reents T, Holmgren E, Semmler V, Deiss M, et al. Identification of predictors for atrial fibrillation-free survival after catheter ablation of persistent atrial fibrillation: results from a large prospective cohort. *Eur Heart J.* 2017;38 (Suppl 1):202.
9. Ad N. Decision-making in surgical treatment for stand-alone atrial fibrillation: minimally invasive Cox Maze procedure. *Innovations* (Phila). 2019;14:487–492.
10. Boersma L, Castella M, van Boven W, Berruezo A, Yilmaz A, Nadal M, et al. Atrial fibrillation catheter ablation versus surgical ablation treatment (FAST): a 2-center randomized clinical trial. *Circ.* 2012;125:23–30.
11. DeLurgio DB, Crossen KJ, Gill J, Blauth C, Oza SR, Magnano AR, et al. Hybrid convergent procedure for the treatment of persistent and long-standing persistent atrial fibrillation: results of CONVERGE clinical trial. *Circ Arrhythm Electrophysiol.* 2020;13:e009288.
12. Dunnington GH, Pierce CL, Eisenberg S, Bing LL, Chang-Sing P, Kaiser DW, et al. A heart-team hybrid approach for atrial fibrillation: a single-centre long-term clinical outcome cohort study. *Eur J Cardiothorac Surg.* 2021;60:1343–1350.
13. Henry L, Durrani S, Hunt S, Friehling T, Tran H, Wish M, et al. Percutaneous catheter ablation treatment of recurring atrial arrhythmias after surgical ablation. *Ann Thorac Surg.* 2010;89: 1227–1231.
14. Bianchini L, Schiavone M, Vettor G, Gasperetti A, Penza E, Ballotta A, et al. Hybrid convergent procedure or pulsed field ablation in long-standing persistent atrial fibrillation. *JACC Clin Electrophysiol.* 2024;10:1700–1710.
15. Je HG, Shuman DJ, Ad N. A systematic review of minimally invasive surgical treatment for atrial fibrillation: a comparison of the Cox-Maze procedure, beating-heart epicardial ablation, and the hybrid procedure on safety and efficacy. *Eur J Cardiothorac Surg.* 2015;48:531–541.
16. Melby SJ, Schuessler RB, Damiano RJ. Ablation technology for the surgical treatment of atrial fibrillation. *ASAIO J.* 2013;59: 461–468.
17. Baust JG, Snyder KK, Santucci KL, Robilotto AT, Van Buskirk RG, Baust JM. Cryoablation: physical and molecular basis with putative immunological consequences. *Int J Hyperthermia.* 2019;36:10–16.
18. Cox JL, Malaisrie SC, Churyla A, Mehta C, Kruse J, Kislitsina ON, McCarthy PM. Cryosurgery for Atrial fibrillation: physiologic basis for creating optimal cryolesions. *Ann Thor Surg.* 2021;112:354–362.
19. Ad N, Massimiano PS, Shuman DJ, Pritchard G, Holmes SD. New approach to exclude the left atrial appendage during minimally invasive cryothermic surgical ablation. *Innovations* (Phila). 2015;10:323–327.
20. Cox JL, Ad N, Palazzo T, Fitzpatrick S, Suyderhoud JP, DeGroot KW, et al. Current status of the Maze procedure for the treatment of atrial fibrillation. *Semin Thorac Cardiovasc Surg.* 2000;12:15–19.
21. Holman WL, Ikeshita M, Ungerleider RM, Smith PK, Ideker RE, Cox JL. Cryosurgery for cardiac arrhythmias: acute and chronic effects on coronary arteries. *Am J Cardiol.* 1983;51:149–155.
22. Cheema FH, Pervez MB, Mehmood M, Younus MJ, Munir MB, Bisleri G, et al. Does CryoMaze injure the circumflex artery? A preliminary search for occult postprocedure stenoses. *Innovations (Phila).* 2013;8:56–66.
23. Cox JL, Malaisrie SC, Kislitsina ON, McCarthy PM: The electrophysiologic basis for lesions of the contemporary Maze operation in a series of 133 patients. *J Thorac Cardiovasc Surg.* 2019;157:584–590.
24. Ad N, Holmes SD, Ali R, Pritchard G, Lamont D. A single center's experience with pacemaker implantation after the Cox Maze procedure for atrial fibrillation. *J Thorac Cardiovasc Surg.* 2017;154:139–146.

39

A Cardiac Surgeon and Interventional Electrophysiologist's Perspective on the Treatment of Long-Standing Persistent Atrial Fibrillation

Amiran Sh, Revishvili

CHAPTER OUTLINE

One of the most perplexing problems facing electrophysiologists (EPs) and cardiac surgeons is how best to treat patients with long-standing persistent atrial fibrillation (LSpAF). EPs believe that we can treat those with LSpAF by catheter ablation with acceptable results while recognizing that we are far better at treating patients with paroxysmal atrial fibrillation (PAF). Non-surgeon physicians understandably try to avoid surgery whenever possible, but this choice can sometimes result in patients receiving suboptimal treatment because of an inherent bias against surgery. On the other hand, some surgeons believe that catheter ablation for patients with LSpAF is simply a waste of time because of poor results and that LSpAF should be treated from the outset by either a hybrid procedure or a minimally invasive CryoMaze-III procedure.

This dilemma provides the author with a rather unique opportunity to address the problem objectively because I am both a practicing interventional EP and a practicing cardiac surgeon. Indeed, over the past several decades, I have performed some 6500 catheter interventional procedures and approximately 1760 surgical procedures for atrial fibrillation (AF), most of which have been for LSpAF. Thus, there is no reason for me to favor either catheter intervention or cardiac arrhythmia surgery because I do both on a regular basis. In this chapter, I offer my objective opinion about how LSpAF should be treated and describe my personal technique for its surgical treatment. I would hope that both my fellow EPs and my fellow arrhythmia surgeons would agree with my approach, but more than likely, both will disagree with significant aspects of it. However, as the great philosopher, Paul Tillich, said "Decision is a risk rooted in the courage of being free." The fact that I enjoy the privilege of being both an interventional EP and a cardiac arrhythmia surgeon frees me from any personal, professional, or financial ramifications that might otherwise influence the choice of the best procedure for a given patient.

MAKING THE DECISION: CATHETER ABLATION OR SURGERY?

Regardless of whether we are dealing with coronary artery disease, aortic valve stenosis, or AF, the decision to treat a problem by catheter intervention or surgery must consider the risk-to-benefit ratio of the two approaches. However, the risk-to-benefit ratio of an interventional procedure depends on more than the safety and efficacy of the two approaches, and generally, safety far outweighs efficacy in the decision-making process (see Chapter 10). In addition, different patients have different goals and may prefer one approach even if the risk-to-benefit ratio favors the alternative approach. Some patients prioritize the relative levels of invasiveness above all else, but others seek only better outcomes regardless of the level of invasiveness.

In the case of LSpAF, the most reliable and well-documented information available are the outcomes of catheter ablation and surgical ablation. There are two seminal studies on the results of catheter ablation specifically for the treatment of patients with LSpAF, the 2012 Hamburg Study[1] and the 2023 Winkle and coworkers study.[2] The Hamburg Study showed that the 5-year success rate after a single catheter ablation for LSpAF is 20%, and after multiple catheter ablations for LSpAF, it is 45%. Winkle et al.'s recent 16-year study showed precisely the same 5-year success rate of 45% after multiple catheter ablations for LSpAF. This means that nearly half of all patients with LSpAF can be relieved of their arrhythmia for 5 years by catheter ablation, a sound reason for performing catheter ablation first before subjecting the patient to a more invasive surgical procedure. If multiple catheter ablations fail, the patients can then be referred for surgery either using an off-pump hybrid procedure, an on-pump minimally invasive CryoMaze-III procedure, or an open Maze-III/IV procedure.

The long-term results for patients with LSpAF with the minimally invasive CryoMaze-III procedure and Maze-III/IV procedures, all of which require cardiopulmonary bypass, are 85% to 90%, or roughly twice the success rate achieved with multiple catheter ablations.[3–6] The 3-year success rates for off-pump hybrid procedures for LSpAF vary from roughly 60% to 80%,[7–12] thus falling between the catheter results and the surgical results (Fig. 39.1). These results of off-pump hybrid procedures and on-pump CryoMaze-III and Maze-III/IV procedures argue in favor of treating LSpAF with surgery as the *initial* option and after being appropriately informed, patients should be allowed to participate in the decision. The critical phrase here is "appropriately informed." It is difficult to convey a true comparison of catheter ablation and surgical ablation of AF to a patient because, of course, all patients would naturally prefer to avoid surgery if possible. The inherent difficulty of providing true "informed consent" can perhaps be better appreciated by the following analogy.

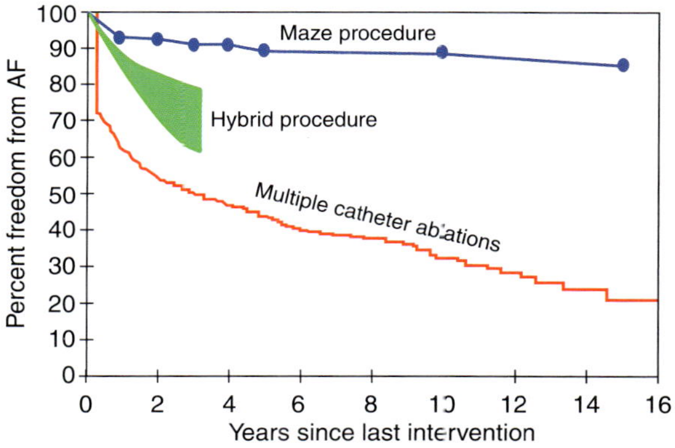

Fig. 39.1 Results of Maze procedures, hybrid procedures, and multiple catheter ablations for the treatment of patients with long-standing persistent atrial fibrillation (AF). See text for further discussion.

"INFORMED CONSENT" – THE ORANGE PILL ANALOGY

Many years ago, Dr. Cox and I were discussing how one might negate the stigma of surgery when explaining to patients their two treatment choices, and he suggested that we might consider using his "orange pill analogy" as a means of presenting an objective comparison of catheter ablation to surgical ablation.

Cardiac surgeons depend almost solely on cardiologists for patient referrals. This means that surgeons depend on the cardiology "gatekeepers" to present the truth, the whole truth, and nothing but the truth to patients when they describe the treatment options that are available. Unfortunately, this does not always happen because catheter ablation for AF is usually presented by cardiologists as being simple (false), safe (true), and effective (misleading), while surgery for AF is presented as being far more dangerous than catheter ablation (false), more painful and debilitating than catheter ablation (true), and no more effective than catheter ablation (false). So, in order to eliminate the stigma of surgery from the discussion, one can "catheter ablation" with a white pill and "surgical ablation" with an orange pill. Table 39.1 shows the relevant numbers for LSpAF.

So here is what I would like our cardiology colleagues to tell their patients when they are counseling them on their various therapeutic options for the treatment of LSpAF: "You have two options here. You can take either a white pill or an orange pill."

Option 1: If you take the white pill, you will feel mild discomfort in your groin for few hours and soreness for a few days, but you can probably go home the day after you take the pill. However, there is only a small chance that the white pill will have any immediate effect on your AF, and there is a slight chance that you will have a stroke as soon as you swallow it. In addition, there is also a chance that this white pill will permanently narrow the blood vessels draining blood from the lungs into your heart, causing you to have breathing difficulties unless you have an open-heart operation to fix the problem. Incidentally, the white pill contains enough radiation to cause 1 in every 1000 patients to develop cancer. Because we administered 2000 white pills last year, we caused 2 people to have cancer. Finally, because this white pill works in only about 20% of patients, you will likely have to take a second white pill within the next year, and all of the potential side effects that I just described will occur at exactly the same rate with the second pill. If two white pills don't work, we can give you a third one, but again, the pill will cause the same initial discomfort during your 2 days in the hospital as well as the same incidence of stroke, lung vessel problems, and risk of cancer that the first two pills did. After all this, you will have a 45% chance of being free of your AF after 5 years.

TABLE 39.1 Comparison of White Pill Versus Orange Pill

	White Pill	Orange Pill
Anesthesia time (hours)	4–8	5–6
Time in hospital (days)	1–2	2–3
Level of discomfort (scale of 1–10)	1	5
Stroke risk during procedure (%)	<1	<1
Risk of pulmonary vein stenosis (%)	<1	0
Cancer from radioactive pill	1 per 1000	N/A
1 pill: AF free after 5 years (%)	20	90
2–3 pills: AF free after 5 years (%)	45	N/A

AF, Atrial fibrillation; *N/A*, not applicable.

Option 2: If you decide to take the orange pill, you will go to sleep immediately upon swallowing it. When you awaken, you will be sore in your chest, and it will hurt to breathe deeply and cough, but the discomfort will be treated with pain medications and will improve rapidly over the following day or two. However, this orange pill has a 90% to 95% chance of stopping your AF immediately so that we only offer the orange pill to patients once. Even 15 years after you take the orange pill, there is an 85% chance that you will still not have AF. In addition, the risk of stroke or death is the same with the orange pill as with the white pill, but the orange pill will not cause any problems with drainage of blood from your lungs, either now or ever. Oh, and the orange pill is not radioactive.

After hearing this description of the consequences of taking the two different pills, many patients would initially choose to take the orange pill. However, when they later learn that the orange pill is actually surgery, most would likely opt for the white pill. The point of this orange pill analogy isn't just to make things simpler; — it's to call out the bias that often shapes how treatment options are presented to patients by their physicians. By translating catheter and surgical ablation into terms with similar levels of stigma (white pills and orange pills), we remove the procedural language that often overwhelms patients and present the decision in terms they can truly understand. The white pill, representing catheter ablation, naturally seems more appealing due to its minimally invasive nature and faster recovery, but it provides significantly lower rates of sustained sinus rhythm and long-term freedom from AF. This difference becomes even more important with age, as the progression of atrial remodeling can lead to structural changes that make AF more resistant to catheter-based treatment. In this context, the surgical option offers not only a more durable solution but also a more complete elimination of the arrhythmogenic substrate.

Truly "informed" consents are tricky and cannot always be perfectly accurate. However, as a person who routinely performs both catheter ablation and surgical ablation for AF, here is my recommendation on how new patients with LSpAF should be treated. Although the "cure rate" of LSpAF after multiple catheter ablations is only 45%, another way of looking at that figure is that nearly half of this most complex and dangerous form of AF can be cured without surgery. Therefore, I believe that at least two attempts at catheter ablation should be tried before sending the patient for surgery. If both procedures fail, there are several options available:

1. Leave the patient in AF and continue to treat medically, focusing on rate control. This leaves the patient without the benefit of the atrial contribution to cardiac output, and it leaves the patient vulnerable to stroke. The latter should be treated by permanent oral anticoagulation or left atrial appendage occlusion (LAAO).

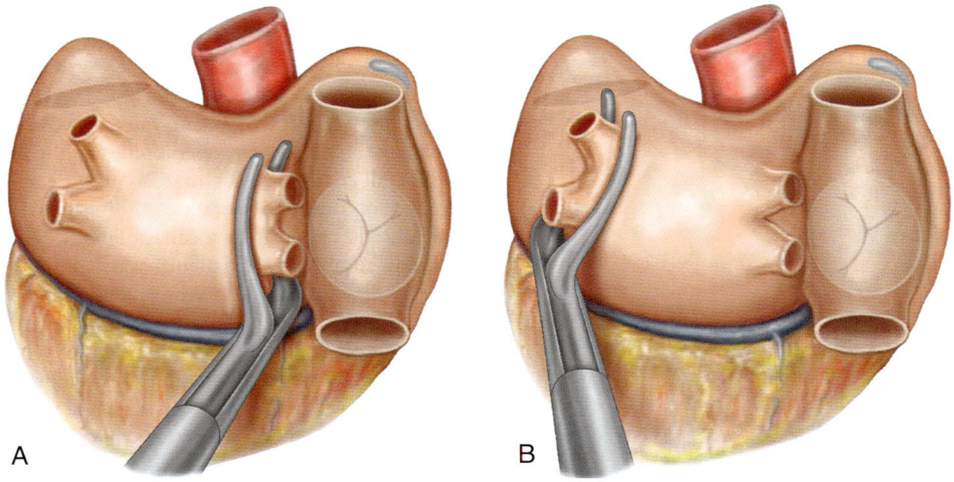

Fig. 39.2 Maze-V procedure: isolation of the pulmonary veins (PVs.) (A) Isolation of the right PVs using a bipolar radiofrequency clamp. (B) Isolation of the left PVs using a bipolar radiofrequency clamp.

2. "Pace and ablate," that is, ablate the His bundle and implant a permanent pacemaker. This also leaves the patient without the benefit of the atrial contribution to cardiac output and it also leaves the patient vulnerable to stroke.
3. Perform a hybrid procedure in which the EP and the surgeon perform a combined off-pump, thoracoscopic surgical procedure and endocardial catheter ablation procedure in an effort to control the arrhythmia. The results of this approach for LSpAF vary between 60% and 80% at 3 years.
4. Perform a minimally invasive on-pump CryoMaze-III or open Maze-III/IV procedure. Both of these procedures yield success rates of around 90% at 5 years. Sinus rhythm with return of atrial function occurs in the vast majority of patients, and the incidence of long-term stroke is virtually eliminated because of the combination of a normal rhythm and LAAO.
5. Perform a median sternotomy for a CryoMaze-III or Maze-III/IV procedure. This is recommended only for patients who are not candidates for the minimally invasive approach (number 4).

In my opinion, the biggest mistake that is made in terms of patient care after two or more failed catheter ablations is to choose options 1 or 2. The fact that patients have subjected themselves to multiple catheter ablations to be relieved of their AF is sufficient evidence that they seriously desire to be free of it. Therefore, there is little justification for simply surrendering to the disease without offering surgery to a patient like this. Unfortunately, some patients who have failed multiple catheter ablations are never even told that surgical therapy for AF is available, much less that it is safe and highly successful. It is also common practice for some physicians to routinely recommend "pace and ablate" to patients who have failed multiple catheter ablations. Unfortunately, this approach leaves the patient with no synchronous atrial function and at risk of stroke unless the pace and ablate approach is accompanied by LAAO. Furthermore, pace and ablate does not always relieve the symptoms of AF and because these patients are so symptomatic, they require surgery for relief of their symptoms. I believe that the best option for patients who have failed multiple catheter ablations for LSpAF is a Maze procedure or a simple LAAO.

THE MAZE-V PROCEDURE

In these patients, I perform what I call the "Maze-V" procedure that I believe creates a more reliable left atrial "box lesion" around the four pulmonary veins (PVs) and the left atrial posterior wall than the CryoMaze-III or the Maze-IV procedure. After isolating the right and left PVs with bipolar radiofrequency (RF) clamps as in the Maze-IV procedure (Fig. 39.2), I place a pursestring suture near the right superior PV and within the cuff of tissue isolated by the right pulmonary vein isolation. The purse-string suture is controlled with a Rumel tourniquet. One arm of the bipolar RF clamp is then passed through this purse-string suture to the inside of the atrium and the other arm is outside the atrium (Fig. 39.3). The clamp is positioned across the top of the LA just posterior to Bachmann's bundle to a location near the left superior PV inside the isolated cuff of the left pulmonary vein isolation lesion. This provides the ability to create the roof lesion using bipolar RF ablation rather than the far less reliable unipolar RF devices that are used in the Maze-IV procedure.

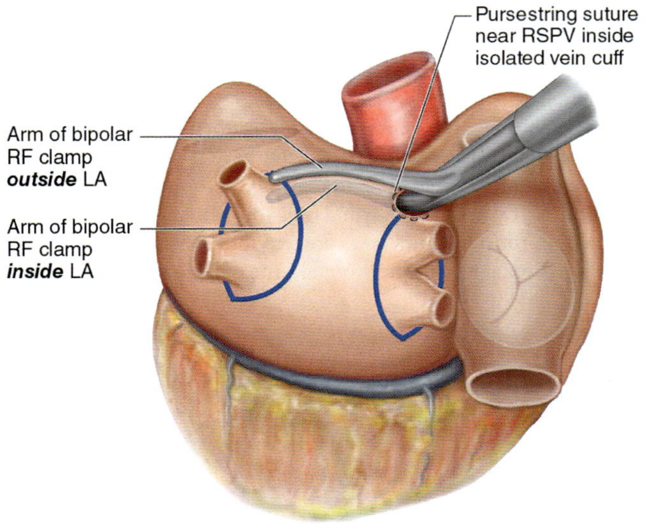

Fig. 39.3 Maze-V procedure: roof lesion. A purse-string suture is placed near the right superior pulmonary vein (RSPV) inside the isolated cuff created by the right pulmonary vein isolation. One arm of a bipolar radiofrequency (RF) clamp is inserted through the purse-string suture and passed across the top of the left atrium (LA) posterior to Bachmann's bundle to a site near the left superior pulmonary vein inside the lesion created to isolate the left pulmonary veins. The roof lesion is then created using the bipolar RF clamp.

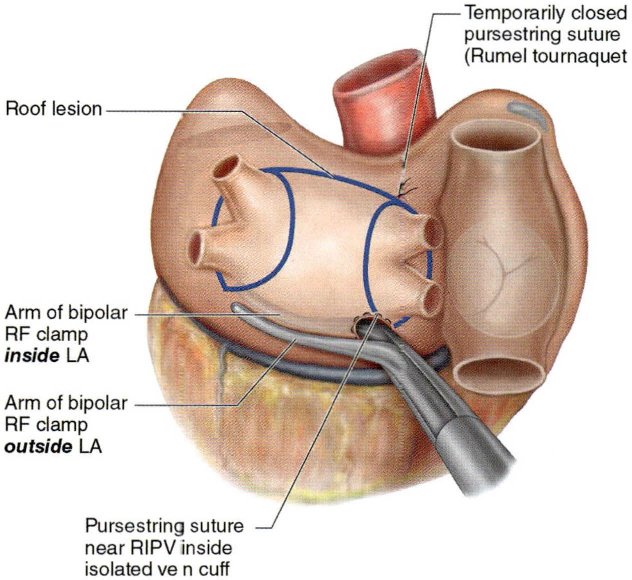

Fig. 39.4 Maze-V procedure: floor lesion. A purse-string suture is placed near the right inferior pulmonary vein (RIPV) inside the lesion created to isolate the right pulmonary veins. One arm of a bipolar radiofrequency (RF) clamp is inserted through the purse-string suture and passed across the posteroinferior left atrium (LA) to a site near the left inferior pulmonary vein inside the lesion created to isolate the left pulmonary veins. This completes the "box lesion" of the Maze-V procedure.

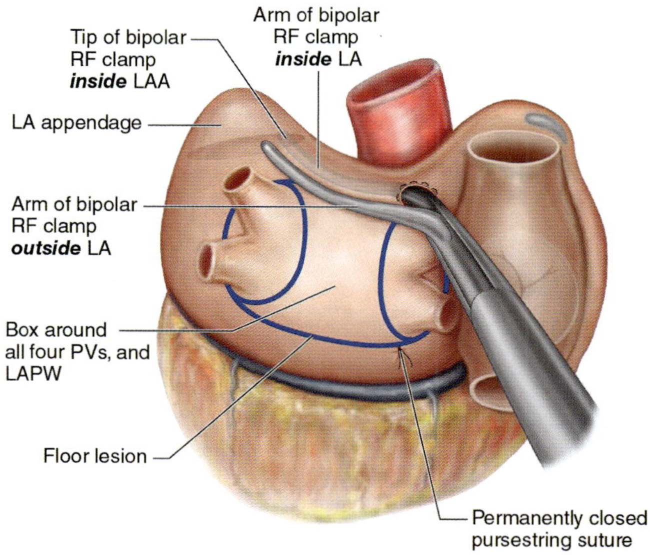

Fig. 39.5 Maze-V procedure: left atrial appendage (LAA) lesion across the coumadin ridge. The upper purse-string is used a second time to position the bipolar radiofrequency (RF) clamp across the top of the left atrium (LA) into the orifice of the LAA. *LAPW,* Left atrial posterior wall.

A second purse-string is then placed near the right inferior PV inside the isolated the lesion created to isolate the right pulmonary veins. Again, one arm of the bipolar clamp is placed inside the LA through the purse-string suture while the other arm is positioned outside the LA. The clamp is placed across the bottom of the LA to a location near the left inferior PV inside the isolated cuff of the left pulmonary veins (Fig. 39.4). This allows the floor lesion of the box to be created using bipolar RF rather than unipolar RF.

Finally, one arm of the bipolar RF clamp is then inserted again through the upper purse-string suture and positioned over to the inside of the left atrial appendage (LAA) being careful to stay posterior to Bachmann's bundle (Fig. 39.5). This creates a bipolar RF lesion across the coumadin ridge between the left superior PV and the LAA. The LAA is then closed by double suture ligatures and its base is ablated between the two ligatures to achieve complete electrical isolation of the remaining LAA stump (Fig. 39.6, *left panel and middle panel*). In 50% of our cases, the left atrial appendage was amputated using a stapling device (Fig. 39.6, right panel).

The LA lesions of the Maze-V procedure most closely resemble those of the Maze-IV procedure, but in my opinion, they are easier and more reliable to perform because of the use of bipolar RF clamps to create the roof and floor lines of the left atrial box lesion (Fig. 39.7). The major difference in the Maze-V procedure is that no mitral line, coronary sinus cryolesion, or anterior trigone lesion is performed to prevent postoperative peri-mitral flutter. I am aware that the deletion of these two lesions will result in a 10% to 15% failure rate due to postoperative peri-mitral atrial flutter (see Chapter 48). In addition, the right atrial lesions in the Maze-V procedure (Figs. 39.8 to 39.10) are slightly different from both the Maze-III and Maze-IV procedures. However, I agree with the patterns and principles recommended for the RA lesions elsewhere in this book, best defined in Chapter 13.

In addition to the possibility of postoperative peri-mitral flutter, one other concern with the Maze-V procedure is the fact that the right atrial lesions include a combination of the "T" lesion to the tricuspid

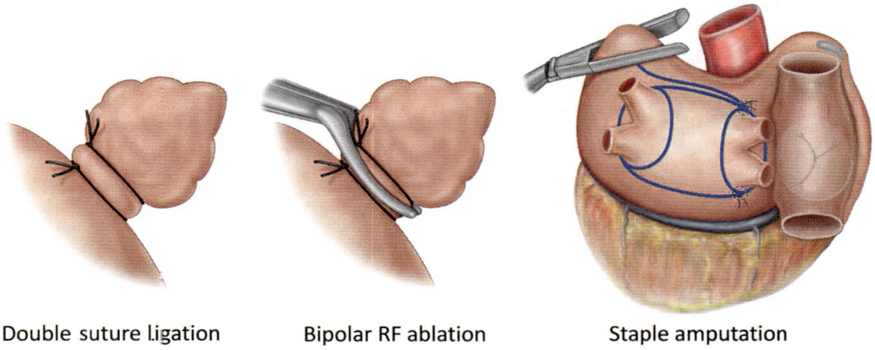

Fig. 39.6 Maze-V procedure: amputation of the left atrial appendage (LAA). The LAA is occluded epicardially by double suture ligatures *(left panel),* and then the tissue between the two ligatures is ablated with a bipolar radiofrequency clamp *(middle panel).* Another options is amputation of the LAA using a stapling device *(right panel). RF,* Radiofrequency.

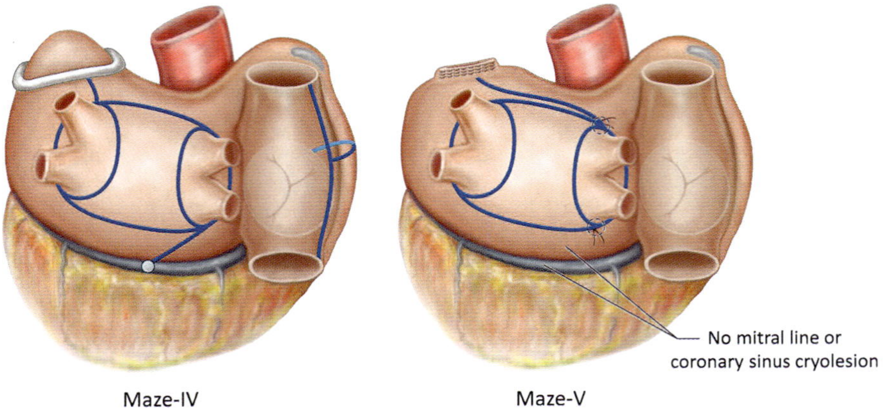

Fig. 39.7 Comparison of the left atrial lesions of the Maze-IV and Maze-V procedures. There are four differences in the Maze-IV and Maze-V procedures. The first is that the roof and floor lesions are created with unipolar radiofrequency (RF) devices in the Maze-IV procedure and with a bipolar RF clamp in the Maze V procedure. The second is that there are no lesions such as the mitral line, coronary sinus cryolesion, or anterior trigone lines created in the Maze-V procedure to prevent the development of postoperative peri-mitral flutter. The third is that the RA lesions of the Maze-V procedure can isolate the lower third of the right atrium where the sinus bradycardia site of the atrial pacemaker complex resides. The fourth is that the tip of the right atrial appendage is excised in the Maze-V procedure but not in the Maze-IV procedure.

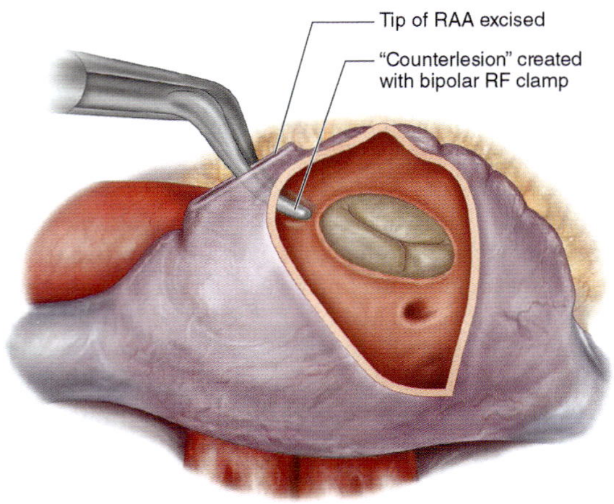

Fig. 39.8 Maze-V procedure: right atriotomy and "counterlesion." After a right atriotomy is created in the location illustrated, the tip of the right atrial appendage (RAA) is excised. A lesion is created from the open RAA to the anterior tricuspid annulus using a bipolar radiofrequency (RF) clamp. A cryolesion is then placed at the terminal end of this lesion at the level of the tricuspid valve annulus. This lesion corresponds to the original "counterlesion" of the Maze-II and Maze-III procedures described in Chapter 12.

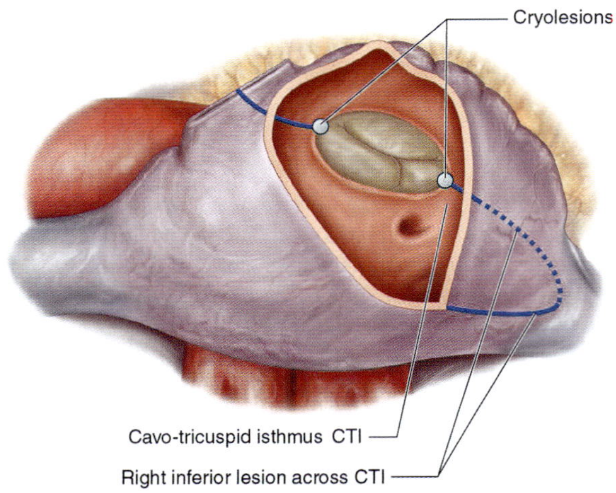

Fig. 39.9 Maze-V procedure: right inferior atrial lesion across the cavotricuspid isthmus (CTI). A lesion is created with a combination of bipolar RF and cryosurgery from the lower end of the atriotomy to the inferior vena cava orifice and then across the CTI to the posterior tricuspid annulus. A cryolesion is then placed at the terminal end of this lesion at the level of the tricuspid valve annulus. See text for further discussion.

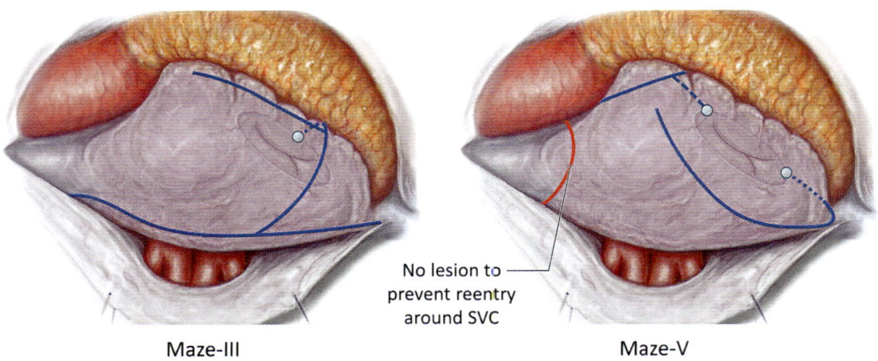

Fig. 39.10 Comparison of the right atrial lesions of the Maze-III and Maze-V procedures. The lesions of the Maze-V procedure prevent the development of all of the right atrial macro-reentrant drivers of atrial fibrillation except the one around the orifice of the superior vena cava (SVC). Fortunately, this is a rare site of right atrial macro-reentry.

valve annulus, an inferior vena cava lesion, and a *cavotricuspid isthmus lesion* in the right atrium (RA). As described in Chapter 13, this combination of lesions results in the electrical isolation of the lower portion of the RA where the sinus bradycardia area of the atrial pacemaker complex resides (see Chapter 13, Fig. 13.18). Whether or not patients become incapable of developing an appropriate sinus bradycardia after a Maze-V procedure (e.g., when they are asleep) is unknown but is probably worth investigating.

Eighty-two coronary artery bypass graft patients with AF have undergone a Maze-V procedure at our institution.[13] The in-hospital mortality rate was 2.4% (two patient fatalities), and in both instances, the cause of death was multiple-organ failure in older adult patients with significant comorbidities, including generalized atherosclerosis, diabetes mellitus, and chronic kidney disease. During hospitalization, there were no major cardiovascular or cerebrovascular events and no new permanent pacemaker requirements. At the time of hospital discharge, 92.4% of patients were in sinus rhythm, which was maintained in 91% of patients at 12 months, 88% at 24 months, 83% at 36 months, and 77% of patients at 48 months after surgery. Only 4.9% of patients underwent redo catheter ablation for postoperative peri-mitral flutter. Thus, these Maze-V procedure results are comparable to those attained by the Maze-III and Maze-IV procedures.

REFERENCES

1. Tilz RR, Rillig A, Thum AM, et al. Catheter ablation of long-standing persistent atrial fibrillation: 5-year outcomes of the Hamburg Sequential Ablation Strategy. *J Am Coll Card.* 2012;60(19):1921-1929.
2. Winkle RA, Mead RH, Engel G, et al. Very long term outcomes of atrial fibrillation ablation. *Heart Rhythm.* 2023;20:680–688.
3. Prasad SM, Maniar HS, Camillo CJ, et al. The Cox maze III procedure for atrial fibrillation: long-term efficacy in patients undergoing lone versus concomitant procedures. *J Thorac Cardiovasc Surg.* 2003;126(6):1822–1827.
4. Ad N, Holmes SD, Friehling T. Minimally invasive stand-alone Cox Maze procedure for persistent and long-standing persistent atrial fibrillation: perioperative safety and 5-year outcomes. *Circ Arrhyth Electrophysiol.* 2017;10(11):e005352.
5. Ruaengsri C, Schill MR, Khiabani AJ, Schuessler RB, Melby SJ, Damiano RJ Jr. The Cox-Maze IV procedure in its second decade: still the gold standard? *Eur J Cardiothorac Surg.* 2018;53(1): i19–i25.
6. Khiabani AJ, MacGregor RM, Bakir NJ, et al. The long-term outcomes and durability of the Cox-Maze IV procedure for atrial fibrillation. *J Thorac Cardiovasc Surg.* 2022;163(2):629–641.
7. Van der Heijden CAJ, Vroomen M, Luemans JG, et al. Hybrid versus catheter ablation in patients with persistent and longstanding persistent atrial fibrillation: a systematic review and meta-analysis. *Eur J Cardio-Thorac Surg.* 2019;56:433–443.
8. Van der Heijden CAJ, Weberndorfer V, Vroomen M, et al. Hybrid ablation versus repeated catheter ablation in persistent atrial fibrillation: A Randomized Controlled Trial. *JACC Clin Electrophysiol.* 2023;Jul;9(7Pt2):1013–1023.
9. Umbrain V, Verborgh C, Chierchia G-B, de Asmundis C, Brugada P, La Meir M. One-stage approach for hybrid atrial fibrillation treatment. *Arrhythm Electrophysiol Rev.* 2017;6(4):210–216.
10. Maesen B, Luermans JGLM, Bidar E, et al. A hybrid approach to complex arrhythmias. *Europace.* 2021;23:ii28–ii33.
11. Dunnington GH, Pierce CL, Eisenberg S, et al. A heart-team hybrid approach for atrial fibrillation: a single-centre long-term clinical outcome cohort study. *Eur J Cardiothorac Surg.* 2021. https://doi.org/10.1093/ejcts/ezab197.
12. Delurgio DB, Crossen KJ, Gill J, et al. Hybrid convergent procedure for the treatment of persistent and long-standing persistent atrial fibrillation: results of the converge clinical trial. *Circ Arrhythm Electrophysiol.* 2020;13(12):e009288.
13. Revishvili A.Sh., Popov VA, Malyshenko ES, Anishchenko MM. Surgical treatment of atrial fibrillation concomitant to coronary artery bypass grafting: in-hospital and long-term results of Maze V procedure. *Min Invas Cardiovasc Surg.* 2022;1:40–52 (In Russ.).

40

Overview of the Surgical Management of the Left Atrial Appendage

James L. Cox, S. Chris Malaisrie, Olga N. Kislitsina

CHAPTER OUTLINE

BACKGROUND

Surgical closure of the left atrial appendage (LAA) was first reported by John Madden in 1949 (Fig. 40.1)[1] In that publication, Madden stated, "*Since a thrombus is the precursor of every arterial embolus, the ideal prophylaxis for recurrent arterial emboli should be the removal of the thrombus together with its site of origin.*" Despite Madden's recommendation, little interest was shown in the LAA or its relation to strokes for the next five decades (Fig. 40.2).[2] In 1996, Blackshear and Odell[3] reported that the left atrium (LA) was involved in up to 57% of strokes in patients with AF with rheumatic heart disease and in up to 91% of patients with AF without rheumatic heart disease.

In 1999, we reported the first large clinical series of LAA occlusions (LAAOs) by either surgical amputation or endocardial surgical closure as a part of the Maze-I, -II, and -III procedures.[4] The LAA occlusions

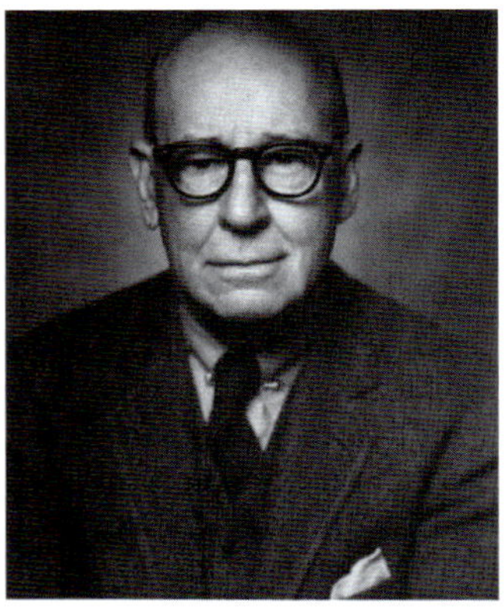

Fig. 40.1 John L. Madden, who in 1949 published the first report on surgical closure of the left atrial appendage to prevent systemic thromboembolism.

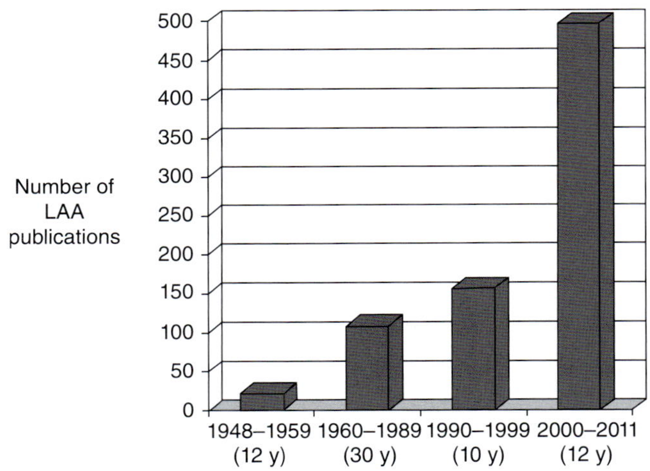

Fig. 40.2 The number of scientific publications on the left atrial appendage (LAA) from Madden's 1949 article through 2011. Note that the *bars* do not represent the same timeframes. (Modified from Chatterjee S, Alexander JC, Pearson PJ, Feldman T. Left atrial appendage occlusion: lessons learned from surgical and transcatheter experiences. *Ann Thorac Surg*. 2011;92(6):2283–2292.)

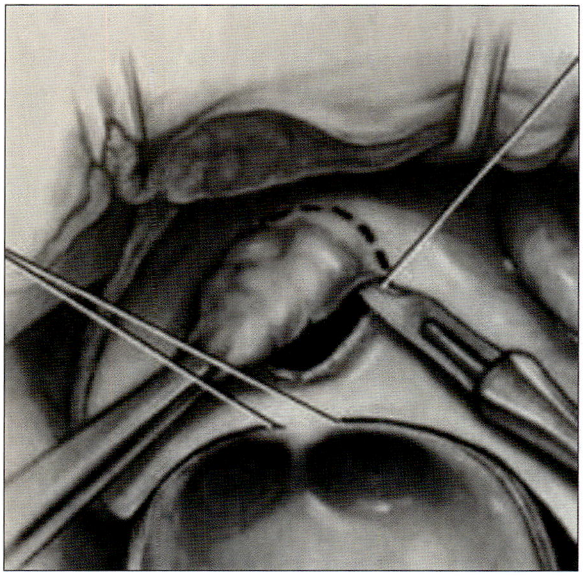

Fig. 40.3 In the original cut-and-sew Maze-I I procedure, forceps were inserted into the orifice of the left atrial appendage (LAA) to grasp its endocardial tip and invert it into the left atrium for better visualization and determination of the exact location of its base. The LAA was then excised at its base, and the defect was closed in two layers with sutures.

were accomplished in the Maze-I, Maze-II, and the cut-and-sew version of the Maze-III procedure by surgical amputation (Fig. 40.3) and by cryosurgical isolation and endocardial suture closure in the minimally invasive cryosurgical version of the Maze-III (CryoMaze-III) procedure (Fig. 40.4). Surprisingly, we found that *perioperative* strokes

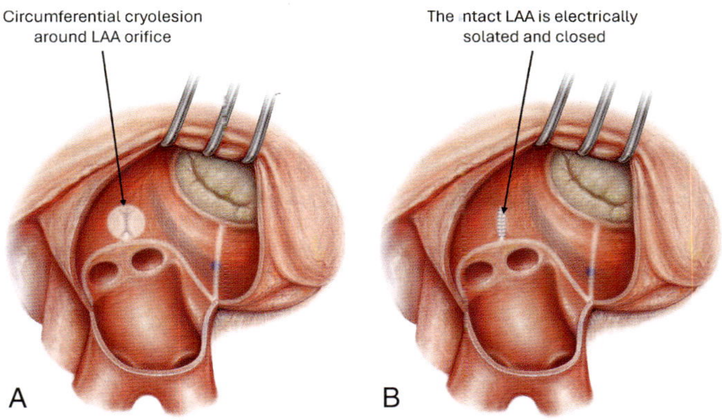

Fig. 40.4 In the minimally invasive CryoMaze-III procedure that replaced the cut-and-sew Maze procedure in 1997, the left atrial appendage (LAA) was first inverted to check for thrombi and then returned to its normal position. A cryolesion was placed around the circumference of the LAA orifice with a 2-cm-diameter nondisposable cryoprobe to electrically isolate the entire LAA from the remainder of the heart *(left panel)*. The LAA was left intact, and its orifice was closed in two layers of sutures *(right panel)*. Thus, after both procedures, not only was the LAA excluded from the systemic circulation, but the myocardium of the LAA was also electrically isolated from the myocardium of the left atrium (LA). In some of the early minimally invasive CryoMaze-III procedures, the cryolesion around the LAA orifice was replaced by a single linear lesion out into the LAA. In retrospect, this was a mistake because even though the LAA was excluded from the systemic circulation by suture closure, the suture line alone did not electrically isolate the LAA from the LA. Fortunately, this alteration did not change the efficacy of the CryoMaze-III procedure.

Surgical procedure	Permanent stroke (%)	Transient stroke (%)	Total strokes (%)
CABG + MVR	4.17	1.73	5.90
CABG + AVR	3.40	1.60	5.00
CABG + MV repair	3.12	1.41	4.53
AVR + MVR	2.73	1.51	4.24
MV repair	1.85	1.45	3.30
MVR	2.28	0.98	3.26
AVR	1.73	1.23	2.96
CABG	1.69	0.75	2.44
Maze ± other	0.65	0	0.65

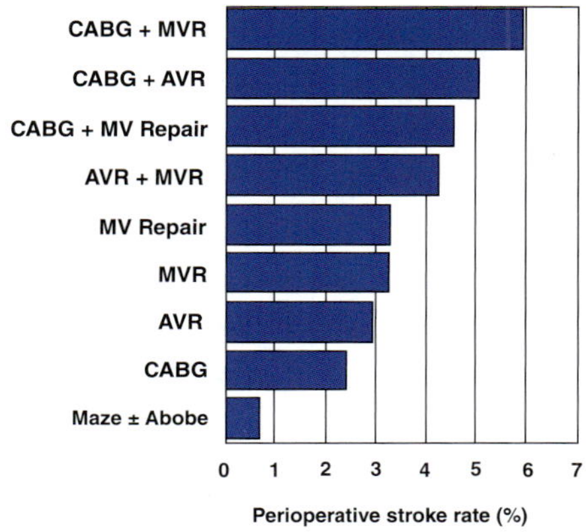

Fig. 40.5 *Upper panel,* Perioperative stroke rates after the most common cardiac surgical procedures according to the 1998 Society of Thoracic Surgeons National Cardiac Surgery Database plus the stroke rate when the Maze procedure was performed with or without these procedures. *Lower panel,* Same information in bar graph form. See text for further discussion. *AVR,* aortic valve replacement; *CABG,* coronary artery bypass grafting; *MV,* mitral valve; *MVR,* mitral valve replacement.

associated with both routine and complex cardiac surgical procedures were virtually eliminated when the Maze procedure was performed concomitantly with those procedures (Fig. 40.5). It was well documented that postoperative atrial fibrillation (POAF) was associated with an increase in perioperative strokes,[5,6] so one might attribute this dramatic reduction in perioperative stroke rate to the Maze procedure having prevented POAF. However, the Maze procedure does *not* prevent POAF as evidenced by 37% of the 265 patients who had either type of Maze-III procedure experienced POAF within the first 2 weeks after surgery, peaking at 4 days. Thus the Maze procedure alone could not have been responsible for the lack of perioperative strokes. The only plausible explanation for the dramatic decrease in perioperative stroke was amputation or closure of the LAA during the procedure.

The $CHADS_2$ and the CHA_2DS_2-VASc scoring systems for stroke risk in patients with atrial fibrillation (AF) had not been devised at the time of our 1999 report. However, the risk of stroke associated with AF was well established at that time based on a number of clinical trials, a history of previous stroke or transient ischemic attack (TIA) and anticoagulation status.[7–10] Therefore, the number of long-term strokes expected over the 12-year follow-up period if these patients had not undergone a Maze procedure could be calculated. By categorizing the patients into groups with different stroke risks, it was predicted that 68 strokes would have occurred over the ensuing 12 years in these 265 patients if they not undergone a Maze procedure (Fig. 40.6). In reality, only one stroke occurred during that time even though 65% of the patients were not anticoagulated. In 2003, Prasad et al.[11] reported a longer follow-up of the same cohort of patients showing that after 15 years, 99.3% of the

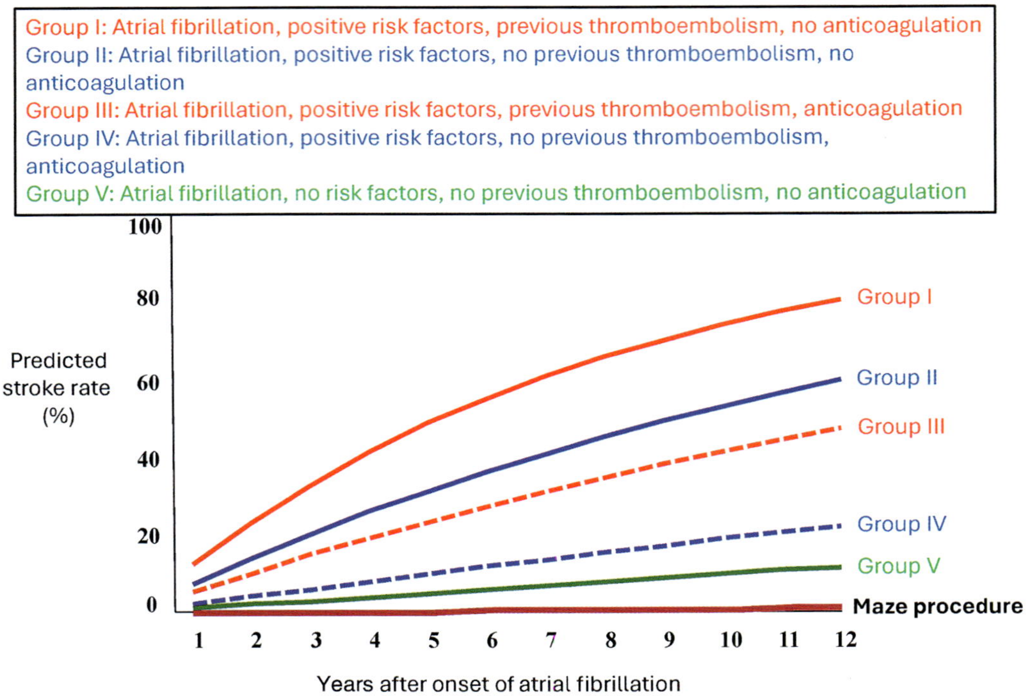

Fig. 40.6 The predicted stroke curves for the patients in our original Maze series divided into five groups based on their known risk factors and thus the predicted incidence of stroke over the ensuing 12 years had they *not* undergone a Maze procedure. The high-risk patients were subdivided on the basis of those who were not anticoagulated (group I) and those who were anticoagulated (group III). The lower-risk patients were also subdivided into those who were not anticoagulated (group II) and those who were anticoagulated (group IV). Group V represented patients with "lone atrial fibrillation" (AF) representing the lowest-risk group for having a stroke. The actual observed stroke rate for all of these patients after the Maze procedure is the lowest line on the graph. Overall, the contemporary knowledge of stroke risks at that time predicted that 68 strokes would have occurred over the ensuing 12 years had their AF not been ablated. The total number of strokes that actually occurred in all five combined groups after the Maze procedure was one stroke in 12 years. See text for further discussion. (Modified from Cox JL, Ad N, Palazzo T. Impact of the Maze procedure on the stroke rate in patients with atrial fibrillation. *J Thor Cardiovasc Surg*. 1999;118:833–840.)

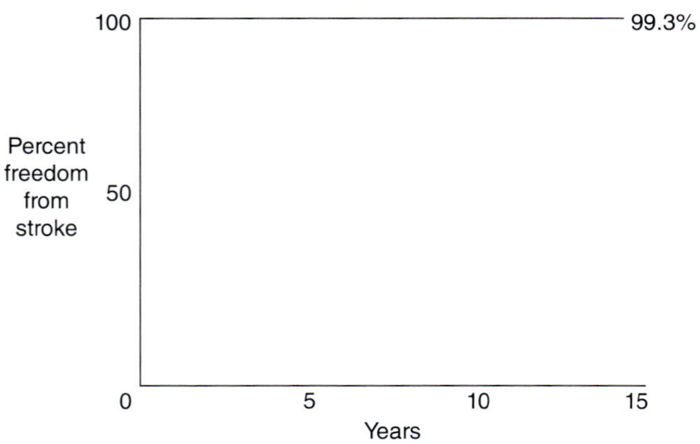

Fig. 40.7 The 15-year freedom from stroke after the Maze procedure was 99.3%.[11] See text for further discussion.

patients were free of stroke after a Maze procedure (Fig. 40.7). Again, many attributed this low incidence of long-term stroke to the success of the Maze procedure in preventing AF.[2] Although LAA closure was clearly responsible for the decrease in *perioperative* strokes, the decrease in *long-term* strokes could have been due to the low recurrence rate of AF, LAA occlusion, or a synergistic combination of both. See Chapter 43 for a detailed update on this subject.

EVOLUTION OF THE SURGICAL MANAGEMENT OF THE LEFT ATRIAL APPENDAGE

Interest in the LAA increased in the second decade of the 21st century as cardiologists and particularly surgeons came to appreciate the relationship between LAA thrombosis and strokes associated with AF as evidenced by the rapid growth in the number of annual LAA publications (Fig. 40.8).[12] It had already been established that approximately 20% of all strokes are associated with AF[13] and that most of the thrombi responsible for strokes in patients with AF originate in the LAA.[14] As a result, surgeons were encouraged to become more aggressive in amputating or closing the LAA in patients with AF undergoing cardiac surgery.[15]

In 2005, Healey et al.[16] published the first randomized controlled trial (now referred to as the LAAOS-I trial) to evaluate whether surgeons could reliably close the LAA surgically. There were two arms in the trial, one in which the LAA was closed with sutures placed epicardially using the surgeon's preferred technique and the other in which the LAA was closed using an epicardial stapling device. The LAAOS trial showed that surgeons could *not* close the LAA safely and reliably by either of these techniques. In the epicardial suture closure group, 57% of the patients had a residual connection between the LAA and the LA, and in the surgical stapling group, there was a residual pouch greater than 1 cm in depth at the base of the LAA in 28% of patients that proved to be thrombogenic. Interestingly, in patients who had

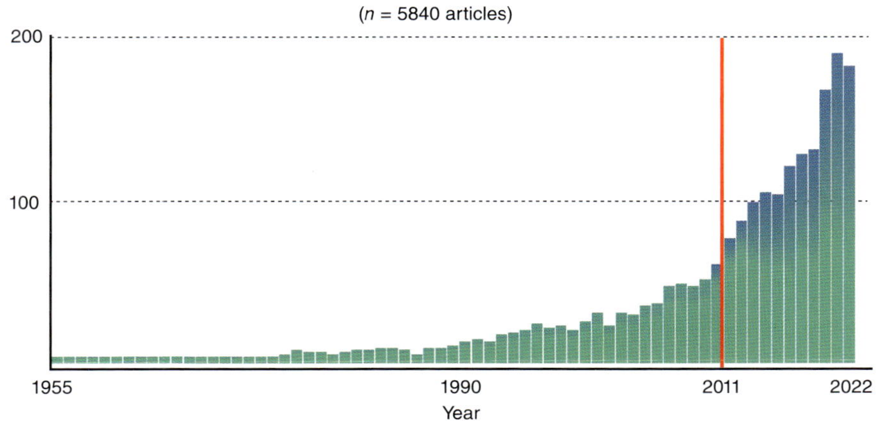

Fig. 40.8 Annual number of scientific publications on the left atrial appendage (LAA) from 1955 through 2022. Note the continued increased interest in the LAA after 2011 illustrated in Fig. 40.2.

successful LAA closures by either technique (i.e., complete closure without residual pouches >1 cm), the stroke rate was reduced, though those patients could not be subjected to statistical analysis because of the structure of the trial. The LAAOS-I trial demonstrated definitively that surgeons could not close the LAA reliably even when using their best direct surgical techniques.

The findings of the LAAOS-I trial were confirmed by Kanderian and coworkers'[17] 2008 Cleveland Clinic trial and Cullen and coworkers'[18] 2016 Mayo Clinic trial. In the latter, LAA surgical amputation was included in the study, and interestingly, there was roughly a 20% postoperative thrombus rate along the LAA suture line closure with approximately 12% of the thrombi being in actual contact with the systemic circulation. This study in particular showed that although amputation of the LAA is obviously simple and cheap, it may not be as safe as most surgeons believe it to be. Fortunately, these problems were overcome with the introduction of the surgical AtriClip (AtriCure, Inc.), which is discussed in detail in Chapters 44 and 45.

LEFT ATRIAL APPENDAGE CLOSURE IN CARDIAC SURGERY PATIENTS WITH ATRIAL FIBRILLATION

The question of whether or not patients undergoing cardiac surgery with a history of AF should have their LAAs closed was addressed in a 2017 report from the Society of Thoracic Surgeons Adult Cardiac Surgery Database by Friedman et al.[19] The study included 10,524 patients, 37% of whom had LAA occlusion at the time of surgery and 63% of whom did not. The study showed superior results for thromboembolism (TE), an end point that included TE, hemorrhagic stroke, or death, and for all-cause mortality in the patients with AF who had LAA closure at the time of surgery (Fig. 40.9). Likewise, a 2019 study

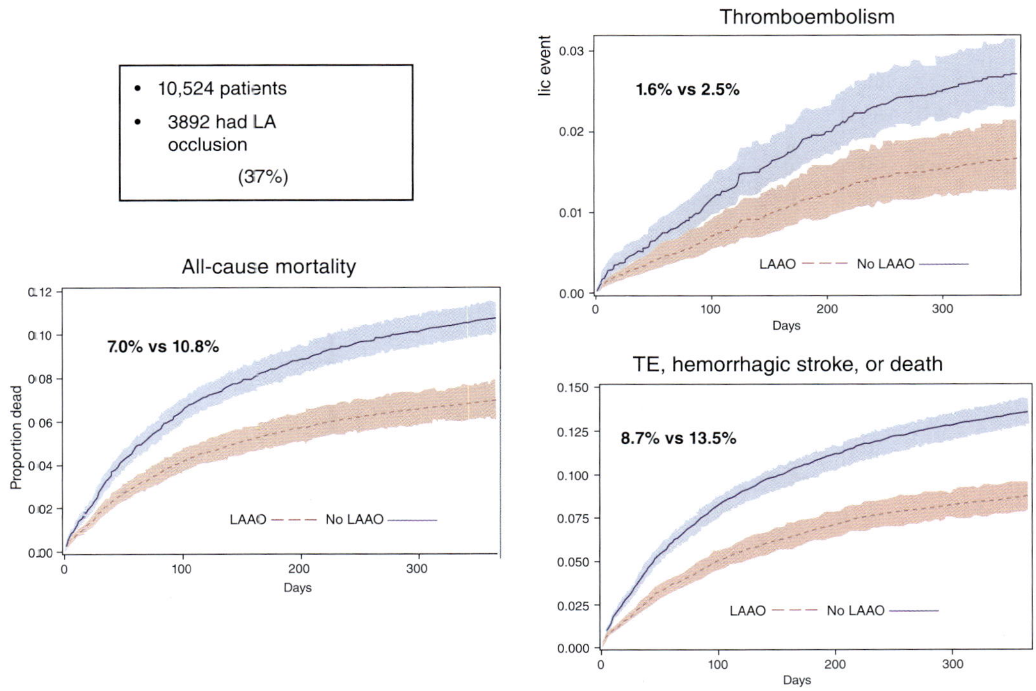

Fig. 40.9 Graphs from Friedman and coworkers'[19] study demonstrating the benefit of closing the left atrial appendage in patients with atrial fibrillation who were undergoing cardiac surgery. *LAAO,* Left atrial appendage occlusion; *TE,* thromboembolism. See text for further discussion. (Modified from Friedman DJ, Piccini JP, Wang T, et al. Association between left atrial appendage occlusion and readmission for thromboembolism among patients with atrial fibrillation undergoing concomitant cardiac surgery. *J Am Med Assoc.* 2018;319(4):365–374.)

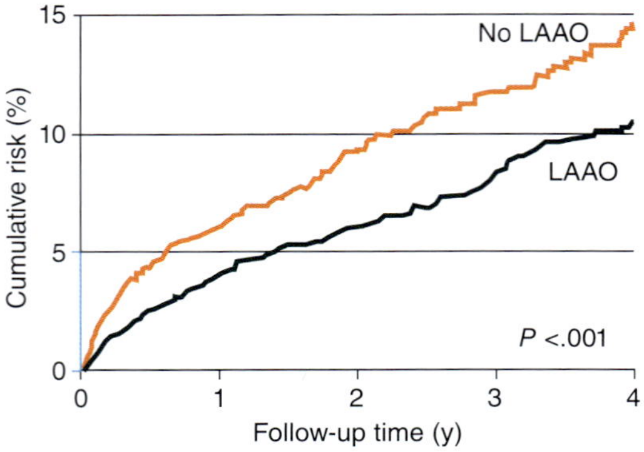

Fig. 40.10 Graphs from Yao and coworkers'[20] study demonstrating the benefit of closing the left atrial appendage in patients with atrial fibrillation who were undergoing cardiac surgery. See text for further discussion. *LAAO,* Left atrial appendage occlusion. (Modified from Yao X, Gersh BJ, Holmes DR, et al. Association of surgical left atrial appendage occlusion with subsequent stroke and mortality among patients undergoing cardiac surgery. *J Am Med Assoc.* 2018;319(20):2116–2126.)

by Yao et al.[20] of 75,782 patients also demonstrated an advantage in cumulative risk by closing the LAA in cardiac surgery patients with AF (Fig. 40.10). A meta-analysis of 280,585 patients by Gutierrez et al.[21] also showed results that favored closure of the LAA in cardiac surgery patients who had preoperative AF. Finally, the issue of whether to close the LAA in cardiac surgery patients with AF was settled by the multicenter, prospective, randomized LAAOS-III trial reported by Whitlock et al.[22] in 2021. The LAAOS-III trial documented that LAA occlusion in cardiac surgery patients with AF decreases subsequent strokes over a mean of 3.8 years (Fig. 40.11). This seminal trial is discussed in detail by Whitlock in Chapter 46.

LEFT ATRIAL APPENDAGE OCCLUSION CLOSURE IN CARDIAC SURGERY PATIENTS WITHOUT ATRIAL FIBRILLATION

The safety and efficacy of closing the LAA in patients with AF led many to believe that *all* patients undergoing cardiac surgery should have their LAAs either closed or amputated at the time of surgery whether or not they have a history of AF. However, Yao and coworkers'[20] study showed that there was no advantage in closing the LAA rather than leaving it intact in patients without a history of AF (Fig. 40.12). On the other hand, a meta-analysis by Ibrahim et al.[23] that included 13,352 patients from 10 studies showed that surgical closure of the LAA during

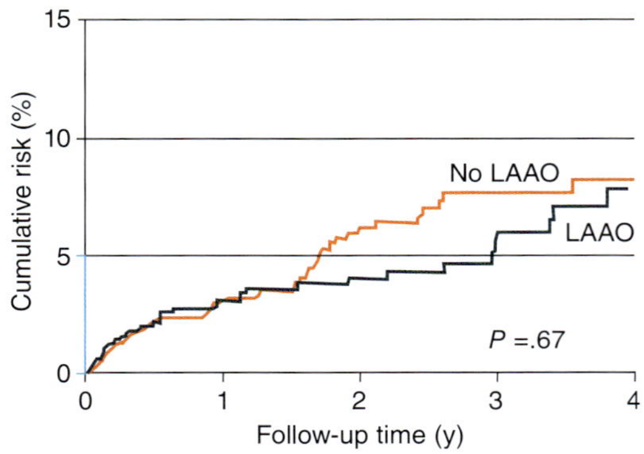

Fig. 40.12 Graphs from Yao and coworkers'[20] study demonstrating lack of benefit in closing the left atrial appendage in patients without atrial fibrillation who were undergoing cardiac surgery. See text for further discussion. *LAAO,* Left atrial appendage occlusion. (Modified from Yao X, Gersh BJ, Holmes DR, et al. Association of surgical left atrial appendage occlusion with subsequent stroke and mortality among patients undergoing cardiac surgery. *J Am Med Assoc.* 2018;319(20):2116–2126.)

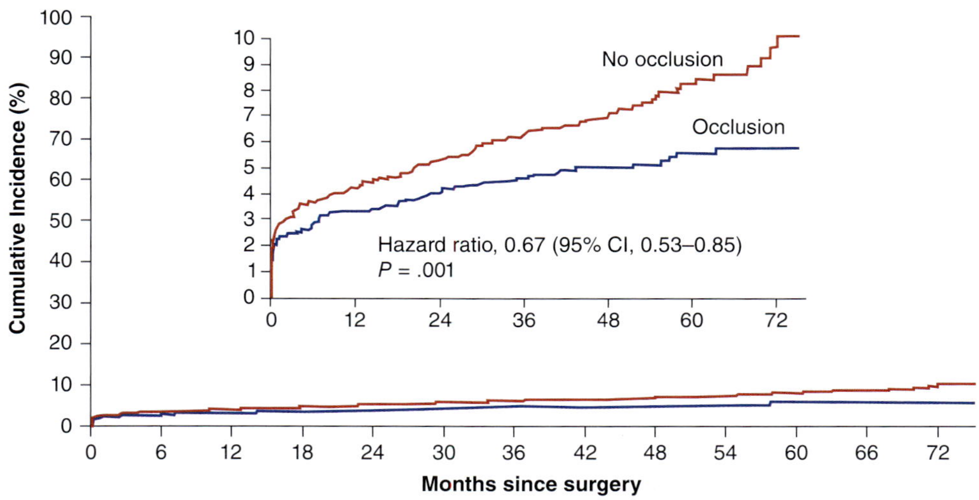

No. at risk													
No occlusion	2391	2134	2081	2030	1981	1897	1607	1291	1016	751	540	348	205
Occlusion	2379	2163	2105	2059	2020	1948	1642	1322	1046	781	550	349	199

Fig. 40.11 Graphs from the prospective, randomized LAAOS-III trial documenting the benefit of closing the left atrial appendage in patients with atrial fibrillation who were undergoing cardiac surgery. See text for further discussion. *CI,* Confidence interval. (Reproduced from Whitlock RP, Belley-Cote EP, Paparella D, et al. Left atrial appendage occlusion during cardiac surgery to prevent stroke. *N Engl J Med.* 2021;384(22):2081–2091.)

cardiac surgery decreased ischemic stroke, systemic embolism, and all-cause mortality compared with the patients who did not have their LAAs closed.

Clearly, the question of closing the LAA in all patients undergoing cardiac surgery whether or not they have a history of AF is controversial. In preparation for a definitive prospective randomized trial to address this issue, two trials were designed. First, Gerdisch et al.[24] demonstrated the safety and efficacy of the surgical AtriClip in the prospective, multicenter ATLAS feasibility trial.[24] This set the stage for the prospective randomized LeAAPS trial, which seeks to determine if all cardiac surgical patients should have their LAAs closed regardless of whether or not they have AF.[25] Whitlock is the principal investigator of the LeAAPS trial, and he discusses it in greater detail in Chapter 46. However, as of this writing, there are no conclusive data to justify closing the LAA in patients undergoing cardiac surgery who have no history of AF.

SYSTEMIC EMBOLISM VERSUS PULMONARY EMBOLISM

During AF, both atria are fibrillating. This raises the question of why AF is often associated with systemic embolism from the LA but rarely with pulmonary embolism (PE) from the right atrium (RA). The three components of Virchow's triad responsible for spontaneous intravascular thrombosis are hypercoagulability, endothelial injury, and stasis of blood flow.[26] Lim et al.[27] documented that AF itself can induce hypercoagulability that is more severe in the atria than in the peripheral circulation. However, patients with hypercoagulation syndromes have the same problem inside the fibrillating RA that they have inside the fibrillating LA. Therefore, if hypercoagulability were the primary culprit in cardiac TE, PE from the right heart would be as common as systemic embolism from the left heart.

The study by Lim et al.[27] also suggested that AF-induced endothelial injury in the atria is a factor in promoting atrial thrombogenesis. However, the study did not differentiate between endothelial injury in the RA and the LA. Atrial stretching and fibrosis, with potential endothelial injury, would be expected to be more prominent in the LA than in the RA in patients with concomitant AF because most of these patients have left-sided heart problems such as hypertension, ischemic heart disease, and mitral and/or aortic valve disease. Thus it is possible that a disparity in endothelial injury could be one reason thromboemboli originate more commonly in the LA than in the RA, but it is likely to be less important than the marked disparity in the degree of stasis in the two atria during AF.

Both the right atrial appendage (RAA) and the LAA are heavily trabeculated in their distal portions. However, the orifice of the RAA is broad, and the RAA itself is shallow, whereas the LAA orifice is narrow, and the LAA itself is deep (Fig. 40.13). In addition, the wide orifice of

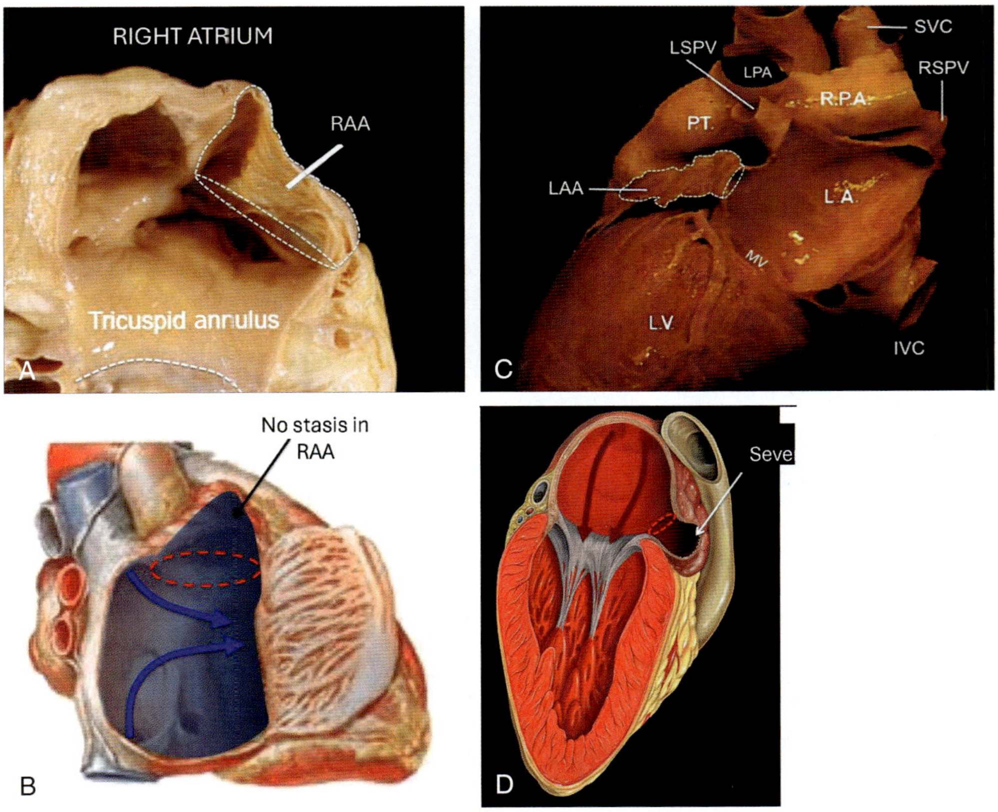

Fig. 40.13 (A) The right atrial appendage (RAA) has a broad orifice *(dashed oval)* and is shallow from its orifice to its tip. (B) Blood returning from the superior vena cava *(blue arrows)* to the tricuspid valve passes close by the large RAA orifice and continuously washes the RAA cavity throughout each cardiac cycle even during atrial fibrillation (AF). Therefore, stasis in the RAA during AF is kept at a minimum. (C) The left atrial appendage (LAA) orifice is small *(dotted oval)*, and the LAA cavity is deep compared with the RAA. (D) The combination of a small LAA orifice and a deep LAA cavity results in severe stasis of flow in the LAA during AF, especially in its trabeculae and its tip. *IVC,* Inferior vena cava; *LA,* left atrium; *LPA,* left pulmonary artery; *LSPV,* left superior pulmonary vein; *LV,* left ventricle; *MV,* mitral valve; *PT,* pulmonary trunk; *RPA,* right pulmonary artery; *RSPV,* right superior pulmonary vein; *SVC,* superior vena cava.

the RAA is positioned adjacent to the predominant path of blood flow from the superior and inferior vena cavae to the tricuspid valve, causing the interior of the RAA to be continuously washed even during AF. In contrast, blood from the pulmonary veins (PVs) actually flows away from the LAA orifice on its way to the mitral valve. Thus the LAA is not washed as thoroughly during AF as is the RA, so the degree of stasis in the LAA is substantially worse than that in the RAA. The tip of the LAA is the only place in the entire cardiovascular system where blood flow is normal during sinus rhythm and essentially stops the instant AF occurs.

RESIDUAL POUCHES AND RESIDUAL LEAKS

The specific site of thrombus formation within the LAA is important clinically because it determines the level at which the appendage can be safely excluded. It has been documented that if a pouch more than 1 cm deep remains at the base of the LAA after closure, it is thrombogenic (i.e., it increases the likelihood of thrombus formation).[16] However, there is no evidence that a small residual pouch smaller than 1 cm has any negative effect or that it is thrombogenic.[16,28]

A more common problem, especially with catheter-based closure devices, is that after endocardial LAA closure, a residual connection ("leak") sometimes remains between the body of the LA and the LAA itself. Small (0–5 mm) leaks are associated with modestly higher incidences of thromboembolic and bleeding events.[29] Surprisingly however, large leaks (>5 mm) are not associated with adverse events, although higher proportions of these patients require anticoagulation. Although epicardial suture closure or staple closure of the LAA results in a high rate of residual connections between the LAA and the LA,[16–18] there are virtually no post-application residual connections between the LAA and the LA after LAA closure with the surgical AtriClip device (Fig. 40.14).[30] The AtriClip LAA occluding device has now been implanted in more than 700,000 patients with excellent results. It is too early to comment on the new surgical epicardial LAA clip called the Penditure that was recently introduced (Medtronic, Inc.) (Fig. 40.15) because there is only one case report of LAA occlusion at the time of this writing.[31]

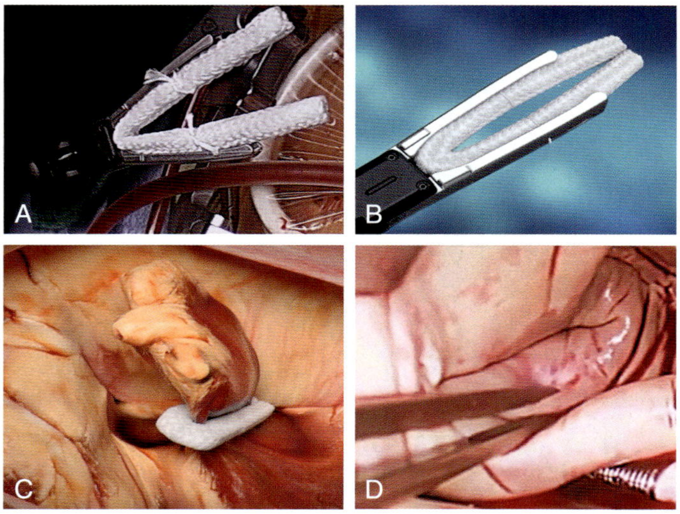

Fig. 40.14 The AtriCure AtriClip device for left atrial appendage (LAA) occlusion. (A) This is the most recent version of the AtriClip with open ends to enhance placement. It is constructed of nitinol springs that produce a continuous dynamic inward force to ensure permanent closure of the LAA. (B) A unique feature of the open-ended version of the AtriClip is that it closes first at the tip and then in the middle of the clip for uniform pressure on the LAA. (C) The AtriClip at the base of the LAA with no residual pouch. (D) The endocardial view of the orifice of the LAA following epicardial closure of the LAA with an AtriClip.

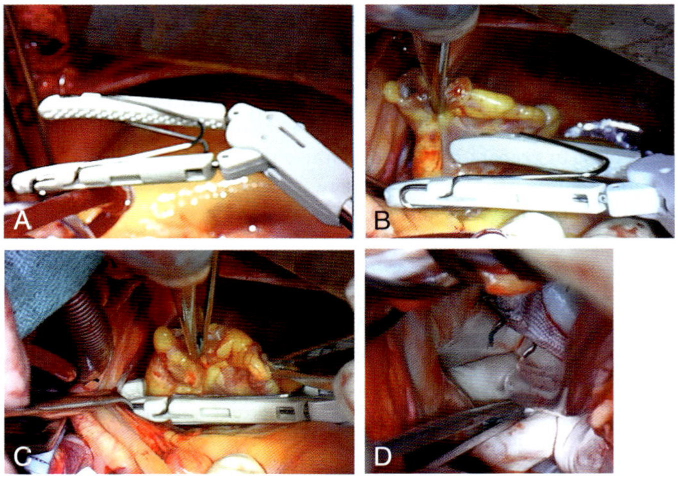

Fig. 40.15 The Medtronic Penditure device for left atrial appendage (LAA) occlusion. (A) The Penditure device is also open ended to enhance LAA closure. (B) There is no cloth covering over the Penditure device, so that there is only a double-row metal spring left behind after LAA occlusion. (C) The Penditure at the base of the LAA with no residual pouch. (D) The endocardial view of the orifice of the LAA after epicardial closure of the LAA with a Penditure.

LEFT ATRIAL APPENDAGE THROMBOSIS

The generally accepted notion of the pathophysiology of TE associated with AF is that a fixed thrombus forms in the LAA and then either the entire thrombus or a portion of it breaks off and embolizes systemically. In the original cut-and-sew Maze-I, -II, and -III procedures, the excised LAA was immediately examined for thrombi at surgery by opening it longitudinally from base to tip. When the original cut-and-sew Maze-III procedure was supplanted by the minimally invasive CryoMaze-III procedure in the mid-1990s, the LAA was no longer excised but rather, it was inverted into the left atrial cavity, directly examined for thrombi, and returned to its normal position. The orifice of the LAA was then cryoablated circumferentially to isolate it electrically from the LA and then closed endocardially. Direct visual examination of the LAA in 360 patients, 19% of whom had previously experienced either a stroke or TIA, revealed small thrombi in the trabeculated LAA in only 2 patients. Both patients were experiencing recurring strokes during the week before undergoing an emergency Maze procedure. Clearly, these patients had a LAA thrombus that was repeatedly embolizing flecks of the thrombus to the brain. No thrombi were found in the LAA, LA, PVs, or left ventricle in any of the 360 patients.[15] These unique premortem observations of the inside of the LAA in the Maze patients suggested that thrombi do not always attach to the trabeculae of the LAA and then embolize to the brain as occurred in the two patients in whom we found LAA thrombi. We believe that a more common scenario is that severely static blood in the LAA congeals into a free-floating thrombus and, after forming, quickly embolizes to the systemic circulation, leaving no trace of its former, rather fleeting, existence. This view is most consistent with the absence of thrombi noted on premortem examination of the left heart and LAA in the vast majority of patients known to have had thromboembolic events associated with AF.

REFERENCES

1. Madden JL. Resection of the left auricular appendix: a prophylaxis for recurrent arterial emboli. *J Am Med Assoc.* 1949;140(9):767–772.
2. Chatterjee S, Alexander JC, Pearson PJ, Feldman T. Left atrial appendage occlusion: lessons learned from surgical and transcatheter experiences. *Ann Thor Surg.* 2011;92(6):2283–2292.
3. Blackshear JL, Odell JA. Appendage obliteration to reduce stroke in cardiac surgical patients with atrial fibrillation. *Ann Thor Surg.* 1996;61(2):755–759.
4. Cox JL, Ad N, Palazzo T. Impact of the Maze procedure on the stroke rate in patients with atrial fibrillation. *J Thor Cardiovasc Surg.* 1999;118:833–840.
5. Creswell LL, Schuessler RB, Rosenbloom M, Cox JL. Hazards of postoperative atrial arrhythmias. *Ann Thor Surg.* 1993;56(3):638–641.
6. Almassi GH, Schowalter T, Nicolosi AC, et al. Atrial fibrillation after cardiac surgery: a major morbid event? *Ann Surg.* 1997;226(4):501–511.
7. The Boston Area Anticoagulation Trial for Atrial Fibrillation Investigators. The effect of low dose warfarin on the risk of strokes in patients with non-rheumatic atrial fibrillation. *N Engl J Med.* 1990;323:1505–1511.
8. Stroke Prevention in Atrial Fibrillation Investigators. Stroke prevention in atrial fibrillation study: final results. *Circulation.* 1991;84:527–539.
9. Stroke Prevention in Atrial Fibrillation Investigators. Warfarin versus aspirin for prevention of thromboembolism in atrial fibrillation: stroke prevention in atrial fibrillation II study. *Lancet.* 1994;343:687–691.
10. Atrial Fibrillation Investigators, et al: Risk factors for stroke and efficacy of antithrombotic therapy in atrial fibrillation. Analysis of pooled data from five randomized controlled trials. *Arch Intern Med.* 1994;154:1449–1457.
11. Prasad SM, Maniar HS, Camillo CJ, et al. The Cox Maze III procedure for atrial fibrillation: long-term efficacy in patients undergoing lone versus concomitant procedures. *J Thor Cardiovasc Surg.* 2003;126(6):1822–1828.
12. National Library of Medicine. Pubmed.ncbi.nlm.nih.gov
13. Wolf PA, Abbott RD, Kannel WB. Atrial fibrillation as an independent risk factor for stroke: the Framingham study. *Stroke.* 1991;22(8):983–988.
14. Rey RC, Monteverde DA, Sica RE. Cardiac sources of cerebral embolism. *Arch Neurol.* 1991;48(4):359–360.
15. Cox JL. Mechanical closure of the left atrial appendage: is it time to be more aggressive? *J Thor Cardiovasc Surg.* 2013;146(5): 1018–1027.
16. Healey JS, Crystal E, Lamy A, et al. Left atrial appendage occlusion study (LAAOS): results of a randomized controlled pilot study of left atrial appendage occlusion during coronary bypass surgery in patients at risk for stroke. *Am Heart J.* 2005;130(2):288–293.
17. Kanderian AS, Gillinov AM, Pettersson GB, Blackstone E, Klein AL. Success of surgical left atrial appendage closure: assessment by transesophageal echocardiography. *J Am Coll Cardiol.* 2008;52(11):924–929.
18. Cullen MW, Stulak JM, Powell BD, White RD, Ammash NM, Nkomo VT. Left atrial appendage patency at cardioversion after surgical left atrial appendage intervention. *Ann Thor Surg.* 2016;101(2):675–681.
19. Friedman DJ, Piccini JP, Wang T, et al. Association between left atrial appendage occlusion and readmission for thromboembolism among patients with atrial fibrillation undergoing concomitant cardiac surgery. *J Am Med Assoc.* 2018;319(4):365–374.
20. Yao X, Gersh BJ, Holmes DR, et al. Association of surgical left atrial appendage occlusion with subsequent stroke and mortality among patients undergoing cardiac surgery. *J Am Med Assoc.* 2018;319(20):2116–2126.
21. Gutierrez EM, Castano M, Gualis J, et al. Beneficial effect of left atrial appendage closure during cardiac surgery: a meta-analysis of 280,585 patients. *Eur J Cardio-Thorac Surg.* 2020;57:252–262.
22. Whitlock RP, Belley-Cote EP, Paparella D, et al. Left atrial appendage occlusion during cardiac surgery to prevent stroke. *N Engl J Med.* 2021;384(22):2081–2091.
23. Ibrahim AM, Tandan N, Koester C, et al. Meta-analysis evaluating the outcomes of surgical left atrial appendage occlusion during cardiac surgery. *Am J Cardiol.* 2019;124(8):1218–1225.
24. Gerdisch MW, Garrett HE Jr, Mumtaz MA, et al. Prophylactic left atrial appendage exclusion in cardiac surgery patients with elevated CHA2DS2-VASc score: results of the randomized ATLAS trial. *Innovations.* 2022;17(6):463–470.
25. Left Atrial Appendage Exclusion for Prophylactic Stroke Reduction Trial (LeAAPS). Accessed September 3, 2022. https://clinicaltrials.gov/ct2/show/NCT05478304
26. Lowe GD. Virchow's triad revisited: abnormal flow. *Pathophysiol Haemost Thromb.* 2003;33:455–457.
27. Lim HS, Willoughby SR, Schultz C, et al. Effect of atrial fibrillation on atrial thrombogenesis in humans: impact of rate and rhythm. *J Am Coll Cardiol.* 2013;61:852–860.
28. Bartus K, Han FT, Bednarek J, et al. Percutaneous left atrial appendage suture ligation using the LARIAT device in patients with atrial fibrillation: initial clinical experience. *J Am Coll Cardiol.* 2013;62:108–118.
29. Alkhouli M, Du C, Killu A, et al. Clinical impact of residual leaks following left atrial appendage occlusion: insights from the NCDR LAAO Registry. *JACC Clin Electrophysiol.* 2022;8(6):766–778.
30. Toale C, Fitzmaurice GJ, Eaton D, Lyne J, Redmond KC. Outcomes of left atrial appendage occlusion using the AtriClip device: a systematic review. *Interact Cardiovasc Thorac Surg.* 2019;29(5):655–662.
31. Torregrossa G, Baudo M, Yakobitis A, Murray C, Kappetein AP. (Case Report) Surgical implant of Medtronic Penditure left atrial appendage exclusion clip during off-pump bilateral internal thoracic coronary artery bypass grafting. *Ann Cardiothorac Surg.* 2024;13(2):182–183.

41

Anatomy and Physiology of the Left Atrial Appendage

Manuel Castella

CHAPTER OUTLINE

EMBRYOLOGIC ORIGIN OF THE LEFT ATRIAL APPENDAGE

The left atrial appendage (LAA) is a special structure of the heart, with important differences in anatomic structure and physiology from the left atrium (LA). Embryologically, the LAA has a different origin from the rest of the LA. On day 22 of gestation, the cardiac tube is formed and starts to fold. Its caudal part folds posteriorly, cranially, and to the left, creating the common atria. The septum primum and secundum create the interatrial septum between days 27 and 35. Beginning at day 35, there is intimate contact of the LA with developing pulmonary buds. From days 35 to 50, fusion of the pulmonary veins (PVs) in the LA evolves into what will become the posterior wall of the adult LA that is formed adjacent to the PV tissue. The primary remnant of the original common atria in the LA is the LAA.[1] This separate origin explains the difference in anatomy in the LA and the LAA. It also explains the prominent trabeculations in the LAA and in the right atrial appendage that are not present in the main body of the LA, right atrium (RA), or interatrial septum. This anatomic difference is also seen at the cellular level and in the relative degree of innervation by the automatic nervous system.[2] There is also an important difference between the functions of the body of the LA and its appendage (LAA), especially in atrial peptide secretion.

ANATOMY OF THE LEFT ATRIAL APPENDAGE

The LAA is an extension on the left side of the LA and normally represents approximately 6% to 7% of the total left atrial volume. The normal size of the LAA is around 44.4 ± 10.9 mm in length, 4.5 ± 2.3 mm in width and 6.9 ± 2.7 mL in internal volume.[3] Externally, the LAA overlaps the left atrioventricular (AV) groove, and its tip usually reaches the right ventricular outflow track. In rare instances, the LAA tip may be oriented toward the transverse sinus in close contact with the left main coronary artery. Commonly, the LAA has small, thin fat pads on the outer surface. Its shape varies and may have one to three lobes. The most common configurations are either one lobe (51%) or two lobes (41%), with the three-lobe configuration being the least common (8%),[4] though the three-lobe configuration is more often associated with thrombus formation independent of clinical risk and stasis.[5] The LAA shape has been defined over the years in types, subtypes, or different shapes. It has been described as being as a horseshoe, cockscomb, paper fan, wing, mountain, hook, or swan.[4] However, the most accepted morphologic classification has categorized the LAA into four anatomic groups: chicken wing, windsock, cauliflower, and cactus. There is a certain overlapping between these shapes, and on occasion the same appendage can be defined in a different shape depending on the perspective from which it is viewed (Fig. 41.1).[6] As an example, the

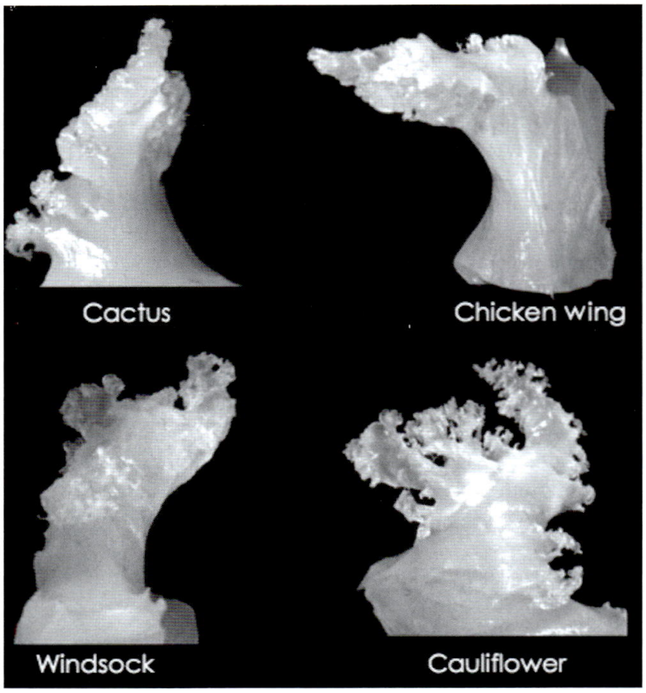

Fig. 41.1 The four anatomic shapes of the left atrial appendage (LAA) based on common cardiac imaging techniques. Surprisingly, the apparent differences in the anatomic shapes displayed here were created from a silastic mold of the same LAA that was simply rotated for photographic purposes in four different planes of view. In other words, this is the same LAA. See text for further discussion. (Courtesy Professor Andrew Cook, University College London, United Kingdom.)

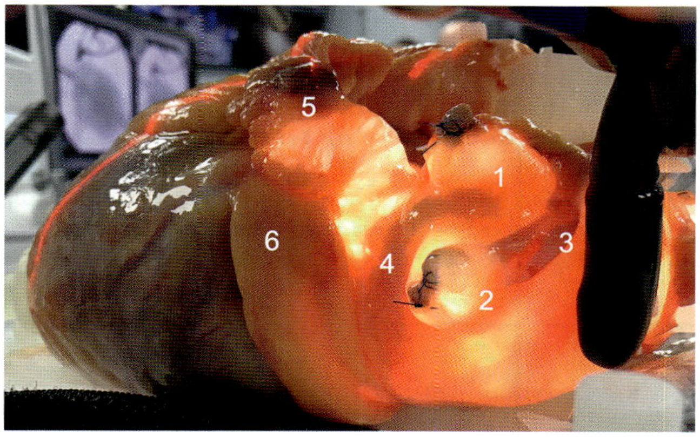

Fig. 41.2 Retroillumination of the human left atrium highlighting variations in atrial wall thickness. The numbers correspond to the *(1)* left superior pulmonary vein (PV), *(2)* left inferior PV, *(3)* pericardial recession, *(4)* coumadin ridge between the left superior PV and the left atrial appendage, *(5)* left atrial appendage, and *(6)* fat pad in the atrioventricular groove.

four "anatomic types" of LAA shown in Fig. 41.1 are actually different imaging angles of the *same* LAA! Such apparent variations in anatomy based on imaging angles, rather than actual anatomic differences, calls into question the use of this classification system in deciding whether or not to close the LAA at the time of catheter ablation or cardiac surgery.

The LAA has important muscular trabeculations that are largely responsible for the force of its brief active contraction (Fig. 41.2). Indeed, large LAA pectinate muscles seen on echocardiograms are often difficult to differentiate from LAA thrombi. The orifice of the LAA varies in size, shape, and position. It is usually located between the orifices of the left PVs and the mitral valve at the level of P1. The LAA orifice can be above the left superior PV (LSPV) (type I, 9%), anterior to the LSPV (type II, 78%), or below the LSPV (type III; 13%).[4] The shape of the orifice can be round, oval (69%), triangular, tear-drop shaped, or footlike.[7]

The area of the LAA orifice changes significantly during each cardiac cycle, becoming smaller during the atrial contractile (pump) phase. The primary reason is the specific anatomy of the distal end of Bachmann's bundle. This important bundle of muscle fibers is located on the superior surface of the atrial muscle mass and extends from the top of the RA to the top of the LA. Although its primary purpose is to convey sinus impulses rapidly from the RA to the LA, its distal muscle fibers diverge at the base of the LAA, resulting in their surrounding the orifice of the LAA (see Chapter 3, Fig. 3.12). One limb of these distal fibers of Bachmann's bundle pass between the LSPV and the LAA, where the atrial wall is particularly thick. This thickened area of the LA between the LSPV and the LAA is commonly called the "coumadin ridge" (Figs. 41.2 and 41.3). In Chapter 48, which describes postoperative peri-mitral atrial flutter, this area is called the "LAA–LSPV isthmus" (see Chapter 48, Figs. 48.7 and 48.10). Because of its thickness, it is quite difficult to create a transmural lesion across the coumadin ridge using unipolar radiofrequency (RF), whether it is delivered endocardially with a catheter or epicardially with a unipolar RF pen.

The anterior limb of the distal Bachmann's bundle lies between the LAA orifice and the mitral valve at the level of P1, an area called the "mitral vestibule" (Fig. 41.4). In Chapter 48 describing postoperative peri-mitral atrial flutter, this mitral vestibule is called the "LAA–MV isthmus" (see Chapter 48, Figs. 48.7 and 48.11). The mitral vestibule is a continuation of what was the embryologic LAA and harbors extrapectinate trabeculations with very thin atrial walls between the thick

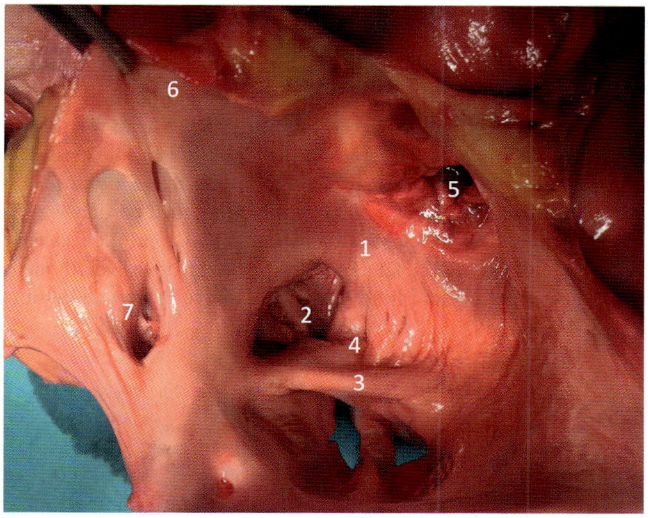

Fig. 41.3 Internal view of the human left atrium. The numbers correspond to the *(1)* mitral vestibule (LAA-MV isthmus), *(2)* left atrial appendage, *(3)* coumadin ridge, *(4)* extrapectineal trabeculations that can be seen in 30% of patients, *(5)* mitral valve, *(6) fossa ovalis, and (7)* assorted other endocardial pouches.

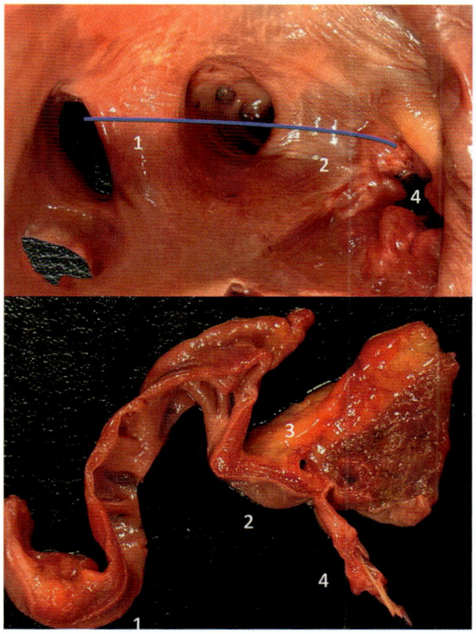

Fig. 41.4 Two views of the same human heart with the *blue line* in the *upper panel* indicating the plane of the photo in the *lower panel*. The differences in thickness of the atrial wall can be appreciated. *(1)* Coumadin Ridge ("LAA-LSPV isthmus"), *(2)* left atrial appendage and mitral vestibule ("LAA-MV isthmus), *(3)* circumflex artery, *(4)* mitral valve at the level of P1.

trabeculations in approximately 30% of patients.[7,8] The relative locations of the anterior and posterior limbs of Bachmann's bundle result in the LAA orifice being surrounded by its distal muscle fibers. In patients with atrial fibrillation (AF), the orifice tends to dilatate and becomes more round with no variation during most of the cardiac cycle.[6] It is important to note that two-dimensional transesophageal echocardiography (TEE) usually underestimates the diameter and circumference of the LAA orifice compared with three-dimensional TEE.

ANATOMIC RELATIONSHIPS OF THE LEFT ATRIAL APPENDAGE

The left phrenic nerve and its accompanying pericardiophrenic vessels are located on the outer side of the pericardial layer from the thoracic inlet to the diaphragm. The left phrenic nerve usually resides at the level of the tip of the LAA (59%) and less commonly at the LAA base (23%).[9]

The LAA lies in close proximity to the circumflex coronary artery in the fat pad of the left AV groove (Fig. 41.5). The circumflex coronary artery is located within the fat pad of the left AV groove, which may be from 1 to 4 mm thick and lies immediately above the mitral vestibule between the LAA and the posterior leaflet of the mitral valve. The distances between the LAA and the circumflex coronary artery may vary. For example, in some patients, the orifice of the LAA can be located closer than normal to the mitral valve annulus and circumflex coronary artery (Fig. 41.6). It is particularly hazardous if such a patient also has a circumflex coronary artery that is located higher than normal in the AV groove (Fig. 41.7). In such rare instances, the proximal circumflex coronary artery can be injured during endocardial suture closure of the LAA (Fig. 41.8).

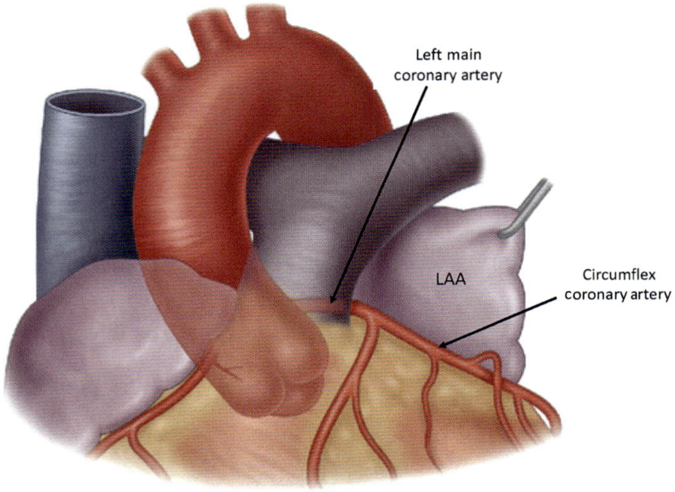

Fig. 41.5 Illustration showing the close proximity between the circumflex coronary artery and the left atrial appendage (LAA).

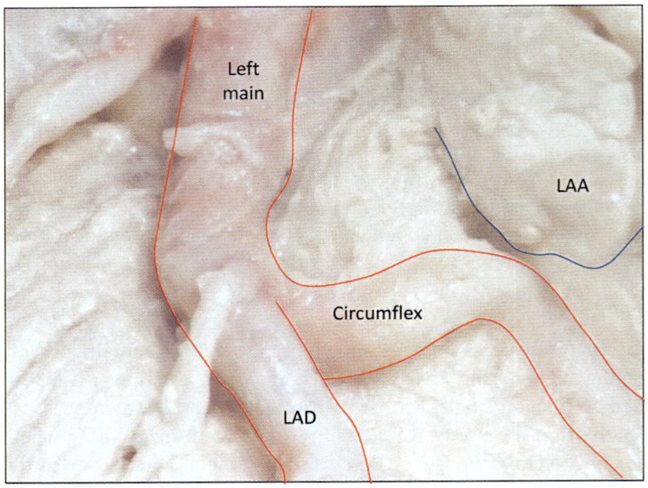

Fig. 41.7 Although the circumflex coronary artery is usually located well away from the orifice of the left atrial appendage (LAA), it can be in a higher than normal location, and in some patients this is attributed to its tortuosity, which causes the artery to be immediately adjacent to the LAA orifice. *LAD,* Left anterior descending coronary artery.

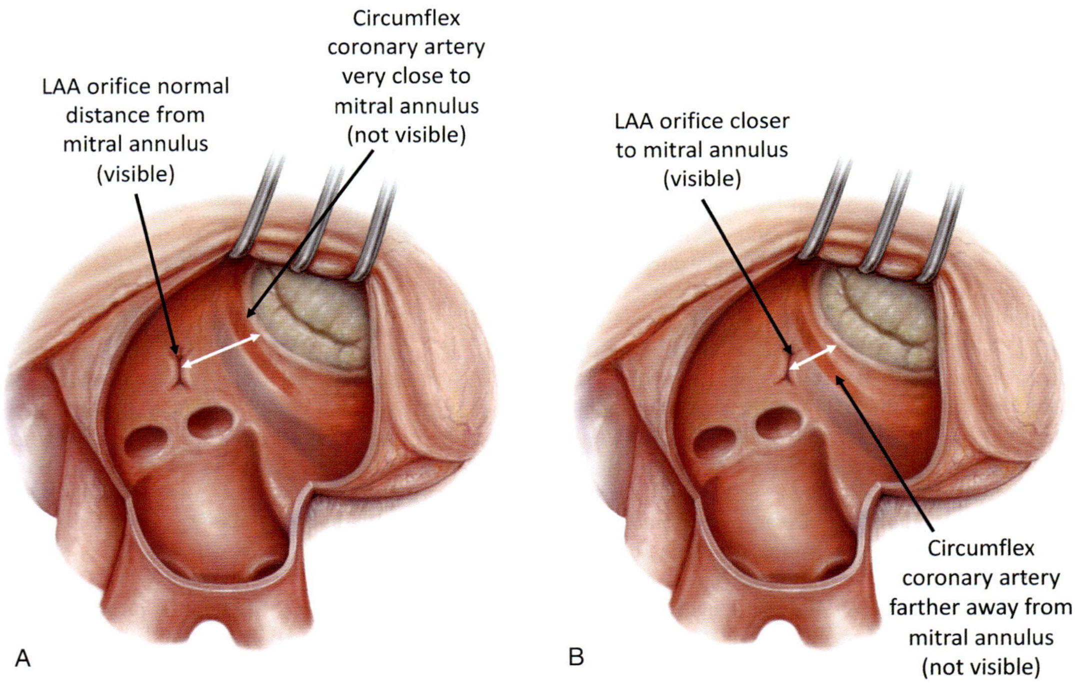

Fig. 41.6 (A) The orifice of the left atrial appendage (LAA) is usually at about the level of the frenulum between the two left pulmonary veins, which puts it well away from the mitral annulus and more important, the circumflex coronary artery. (B) In some patients, the orifice of the LAA is much closer to the mitral annulus and circumflex coronary artery. Thus one must be careful not to injure the coronary artery when closing the LAA orifice with endocardial sutures.

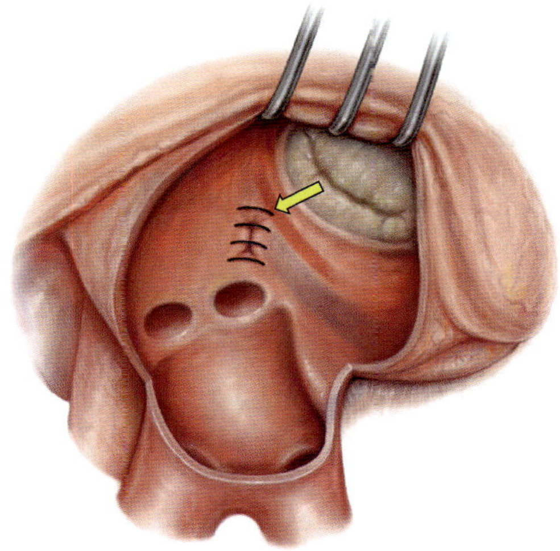

Fig. 41.8 The combination of an abnormally low location of the orifice of the left atrial appendage (LAA) and an abnormally high location of the circumflex coronary artery is insignificant unless the LAA needs to be amputated and its base closed during cardiac surgery. In this case, it is easy to place one of the endocardial closure sutures through the coronary artery (*yellow arrow*). This iatrogenic injury occurs approximately 1.5 cm distal to the origin of the circumflex coronary artery.

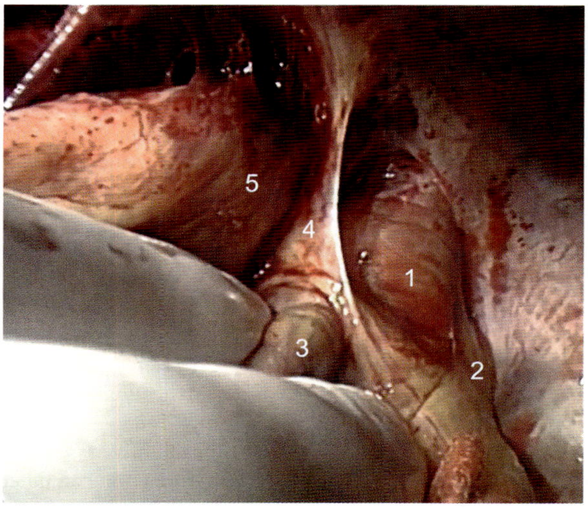

Fig. 41.9 External view of the left atrium showing the *(1)* left superior pulmonary vein (PV), *(2)* left inferior PV, *(3)* left atrial appendage, *(4)* ligament of Marshall, and *(5)* left pulmonary artery.

The ligament of Marshall lies between the left superior PV and the LAA (Fig. 41.9). In most cases, this ligament is simply a reflection of the pericardium that extends from the parietal pericardium. It usually harbors the vein of Marshall, a small vestige of the embryologic left superior vena cava (SVC). In two-thirds of patients, there is a left intermediate atrial artery that originates from the circumflex coronary artery next to the inferior border of the LAA. This artery runs parallel to the coumadin ridge to reach the superior wall of the LA. Its diameter ranges from 0.5 to 1.6 mm.[7] In fewer than 0.1% of the human population, the ligament of Marshall persists as a left SVC.

The autonomic nervous system of the heart has a close relationship with the LA. In the dog model, both sympathetic and parasympathetic fibers are numerous around the left atrial structures, with more density on the epicardium and less in the endocardium. The highest density of autonomic fibers is in the posterior left atrial wall, followed in decreasing order by the PVs, interatrial septum, anterior roof of the LA, and finally the LAA, which has the least neuronal tissue. Of particular interest is the epicardial fat of the coumadin ridge, the richest zone of parasympathetic ganglia near the LAA.[7] A higher density of neuronal elements is found in the epicardial region of the coumadin ridge on top of the left superior PV.

PHYSIOLOGY OF THE LEFT ATRIAL APPENDAGE

Because of its important muscular structure, the LAA is the most expansive and moveable part of the LA. Normally, it has a mean maximum volume of 8.7 ± 2.9 mL and mean minimum volume of 3.2 ± 1.2 mL. The emptying volume is estimated at a mean of 5.55 ± 1.9 mL. There is no significant difference in the normal LA volume index between males and females, but the maximal, minimal, and emptying volumes have been positively correlated with the body weight, height, and surface area.[4]

As is the case with both atria, the LAA follows the three main phases of the cardiac cycle, the reservoir, conduit, and active contraction phases. The passive reservoir phase is the time during ventricular systole, in which the mitral valve closes, the mitral annulus moves toward the apex because of ventricular contraction, and both atria quickly increase their volumes partially because of this piston effect of the mitral valve. The conduit phase occurs with the relaxation of the ventricles. The mitral valve opens, and its annulus moves away from the apex. This is the fast-filling phase of the ventricles, and the atria lose volume passively. This phase is responsible for approximately 80% of the ventricular filling in normal sinus rhythm.

Finally, the contraction of the atria further enhances ventricular filling as the mitral annulus moves still farther away from the ventricular apex. The LAA follows the same pattern, participating importantly in the reservoir phase by increasing its volume proportionally more than the rest of the LA. In contrast, most of its volume decrease is not in the passive conduit phase as it is in the rest of the LA but in the active contractile phase (Fig. 41.10).[10] The potential importance of this contractile component of LAA is unknown, even in young athletes who can increase their cardiac output during exercise up to four times with a sinus tachycardia of greater than 200 beats/min. Such an exercise-induced state shortens atrial diastole and is almost certainly an important component of the decrease cardiac output in patients with AF.

Doppler echocardiography is useful to assess LAA function by providing a means of quantitating flow velocities and color flow analysis. The velocity and color flow of the LAA are concordant to reduction in size during contraction in sinus rhythm. Flow velocity during LAA contraction ranges between 50 ± 6 cm/s and 83 ± 19 cm/s with filling velocities ranging from 46 ± 12 cm/s to 60 cm/s in normal human in sinus rhythm.[6] Flow velocities below 40 cm/s are associated with a higher risk of stroke and the appearance of spontaneous echocardiographic contrast.[11]

THE LEFT ATRIAL APPENDAGE AS A NEUROENDOCRINE ORGAN

Both atrial and ventricular myocytes have neuroendocrine capabilities. The atrial myocardium is the main source of type A, or atrial natriuretic peptide (ANP), and the right and the LAAs are responsible for more than 30% of its production. Type B, or brain natriuretic peptide (BNP),

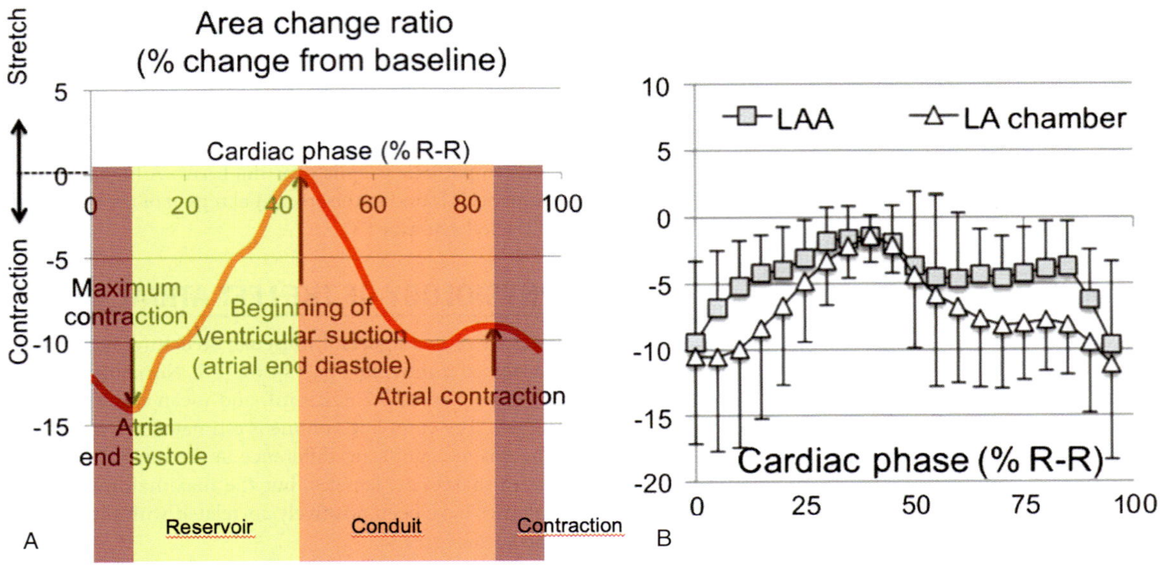

Fig. 41.10 (A) The three phases of atrial function during a single cardiac cycle including the reservoir phase *(yellow)*, conduit phase *(orange)*, and pump phase *(maroon)*. (B) Differences in left atrial function and left atrial appendage (LAA) function during one cardiac cycle. *LA*, Left atrium. (Reproduced from Ashikaga H, Cammin J, Tang Q, et al. Quantitative assessment of atrial regional function using motion estimation computed tomography. *J Comput Assist Tomogr*. 2014;38(5):773–778.)

is released primarily by the ventricular myocardium, although the atria can also produce BNP, especially in patients with heart failure and AF. Both ANP and BNP promote diuresis, natriuresis, and vasodilation, and they both help prevent cardiac hypertrophy. The main stimulus for the production of ANP is myocardial stretch.[12,13] It is important to note that most of the studies in humans tying ANP levels to the LAA have been performed in AF patients, in which not only the LAA is constantly distended, but there is also stretching of both atria and a certain degree of atrial substrate deterioration. It is known that patients with long-standing AF have increased levels of ANP and BNP that are largely independent of the LAA production and that do not correlate with left atrial pressure.[14,15]

REFERENCES

1. DeSimone CV, Prakriti BG, Tri J, Syed F, Sm AN, Asirvatham SJ. A review of the relevant embryology, pathohistology, and anatomy of the left atrial appendage for the invasive cardiac electrophysiologist. *J Atr Fibrillation*. 2015;8(2):1129.
2. Leinonen JV, Emanuelov AK, Platt Y, et al. Left atrial appendages from adult hearts contain a reservoir of diverse cardiac progenitor cells. *PLoS One*. 2013;8(3):e59228.
3. Wang Y, Di Biase L, Horton RP, Nguyen T, Morhanty P, Natale A. Left atrial appendage studied by computed tomography to help planning for appendage closure device placement. *J Cardiovasc Electrophysiol*. 2010;21(9):973–982.
4. Li CY, Gao BL, Liu XW, et al. Quantitative evaluation of the substantially variable morphology and function of the left atrial appendage and its relation with adjacent structures. *PLoS One*. 2015;10(7):e0126818.
5. Yamamoto M, Seo Y, Kawamatsu N, et al. Complex left atrial appendage morphology and left atrial appendage thrombus formation in patients with atrial fibrillation. *Circ Cardiovasc Imaging*. 2014;7(2):337–343.
6. Beigel R, Wunderlich NC, Ho SY, Arsanjani R, Siegel RJ. The left atrial appendage: anatomy, function, and noninvasive evaluation. *JACC Cardiovasc Imaging*. 2014;7(12):1251–1265.
7. Cabrera JA, Ho SY, Climent V, Sanchez-Quintana D. The architecture of the left lateral atrial wall: a particular anatomic region with implications for ablation of atrial fibrillation. *Eur Heart J*. 2008;29(3):356–362.
8. Cabrera J. Left atrial appendage: anatomy and imaging landmarks pertinent to percutaneous transcatheter occlusion. *Heart*. 2014;100(20):1636–1650.
9. Sanchez-Quintana D, Ho SY, Climent V, Murillo M, Cabrera JA. Anatomic evaluation of the left phrenic nerve relevant to epicardial and endocardial catheter ablation: implications for phrenic nerve injury. *Heart Rhythm*. 2009;6(6):764–768.
10. Ashikaga H, Cammin J, Tang Q, et al. Quantitative assessment of atrial regional function using motion estimation computed tomography. *J Comput Assist Tomogr*. 2014;38(5):773–778.
11. Fatkin D, Kelly RP, Feneley MP. Relations between left atrial appendage blood flow velocity, spontaneous echocardiographic contrast and thromboembolic risk in vivo. *J Am Coll Cardiol*. 1994;23(4):961–969.
12. Song W, Wang H, Wu Q. Atrial natriuretic peptide in cardiovascular biology and disease (NPPA). *Gene*. 2015;569(1):1–6.
13. Tabata T, Oki T, Yamada H, Abe M, Onose Y, Thomas JD. Relationship between left atrial appendage function and plasma concentration of atrial natriuretic peptide. *Eur J Echocardiogr*. 2000;1(2):130–137.
14. Sramko M, Wichterle D, Melenovsky V, et al. Independent effect of atrial fibrillation on natriuretic peptide release. *Clin Res Cardiol*. 2019;108(2):142–149.
15. Grieshaber P, Arneth B, Steinsberger F, et al. Influence of left atrial appendage amputation on natriuretic peptides—a randomized controlled trial. *Thorac Cardiovasc Surg*. 2021;69(2):117–123.

42

Neurohormonal Consequences of Left Atrial Appendage Closure

Manuel Castella

CHAPTER OUTLINE

Both the left atrium (LA) and the right atrium secrete natriuretic peptides in response to atrial stretch and elevated atrial pressure and thereby participate actively in the maintenance of systemic homeostasis. The most important natriuretic peptide secreted by the atria is A-type or atrial natriuretic peptide (ANP). The atria are also capable of secreting B-type natriuretic peptide, which is known as brain natriuretic peptide (BNP), but the ventricular endocardium, not the atrium, is the main cardiac source for BNP. ANP and BNP exhibit antagonistic effects against angiotensin II via diuretic and natriuretic actions, vasodilatory actions, and inhibition of aldosterone secretion.[1] C-type, or cerebral natriuretic peptide (CNP), was first identified in the porcine brain and is produced by multiple different cell types throughout the body. CNP helps regulate systemic homeostasis by impacting vascular tone, blood pressure, and the immune system.[2,3]

Although both the right atrial appendage (RAA) and left atrial appendage (LAA) secrete ANP, the LAA is responsible for up to 30% of all cardiac ANP production.[4] Active secretion of ANP by both appendages is likely attributable to their origin from the common primitive atrium, while the main body of the LA originates from the pulmonary vein buttons and the endocardial cushions. Because the LAA is relatively more compliant than the rest of the LA, it serves as an excellent reservoir that is especially sensitive to changes in systemic volume, exercise, and atrial stretch.[5] However, the LAA has fewer autonomic nervous system fibers than the rest of the LA, suggesting that ANP production is primarily the result of mechanical stretch and volume overload of the LA rather than a result of neurologic influences.[6]

ATRIAL NATRIURETIC PEPTIDE SECRETION DURING ATRIAL FIBRILLATION

Atrial fibrillation (AF) significantly alters the neurophysiology of the atrial wall. Because the LA is continuously stimulated electrically during AF, it is also constantly stretched. A 20% to 100% increase in ANP and BNP secretion can occur during AF in response to an increase in left atrial pressure of only 5 mm Hg. However, in hemodynamically stable patients with preserved left ventricular ejection fraction, ANP production and BNP production are not significantly influenced by changes in left atrial pressure during AF. Whereas ANP and BNP levels double when atrial pressure increases from 5 to 25 mm Hg in sinus rhythm patients, their levels remain essentially the same during AF regardless of pressure overload (Fig. 42.1). This explains how patients in AF can lose the capability of atrial-induced diuresis and natriuresis secondary to volume overload.[7] The increase in both ANP and BNP independent of left atrial pressure has been described in patients even after 20 minutes of AF induced by rapid atrial pacing. This suggests that the increase in both of the natriuretic peptides during AF is caused by the activation of atrial mechano-receptors and mechano-sensitive ion channels that are activated by permanent atrial stretch rather than by hemodynamic changes or atrial remodeling.[8,9]

Although the rapid increase in natriuretic peptide secretion occurs shortly after the initiation of AF, serum levels are higher in persistent

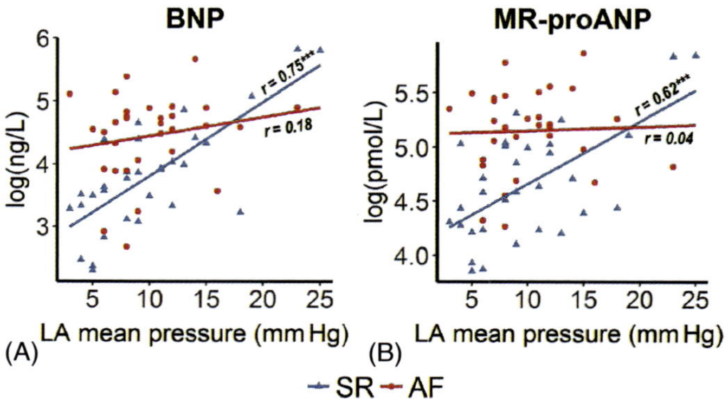

Fig. 42.1 Correlation of mean left atrial (LA) pressure and natriuretic peptide plasma concentrations in patients in atrial fibrillation (AF; *red*) or sinus rhythm (SR; *blue*).[7] (A) Brain natriuretic peptide (BNP), (B) Midregional proatrial natriuretic peptide (MR-proANP).

AF than in paroxysmal AF.[10] Paradoxically, serum ANP levels are often *lower* in patients with long-standing persistent AF (LSpAF), though they are consistently higher than ANP levels during sinus rhythm. The most likely reason for this apparent paradox is that patients with LSpAF tend to have more atrial scarring and therefore fewer active atrial myocytes that produce ANP.[11]

AF is present in 60% of patients diagnosed with heart failure and preserved ejection fraction. However, the use of serum ANP and BNP levels alone as surrogates for left-sided pressure overload can result in an overdiagnosis of heart failure in patients with AF and an underdiagnosis of heart failure in patients who are in normal sinus rhythm.[12]

USE OF BRAIN NATRIURETIC PEPTIDE OR N-TERMINAL PROHORMONE OF BRAIN NATRIURETIC PEPTIDE FOR ATRIAL FIBRILLATION SCREENING

The secretion of both ANP and BNP is increased during AF, but the variation in the degree of increased ANP secretion prevents the use of ANP serum level as a screening test for AF detection. In contrast, several studies have suggested that serum BNP and N-terminal prohormone of BNP (NT-proBNP) levels can be used to detect subclinical AF.[13–15] If true, elevated serum levels of BNP and NT-proBNP could prove to be useful in identifying AF as the source of stroke in patients who are in sinus rhythm at the time they have the stroke. Although there is no current consensus on which peptide is better for predicting AF, BNP has a shorter half-life than ANP, so higher BNP levels may better reflect episodes of AF. Also, other noncardiac conditions, such as renal failure, have less effect on serum BNP levels than on serum ANP levels. Although further studies are essential for confirmation, some contemporary studies suggest that serum BNP levels are more sensitive, but serum NT-proBNP levels are more specific for the detection of AF.[16,17]

INFLUENCE OF LEFT ATRIAL APPENDAGE CLOSURE OR EXCLUSION ON ATRIAL NATRIURETIC PEPTIDE SECRETION

Endocardial LAA occlusion (LAAO) devices implanted by catheters and endocardial suture closure of the LAA do not devascularize the myocardium of the LAA and therefore would not be expected to have a significant effect on serum ANP and BNP levels. However, in patients with AF, epicardial closure of the LAA with a clip, ligature, or stapling device, as well as LAA amputation, eliminates the production of ANP and BNP by the myocardium of the LAA. Therefore, these epicardial LAA closure techniques would be expected to decrease the serum levels of ANP and BNP. However, neither endocardial closure nor epicardial exclusion or amputation of the LAA in patients with AF results in a permanent decrease in serum ANP and BNP levels.[18] After endocardial device implantation, ANP and BNP levels increase slightly in the first few hours and then normalize within 24 hours. Epicardial LAA exclusion and LAA amputation are followed by an immediate decrease in serum ANP and BNP levels and then by an increase in their levels that can last up to 30 days after LAA exclusion. However, after approximately 3 months, serum ANP and BNP levels have returned to pre-LAA exclusion levels (Fig. 42.2).[19]

	Post-procedure with an epicardial device					Post-procedure after an endocardial device			
	0 hours	24 hours	3 months	12 months	24 months	0 hours	24 hours	3 months	12 months
Adrenaline	—	↓	↓	↓	↓	—	—	—	—
Noradrenaline	↓	↓	↓	↓	↓	—	—	—	
Renin	—	—	↓	↓	↓	—	—	—	
Aldosterone	—	↓	↓	↓	↓	—	—	—	↓
Insulin	—	↑	↑			—	↑	—	
ANP and BNP	↓	↑	—/↓	—	—	↑	—	—	—
Vasopressin		↓		↓	↓				
Systemic blood pressure	↓	↓	↓	↓	↓	↓	—	—	
Sodium		↓	—	—	—			—	
Potassium		—	—	—	—				

Fig. 42.2 Plasma levels of different hormones and blood pressure after endocardial or epicardial left appendage closure in patients who remain in atrial fibrillation (no ablation). *Arrows* indicate increased or decreased plasma levels compared with before the procedure. — indicates no significant change. The *blank box* represents no data available.[18–21] *ANP,* Atrial natriuretic peptide; *BNP,* brain natriuretic peptide.

In patients with AF, serum sodium levels decrease within 24 hours and normalize within 7 days after epicardial LAA exclusion or amputation, but the changes in absolute levels of sodium are minimal and do not significantly impact fluid balance. No significant changes in serum potassium or chloride levels have been described for up to 2 years after LAAO, LAA exclusion, or LAA amputation in patients with AF.[20] Finally, no information is currently available regarding the impact of LAAO, LAA exclusion, or LAA amputation on ANP secretion in patients without a history of AF who are in sinus rhythm.

LEFT ATRIAL APPENDAGE CLOSURE AND THE RENIN–ANGIOTENSIN–ALDOSTERONE SYSTEM

The relationship between the LAA and the renin–angiotensin–aldosterone system (RAAS) is not well defined in patients with AF. Epicardial LAA closure in patients with AF has been shown to lower serum renin and aldosterone levels for 3 months, and this effect is sustained for at least 2 years.[20] Also, LAA closure has also been shown to decrease adrenaline and noradrenaline levels, resulting in improved blood pressure control in patients with hypertension.[19,20] These effects suggest that in patients with AF, the relationship between the LAA and the RAAS may not be entirely dependent on natriuretic peptide levels because the effect on RAAS goes beyond the normalization of ANP and BNP levels. The RAAS is either downregulated directly by some unknown action of the LAA or by permanent damage to the afferent and efferent autonomic nervous system. In contrast, endocardial LAA closure has not been shown to decrease adrenaline levels, though it does result in a significant decrease in serum aldosterone levels at 1 year (see Fig. 42.2).[18]

These observations clearly indicate that LAA exclusion or amputation in patients with AF causes a downregulation of the RAAS that may explain the improved systolic and diastolic blood pressure control that is maintained over time. Clinical trials have demonstrated that RAAS antagonism reduces the incidence of AF in patients after myocardial infarction and heart failure.[22] This suggests that LAA exclusion or amputation in patients with AF can help avoid AF recurrence after initial ablation not only by isolating atrial AF triggers and/or interrupting macro-reentrant AF drivers but also by RAAS downregulation.

NEUROENDOCRINE CHANGES AFTER LEFT ATRIAL APPENDAGE CLOSURE AND ATRIAL FIBRILLATION ABLATION

There are limited data on neurohormone atrial expression comparing patients undergoing AF ablation with and without LAA exclusion. However, from the evidence described earlier, one might conclude that the decrease in serum ANP and BNP levels after AF ablation and LAAO is caused as much by restoring sinus rhythm as by the LAA closure. This notion is compatible with the findings of one study in which patients with endocardial catheter AF ablation were randomized for endocardial exclusion or nonexclusion of the LAA. Both groups showed lower serum BNP levels at 3 months in exactly the same proportion. The recurrence rates of AF or atrial flutter at 3 months were 24.2% without LAAO and 21.0% with LAAO (P >.05).[23]

CONCLUSIONS

ANP and BNP are both secreted by the entire atrial myocardium as well as by the two atrial appendages, especially the LAA. In patients with AF, the expected impact of removing or excluding the LAA on serum ANP and BNP levels is modulated by the restoration of sinus rhythm. In addition, LAA exclusion or amputation downregulates the RAAS, which helps control systemic hypertension that in turn can favorably impact the recurrence of AF.

REFERENCES

1. Kuwahara K. The natriuretic peptide system in heart failure: diagnostic and therapeutic implications. *Pharmacol Ther.* 2021;227:107863.
2. Liu C, Long Q, Yang H, et al. Sacubitril/Valsartan inhibits M1 type macrophages polarization in acute myocarditis by targeting C-type natriuretic peptide. *Biomed Pharmacother.* 2024;174:116535.
3. Cabiati M, Sabatino L, Caruso R, et al. Gene expression of C-type natriuretic peptide and of its specific receptor NPR-B in human leukocytes of healthy and heart failure subjects. *Peptide.* 2012;37(2):240–246.
4. Al-Saady NM, Obel OA, Camm AJ. Left atrial appendage: structure, function, and role in thromboembolism. *Heart.* 1999;82(5):547–554.
5. DeSimone CV, Prakriti BG, Tri J, Syed F, Sm AN, Asirvatham SJ. A review of the relevant embryology, pathohistology, and anatomy of the left atrial appendage for the invasive cardiac electrophysiologist. *J Atr Fibrillation.* 2015;8(2):1129.
6. Cabrera JA, Ho SY, Climent V, Sanchez-Quintana D. The architecture of the left lateral atrial wall: a particular anatomic region with implications for ablation of atrial fibrillation. *Eur Heart J.* 2008;29(3):356–362.
7. Sramko M, Wichterle D, Melenovsky V, et al. Independent effect of atrial fibrillation on natriuretic peptide release. *Clin Res Cardiol.* 2019;108(2):142–149.
8. De Jong AM, Maass AH, Oberdorf-Maass SU, Van Veldhuisen DJ, Van Gilst WH, Van Gelder IC. Mechanisms of atrial structural changes caused by stretch occurring before and during early atrial fibrillation. *Cardiovasc Res.* 2011;89(4):754–765.
9. Zhang YH, Youm JB, Earm YE. Stretch-activated non-selective cation channel: a causal link between mechanical stretch and atrial natriuretic peptide secretion. *Prog Biophys Mol Biol.* 2008;98(1):1–9.
10. Hijazi Z, Wallentin L, Siegbahn A, et al. N-terminal pro-B-type natriuretic peptide for risk assessment in patients with atrial fibrillation: insights from the ARISTOTLE Trial (Apixaban for the Prevention of Stroke in Subjects With Atrial Fibrillation). *J Am Coll Cardiol.* 2013;61(22):2274–2284.
11. Zografos TA, Katritsis DG. Natriuretic peptides as predictors of atrial fibrillation recurrences following electrical cardioversion. *Arrhythm Electrophysiol Rev.* 2013;2(2):109–114.
12. Morbach C, Buck T, Rost C, et al. Point-of-care B-type natriuretic peptide and portable echocardiography for assessment of patients with suspected heart failure in primary care: rationale and design of the three-part Handheld-BNP program and results of the training study. *Clin Res Cardiol.* 2018;107(2):95–107.
13. Ghazal F, Theobald H, Rosenqvist M, Al-Khalili F. Assessment of N-terminal pro-B-type natriuretic peptide level in screening for atrial fibrillation in primary health care. *PLoS One.* 2019;14(2):e0212974.
14. Wasser K, Weber-Kruger M, Groschel S, et al. Brain natriuretic peptide and discovery of atrial fibrillation after stroke: a subanalysis of the find-AF(RANDOMISED) trial. *Stroke.* 2020;51(2):395–401.
15. Fonseca AC, Brito D, Pinho e Melo T, et al. N-terminal pro-brain natriuretic peptide shows diagnostic accuracy for detecting atrial fibrillation in cryptogenic stroke patients. *Int J Stroke.* 2014;9(4):419–425.

16. Bai J, Sun H, Xie L, Zhu Y, Feng Y. Detection of cardioembolic stroke with B-type natriuretic peptide or N-terminal pro-BNP: a comparative diagnostic meta-analysis. *Int J Neurosci.* 2018;128(11):1100–1108.
17. Pala E, Pagola J, Juega J, et al. B-type natriuretic peptide over N-terminal pro-brain natriuretic peptide to predict incident atrial fibrillation after cryptogenic stroke. *Eur J Neurol.* 2021; 28(2):540–547.
18. Wang F, Ruan ZB, Chen GC, Zhu JG, Zhu L. Effects of left atrial appendage closure on neuroendocrine function in patients with nonvalvular atrial fibrillation. *Med Sci Monit.* 2022;28:e937586.
19. Lakkireddy D, Turagam M, Afzal MR, et al. Left atrial appendage closure and systemic homeostasis: the Laa Homeostasis study. *J Am Coll Cardiol.* 2018;71(2):135–144.
20. Bartus K, Kanuri SH, Litwinowicz R, et al. Long term impact of epicardial left atrial appendage ligation on systemic Hemostasis: LAA HOMEOSTASIS-2. *J Clin Med.* 2022;11(6):1495–1504.
21. Luani B, Rauwolf T, Groscheck T, et al. Serial assessment of natriuretic peptides in patients undergoing interventional closure of the left atrial appendage. *Heart Lung Circ.* 2018;27(7):828–834.
22. Maggioni AP, Latini R, Carson PE, et al. Valsartan reduces the incidence of atrial fibrillation in patients with heart failure: results from the Valsartan Heart Failure Trial (Val-HeFT). *Am Heart J.* 2005;149(3):548–557.
23. Yang J, You L, Liu M, et al. Impact of left atrial appendage closure combined with catheter ablation on endocrine and mechanical cardiac function in patients with atrial fibrillation. *J Interv Cardiol.* 2022;2022:3932912.

43

Effect of Left Atrial Appendage Occlusion on Left Atrial Function and Electrophysiology

James L. Cox, Olga N. Kislitsina

CHAPTER OUTLINE

NORMAL LEFT ATRIAL FUNCTION

The major contribution of the left atrium (LA) to forward cardiac output is its function as a passive *capacitance* chamber, not as a *contracting* pumping chamber like the ventricles. Most of the changes in LA size and volume during a cardiac cycle are passive, and the left atrial muscle contracts only very briefly at the end of ventricular diastole, more like a "twitch" than a smooth prolonged contraction (Fig. 43.1). The mitral valve is fully open when the LA contracts, meaning that the afterload against which the LA contracts is minimum and corresponds to the earliest level of left ventricular diastolic pressure. This is not to imply that left atrial function is unimportant to cardiac hemodynamics, only that its importance is not primarily as a pump.

The physiologic relationship of atrial contraction to forward cardiac output is analogous to that of pushing a child on a swing (Fig. 43.2). Each time the swing reaches its apogee, a small tap on the back is sufficient to keep the swing in motion indefinitely. There is only a very light push ("tap") on the person on the swing, just as there is a very light push ("tap") of left atrial blood into the left ventricle during normal sinus rhythm. The critical component of keeping the child swinging is the precise *timing* of the tap on the back, not the forcefulness of the tap. Likewise, the critical component of optimizing the blood flow through the heart is the atrium's *synchrony* with the ventricle, not the strength of atrial contraction.

The misperception that a forceful atrial "kick" propels LA blood into the ventricle derives from the appearance of the emptying ("conduit") phase of the LA during early ventricular diastole. During left ventricular systole, the LA fills passively (reservoir phase) and therefore increases in size. When left ventricular diastole begins and the mitral valve opens, the blood in the LA reservoir is sucked into the left ventricle by contraction of the ventricle's spiral musculature,

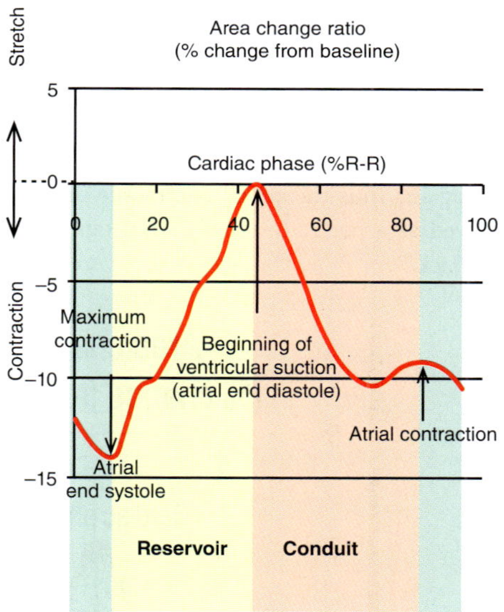

Fig. 43.1 Volume-time curve of normal left atrial function *(red line)*. Left atrial function is divided into three phases: reservoir phase *(yellow)*, conduit phase *(orange)*, and pump or contraction phase *(green)*. The reservoir phase of left atrial function begins when the mitral valve closes at the beginning of left ventricular systole and the end of left atrial systole. As the left atrium fills with blood from the pulmonary veins, it expands passively (upward slope of curve) until the end of atrial diastole (peak of curve). At that point, the mitral valve opens in response to left ventricular diastole. The LA passively decreases in size because of its blood being sucked into the ventricle during left ventricular diastole (conduit phase). Near the end of the passive conduit phase, the atrial muscle briefly contracts (pump phase) immediately before the beginning of left ventricular systole. *LV*, Left ventricle.

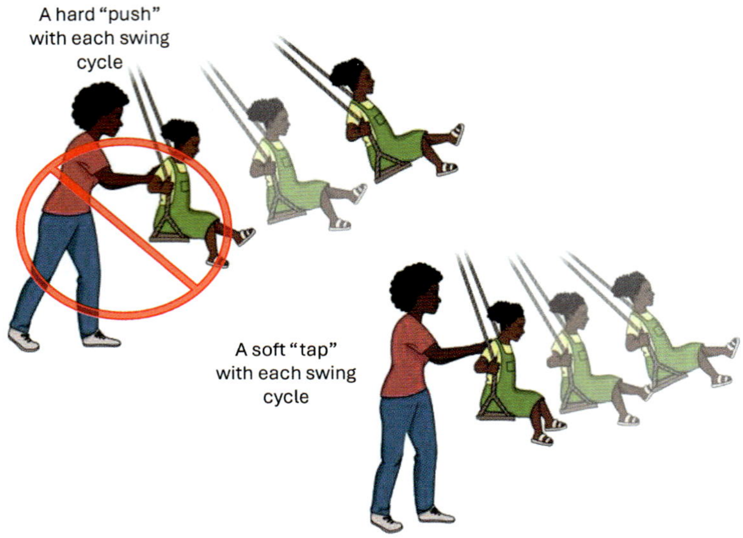

Fig. 43.2 The left atrium (LA) functions much like a person pushing a swing to keep it in motion. It is not necessary to push a swing hard with each swing cycle to keep it going *(upper panel)*. Rather, a perfectly timed light "tap" on the back of the person swinging is all that is required *(lower panel)*. Similarly, the LA does not create a forceful "kick" that propels blood from the LA into the left ventricle (LV) during a normal cardiac cycle. Rather, the LA provides a perfectly timed light "tap" just before closure of the mitral valve to optimize the delivery of blood from the LA into the LV. The vast majority of LA movement during normal sinus rhythm is passive.

so the LA passively and rapidly decreases in size (conduit phase). This dramatic visual movement of the atrium is commonly mistaken for "atrial systole," which implies forceful contraction of the atrium. However, the entire reservoir phase and the entire conduit phase of atrial function are passive. At the very end of the conduit phase, the left atrial muscle briefly contracts (the "tap") just before ventricular systole begins again. Thus the actual contractile function of the LA should be viewed as a perfectly timed "atrial tap" rather than as a forceful "atrial kick."

NORMAL LEFT ATRIAL APPENDAGE FUNCTION

The LA appendage (LAA) also participates in all three phases of overall left atrial function (Fig. 43.3). First, the appendage serves as an additional reservoir by passively expanding simultaneously with the body of the LA itself as blood enters the left heart from the pulmonary veins during ventricular systole (Fig. 43.4). Its contribution to the conduit function of the LA is less dramatic because its size usually changes little during the conduit phase (Fig. 43.5). Finally, the LAA contracts simultaneously with the body of the LA at the end of ventricular diastole (Fig. 43.6).

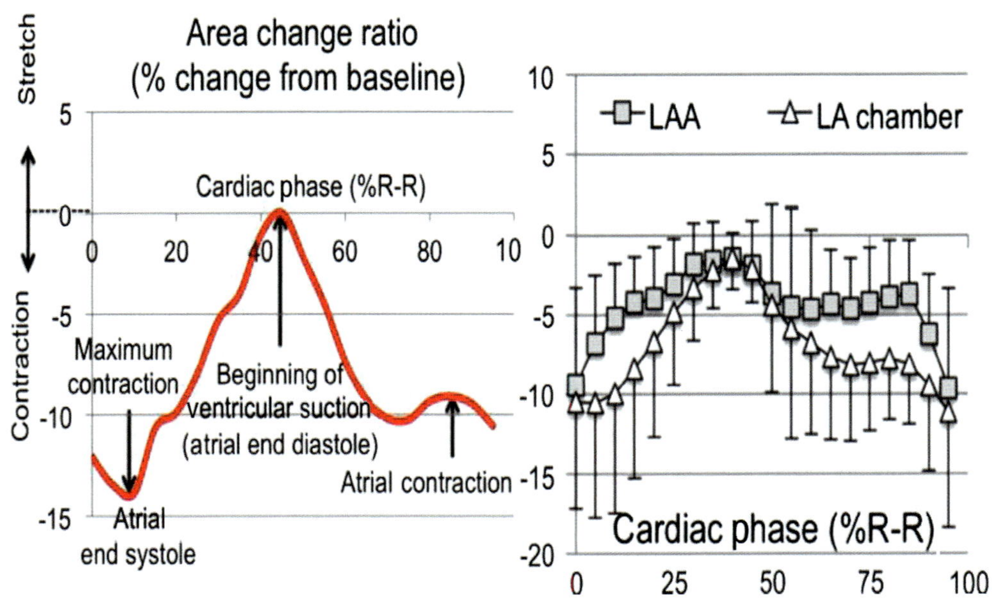

Fig. 43.3 *Left panel,* Normal volume-time curve of normal left atrial function during sinus rhythm including contributions from both the body of the left atrium (LA) and from the left atrial appendage (LAA). *Right panel,* Volume-time curves of both the body of the LA *(triangles)* and the LAA (squares). Note that the LAA contributes to all three phases of overall left atrial function.

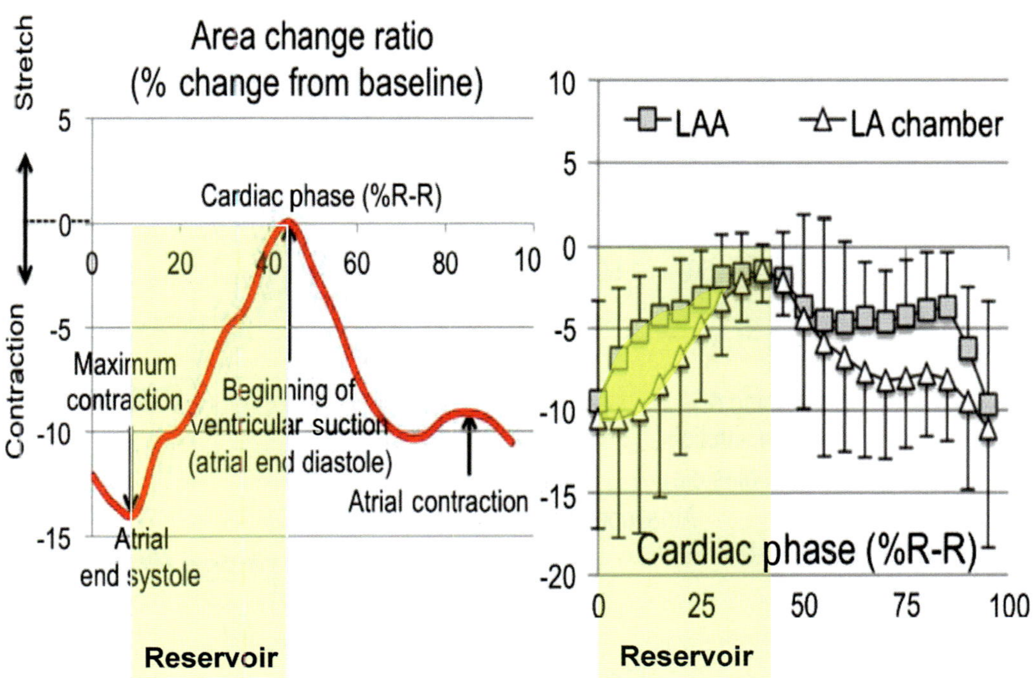

Fig. 43.4 *Left panel,* The reservoir phase of a normal volume-time curve of overall left atrial function is highlighted in *pale yellow. Right panel,* The reservoir phases of normal volume-time curves of the left atrium (LA) and LAA are highlighted in *pale yellow.* The additional contribution of the left atrial appendage (LAA) to overall left atrial reservoir function is denoted in *bright yellow.* This confirms that although the left atrial body is normally the most important capacitance chamber in the left heart, the LAA also functions normally as an additional capacitance chamber.

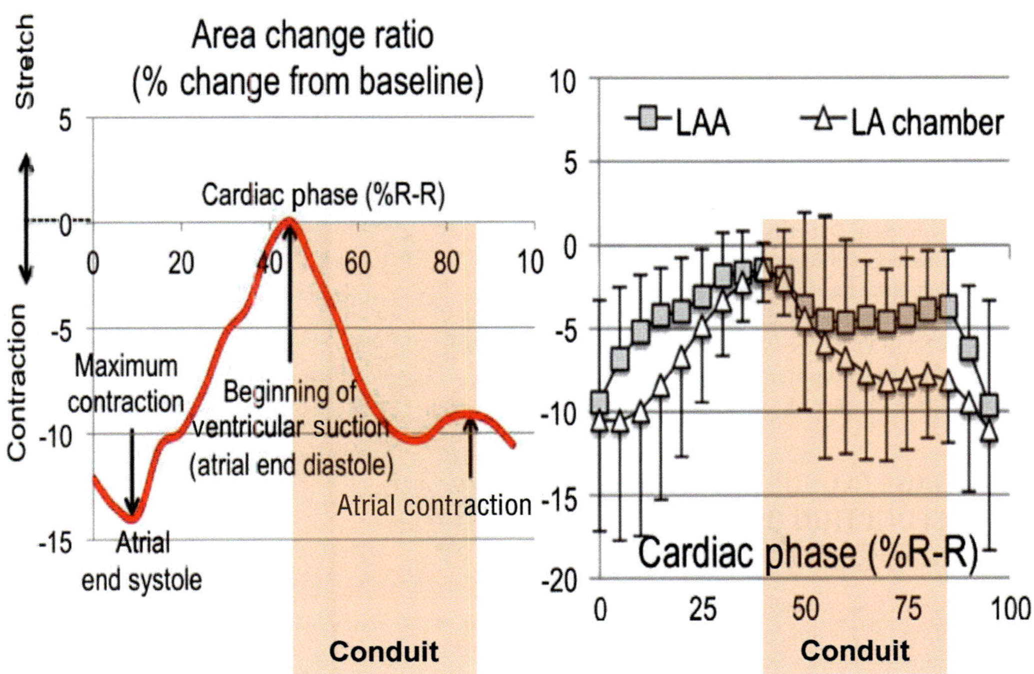

Fig. 43.5 *Left panel,* The conduit phase of a normal volume-time curve of overall left atrial function is highlighted in *orange. Right panel,* The conduit phases of normal volume-time curves of the left atrium (LA) and t atrial appendage (LAA) are highlighted in *orange.* The impact of the LAA on the conduit phase is less dramatic than it is on the reservoir phase of left atrial function as evidenced by the flattening of the volume-time curve of the LAA during the conduit phase.

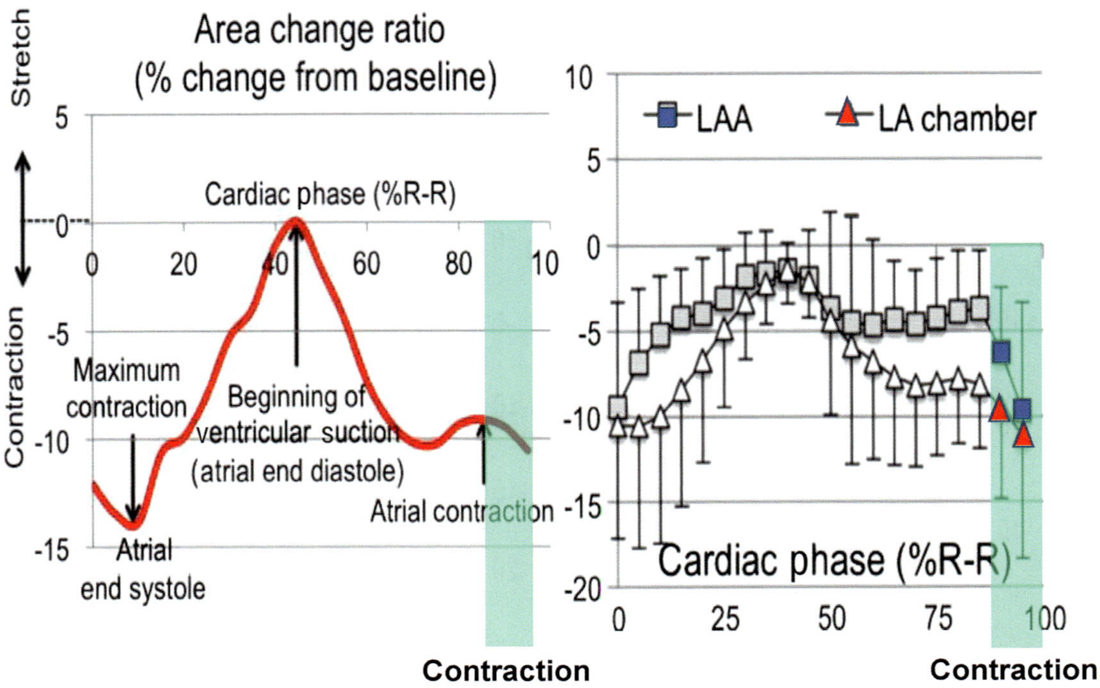

Fig. 43.6 *Left panel,* The pump (contraction) phase of a normal volume-time curve of overall left atrial function is highlighted in *green*. *Right panel,* The pump (contraction) phases of normal volume-time curves of the left atrium (LA) and the atrial appendage (LAA) are highlighted in *green*. Both the LA *(red triangles)* and the LAA *(blue squares)* actively contract very briefly after completion of the conduit phase, both serving as synchronized "taps" on the blood just before the mitral valve closes.

IMPACT OF LEFT ATRIAL APPENDAGE EXCLUSION ON LEFT ATRIAL FUNCTION

When catheter and surgical LAA occlusion (LAAO) became more routine for the prevention of strokes, there was concern that occlusion of the LAA would have a negative impact on postocclusion left atrial function. However in 2017, Coisne et al.[1] showed that percutaneous LAA endocardial closure with the Watchman device in a subset of patients in the PROTECT AF trial actually *improved* left atrial mechanical function by the Frank-Starling mechanism because of a modification of the LA loading conditions. The following year, Dar et al.[2] using two-dimensional speckle-tracking echocardiography to measure left atrial strain (see Chapter 7), showed that the left atrial reservoir function, conduit function, and booster function were all increased after epicardial closure of the LAA with a percutaneous LARIAT device (SentreHEART). In addition, these positive changes in LA function after LAA closure resulted in reverse remodeling of the LA (see Chapter 8).

LEFT ATRIAL APPENDAGE CLOSURE IN PATIENTS WITH DIASTOLIC DYSFUNCTION OF THE LEFT VENTRICLE

The effectiveness of LAA closure in decreasing the incidence of stroke in patients with atrial fibrillation (AF) is now settled science, although a stroke benefit of LAA closure in patients without AF has not been documented definitively (see Chapter 40). Nevertheless, documentation of the many benefits of LAA closure and easy access to the LAA during cardiac surgery has promoted the practice among some surgeons of amputating or closing the LAA in virtually all patients undergoing cardiac surgery.[3] However, in addition to the specific detrimental side-effects of amputating or closing the LAA described in Chapters 41 and 42, patients with significant diastolic dysfunction of the left ventricle can theoretically be permanently harmed by LAA closure. For example, in patients with giant LAAs (Fig. 43.7), the LA is often quite stiff and incapable of passive expansion during the reservoir phase. In such patients, the LAA may be the primary capacitance chamber, rather than the LA itself, and its amputation or closure can result in increased

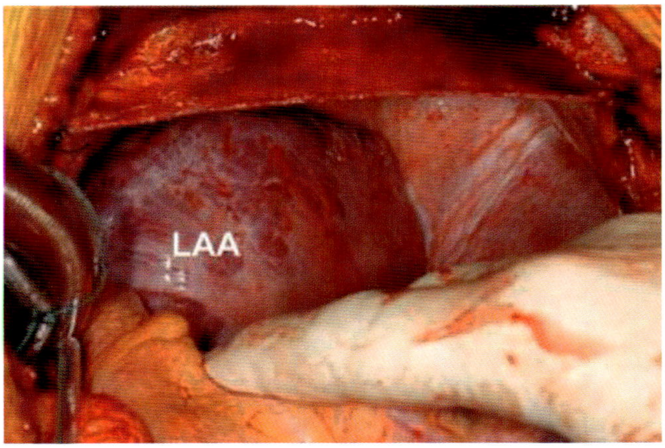

Fig. 43.7 Intraoperative photograph of a giant left atrial appendage (LAA). Because such large LAAs are often associated with stiff left atria, the LAA may be a more important capacitance chamber than the left atrium itself (LA). Therefore, one should be wary of amputating such a large LAA until the body of the LA alone has been documented to be sufficiently compliant. Otherwise, left atrial and pulmonary vasculature pressures may increase after LAA amputation, causing detrimental and irreversible cardiopulmonary sequelae. See text for further discussion.

pressure in the LA and the pulmonary vasculature. These patients can become profoundly short of breath after LAAO, and if they do, there is little that can be done to treat it.

The so-called "stiff LA syndrome" can be caused by infiltrative restrictive cardiomyopathies such as cardiac amyloidosis, cardiac sarcoidosis, and cardiac hemochromatosis, by hypertrophic obstructive cardiomyopathy, and by systemic hypertension.[4] All of these conditions affecting the left heart can cause diastolic dysfunction of the left ventricle, which can lead to loss of compliance in the LA. Amputation or closure of the LAA in these patients can lead to the same detrimental sequelae described earlier and should be done only sparingly if at all. In addition, patients who have undergone extensive radiofrequency catheter ablation for AF can develop a stiff LA[5] that can be problematic for subsequent LAA closure.

One should be particularly mindful of similar problems that can arise from closing the LAA in patients with AF and heart failure with preserved ejection fraction (HFpEF). It has been suggested that the same underlying cardiomyopathy may be causing fibrillation in the atria and HFpEF in the ventricles.[6] It is important to restore atrioventricular synchrony in patients with AF and heart failure with reduced EF (HFrEF) in which the primary problem is *left ventricular systolic dysfunction*. However, it is especially important to restore sinus rhythm in patients who have HFpEF in whom the primary problem is *left ventricular diastolic dysfunction*. However, LAAO should not be a part of AF treatment in patients with HFpEF unless it is deemed absolutely essential because the results can be especially detrimental in the presence of left ventricular diastolic dysfunction.

IMPACT OF LEFT ATRIAL APPENDAGE EXCLUSION ON THE RESULTS OF ATRIAL FIBRILLATION ABLATION

Percutaneous endocardial LAAO devices such as the Watchman (Boston Scientific) and Amulet (Abbott) occlude the LAA, but they do not electrically isolate the LAA myocardium. These devices that *occlude* the LAA but do not *exclude* the LAA myocardium have no effect on the results of catheter ablation for AF.[7] The only commercial devices that electrically isolate the LAA are the surgical AtriClip, the percutaneous LARIAT, and stapling devices, all of which are applied at the base of the LAA epicardially (Fig. 43.8).

Electrical isolation of the LAA

- Percutaneous LARIAT Device (Epicardial)
- Percutaneous Cryoballoon Ablation of LAA Base (Endocardial)
- Surgical AtriClip (Epicardial)
- Surgical Stapling Device (Epicardial)
- Surgical Cryoablation of LAA Base (Endocardial)
- Surgical Amputation

No electrical isolation of the LAA

- WATCHMAN Device (Endocardial)
- Amplatzer/Amulet Plug (Endocardial)
- All Other Percutaneous Endocardial Devices
- Surgical Endocardial Suture Closure

Fig. 43.8 There are multiple ways to close the left atrial appendage (LAA) for stroke prevention, but not all of them electrically isolate the LAA from the left atrium (LA). The only commercially available LAA closure devices that isolate the LAA electrically are the surgical AtriClip device, the percutaneous LARIAT device, and stapling devices. All of these devices are placed epicardially across the base of the LAA. None of the commercially available percutaneous endocardial closure devices electrically isolate the LAA from the LA.

Impact of Left Atrial Appendage Occlusion on the Results of Paroxysmal Atrial Fibrillation Ablation

In 2010, Di Biase and colleagues[8] demonstrated that up to 27% of patients presenting for repeat catheter ablation procedures had triggers in the LAA that were responsible for their recurrent AF. During either the initial or repeat AF catheter ablation procedure, they used an endocardial cryoballoon catheter to isolate the LAA in some of their patients by circumferential ablation of its base. Electrical isolation of the LAA in this manner resulted in a dramatic improvement in the success rate of AF ablation (Fig. 43.9).

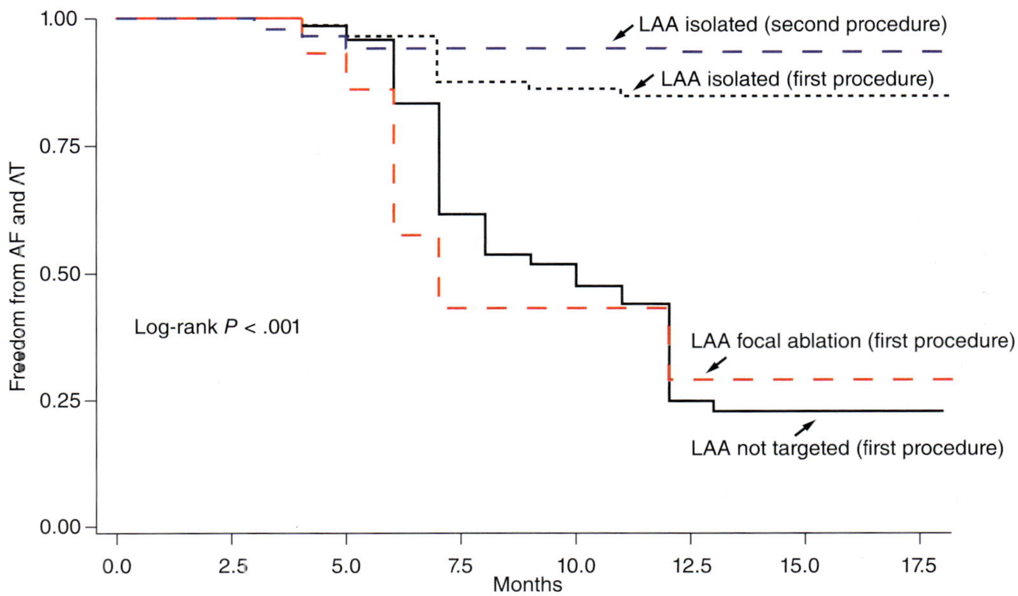

Fig. 43.9 Kaplan-Meier curves showing an improvement in the results of catheter ablation for atrial fibrillation (AF) when the ablation procedure is accompanied by electrical isolation of the left atrial appendage (LAA). See text for further discussion. *AT*, atrial tachycardia. (Reproduced from Di Biase L, Burkhardt JD, Mohanty P, et al. Left atrial appendage; an underrecognized trigger site of atrial fibrillation. *Circulation*. 2010;122(2):109–118.)

Experience has demonstrated that at least 10%, and perhaps more, of the atrial triggers that induce AF reside in the LAA (see Chapter 25). The LARIAT ligature is placed epicardially and therefore, it devascularizes the myocardium of the LAA (Fig. 43.10), causing ischemic myocardial necrosis and ultimate absorption of the dead appendage (Fig. 43.11).[9] The epicardial surgical AtriClip also devascularizes the myocardium of the LAA (Fig. 43.12), resulting in ischemic myocardial necrosis and absorption of the dead appendage (Fig. 43.13).[10] Therefore, it is to be expected that LAA amputation or LAA exclusion with either of the epicardial closure devices (percutaneous LARIAT or surgical AtriClip) would improve the results of the treatment of paroxysmal AF (PAF).

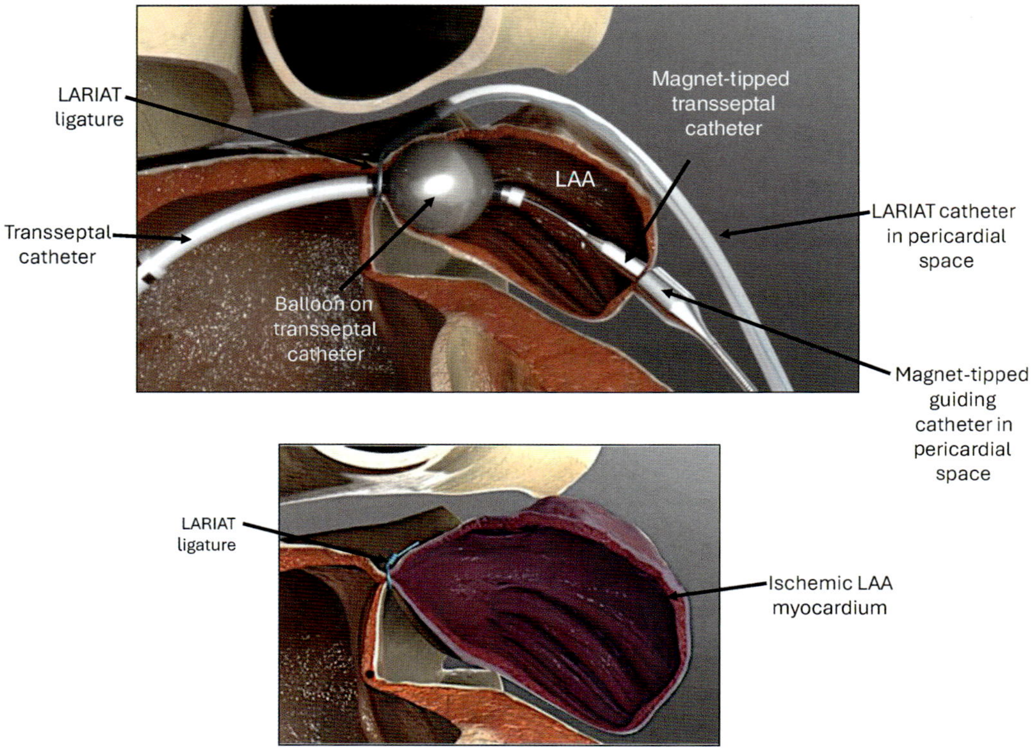

Fig. 43.10 *Upper panel,* LARIAT device for closing the left atrial appendage (LAA). A transseptal catheter with a magnetized tip and an inflatable balloon is placed across the atrial septum and positioned into the tip of the LAA. A catheter with a magnetized tip is then placed into the pericardial space by a "dry stick" of the pericardium in the subxiphoid area and guided into place by the magnetized catheter in the LAA. The balloon on the transseptal catheter is then inflated, and a second pericardial catheter with a loop (LARIAT) is guided over the LAA and positioned at the base of the LAA by closing it over the inflated balloon. *Lower panel,* After the ligature is secured, the LAA is electrically isolated from the left atrium because the LAA myocardium is ischemic. The myocardium of the LAA is devascularized *(purple)* by the epicardial LARIAT ligature.

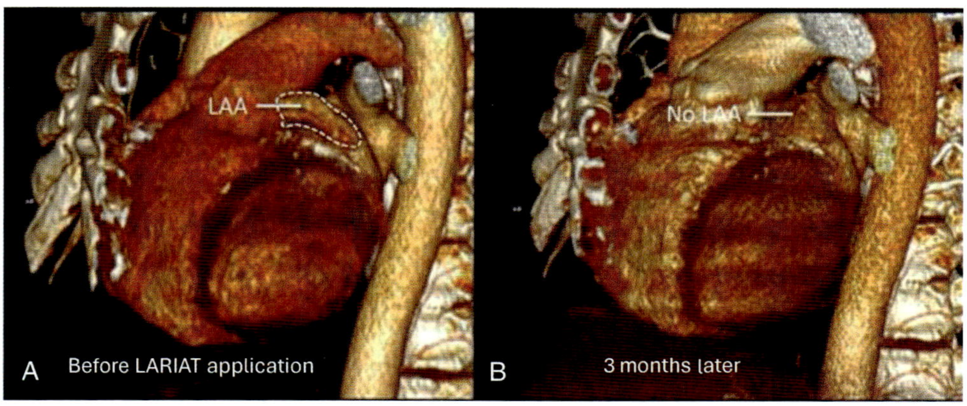

Fig. 43.11 (A) Image of the heart showing the left atrial appendage (LAA) before being closed with a percutaneous epicardial LARIAT device. The LAA is outlined by the *white dashed line.* (B) Three months after closing the LAA with the LARIAT device, the LAA has been completely resorbed. (Reproduced from Girota S, Murarka S, Eddin M, et al. Percutaneous suture ligation of left atrial appendage using the LARIAT device: a review of technique and current data. *Intervent Cardiol.* 2014;6(5):477–487.)

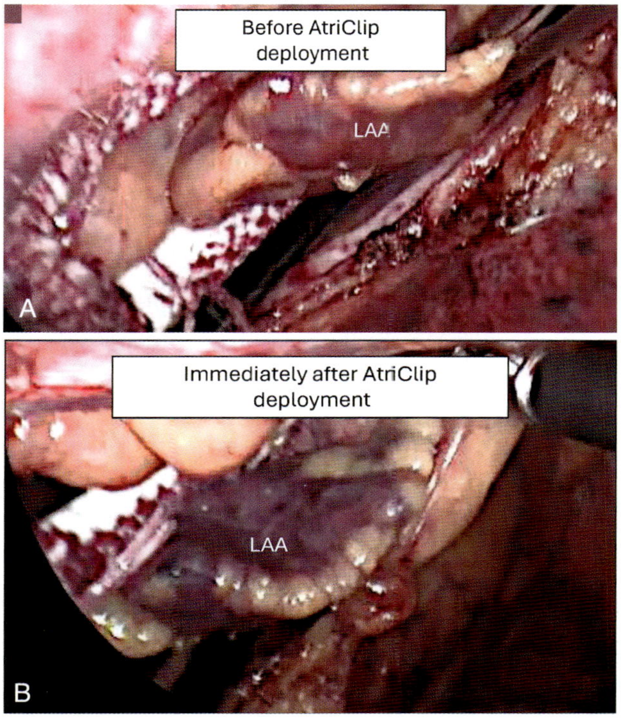

Fig. 43.12 Operative photographs during thoracoscopic closure of the left atrial appendage (LAA) with a surgical AtriClip. (A) The AtriClip device is in position but has not yet been deployed. Note the normal pink color of the LAA. (B) Immediately after deployment of the AtriClip, the LAA changes to a dark blue color, indicating that the LAA myocardium has been made ischemic by the AtriClip. The LAA is not only occluded but is now electrically isolated from the left atrium as well.

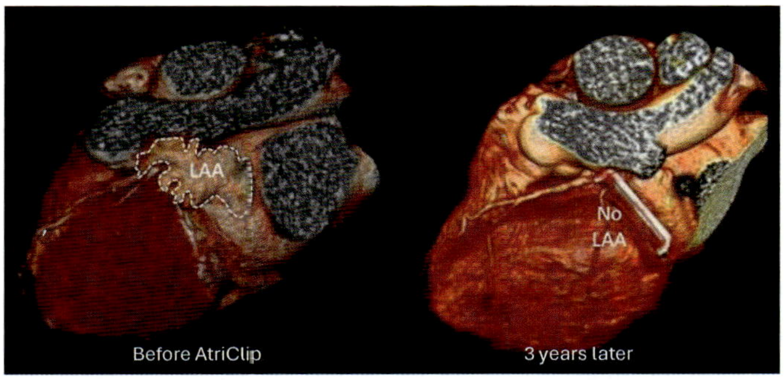

Fig. 43.13 *Left panel,* Image of a large left atrial appendage (LAA) before closing it epicardially with a surgical AtriClip device. The LAA is outlined by the *white dashed line. Right panel,* Three years after the LAA shown in the *left panel* was closed with an AtriClip device. The LAA has undergone necrosis and has been completely resorbed. (Modified from Ailawadi G, Gerdisch MW, Harvey RL, et al. Exclusion of the left atrial appendage with a novel device: early results of a multicenter trial. *J Thor Cardiovasc Surg.* 2011;142:1002–1009.)

Impact of Left Atrial Appendage Occlusion on the Results of Nonparoxysmal Atrial Fibrillation Ablation

Yorgun et al.[11] reported a 20% improvement in the results of pulmonary vein isolation (PVI) for persistent AF when electrical isolation of the LAA was added. In 2015, a report on the LAALA-AF Registry showed that in patients with persistent AF, the addition of LAA ligation with the LARIAT device to conventional AF ablation improved the success rate of AF ablation by approximately 25% (Fig. 43.14).[12] It

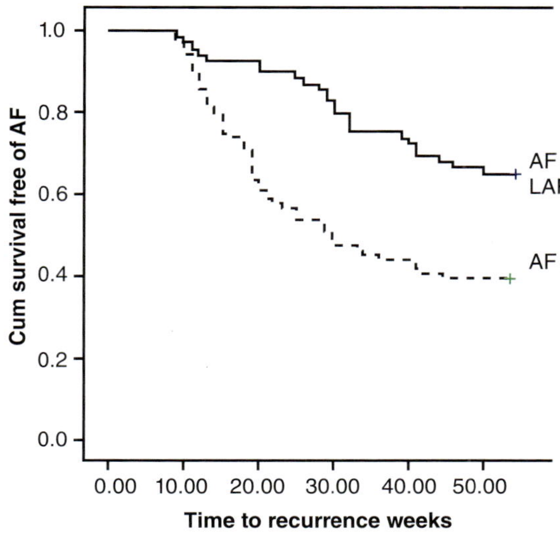

Fig. 43.14 Graph showing the freedom from atrial fibrillation (AF) after catheter ablation for AF when the ablation procedure is accompanied by electrical isolation of the left atrial appendage (LAA) using a percutaneous epicardial LARIAT device. See text for further discussion. (Reproduced from Lakkireddy D, Mahankali AS, Kanmanthareddy A, et al. Left atrial appendage ligation and ablation for persistent atrial fibrillation: the LAALA-AF registry. *JACC Clin Electrophysiol.* 2015;1(3):153–160.)

is critical to recall that nonparoxysmal AF (non-PAF) is dependent on macro-reentrant drivers to sustain it, not on the AF triggers that induce it. Therefore, the increased success rates for non-PAF ablation after LAAO or LAA exclusion reported in these two observational studies suggest that 20% to 25% of the macro-reentrant drivers of non-PAF use the LAA as at least a part of their reentrant circuit. Undoubtedly, some of the AF drivers do use the LAA, but there is no evidence other than these observational studies that 20% to 25% of the macro-reentrant drivers of AF are dependent on the LAA.

Because these observations were somewhat suspect, a multicenter, prospective, open label, randomized clinical trial (the aMAZE trial) was designed to determine definitively whether or not LAA exclusion with the LARIAT device improved the results of non-PAF ablation.[13] The study included 404 patients randomized to undergo PVI plus LAAO with the percutaneous LARIAT device, and 206 patients were randomized to undergo PVI only for the treatment of *non-PAF.* The trial showed that there was no significant difference in the success rates for the ablation of *non-PAF* between the two groups. In other words, LAAO with the LARIAT device did not improve the results of the ablation of non-PAF.

Unfortunately, the misinterpretation of the results of this clinical trial was that "LAAO with an epicardial LARIAT device does not improve the results of AF ablation." Again, confusion has resulted because so many practitioners fail to distinguish between the treatment of PAF and non-PAF in analyzing the results of AF intervention. It is critical to note that *the aMAZE trial did not include any patients with PAF,* which is the only group in which LAAO enhancement of AF ablation results should be expected.

The reason that LAA isolation by either amputation or epicardial device exclusion improves the results of PAF ablation is that it eliminates at least 10%, and more in some patients, of the atrial triggers responsible for PAF (Fig. 43.15). The reason that LAA isolation by either amputation or epicardial device exclusion does *not* improve the results of non-PAF ablation is that few, if any, of the macro-reentrant drivers that sustain non-PAF involve the LAA (Fig. 43.16).

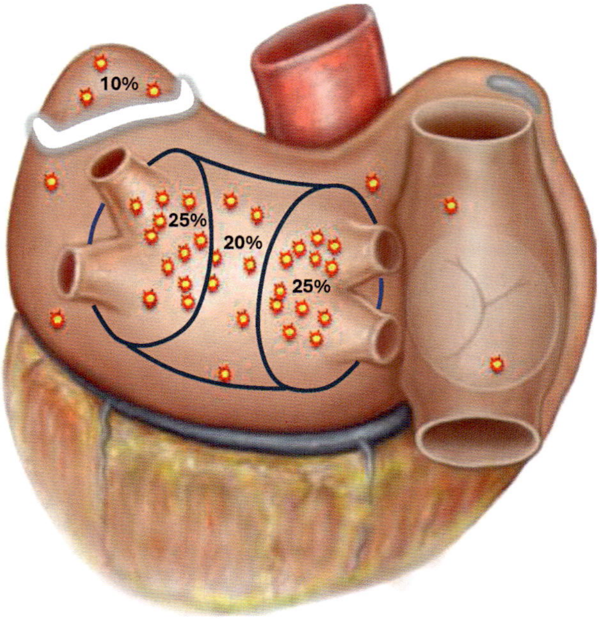

Fig. 43.15 Relative distribution of atrial triggers that induce repeated episodes of atrial fibrillation (AF) in patients with paroxysmal AF (PAF). The left atrial appendage (LAA) harbors at least 10% of these AF triggers and may harbor many more in some patients. Amputation or exclusion of the left atrial appendage (LAA) with an epicardial occlusion device decreases the episodes of AF in proportion to the number of AF triggers residing in the LAA in a given patient with PAF. This is why LAA amputation or LAA closure with an AtriClip or LARIAT device improves the results of PAF ablation.

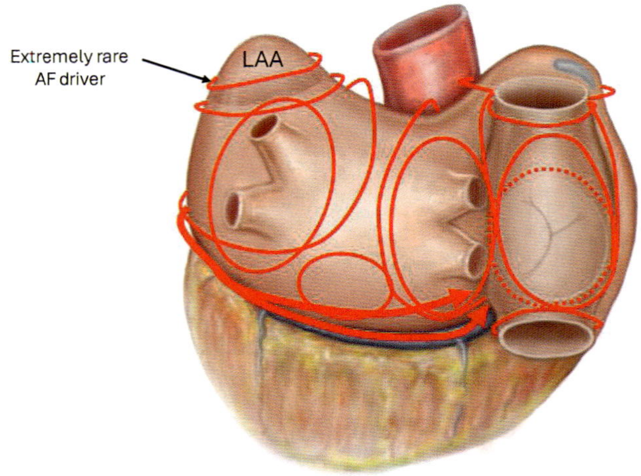

Fig. 43.16 Locations of atrial macro-reentrant drivers in nonparoxysmal atrial fibrillation (non-PAF). In contrast to potential left atrial appendage (LAA) triggers in patients with paroxysmal AF (PAF), the macro-reentrant drivers that sustain non-PAF can occur only in certain areas of the heart depending on their size, wavefront conduction velocity, and local atrial refractory periods. This diagram depicts the locations in the atria where these macro-reentrant drivers have been mapped or can theoretically occur. Very few of these macro-reentrant drivers are located in the LAA or use it as a part of their reentrant circuit. This is the reason why epicardial exclusion with an AtriClip or LARIAT device, or amputation cannot be expected to decrease the likelihood that AF will be sustained in patients with non-PAF. Despite several observational studies suggesting otherwise, the multicenter, prospective, randomized, controlled aMAZE trial showed that epicardial exclusion of the LAA did not improve the results of non-PAF ablation.

Atrial Fibrillation Ablation Only Versus Left Atrial Appendage Occlusion Only Versus Atrial Fibrillation Ablation Plus Left Atrial Appendage Occlusion

Some respected authorities have suggested that because LAAO not only excludes the LAA from the systemic circulation but also electrically isolates it from the rest of the heart, LAAO is as effective in reducing stroke and improving survival as the surgical ablation of AF (see Chapter 46).[14,15] This suggests that once the LAA has been excluded, it no longer matters if the patient is in sinus rhythm or in AF in terms of subsequent stroke rate and survival. This logic rests on the erroneous notion that patients who are in AF with nonoccluded LAAs but who do not have a stroke (which is the vast majority of patients with AF) have the same stroke rates and survival rates as patients in sinus rhythm who do not have strokes. Of course, this is not true because in the case of stoke rates, this would mean that every stroke that occurs in a patient with AF would have to be caused by thromboembolism from the LAA. In the case of survival rates, it would mean that the only way AF can cause death is by a stroke caused by thromboembolism from the LAA. Obviously, neither of those concepts is correct because the basic suggestion is incorrect. Thus it is potentially harmful to patients to perpetuate the misconception that the only surgical procedure that impacts the stroke rate and survival rate in patients with AF is closure of the LAA.

Two recent studies have compared the relative impact of surgical AF ablation and LAAO on 5-year survival rates. The first was by a 2023 study by Mehaffey and colleagues[16] at West Virginia University, who compared the survival results of the surgical ablation of AF without LAAO (surgical ablation only), with LAAO only, with surgical ablation plus LAAO in 100,000 Medicare patients. Their study clearly refutes the suggestion that simply closing the LAA is the procedure of choice for treating patients with AF because it showed the clear superiority of combined surgical AF ablation and LAAO. The 3-year survival rate after surgical ablation of AF combined with LAAO was superior to either surgical ablation alone or LAAO alone (Fig. 43.17). It is noteworthy that all iterations of the Maze procedure fall into this surgical ablation plus LAAO category. The second study came from the KROK Polish Registry that compared the 6-year survival rates after the same three interventions in nearly 34,000 patients.[17] Again, the combination of surgical AF ablation and LAAO was superior to both LAAO only and surgical ablation only (Fig. 43.18).

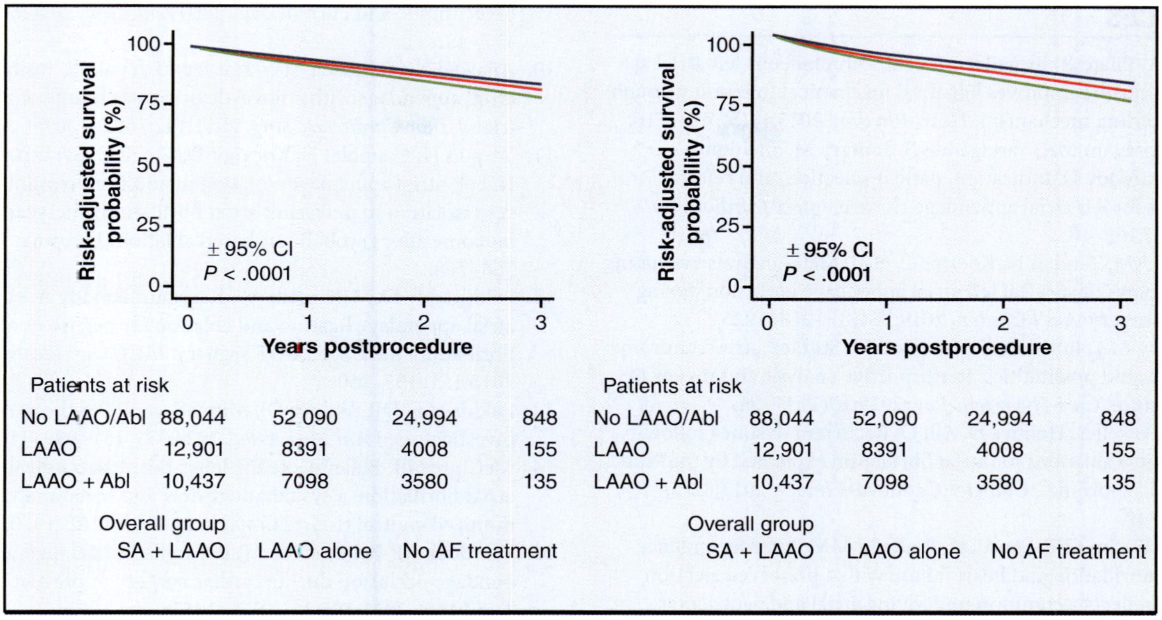

Fig. 43.17 In a large registry-based analysis, atrial fibrillation (AF)–directed interventions (isolated surgical ablation [SA], isolated left atrial appendage occlusion [LAAO], and combined SA plus LAAO) surpassed no treatment in 6-year survival rate. The strongest benefit was associated with combined treatment trailed by SA only and LAAO only. This study advocates SA plus LAAO for preoperative AF in cardiac surgery. (Reproduced from Mehaffey JH, Hayanga A, Wei L, Mascio C, Rankin JS, Badhwar V. Surgical ablation of atrial fibrillation is associated with improved survival compared with appendage obliteration alone: an analysis of 100,000 Medicare beneficiaries. *J Thor Cardiovasc Surg*. 2023;168(1):104–116.)

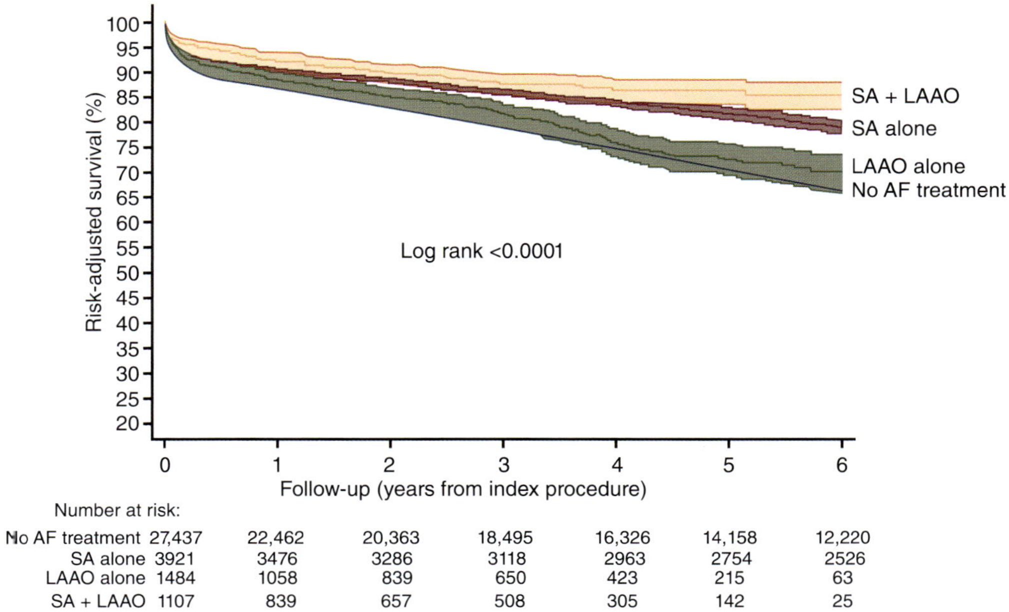

Fig. 43.18 The KROK Polish Registry comparison of the survival of concomitant atrial fibrillation (AF) surgical patients in whom the AF was treated by surgical ablation (SA) alone, left atrial appendage occlusion (LAAO) alone, SA plus LAAO, or no treatment. Note that the combination of SA plus LAAO was superior to either SA alone or LAAO alone. (Reproduced from Pasierski M, Batko J, Kuxma L, et al. Surgical ablation, left atrial appendage occlusion or both? Nationwide registry analysis of cardiac surgery patients with underlying atrial fibrillation. *Eur J Cardio-Thorac Surg*. 2024;65(3):ezae014.)

REFERENCES

1. Coisne A, Pilato R, Brigadeau F, et al. Percutaneous left atrial appendage closure improves left atrial mechanical function through Frank-Starling mechanism. *Heart Rhythm*. 2017;14(5):710–716.
2. Dar T, Turagam MK, Yarlagadda B, Tantary M, Sheldonn SH, Lakkireddy D. Indication, patient selection, and referral pathways for left atrial appendage closure. *Interv Cardiol Clin*. 2018;7(2):169–183.
3. Ibrahim AM, Tandan N, Koester C, et al. Meta-analysis evaluating the outcomes of surgical left atrial appendage occlusion during cardiac surgery. *Am J Cardiol*. 2019;124(8):1218–1225.
4. Chaudhry MA, Johnson A, Heywood JT. Stiff left atrial syndrome: prospects and possibilities. Retrospective analysis and review of the literature. *Curr Hypertens Rev*. 2019;15(1):17–21.
5. Witt C, Powell B, Holmes D, Alli O. Recurrent dyspnea following multiple ablations for atrial fibrillation explained by the "stiff left atrial syndrome.". *Catheter Cardiovasc Interv*. 2013;82(5): E747–E749.
6. Packer M, Lam CSP, Lund LH, Redfield MM. Interdependence of atrial fibrillation and heart failure with a preserved ejection fraction reflects a common underlying atrial and ventricular myopathy. *Circulation*. 2020;141:4–6.
7. Lakkireddy D, Turagam M, Afzai MR, et al. Left atrial appendage closure and systemic homeostasis: the LAA HOMEOSTASIS study. *J Am Coll Card*. 2018;71:135–144.
8. Di Biase L, Burkhardt JD, Mohanty P, et al. Left atrial appendage: an underrecognized trigger site of atrial fibrillation. *Circulation*. 2010;122(2):109–118.
9. Girota S, Murarka S, Eddin M, et al. Percutaneous suture ligation of left atrial appendage using the LARIAT device: a review of technique and current data. *Intervent Card*. 2014;6(5): 477–487.
10. Ailawadi G, Gerdisch MW, Harvey RL, et al. Exclusion of the left atrial appendage with a novel device: early results of a multicenter trial. *J Thor Cardiovasc Surg*. 2011;142:1002–1009.
11. Yorgun H, Canpolat U, Kocyigit D, Coteli C, Evranos B, Aytemir K. Left atrial appendage isolation in addition to pulmonary vein isolation in persistent atrial fibrillation: one-year clinical outcome after cryoballoon-based ablation. *Europace*. 2017;19: 758–768.
12. Lakkireddy D, Mahankali AS, Kanmanthareddy A, et al. Left atrial appendage ligation and ablation for persistent atrial fibrillation: the LAALA-AF registry. *JACC Clin Electrophysiol*. 2015;1(3):153–160.
13. Lakkireddy DR, Wilber DJ, Mittal S, et al. For the amaze investigators. *J Am Med Assoc*. 2024;331(13):1099–1108.
14. McClure GR, Belley-Cote EP, Jaffer IH, et al. Surgical ablation of atrial fibrillation: a systematic review and meta-analysis of randomized control trials. *Europace*. 2018;20:1442–1450.
15. Whitlock RP, Belley-Cote EP, Paparella D, et al. Left atrial appendage occlusion during cardiac surgery to prevent stroke. *N Eng J Med*. 2021;385(11):1054–1055.
16. Mehaffey JH, Hayanga A, Wei L, Mascio C, Rankin JS, Badhwar V. Surgical ablation of atrial fibrillation is associated with improved survival compared with appendage obliteration alone: an analysis of 100,000 Medicare beneficiaries. *J Thor Cardiovasc Surg*. 2023;168(1):104–116.
17. Pasierski M, Batko J, Kuxma L, et al. Surgical ablation, left atrial appendage occlusion or both? Nationwide registry analysis of cardiac surgery patients with underlying atrial fibrillation. *Eur J Cardio-Thorac Surg*. 2024;65(3):ezae014.

The AtriClip Device and Long-Term Results of Left Atrial Appendage Closure

Sacha P. Salzberg, Etem Caliskan, Maximilian Y. Emmert

CHAPTER OUTLINE

Left atrial appendage (LAA) amputation for stroke prevention in atrial fibrillation (AF) was initially described by Madden et al. in 1948.[1] Since then, surgeons have used different approaches to deal with the LAA over time. However, it was not until the early 2000s that a team at the Cleveland Clinic developed an epicardial device specifically for mechanical closure of the LAA, a device that was initially known as the CG-Clip.[2] This clip went through several changes during its development phase, eventually evolving into the AtriClip device (AtriCure, Inc., Mason, OH).

The complete LAA Clip System includes a self-closing, implantable clip and a disposable measuring guide to determine the optimal clip size to use clinically from a choice of four options (35, 40, 45, or 50 mm). When deployed in its fully closed position, the epicardial AtriClip applies uniform and continuous pressure to the LAA throughout its length to ensure consistent, reproducible, secure occlusion of the base of the LAA (Fig. 44.1).[3] Because the AtriClip is applied epicardially, it devascularizes the myocardium of the LAA and therefore accomplishes not only mechanical closure of the LAA but also electrical isolation of the LAA from the remainder of the heart. The AtriClip can be applied during open cardiac surgery via a median sternotomy, thoracotomy, or thoracoscopically during minimally invasive cardiac surgery (Fig. 44.2).

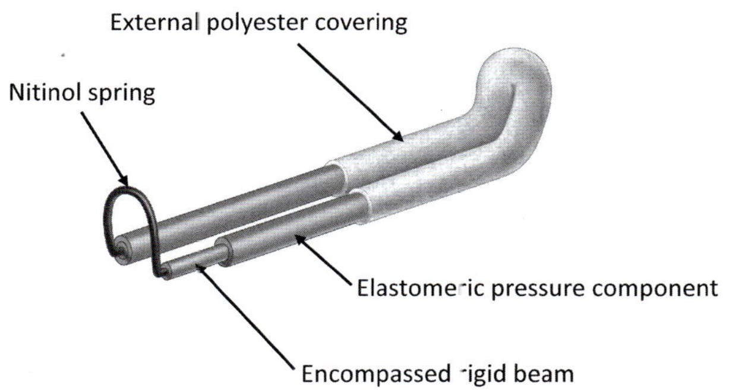

Fig. 44.1 AtriClip construction. The AtriClip consists of two rigid components facing each other that are kept closed by continuous dynamic inward pressure caused by a nitinol spring mechanism and the elastomeric pressure components. The encompassed rigid beams and the rigid elastomeric beams combine to aid in the remodeling of the closed left atrial appendage orifice inside the left atrium. Additionally, the external polyester covering adds friction and promotes full encapsulation by the surrounding structures to ensure that the AtriClip stays anchored at its original implantation site and does not migrate over time.

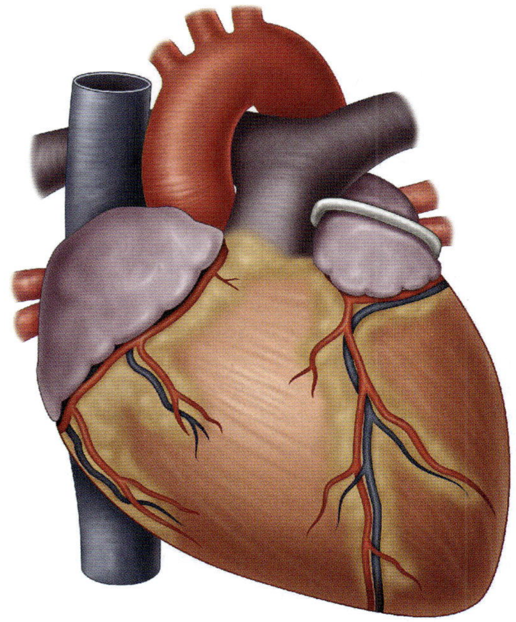

Fig. 44.2 An AtriClip properly deployed across the base of the left atrial appendage.

LONG-TERM RESULTS OF ATRICLIP CLOSURE OF THE LEFT ATRIAL APPENDAGE

Extensive preclinical evaluation showed that the AtriClip device was safe and effective for LAA occlusion (LAAO), and this led to the first human application of the AtriClip device, which we performed in Zurich in 2009.[3,4] The AtriClip device was subsequently deployed successfully as a concomitant procedure in our series of 34 patients undergoing elective open cardiac surgery who had a prior history of AF and ongoing stroke prevention treatment with oral anticoagulants.[5] Serial 3-month computed tomography (CT) scans after LAAO with the AtriClip confirmed that the LAA was completely closed in all patients with no evidence of residual reperfusion of the LAA. In addition, all AtriClips remained at their original site of implantation with no interim migration, and no patient had a stroke or transient ischemic attack (TIA) during or after LAA closure.

In 2011, Ailawadi et al.[6] reported a multicenter US Food and Drug Administration trial to determine the safety and efficacy of the AtriClip device in 71 patients undergoing elective cardiac surgery.[6] At 3-month follow-up, no adverse events or device-related perioperative deaths had occurred. Complete closure of the LAA, confirmed by either CT angiography (CTA) or transesophageal echocardiography, was accomplished in 98.4% (60 of 61) of patients with the AtriClip device. This study again showed that the AtriClip device was safe and atraumatic with a greater than 95% successful closure rate and excellent short-term durability.

In 2018, our group reported the long-term AtriClip data on 251 consecutive patients, including all patients from our first-in-human prospective trial and our institutional registry.[7] We used CT scans to assess the safety, efficacy, and long-term durability of epicardial AtriClip LAA closure and its subsequent impact on stroke prevention in patients with AF undergoing cardiac surgery. The LAA was successfully excluded in all patients during a mean follow-up of 36 ± 23 months. No device-related complications occurred, and CT imaging in patients 5 years or more after implant revealed complete LAAO with no signs of residual reperfusion or significant residual LAA pouches. Patients with discontinued oral anticoagulation (n = 166) experienced a relative risk reduction of 87.5% with an observed ischemic stroke rate of 0.5 per 100 patient-years compared with an expected ischemic stroke rate of 4.0 per 100 patient-years in patients with similar CHA_2DS_2-VASc scores. In a subsequent retrospective analysis of 291 patients from this study cohort, 43 patients had available postoperative short-term and long-term follow-up by CTA. Both residual LAA patency and the presence of residual LAA pouches were assessed by two-dimensional multiplanar reconstructions, maximum intensity projection images, and volume as determined by three-dimensional CT reconstructions.[8] At a mean follow-up period of 7.1 ± 0.8 years after AtriClip LAAO, there was no residual connection between the left atrium and the LAA in any patient. CTA revealed no residual LAA pouch in 72% (31 of 43) of patients, insignificant (<10 mm) residual pouches in 26% (11 of 43) of patients, and a significant residual pouch (>10 mm) in one patient (2%) with a residual pouch that measured 12 mm in depth.

Ellis et al.[9] used CTA to assess long-term outcomes when the AtriClip was applied via a totally thoracoscopic approach. They reported a complete occlusion rate of 93.9% and no major complications during a mean follow-up period of 34.3 months after thoracoscopic AtriClip closure of the LAA.[9] Kurfirst et al.[10] reported a successful AtriClip LAA closure rate of 98% in 101 patients over a follow-up period of 18 ± 11 months. In that series, the AtriClip was applied via a sternotomy, thoracotomy, or thoracoscopically. There were no clip migration, no leakage around the clip, and no thrombus formation near any small remnant pouch. Toale et al.[11] performed a metaanalysis of 11 studies that included 922 patients who underwent LAA closure with an AtriClip device. Successful closure was accomplished in 97.8% (902 of 922) of patients with no device-related adverse events. The incidence of stroke or TIA after AtriClip LAA closure ranged from 0.2 to 1.5 per 100 patient-years. The authors concluded that the concomitant or stand-alone application of an AtriClip device is safe and effective for the management of patients with AF undergoing cardiac surgery. In 2012, Starck et al.[12] reported that epicardial LAAO with an AtriClip device leads to the acute electrical isolation of the LAA and suggested additionally that it may reduce the recurrence of AF.

The AtriClip device has now been successfully deployed in more than 500,000 patients worldwide. However, the largest cohort yet published consisted of only 291 patients, reflecting the problematic lack of available long-term data in large patient cohorts. Unfortunately, the largest randomized controlled trial assessing surgical LAA closure to date, the LAAOS III trial, did not include detailed information on the deployment rate of the AtriClip device within the surgical arm of the study, so its long-term outcomes could not be compared with other LAAO strategies.[13,14]

SUMMARY

The AtriClip provides safe, durable, and reproducible electrical and mechanical exclusion of the LAA. Recent milestone advances in the field of LAA closure have led to its incorporation into both the 2020 European Society of Cardiology/European Association for Cardio-Thoracic Surgery and the 2023 American College of Cardiology/American Heart Association/American College of Clinical Pharmacy/Heart Rhythm Society Guidelines for the Diagnosis and Management of Atrial Fibrillation.[15,16]

REFERENCES

1. Madden JL. Resection of the left auricular appendix: a prophylaxis for recurrent arterial emboli. *J Am Med Assoc.* 1949;140(9):769–772.
2. Kamohara K, Fukamachi K, Ootaki Y, et al. A novel device for left atrial appendage exclusion. *J Thorac Cardiovasc Surg.* 2005;130(6):1639–1644.
3. Fumoto H, Gillinov AM, Ootaki Y, et al. A novel device for left atrial appendage exclusion: the third-generation atrial exclusion device. *J Thorac Cardiovasc Surg.* 2008;136(4):1019–1027.
4. Salzberg SP, Gillinov AM, Anyanwu A, Castillo J, Filsoufi F, Adams DH. Surgical left atrial appendage occlusion: evaluation of a novel device with magnetic resonance imaging. *Eur J Cardio-Thorac Surg.* 2008;34(4):766–770.
5. Salzberg SP, Plass A, Emmert MY, et al. Left atrial appendage clip occlusion: early clinical results. *J Thorac Cardiovasc Surg.* 2010;139(5):1269–1274.
6. Ailawadi G, Gerdisch MW, Harvey RL, et al. Exclusion of the left atrial appendage with a novel device: early results of a multicenter trial. *J Thorac Cardiovasc Surg.* 2011;142(5):1002–1009.
7. Caliskan E, Sahin A, Yilmaz M, et al. Epicardial left atrial appendage AtriClip occlusion reduces the incidence of stroke in patients with atrial fibrillation undergoing cardiac surgery. *Europace.* 2018;20(7):e105–e114.
8. Caliskan E, Eberhard M, Falk V, Alkadhi H, Emmert MY. Incidence and characteristics of left atrial appendage stumps after device-enabled epicardial closure. *Interact Cardiovasc Thorac Surg.* 2019;29(5):663–669.
9. Ellis CR, Aznaurov SG, Patel NJ, et al. Angiographic efficacy of the AtriClip left atrial appendage exclusion device placed by minimally invasive thoracoscopic approach. *JACC Clin Electrophysiol.* 2017;3(12):1356–1365.
10. Kurfirst V, Mokracek A, Canadyova J, Frana R, Zeman P. Epicardial clip occlusion of the left atrial appendage during cardiac surgery provides optimal surgical results and long-term stability. *Interact Cardiovasc Thorac Surg.* 2017;25(1):37–40.

11. Toale C, Fitzmaurice GJ, Eaton D, Lyne J, Redmond KC. Outcomes of left atrial appendage occlusion using the AtriClip device: a systematic review. *Interact Cardiovasc Thorac Surg.* 2019;29(5):655–662.
12. Starck CT, Steffel J, Emmert MY, et al. Epicardial left atrial appendage clip occlusion also provides the electrical isolation of the left atrial appendage. *Interact Cardiovasc Thorac Surg.* 2012;15(3):416–418.
13. Whitlock RP, Belley-Cote EP, Paparella D, et al. Left atrial appendage occlusion during cardiac surgery to prevent stroke. *N Eng J Med.* 2021:2081–2091.
14. Caliskan E, Falk V, Emmert MY. Left atrial appendage occlusion during cardiac surgery to prevent stroke. *N Engl J Med.* 2021;385(11):1054.
15. Hindricks G, Potpara T, Dagres N, et al. 2020 ESC guidelines for the diagnosis and management of atrial fibrillation developed in collaboration with the European Association for Cardio-Thoracic Surgery (EACTS). *Eur Heart J.* 2021;42(5):373–498.
16. Joglar JA, Chung MK, Armbruster AL, et al. 2023 ACC/AHA/ACCP/HRS guideline for the diagnosis and management of atrial fibrillation: a report of the American College of Cardiology/American Heart Association Joint Committee on clinical practice guidelines. *Circulation.* 2024;149(1):e1–e156.

45

Totally Thoracoscopic Left Atrial Appendage Occlusion

Stefano Benussi, Fabrizio Rosati, Stefano Branzoli, Giuseppe D´Ancona

CHAPTER OUTLINE

The unique anatomic configuration of the left atrial appendage (LAA) inherently increases the risk of thrombus formation in patients with atrial fibrillation (AF), with nearly 90% of left atrial thrombi being discovered within its intricate trabeculations.[1] Oral anticoagulation (OAC) is the first-line therapy for thromboembolic prevention, although the increased risk of bleeding is considered a potential contraindication to long-term anticoagulation in high-risk patients.[2] Thus mechanical LAA closure, either via a percutaneous or surgical approach, has gained popularity over the past decade not only for thromboembolic risk control but also for its possible impact on AF ablation.

Although the overall evidence has yielded mixed results and professional guidelines continue to evolve based on emerging data, percutaneous approaches to LAA closure have thus far failed to show a clear benefit in preventing thromboembolic cerebrovascular events compared with OAC. The combined 5-year outcomes of the two landmark trials, PREVAIL and PROTECT AF, have demonstrated that percutaneous LAA occlusion (LAAO) with the Watchman device (Boston Scientific) provides a level of overall stroke prevention in non-valvular AF that is comparable to that of warfarin. This includes, however, a reduction in hemorrhagic stroke, other significant bleeding, and mortality with the percutaneous Watchman device.[3] The recent randomized trial PRAGUE-17 compared percutaneous LAAO with the Watchman and Amulet (Abbott Medical) devices with the most updated direct AOC treatment.[4] The 4-year outcomes confirm non-inferiority of composite ischemic and bleeding outcomes, albeit with a limited sample size.

Apart from its persistently unclear benefits compared with medical therapy, percutaneous occlusion of the LAA is achieved endocardially and for this reason requires OAC, dual antiplatelet therapy (DAPT), or single antiplatelet therapy early after implant to allow time for neo-endothelization to occur. Although a "bridge therapy" with DAPT seems to offer the best risk-to-benefit ratio, it may not be ideal in patients at high risk of bleeding, as is typically the case in those who are referred for LAAO.[5] Moreover, certain specific anatomic features of the LAA ostium can often pose a technical limitation for percutaneous approaches.[3]

There has been renewed interest in the surgical field to respond to the limitations of percutaneous LAAO. The LAAOS III prospective randomized trial clearly showed that in patients with AF undergoing cardiac surgical procedures for another indication, the risk of long-term follow-up ischemic stroke or systemic embolism is lower with concomitant LAAO performed during the surgery than without it.[6] In this complex and evolving scenario, there has been a rapid evolution of techniques and technologies aimed at performing a totally thoracoscopic (TT) surgical exclusion of the LAA with the specific goal of establishing a tailored treatment to permanently exclude any anatomic variable of the LAA epicardially and to eliminate the need for anticoagulation and anti-platelet aggregation unless required for other medical reasons. This ambitious surgical goal should be achieved while maintaining peri-procedural complications at a negligible level.

The present chapter aims to give a synoptic overview of different approaches for TT LAA exclusion performed as a combined or stand-alone procedure. We summarize the evolution of this still-evolving technique, emphasizing the crucial steps that have evolved into a standardized, simplified, and consistently reproducible TT approach.

THE PATH

Before adopting a TT approach, surgical closure of the LAA was performed primarily as a concomitant procedure that achieved variable levels of success using different strategies and closure devices. Indeed, different surgical techniques for LAAO have been proposed, including LAA stapling, suturing, and amputation, using different surgical approaches, including full sternotomy, mini-thoracotomy, and thoracoscopy.[6–14] Surgical success is typically defined by the absence of echocardiographic residual flow between the LA and LAA and a residual LAA stump smaller than 10 mm.[8,9] Incomplete LAAO is correlated with a higher incidence of stroke regardless of the type of surgical technique used.[10] In a prospective pilot comparison, the overall failure of complete LAA exclusion was more than 50%, 63% for the endocardial suturing and ligation, 60% for the stapler excision, and 50% for the surgical amputation.[7] Because of these drawbacks, safer and more effective options for LAAO were required. Thus, surgical devices have been developed, and most of them are designed to occlude the LAA rather than excise it. The effectiveness of these epicardial devices depend on their ability to occlude the LAA parallel to the LAA ostium without tearing it or causing embolization while providing electrical isolation of the LAA with a negligible rate of complications. The introduction and regulatory approval of specifically designed LAA clip occlusion devices[15] have simplified LAA surgical management, providing consistently permanent and reliable occlusion and electrical isolation of the LAA compared with previous surgical strategies.

EVOLUTION OF TOTALLY THORACOSCOPIC LEFT ATRIAL APPENDAGE OCCLUSION

TT LAA occlusion (LAAO) was first described in 1996 as a stand-alone procedure by Odell et al.,[11] who used a stapler and an endo-loop in a canine model. This was followed in 2003 by a report from the same group on 14 patients who were treated using two customized endo-loops and a series of row staplers (the so-called "LAPTONI procedure") with one emergent surgical conversion and no late neurologic events at follow up.[12]

The first experience of LAA stapling was reported in 1988 by DiSesa and coworkers[13] in a sheep model. However, because the staplers were designed for intestinal stapling procedures, using them for LAAO was often complicated by serious bleeding. Unfortunately, the latest generation of staplers has not yet overcome these limitations.[13] Moreover, when assessed with transesophageal echocardiography (TEE), LAA stapling was noted to have a significant rate of incomplete LAA exclusion as well residual pouches deeper than 1 cm.[7-9] The authors suggested that a thoracoscopic approach could facilitate a more suitable angle of instrumentation of the stapling device along the long axis of the oval-shaped shape of the base of the LAA. In this way, a complete exclusion of the LAA can be achieved more quickly.[16]

The first feasible epicardial LAA clip was reported by Fumoto and colleagues[17] in 2008 when an early prototype of an epicardial LAA excluding device consisting of two parallel, straight, rigid titanium tubes and two nitinol springs with a knit-braided polyester fabric was implanted using a median sternotomy approach. In subsequent years, the AtriClip device (AtriCure, Inc., Mason, OH) emerged as a safe, effective, and reproducible way to deal with the LAA during open concomitant surgery.[15] The device resulted in a watertight proximal LAA exclusion, and no residual leaks were reported through the line of LAA closure. AtriCure received US Food and Drug Administration 510(k) clearance for the AtriClip device in June 2010 based on the successful results of the EXCLUDE trial.[15] At that point, surgeons had a new addition to their armamentarium that could safely and completely exclude the LAA and support a safe transition to a TT approach.[18]

As experience with the stand-alone TT LAAO increased, it became clear that the AtriClip provided complete anatomic and electrical isolation of the LAA,[19] consistently decreasing the AF burden in patients for whom rhythm control was also needed.[20-22] In the ensuing years, emerging series of combined or stand-alone TT LAA exclusion procedures were described. Different surgical techniques, including robotically assisted approaches, and evolving indications for LAAO have been proposed and are discussed briefly in the following sections of this chapter.[22-26]

TIPS FOR TOTALLY THORACOSCOPIC LEFT ATRIAL APPENDAGE OCCLUSION

The LAA is a remnant of the embryonic left atrium (LA) that forms during the third week of gestation.[27] It is located on the lateral wall of the heart near the circumflex coronary artery and the great cardiac vein. On the endocardial surface, the LAA orifice is within 1 cm of the mitral valve annulus, and the orifice of the left superior pulmonary vein,[28] forms a narrow junction with the LA, and angles downward from its origin. However, it may also project into the transverse sinus with one or more lobes.[29] The LAA rests freely within the pericardial sac, with the left phrenic nerve having a variable superimposed course as part of the pericardiophrenic neurovascular bundle.[30,31] Endocardially, the LAA is differentiated from the surrounding atrium by rich endocardial trabeculations, which contribute to thrombus formation, formed by parallel muscle bars termed pectinate muscles.[32] In approximately 30% of individuals, muscular trabeculations can be found extending inferiorly from the appendage to the vestibule of the mitral valve.[33] The LAA ostium shares an essential relationship with the left superior pulmonary vein endocardially and the coronary vessels epicardially, with the left aortic sinus and the left main coronary artery lying posterior and medial and the greater cardiac vein and circumflex artery lying inferiorly less than 2 mm from the LAA ostium. The left anterior descending coronary artery runs underneath the LAA body, emerging at a point immediately below the LAA tip, although the tip's position may vary.[28,33,34] The LAA ostium is oval in 70%, ovaloid in 18 %, triangular in 8%, and round in 6% of patients.[35] As previously elucidated, such variability in the shape of the LAA orifice shape is one of the critical aspects of endovascular occlusion devices, which are generally quite compliant, with an LAA that has a round, symmetrically shaped orifice. In a minority of patients, the sinus node artery arises from the circumflex artery and runs near the LAA where it can assume an S-shape as it courses between the LAA and the left superior pulmonary vein. Coronary vessels should be visualized before epicardial closure of the LAA (Fig. 45.1).[28,33] The number of LAA lobes may vary, and their shape has been associated with different risks of thrombosis, according to four prevalent morphologies, namely "windsock," "chicken wing," "cauliflower," and "cactus-like."[36]

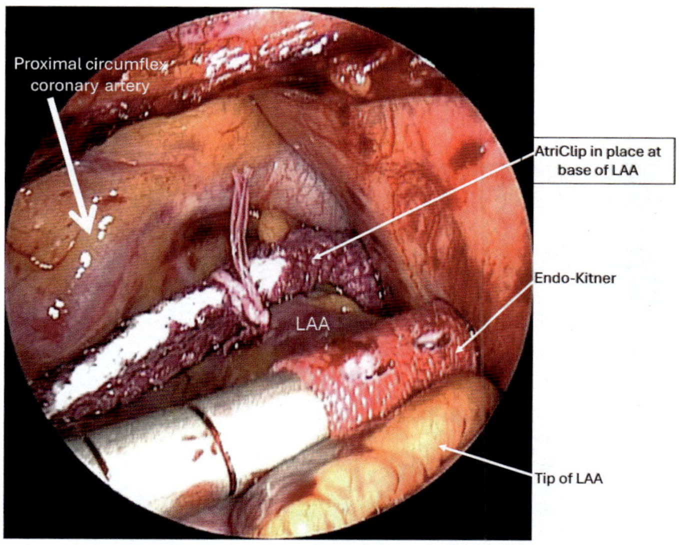

Fig. 45.1 Intraoperative visualization of the circumflex artery and its relationship to the base of the left atrial appendage (LAA).

Electrophysiologically, an underappreciated role of the LAA is its function as a trigger for recurrent AF.[37] Therefore, in the setting of a rhythm control strategy, successful management of the LAA should include its complete electrical isolation to enhance the efficacy of AF ablation (see Chapter 43).[38] Finally, the LAA and the right atrial appendage (RAA) are the primary sources of atrial natriuretic peptide, with concentrations in the appendage walls being 40-fold higher than in the left atrial free wall and ventricles.[39] It is postulated that atrial natriuretic peptide is released in response to the stretch of the LAA wall and stimulates diuresis, thus playing a role in volume control and arterial pressure homeostasis (see Chapter 42).[40,41]

LEFT-SIDED TOTALLY THORACOSCOPIC LEFT ATRIAL APPENDAGE OCCLUSION

Patient and Port Positioning

The most common approach to perform TT LAAO is via the left chest as a stand-alone procedure or concomitantly with AF thoracoscopic ablation. Under general anesthesia, a double-lumen tube for selective lung ventilation is positioned, and external defibrillation pads are placed (parasternal right and posterior paravertebral left). The patient is positioned supine, and an inflatable bag is placed vertically along the left scapula to gently lift the left thorax by approximately 30 degrees, thus enhancing exposure. Both arms are positioned next to the thorax and a TEE probe is inserted to confirm that both the LA and the LAA are free of thrombi. The presence of thrombi involving the proximal part of the LAA and its ostium supports aborting the procedure. If the presence of thrombi is excluded by TEE, a camera port (5 or 10 mm) is positioned through the third intercostal space at the midaxillary line. CO_2 is then delivered into the pleural space at a pressure of 8 to 10 cm H_2O to achieve left lung collapse and a convenient rightward shift of the mediastinum and heart. As an option to minimize the risk of lung injury, a left pneumothorax can be induced by delivering CO_2 into the pleural space with a needle before positioning the camera port, but close attention must be paid to the patient's hemodynamics if this is done. Therefore, two working ports (5 mm) are placed through the second and fifth or sixth intercostal spaces (12 mm, for the clip insertion) between the mid- and anterior axillary lines. A 5- or 10-mm 0-degree standard camera is then inserted through the central port (Fig. 45.2).

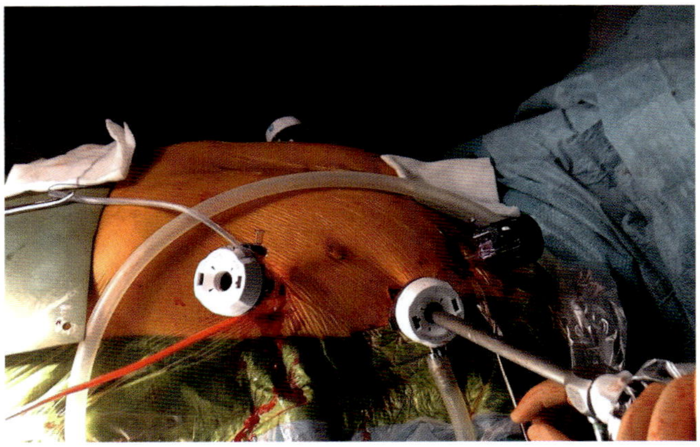

Fig. 45.2 Ports setup for left-sided thoracoscopy. See text for further description.

Pericardiotomy

The left phrenic nerve pedicle should be visualized before opening the pericardium (Fig. 45.3). The pericardium distal to the left pulmonary vein hilum is retracted, and a longitudinal pericardiotomy is placed at least 2 cm posterior and parallel to the phrenic nerve bundle (Fig. 45.4). The pericardiotomy is usually extended from the level of the ligament of Marshall to the base of the left ventricle just caudal to the circumflex coronary artery. This provides exposure of the entire LAA (lobes, base, and surrounding structures), reducing the risk of incomplete closure and peri-procedural complications. Pericardial stay sutures are generally not needed but may be used if necessary to optimize the exposure.

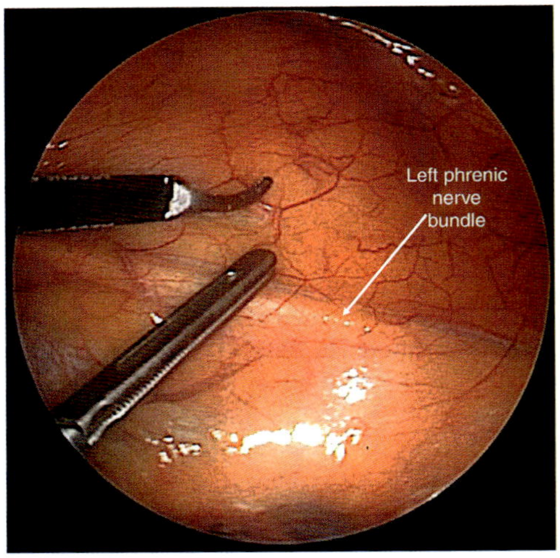

Fig. 45.3 Thoracoscopic view of the left phrenic nerve bundle.

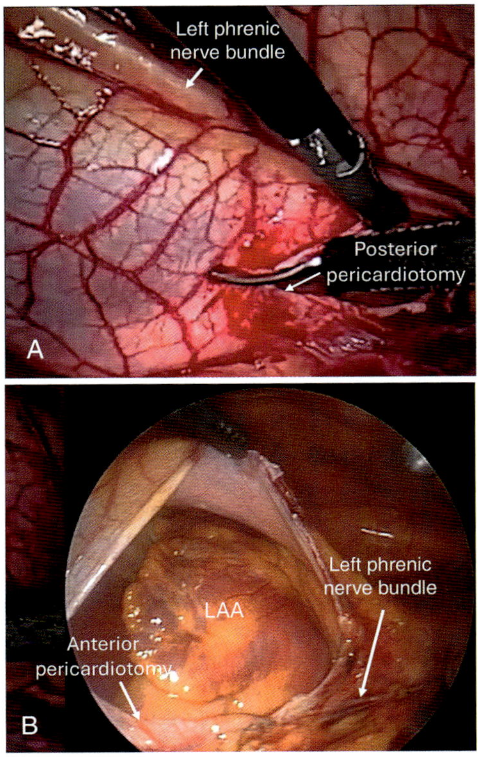

Fig. 45.4 Thoracoscopic pericardiotomy from the left side. (A) Subphrenic posterior approach. (B) Antephrenic anterior approach. *LAA,* Left atrial appendage.

Left Atrial Appendage Clip Placement

After being exposed, the base of the LAA is measured along its long axis (Fig. 45.5). An AtriClip epicardial LAAO device (AtriCure, Inc., Mason, OH) is passed through the lower port and positioned around the base of the LAA. The whole LAA is gently teased into a position within the open clip using an Endo-Kittner to avoid excessive manipulation while simultaneously position the clip softly all the way down to the LAA base (Fig. 45.6A). Only after the LAA is fully engaged within the clip can forceps be used to enhance the positioning of the clip at the true base of the LAA (Fig. 45.6B). Before triggering the clip device to close, one should visually confirm that the two ends of the clip in the transverse sinus include all lobes of the LAA. The final landing of the device should entail a clockwise rotation of the whole delivery system to prevent a residual pouch on the left pulmonary vein side of the clip. This last step before final clip closure is necessary because the anatomic base of the LAA is at the side of the heart, not in front of it (Fig. 45.7).

With the LAA clip in a closed position but before its final release, the TEE image is checked for completeness of the LAA exclusion with no residual stump (Fig. 45.8). An electrocardiogram (ECG) is checked to detect any signs of myocardial ischemia resulting from compression or kinking of the circumflex coronary artery. If the ECG shows any ischemic changes or if TEE shows a significant residual stump, the LAA clip is reopened. If bleeding occurs during LAA manipulation, we advise closing the device proximal to the tear and using it as a hemostatic tool. At the end of the procedure, the left pericardium is partially closed, and a chest tube is placed in the chest cavity.

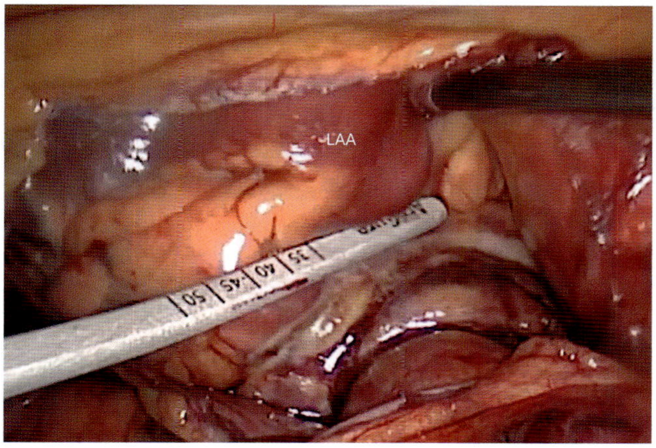

Fig. 45.5 Thoracoscopic sizing of the left atrial appendage base.

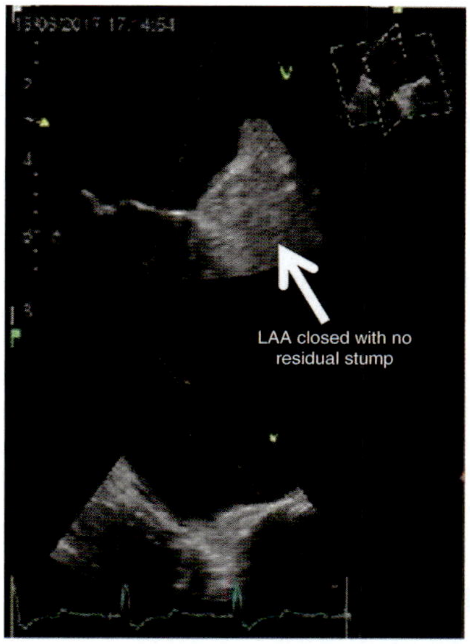

Fig. 45.8 Intraoperative transesophageal echocardiography confirming the absence of any residual stump greater than 1 cm in depth after left atrial appendage (LAA) occlusion.

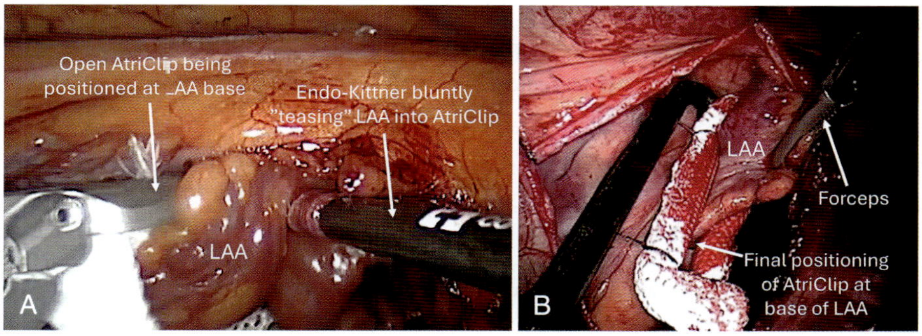

Fig. 45.6 Engagement of the left atrial appendage (LAA) within the AtriClip exclusion system. (A) The tip of the LAA is smoothly accommodated by means of an atraumatic tool ("Endo-Kittner"). (B) After being engaged, the LAA is manipulated for final positioning by means of forceps.

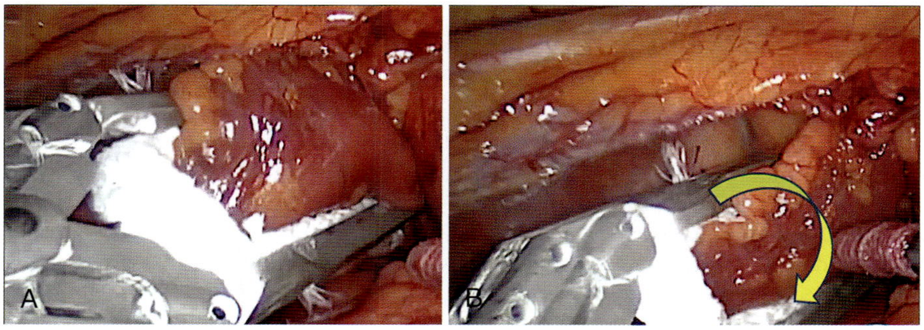

Fig. 45.7 Before releasing the exclusion device (A), a clockwise rotation (B) may be useful to engage the left atrial appendage all the way to its base.

Epicardial LAAO can also be safely and effectively achieved using robotic-assisted video-thoracoscopy. The patient is positioned and prepped as previously described for a TT left-sided approach. Three dedicated ports (12 mm) for robotic arms are positioned at the level of the second (mid-clear line), sixth (anterior axillary line), and fourth (mid-clear line, camera port) intercostal spaces. An accessory working port close to the posterior axillary line in the seventh intercostal space may be helpful for introduction of the clip device. A robotic platform supports improved visibility and manoeuvrability. The patient's body size and habitus seem to have a lesser effect on procedure execution when adopting a robotically enhanced approach.[42]

RIGHT-SIDED TOTALLY THORACOSCOPIC LEFT ATRIAL APPENDAGE OCCLUSION

Although the left-sided approach has been suggested as the most direct way to address the LAA thoracoscopically, a right-sided TT approach has also been proposed for LAAO by van Putte's group.[25,43] A detailed description of their AF ablation technique is described in Chapter 32. At the end of the AF ablation, an AtriClip is introduced into the transverse sinus via the lower or upper right-sided working port. The LAA is gently manipulated between the two arms of the AtriClip using a suction device, and complete closure with no residual stump is confirmed by TEE. An ECG is used to rule out any disturbance of blood flow through the circumflex coronary artery.

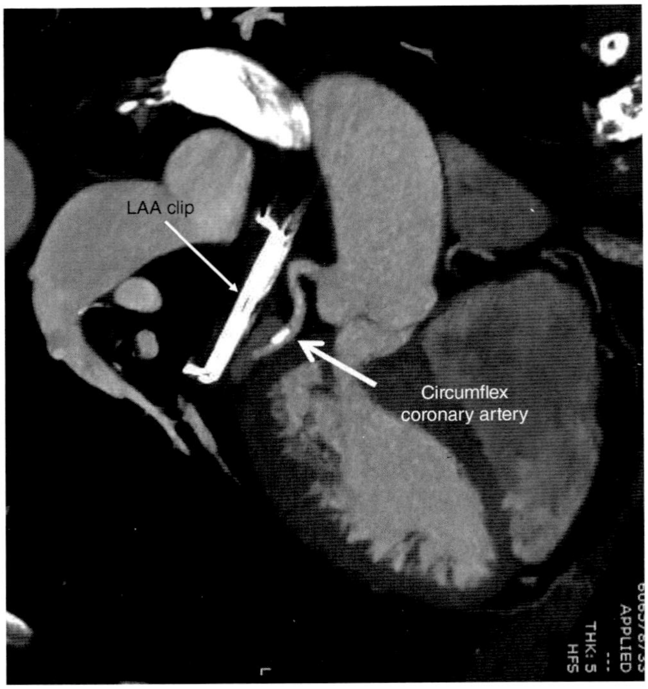

Fig. 45.9 Postoperative computed tomography scan confirming complete occlusion of the left atrial appendage (LAA) highlights the close proximity of the exclusion device to the circumflex artery.

IMAGING FOR TOTALLY THORACOSCOPIC LEFT ATRIAL APPENDAGE OCCLUSION

Transesophageal Echocardiography

TEE remains the gold-standard tool for detecting LAA thrombus[44,45] and is considered the standard imaging modality to guide all phases of LAA management. TEE accuracy is operator dependent and relies on the quality of the acquired images.[44] Intraoperatively, TEE is essential to confirm the absence of thrombi and to guide the proper placement of the epicardial clip device for LAAO.

Computed Tomography Scanning

Although a computed tomography (CT) scan is not mandatory, it can be a valuable tool for effective surgical planning and post-procedural monitoring in all TT LAAO procedures.

Indeed, advanced CT imaging facilitates the creation of a virtual patient avatar that displays the LAA and its topographic relationship to the surrounding cardiac, thoracic, and skeletal anatomy.[46] Furthermore, the ability of CT scans to detect thrombi may improve with the use of delayed acquisition protocols. This approach optimizes test specificity for intracardiac thrombosis, reducing false positives and avoiding unnecessary cancellations of prescheduled procedures.[47]

The LAA has complex and varying morphology that can be accurately identified by CT imaging (Fig. 45.9), and it can impact not only periprocedural management but also follow-up outcomes. Whereas TEE is used for intra-procedural guidance, CT angiography can serve as an adjunct for pre- and post-procedural assessment. It has been suggested that a combined approach using both modalities can identify anatomic characteristics of the LAA and the LA that predispose patients to a post-procedural residual stump.[48,49]

CT scans can also help identify rare anatomic variants that could preclude specific treatment approaches. For example, the detection of an LAA lobe projecting into the transverse sinus is a deterrent for transcatheter LAAO with the LARIAT device.[50] Furthermore, preprocedural CT scans can help identify a persistent superior vena cava or rare coronary variants that can impact the percutaneous delivery technique.

CT scans have proven to be valuable for measuring the size (depth) of a residual stump after LAAO,[48] and they are a sensitive modality for detecting potential device-related thrombosis. However, no definitive comparison between CT and TEE has been conducted after TT exclusion of the LAA.[49,50]

INDICATIONS FOR TOTALLY THORACOSCOPIC LEFT ATRIAL APPENDAGE OCCLUSION

Surgical LAAO as a stand-alone procedure was not explicitly addressed in either the 2020 European Society of Cardiology/European Heart Rhythm Association/European Association for Cardio-Thoracic Surgery European guidelines[51] or in the 2023 American College of Cardiology/American Heart Association/American College of Clinical Pharmacy/Heart Rhythm Society US guidelines.[52] The US guidelines recommend percutaneous LAAO (Class 2, level A) in patients with a moderate to high risk of stroke (CHA_2DS_2-VASc score ≥2) and a contraindication to long-term OAC from a nonreversible cause. In patients with no absolute contraindication to anticoagulation but with a high risk of significant bleeding on OAC, percutaneous LAAO is recommended (Class 2b, level B). The 2020 European guidelines recommended percutaneous LAAO only in patients with contraindications to long-term anticoagulation (Class 2b, level B).

In patients with AF undergoing cardiac surgery with a CHA_2DS_2-VASc score of 2 or less or equivalent stroke risk, surgical LAAO with continued anticoagulation is recommended by the 2023 US guidelines (Class 1, level A). These guidelines specify that a surgical technique that blocks blood flow across the line of occlusion with a stump smaller 1 cm as determined by intraoperative TEE should be used as the criterion for successful LAAO. However, the guidelines also state that the benefit of surgical LAAO in the absence of continued anticoagulation to reduce the risk of stroke and systemic embolism is uncertain (Class 2b, level of evidence A). The European 2020 AF guidelines remain less specific on the surgical occlusion of the LAA that may be considered for stroke prevention in patients with AF undergoing cardiac surgery (Class 2b, level of evidence C).

It should be emphasized that there is a need for adequately powered clinical trials to determine the best treatment strategy in patients with absolute or relative contraindication to OACs. The COMPARE LAAO trial will assess the safety and efficacy of percutaneous LAAO in patients with AF who are ineligible to use OAC.[53] Moreover, evidence is needed concerning the most appropriate treatment in patients experiencing a stroke of ischemic origin despite OAC and to define the best regimen and duration of antithrombotic therapy after either percutaneous or surgical LAA management.

Surgical LAA exclusion is supported in the guidelines mainly because of the prospective randomized trial LAOOS III (see Chapter 46).[6] According to the most recent European Guidelines on Valvular Heart Disease, occlusion of the LAA should be included with the Maze procedure when performing concomitant valve or coronary artery bypass graft surgery to decrease the risk of stroke in patients with AF (Class 2a, level B).[54] The LAOOS III trial investigated nonthoracoscopic procedures, and it seems reasonable to extrapolate these results to TT procedures as the epicardial LAA clip has the same features.

Sparse real-world data support the fact that surgical LAAO via a minimally invasive TT approach could eventually be seen as the preferred strategy, particularly in patients with increased cerebrovascular ischemic or hemorrhagic risk, in those with previous major or recurrent bleeding (mainly gastrointestinal followed by cerebral hemorrhage), and in other situations including prohibitive LAA and access anatomy.[16,55,56]

PROCEDURAL SUCCESS: COMPLETE LEFT ATRIAL APPENDAGE CLOSURE AND "THE STUMP"

Since the first seminal report of LAA surgical excision by Dr. John L Madden in 1948,[57] there has been an evolution of techniques and technologies aimed at epicardial LAA exclusion. The last US guidelines state that a residual LAA stump after LAAO is thought to expose patients to increased thromboembolic events if it is more than 1 cm deep as determined by intraoperative TEE.[52] It should be noted that after percutaneous LAAO, the issue of residual stump is of a different nature than LAA stumps after epicardial LAAO using an epicardial clip. After epicardial clip LAAO, a stump may remain, but no blood will flow between the LA and LAA.[58] Moreover, LAA stump measurements are based on CT scan reconstructions and are affected by observer variability. Consequently, the implications of a residual stump and the thrombogenic threshold for its size are uncertain. Therefore, most clinicians continue anticoagulation whenever any LAA stump is detected after LAAO.[58–60]

The 1-cm threshold for thrombogenicity was adopted arbitrarily in the past, and as a result, investigators such as Suwalski et al.[59] and Osmancik et al.[60] have attempted to standardize the relationship between the size of the residual LAA stump after epicardial LAAO and its thrombogenic threshold. A stump depth of 0 mm may not be achievable after clip exclusion, and technically speaking, stump incidence may be as high as 100%. Ailawadi et al.[15] stated that voluminous LAAs with a large ostium are prone to stump development, especially those with fundic irregularities, which are an anatomic predisposing factor for thrombosis. Ellis et al.[61] have suggested that exposed trabeculations in the stump may be more important than stump depth as a risk factor for thrombosis. In addition, thrombus formation in patients with AF also depends on LAA shape, LAA take-off, and a combination of other factors, including endothelial dysfunction and hypercoagulability. Thus, a standardized definition is needed for precisely delineating what constitutes a thrombogenic LAA stump, and stump size thresholds connected with thromboembolic events after epicardial LAAO should be defined.

PROCEDURAL SAFETY AND CLINICAL EFFICACY

The safety and efficacy of TT LAAO using an epicardial LAA clip can now be compared with the safety and efficacy of percutaneous endocardial LAAO. Sufficient evidence has recently been reported by meta-analyses and large observational series to confirm that after TT LAA clipping, no significant epicardial LAA clip-related complications have been reported, which compares favorably with any other devices available for thoracoscopic approaches.[16,55,56,62] Intra-procedural conversion to thoracotomy or sternotomy or surgical revision for bleeding has been reported mainly because of lung injuries during the early phases of the operation or for LAA tears at the base of the LAA related to inappropriate surgical exposure and rough manipulation of the fragile LAA tissue. Pleural effusion and pericarditis are the most common complications after epicardial clip LAAO and are usually treated effectively with anti-inflammatory drugs and diuretics.

Even many years after its first introduction, percutaneous endocardial LAAO is still burdened by important challenges such as peri-device leaks and device thrombosis, which impose the necessity of continuing anticoagulant therapy even after device implant.[51,52] These unresolved issues may lead to increased rates of late bleeding, particularly in patients who receive percutaneous LAAO because of an absolute contraindication to anticoagulation.[63] Conversely, to our knowledge, residual flow across an AtriClip device has never been reported. Thus, when we use an epicardial device for LAA exclusion, we immediately discontinue all antithrombotic therapy. Because most thoracoscopic LAAO clipping procedures have been performed concomitantly with other cardiac surgical procedures, some antithrombotic therapy is mandatory because of the primary surgical procedure.[43,64–66] Emerging large series on stand-alone TT LAAO have shown a tendency toward an increasing number of patients being discharged without any anti-platelet therapy after LAAO with an epicardial clip or stapler, thus decreasing the relative hemorrhagic risk in patients with absolute contraindications to anticoagulation.[18,55,56]

Although the definition of procedural success remains the absence of a residual stump larger than 1 cm, the definition of what constitutes a thrombogenic LAA stump remains unclear. The actual risks of thromboembolism should be defined not only by the presence of a residual stump and its eventual size but also for the presence of residual blood flow between the LA and the LAA stump. The most important aspect related to the use of an epicardial LAAO device is the extraordinarily high incidence of complete exclusion of the LA without a significant residual stump, resulting in the possibility of avoiding long-term OAC. This point is of particular importance in patients with relative or absolute contraindications to OAC, considering their high risk of bleeding.

TT LAAO has shown an overall freedom from stroke of 80.9% to 99.1%, which compares most favorably with the success rate reported for endovascular devices.[16,55,56] A recent meta-analysis compared the safety and efficacy of TT LAAO and concomitant AF ablation using any device or technique with percutaneous LAAO using any device.[67] The primary endpoint was the 1-year follow-up stroke rate, and the secondary end-points were an acute success rate of complete LAA closure, postprocedural mortality and complications, and all-cause mortality at 1 year. Twenty-five studies comprising 1958 patients were included in the analysis, which showed no significant difference in stroke rate or all-cause mortality. The percutaneous group had a significantly higher acute success rate of complete LAAO. It must be noted, however, that only a portion of the TT studies included epicardial LAA clipping. Moreover, percutaneous LAAO resulted in a higher risk of hemorrhage during post-procedural management. Other post-procedural complications (stroke or transient ischemic attack, pericardial effusion) and deaths occurred at a similar rate when using the two techniques.[67]

Wang et al.[68] reported a prospective randomized trial comparing percutaneous LAAO using the WATCHMAN device with TT LAAO using a stapling device. More than 200 patients were followed for 1.8 years and evaluated for perioperative complications, efficacy endpoints (thromboembolism and death), and a safety endpoint (bleeding events). The results confirmed that TT and transcatheter LAA closure had similar efficacy in preventing stroke. The TT group had significantly fewer bleeding events but required significantly longer hospitalization.

CONCLUSIONS

OAC remains the first-line treatment for the prevention of thromboembolic events in patients with AF. It remains the most effective, most ubiquitously applicable, best tolerated, least invasive, and most economically sustainable form of treatment for the majority of patients affected worldwide by AF. Pharmacologic therapy is advancing, possibly at a faster pace than device therapy. For this reason, its applicability and "user-friendliness" will likely be further improved in the years to come. That said, there has been an increase in the referral pattern of patients with AF that nowadays, like never before, present a higher and more complex comorbid burden that exposes them to high risks of complications, even when the most advanced forms of OAC are applied. In this specific context, the past years have seen an exponential increase in the application of device-supported treatments to exclude the most important and documented source of thromboembolism in patients with AF, the LAA, from the blood circulation. Percutaneous LAAO is a valid therapeutic method for excluding the LAA. It is at least as good as OAC and may add benefits such as reducing overall bleeding events and hemorrhagic strokes. It remains unclear if, after percutaneous LAAO, anticoagulation and anti-aggregation drugs can be safely withheld immediately and permanently. Epicardial LAAO was proposed much earlier than percutaneous LAAO. However, it has only recently become popular thanks to the development of structured programs for a TT approach supported by the development of tailored instruments. Epicardial TT LAAO in patients with AF is clearly an effective and durable stroke prevention tool in selected patients with AF. The combined benefit of electrical isolation and hemodynamic occlusion of the LAA provided by epicardial LAAO clipping has now been thoroughly documented.

There is growing evidence that percutaneous LAAO and TT LAAO have similar efficacy in terms of stroke prevention. However, epicardial LAAO has the additional advantage of electrically isolating the LAA from the LA, an important trait of epicardial devices, that does not exist with percutaneous endocardial catheter LAA closure devices. A percutaneous approach can be performed without general anesthesia and endotracheal intubation, even in the presence of mediastinal adhesions resulting from previous surgery, and requires shorter hospitalization. However, the TT approach results in fewer follow-up bleeding complications. Epicardial LAAO using a clip does not require intraprocedural anticoagulation and can be applied even in the presence of the most complex LAA anatomy and in the case of vascular access variations that preclude a percutaneous approach (e.g., anomalous venous return, interrupted inferior vena cava).

Devices, techniques, and indications for TT LAAO will likely continue evolving as more data become available from future studies.

REFERENCES

1. Al-Saady NM, Obel OA, Camm AJ. Left atrial appendage: structure, function, and role in thromboembolism. *Heart.* 1999;82:547–554.
2. Pisters R, Lane DA, Nieuwlaat R, et al. A novel user-friendly score (HAS-BLED) to assess 1-year risk of major bleeding in patients with atrial fibrillation: the Euro Heart Survey. *Chest.* 2010;138:1093–1100.
3. Reddy VY, Doshi SK, Kar S, et al. 5-year outcomes after left atrial appendage closure: from the prevail and protect aftrials. *J Am Coll Cardiol.* 2017;70(24):2964–2975.
4. Osmancik P, Herman D, Neuzil P, et al. 4-year outcomes after left atrial appendage closure versus nonwarfarin oral anticoagulation for atrial fibrillation. *J Am Coll Cardiol.* 2022;79(1):1–14.
5. Carvalho PEP, Gewehr DM, Miyawaki IA, et al. Network meta-analysis of initial antithrombotic regimens after left atrial appendage occlusion. *J Am Coll Cardiol.* 2023;82(18):1765–1773.
6. Whitlock RP, Belley-Cote EP, Paparella D, et al. Left atrial appendage occlusion during cardiac surgery to prevent stroke. *N Engl J Med.* 2021;384(22):2081–2091.
7. Lee RL, Vassallo P, Kruse J, et al. A randomized, prospective pilot comparison of three atrial appendage elimination techniques: internal ligation, stapled excision, and surgical excision. *J Thorac Cardiovasc Surg.* 2016;152:1075–1080.
8. Gillinov AM, Patterson G, Cosgrove DM. Stapled excision of the left atrial appendage. *J Thorac Cardiovasc Surg.* 2005;129:679–680.
9. Kanderian AS, Gillinov AM, Pettersson GB, et al. Success of surgical left atrial appendage closure: assessment by transesophageal echocardiography. *J Am Coll Cardiol.* 2008;52(11):924–929.
10. Garcia-Fernandez MA, Perez-David E, Quiles J, et al. Role of left atrial appendage obliteration in patients with mitral valve prosthesis. *J Am Coll Cardiol.* 2003;42:1253–1258.
11. Odell J, Blackshear JL, Davies E, et al. Thoracoscopic obliteration of the left atrial appendage: potential for stroke reduction? *Ann Thorac Surg.* 1996;61:565–569.
12. Blackshear JL, Johnson WD, Odell JA. Thoracoscopic extracardiac obliteration of the left atrial appendage for stroke risk reduction in atrial fibrillation. *J Am Coll Cardiol.* 2003;42:1249–1252.
13. DiSesa V, Tam S, Cohn LH. Ligation of left atrial appendage using an automatic surgical stapler. *Ann Thorac Surg.* 1988;46:652–653.
14. Wehbe MS, Doll N, Merk DR. Fatal complications associated with surgical left atrial appendage exclusion. *J Thorac Cardiovasc Surg.* 2018;156:e207–e208.
15. Ailawadi G, Gerdisch MW, Harvey L, et al. Exclusion of the left atrial appendage with a novel device: early results of a multicenter trial. *J Thorac Cardiovasc Surg.* 2011;142(5):1002–1009.
16. Ohtsuka T, Ninomiya M, Nonaka T, Hisagi M, Ota T, Mizutani T. Thoracoscopic stand-alone left atrial appendectomy for thromboembolism prevention in nonvalvular atrial fibrillation. *J Am Coll Cardiol.* 2013;62(2):103–107.
17. Fumoto H, Gillinov AM, Ootaki Y, et al. A novel device for left atrial appendage exclusion: the third-generation atrial exclusion device. *J Thorac Cardiovasc Surg.* 2008;136(4):1019–1027.
18. Ramlawi B, Bedeir K, Edgerton JR. Totally thoracoscopic closure of the left atrial appendage. *Ann Thorac Surg.* 2019;107(1):e71–e73.
19. Benussi S, Mazzone P, Maccabelli G, et al. Thoracoscopic appendage exclusion with an AtriClip device as a solo treatment for focal atrial tachycardia. *Circulation.* 2011;123(14):1575–1578.

20. Di Biase L, Burkhardt JD, Mohanty P, et al. Left atrial appendage isolation in patients with longstanding persistent AF undergoing catheter ablation: BELIEF trial. *J Am Coll Cardiol.* 2016;68(18):1929–1940.
21. Starck CT, Steffel J, Emmert MY, et al. Epicardial left atrial appendage clip occlusion also provides the electrical isolation of the left atrial appendage. *Interact Cardiovasc Thorac Surg.* 2012;15(3):416–418.
22. Lakkireddy D, Sridhar Mahankali A, Kanmanthareddy A, et al. Left atrial appendage ligation and ablation for persistent atrial fibrillation. The LAALA-AF registry. *JACC Clin Electrophysiol.* 2015;1(3):153–160.
23. Branzoli S, Marini M, Guarracini F, et al. Standalone totally thoracoscopic left appendage clipping: safe, simple, standardized. *Ann Thorac Surg.* 2021;111(1):e61–e63.
24. Maesen B, La Meir M. Unilateral Left-sided thoracoscopic ablation of atrial fibrillation. *Ann Thorac Surg.* 2020;110(1):e63–e66.
25. Fleerakkers J, Hofman FN, van Putte BP. Totally thoracoscopic ablation: a unilateral right-sided approach. *Eur J Cardiothorac Surg.* 2020;58(5):1088–1090.
26. Lewis CT, Stephens RL, Horst VD, Angelillo M, Tyndal CM. Application of an epicardial left atrial appendage occlusion device by a robotic-assisted, right chest approach. *Ann Thorac Surg.* 2016;101(5):e177–e178.
27. Ho SY, Cabrera JA, Sanchez-Quintana D. Left atrial anatomy revisited. *Circ Arrhythm Electrophysiol.* 2012;5:220–228.
28. Su P, McCarthy KP, Ho SY. Occluding the left atrial appendage: anatomical considerations. *Heart.* 2008;94(9):1166–1170.
29. Veinot JP, Harrity PJ, Gentile F, et al. Anatomy of the normal left atrial appendage. *Circulation.* 1997;96:3112–3115.
30. Matsumoto Y, Krishnan S, Fowler SJ, et al. Detection of phrenic nerves and their relation to cardiac anatomy using 64-slice multidetector computed tomography. *Am J Cardiol.* 2007;100(1):133–137.
31. Lachman N, Syed FF, Habib A, et al. Correlative anatomy for the electrophysiologist, part II: cardiac ganglia, phrenic nerve, coronary venous system. *J Cardiovasc Electrophysiol.* 2011;22(1):104–110.
32. Al Saady NM, Obel OA, Camm AJ. Left atrial appendage: structure, function, and role in thromboembolism. *Heart.* 1999;82(5):547–554.
33. Cabrera JA, Saremi F, Sánchez-Quintana D. Left atrial appendage: anatomy and imaging landmarks pertinent to percutaneous transcatheter occlusion. *Heart.* 2014;100(20):1636–1650.
34. Wongcharoen W, Tsao HM, Wu MH, et al. Morphologic characteristics of the left atrial appendage, roof, and septum: implications for the ablation of atrial fibrillation. *J Cardiovasc Electrophysiol.* 2006;17(9):951–956.
35. Wang Y, Di Biase L, Horton RP, Nguyen T, Morhanty P, Natale A. Left atrial appendage studied by computed tomography to help planning for appendage closure device placement. *J Cardiovasc Electrophysiol.* 2010;21(9):973–982.
36. Di Biase L, Santangeli P, Anselmino M, et al. Does the left atrial appendage morphology correlate with the risk of stroke in patients with atrial fibrillation? Results from a multicenter study. *J Am Coll Cardiol.* 2012;60(6):531–538.
37. Di Biase L, Burkhardt JD, Mohanty P, et al. Left atrial appendage: an underrecognized trigger site of atrial fibrillation. *Circulation.* 2010;122(2):109–118.
38. Romero J, Michaud GF, Avendano R, et al. Benefit of left atrial appendage electrical isolation for persistent and long-standing persistent atrial fibrillation: a systematic review and meta-analysis. *Europace.* 2018;20(8):1268–1278.
39. Tabata T, Oki T, Yamada H, Abe M, Onose Y, Thomas JD. Relationship between left atrial appendage function and plasma concentration of atrial natriuretic peptide. *Eur J Echocardiogr.* 2000;1(2):130–137.
40. Bartus K, Kanuri SH, Litwinowicz R, et al. Long term impact of epicardial left atrial appendage ligation on systemic hemostasis: LAA HOMEOSTASIS-2. *J Clin Med.* 2022;11(6):1495.
41. Park HC, Shin J, Ban JE, Choi JI, Park SW, Kim YH. Left atrial appendage: morphology and function in patients with paroxysmal and persistent atrial fibrillation. *Int J Cardiovasc Imaging.* 2013;29(4):935–944.
42. Antaki T, Michaelman J, McGroarty J. Robotics-assisted epicardial left atrial appendage clip exclusion. *J Thorac Cardiovasc Surg Tech.* 2021;9:59–68.
43. Vos LM, Fleerakkers J, Hofman FN, van Putte BP. Closed-chest unilateral thoracoscopic ablation: box lesion with radiofrequency clamps only. *Eur J Cardiothorac Surg.* 2022;62(1):ezac316. https://doi.org/10.1093/ejcts/ezac316.
44. Wunderlich NC, Beigel R, Swaans MJ, Ho SY, Siegel RJ. Percutaneous interventions for left atrial appendage exclusion: options, assessment, and imaging using 2D and 3D echocardiography. *JACC Cardiovasc Imaging.* 2015;8(4):472–488.
45. Yu S, Zhang H, Li H. Cardiac computed tomography versus transesophageal echocardiography for the detection of left atrial appendage thrombus: a systemic review and meta-analysis. *J Am Heart Assoc.* 2021;10(23):e022505.
46. Prosper A, Shinbane J, Maliglig A, Saremi F, Wilcox A, Lee C. Left atrial appendage mechanical exclusion: procedural planning using cardiovascular computed tomographic angiography. *J Thorac Imaging.* 2020;35(4):W107–W118.
47. Spagnolo P, Giglio M, Di Marco D, et al. Diagnosis of left atrial appendage thrombus in patients with atrial fibrillation: delayed contrast-enhanced cardiac CT. *Eur Radiol.* 2021;31(3):1236–1244.
48. Mochen M, Branzoli S, D'Onghia G, et al. The role of cardiac imaging before and after left atrial appendage standalone thoracoscopic exclusion. *Cardiovasc Med.* 2023;24(3):191–199.
49. Korsholm K, Jensen JM, Nørgaard BL, Nielsen-Kudsk JE. Detection of device-related thrombosis following left atrial appendage occlusion: a comparison between cardiac computed tomography and transesophageal echocardiography. *Circ Cardiovasc Interv.* 2019;12(9):e008112.
50. Laura DM, Chinitz LA, Aizer A, et al. The role of multimodality imaging in percutaneous left atrial appendage suture ligation with the LARIAT device. *J Am Soc Echocardiogr.* 2014;27(7):699–708.
51. Hindricks G, Potpara T, Dagres N, et al. 2020 ESC guidelines for the diagnosis and management of atrial fibrillation developed in collaboration with the European Association for Cardio-Thoracic Surgery (EACTS): the task force for the diagnosis and management of atrial fibrillation of the European Society of Cardiology (ESC) Developed with the special contribution of the European Heart Rhythm Association (EHRA) of the ESC. *Eur Heart J.* 2021;42(5):373–498.
52. Joglar JA, Chung MK, Armbruster AL, et al. 2023 ACC/AHA/ACCP/HRS guideline for the diagnosis and management of atrial fibrillation: a report of the American College of Cardiology/American Heart Association Joint Committee on clinical practice guidelines. *J Am Coll Cardiol.* 2024;83(1):109–279.
53. Huijboom M, Maarse M, Aarnink E, et al. Rationale and design of the randomized controlled trial comparing effectiveness and safety of left atrial appendage occlusion to standard of care for atrial fibrillation patients at high stroke risk and ineligible to use oral anticoagulation therapy. *Am Heart J.* 2022;250:45–56.

54. Vahanian A, Beyersdorf F, Praz F, et al. ESC/EACTS scientific document group: 2021 ESC/EACTS guidelines for the management of valvular heart disease. *Eur Heart J*. 2022;43(7): 561–632.
55. Branzoli S, Guarracini F, Marini M, et al. Heart team for left appendage occlusion without the use of antithrombotic therapy: the epicardial perspective. *J Clin Med*. 2022;11(21):6492.
56. Cartledge R, Suwalski G, Witkowska A, et al. Standalone epicardial left atrial appendage exclusion for thromboembolism prevention in atrial fibrillation. *Interact Cardiovasc Thorac Surg*. 2022;34(4):548–555.
57. Madden JL. Resection of the left auricular appendix: a prophylaxis for recurrent arterial emboli. *J Am Med Assoc*. 1949;140(9):769–772.
58. Caliskan E, Eberhard M, Falk V, Alkadhi H, Emmert MY. Incidence and characteristics of left atrial appendage stumps after device-enabled epicardial closure. *Interact Cardiovasc Thorac Surg*. 2019;29(5):663–669.
59. Suwalski G, Emery R, Gryszko L, Kaczejko K, Mroz J, Skrobowski A. Intraoperative assessment of left atrial diverticulum and remnant stump after left atrial appendage epicardial occlusion. *Echocardiography*. 2016;33:1368–1373.
60. Osmancik P, Budera P, Zdarska J, et al. Residual echocardiographic and computed tomography findings after thoracoscopic occlusion of the left atrial appendage using the AtriClip PRO device. *Interact Cardiovasc Thorac Surg*. 2018;26(6):919–925.
61. Ellis CR, Aznaurov SG, Patel NJ, et al. Angiographic efficacy of the atriclip left atrial appendage exclusion device placed by minimally invasive thoracoscopic approach. *JACC Clin Electrophysiol*. 2017;3(12):1356–1365.
62. Toale C, Fitzmaurice GJ, Eaton D, Lyne J, Redmond KC. Outcomes of left atrial appendage occlusion using the AtriClip device: a systematic review. *Interact Cardiovasc Thorac Surg*. 2019;29(5):655–662.
63. Alkhouli M, Ellis CR, Daniels M, Coylewright M, Nielsen-Kudsk JE, Holmes DR. Left atrial appendage occlusion: current advances and remaining challenges. *JACC*. 2022;1:1–18.
64. Doll N, Weimar T, Kosior DA, et al. Efficacy and safety of hybrid epicardial and endocardial ablation versus endocardial ablation in patients with persistent and longstanding persistent atrial fibrillation: a randomised, controlled trial. *EClin Med*. 2023;61:102052. https://doi.org/10.1016/j.eclinm.2023.102052.
65. van der Heijden CAJ, Weberndörfer V, Vroomen M, et al. Hybrid ablation versus repeated catheter ablation in persistent atrial fibrillation: a randomized controlled trial. *JACC Clin Electrophysiol*. 2023;9(7):1013–1023.
66. Castellá M, Kotecha D, van Laar C, et al. Thoracoscopic vs. catheter ablation for atrial fibrillation: long-term follow-up of the FAST randomized trial. *Europace*. 2019;21(5):746–753.
67. Zhang S, Cui Y, Li J, et al. Concomitant transcatheter occlusion versus thoracoscopic surgical clipping for left atrial appendage in patients undergoing ablation for atrial fibrillation: a meta-analysis. *Front Cardiovasc Med*. 2022;9:970847.
68. Wang JL, Zhou K, Qin Z, Cheng WJ, Zhang LZ, Zhou YJ. Minimally invasive thoracoscopic left atrial appendage occlusion compared with transcatheter left atrial appendage closure for stroke prevention in recurrent nonvalvular atrial fibrillation patients after radiofrequency ablation: a prospective cohort study. *J Geriatr Cardiol*. 2021;18(11):877–885.

46

Randomized Trials of Left Atrial Appendage Occlusion

Richard Whitlock, Emilie Belley-Côté

CHAPTER OUTLINE

Atrial fibrillation (AF) affects 1% of the general population[1] and about 11% of patients undergoing cardiac surgery, and it is an important risk factor for stroke.[2–4] Most ischemic strokes in patients with AF are cardio-embolic in nature,[5] with the majority originating in the left atrial appendage (LAA).[6] Anticoagulation is an effective approach to stroke prevention, but it requires lifelong adherence and its use is limited by bleeding. Surgical occlusion of the LAA has been shown to be an effective complement to antithrombotic therapy and is also effective as a stand-alone treatment.

Oral anticoagulation (OAC) reduces the risk of stroke in patients with AF, and therefore it is recommended for most patients with AF.[7] Nonetheless, contemporary registries show that only about half of high-risk patients with AF receive OAC.[8] For those started on anticoagulation, discontinuation rates exceed 50% at 3 years.[9] Temporary and permanent anticoagulation discontinuation occurs for a variety of reasons, including surgery, illness, bleeding, and so on. The main shortcoming of anticoagulation is that maintaining anticoagulation treatment over long periods for a lifelong stroke risk is difficult and inconvenient.

Physical elimination or exclusion of the LAA is an alternative approach to stroke prevention in AF that does not suffer from the limitations of pharmacologic therapy, including noncompliance, discontinuation, and ongoing risk of bleeding. After it has been performed, the effects of the occlusion are permanent and do not require patient compliance. Despite first being described in 1948,[10] randomized trials did not begin until 2001.[11]

PERCUTANEOUS LEFT ATRIAL APPENDAGE OCCLUSION TRIALS

The first randomized trials that informed clinical practice were completed in the transcatheter LAA occlusion (LAAO) field. We limit our discussion to the trials using the Watchman device because these trials have most advanced the evidence in that field. We have learned that LAAO is likely beneficial as an alternative to warfarin in patients with AF from randomized controlled trials (RCTs) of percutaneous device closure (PROTECT-AF[12] and PREVAIL[13]). A meta-analysis of these trials shows noninferiority of the device compared with warfarin.[14] However, much of the benefit of LAAO with a device compared with warfarin is due to the absence of intracranial bleeding, which is often seen with warfarin. The effect of LAAO on ischemic stroke remained to be determined and was suggested to be inferior to warfarin based on that meta-analysis.[14] Important differences exist between device-based and surgical LAAO, which can be performed at the same time as cardiac surgery for another indication or as a stand-alone procedure. Device-based LAAO is costly and associated with procedural risk. As such, it is mostly used for the subset of patients who cannot receive anticoagulation because of very high bleeding risk. Furthermore, patients enrolled in device trials were very different from the surgical patients with AF who have higher CHA_2DS_2-VASc scores and who often have valvular heart disease. (These patients were excluded in the percutaneous trials, and they may have more frequent thrombi outside of the LAA.[6]) Finally, whereas surgical occlusion is an extravascular procedure, endovascular device occlusion carries the risk of device-related thrombus formation and embolism. Therefore, the results from percutaneous LAA closure cannot be extrapolated to surgical LAAO and vice versa. In summary, the device-based trials provided proof of concept that LAAO may be beneficial but did not address patients with AF who undergo cardiac surgery, did not inform on the combination of LAAO and medical prophylaxis, and did not evaluate a surgical intervention that can be offered to millions of patients as concomitant therapy with cardiac surgery at virtually no additional cost or risk.

SURGICAL LEFT ATRIAL APPENDAGE OCCLUSION TRIALS

The RCT evidence that LAAO reduces the risk of ischemic stroke in AF comes from the surgical trial Left Atrial Appendage Occlusion Study (LAAOS) III. This seminal trial was part of a program established by researchers at McMaster University, Hamilton, Canada.

Left Atrial Appendage Occlusion Study I

The LAAOS research program started with LAAOS I, which was a two-center pilot trial to demonstrate the safety of surgical LAAO. The trial randomized 77 patients to LAAO at the time of cardiac surgery versus no occlusion and reported that surgical occlusion could be performed with a low rate of adverse events.[11] LAAOS I included patients with and without AF at increased risk of stroke. This trial also established a commonly used definition of LAAO success based on transesophageal echocardiography (TEE) parameters: a residual stump smaller than 1 cm and no leak across the occlusion line. Based on this definition, LAAOS I suggested that complete removal of the appendage is preferred to oversewing.

Left Atrial Appendage Occlusion Study II

LAAOS II was a pilot study at four Canadian centers designed to establish the feasibility of a trial of LAAO versus OAC in patients undergoing cardiac surgery with a preexisting history of AF.[4] Specifically, it compared LAAO plus aspirin with guideline-directed oral anticoagulant therapy in 51 patients. LAAOS II struggled with recruitment outside of the lead center in Hamilton, Ontario, Canada. Furthermore, the use of OAC in both arms converged over time, suggesting a lack of buy-in of physicians regarding the ethics of withholding OAC despite LAAO. The study confirmed the effectiveness and safety of amputation and closure for occlusion with a 100% success rate and no instances of left atrial tears deemed to be life-threatening. The addition of amputation and closure to a cardiac surgical procedure for another indication added approximately 10 minutes of surgical time. Last, a cross-sectional study performed during LAAOS II better defined the prevalence of preexisting AF and related risk factors in the cardiac surgical population, further informing the final design of LAAOS III.

Left Atrial Appendage Occlusion Study III

The rationale and design of LAAOS III have been published.[15] In summary, it was a multicenter, prospective, blinded, randomized trial of concomitant surgical LAAO in patients with AF and CHA_2DS_2-VASc scores of 2 or less undergoing cardiac surgery for other reasons. In the trial, LAAO could be performed using the following techniques: (1) amputation and closure (promoted as the preferred technique, (2) stapler closure, (3) double-layer linear closure from within the atrium (for mini-thoracotomy cases if successful occlusion could be confirmed by TEE), or (4) use of a surgical LAAO device that was approved by applicable regulatory authorities (i.e., AtriClip, AtriCure Inc.). The Trial Operations Committee approved other techniques on a case-by-case basis. Percutaneous closure was not permitted, nor was surgical purse-string suture closure. Intraoperative TEE was recommended to demonstrate successful closure of the appendage defined as the absence of flow across the suture line and a residual stump smaller than 1 cm. If the initial closure was not successful, the surgeons were expected to perform additional maneuvers to rectify. In patients with preoperative LAA thrombus, the LAA was opened to remove the thrombus before LAAO. In the LAAOS III, the patients and health care workers outside of the operating room were blinded. All patients were expected to receive best care for stroke prevention. The LAAOS III investigators actively promoted ongoing adherence to guidelines for antithrombotic therapy for stroke prevention during follow-up. The medical team or family physician, without knowledge of whether the patient had had occlusion of the LAA, oversaw antithrombotic management. The operating surgeon was recused from managing antithrombotic therapy after surgery. Patients in the control arm did not have surgical LAAO but otherwise were treated identically.

The primary question of LAAOS III was whether or not concomitant LAAO at the time of other cardiac surgery would reduce ischemic stroke in patients with AF. In the context of cardiac surgery for other indications, LAAO was tested in addition to usual stroke prevention care. The alternate approach of testing LAAO as an alternative to OAC was not only impractical as learned in LAAOS II, but it did not align with the idea that anticoagulation and LAAO should work well together. OAC is remarkably effective in those with AF but has limitations inherent in many long-term prophylactic medications (e.g., bleeding risk, failure to prescribe, failure to adhere and necessary discontinuations). It was hypothesized that the addition of LAAO to anticoagulation would mitigate the risk from those limitations.

LAAOS III enrolled 4811 patients from 105 centers in 27 countries. The surgical LAAO techniques used were as follows: amputation and closure, 56%; surgical LAAO device, 15%; linear closure from within atrium, 14%; stapler, 11%; and other approved techniques, 4%. After the second formal interim analysis of efficacy, the data safety monitoring board recommended termination of follow-up and reporting of the trial; the mean duration of follow-up was 3.8 years. The results showed clearly that LAAO reduces ischemic stroke by about 33% (Fig. 46.1).

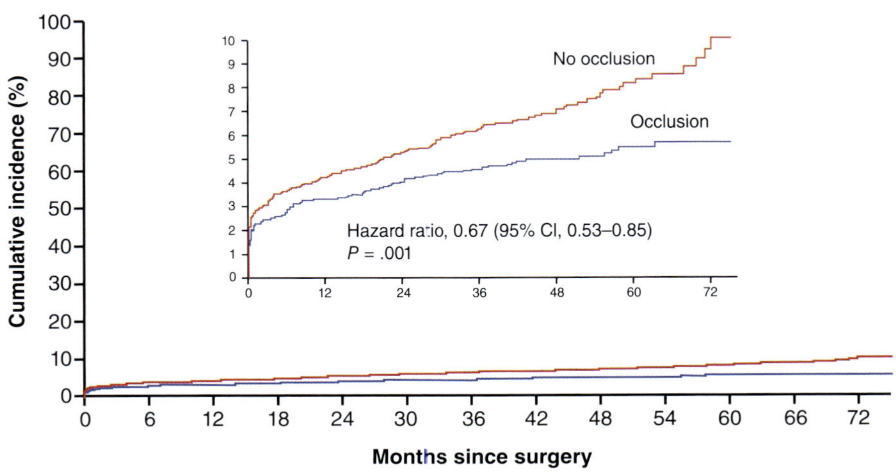

No. at risk													
No occlusion	2391	2134	2081	2030	1981	1897	1607	1291	1016	751	540	348	205
Occlusion	2391	2163	2105	2059	2020	1948	1642	1322	1046	781	550	349	199

Fig. 46.1 Cumulative incidence of stroke or systemic arterial embolism. The participants in the occlusion group underwent left atrial appendage occlusion (LAAO) at the time of cardiac surgery for another indication, and those in the no-occlusion group did not undergo LAAO at the time of cardiac surgery; all participants were expected to receive usual care. The inset shows the same data on an enlarged *y*-axis. *CI*, Confidence interval. (Reproduced from Whitlock RP, Belley-Cote EP, Paparella D, et al. Left atrial appendage occlusion during cardiac surgery to prevent stroke. *N Eng J Med.* 385(11):1054–1055.)

The hazard ratio in favor of LAAO was 0.67 (95% confidence interval, 0.53–0.85; $P = .001$). Thus LAAOS III was the largest RCT to demonstrate the benefit of LAAO on ischemic events. Importantly, most patients (>75%) in LAAOS III received OAC.

Surgical LAAO was also demonstrated to be safe. The mean cross-clamp and cardiopulmonary bypass times were increased by an average of 4 minutes and 6 minutes, respectively, which are not clinically meaningful increases. Perioperative bleeding as assessed by chest tube output, transfusion, and surgical reexploration did not differ between the groups. The 30-day mortality rates were 3.7% and 4.0% for the LAAO and no occlusion groups, respectively. Finally, the rate of readmission for heart failure was not increased by LAAO. Therefore, concomitant surgical LAAO in patients with a history of AF provides ongoing stroke prevention on top of anticoagulation without increasing perioperative or long-term adverse events.

Other trials have evaluated surgical LAAO but without providing the definitive evidence LAAOS III provided, mainly because the trials were too small and underpowered to assess definitive differences in clinical outcomes.

Left Atrial Appendage Closure by Surgery 2 Trial

The Left Atrial Appendage Closure by Surgery (LAACS)-2 trial is a multicenter randomized trial examining the impact of surgical LAAO on stroke in patients undergoing cardiac surgery irrespective of AF status and CHA_2DS_2-VASc score. The trial enrolled participants 18 years or older scheduled for first-time elective open-heart surgery from cardiac surgery centers in Denmark, Spain, and Sweden. Patients for whom AF ablation or LAA closure during surgery were already planned, with current endocarditis, or in whom follow-up was not possible were considered ineligible. Participants were randomized 1:1 to either concomitant LAA closure or standard care (i.e., no LAA closure). The primary outcome of the trial is stroke, including transient ischemic attack, as assigned by two independent neurologists blinded to the treatment allocation. The LAACS-2 trial completed enrollment in October 2023 with 1500 patients entered. The trial will follow participants until 55 primary outcome events have occurred and then report its results.

Left Atrial Appendage Exclusion for Prophylactic Stroke Reduction

The Left Atrial Appendage Exclusion for Prophylactic Stroke Reduction (LeAAPS) trial seeks to assess the role of LAA exclusion using the AtriClip device for stroke prevention in patients who do not have AF but who have atrial cardiomyopathy. In LAAOS III, the benefit of surgical LAAO was clearly shown for patients with AF, and this occurred in addition to OAC in most patients. A high percentage of cardiac surgery patients do not have preexisting AF, but many of them still have a substantial risk of developing AF and a stroke. It is well known that electrical and structural remodeling of the left atrium precedes the development of clinical AF by many years in many patients (see Chapter 8). This electrical and structural remodeling of the atrium, which can be detected by simple tests, is now termed *atrial cardiomyopathy* and is recognized as a precursor of clinical AF. Heart rhythm societies have defined and characterized atrial cardiomyopathy as "any complex of structural, architectural, contractile or electrophysiological changes affecting the atria with the potential to produce clinically-relevant manifestations."[16] Diseases such as hypertension, diabetes, and valve dysfunction, as well as aging itself, predispose to atrial cardiomyopathy with similar pathological changes that progress with time. Atrial cardiomyopathy without documented occurrence of AF is often present in patients undergoing cardiac surgery. Echocardiographic and biochemical markers can readily identify atrial cardiomyopathy in patients at high risk of developing AF. It is currently unknown if exclusion or removal of the LAA is beneficial in patients at risk of developing AF but who have not yet been diagnosed with AF.

As demonstrated in LAAOS III, cardiac surgery provides an excellent opportunity to exclude the LAA at very low risk. During most cardiac surgical procedures, the LAA is exposed and readily accessible, and LAAO can be performed without significantly prolonging the cardiac surgery. The ATLAS trial was a prospective, randomized multicenter feasibility trial of 562 cardiac surgery patients without a history of AF randomized 2:1 for AtriClip versus no LAA exclusion.[17] ATLAS demonstrated that prophylactic occlusion appeared safe and reported a trend in reduction of stroke and systemic embolism (19%) at 1 year in patients who received AtriClip versus those who did not have their LAA excluded. Based on LAAOS III and the ATLAS trial, the unmet medical need was for a robust randomized trial to evaluate if exclusion of the LAA at the time of other routine cardiac surgery can reduce the incidence of stroke during long-term follow-up in patients with atrial cardiomyopathy (the LeAAPS trial). The total sample size of 6500 patients will have at least 84% power to detect 25% relative reduction in ischemic stroke or systemic embolism. LeAAPS opened to enrollment in February 2023 and randomized approximately 1600 patients in the first year.

The Anticoagulant Therapy in Patients With Atrial Fibrillation After Surgical Left Atrial Appendage Closure Trial

Surgical LAAO has been proven to be beneficial as an adjunct to OAC, but the question of whether surgical LAAO renders anticoagulation unnecessary remains unanswered. The Anticoagulant Therapy in Patients with Atrial Fibrillation after Surgical Left Atrial Appendage Closure (ATLAAC) trial is a randomized trial of 1220 patients who have previously undergone surgical LAAO to determine if anticoagulation can be safely discontinued in these patients. First, potential participants will undergo a cardiac computed tomography scan to determine whether LAAO was successful. Patients with successful closure who consent to participate will be randomized to either continue or discontinue anticoagulation. Participants will be followed every 6 months using national Scandinavian registries. The trial will assess whether stopping anticoagulation after surgical LAAO is noninferior to continuing anticoagulation for the occurrence of ischemic stroke, peripheral arterial embolism, and major bleeding. Enrollment is expected to take 12 to 18 months. The duration of follow-up will be event driven (128 events) with an expected follow-up period of about 4 years. The trial opened to enrollment in February 2024. The ATLAAC trial is proposed as a national Danish trial, but if the required number of patients cannot be achieved from the Danish population, the trial will expand to enroll in other countries.

CONCLUSIONS

Evidence from a large, randomized trial of LAAO in patients with AF having cardiac surgery showed that concomitant LAAO reduces the risk of stroke over long-term follow-up. The impact of LAAO in patients undergoing cardiac surgery who do not have a history of AF but are at risk of stroke and AF is currently being assessed. The LeAAPS trial could extend the benefit of LAAO to a much broader population. Finally, the ATLAAC trial should answer the question of whether anticoagulation can be discontinued after surgical LAAO.

REFERENCES

1. Go AS, Hylek EM, Phillips KA, et al. Prevalence of diagnosed atrial fibrillation in adults: national implications for rhythm management and stroke prevention: the AnTicoagulation and

Risk Factors in Atrial Fibrillation (ATRIA) study. *J Am Med Assoc.* 2001;285:2370–2375.
2. Wolf PA, Abbott RD, Kannel WB. Atrial fibrillation as an independent risk factor for stroke: the Framingham Study. *Stroke.* 1991;22:983–988.
3. Gage BF, van Walraven C, Pearce L, et al. Selecting patients with atrial fibrillation for anticoagulation: stroke risk stratification in patients taking aspirin. *Circulation.* 2004;110:2287–2292.
4. Whitlock RP, Vincent J, Blackall MH, et al. Left atrial appendage occlusion study II (LAAOS II). *Can J Cardiol.* 2013;29:1443–1447.
5. Stroke prevention in atrial fibrillation investigators. Final results. *Circulation.* 1991;84:527–539.
6. Blackshear JL, Odell JA. Appendage obliteration to reduce stroke in cardiac surgical patients with atrial fibrillation. *Ann Thor Surg.* 1996;61:755–759.
7. Fuster V, Ryden LE, Cannom DS, et al. Guidelines for the management of patients with atrial fibrillation: executive summary. *Revista Espanola de Cardiologia.* 2006;59:1329.
8. Apenteng PN, Gao H, Hobbs FR, Fitzmaurice DA, Investigators UG-A, Committee G-AS. Temporal trends in antithrombotic treatment of real-world UK patients with newly diagnosed atrial fibrillation: findings from the GARFIELD-AF registry. *BMJ Open.* 2018;8:e018905.
9. Gallagher AM, Rietbrock S, Plumb J, van Staa TP. Initiation and persistence of warfarin or aspirin in patients with chronic atrial fibrillation in general practice: do the appropriate patients receive stroke prophylaxis? *J Thromb and Haemostas.* 2008;6:1500–1506.
10. Madden JL. Resection of the left auricular appendix; a prophylaxis for recurrent arterial emboli. *J Am Med Assoc.* 1949;140:769–772.
11. Healey JS, Crystal E, Lamy A, et al. Left Atrial Appendage Occlusion Study (LAAOS): results of a randomized controlled pilot study of left atrial appendage occlusion during coronary bypass surgery in patients at risk for stroke. *Am Heart J.* 2005;150:288–293.
12. Holmes DR, Reddy VY, Turi ZG, et al. Percutaneous closure of the left atrial appendage versus warfarin therapy for prevention of stroke in patients with atrial fibrillation: a randomised non-inferiority trial. *Lancet.* 2009;374:534–542.
13. Holmes DR Jr, Kar S, Price MJ, et al. Prospective randomized evaluation of the watchman left atrial appendage closure device in patients with atrial fibrillation versus long-term warfarin therapy: the prevail trial. *J Am Coll Cardiol.* 2014;64:1–12.
14. Holmes DR Jr, Doshi SK, Kar S, et al. Left atrial appendage closure as an alternative to warfarin for stroke prevention in atrial fibrillation: a patient-level meta-analysis. *J Am Coll Cardiol.* 2015;65:2614–2623.
15. Whitlock R, Healey J, Vincent J, et al. Rationale and design of the Left Atrial Appendage Occlusion Study (LAAOS) III. *Ann Cardiothorac Surg.* 2014;3:45–54.
16. Goette A, Kalman JM, Aguinaga L, et al. EHRA/HRS/APHRS/SOLAECE expert consensus on atrial cardiomyopathies: definition, characterization, and clinical implication. *Europace.* 2016;18:1455–1490.
17. Gerdisch MW, Garrett Jr HE, Mumtaz MA, et al. Prophylactic left atrial appendage exclusion in cardiac surgery patients with elevated CHA(2)DS(2)-VASc score: results of the randomized ATLAS trial. *Innovations.* 2022;17:463–470.

47

New-Onset Postoperative Atrial Fibrillation

James L. Cox, Patrick M. McCarthy, Olga N. Kislitsina

CHAPTER OUTLINE

New-onset postoperative atrial fibrillation (POAF) is a serious complication of adult cardiac surgery that occurs in 20% to 55% of cases.[1] It should be differentiated from recurrent atrial fibrillation (AF) after surgical ablation for preoperative AF because patients with new-onset POAF after cardiac surgery had no history of ever having AF before the surgery. New-onset POAF is associated with an increase in perioperative stroke, myocardial infarction, ventricular tachycardia or fibrillation (cardiac arrest), need for new pacemakers, intensive care unit days, hospital stay, and 30-day operative mortality.[2,3] In addition, long-term survival is less in patients who develop new-onset POAF after coronary artery bypass grafting (CABG) than in those who do not develop new-onset POAF (Fig. 47.1).[4] In 90% of these patients, new-onset POAF manifests within the first 6 days after surgery, coinciding with the peak of the postoperative systemic inflammatory response. This condition imposes a substantial clinical and financial burden in the United States, with annual health care costs exceeding $1 billion, prolonged hospital stays, and increased stress on patients and their families. Thus, there is a clear need for effective preventative strategies and management to mitigate the impact of new-onset POAF.[5]

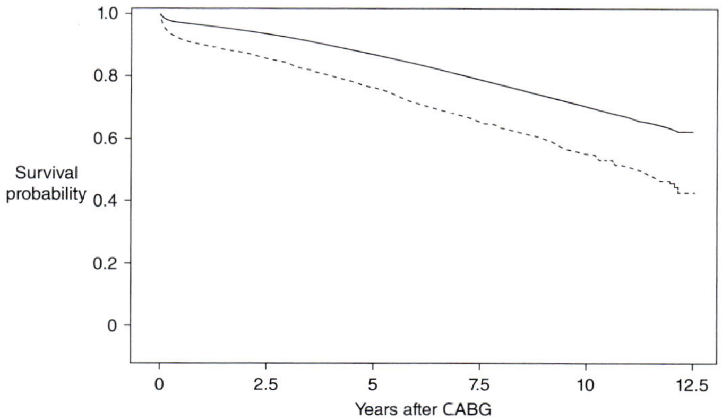

Fig. 47.1 Scope of postoperative atrial fibrillation (POAF). The development of postoperative atrial fibrillation (POAF) after coronary artery bypass grafting (CABG) is associated with decreased long-term survival compared with patients who do not develop POAF. (Reproduced from Almassi GH, Schowalter T, Nicolosi AC, et al. Atrial fibrillation after cardiac surgery: a major morbid event? *Ann Surg*. 1997;226(4):501–513.)

Currently, there is no way to predict which patients will develop new-onset POAF after cardiac surgery, and there is no prophylactic strategy that is universally agreed on to prevent it. Furthermore, it is virtually impossible to assess the true efficacy of any prophylactic regimen designed to prevent new-onset POAF because it is impossible to control for all of the variables in a cardiac surgical procedure that can impact the development of new-onset POAF. Therefore, designing randomized controlled clinical trials to determine the efficacy of prophylactic measures to prevent new-onset POAF after cardiac surgery is difficult at best and usually a futile endeavor.

PREOPERATIVE VULNERABILITY TO THE DEVELOPMENT OF NEW-ONSET POSTOPERATIVE ATRIAL FIBRILLATION

Why do some patients develop new-onset POAF after cardiac surgery while others do not? Perhaps the most interesting aspect of new-onset POAF is that it does *not* develop in roughly two-thirds of cardiac surgery patients regardless of how complex the surgical procedure might be. The reported incidence of new-onset POAF after cardiac surgery varies widely because of a variety of factors, including, among others, the unknown number of patients receiving new-onset POAF prophylaxis in the studies.[6]

New-onset POAF risk factors can be categorized into two groups: modifiable and nonmodifiable. Nonmodifiable factors include age, race, gender, heart failure, and valvular heart disease. Among these, age has been most strongly associated with the development of new-onset POAF after cardiac surgery, likely because of age-related slowing of conduction and an increase in myocardial fibrosis. A large retrospective study involving more than 140,000 patients undergoing *noncardiac* surgery revealed that the incidence of new-onset POAF varies by both age and sex. Although no significant difference in new-onset POAF risk was observed between sexes in patients younger than 40 years, male patients in older age groups had a significantly higher risk compared with female patients.[7] Additionally, a comparative study demonstrated that men exhibited higher postoperative peak lactate levels and a greater incidence of death during a 4-year follow-up period.[8] Racial disparities have also been reported, with White patients undergoing CABG shown to have a higher incidence of new-onset POAF compared to non-White patients. However, studies assessing the impact of race on new-onset POAF are often limited by a significantly lower representation of non-White patients.[9]

In contrast, modifiable factors, such as obesity and high body mass index (BMI), present opportunities for intervention. Obesity and elevated BMI predispose patients to hypertension and diabetes, which serve as secondary risk factors for new-onset POAF.[10] Another modifiable risk factor is lifestyle choices, which significantly impact the risk of new-onset POAF after cardiac surgery. Maintaining a healthy weight, engaging in regular exercise, limiting alcohol intake, smoking cessation, stress management, adequate sleep, and a balanced diet can help regulate blood pressure, cholesterol levels, and overall heart health, potentially reducing the likelihood of developing new-onset POAF. In this context, patient education is crucial to empower individuals to make informed decisions and adopt heart-healthy habits.

If all cardiac surgery patients, regardless of age, sex, type of surgery, comorbidities, and with no new-onset POAF prophylaxis are included, an average of approximately 35% of them will develop new-onset POAF (Fig. 47.2).[11] Thus if 100 patients undergo cardiac surgery without any prophylaxis, an average of 65 of them will not develop POAF, and 5 of them will develop new-onset POAF even after having the simplest noncardiac surgery. This indicates that these latter 5 patients are far more vulnerable to the development of new-onset POAF than either the 30 patients who develop new-onset POAF only after cardiac surgery or the 65 patients who do not develop new-onset POAF at all. The reason for this variability in the preoperative vulnerability of patients to the development of new-onset POAF after cardiac surgery is unknown.

All arrhythmias, including new-onset POAF, require two factors to develop: (1) abnormal dispersion of refractoriness (nonuniform recovery) and (2) a trigger. The possible triggers for new-onset POAF are numerous and can include inflammation from postoperative pericarditis, surgical trauma, general anesthesia, elevated circulating catecholamines, autonomic nervous system imbalance, and many other perioperative factors. However, those factors occur with similar frequency in the extremely vulnerable 5% group, the somewhat vulnerable 30% group, and the invulnerable 65% groups described. Therefore, differences in the presence of triggers cannot explain the differences in the vulnerability of the three groups to the development of new-onset POAF. Instead, it is obvious that some abnormality in the pattern of electrical recovery (repolarization) in the atria renders some patients vulnerable and other patients invulnerable to the development of new-onset POAF.

In the 1990s we identified experimentally at least one abnormality to explain why some patients present for cardiac surgery with atria that are more vulnerable than others to developing new-onset POAF, *the distribution of local refractory periods in the atria*.[12] The construction of "refractory period distribution maps" of local refractory periods is laborious and time consuming and therefore, it is feasible only under experimental conditions. Local refractory period maps require that the local refractory period be determined for each single site in the atrium by repeatedly pacing at that single site with a progressively decreasing pacing interval until failure of capture occurs. The longest cycle length at which the pacing fails to capture is the local refractory period for that particular site but only for that particular site. To construct the global pattern of local refractory period distribution, this same pacing process must be repeated at multiple sites in the atria.

As explained in Chapter 4, the local refractory periods are shorter in the left atrium (LA) than in the right atrium (RA; see Fig. 4.15). The distribution of local refractory periods normally exhibits a smooth transition from the shorter ones in the LA to the longer ones in the RA (Fig. 47.3). If a patient has this distribution of local refractory periods in the atria, it is highly unlikely that any perioperative trigger can induce AF. This is analogous to the inability of premature atrial beats (triggers) to induce AF in an atrium that is incapable of sustaining a macro-reentrant circuit (see Chapter 5, Fig. 5.33). Thus this is the normal pattern of refractory period distribution in the atria that can be expected in the 65% of cardiac surgery patients who do not develop new-onset POAF.

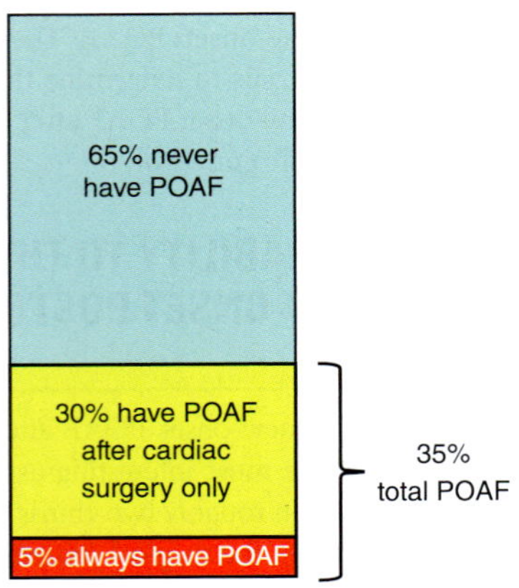

Fig. 47.2 Scope of postoperative atrial fibrillation (POAF). After adult cardiac surgery of all types, if prophylactic measures against POAF are not instituted preoperatively, an average of approximately 35% will develop POAF. This includes 30% who develop POAF only after undergoing cardiac surgery and 5% who have POAF after any cardiac or noncardiac surgery. The incidence of POAF varies between types of cardiac surgery performed. Interestingly, approximately 65% of patients will *not* develop POAF no matter how complex the surgical procedure.

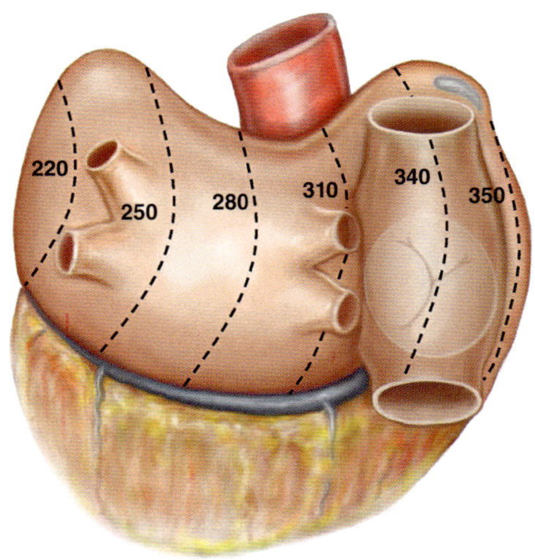

Fig. 47.3 Normal distribution of local refractory periods in the 65% of patients who never have postoperative atrial fibrillation (POAF). The refractory periods at specific local sites in the atria are shorter in the left atrium than in the right atrium and the transition from short refractory periods to longer refractory periods is smooth and sequential. Patients with this normal distribution of local refractory periods are unlikely to develop POAF after cardiac surgery. (See text for further discussion.)

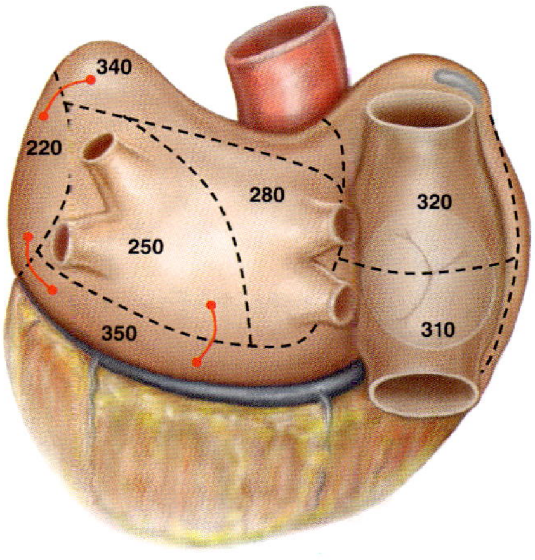

Fig. 47.4 **Mild dispersion of refractoriness in the 30% of patients who have postoperative atrial fibrillation (POAF) only after cardiac surgery.** If the distribution of local refractory periods is not smooth and sequential ("dispersion of refractoriness"), several areas can exist adjacent to one another where there is great disparity between the refractory periods *(curved red bars)*. This abnormality can result in POAF. If the dispersion of refractoriness is mild (i.e., there are not too many of these adjacent areas), the patient may or may not have POAF, and prophylactic measures to prevent it are likely to be beneficial. We believe that the 30% of patients who develop POAF only after a cardiac surgical procedure most likely have this type of mild dispersion of refractoriness.

If the dispersion of refractoriness in the atria is such that areas of long refractoriness are occasionally located adjacent to areas of much shorter refractoriness (Fig. 47.4), the patient is more vulnerable to the development of new-onset POAF. We know that an abnormal distribution of atrial refractory periods makes patients vulnerable to the development of AF (see Chapters 4 and 5). Therefore, we surmise that this AF vulnerability, coupled with the multiple potential AF triggers that exist after cardiac surgery, results in the 30% of patients who develop new-onset POAF only after cardiac surgery. If the dispersion of atrial refractoriness is even greater so that there are *multiple* areas of short refractoriness adjacent to areas of long refractoriness (Fig. 47.5), the

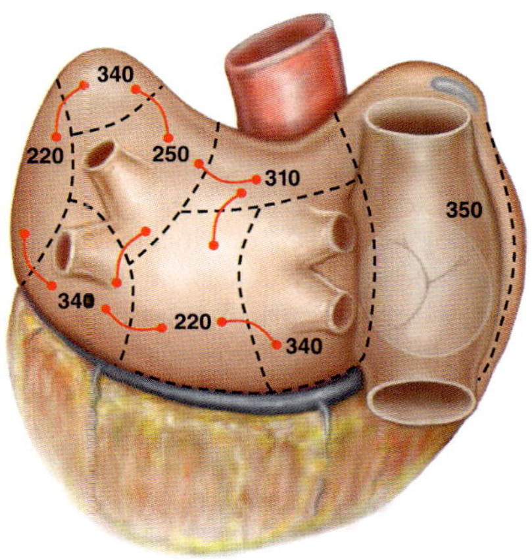

Fig. 47.5 **Severe dispersion of refractoriness in the 5% of patients who always have postoperative atrial fibrillation (POAF).** If atrial repolarization is such that the dispersion of refractoriness results in numerable adjacent areas in the atria with widely varying local refractory periods (curved red bars), the patient will be extremely vulnerable to developing POAF. This is the problem that likely exists in the 5% of patients who will develop POAF no matter what surgical procedure they undergo.

atrium is extremely vulnerable to the development of AF. These highly vulnerable patients represent the 5% who will develop new-onset POAF after most *any* type of surgery, cardiac or noncardiac.

THE PROBLEM OF PROPHYLAXIS FOR NEW-ONSET POSTOPERATIVE ATRIAL FIBRILLATION

A major problem with studies designed to assess the risk-to-benefit ratio of prophylactic drugs is related to the confounding clinical characteristics of new-onset POAF described in the preceding section. POAF prophylaxis is not needed in approximately two-thirds of patients because regardless of the surgical procedure, they will not develop POAF. In addition, no prophylaxis can prevent POAF from developing in the 5% of patients who will always have POAF no matter how minor the surgical procedure. That leaves only about 30% of cardiac surgery patients who will potentially respond to prophylactic therapy. Unfortunately, 100% of the patients have to be exposed to the side effects of a prophylactic drug (Fig. 47.6). In effect, this triples the potential risk-to-benefit ratio of drug prophylaxis for new-onset POAF and is a major reason why many drugs that are known to reduce new-onset POAF simply cannot be used clinically because their side effects outweigh their benefits.

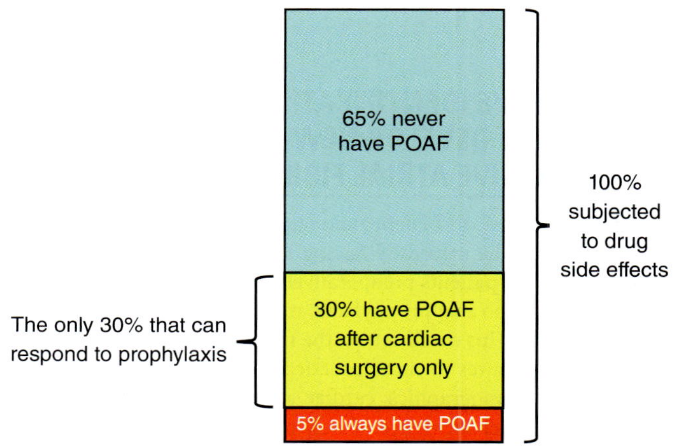

Fig. 47.6 **The risk-to-benefit problem with postoperative atrial fibrillation (POAF) prophylaxis.** The unique problem that exists with prophylactic measures, especially drugs, to decrease the incidence of POAF relates to the risk-to-benefit ratio of POAF prophylaxis. Because 65% of patients do not need any prophylaxis and 5% will not respond to it, only 30% of patients have any potential of responding to POAF prophylaxis. However, 100% of them are exposed to the side effects of the prophylactic drug. This effectively *triples* the risk-to-benefit ratio of prophylactic drugs for POAF.

IS NEW-ONSET POSTOPERATIVE ATRIAL FIBRILLATION THE SAME AS "NATURALLY OCCURRING" ATRIAL FIBRILLATION?

If one mapped new-onset POAF, the electrophysiologic pattern would be the same as any other AF, but there are several differences between new-onset POAF and AF that occurs spontaneously or that develops secondary to left-heart disorders. As described earlier, numerous triggers occur after cardiac surgery that are not at play in "naturally occurring" AF. In addition, some of these same triggers, such as inflammation and increased catecholamines, not only increase the postoperative triggers but also shorten the refractory periods in the atria and aggravate the dispersion of refractoriness that would not have been "unmasked" except by the surgical procedure. For example, one of the unexpected findings in the original series of Maze patients was that 37% of them had POAF despite having just undergone an operation that we thought rendered the atrium incapable of fibrillating! When this surprising and disappointing occurrence was studied, we found that the most consistent new abnormality after cardiac surgery was a generalized shortening of the atrial refractory periods. For example, we had 9 patients who had preoperative atrial flutter in addition to AF who underwent the Maze procedure. Their preoperative atrial flutter had the typical cycle length of 200 ms, resulting in an atrial rate of 300 beats/min and a ventricular rate of 150 beats/min (see Chapter 5, Fig. 5.15). Postoperatively, atrial flutter could still be induced in these 9 patients but their atrial flutters all had shorter cycle lengths than they had preoperatively. We interpreted this to mean that despite a successful Maze procedure, the atrial refractory periods were temporarily shortened to the extent that smaller macro-reentrant circuits (drivers) could form between the lesions of the Maze procedure, resulting in what amounted to a new-onset POAF even though the patients had a long history of preoperative AF (see Chapter 4, Fig. 4.14). After the atria had sufficient time to heal postoperatively, the atrial refractory periods lengthened back to normal, the new-onset POAF subsided, and the long-term success of the Maze procedure for the "naturally occurring" AF was the same in these patients as in the ones who did not develop new-onset POAF.

PREOPERATIVE IDENTIFICATION OF PATIENTS DESTINED TO DEVELOP NEW-ONSET POSTOPERATIVE ATRIAL FIBRILLATION

The unfavorable risk-to-benefit ratio of prophylaxis against new-onset POAF could best be solved by having the ability to identify the 30% of cardiac surgery patients preoperatively who are destined to develop new-onset POAF so that prophylactic measures could be applied only in these patients. This could return the risk-to-benefit ratio of prophylactic POAF measures to more practical levels. It is well known that certain patient demographics, cardiac abnormalities, and comorbidities lead to a higher incidence of new-onset POAF, but this information is not particularly helpful in deciding which patients should be subjected to POAF prophylaxis and perhaps more important, which patients should *not* be subjected to the side effects of unnecessary drugs. For example, all older adult patients with poor cardiac function and preoperative renal failure do not develop new-onset POAF, and the avoidance of POAF prophylaxis in such patients is desirable. However, it is usually these very patients who are most likely to be subjected to POAF prophylaxis that in many cases is unnecessary.

Unfortunately, it is still not possible to identify patients before surgery who are destined to develop new-onset POAF with sufficient specificity to limit POAF prophylaxis to those patients only despite long and continuing efforts to do so.[13–18] However, conventional echocardiographic studies have demonstrated that hypertension and LA diameter are independent preoperative predictors of POAF.[19] Left atrial volume (LAV) has also been explored, but it is not an ideal predictor of POAF because of variability related to individual body size and composition. For instance, comparing LAV between a 150-lb man and a 200-lb, 6-ft-tall man may lead to inaccurate conclusions because obesity is an independent risk factor for the recurrence of the "natural" types of AF.

In this context, the left atrial volume index (LAVI), which normalizes LA volume to body surface area, offers a more reliable metric than unadjusted left atrial size or volume. LAVI can be determined without advanced speckle-tracking analysis and has been shown to be associated with an increase in AF, including new-onset POAF after cardiac surgery. Osranek and colleagues[20] showed that a LAVI greater than 32 mL/M^2 was associated with a fivefold increase in the risk of developing POAF independent of age and other clinical risk factors. However, it should be noted that no matched comparisons were performed in the study.

We showed in a matched group study that LAVI was significantly larger in patients who developed new-onset POAF compared with those who did not.[21] Interestingly, however, the absolute value for LAVI in the POAF group was 29.8 mL/M^2, which is still within the normal range according to current guidelines.[22] This finding suggests that although LAVI can be a helpful echocardiographic parameter, it may not serve as an ideal stand-alone marker for predicting new-onset POAF, highlighting the need for more comprehensive and individualized risk assessment approaches.

Preoperative Left Atrial Strain and New-Onset Postoperative Atrial Fibrillation

Several small observational studies have suggested that preoperative compliance abnormalities of the LA, detected by calculating left atrial strain using speckle-tracking analysis of preoperative echocardiograms, might be able to predict new-onset POAF after cardiac surgery. Left atrial strain measured by speckle tracking echocardiography is a quick, sensitive, and objective parameter that assesses left atrial deformation, providing insights into its reservoir, conduit, and contraction phases (Fig. 47.7). This technique has gained recognition as a valuable predictor of AF recurrence and persistence after various medical and interventional therapies for AF. Moreover, left atrial strain has been identified as a marker of left atrial fibrosis. Previous studies have explored left atrial strain across different clinical scenarios. For instance, peak atrial contraction strain (PACS) was identified as an independent predictor of AF development in patients with cryptogenic stroke. Additionally, both peak atrial longitudinal strain (PALS) and PACS were associated with the occurrence of new-onset POAF in patients undergoing surgical treatment for aortic stenosis.[23]

In 2011, Haffajee and colleagues[24] reported that in 40 patients with new-onset POAF, the preoperative mechanical function of the LA as determined by the left atrial total emptying fraction was an independent predictor of new-onset POAF. In 2013, Candan et al.[25] found that in 15 patients with new-onset POAF, both peak left atrial longitudinal strain and LAVI predicted the POAF, though LAVI does not require speckle-tracking analysis and is not a left atrial strain parameter. Other small studies have suggested that age, the degree of atrial scarring, and decreased preoperative left atrial reservoir strain are all associated with new-onset POAF.[26,27]

In 2022, our group evaluated 211 patients with normal preoperative left ventricular function who underwent isolated CABG. Left atrial, left ventricular, and right ventricular strain were calculated before and after CABG and 94 patients were subjected to propensity score matching of the groups with ($n = 47$) and without ($n = 47$) POAF.[21] The standard echocardiographic measures of left atrial function were not predictive of new-onset POAF. In addition, neither left ventricular nor right ventricular strain parameters were predictive of new-onset POAF. However, the preoperative left atrial fractional area change, left atrial emptying fraction, left atrial reservoir strain, and left atrial pump strain were all predictive of new-onset POAF after CABG (see Fig. 47.7).

Another recently published study involving 310 patients demonstrated that new-onset POAF occurred in 103 patients (33%). Lower global PALS values were found to significantly increase the risk of new-onset POAF and optimal cutoff value for arrhythmia prediction was identified

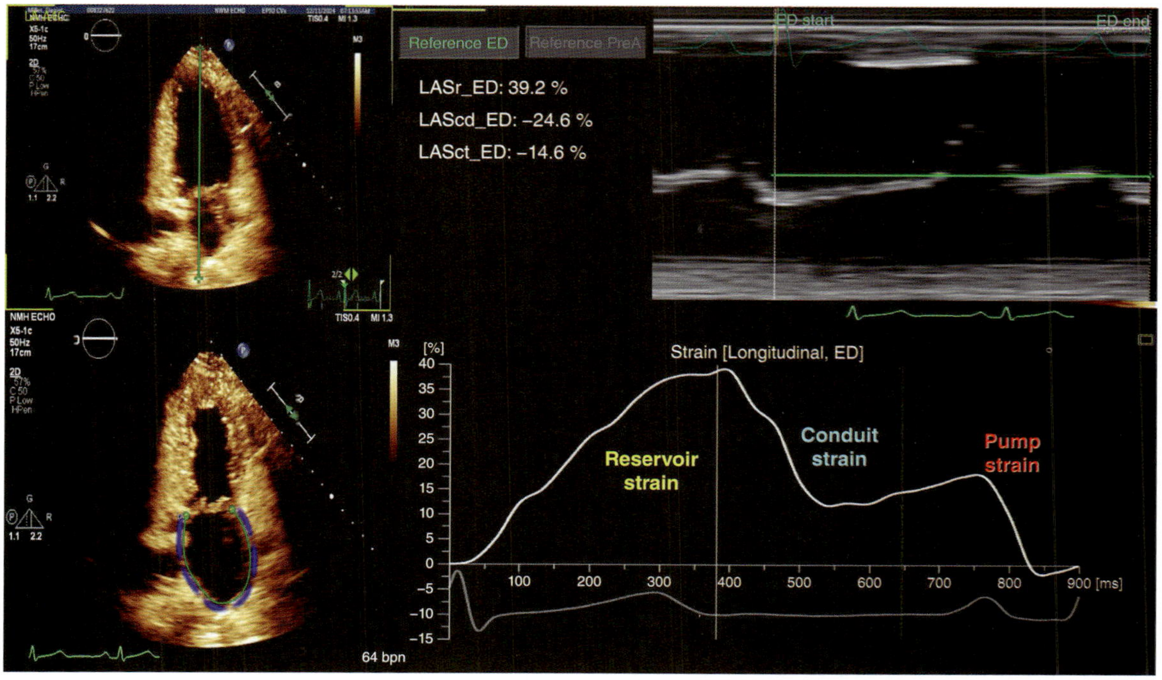

Fig. 47.7 Left atrial strain. There are three phases of left atrial function: the reservoir, conduit, and pump phases. Measurement of left atrial strain is determined by speckle-tracking analysis of echocardiograms. *Left panel,* A four-chamber echocardiographic view shows the left atrium (LA) with endocardial borders traced for strain calculation. The strain measurements correspond to different LA phases: reservoir strain (LASr), conduit strain (LAScd), and pump (contraction) strain (LASct). Recorded strain values in this patient are:
Reservoir strain (LASr-ED): 39.2%
Conduit strain (LAScd-ED): −24.6%
Pump strain (LASct-ED): −14.6%
Right upper panel, Spectral Doppler analysis synchronized with the echocardiographic strain waveforms demonstrating the timing of atrial strain phases relative to the cardiac cycle (end-diastole and pre-atrial contraction).
Left lower panel, Magnified image of the left atrial region with strain tracking lines applied to monitor myocardial deformation.
Right lower panel, The left atrial strain curve, with its phasic components labeled.

- Reservoir strain *(yellow)*: represents left atrial stretching during left ventricular systole, reflecting atrial compliance and storage of pulmonary venous return
- Conduit strain *(blue)*: occurs during early left ventricular diastole, reflecting the passive transfer of blood from the LA to the left ventricle (LV)
- Pump strain *(red)*: represents active left atrial contraction during late left ventricular diastole, reflecting atrial booster function

The strain values align with normal physiological ranges for the LA. The LASr reflects optimal atrial compliance, and the conduit and LASct values highlight balanced atrial function, indicating effective volume accommodation, passive emptying, and active contraction.
This comprehensive depiction of left ventricular strain phases provides key insights into atrial function, particularly in assessing conditions such as atrial fibrillation, diastolic dysfunction, or valvular heart disease. (Reproduced from Kislitsina ON, Cox JL, Shah SJ, et al. Preoperative left atrial strain abnormalities are associated with the development of postoperative atrial fibrillation following isolated coronary artery bypass surgery. *J Thorac Cardiovasc Surg.* 2022;164(3):917–924.)

as a global PALS value less than 28%, which showed a specificity of 86% and a sensitivity of 36%. The incidence of new-onset POAF was notably higher in patients with global PALS less than 28% (51%) compared with those with PALS of 28% or greater (14%; $P < .001$).[28]

Additionally, Parwani et al.[29] focused on the prediction of recurrent postoperative AF after catheter ablation for AF. Although these patients with preoperative AF requiring intervention have no obvious connection to patients with no history of AF who develop new-onset POAF after cardiac surgery, there may be some common value in knowing what causes recurrent AF after AF ablation. Parwani and colleagues' study indicated that lower PALS values, particularly below 15%, were associated with a moderate risk of AF recurrence after catheter AF ablation, with the risk increasing as PALS values decreased further. This highlights the critical role of PALS as a prognostic marker in managing patients at risk of AF recurrence after interventional ablation.[29] Thus, it would be interesting to know if preoperative LA compliance and mechanical function as determined by speckle-tracking strain analysis might provide the sensitivity and specificity needed to identify the 35% of patients who are destined to develop new-onset POAF after cardiac surgery. If these findings regarding postprocedure AF recurrence can be shown to relate to new-onset POAF and confirmed prospectively, we may eventually be able to administer prophylaxis for new-onset POAF only in patients who are certain to develop it, thereby improving our ability to prevent new-onset POAF in a safer and more effective manner.

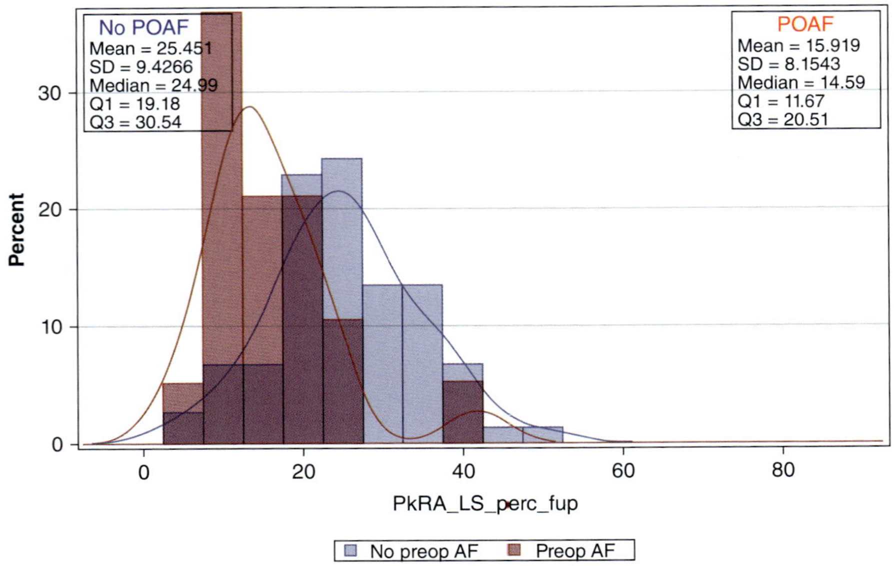

Fig. 47.8 Distribution of right atrial peak longitudinal strain percentage (PkRA_LS_perc_fup) during follow-up in patients categorized into two groups: those with postoperative atrial fibrillation (POAF) and those without (no POAF). Patients in the POAF group had significantly reduced right atrial strain values compared with the no POAF group, suggesting impaired atrial function in patients who developed POAF. The lower right atrial longitudinal strain in the POAF group may reflect preexisting atrial remodeling or dysfunction, which predisposes these patients to the development of atrial fibrillation after surgery. This figure underscores the importance of right atrial function as a potential marker for predicting POAF in the postoperative period.

Preoperative Right Atrial Strain and New-Onset Postoperative Atrial Fibrillation

Several recent studies have shown that pre-interventional right atrial structural remodeling and the ratio of right atrial volume index (RAVI) to LAVI are independently associated with a higher AF recurrence after catheter ablation for AF.[30,31] Our group investigated 322 patients with degenerative mitral valve regurgitation and paroxysmal AF who underwent successful mitral valve repair procedures.[32] At 1-year follow-up, the right atrial reservoir strain remained significantly lower, as did the right atrial contraction (pump) strain. This indicated that even after the Maze procedure and restoration of sinus rhythm, both left atrial function and right atrial function can be slow to return to normal (Fig. 47.8). Importantly, we found that the right atrial reservoir strain was as strong a predictor of late AF recurrence as the left atrial reservoir strain. These observations suggest the possibility that preoperative right atrial structural remodeling and right atrial functional abnormalities as determined by right atrial strain might also serve as preoperative markers for the development of new-onset POAF after cardiac surgery. Clearly, that possibility should be high on the agenda of subjects to study in the future.

INTRAOPERATIVE MEASURES TO DECREASE NEW-ONSET POSTOPERATIVE ATRIAL FIBRILLATION

Atrial Septal Cooling During Cardioplegic Arrest

Surgeons have tried multiple intraoperative measures in the past to decrease the likelihood that patients with no history of AF will develop new-onset POAF after cardiac surgery. Several years ago, we noticed that the atria often started to beat during the period of cardioplegic arrest. Because the atrial muscle depends on a blood supply from the coronary arteries just as the ventricular muscle does, it occurred to us that perhaps the atria were becoming ischemic during the cross-clamp period, in which atrial ischemia might be one of the triggers that caused POAF. We first evaluated this concept in the experimental laboratory, where we inserted needle thermistors into both the atrial septum and the ventricular septum of dogs to monitor their respective myocardial temperatures continuously during cardioplegic arrest.[33] The experimental studies clearly showed that although the ventricular septum remained at satisfactorily low temperatures during the cross-clamp period, the atrial septum did not. In fact, within 5 minutes after stopping cardioplegia infusion, the atrial septal temperature returned to the systemic perfusion temperature and remained there until the next dose of cardioplegia (Fig. 47.9A). Several adverse sequelae resulted from the uncontrolled warming of the atrial septum during cardioplegic arrest, the most important of which was varying degrees of atrioventricular (AV) node dysfunction, including complete heart block. Subsequent measures were taken to prevent the atrial septum from rewarming including double venous cannulation using vena cava tapes to prevent systemic blood from reaching the RA and atrial septum as well as topical iced saline slush on both atria. These measures resulted in the atrial septal temperature remaining within acceptable temperature ranges during cardioplegic arrest (Fig. 47.9B), disappearance of atrial mechanical activity during the cross-clamp period, and amelioration of the postoperative AV node conduction abnormalities.

On the basis of these experimental findings, we began routinely monitoring both atrial septal and ventricular septal temperatures in patients undergoing cardiac surgery. When using a dual-stage venous return cannulae, similar warming of the atrial septum occurred during cardioplegic arrest clinically,[34] and it could be negated by double venous cannulation and frequent applications of topical iced saline slush between separate doses of cardioplegia (Fig. 47.10). Unfortunately, this attention to atrial septal temperature did not significantly affect the incidence of postoperative new-onset POAF.

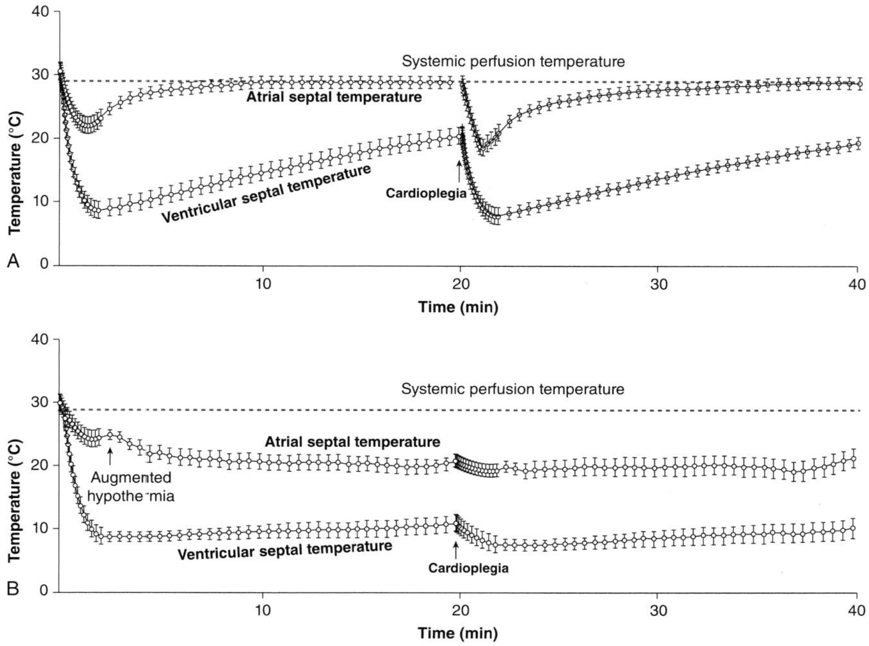

Fig. 47.9 Atrial septal and ventricular septal temperatures measured continuously with needle thermistors during aortic cross-clamping and cold cardioplegic arrest of the heart in animals on cardiopulmonary bypass (CPB). The systemic perfusion temperature was held constant at 28°C. (A) A dual-stage venous return cannula was used for CPB, and no topical hypothermic measures were used on the heart. Antegrade cold crystalloid cardioplegia was administered immediately after aortic cross-clamping and repeated 20 minutes later. The total aortic cross-clamp time was 40 minutes. Note that although the ventricular septal temperature remained below 20°C following both cycles of cardioplegia delivery, atrial septal temperature increased to that of the systemic perfusion temperature (28°C) within 5 minutes of completion of cardioplegia delivery. This suggests that one cause of atrial septal warming during the cross-clamp time was the systemic blood returning to the right atrium before being directed to the heart–lung machine because of the use of a dual-stage venous return cannula. These animals had a variety of postoperative electrophysiologic anomalies, including atrioventricular (AV) node dysfunction and heart block. These studies suggested to us that atrial ischemia during cardioplegic arrest might be a trigger for the development of new-onset POAF in vulnerable atria after cardiac surgery. (B) Identical experimental setup except that the vena cavae were cannulated separately to prevent systemic blood from reaching the right atrium, and topical iced saline slush was used to cover the atria throughout the 40 minute aortic cross-clamp period. Note that not only did the left ventricular septum remain below 10°C, but the atrial septal temperature remained below 20°C throughout the 40-minute cross-clamp period. These animals exhibited no postoperative AV node dysfunction. (Reproduced from Smith PK, Buhrman WC, Ferguson Jr. TB, Levett JM, Cox JL. Conduction block after cardioplegic arrest: prevention by augmented atrial hypothermia. *Circulation.* 1983;68(3):1141–1148.)

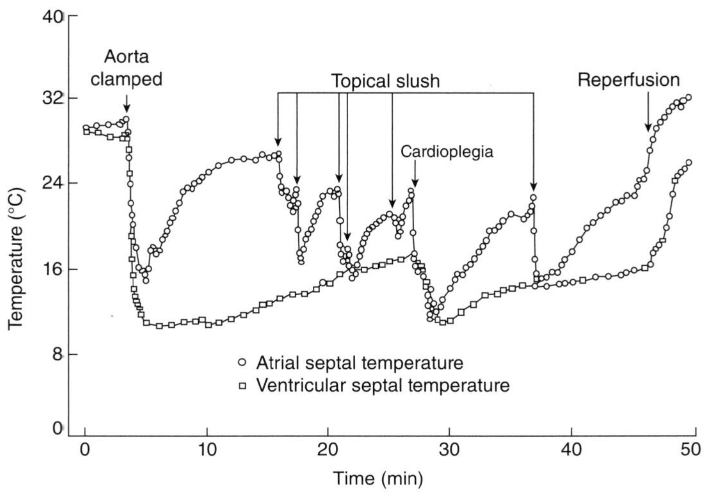

Fig. 47.10 Atrial septal and ventricular septal temperatures measured continuously with needle thermistors during aortic cross-clamping and cold cardioplegic arrest of the heart a patient undergoing quadruple coronary artery bypass grafting. The systemic perfusion temperature was held constant at 28°C. A dual-staged venous return cannula was used for cardiopulmonary bypass, and antegrade cold blood cardioplegia was used to arrest the heart. The total cross-clamp time was 45 minutes. Note the rapid rewarming of the atrial septum between cardioplegia administrations and between topical iced saline slush applications. (Reproduced from Smith PK, Buhrman WC, Ferguson Jr. TB, Levett JM, Cox JL. Conduction block after cardioplegic arrest: prevention by augmented atrial hypothermia. *Circulation.* 1983;68(3):1141–1148.)

Left Posterior Pericardiotomy

Another intraoperative measure that surgeons have used to decrease new-onset POAF is the removal of retained blood from the pericardium after cardiac surgery.[35] The hypothesis was that pericardial inflammation or oxidative stress derived from retained blood served as a trigger for new-onset POAF. One of the most common techniques to potentially mitigate this problem is to perform a posterior pericardiotomy (PP) to drain retained pericardial blood into the pleural spaces where it is then removed through the chest tubes.

A meta-analysis of 10 randomized trials of patients undergoing CAB found a significant reduction in the risk of developing new-onset POAF in the group undergoing PP (risk ratio, 0.45; 95% confidence interval [CI], 0.29–0.64; P <.0001).[36] The incidences of new-onset POAF were 10.3% (94/910) in the PP group and 25.7% (236 /919) in the control group. A random-effects model indicated that the incidence of new-onset POAF after CABG was significantly lower in the PP group than in the control group (risk ratio, 0.45; 95% CI, 0.29–0.64; P <.0001). In a separate randomized controlled trial, 3601 patients were screened, and 420 were included and randomly assigned to the posterior left pericardiotomy group ($n = 212$) or the no intervention group ($n = 208$).[37] No patients were lost to follow-up, and data completeness was 100%. The incidence of new-onset POAF was significantly lower in the posterior left pericardiotomy group than in the no intervention group (17% vs 32%, $P = 0.0007$; odds ratio adjusted for the stratification variable, 0.44 [95% CI, 0.27–0.70; $P = 0.0005$]). No posterior left pericardiotomy–related complications were seen. PP was subsequently elevated to a Class IIa recommendation in the American Heart Association AF Guidelines based on these studies.[38]

Another technique that showed initial promise of decreasing new-onset POAF was the use of active chest tube clearance (ClearFlow, Inc.) to keep the chest tubes open after cardiac surgery to actively evacuate postoperative pericardial blood. However, our group conducted a prospective study of 1367 patients in which 1113 served as control participants and 254 received active chest tube clearance (ACT group). The incidences of new-onset POAF were 20.8% (52 of 254) in the ACT group and 20.2% (221 of 1113) in the control group ($P = .837$).[39] Thus, while the prevention of pericardial blood accumulation by a PP has had a positive effect on new-onset POAF, the removal of retained pericardial blood after cardiac surgery using commercially available active draining devices has not held up to strenuous clinical testing.

REFERENCES

1. Albini A, Malavasi VL, Vitolo M, et al. Long-term outcomes of postoperative atrial fibrillation following non cardiac surgery: a systematic review and metanalysis. *Eur J Int Med.* 2021;85:27–33.
2. Creswell LL, Schuessler RB, Rosenbloom M, Cox JL. Hazards of postoperative atrial arrhythmias. *Ann Thor Surg.* 1993;56:539–549.
3. Almassi GH, Schowalter T, Nicolosi AC, et al. Atrial fibrillation after cardiac surgery: a major morbid event? *Ann Surg.* 1997;226(4):501–513.
4. El-Chami MF, Kilgo P, Thourani V, et al. New-onset atrial fibrillation predicts long-term mortality after coronary artery bypass graft. *J Am Coll Card.* 2010;55(13):1370–1376.
5. Almassi GH. Postoperative atrial fibrillation; the search goes on. *J Surg Res.* 2015;198:57–58.
6. Eikelboom R, Sanjanwala R, Le M-L, Yamashita MH, Arora RC. Postoperative atrial fibrillation after cardiac surgery: a systematic review and meta-analysis. *Ann Thor Surg.* 2021;111:544–555.
7. Oh AR, Kwon JH, Park J, Lee JH. Age-related association between sex and postoperative atrial fibrillation in non-cardiac surgery patients: observational cohort study. *Rev Cardiovasc Med.* 2023;24(9):271.
8. Fragão-Marques M, Mancio J, Oliveira J, et al. Gender differences in predictors and long-term mortality of new-onset postoperative atrial fibrillation following isolated aortic valve replacement surgery. *Ann Thorac Cardiovasc Surg.* 2020;26:342–351.
9. Efird JT, Gudimella P, O'Neal WT, et al. Comparison of risk of atrial fibrillation in black versus white patients after coronary artery bypass grafting. *Am J Cardiol.* 2016;117:1095–1100.
10. Phan K, Khuong JN, Xu J, et al. Obesity and postoperative atrial fibrillation in patients undergoing cardiac surgery: systematic review and meta-analysis. *Internat J Cardiol.* 2016;217:49–57.
11. Cox JL. A perspective of postoperative atrial fibrillation in cardiac operations. *Ann Thor Surg.* 1993;56:405–409.
12. Sato S, Yamauchi S, Schuessler RB, Boineau JP, Matsunaha Y, Cox JL. The effect of augmented atrial hypothermia on atrial refractory period, conduction, and atrial flutter/fibrillation in the canine heart. *J Thor Cardiovasc Surg.* 1992;104:297–306.
13. Lowe JE, Hendry PJ, Hendrickson SC, Wells R. Intraoperative identification of cardiac patients at risk to develop postoperative atrial fibrillation. *Ann Surg.* 1991;213(5):388–392.
14. Vesela J, Osmancik P, Herman D, et al. Prediction of post-operative atrial fibrillation in patients after cardiac surgery using heart rate variability. *BMC Cardiovasc Disord.* 2023;23(1):290.
15. Pandey A, Okaj I, Ichhpuniani S, et al. Risk scores for prediction of postoperative atrial fibrillation after cardiac surgery: a systematic review and meta-analysis. *Am J Cardiol.* 2023;209:232–240.
16. Qian SS, Crandell I, Hanlon A, Joseph M, Poelzing S. Predictive capability of metabolic panels for postoperative atrial fibrillation in cardiac surgery patients. *J Surg Res.* 2022;278:271–281.
17. Turagam MK, Mirza M, Werner PH, et al. Circulating biomarkers predictive of postoperative atrial fibrillation. *Cardiol Rev.* 2016;24(2):76–87.
18. El-Sherbini AH, Shah A, Cheng R, et al. Machine learning for predicting postoperative atrial fibrillation after cardiac surgery: a scoping review of current literature. *Am J Cardiol.* 2023;209:66075.
19. Berruezo A, Tamborero D, Mont L, et al. Pre-procedural predictors of atrial fibrillation recurrence after circumferential pulmonary vein ablation. *Eur Heart J.* 2007;28(7):836–841.
20. Osranek M, Fatema K, Qaddoura F, et al. Left atrial volume predicts the risk of atrial fibrillation after cardiac surgery: a prospective study. *J Am Coll Cardiol.* 2006;48:779–786.
21. Kislitsina ON, Cox JL, Shah SJ, et al. Preoperative left atrial strain abnormalities are associated with the development of postoperative atrial fibrillation following isolated coronary artery bypass surgery. *J Thorac Cardiovasc Surg.* 2022;164(3):917–924.
22. Cheitlin MD, Armstrong WF, Aurigemma GP, et al. ACC/AHA/ASE 2003 guideline update for the clinical application of echocardiography: summary article. A report of the American College of Cardiology/American Heart Association Task Force on practice guidelines (ACC/AHA/ASE Committee to update the 1997 guidelines for the clinical application of echocardiography). *J Am Soc Echocardiogr.* 2003;16:1091–1110.
23. Bufano G, Radico F, D'Angelo C, et al. Predictive value of left atrial and ventricular strain for the detection of atrial fibrillation in patients with cryptogenic stroke. *Front Cardiovasc Med.* 2022;9:869076.
24. Haffajee JA, Lee Y, Alsheikh-Ali AA, Kuvin JT, Pandian NG, Patel AR. Pre-operative left atrial mechanical function predicts risk of atrial fibrillation following cardiac surgery. *JACC Cardiovasc Imaging.* 2011;4:833–840.
25. Candan O, Ozdemir N, Aung SM, et al. Left atrial longitudinal strain parameters predict postoperative persistent atrial fibrilla-

tion following mitral valve surgery: a speckle tracking echocardiography study. *Echocardiography*. 2013;30:1061–1068.

26. Ozben B, Akaslan D, Sunbul M, et al. Postoperative atrial fibrillation after coronary artery bypass grafting surgery: a two-dimensional speckle tracking echocardiography study. *Heart Lung Circ*. 2016;25:993–999.
27. Verdejo HE, Becerra E, Zalaquet R, et al. Atrial function assessed by speckle tracking echocardiography is a good predictor of postoperative atrial fibrillation in elderly patients. *Echocardiography*. 2016;33:242–248.
28. Pastore MC, Degiovanni A, Grisafi L, et al. Left atrial strain to predict postoperative atrial fibrillation in patients undergoing coronary artery bypass grafting. *Circ Cardiovasc Imaging*. 2024;17(1):e015969.
29. Parwani AS, Morris D-A, Blaschke F, et al. Left atrial strain predicts recurrence of atrial arrhythmias after catheter ablation of persistent atrial fibrillation. *Open Heart*. 2017;4(1):e000572.
30. Takagi T, Nakamura K, Asami M, et al. Impact of right atrial structural remodeling on recurrence after ablation for atrial fibrillation. *J Arrhythm*. 2021;37(3):597–606.
31. Sasaki T, Nakamura K, Naito S, et al. The right to left atrial volume ratio predicts outcomes after circumferential pulmonary vein isolation of longstanding persistent atrial fibrillation. *Pacing Clin Electrophysiol*. 2016;39:1181–1190.
32. Kislitsina ON, Thomas J, Rigolin V, et al. Impact of preoperative paroxysmal atrial fibrillation on postoperative strain in patients with degenerative mitral regurgitation following mitral valve surgery. *J Am Coll Cardiol*. 2021;77(18):1777.
33. Smith PK, Buhrman WC, Ferguson Jr TB, Levett JM, Cox JL. Conduction block after cardioplegic arrest: prevention by augmented atrial hypothermia. *Circulation*. 1983;68(3):1141–1148.
34. Smith PK, Buhrman WC, Levett JM, Ferguson Jr TB, Holman WL, Cox JL. Supraventricular conduction abnormalities following cardiac operations. *J Thor Cardiovasc Surg*. 1983;65(1):105–115.
35. St-Onge S, Perrault LP, Demers P, et al. Pericardial blood as a trigger for postoperative atrial fibrillation after cardiac surgery. *Ann Thor Surg*. 2018;105(1):321–328.
36. Xiong T, Pu L, Ma YF, et al. Posterior pericardiotomy to prevent new-onset atrial fibrillation after coronary artery bypass grafting: a systematic review and meta-analysis of 10 randomized controlled trials. *J Cardiothorac Surg*. 2021;16:233.
37. Gaudino M, Sanna T, Ballman KV, et al. Posterior left pericardiotomy for the prevention of atrial fibrillation after cardiac surgery: an adaptive, single-centre, single-blind, randomised, controlled trial. *Lancet*. 2021;398:2075–2083.
38. Joglar JA, Chung MK, Armbruster AL, et al. 2023 ACC/AHA/ACCP/HRS guideline for the diagnosis and management of atrial fibrillation: a Report of the American College of Cardiology/American Heart Association Joint Committee on clinical practice guidelines. *Circulation*. 2024;149(1):e1–e156. https://doi.org/10.1161/CIR.0000000000001193.
39. Churyla A, Kruse J, Fiehler M, et al. Does active chest tube clearance after cardiac surgery provide any clear benefits? *Ann Thor Surg*. 2022;114(4):1334–1340.

48

Postoperative Peri-Mitral Flutter

James L. Cox

CHAPTER OUTLINE

Peri-mitral atrial flutter is a common postoperative arrhythmia that often occurs after isolation of the pulmonary veins (PVs), especially when the posterior wall of the left atrium (LA) is also encompassed to create a so-called "box lesion" around all four PVs (Fig. 48.1). Unlike classic right atrial flutter, which occurs spontaneously in the clinical setting, peri-mitral atrial flutter does not occur clinically except after catheter or surgical ablation. Indeed, peri-mitral atrial flutter is a classic example of an iatrogenic arrhythmia defined as "an adverse condition that results from treatment by a physician, nurse, or allied health professional."

Peri-mitral atrial flutter was called "atypical left atrial flutter" from the first time it was ever diagnosed following the second Maze procedure in 1988[1] until catheter ablation for atrial fibrillation (AF) was introduced some 10 years later. There was no apparent reason for changing the name of the arrhythmia, but historically, it has been a common practice for electrophysiologists (EPs) to change the names of electrophysiological events for no particular reason. Thus, readers should be neither confused nor surprised by the fact that "peri-mitral flutter," "atypical flutter," "atypical atrial flutter," and "atypical left atrial flutter" all refer to the same iatrogenic arrhythmia. However, as readers will learn in this chapter, the moniker "atypical left atrial flutter" is a more accurate description of the arrhythmia than "peri-mitral flutter" because of the multiple anatomic routes the macro-reentrant circuit of this arrhythmia can take to complete one cycle. Much like the three potential macro-reentrant drivers of classic right atrial flutter (see Chapter 12, Fig. 12.3), the macro-reentrant driver of atypical left atrial flutter can use different anatomic structures that have nothing to do with the mitral valve (MV). These structures include the isthmus between the left atrial appendage (LAA) orifice and the left superior PV (LSPV; commonly called the "coumadin ridge") the isthmus between the LAA orifice and the MV annulus, the coronary sinus, and the myocardium of the posteroinferior portion of the left atrial isthmus between the lower PVs and the MV annulus. Nevertheless, because "peri-mitral flutter" has been adopted by our electrophysiology colleagues and is perhaps easier to remember, we will use this designation for the remainder of this chapter.

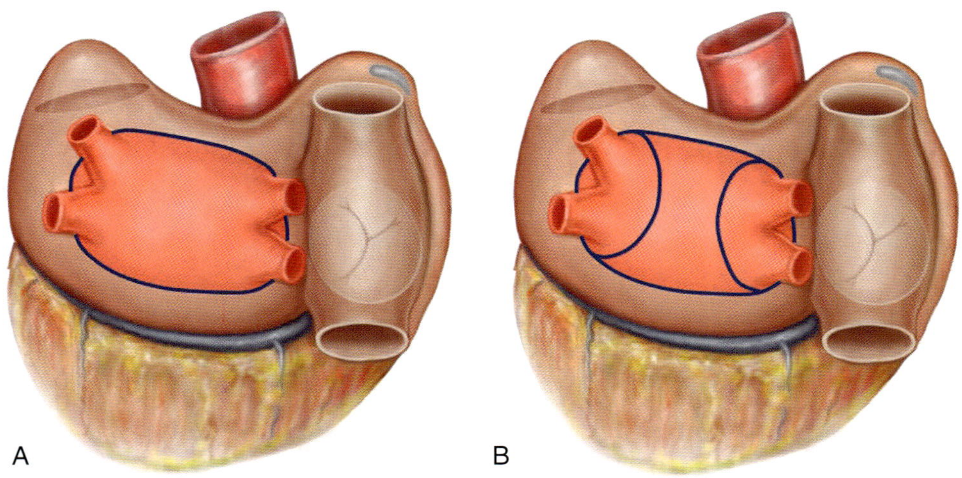

Fig. 48.1 The box lesions in both the Maze-III procedure (A) and the Maze-IV procedure (B) encompass the orifices of all four pulmonary veins (PVs) and the intervening posterior left atrial wall between the right and left PVs. From an electrophysiological standpoint, they are identical. However, they are created by different ablation techniques in the two iterations of the Maze procedure. Ironically, the creation of a perfect box lesion in the left atrium appears to be the essential component necessary for the development of iatrogenic postoperative peri-mitral flutter.

ELECTROPHYSIOLOGY OF PERI-MITRAL ATRIAL FLUTTER

The macro-reentrant circuit that drives peri-mitral flutter following a simple box lesion in the LA uses the atrial septum, anterior left atrial wall, lateral left atrial wall, and posterior left atrial isthmus (Fig. 48.2). In the left atrial isthmus, the peri-mitral flutter wave can propagate across either the posteroinferior left atrial myocardium or through the coronary sinus. The macro-reentrant circuit is physically larger than that of classic atrial flutter in the right atrium (RA), and as a result, it takes longer for electrical activity to complete one complete cycle around the circuit. Thus peri-mitral flutter is said to have a longer "cycle length" than that of classic right atrial flutter.

The cycle length of classic right atrial flutter is 200 ms, meaning that electrical activity propagates around the circuit five times per second, or 300 times per minute (Table 48.1). This results in a regular atrial rate of 300 beats/min, which is blocked 2:1 in the atrioventricular node, resulting in a regular ventricular rate of 150 beats/min. However, the cycle length of peri-mitral flutter is approximately 250 ms, meaning that electrical activity propagates around the peri-mitral circuit only four times per second, resulting in a regular atrial rate of 240 beats/min and a regular ventricular rate of 120 beats/min.

A common pitfall relating to peri-mitral flutter is that it can be easily mistaken for sinus tachycardia immediately after AF surgery or catheter ablation. As an example, imagine that you are performing an off-pump thoracoscopic procedure to ablate AF that has been present for the past 5 years. During the ablation procedure, the AF suddenly breaks into a stable, regular tachycardia of 120 beats/min. Chances are that you and your surgical team will be elated at the successful ablation because it appears that the patient is now in a sinus tachycardia that will be expected to slow down and stabilize with time. However, it is extremely rare for a patient to have sinus tachycardia immediately after surgical ablation of long-standing persistent AF because the sinoatrial node has been suppressed for so long that it takes quite some time to recover. Thus, *sinus bradycardia* is far more common during the early post-ablation period in patients who have had AF for long periods of time. Therefore, one should be aware that any time a stable heartbeat of around 120 beats/min is seen in the operating room immediately after AF ablation, it is likely that the patient has peri-mitral flutter, not sinus tachycardia.

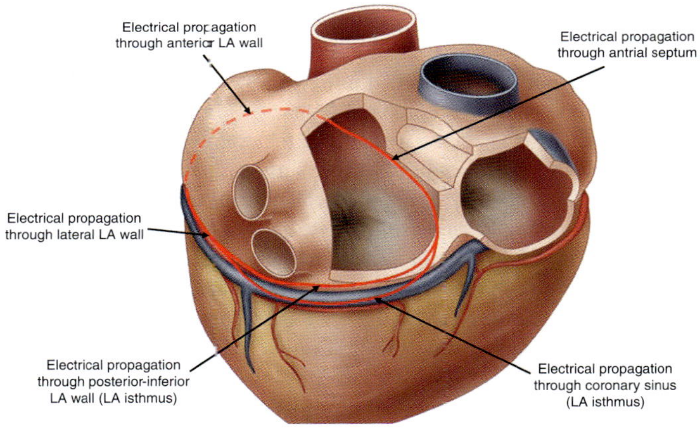

Fig. 48.2 The macro-reentrant circuit of peri-mitral atrial flutter after a simple box lesion in the left atrium (LA) (not shown) uses all sides of the LA. Posteriorly, it can also use the coronary sinus. (See text for further discussion.)

TABLE 48.1 Differences in the Cycle Length of the Macro-reentrant Driver of Classic Right Atrial Flutter and Postablation Peri-Mitral Flutter

Electrophysiology	Classic RA Flutter	Peri-Mitral Flutter
Cycle length (ms)	200	250
Cycles/s	5	4
Atrial rate (beats/min)	300	240
Atrioventricular node block	2:1	2:1
Ventricular rate (beats/min)	150	120

LESIONS OF THE MAZE PROCEDURE THAT PREVENT POSTOPERATIVE PERI-MITRAL ATRIAL FLUTTER

As with any reentrant circuit, the macro-reentrant circuit that drives peri-mitral flutter can be ablated by interrupting it in only one place. In the Maze procedure, we chose to preclude postoperative peri-mitral flutter by interrupting conduction across the left atrial isthmus because we believed this isthmus to be the narrowest and most accessible common anatomic pathway in all the different reentrant circuits that can cause the arrhythmia (Fig. 48.3). However, we learned during the development of the left atrial isolation procedure nearly a decade before the first Maze procedure (see Chapter 9, Fig. 9.14) that electrical conduction across the left atrial isthmus can occur through the posteroinferior left atrial myocardium or through the walls of the coronary sinus (Fig. 48.4). Therefore, to block conduction across the left atrial isthmus, it is necessary to create lesions in both the atrial muscle (the endocardial "mitral line") and in the coronary sinus with a circumferential cryolesion (Fig. 48.5). *It is critical to place the mitral line and the coronary sinus cryolesion in the same plane.* Otherwise, the electrical activity can skirt

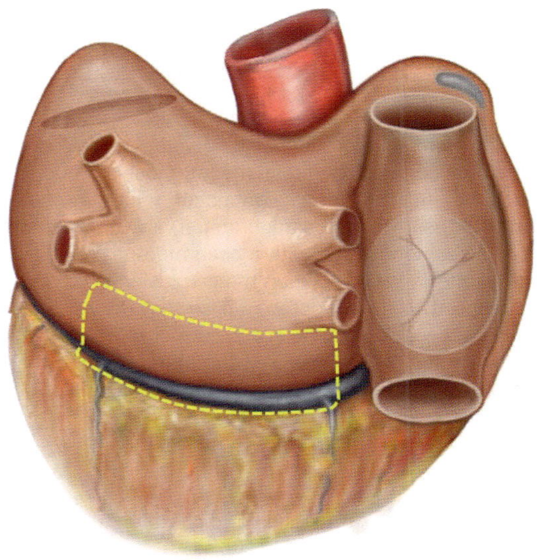

Fig. 48.3 Left atrial isthmus. The left atrial isthmus *(yellow dashed rectangle)* is the part of the left atrium between the inferior pulmonary veins and the posterior mitral valve annulus and includes the left atrioventricular groove that harbors the coronary sinus.

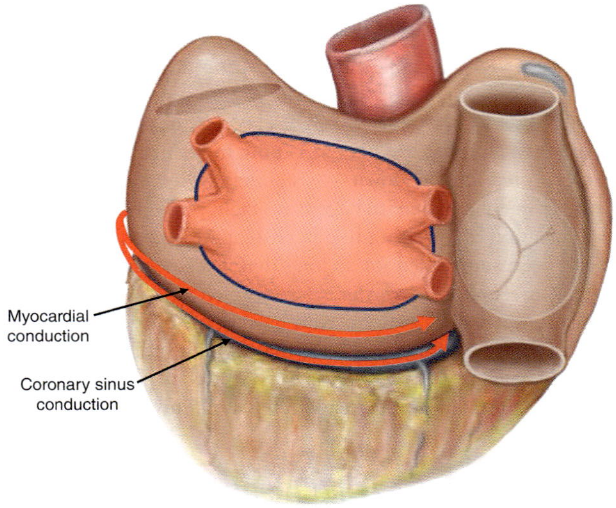

Fig. 48.4 Both the left atrial myocardium and the coronary sinus in the left atrial isthmus are capable of conducting electrical activity, and they can both be a part of the macro-reentrant peri-mitral atrial flutter (see Fig. 48.2).

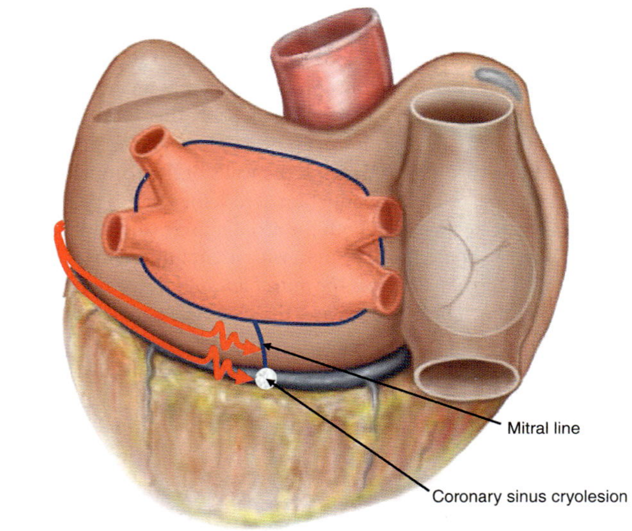

Fig. 48.5 Mitral line and coronary sinus cryolesion block of peri-mitral flutter. To block all conduction across the left atrial isthmus, it is necessary to block the atrial myocardial conduction with a transmural mitral line from the box lesion to the posterior mitral valve annulus and to block the coronary sinus conduction with a circumferential cryolesion in the same plane as the mitral line. When the cryolesion is created, external pressure is applied to the cryoprobe tip so that the coronary sinus is completely collapsed. This results in a circumferential lesion around the entire coronary sinus. It is critical that the mitral line and the coronary sinus lesions be aligned to effect complete conduction block across the left atrial isthmus.

around the coronary sinus cryolesion and continue to propagate across the left atrial isthmus (Fig. 48.6).

It is particularly important to prevent postablation peri-mitral atrial flutter because it is actually more symptomatic than atrial fibrillation itself. As a result, patients are invariably dissatisfied with their surgery if they have had atrial fibrillation replaced by peri-mitral atrial flutter.

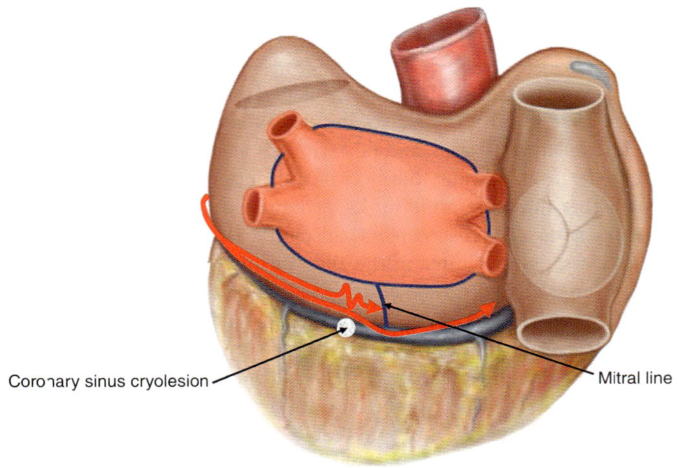

Fig. 48.6 Misalignment of the mitral line and coronary sinus cryolesion. If the coronary sinus cryolesion and the mitral line are not aligned, an electrical impulse can skirt between the two lesions as shown. This allows continued conduction across the left atrial isthmus and perpetuation of the peri-mitral flutter.

HYBRID PROCEDURES: THE EXCEPTION TO THE RULE

The fact that 10% to 15% of patients are destined to develop peri-mitral flutter after AF surgical ablation means that 85% to 90% of them will *not* have it after AF ablation. This means that the mitral line–coronary sinus lesion is not actually needed in 85% to 90% of patients undergoing a Maze procedure. The problem is that it is impossible to identify preoperatively which patients are destined to develop postoperative peri-mitral flutter and which are not. Because surgeons have only one chance at success with an open-heart approach, all patients undergoing an open Maze procedure should get these lesions to avoid a 10% to 15% obligatory failure rate. However, it is not necessary to create the mitral line–coronary sinus lesions to prevent peri-mitral atrial flutter in patients undergoing the initial thoracoscopic surgery in hybrid procedures because the 10% to 15% of patients who develop it can be treated at the time of the obligatory follow-up catheter ablation. This is fortuitous because the mitral line–coronary sinus cannot be performed thoracoscopically from the epicardium.

Unfortunately, there is a major problem with the creation of the mitral line–coronary sinus lesions using a catheter ablation approach. Interventional EPs claim that the mitral line is especially difficult to create with a catheter because the left atrial wall is *thicker* in the left atrial isthmus than in other areas of the atrium. Having surgically divided the left atrial wall in this specific area to create the mitral line during the performance of approximately 250 cut-and-sew Maze procedures, I can say with some assurance that the atrial wall is *not* thicker in this area than in other areas of the LA. In fact, the left atrial wall is more commonly *thinner* in the left atrial isthmus than it is in other areas of the atrium such as the left atrial free walls and the atrial septum.

The problem that EPs have in creating the mitral line is primarily because they ignore the role of the coronary sinus in conducting electrical activity across the left atrial isthmus. EPs create the endocardial mitral line with the same catheter that they use to isolate the PVs, but in order to create the CS lesion, they have to switch catheters. Therefore, as soon as they have isolated the PVs, they try to create the mitral line *first* because they still have the appropriate catheter inside the LA to do so. Their practice therefore, is to try to create the mitral line *without having ablated the coronary sinus first*. For some reason, many of them do not seem to accept the fact that as long as the CS is intact, it can conduct electrical activity across the left atrial isthmus no matter how much time they spend or energy they deliver to the myocardium in trying to create the mitral line. This "problem" with creating the mitral line with a catheter can be easily overcome by simply creating the CS lesion *before* attempting to create the mitral line. However, this means that after the PVs have been isolated, the EP would have to remove the catheter, replace it with one they can use in the CS, and then remove the CS catheter and replace it with their original catheter to create the mitral line. Most EPs are unwilling to change catheters so frequently, so they struggle with trying to create the mitral line and explain their difficulty by stating that the atrial wall is too thick in that region, which is not true.

LESIONS OTHER THAN THE MITRAL LINE–CORONARY SINUS LESIONS THAT CAN PREVENT POSTOPERATIVE PERI-MITRAL ATRIAL FLUTTER

Peri-mitral atrial flutter occurs in 10% to 15% of patients undergoing surgery for AF if nothing is done to prevent it.[2] Historically, surgeons have believed that creating both a mitral line and a cryolesion as described earlier is either unnecessary or too difficult to perform correctly. Most of the modifications of the Maze procedure that have been introduced and applied in significant numbers of patients over the past two to three decades have ignored the frequency and importance of postoperative peri-mitral flutter. These include the so-called Wolf mini-Maze procedure,[3] the five-box procedure,[4] and many others. In addition, even when the mitral line was performed in the so-called "left atrial Maze procedure"[5] or in procedures that claimed to be a biatrial Maze procedure but were not,[6] the coronary sinus lesion was typically not included. The most successful iterations of the Maze procedure have been the Maze-III and the Maze-IV techniques, both of which include the mitral line and the coronary sinus lesions to prevent postoperative peri-mitral flutter (see Chapters 12 and 17).

ANTERIOR LIMB VERSUS POSTERIOR LIMB OF THE PERI-MITRAL FLUTTER WAVE

It is worth mentioning that the so-called "simple" atrial flutter waves in both atria are actually more complex and variable than one appreciates at first glance. For example, we thought for many years that classic right atrial flutter was invariably caused by the same flutter wave, a macroreentrant circuit that rotated around an area of functional block along the crista terminalis, because this was its location in the first patient ever globally mapped simultaneously with multiple electrodes during an episode of atrial flutter (see Chapter 5, Fig. 5.4). However, it was later learned that the right atrial flutter wave always uses the cavotricuspid isthmus (CTI), and that therefore a CTI lesion is extremely successful in ablating classic right atrial flutter. As noted earlier, Santucci showed that although right atrial flutter invariably involved the CTI, there are actually three different macro-reentrant circuits in the RA that can result in classic right atrial flutter (see Chapter 12, Fig. 12.3).

Likewise, when we first inadvertently caused "atypical left atrial flutter" ("peri-mitral flutter") in the second patient to ever undergo a Maze procedure in 1988, we were aware that the posterior portion of the flutter wave was conducting across the left atrial isthmus and potentially propagating through both the left atrial myocardium and the coronary sinus. However, we assumed that the remainder of the flutter wave was simply propagating through the atrial septum, the broad anterior portion of the LA, and the lateral left atrial wall to complete the circuit (see Fig. 48.2). Because our attention was focused on preventing this peri-mitral flutter wave by focusing on its posterior limb involving the left atrial isthmus, this simplified concept was sufficient for our purposes and has remained so to the present time.

Our simplified concept of peri-mitral flutter waves was broadened in 2008 when we were trying to develop a variant of the Maze procedure that could be done off pump entirely through the LAA using updated techniques and tools that we referred to at the time as the "Maze-VII" procedure. The term "Maze V" had been reserved for Revishvilli's technique (see Chapter 39), and I promised Jimmy Edgerton that if he would add the right atrial lesions to the Dallas lesion set, I would thereafter refer to it as the "Maze-VI" procedure because the combination of the Dallas lesion set (all in the LA) with the right atrial Maze lesions actually adhered to the concept and principles of a Maze procedure.

Key to the proposed "Maze-VII" procedure, which was never used clinically, was the realization that the orifice of the LAA dictates the only possible pathways of conduction for the *anterior* limb of a peri-mitral flutter wave. There are only two potential pathways around the base of the LAA, the LAA–LSPV isthmus made up primarily of the coumadin ridge and the small band of atrium between the base of the LAA and the MV that we call the LAA–MV isthmus (Fig. 48.7). Because all Maze procedures include a LAA–LSPV lesion to prevent reentry around the base of the LAA (Fig. 48.8), we realized that if we simply added to that LAA-LSPV lesion, another blocking lesion across the LAA–MV isthmus, by ablating it with a right-angle cryoprobe placed through the tip of the LAA (Fig. 48.9), the two combined lesions would prevent postoperative peri-mitral flutter. By blocking all of the potential pathways for this *anterior* limb of the peri-mitral flutter wave, the posterior mitral line–coronary sinus lesions would not be necessary.

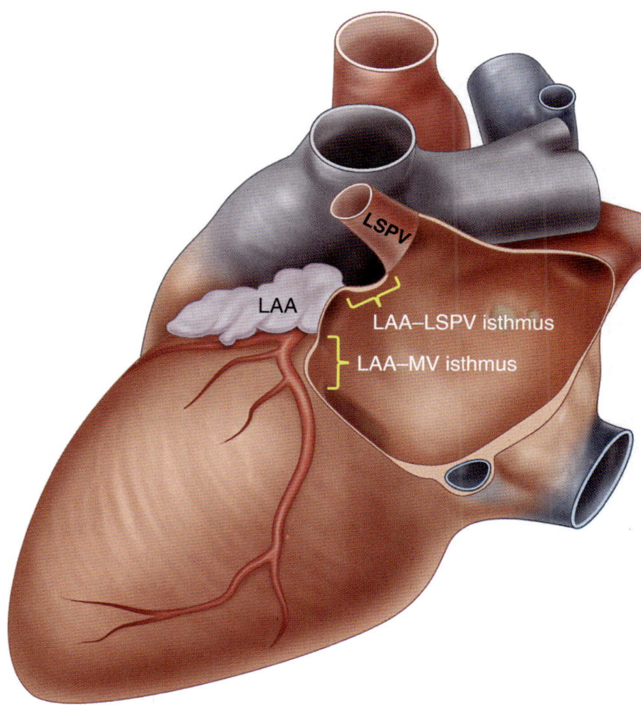

Fig. 48.7 The orifice of the left atrial appendage (LAA) is bordered superiorly by the isthmus of atrial muscle between the left superior pulmonary vein (LSPV) and the LAA orifice (the LAA–LSPV isthmus). This is also called the coumadin ridge. Inferiorly, it is bordered by the narrow band of atrial muscle between the LAA orifice and the mitral valve (MV) annulus (the LAA–MV isthmus).

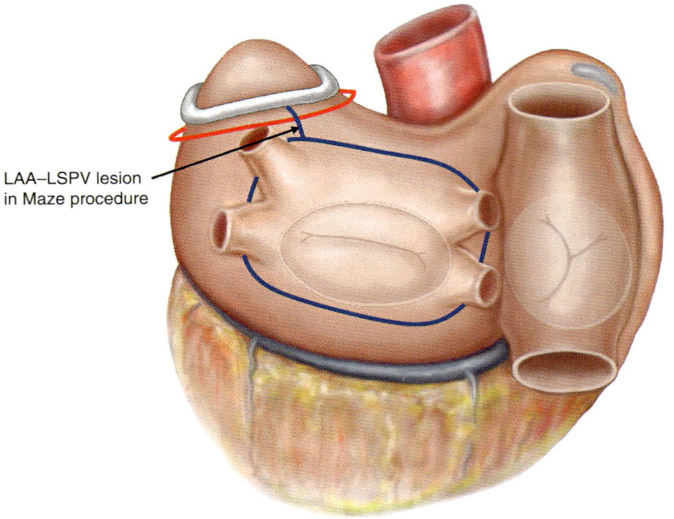

Fig. 48.8 Left atrial appendage (LAA)–left superior pulmonary vein (LSPV) lesion to prevent reentry around the LAA base. In all Maze procedures, conduction across the LAA–LSPV isthmus harboring the coumadin ridge is routinely blocked by the LAA–LSPV lesion that is created in the Maze procedure to prevent postoperative reentry around the base of the occluded LAA.

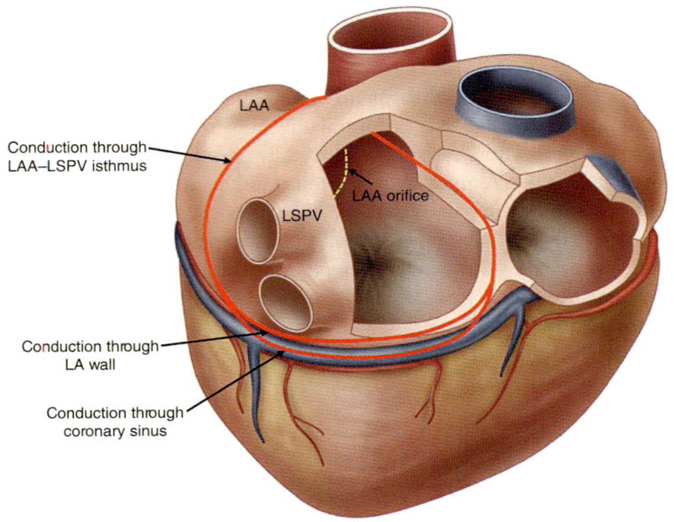

Fig. 48.10 Peri-mitral flutter wave using the left atrial appendage (LAA)–left superior pulmonary vein (LSPV) isthmus. The most common macro-reentrant circuit that can result in postoperative peri-mitral flutter following creation of a simple box lesion (not shown) uses the isthmus between the orifice of the LAA and the LSPV as the anterior part of its circuit.

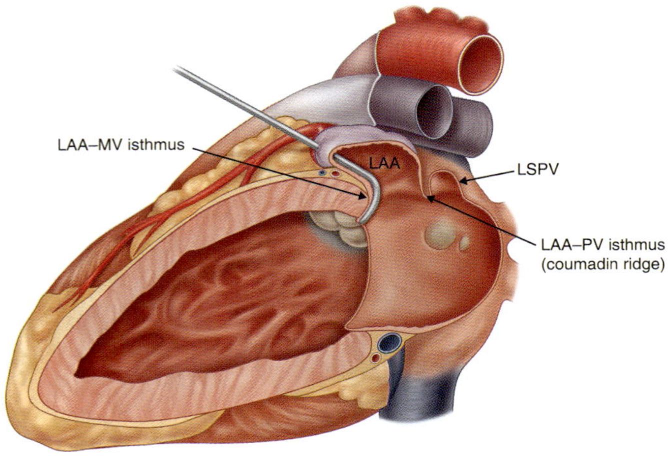

Fig. 48.9 One method of ablating the left atrial appendage (LAA)-mitral valve (MV) isthmus off pump is by passing a right-angle cryoprobe through a pursestring suture in the LAA. (See text for further discussion.) *MV,* Mitral valve; *PV,* pulmonary vein.

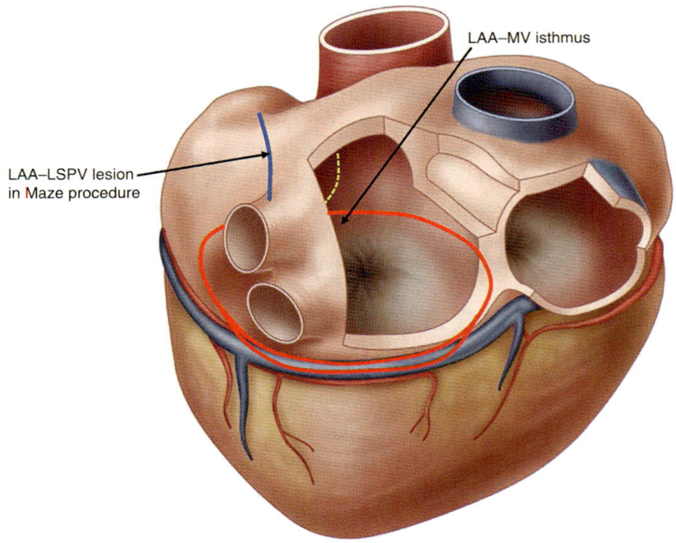

Fig. 48.11 Peri-mitral flutter wave using the left atrial appendage (LAA)–mitral valve (MV) isthmus. If the patient has a LAA–left superior pulmonary vein (LSPV) lesion as a part of the Maze procedure, peri-mitral flutter can persist by using the LAA–MV isthmus between the orifice of the LAA *(yellow dashed line)* and the MV annulus.

The major prerequisite for the development of postoperative peri-mitral flutter is a perfectly performed box lesion in the posterior LA, a critical component of all interventional therapy for AF. After the creation of a box lesion without other associated lesions, the most common macro-reentrant circuit that can result in postoperative peri-mitral flutter uses the LAA–LSPV isthmus as the anterior part of its circuit (Fig. 48.10). However, because the LAA–LSPV isthmus is always a part of the Maze procedure, it would also prevent a postoperative peri-mitral flutter wave from using this isthmus as the anterior part of its macro-reentrant circuit. However, this would leave the possibility of the peri-mitral flutter wave using the LAA–MV isthmus as the anterior part of its circuit (Fig. 48.11). Therefore, in the presence of the LAA–LSPV lesion of a Maze procedure, it is still necessary to create a lesion across the LAA–MV isthmus (Fig. 48.12) to prevent postoperative peri-mitral flutter if one is to avoid the necessity of performing the posterior mitral line–coronary sinus lesion.

In 2021 I spoke by phone with two surgeons who by that time had performed more than 20 AF ablations in patients using this combination of the LAA–LSPV lesion plus the LAA–MV lesion (Fig. 48.13) in lieu of performing the traditional mitral line–coronary sinus lesion to prevent postoperative peri-mitral flutter with excellent early results. In addition, Drs. Kevin Makati and Andrew Sherman in Tampa, Florida, have been performing the same procedure recently with

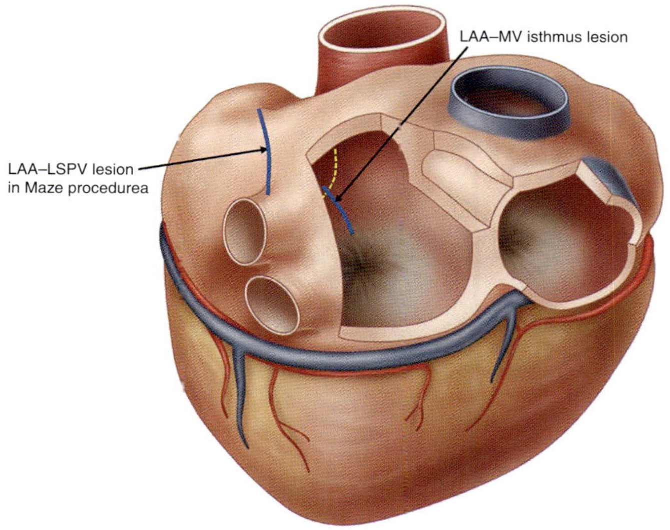

Fig. 48.12 Peri-mitral flutter wave using the left atrial appendage (LAA)–mitral valve (MV) isthmus. An additional lesion across the LAA–MV isthmus, combined with the LAA–left superior pulmonary vein (LSPV) lesion of a Maze procedure, will prevent postoperative peri-mitral flutter without the need to create the posterior mitral line–coronary sinus lesions.

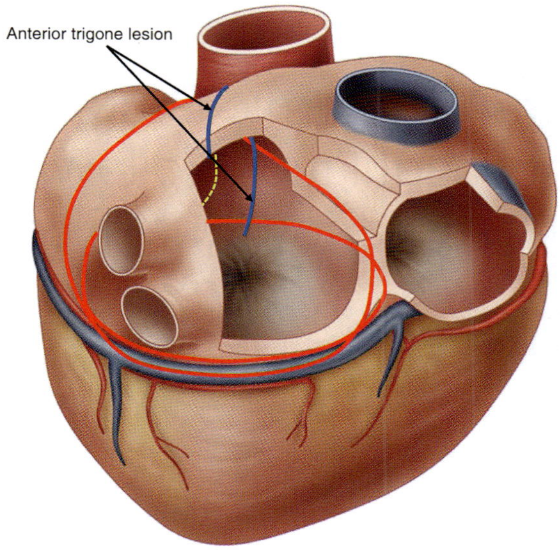

Fig. 48.14 Anterior trigone lesion for peri-mitral flutter. An anterior trigone lesion from the top of the box lesion, across Bachmann's bundle down to the anterior annulus of the mitral valve, prevents the development of postoperative flutter waves regardless of which anterior isthmus it uses. Therefore, if contiguous and uniformly transmural, an anterior trigone lesion will prevent postoperative peri-mitral flutter and negate the need for a traditional mitral line–coronary sinus lesion posteriorly.

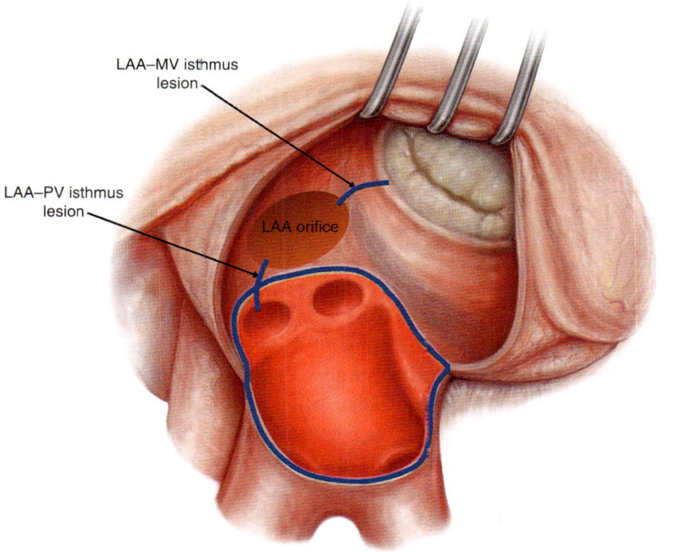

Fig. 48.13 Surgeon's view of the lesions across the left atrial appendage (LAA)–left superior pulmonary vein (LSPV) isthmus and the LAA–mitral valve (MV) isthmus that in combination prevents postoperative peri-mitral flutter.

similar early results. They have dubbed their approach the "Tampa Two" procedure after the famed defensive formation developed by Monty Kiffen and Tony Dungy and first deployed by the Tampa Bay Buccaneers professional football team that won Super Bowl XXXVII in 2003. Hopefully, the surgery will be equally successful and last more than 1 year. Neither surgical group has reported the full follow-up results of their series to date.

Finally, the first effort to prevent postoperative peri-mitral atrial flutter with a lesion other than the combined mitral line–coronary sinus lesions was part of the "Dallas Lesion Set" described by Edgerton and coworkers[7] in 2009. Their approach was to replace the mitral line–coronary sinus lesions with an "anterior trigone lesion," which if complete and placed in the proper location, is theoretically as effective in preventing postoperative peri-mitral flutter as the mitral line–coronary sinus lesions (Fig. 48.14). Anterior trigone lesions are usually used for off-pump surgery. Therefore, they are created with unipolar ablation devices applied to the epicardium in the beating, working heart. Unfortunately, it is extremely difficult to create contiguous, uniformly transmural anterior trigone lesions from the epicardium with a unipolar ablation device off-pump because of the thickness of Bachmann's bundle (see Chapter 19, Fig. 19.8).

REFERENCES

1. Cox JL. The first Maze procedure. *J Thor Cardiovasc Surg.* 2011;141(5):1093–1097.
2. Cox JL, Malaisrie SC, Kislitsina ON, McCarthy PM. The electrophysiologic basis for lesions of the contemporary Maze operation. *J Thor Cardiovasc Surg.* 2019;157(2):584–590.
3. Wolf RK, Schneeberger EW, Osterday R, et al. Video-assisted bilateral pulmonary vein isolation and left atrial appendage exclusion for atrial fibrillation. *J Thorac Cardiovasc Surg.* 2005;130(3):797–802.
4. Sirak J, Jones D, Schwartzman D. The five-box thoracoscopic Maze procedure. *Ann Thorac Surg.* 2012;95(3):986–989.
5. Cox JL, Churyla A, Malaisrie SC, et al. When is a Maze procedure a Maze procedure? *Can J Cardiol.* 2018;34(11):1492–1491.
6. Gillinov AM, Gelijns AC, Parides MK, et al. Surgical ablation of atrial fibrillation during mitral-valve surgery. *N Eng J Med.* 2015;372(15):1399–1409.
7. Edgerton JR, Jackman WM, Mack MJ. A new epicardial lesion set for minimal access left atrial Maze: the Dallas Lesion Set. *Ann Thorac Surg.* 2009;88:1655–1657.

49

Anti-Arrhythmic Drug Therapy and Anticoagulation Following the Maze Procedure for Atrial Fibrillation

Jane Kruse, Patrick M. McCarthy, James Edgerton, James L. Cox

CHAPTER OUTLINE

The objective of the Maze procedure is to render the atria incapable of fibrillating by precluding or interrupting the development of macro-reentrant circuits (drivers) that sustain atrial fibrillation (AF) drivers and to restore the ability of a sinus-generated impulse to activate both atria and the ventricles in a shychronous fashion.[1] Therefore, it reasonable to expect that the procedure would also prevent early perioperative AF, but this has never been the case.[2,3] The atria have shorter refractory periods in the milieu of the postoperative inflammatory state, meaning that smaller macro-reentrant circuits can develop *between* the lesions of the Maze procedure, resulting in early perioperative AF (see Chapter 4). Efforts to control early postoperative AF (POAF) in following a Maze procedure center around the use of drugs that either prolong the atrial refractory periods (rhythm control) or control the ventricular rate (rate control) until the inflammatory response subsides and the atrial refractory periods return to normal. After the refractory periods return to their preoperative status with time, only large reentrant circuits can develop in the atria, and the lesions of the Maze procedure usually prevent them from developing without the need for continuing the antiarrhythmic drugs. This practice of allowing for tissue healing (maturation of the atrial lesions) and electrophysiologic recovery of the atria from surgery is the basis of the standard 90-day blanking period observed after both surgical and catheter ablation.

Reports on the original series of Maze procedure patients[2–5] and many of the large clinical series reports that followed[6–8] included the incidence of early perioperative AF but offered little useful information regarding how it should be treated. Despite the availability of guideline recommendations,[9] there is still no universally accepted prophylactic protocol for preventing early POAF after any type of cardiac surgery, including the Maze procedure, and its incidence has changed little over the past four decades. Likewise, there is no generally accepted anticoagulation regimen for patients after Maze procedures either with or without POAF. All iterations of the Maze procedure include removal or occlusion (LAAO) of the left atrial appendage (LAA) because it is believed that the LAA is the site of origin of the vast majority of thromboembolic strokes associated with AF. However, some of the non-Maze surgical procedures currently used for the treatment of patients with AF include LAAO and others do not.[10] There are general guidelines from various societies about new-onset POAF in patients after cardiac surgery, and most surgeons treat POAF following the Maze procedure in the same way.[11] In addition, the importance and validity of the $CHADs_2VASC$ score remains unclear after AF is ablated and/or the LAA is closed. Therefore, the need for anticoagulation, what type, and for how long remain unanswered questions.

TREATMENT OF EARLY POSTOPERATIVE ATRIAL FIBRILLATION AFTER SURGICAL ATRIAL FIBRILLATION ABLATION PROCEDURES

The treatment of new-onset POAF after cardiac surgery in patients with no history of preoperative AF is based on either rate control or rhythm control with a variety of antiarrhythmic medications.[11] Meta-analyses and randomized trials have failed to show a treatment advantage of one strategy over the other.[12,13] However, patients who develop postoperative AF after cardiac surgery that was performed specifically to ablate preoperative AF are like no other patients. Are they to be considered in the same category as patients with no history of preoperative AF who develop new-onset POAF after cardiac surgery? Should the treatment of the two be the same? We do not know the answer to these questions, but the patients should probably be considered to be in two different groups. As discussed in Chapter 47, patients who have no history of AF but then develop new-onset POAF after cardiac surgery most likely have a preoperative maldistribution of their local atrial refractory periods.[14] However, patients with a history of preoperative AF who undergo a Maze procedure for that AF are thought to develop early POAF because of a shortening of their refractory periods caused by the general perioperative inflammatory response to the surgery.[2] Despite these potential differences in the underlying electrophysiologic derangements responsible for early POAF in patients with and without preoperative AF, we have little choice currently but to treat them in the same manner. Cardioversion during the postoperative period may be required depending on the patient's clinical status.[13,15] Recommendations for treatment of new-onset POAF from the joint guidelines of the American College of Cardiology (ACC), American Heart Association (AHA), American College of Clinical Pharmacy (ACCP), and Heart Rhythm Society (HRS) are shown in Table 49.1.[9]

TABLE 49.1 Joint Guideline Recommendations of the American College of Cardiology, American Heart Association, American College of Clinical Pharmacy, and Heart Rhythm Society for the Treatment of Patients with New-Onset Postoperative Atrial Fibrillation After Cardiac Surgery

Guidelines: ACC/ AHA/ACCP/HRS	Recommendations: Treatment of AF After Cardiac Surgery	Class of Recommendation	Level of Recommendation
Joglar et al.[9]	In postoperative cardiac surgery patients, beta-blockers are recommended to achieve rate control for AF unless contraindicated or ineffective, in which case a nondihydropyridine calcium channel blocker is recommended.	I	A (beta-blocker) B-R (nondihydropyridine calcium channel blocker)
	In hemodynamically stable cardiac surgery patients with postoperative AF, rate-control (target heart rate, <100 beats/min) and/or rhythm-control medications are recommended as initial therapy, with the choice of strategy according to patient symptoms, hemodynamic consequences of the arrhythmia, and physician preference.	I	B-R
	In patients who develop poorly tolerated AF after cardiac surgery, direct current cardioversion in combination with antiarrhythmic drug therapy is recommended, with consideration of imaging to rule out LAA thrombus before cardioversion in patients in whom AF has been present >48 hours and who have not been on anticoagulation.	I	B-R
	In patients who develop postoperative AF after cardiac surgery, it is reasonable to administer anticoagulation when deemed safe in regard to surgical bleeding for 60 days after surgery unless complications develop and to reevaluate the need for longer term anticoagulation at that time.	IIa	B-R
	In patients who develop AF after cardiac surgery and who are treated with rate-control strategy, at 30- to 60-day follow-up, it is reasonable to perform rhythm assessment, and if AF does not revert to sinus rhythm spontaneously, consider cardioversion after an adequate duration of anticoagulation.	IIa	B-R

ACC, American College of Cardiology; *ACCP*, American College of Clinical Pharmacy; *AF*, atrial fibrillation; *AHA*, American Heart Association; *HRS*, Heart Rhythm Society; *LAA*, left atrial appendage.
Class of recommendations: Class I: recommended or indicated Class IIa: should be considered Level of Recommendation: A: high quality evidence from randomized clinical trials B-R: Moderated-quality evidence from randomized clinical trials.

ANTICOAGULATION FOR EARLY POSTOPERATIVE ATRIAL FIBRILLATION AFTER SURGICAL ATRIAL FIBRILLATION ABLATION PROCEDURES

There are no studies that definitively establish best practices for short-term or long-term oral anticoagulation (OAC) management for patients undergoing surgical AF ablation with or without LAAO. Postoperative anticoagulation for a minimum of 60 days after AF surgery was found to have a protective effect against stroke in a review of eight observational studies comprising 15,335 patients.[16] Perhaps the data most relevant for these patients come from a meta-analysis of almost 1.7 million coronary artery bypass graft patients examining thromboembolic events, mortality, and bleeding differences in patients treated with OAC versus those who were not. Over multiple different time frame comparisons, there was no reduction in mortality or thromboembolism for patients on OAC. However, there were a greater number of bleeding events in that group. This large meta-analysis relied on best evidence but had many limitations, and it included no randomized studies.[17]

The joint guidelines of the ACC, AHA ACCP, and HRS recommend 3 months of anticoagulation therapy for patients after surgical ablation for AF.[9] The Society of Thoracic Surgeons guidelines and those of the European Society of Cardiology/European Association for Cardio-Thoracic Surgery do not make a specific recommendation for anticoagulation after the surgical ablation of AF.[11,18] All of these guidelines agree that more data are needed for improved decision making regarding the time frame for screening AF episodes and discontinuing anticoagulation postoperatively.

Many unanswered questions remain regarding the need for long-term anticoagulation after catheter and surgical ablation of AF, especially when the LAA has been closed. It is unclear whether the $CHADs_2VASC$ score should be used to guide this decision. In addition, the preferred type of OAC to use is unclear. Should it be aspirin only, warfarin, direct OACs, or non–vitamin K antagonist OACs? And when or if should OAC be discontinued? Plenty of opinions are available, but they are usually based on single-center studies, and there have been no randomized clinical trials (RCTs) to answer these questions. Many surgeons and cardiologists involved in the late management of these patients are uncomfortable discontinuing OAC, partly because of vague guideline recommendations such as continuing OAC indefinitely after catheter ablation for AF even if it is successful. There are no RCTs to guide the use of OAC in patients undergoing surgical AF ablation. In the LAAOS III trial, the benefit of LAAO was present whether or not patients received OACs.[19]

REFERENCES

1. Cox JL, Schuessler RB, D'Agostino HJ Jr, et al. The surgical treatment of atrial fibrillation: III. Development of a definitive surgical procedure. *J Thorac Cardiovasc Surg*. 1991;101:569–583.
2. Cox JL, Boineau JP, Schuessler RB, Kater KM, Lappas DG. Five-year experience with the maze procedure for atrial fibrillation. *Ann Thorac Surg*. 1994;56:814–824.
3. Cox JL, Schuessler RB, Lappas DG, Boineau JP. An 8½ year clinical experience with surgery for atrial fibrillation. *Ann Surg*. 1996;224(3):267–275.

4. Prasad SM, Maniar HS, Camillo CJ, et al. The Cox Maze III procedure for atrial fibrillation: long-term efficacy in patients undergoing lone versus Cox JL, Boineau JP, Schuessler RB, Kater KM, Lappas DG: Five-year experience with the Maze procedure for atrial fibrillation. *Ann Thorac Surg.* 1994;56:814–824.
5. Weimar T, Schena S, Bailey MS, et al. The Cox-Maze procedure for lone atrial fibrillation. *Circ Arrhythm Electrophysiol.* 2012;5(1):8–14.
6. Ruaengsri C, Schill MR, Khiabani AJ, Schuessler RB, Melby SJ, Damiano RJ Jr. The Cox-Maze iv procedure in its second decade: still the gold standard? *Eur J Cardio-Thorac Surg.* 2018;53(suppl_1):i19–i25.
7. Ad N, Holmes SD, Massimiano PS, Rongione AJ, Fornaresio LM. Long-term outcome following concomitant mitral valve surgery and cox Maze procedure for atrial fibrillation. *J Thorac Cardiovasc Surg.* 2018;155(3):983–994.
8. McCarthy PM, Cox JL, Kruse J, Elenbaas C, Andrei A-C. One hundred percent utilization of a modified CryoMaze III procedure for atrial fibrillation with mitral surgery. *J Thorac Cardiovasc Surg.* 2024;167(4):1278-1289.
9. Joglar JA, Chung MK, Armbruster AL, et al. 2023 ACC/AHA/ACCP/HRS guideline for the diagnosis and management of atrial fibrillation: a report of the American College of Cardiology/American Heart Association Joint Committee on clinical practice guidelines. *Circulation.* 2024;149(1):e1–e156.
10. Whitlock RP, Belley-Cote EP, Paparella D, et al. Left atrial appendage occlusion during cardiac surgery to prevent stroke. *N Engl J Med.* 2021;384(22):2081–2091.
11. Wyler von Ballmoos MC, Hui DS, Mehaffey JH, et al. The Society of Thoracic Surgeons 2023 clinical practice guidelines for the surgical treatment of atrial fibrillation. *Ann Thorac Surg.* 2024;118(2):291–310.
12. Ahmed M, Belley-Cote EP, Qiu Y, et al. Rhythm vs. rate control in patients with postoperative atrial fibrillation after cardiac surgery: a systematic review and meta-analysis. *J Clin Med.* 2023;12(13):4534.
13. Gillinov AM, Bagiella E, Moskowitz AJ, et al. Rate control versus rhythm control for atrial fibrillation after cardiac surgery. *N Eng J Med.* 2016;374(20):1911–1921.
14. Sato S, Yamauchi S, Schuessler RB, Boineau JP, Matsunaha Y, Cox JL. The effect of augmented atrial hypothermia on atrial refractory period, conduction, and atrial flutter/fibrillation in the canine heart. *J Thor Cardiovasc Surg.* 1992;104:297–306.
15. Rezk M, Taha A, Nielsen SJ, et al: Clinical course of postoperative atrial fibrillation after cardiac surgery and long-term outcome. Ann Thorac Surg 114(6):2209-2215.
16. Fragao-Marques M, Teixeira F, Mancio J, et al. Impact of oral anticoagulation therapy on postoperative atrial fibrillation outcomes: a systematic review and meta-analysis. *Thromb J.* 2021;19(1):89.
17. van de Kar MRD, van Brakel TJ, Van't Veer M, et al. Anticoagulation for post-operative atrial fibrillation after isolated coronary artery bypass grafting: a meta-analysis. *Eur Heart J.* 2024;45(29):2620–2630.
18. Van Gelder IC, Rienstra M, Bunting KV, et al. 2024 ESC guidelines for the management of atrial fibrillation developed in collaboration with the European Association for Cardio-Thoracic Surgery (EACTS). *Eur Heart J.* 2024;45(36):3314–3414.
19. Connolly SJ, Healey JS, Belley-Cote EP, et al. Oral anticoagulation use and left atrial appendage occlusion in LAAOS III. *Circulation.* 2023;148(17):1298–1304.

50

The Future of Left Atrial Appendage Management

Marc Gillinov, Edward G. Soltesz

CHAPTER OUTLINE

Surgeons' interest in the left atrial appendage (LAA) dates to 1949, when John L. Madden published a paper titled "Resection of the left auricular appendix: A prophylaxis for recurrent arterial emboli."[1] In that communication, he described two cases in which patients had had embolic events, noting that pathologic examination revealed LAA thrombus in both patients Writing that "*in about 90 per cent of the cases the mural thrombi are located in the auricles, mainly in the left auricle and its appendix*," he concludes his discussion with the comment, "*Resection of the left auricular appendix is suggested as a prophylaxis for recurrent emboli.*" Seventy-five years later, we have data to support this statement. Termed "*our most lethal human attachment*" by Dudley Johnson,[2] the LAA has captured the interest of both surgeons and cardiologists in recent years. With an understanding of the increased stroke risk in those with atrial fibrillation (AF) and the pathogenesis of these events, surgeons and interventionalists have deemed the LAA a target for both primary and secondary stroke prevention in patients with AF.[2–6] There can be no doubt that this interest will grow and that greater numbers of patients with AF will have management plans that address the LAA.

As the number of patients with AF continues to increase, the two questions that surgeons face regarding LAA management are "when" and "how." When should the surgeon treat the LAA? And how should they address this delicate structure?

WHEN SURGEONS SHOULD MANAGE THE LEFT ATRIAL APPENDAGE

When contemplating LAA management, surgeons can divide patients into two groups: (1) those with preexisting AF and (2) those with no known history of AF.

Patients With Preexisting Atrial Fibrillation: Concomitant Procedures

In the concomitant setting, surgeons encounter large numbers of patients who have AF in addition to structural heart disease. Supported by a wide body of literature, the Cox Maze procedure, which includes LAA management, is clearly the best approach to these patients.[3,4,7–9] The risk of embolic stroke after a Cox Maze procedure is remarkably low,[3,4] and restoration of sinus rhythm is achieved in the majority of patients.[4,10] Although there is some controversy concerning the relative impacts of the lesion set versus LAA management in this reduced stroke risk, there can be no doubt that proper management of the LAA plays an important role.[7,11]

Nearly all guidelines recommend surgical ablation, including LAA management, at the time of concomitant surgery in patients with preexisting AF.[12] Nevertheless, historically, a majority of cardiac surgery patients with AF have not received ablation.[12,13] Fortunately, recent data recommend the increased use of ablation plus LAA management in cardiac surgical patients with AF.[12] In the future, this proportion will continue to increase, particularly if concomitant surgical ablation in those with AF becomes a quality metric.

Meanwhile, based on Whitlock's landmark Left Atrial Appendage Occlusion Study (LAAOS)-III trial[14] demonstrating that LAA treatment reduces stroke and systemic thromboembolism in cardiac surgical patients with preexisting AF and risk factors for stroke, surgical management of the LAA as a concomitant procedure in patients with AF has become widespread. It received a Class IA recommendation in the 2023 American College of Cardiology/American Heart Association/American College of Clinical Pharmacy/Heart Rhythm Society Guidelines for the Diagnosis and Management of Atrial Fibrillation[15] and in the 2023 Society of Thoracic Surgeons Clinical Practice Guidelines for the Surgical Treatment of Atrial Fibrillation.[16] This important change in the guidelines will certainly generate an increase in surgical management of the LAA in patients with AF. The danger, though, is that surgeons may deem LAA management to be sufficient in their patients with AF and consequently forego ablation. This would be a mistake because the combination of ablation with LAA management is superior to LAA management alone,[7,11,17] with the former strategy (ablation plus LAA management) associated with improved survival compared with LAA treatment alone.

Patients With Preexisting Atrial Fibrillation: Sole Left Atrial Appendage Management

Thoracoscopic LAA management as an isolated procedure has been reported by several groups over the past two decades.[18,19] With port-based access via the left chest and a posterior pericardiotomy, most procedures involved application of either a suture to snare the appendage or a stapler to excise it. Occasionally, problematic bleeding occurred. Now that surgeons have access to LAA clips designed specifically for thoracoscopic application, procedural safety has been enhanced.[19,20] Although there will likely be an uptick in surgical sole LAA management, the widespread availability of endovascular devices designed to plug or occlude the appendage will limit surgical involvement to those patients who are not candidates for an endovascular approach or who prefer a surgical approach.[5]

Although current endovascular LAA occlusion (LAAO) devices have improved safety and efficacy profiles compared with earlier generations, they can still engender early and late complications. Although early complications are typically procedural (e.g., perforation and pericardial effusion), late complications are generally caused by device-related thrombus or peri-device leaks that increase stroke risk.[21] Here, epicardially placed surgical devices have an advantage because they completely exclude the appendage and do not include an endovascular component that can be a nidus for thrombus formation.

Patients Without Preexisting Atrial Fibrillation

Now that device-based LAA exclusion is simple, quick, and relatively complication free, some surgeons exclude the LAA in all patients who undergo a sternotomy, even if the patient has never experienced AF. Retrospective studies support the safety of this strategy and suggest a possible benefit in terms of early and late thromboembolic risk.[22–24] It is also possible that routine LAA treatment will reduce the risk of stroke in those who develop new-onset postoperative AF.[11] However, at this time, data are insufficient to support LAA management in patients with no history of AF.[24]

The Left Atrial Appendage Exclusion for Prophylactic Stroke Reduction (LeAAPS) trial will clarify the role of LAA management in patients without a history of AF but with risk factors for AF and ischemic stroke. This trial will enroll up to 6500 patients undergoing cardiac surgery at 250 sites. The primary endpoint is occurrence of ischemic stroke or systemic embolism, with a minimum of 5-year follow-up period in all patients. If this trial proves positive, LAA management will likely become a component of nearly all cardiac surgical procedures.

HOW TO CLOSE THE LEFT ATRIAL APPENDAGE

By their very nature, surgeons are adept at the application of a needle holder with a needle and suture. With a single polypropylene suture, surgeons can achieve a secure and permanent aortic closure, coronary artery distal anastomosis, or insertion of a Dacron graft. One would surmise, therefore, that standard surgical techniques should suffice for suture closure of the LAA. Multiple studies refute this hypothesis.[25–27] Suture closure of the LAA, whether with a pursestring suture or two-layered running suture, does not produce reliable secure and long-term exclusion of the appendage. Furthermore, incomplete closure of the LAA leaves patients at increased risk for thromboembolic events.[11] Although it is possible that more involved suture techniques, including inversion of the appendage and incorporation of the appendage into the suture line, may result in more effective obliteration of the orifice, suture closure, in general, has proven disappointing.[28]

Recognizing that suture closure of the LAA is problematic, some surgeons turned to staplers to either exclude or excise the LAA. Incorporation of pericardial strips helped to control staple line bleeding, but treatment was often incomplete because the procedure left a remnant cul-de-sac of LAA larger than 10 mm.[29–31] In addition, noncutting staplers often allowed late recanalization of the LAA.[30] Thus surgical staplers, which were generally designed for other purposes, do not present a reliable option for LAA management.

Excision of the appendage and oversewing its base is certainly effective but comes with an associated risk of bleeding. This is particularly troublesome in older individuals with fragile tissues. Although surgical excision was a mainstay of the original Cox Maze procedure,[11] it has been supplanted by device-based closure.

Device-based closure with a commercially available clip designed specifically for the LAA is the safest and most reliable means of achieving complete and permanent LAA exclusion. The clip has a success rate that exceeds 95%[32] but incorrect placement that is too far distal (i.e., not at the LAA base) represents failure.

Recanalization of a properly occluded appendage is virtually impossible. After clip placement, the LAA scars down and, over the course of months, essentially "disappears." In addition, it becomes electrically "silent."[33] The clip comes in a variety of sizes and configurations, some of which are designed for minimally invasive thoracoscopic application. In patients with AF who are intolerant of anticoagulants and do not have anatomy suitable for an endovascular approach, epicardial thoracoscopic LAAO represents an excellent option. One would expect some growth in this surgical approach to the LAA in the future

SURGICAL LEFT ATRIAL APPENDAGE MANAGEMENT: THE FUTURE

Among patients with AF undergoing concomitant surgery, the use of ablation, coupled with LAA exclusion, will continue to increase. Younger surgeons emerging from residency are well versed in the importance of AF management in their patients, and they will follow the guidelines that strongly endorse ablation with LAA management at the time of cardiac surgery. Even without the results of the LeAPPS trial, surgeons are increasingly embracing the concept of LAA management in patients without a history of AF but who are judged to be at high risk for developing AF or a stroke from atrial myopathy. This practice, too, will likely increase rapidly. The growth of surgical LAA management as a stand-alone procedure will be seen only in centers where surgeons and electrophysiologists collaborate closely. At this time, surgeons are thinking more and more about the LAA, and it is likely that LAA management will grow considerably in the surgical population.

REFERENCES

1. Madden JL. Resection of the left auricular appendix: a prophylaxis for recurrent emboli. *J Am Med Assoc*. 1949;140:769–772.
2. Johnson WD, Ganjoo AK, Stone CD, Srivyas RC, Howard M. The left atrial appendage: our most lethal human attachment! Surgical implications. *Eur J Cardio-Thoracic Surg*. 2000;17:718–722.
3. Cox JL, Ad N, Palazzo T. Impact of the Maze procedure on the stroke rate in patients with atrial fibrillation. *J Thorac Cardiovasc Surg*. 1999;118:833–840.
4. Ad N, Holmes SD, Massimiano PS, Rongione AJ, Fornaresio LM. Long-term outcome following concomitant mitral valve surgery and cox Maze procedure for atrial fibrillation. *J Thorac Cardiovasc Surg*. 2018;155:983–994.
5. Lu MLR, De Lurgio DB. Left atrial appendage closure: the journey today and tomorrow. *Curr Opin Cardiol*. 2024;39:20–26.
6. Moss JD. Left atrial appendage exclusion for prevention of stroke in atrial fibrillation: review of minimally invasive approaches. *Curr Cardiol Rep*. 2014;16:1–10.

7. Mehaffey JH, Hayanga JW, Wei L, Mascio C, Rankin JS, Badhwar V. Surgical ablation of atrial fibrillation is associated with improved survival compared with appendage obliteration alone: an analysis of 100,000 medicare beneficiaries. *J Thorac Cardiovasc Surg*. 2023;168:1–13.
8. Malaisrie SC, McCarthy PM, Kruse J, et al. Ablation of atrial fibrillation during coronary artery bypass grafting: late outcomes in a medicare population. *J Thorac Cardiovasc Surg*. 2021;161:1251–1261.
9. Musharbash FN, Schill MR, Sinn LA, et al. Performance of the cox-Maze IV procedure is associated with improved long-term survival in patients with atrial fibrillation undergoing cardiac surgery. *J Thorac Cardiovasc Surg*. 2018;155:159–170.
10. McCarthy PM, Cox JL, Kruse J, Elenbaas C, Adnin-Cristian A. One hundred percent utilization of a modified CryoMaze III procedure for atrial fibrillation with mitral surgery. *J Thorac Cardiovasc Surg*. 2022;167:1–12.
11. Cox JL. Mechanical closure of the left atrial appendage: is it time to be more aggressive? *J Thorac Cardiovasc Surg*. 2013;146:1018–1027.
12. Badhwar V, Rankin JS, Ad N, et al. Surgical ablation of atrial fibrillation in the United States: trends and propensity matched outcomes. *Ann Thorac Surg*. 2017;104:493–500.
13. McCarthy PM, Davidson CJ, Kruse J, et al. Prevalence of atrial fibrillation before cardiac surgery and factors associated with concomitant ablation. *J Thorac Cardiovasc Surg*. 2020;159:2245–2253.
14. Whitlock RP, Belley-Cote D, Paparella JS, et al. Left atrial appendage occlusion during cardiac surgery to prevent stroke. *N Engl J Med*. 2021;384:2081–2091.
15. Joglar JA, Chung MK, Armbruster AL, et al. 2023 ACC/AHA/ACCP/HRS guideline for the diagnosis and management of atrial fibrillation: a report of the American College of Cardiology/American Heart Association Joint Committee on clinical practice guidelines. *Circulation*. 2024;149:e1–e156.
16. Wyler von Ballmoos MC, Hui DS, Mehaffey JH, et al. The society of thoracic surgeons 2023 clinical practice guidelines for the surgical treatment of atrial fibrillation. *Ann Thorac Surg*. 2024. S0003-4975(24)00057-2. https://doi.org/10.1016/j.athoracsur.2024.01.007.
17. Pasierski M, Batko J, Kuzma L, et al. Surgical ablation, left atrial appendage occlusion or both? Nationwide registry analysis of cardiac surgery patients with underlying atrial fibrillation. *Eur J Cardio-Thorac Surg*. https://doi.org/10.1093/ejcts/ezae014.
18. Ohtsuka T, Ninomiya M, Nonaka T, Hisagi M, Ota T, Mizutani T. Thoracoscopic stand-alone left atrial appendectomy for thromboembolism prevention in nonvalvular atrial fibrillation. *J Am Coll Cardiol*. 2013;62:103–107.
19. Blackshear JL, Johnson WD, Odell JA, et al. Thoracoscopic extracardiac obliteration of the left atrial appendage for stroke risk reduction in atrial fibrillation. *J Am Coll Cardiol*. 2003;42:1249–1252.
20. Ailawadi G, Gerdisch MW, Harvey RL, et al. Exclusion of the left atrial appendage with a novel device: early results of a multicenter trial. *J Thorac Cardiovasc Surg*. 2011;142:1002–1009.
21. Mostafa MR, Eid MM, Abuelazm, et al. Meta-analysis of the outcomes of peri-device leak after left atrial appendage closure. *Am J Cardiol*. 2023;204:325–332.
22. Madsen CV, Park-Hansen J, Holme SJV, et al. Randomized trial of surgical left atrial appendage closure: protection against cerebrovascular events. *Semin Thorac Surg*. 2022;35:664–672.
23. Kim R, Baumgartner N, Clements J. Routine left atrial appendage ligation during cardiac surgery may prevent postoperative atrial fibrillation-related cerebrovascular accident. *J Thorac Cardiovasc Surg*. 2013;145:582–589.
24. Yao X, Gersh BJ, Holmes DR, et al. Association of surgical left atrial appendage occlusion with subsequent stroke and mortality among patients undergoing cardiac surgery. *JAMA*. 2018;319:2116–2126.
25. Dominguez H, Madsen CV, Westh ONJ, et al. Does left atrial appendage amputation during routine cardiac surgery reduce future atrial fibrillation and stroke? *Current Cardiol Rep*. 2018;20:99.
26. Katz ES, Tsiamtsiouris T, Applebaum RM, Schwartzbard A, Tunick PA, Kronzon I. Surgical left atrial appendage ligation is frequently incomplete: a transesophageal echocardiographic study. *J Am Coll Cardiol*. 2000;36:468–471.
27. Lee R, Vassallo P, Kruse J, et al. A randomized prospective pilot comparison of 3 atrial appendage elimination techniques: internal ligation, stapled excision, and surgical excision. *J Thorac Cardiovasc Surg*. 2016;152:1075–1080.
28. Hanke T. Surgical management of the left atrial appendage: a must or a myth. *Eur Jo Cardio-Thorac Surg*. 2018;53:133–138.
29. Badhwar V, Rankin JS, Lee R, McCarthy PM, Wei LM. Contemporary left atrial appendage management during adult cardiac surgery. *J Thorac Cardiovasc Surg*. 2023;165:1398–1404.
30. Gillinov AM, Pettersson G, Cosgrove DM. Stapled excision of the left atrial appendage. *J Thorac Cardiovasc Surg*. 2005;129:679–680.
31. Roth P, Rahimi A, Boening A. The pericardium-reinforced technique of amputation of the left atrial appendage: quick, safe, and simple. *Ann Thorac Surg*. 2010;90:e11–e13.
32. Emmert MY, Puippe G, Baumuller S, et al. Safe, effective and durable epicardial left atrial appendage clip occlusion in patients with atrial fibrillation undergoing cardiac surgery: first long-term results from a prospective device trial. *Eur J Cardio-Thorac Surg*. 2014;45:126–131.
33. Ali Hassan SM, Paleczny S, Yanagawar B, Glover B, Bileri G. Electrical isolation following thoracoxcopic left atrial appendage exclusion during hybrid ablation for longstanding persistent atrial fibrillation. *J Atrial Fibrillation Electrophysiol*. 2022;15(1). http://www.jafib.com/PMC/XML/Inprogress/FullIssue/2022-01-31.pdf#page=51.

51

The Future of Concomitant Atrial Fibrillation Ablation

Patrick M. McCarthy, MD

CHAPTER OUTLINE

The biggest challenge that needs to be addressed in the concomitant surgical treatment of patients with atrial fibrillation (AF) is education. The Society of Thoracic Surgeons (STS) and European Association for Cardio-Thoracic Surgery guidelines made a strong case summarizing the data that support concomitant surgical ablation and all societies support concomitant left atrial appendage occlusion (LAAO).[1–3]

Surgeons should not continue to ignore the evidence demonstrating reductions in mortality, stroke, and AF with manageable perioperative risks.[4–6] The guidelines are meaningless and ineffective if surgeons ignore them, and that is what is happening. Only 34% perform surgical ablation in mitral surgery patients with AF, 18% in aortic valve surgery, and 10% in coronary artery bypass grafting (CABG) patients with AF (see Chapter 23). Compare this with the guideline recommendation for left internal mammary artery (LIMA)– left anterior descending artery (LAD) with near 100% compliance for CABG.

A PRACTICAL APPROACH TO CONCOMITANT SURGICAL ABLATION

We need to listen to the surgeons who ignore AF in their cardiac surgery patients to understand how to improve the situation. According to a survey on barriers to adoption of concomitant AF ablation, almost 90% of surgeons are aware of the guidelines, so there is little room for improvement there.[7] However, only about half of the surgeons learned how and when to perform AF surgical ablation in residency or fellowship or took specialized courses devoted to the surgical ablation of AF. More support from the Thoracic Surgery Directors Association for the inclusion of AF surgery in the training curriculum and more aggressive requirements for AF surgical experience during training by the Thoracic Surgery Residency Review Committee and the American Board of Thoracic Surgery are needed. Improved residency training may require outside visiting surgeon lectures, demonstrations, simulations, and videos to educate the trainees on the "basics" of AF and AF surgery, the benefits of concomitant AF surgery, and the appropriate ablation procedure for an individual patient with AF who requires CABG, valve, or thoracic aortic surgery. Ideally, the visits would be in person, but virtual conferences and prerecorded videos may be a good start for learning the basics.

We also need to address the biggest issue, which is that surgeons believe that the operation is too complex and dangerously increases aortic cross-clamp time. Reports indicate they may be correct, especially if a full Cox-Maze-III or IV procedure is the operation called for in a specific patient and the surgeon has little or no experience with AF surgical ablation (see Chapters 15 and 25).[8] However, numerous studies have consistently documented that in experienced and properly trained hands, the addition of a Maze procedure to CABG and/or valve surgery does not adversely affect the surgical morbidity or mortality rates.[4–6,9–11] Indeed, Badhwar et al.[12] reported a large STS database analysis showing that the addition of AF ablation to MVR, CABG, aortic valve replacement (AVR), or CABG plus AVR procedures actually *decreased* the 30-day operative mortality rate. Both the STS guidelines[13] and the American Association for Thoracic Surgery (AATS) Expert Opinion Consensus[14] confirmed that concomitant AF surgery did not impact operative morbidity and that it either decreased or had no impact on operative mortality rates. Thus, both of these thoracic surgery societies strongly support the addition of concomitant AF ablation to these index surgical procedures and they should have eliminated any safety concern about adding a concomitant Maze procedure in patients with AF undergoing the most common types of cardiac surgery. Of course, the surgical procedures in all of these studies were done by experienced surgeons, again emphasizing the need for improved training in AF ablation techniques.

In the survey, surgeons were also concerned about postoperative arrhythmias and the need for new pacemakers. Therefore, they assumed that patient risk was automatically increased by adding a concomitant AF ablation procedure. We can point to the STS data showing reduced 30-day mortality and stroke rates, but with only 50% of surgeons trained in surgical ablation or who took courses, would that still be true if suddenly large numbers of surgeons were trying to add a full Cox Maze-III or Cox Maze-IV to all operations? Seems unlikely. To keep the 30-day, publicly reported, risk at a low level (trying to get three stars from STS!) many surgeons have opted to just skip the ablation. To reverse this unfortunate practice, we need a change in mindset to a more practical approach and hopefully, new technology.

"The enemy of good is better" (Voltaire; attributed). For years we have preached to surgeons that a full Cox Maze-III or Cox Maze-IV procedure using cryoablation and/or bipolar radiofrequency (RF) is the "best" way to treat patients with concomitant AF, and it is. Some would add it's the "only" way to treat patients with AF. But the non-arrhythmia surgeons are right. It does add aortic cross-clamp time, and in their hands, it could increase the 30-day operative mortality risk. Maybe "less is more" (fewer lesions but more ablation in this case) (Ludwig Mies van der Rohe; attributed). Left atrial ablation alone is acceptable for mitral operations without right-sided involvement in reoperations (see Chapters 25 and 27), and pulmonary vein (PV) isolation alone is a good choice for a recent graduate doing a low ejection fraction CABG with paroxysmal AF on the weekend with no senior partner nearby, an epicardial box lesion with a clamp and left atrial appendage (LAA) closure may be a good choice with surgical aortic valve replacement for an aortic stenosis patient with paroxysmal AF compared with transcatheter aortic valve replacement alone.[8] The options for treatment need to be expanded. A Cox Maze-III or Cox Maze-IV procedure performed by an experienced surgeon is certainly a good option for most patients in most situations, but it should not be considered the only option for all patients.

QUALITY MEASUREMENTS FOR CONCOMITANT TREATMENT OF ATRIAL FIBRILLATION

LAA closure, with complete occlusion and a residual stump of less than 10 mm, is safe, fast, durable, and easy. All surgeons, even new graduates, can do this procedure, especially with the AtriClip. Although suture closure is certainly less expensive than device closure, it has been associated with incomplete occlusion and has some risk of bleeding when the LAA is excised. However, this may be the preferred approach in certain situations, such as in a reoperation mitral valve (MV) procedure (see Chapter 15). There are many commercially available LAA closure devices in various sizes and shapes, and no doubt more are coming in the future. The *Left Atrial Appendage Occlusion Study* (LAAOS) III trial clearly demonstrated the benefit of adding LAAO, and a variety of types of occlusion were used in that trial. LAAO should be considered, whenever possible, in every patient with preexisting AF unless there is a specific contraindication to closing the LAA.[15–18]

An effective way to change surgeon behavior would be to add LAAO as a quality metric, similar to the situation with LIMA–LAD for coronary artery bypass.[19] This seems like a simple step, but there is only one procedure relating to coronary artery bypass, LIMA–LAD, that is a quality metric. Considering that LAAO is simple, safe, and effective, it should be adopted as standard operating procedure. Studies demonstrated low uptake in California (51% in 2019), but this may be "old news" because it increased every year from 2016 through 2019.[20] In Michigan, a concerted effort to increase compliance was put in place, and reported compliance reached 79% at the end of the study.[21] There will need to be exceptions (there are also a few for the use of LIMA–LAD), and reoperations will be the most common exception. Others could include pericardial adhesions, poor tissue quality with a significant risk for bleeding in the judgement of the surgeon, and anatomy unfavorable for LAA closure (rare). Despite these caveats, concomitant LAAO for patients with AF should approach 100% utilization, as does LIMA–LAD grafting in coronary patients.

In view of the universally recognized positive impact of concomitant AF surgical ablation (SA) on postoperative stroke rates and long-term survival, concomitant SA clearly should be performed far more often than it is currently (<25%). Discussion continues to revolve around the best technology, the preferred lesion set (biatrial Maze, LA Maze, PVI, CTI, etc), and which patients should have concomitant AF ablation.[8] Even though there is still no consensus on these issues, *any* of the SA procedures is preferable to ignoring the AF completely (>75%). Thus, while it would be inappropriate to declare a specific lesion pattern (say, a biatrial Maze procedure) as a quality metric, the designation of the general category of "concomitant AF surgical ablation," which would include any of the lesions sets, should be strongly encouraged as a part of every cardiac surgical procedure in a patient with preoperative AF. The surgical societies and guideline committees that mandate near 100% adoption of concomitant SA of AF are responding to the accumulation of a vast body of positive evidence in making their recommendations, and they are on firm ground in doing so with or without declaring it to be a quality metric.

NEW TECHNOLOGY

As of this writing, there are no published clinical data using the latest surgical ablation technology, the EnCompass Bipolar Radiofrequency Clamp (AtriCure, Inc., Mason, OH), which was specifically designed for operations such as CABG and AVR in which the left atrium is not normally opened. Using this new clamp in CABG or AVR patients creates a box lesion with one tissue clamping, and the results in animal studies have been favorable. However currently, the entire electrophysiology community is enamored with pulsed-field ablation (PFA), and this new clamp will likely be adapted to currently available RF and cryosurgical devices in the next few years.[22–25] Surgical devices using PFA instead of bipolar RF have the potential to be much faster, which will be a welcome improvement, but as discussed in Chapter 52, initial reports on the efficacy of PFA compared with RF and cryosurgery are disappointing. Ultra-low-temperature cryoablation (ULTC) cryocatheters using "near-critical nitrogen," which is essentially liquid nitrogen suspended in a gaseous state at −196°C, have met with initial clinical success for the ablation of atrial flutter,[26] AF,[27] and ventricular tachycardia.[28] We expect that this promising new technology will be adapted to surgical devices in the future. Experimental studies with catheters that combine ULTC and PFA (called PFCA) have been promising, but no clinical data on PFCA ablation are currently available. These new single and combined ablation energy sources are discussed in more detail in Chapter 52. Although they are currently being developed for treating patients with stand-alone AF and ventricular tachycardia with catheters, they will undoubtedly be adapted in the future for use in surgical devices as well. Similarly, LAA closure devices ideally will be easier to apply in minimally invasive and robotic procedures in the future.

PROPHYLACTIC LEFT ATRIAL APPENDAGE OCCLUSION AND ATRIAL FIBRILLATION ABLATION PROCEDURES

When surgeons are operating on patients for other reasons, it is a simple procedure to close the LAA, and the potential danger of an open LAA has been recognized for many years.[29] Meta-analyses, single-center studies, and database studies have demonstrated a reduced risk of stroke in patients with no history of AF who undergo LAAO versus those without LAAO.[30,31] This makes sense intuitively, particularly in patients with a significant underlying risk of developing AF and therefore stroke. Such patients may be older, have a CHA_2DS_2-VASc score of 3 or more, have a dilated atrium, or have other markers of "atrial myopathy." The ongoing 6,000-patient randomized clinical LEft Atrial Appendage Exclusion for Prophylactic Stroke reduction (LeAAPS) trial will shed light on this subject.[32] Assuming that this trial is positive and shows that LAAO-treated patients with no history of AF have a lower long-term risk of stroke, it will set the stage for another important question: "Can anticoagulation be withheld in patients with successful LAAO if they develop AF?".

A riskier trial would be to study concomitant surgical ablation to prevent new-onset postoperative AF and/or late recurrent AF.[33] However, the trigger mechanisms for new-onset postoperative AF

(POAF) are not the same as the PV triggers that induce typical AF (see Chapter 47), so prophylactic surgical ablation for AF may not have a significant early impact on new-onset POAF. We do know that Maze surgery does not prevent POAF, but we do not know whether or not the early POAF after a Maze procedure is similar to new-onset POAF in a patient with no preoperative history of AF. However, a reduction in late recurrent AF could be reasonably expected after such a prophylactic surgical ablation depending on the patient population. A patient population with no history of AF but with a high risk for developing AF in the future would be an interesting trial target, but even MV patients with no AF history had only a 22% rate of developing *de novo* AF on 10-year follow-up, so such a trial design may be impractical.[34] These trials have been discussed for many years, but with the success of LAAOS III, there is growing interest in large surgical randomized controlled trials in AF therapy.

WHAT SHOULD THE GOAL BE BY 2035?

The stage is set for significant advancement in the concomitant surgical treatment of patients with AF over the next 10 years. LAAO should become routine with near 100% adoption rate even in patients without previous AF, with a handful of exceptions. New technologies and procedures should lead to effective surgical ablation that is significantly simpler for surgeons. This will be supported by the guidelines and extensive educational efforts, especially early in the surgeons' careers. For open left atrial procedures, concomitant ablation should approach 100%, and for closed left atrial procedures, it should approach 80% to 90%. We are already at these levels at Northwestern University in Chicago, and we hope that this textbook and associated educational efforts will help speed this level of adoption worldwide.

REFERENCES

1. Wyler von Ballmoos MC, Hui DS, Mehaffey JH, et al. The Society of Thoracic Surgeons 2023 clinical practice guidelines for the surgical treatment of atrial fibrillation. *Ann Thor Surg*. 2024. https://doi.org/10.1016/j.athoracsur.2024.01.007.
2. Van Gelder IC, Rienstra M, Bunting KV, et al. 2024 ESC guidelines for the management of atrial fibrillation developed in collaboration with the European Association for Cardio-Thoracic Surgery (EACTS). *Eur Heart J*. 2024;45(36):3314–3414.
3. Joglar JA, Chung MK, Armbruster AL, et al. 2023 ACC/AHA/ACCP/HRS guideline for the diagnosis and management of atrial fibrillation: a report of the American College of Cardiology/American Heart Association Joint Committee on clinical practice guidelines. *Circulation*. 2024;149(1):e1–e156.
4. McCarthy PM, Davidson CJ, Kruse J, et al. Prevalence of atrial fibrillation before cardiac surgery and factors associated with concomitant ablation. *J Thor Cardiovasc Surg*. 2020;159(6):2245–2253.
5. Malaisrie SC, McCarthy PM, Kruse J, et al. Ablation of atrial fibrillation during coronary artery bypass grafting: late outcomes in a Medicare population. *J Thor Cardiovasc Surg*. 2021;161(4):1251–1261.
6. Churyla A, Andrei AC, Kruse J, et al. Safety of atrial fibrillation ablation with isolated surgical aortic valve replacement. *Ann Thor Surg*. 2021;111(3):809–817.
7. Mehaffey JH, Charles EJ, Berens M, et al. Barriers to atrial fibrillation ablation during mitral valve surgery. *J Thor Cardiovasc Surg*. 2021. https://doi.org/10.1016/j.jtcvs.2021.03.039.
8. McCarthy PM, Cox JL. Practical approaches to concomitant surgical ablation of atrial fibrillation: matching the ablation to the patient. *J Thor Cardiovasc Surg*. 2024. https://doi.org/10.1016/j.jtcvs.2024.03.023.
9. Ad N, Henry L, Hunt S, Holmes SD. Do we increase the operative risk by adding the Cox Maze III procedure to aortic valve replacement and coronary artery bypass surgery? *J Thor Cardiovasc Surg*. 2012;143(4):936–944.
10. Saint LL, Damiano Jr RJ, Cuculich PS, et al. Incremental risk of the Cox-Maze IV procedure for patients with atrial fibrillation undergoing mitral valve surgery. *J Thor Cardiovasc Surg*. 2013;146(5):1072–1077.
11. Al-Atassi T, Kimmaliardjuk D-M, Dagenais C, Bourke M, Lam B-K, Rubens FD. Should we ablate atrial fibrillation during coronary artery bypass grafting and aortic valve replacement? *Ann Thor Surg*. 2017;104:515–522.
12. Badhwar V, Rankin JS, Ad N, et al. Surgical ablation of atrial fibrillation in the United States: trends and propensity matched outcomes. *Ann Thor Surg*. 2017;104:493–500.
13. Badhwar V, Rankin JS, Damiano RJ, et al. The Society of Thoracic Surgeons 2017 clinical practice guidelines for the surgical treatment of atrial fibrillation. *Ann Thor Surg*. 2017;103(1):329–341 Erratum in: *J Thor Cardiovasc Surg* 2017;153(6):1330-1354.
14. Ad N, Damiano Jr. RJ, Badhwar V et al., Expert consensus guidelines: examining surgical ablation for atrial fibrillation. *J Thorac Cardiovasc Surg*. 2017;153(6):1330–1354.e1.
15. Yao X, Gersh BJ, Holmes Jr DR, et al. Association of surgical left atrial appendage occlusion with subsequent stroke and mortality among patients undergoing cardiac surgery. *J Am Med Assoc*. 2018;319(20):2116–2126.
16. Friedman DJ, Piccini JP, Wang T, et al. Association between left atrial appendage occlusion and readmission for thromboembolism among patients with atrial fibrillation undergoing concomitant cardiac surgery. *J Am Med Assoc*. 2018;319(4):365–374.
17. Whitlock RP, Belley-Cote EP, Paparella D, et al. Left Atrial appendage occlusion during cardiac surgery to prevent stroke. *N Eng J Med*. 2021;384(22):2081–2091.
18. Mehaffey JH, Rankin JS, Wei LM, Badhwar V. Outcome benefits of surgical ablation and left atrial appendage obliteration for atrial fibrillation during adult cardiac surgery. *J Thor Cardiovasc Surg*. 2024. https://doi.org/10.1016/j.jtcvs 2024.05.008.
19. Shahian DM, Edwards FH, Ferraris VA, et al. Quality measurement in adult cardiac surgery: part 1—conceptual framework and measure selection. *Ann Thor Surg*. 2007;83(4):3–12.
20. Hadaya J, Hernandez R, Sanaiha Y, et al. Left atrial appendage closure during cardiac surgery: safe but underutilized in California. *J Thor Cardiovasc Surg Open*. 2023;13:150–162.
21. Brescia AA, Groskurth JD, Murphy ET, et al. Increasing adoption of left atrial appendage occlusion in isolated coronary artery bypass grafting. *Ann Thor Surg*. 2024;118(4):854–862.
22. Yu J, Yi J, Nikolaisen G, et al. Efficacy of a surgical cardiac ablation clamp using nanosecond pulsed electric fields: an acute porcine model. *J Thor Cardiovasc Surg*. 2024. https://doi.org/10.1016/j.jtcvs.2024.06.009.
23. Iribarne A, DiScipio AW, McCullough JN, et al. Surgical atrial fibrillation ablation improves long-term survival: a multicenter analysis. *Ann Thor Surg*. 2019;107(1):135–142.
24. Willekes CL, Fanning JS, Heiser JC, et al. Randomized feasibility trial of prophylactic radiofrequency ablation to prevent atrial fibrillation after cardiac surgery. *J Thor Cardiovasc Surg*. 2024;167(6):2129–2135.
25. Di Biase L, Diaz JC, Zhang XD, Romero J. Pulsed field catheter ablation in atrial fibrillation. *Trends Cardiovasc Med*. 2022;32(6):378–387.
26. Klaver MN, De Potter TJR, Iliodromitis K, et al. Ultralow temperature cryoablation using near-critical nitrogen for cavotricuspid isthmus-ablation, first-in-human results. *J Cardiovas Electrophysiol*. 2021;32(8):2025–2032.

27. De Potter T, Klaver M, Babkin A, et al. Ultra-low temperature cryoablation for atrial fibrillation: primary outcomes for efficacy and safety: the Cryocure-2 study. *JACC Clin Electrophysiol.* 2022;8(8):1034–1039.
28. Verma A, Essebag V, Neuzil P, et al. Cryocure-VT: the safety and effectiveness of ultra-low-temperature cryoablation of monomorphic ventricular tachycardia in patients with ischaemic and non-ischaemic cardiomyopathies. *Europace.* 2024;26(4). https://doi.org/10.1093/europace/euae076.
29. Johnson WD, Ganjoo AK, Stone CD, Srivyas RC, Howard M. The left atrial appendage: our most lethal human attachment! Surgical implications. *Eur J Cardiothorac Surg.* 2000;17(6):718–722.
30. Baudo M, Sicouri S, Yamashita Y, et al. Stroke prevention with prophylactic left atrial appendage occlusion in cardiac surgery patients without atrial fibrillation: a meta-analysis of randomized and propensity-score studies. *Circ Cardiovasc Interv.* 2024;17(10):e014296.
31. McCarthy PM, Mehran R, Gerdisch M, et al. Left Atrial appendage exclusion during open cardiac surgery in patients without atrial fibrillation reduces 4-year ischemic stroke and mortality. *JTCVS Struct Endovasc.* 2024;4:100032. https://doi.org/10.1016/j.xjse.2024.100032.
32. Whitlock RP, McCarthy PM, Gerdisch MW, et al. The LEft Atrial Appendage Exclusion for Prophylactic Stroke reduction (LeAAPS) trial: rationale and design. *Am Heart J.* 2024. https://doi.org/10.1016/j.ahj.2024.10.006.
33. Dunnington GH, Pierce CL, Eisenberg S, et al. A heart-team hybrid approach for atrial fibrillation: a single-centre long-term clinical outcome cohort study. *Eur J Cardiothorac Surg.* 2021;60(6):1343–1350.
34. Mehta CK, McCarthy PM, Andrei AC, et al. De novo atrial fibrillation after mitral valve surgery. *J Thor Cardiovasc Surg.* 2018;156(4):1515–1525.

52

Future of the Interventional Treatment of Stand-Alone Atrial Fibrillation

James L. Cox

CHAPTER OUTLINE

CURRENT STATUS

During a September 2022 celebration of the 35th anniversary of the first Maze procedure, I was asked if I thought that the Maze procedure would still be around in 35 more years. My immediate answer was "No, of course not!." However, after thinking about that reflexive answer for a few seconds, I added, "But if you had asked me that question 35 years ago, I would have given you the same answer!"

Before the introduction of the surgical Maze procedure,[1] the only way to treat patients with atrial fibrillation (AF) with any degree of success was with drugs. Interestingly, more than 95% of all patients with AF are still treated with drugs. Although the Maze procedure proved to be highly successful, it was too invasive to be used routinely as a first-line therapy for patients with drug-refractory AF. The introduction of catheter ablation for AF by Haïssaguerre and coworkers[2] in 1998 provided a far less invasive intervention to treat patients with AF, but as might be expected, it proved to be substantially less effective than the more invasive surgical Maze procedure. The disappointing results of catheter ablation for the persistent forms of AF (see Chapter 31) led to the ablation of wider areas of the atrium, irrigated catheters, contact-force catheters, cryoballoon catheters, and new guidance systems such as stereotaxis and the Hanson robot. Unfortunately, none of those developments resulted in more than a marginal improvement in the results of catheter ablation for AF. Because the surgical Maze procedure was too invasive to be used routinely, surgeons developed minimally invasive surgical procedures, totally thoracoscopic off-pump approaches, and robotic procedures, but even these less invasive surgical procedures were deemed by most cardiologists to be too invasive to be the first-line therapy for stand-alone AF. A combination of the suboptimal results of catheter ablation for persistent AF and the refinement of off-pump thoracoscopic surgical techniques eventually resulted in the introduction of "hybrid procedures" in which both thoracoscopic surgery and catheter ablation are used to treat the more complex forms of stand-alone AF. Overall, thoracoscopic–catheter hybrid procedures have proven to be superior to catheter ablation for the treatment of patients with long-standing persistent AF (LSpAF).[3]

It was hoped that the continued improvement in clinical electrophysiological mapping systems would improve the interventional results of AF ablation, and certainly, the systems that are now available are far better than the ones we developed in the mid-1980s. However, the ability to perform real-time mapping to identify and ablate complex fragmented atrial electrogram (CFAE) sites, extrapulmonary vein rotors, automatic foci, and micro-reentrant foci has had little effect on the results of catheter ablation for AF and no effect whatsoever on its surgical ablation. Ironically, despite the availability of these sophisticated mapping systems, the two proven interventional procedures for AF treatment remain pulmonary vein isolation (PVI) and the Maze procedure, neither of which requires electrophysiologic mapping. Mapping systems are currently used primarily as a confirmation tool to document the integrity of lesions created around the pulmonary veins (PVs). However, when they have been used to "map guide" the catheter ablation of AF, the clinical results have not improved. Indeed, the STAR AF 2 trial demonstrated no difference in the clinical results of PVI alone versus PVI and additional ablation lines versus PVI and CFAE ablation based on map guidance.[4] Because the multiple extra-pulmonary vein ablation lines of the Maze procedure clearly improve the results of surgical ablation over surgical PVI alone, it seems apparent that the STAR AF 2 trial primarily demonstrated the futility of trying to map guide AF ablation and the difficulty of creating contiguous, uniformly transmural lesions reliably with a catheter. The study confirmed a statement made to me previously on at least two separate occasions by Michel Haïssaguerre that "Trying to create a line of conduction block with the tip of a catheter is like trying to cut off the corner of a sheet of paper with a straight pin. It is possible, but it is very difficult" (Fig. 52.1).

The fact that isolation of the PVs is the main goal of catheter ablation emphasizes the misnomer of the term "catheter ablation." The actual objective of catheter ablation for AF is not to "ablate" AF but rather to isolate as many of the PV triggers that induce AF as possible.

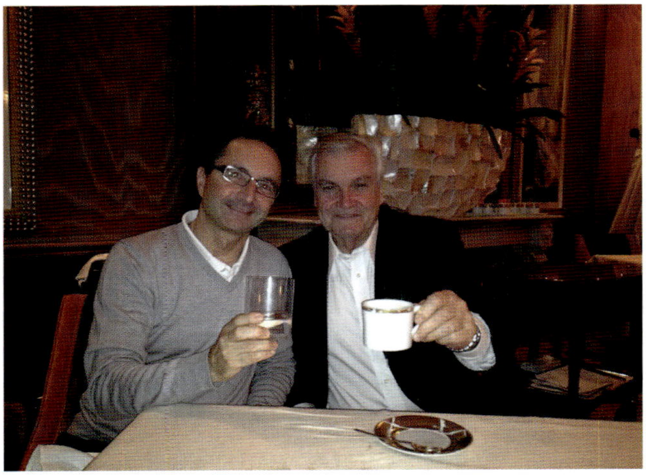

Fig. 52.1 Photograph of Professor Michel Haïssaguerre *(left)* and the author *(right)* at a private dinner in Bordeaux, France, in November 2013. It was at this dinner that Haïssaguerre lamented how difficult it was for interventional electrophysiologists to create a contiguous, uniformly transmural linear lesion in the atrium with the tip of a catheter. (Photo taken by Prof. Meleze Hoccini).

Thus, successful PVI does not "ablate" AF but rather, it simply makes a future episode of AF less likely to be induced. On the contrary, the Maze procedure was designed specifically to ablate AF and preclude its ability to return by rendering the atria incapable of fibrillating. It seems clear that one avenue that should be pursued in the future is to refocus "catheter ablation" on the actual ablation of AF rather than on reducing the likelihood that it will be induced after intervention. However, there remain several seemingly intractable hurdles to making significant progress in catheter or surgical ablation of AF in the future despite the current universal infatuation with pulsed-field ablation (PFA) as the ultimate ablative energy source for arrhythmias (see later discussion).

CURRENT OBSTACLES TO PROGRESS

Inadequate Classification System for Atrial Fibrillation Interventional Therapy

The current clinical classification parameters for AF are fundamentally different from the clinical classification systems for other heart disease because it is based on the single criterion of the *duration* of an AF episode. Classification systems for other structural heart diseases weigh the impact of patient demographics, symptomatology, anatomy, pathophysiology, and comorbidities. All of these factors can impact the outcomes of intervention for AF, but none of them are included in the current classification of AF. The interventional electrophysiologist (EP) and the AF surgeon are likely aware of most of these important preoperative characteristics, but they are not used to categorize the patients into groups that require different specific interventions and have different interventional goals, risks, and expectations. This is of particular importance in patients with AF because without the availability of a meaningful and clinically relevant classification of AF before intervention, the selection of the optimal interventional procedure for a given patient is more difficult to determine, and inappropriate interventional procedures can be the result. The present classification system has served noninvasive cardiologists reasonably well but not interventional EPs and arrhythmia surgeons (i.e., those who treat patients with AF by interventional means rather than with drugs).

When a patient is scheduled to undergo surgical mitral valve (MV) repair for mitral regurgitation (MR), the surgeon knows the magnitude of the preoperative MR, its likely cause, the specific anatomic abnormality of the valve, and the patient's preoperative symptomatology, functional capacity at rest and exercise, quality of life, and relevant comorbidities that could impact the safety and efficacy of the surgery, as well as the functional characteristics of the atria and ventricles as quantitated by preoperative echocardiography and other tests. This information helps determine the optimal surgical intervention for individual patients with any type of structural heart abnormality. A similar level of the preoperative characteristics of AF should be included in a classification system for patients with AF who require catheter or surgical intervention. Such factors include age, sex, the type and duration of AF, AF burden, symptomatology, functional capacity at rest and exercise, quality of life, four-chamber cardiac function, left and right atrial sizes and volumes, the degree of left atrial fibrosis, history of transient ischemic attack or stroke or other systemic thromboembolism, and comorbidities. As noted earlier, we usually know these patient characteristics before surgery for other cardiac disorders, but none of them have anything to do with classifying the AF into paroxysmal AF (PAF), persistent AF, or LSpAF.

Currently, AF seems to be viewed as one large disease that can be divided into these three simple categories to determine the appropriate interventional procedure and to assess its outcomes. This is analogous to classifying all neoplastic disease into the simple categories of head and neck cancer, torso cancer, and limb cancer and then reporting the results of "cancer therapy" for each of those meaningless categories. AF is a spectrum of diseases that varies from simple, classic right atrial flutter to complex forms of LSpAF (see Chapter 5). That spectrum can be subdivided in multiple ways, and each subdivision (say, persistent AF) can be further subdivided based on such characteristics as its response to PVI alone or to a box lesion. It is imperative that a new, clinically relevant classification system be developed for AF that will help us decide on the best interventional therapy to offer each individual patient and improve our ability to determine the actual clinically relevant outcomes of our interventional procedures. Unfortunately, as pointed out throughout this book, intraoperative mapping is not currently capable of defining the optimal interventional approach for each patient.

Dubious Definition of Success or Failure of Atrial Fibrillation Interventions

Even more egregious than the shortcomings of the current AF classification system is the virtually worthless definition that is universally accepted for defining the success or failure of catheter and surgical ablation for AF. Failures of catheter and surgical ablation for AF are currently defined as a documented 30-second episode of AF that recurs more than 3 months after intervention (the "blanking period") in a patient who is on no antiarrhythmic drugs. Yet no adverse sequelae of a 30-second burst of AF have ever been documented, and to make matters worse, no continuous loop recorder is capable of detecting a 30-second episode of AF! Thus a treatment failure in which a patient has episodes of AF lasting less than 2 minutes each could go undetected for years even though the patient's rhythm is being monitored continuously.

Although the definitions of success or failure after surgery for valve disorders or coronary artery disease are objective and meaningful, the success or failure of catheter or surgical ablation for AF can be meaningless clinically. For example, consider a patient who has experienced AF 24 hours per day for years and then undergoes a catheter or surgical intervention. Under the current definition of procedure success or failure, after a 90-day blanking period, one documented 2-minute episode of AF is enough to designate the interventional AF procedure as a failure (Fig. 52.2). This isolated episode of AF is likely asymptomatic, cannot cause tachycardia-induced cardiomyopathy, and does not increase the stroke

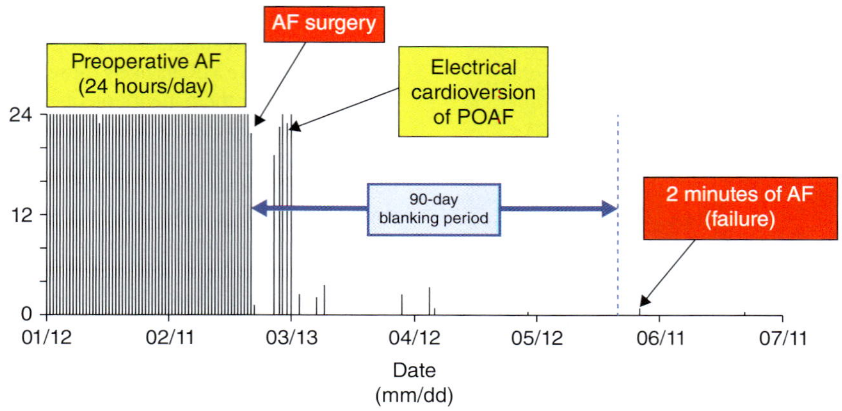

Fig. 52.2 Implanted pacemaker continuous monitoring demonstrating that this patient was in atrial fibrillation (AF) 24 hours per day before having a surgical Maze procedure. He was successfully cardioverted for postoperative AF (POAF), and after a 90-day blanking period, the only episode of AF he had was asymptomatic and lasted only 2 minutes. Nevertheless, under the current definition of success or failure, his surgical procedure is classified as a "failure."

risk, especially if the left atrial appendage has been closed or amputated, so it is of utterly no clinical importance. Nevertheless, the interventional procedure is still deemed to be a failure. Furthermore, the "failure" designation cannot be changed to a "success" later because most follow-up data are reported using Kaplan-Meier *survival* curves that, as the name implies, are based on an irreversible endpoint, death. In addition, the current definition of success or failure for a catheter PVI in a healthy 45-year-old patient with PAF is the same as it is for a surgical Maze procedure in a 75-year-old patient with LSpAF. This nonsensical definition of success versus failure is a major reason why it is virtually impossible to collect accurate and meaningful data on the true clinical effectiveness of either catheter ablation or surgery for AF. It is likely that both catheter and surgical ablation for AF are far more successful clinically than is currently reported. Thus in the future, it is imperative that a new classification system and a new definition of success versus failure be developed for the interventional treatment of patients with AF.

Lack of Collaboration between Electrophysiologists and Cardiac Surgeons

In the Preface to this book, I mentioned the lag time of 10 to 20 years between the development of a surgical treatment for individual cardiac arrhythmias and the catheter ablation of these same arrhythmias. However, this sequence for the development of interventional therapy for cardiac disease is not unique to arrhythmias. For example, the first successful coronary artery bypass grafting for ischemic heart disease was performed in the mid-1960s, but the first percutaneous coronary angioplasty by a non-surgeon was not performed until in the mid-1970s. Closure of a patent ductus arteriosus (PDA) was first performed surgically in 1938, but it was more than 40 years before PDA closure could be accomplished reliably by non-surgeons. Closed MV commissurotomy was first performed for mitral stenosis in 1923 and became routine practice in 1947, but balloon mitral valvotomy by non-surgeons did not become common until some 30 years later. Similar lag times between interventional therapy by surgeons and interventional therapy by nonsurgeons existed for every congenital cardiac anomaly, mitral insufficiency, aortic stenosis, aortic insufficiency, and thoracic aortic disease. One reason why it was surgeons rather than non-surgeons who developed the first interventional procedures for all of these cardiac anomalies is that surgeons are trained to manipulate *anatomy*, but non-surgeons are trained to manipulate *images*. This gives surgeons an obvious advantage over non-surgeons in developing new interventional procedures. However, non-surgeons were the first to understand and explain the pathophysiology of disease processes in depth, especially congenital malformations, coronary artery disease, and cardiac arrhythmias. Without non-surgeons sharing this basic knowledge and including their surgical colleagues in collaborative new approaches, the development of surgical therapy for cardiac disorders would have evolved much more slowly. Thus, the evolution of interventional treatment for all cardiac disease has historically depended on a collaboration between surgeons and non-surgeons.

The evolution of mapping capabilities, surgery, and catheter ablation for cardiac arrhythmias over the past half-century has again demonstrated the importance of surgeon and non-surgeon collaboration. Cardiac surgeons will never know as much electrophysiology as cardiac EPs, but EPs are less capable of designing interventional procedures that are as effective as surgical procedures. Of course, nonsurgical interventions are far less invasive, but they are also less effective. One reason that "hybrid procedures" were developed was so that the talents unique to both surgeons and non-surgeons could be combined to solve the problem of how best to treat patients with stand-alone LSpAF. It is also the reason that the development of better interventional procedures in the future should also depend on that collaboration. Perhaps the best way of putting it from a surgeon's standpoint is a statement that I have repeated hundreds of times over the past several decades: "An arrhythmia surgeon is only as good as his/her electrophysiologist." This remains as true today as it was 50 years ago.

PATHWAYS TO FUTURE IMPROVEMENT

Science usually progresses in small, sequential steps and less often by complete paradigm shifts. Progress in the interventional treatment of patients with AF has been made by gradually improving the understanding of normal and abnormal electrophysiology in general and ultimately, the abnormal electrophysiology of AF. This accrued knowledge provided the scientific basis for the development of the Maze procedure as well as for the catheter ablation of AF. Near-future progress in the treatment of stand-alone AF is likely to continue its historical arc toward less invasive interventional procedures, and at least for the foreseeable future, this means catheter ablation and for a while longer, hybrid procedures. The most important areas of catheter ablation for stand-alone AF depend on the discovery or creation of *new ablative energy sources* and the development of *more manipulative catheters* that are capable of creating contiguous, uniformly transmural linear lesions anywhere inside the heart. Currently, this can be accomplished consistently only with open surgical techniques. Although the most dramatic changes in the treatment of stand-alone AF that should be expected in the near future will likely occur with catheter ablation, it is an unfortunate truth that despite 25 years of experience, millions of patients, billions of development and marketing dollars, and the demonstration of catheter ablation's superiority over pharmacologic therapy but inferiority to surgery, only around 4% of all patients with AF undergo catheter ablation annually,[5] and fewer than half of them are successfully ablated long term (see Chapter 31). One might contemplate that if a new drug had been introduced in 1998 for the treatment of patients with AF that had the same safety, efficacy, and cost profile as catheter ablation for AF, would that drug still be on the market a quarter-century later?

The Future Role of Surgery in Treating Stand-Alone Atrial Fibrillation

Although the concomitant surgical ablation of AF when performing other cardiac surgical procedures will continue to be an important part of cardiac surgery in the future, it is unlikely that surgery for stand-alone AF will ever be performed as primary therapy, even for LSpAF. Surgery has always been considered to be too invasive for the routine treatment of stand-alone AF, though minimally invasive surgical Maze procedures still yield the best results for the treatment of stand-alone LSpAF (see Chapters 17 and 28). If off-pump hybrid procedures can be modified so that the combination of thoracoscopic and catheter lesions create all of the lesions of a surgical Maze procedure, the results can be expected to be the same as they are currently for the on-pump minimally invasive surgical Maze procedures (see Chapter 37). Both robotic Maze procedures and the minimally invasive surgical Maze procedures require cardiopulmonary bypass and therefore are unlikely to ever become first-line therapy for stand-alone AF (see Chapter 16).

Improved Ablative Energy Sources

Before the late 1990s, only two ablative energy sources were available to treat AF, nitrous oxide (N_2O) for cryosurgery and unipolar radiofrequency (RF) energy for catheter ablation. After Haïssaguerre and coworkers' introduction of RF catheter ablation for the treatment of AF in 1998, both unipolar and bipolar RF surgical devices were developed to provide surgeons with the benefits of the speed and ease of use of these new devices. Soon thereafter, several other energy sources were introduced for the surgical ablation of AF, including microwave energy, laser energy, high-intensity focused ultrasound (HIFU), and argon gas cryogen. Unfortunately, none of these new energy sources could be delivered safely and reliably through a catheter, so they were used exclusively by surgeons. For a variety of reasons, microwave, laser, and HIFU energy devices were soon withdrawn from the surgical market, leaving only unipolar RF, bipolar RF, and N_2O and argon gas as viable ablative energy sources that can be used in surgery. Unipolar RF and N_2O cryogen have been the only available ablative energy sources for catheter ablation for several years, but recently, two new energy sources have been made available for catheter ablation: electroporation and near-critical nitrogen. Electroporation is more commonly called "pulsed-field ablation," and near-critical nitrogen is referred to as "ultra-low-temperature cryoablation" (ULTC).

Pulsed-Field Ablation

Interventional EPs have embraced PFA using electroporation more enthusiastically than any ablative energy source since RF ablation was introduced more than 30 years ago. Electroporation is a biophysical technique in which trains of high-voltage electrical pulses are applied to open or enlarge physical holes in the cell membranes of the targeted tissue. The size of the pores that can be created in the cell membranes is related to the amount of current applied to the tissue.

Reversible electroporation has been used for years to treat patients with various types of cancer by opening holes in the cell membrane enough to allow anticancer drugs, genes, or DNA to be "inserted" directly into the cell itself. After this transfer is accomplished, the train of electrical impulses (electroporation) is stopped, and the holes in the cell membrane close, trapping the therapeutic drug, gene, or DNA inside the cell. Reversible electroporation does not create heat in the targeted tissue.

Irreversible electroporation destroys cells by creating holes in the cell membrane that are too large to reclose upon termination of the electroporation, so the cells quickly die and are replaced by fibrocytes. Because irreversible electroporation results in the creation of scars, it can be used to treat patients with AF. The alleged advantage of irreversible electroporation over other ablation energy sources is its safety because there is an energy zone between reversible electroporation and heat-generated irreversible electroporation where irreversible electroporation can be accomplished without heating the targeted tissue (Fig. 52.3).[6] This means that permanent atrial lesions can be created by *nonthermal irreversible electroporation* (or PFA). The tissues of anatomic structures adjacent to the heart, such as the esophagus and phrenic nerves, are not irreversibly ablated at the specific level of energy that is lethal for myocardial cells. Therefore, PFA is said to be a nonthermal, "myocardial-specific" ablation technique that is safer than RF or cryothermia, both of which are temperature-dependent ablative energy sources that can potentially damage surrounding structures.

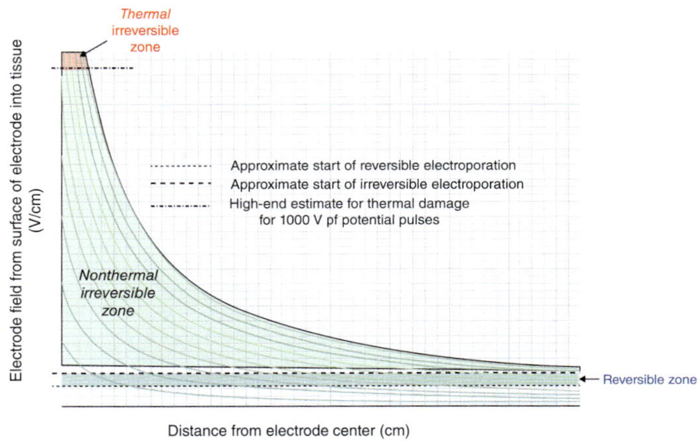

Fig. 52.3 A graph of the electric field of electroporation as a function of the distance from the center of the pulsed-field ablation (PFA) catheter electrode. The *curved lines* represent the electric field for electrode voltages from 100 volts *(lower curved line)* in increments of 100 volts. The three stages of *(1)* reversible electroporation, *(2)* nonthermal irreversible electroporation, and *(3)* thermal electroporation are designated. The objective of PFA for atrial fibrillation is to stay within the nonthermal irreversible stage. If too little energy is applied, the PFA will be reversible, and no permanent lesions will be created. If too much energy is applied, the thermal irreversible stage will be reached, and the PFA catheter will function as a heat-based ablative energy much the same as a radiofrequency catheter. (Reproduced from Daniels CS, Rubinsky B. Cryosurgery with pulsed electric fields. *PLoS One*. 2011;6(11):e26219).

Although PFA is theoretically less likely to damage the phrenic nerves or the esophagus, PFA can cause several problematic side effects even if the current is maintained within the nonthermal irreversible zone. These side effects of PFA include coronary artery spasm (Fig. 52.4),[7,8] which is associated with long-term neointimal hyperplasia and tunica media fibrosis in coronary arteries (Fig. 52.5).[9] Coronary artery spasm and subsequent pathological changes in coronary arteries near the site of PFA catheters has proven to be such a problem that on September 15, 2022, the device company that manufactures the PFA catheter (Farapulse–Boston Scientific, Inc.) issued an "Urgent Field Safety Notice – Product Advisory" in which the following was stated:

"The FARAWAVE PFA Catheter has not been studied clinically in the mitral isthmus or cavotricuspid isthmus areas. Ablations in areas adjacent to coronary arteries may lead to coronary artery spasm and/or injury, and the resulting myocardial injury can be fatal."

The Product Advisory went on to recommend that this PFA catheter not be used to create lesions in either the right atrial isthmus ("flutter line") or the left atrial isthmus ("mitral line") and reemphasized that the PFA catheter was approved only for isolation of the PVs. Thus, regardless of how effective or ineffective PFA is in creating uniformly transmural lesions individually, its clinical utility is limited because of the inability to place lesions in certain areas of the atrium that are critical to the successful treatment of both atrial flutter and non-paroxysmal atrial fibrillation (non-PAF).

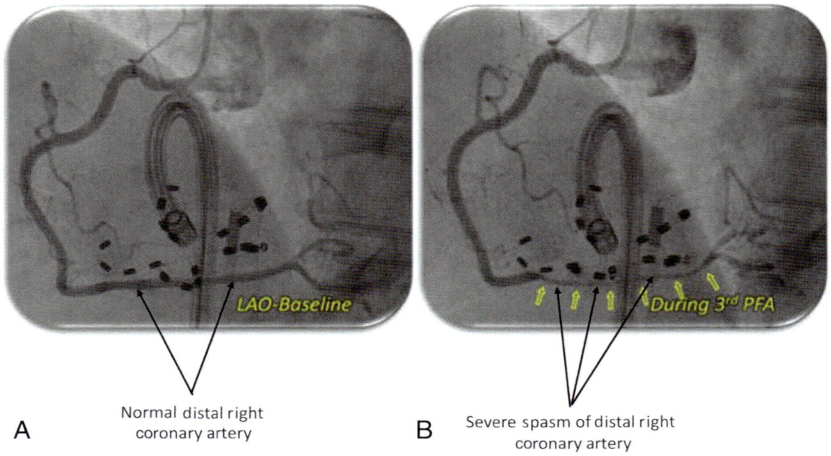

Fig. 52.4 Spasm of the distal right coronary artery during the creation of a cavotricuspid isthmus (CTI) lesion in the right atrium with a pulsed-field ablation (PFA) catheter. (A) Before PFA. (B) During PFA. *LAO,* Left anterior oblique view. (See text for further discussion.)

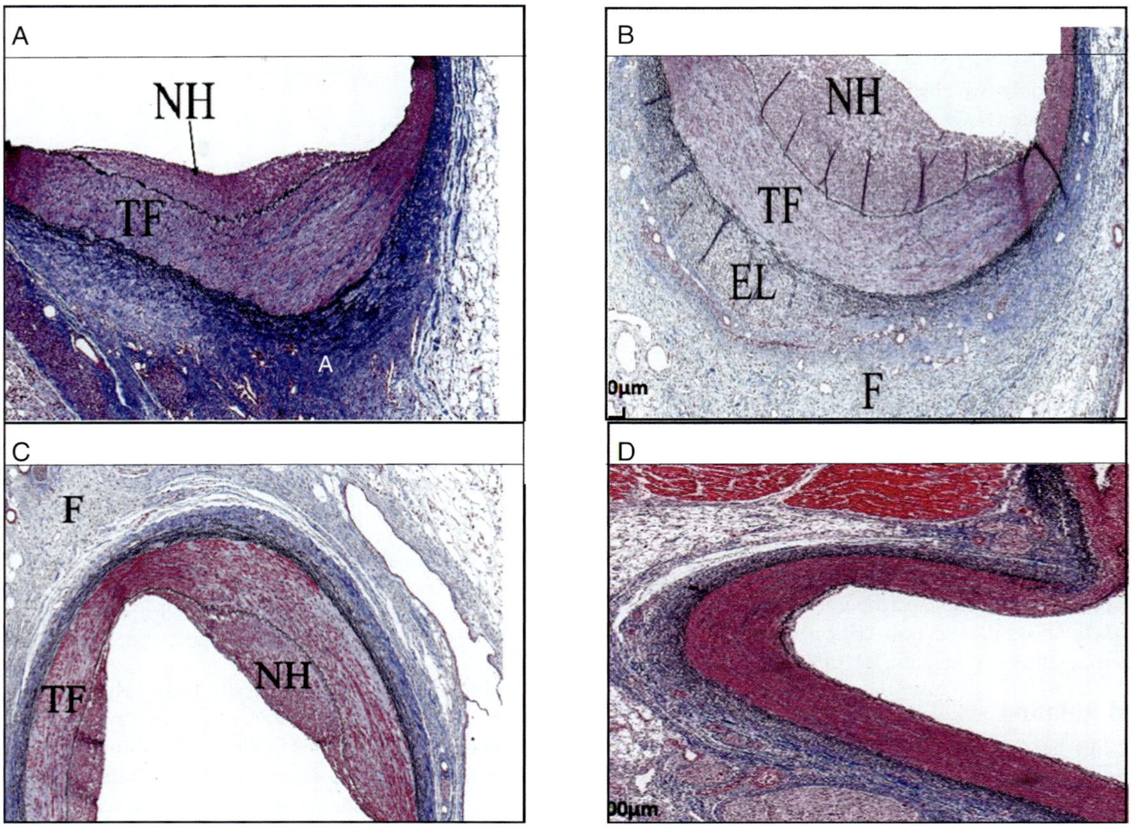

Fig. 52.5 (A) and (B) Neointimal hyperplasia (NH) and tunica media fibrosis (TF) in the left anterior descending (LAD) coronary artery 4 weeks after direct application of pulsed-field ablation (PFA). (C) Neointimal hyperplasia (NH) and tunica media fibrosis (TF) in the LAD coronary artery 8 weeks after direct application of PFA. (D) Normal LAD coronary artery located 1 cm away from the PFA energy source 8 weeks after PFA application. *EL,* Adventitial elastic fiber loss; *F,* adipose tissue fibrosis (Reproduced From Higuchi S, Im SI, Stillson C, et al. Effect of epicardial pulsed field ablation directly on coronary arteries. *JACC Clin Electrophysiol.* 2022;8(12):1486–1496).

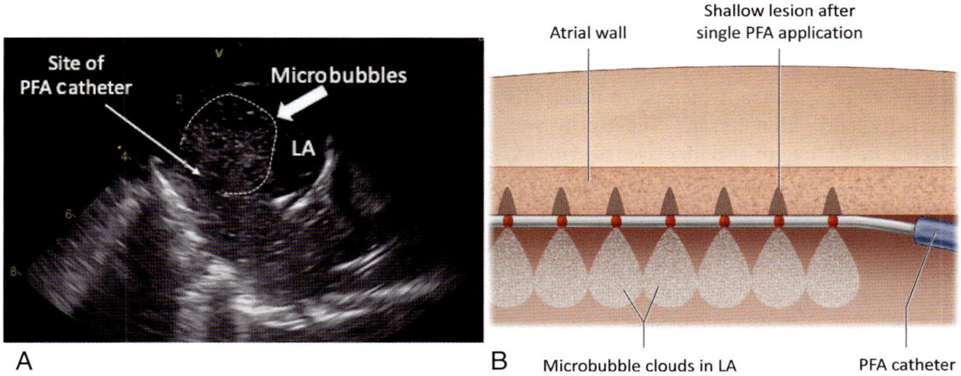

Fig. 52.6 (A) Echocardiogram of the left atrium (LA) during application of pulsed-field ablation (PFA) to the endocardium showing the microbubbles created inside the LA by PFA energy lost into the cavitary blood. (B) Diagrammatic representation of why the current method of applying PFA in the LA is hampered by difficulty in creating transmural lesions. Most of the PFA energy is lost into the cavitary blood of the LA in the form of micro-bubble clouds.

In addition to coronary artery spasm, PFA ablation can cause skeletal muscle contraction that is severe enough in some patients to require general anesthesia for the PFA catheter ablation procedure.[10] Another disconcerting problem is the creation of clouds of bubbles inside the left atrium (LA) during PFA application.[11] The tips of endocardial ablation catheters are not isolated from the cavitary blood because the catheter tip is where the ablative energy is delivered. Thus when PFA energy is applied to the endocardium of the LA, a majority of the electrical current follows the path of least resistance, and blood is less resistant than myocardium. Therefore, a large portion of the PFA ablative energy can escape into the systemic circulation, leaving little energy to ablate the myocardium (Fig. 52.6). This loss of ablative energy into the systemic circulation prevents PFA from penetrating more than a few millimeters into the left atrial wall with a single pulse application, so it is necessary to apply PFA several times in the same location to attain greater lesion depth. Even if a single PFA lesion is transmural, it leaves multiple gaps between the individual lesions (Fig. 52.7A and B). Therefore, it is necessary to rotate the PFA catheter several times (Fig. 52.7C) and repeat the ablation process for a better chance of attaining contiguous, uniformly transmural lesions. PFA has many of the limitations of RF ablation in that even with circular ablation catheters with multiple ablation electrodes along their length, it is still difficult to attain linear (or circular) lesions that are contiguous and uniformly transmural simply because of the physics of trying to create a linear lesion by "connecting the dots" from individual focal ablation sites (Fig. 52.7D).

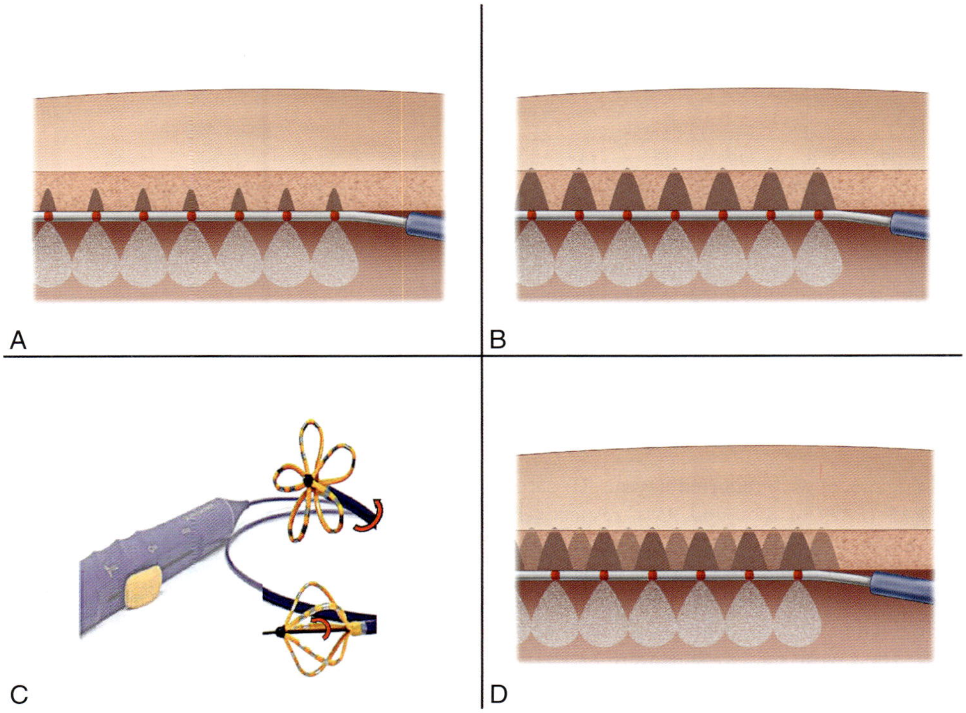

Fig. 52.7 (A) Schematic representation of lesions in the atrial wall delivered from single electrodes along a linear or circular pulsed-field ablation (PFA) catheter. Note that most of the PFA energy goes into the cavitary blood, which limits the depth of myocardial lesion that can be attained with PFA alone. (B) Even if the individual endocardial PFA lesions do extend to the epicardium, they are not contiguous and would therefore be ineffective. (C) The lack of lesion contiguity is the reason that the PFA catheter is typically rotated multiple times *(red arrows)* to try to close the gaps remaining between the individual lesions. (D) This problem of noncontiguity and nontransmurality is not unique to PFA catheters; it is also a problem for the endocardial unipolar radiofrequency catheters that have been used for the past 25 years.

Another way to improve the size and depth of PFA lesions is to increase the electric field strength (V/cm) to drive the myocardial lesion deeper. However, PFA can easily become a heat-based thermal ablative energy source much like RF (see Fig. 52.3), at which point it loses its so-called "myocardial specificity" and with it, its safety superiority over RF. Increasing the PFA electric field strength also increases the volume of left atrial bubbles created as well as the magnitude of coronary artery spasm and skeletal muscle contractions.

Despite the level of enthusiasm for the adoption of PFA because of its alleged safety and ease of use, the reported 1-year success rates for PFA catheter ablation have been no better than those for heat-based RF catheter ablation (Fig. 52.8). As mentioned in Chapter 31, the *overall results* of RF catheter ablation at 1 year in both the Winkle and coworkers series[12] and the CABANA trial[13] were almost identical at 80% and 79%, respectively. The inspIRE Trial[14] across 13 European centers (226 patients) showed a 1-year success rate of 79% with PFA ablation for AF. The MANIFEST-PF registry[15] that included 24 European centers using PFA had an overall success rate of 78% using PFA for AF ablation.

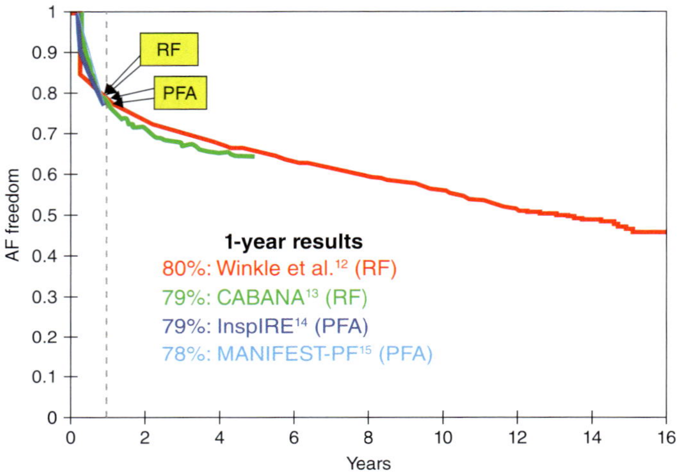

Fig. 52.8 Catheter ablation at 1 year for all patients with atrial fibrillation (AF). In all patients with AF combined (paroxysmal, persistent, and long-standing persistent), the 1-year results of pulsed-field ablation (PFA) catheter ablation are virtually identical to those for radiofrequency (RF) catheter ablation. The success rates for RF catheter ablation were 80% in Winkle and coworkers' series[12] and 79% in the CABANA trial.[13] The 1-year success rates for PFA were 79% in the InspIRE trial[14] and 78% in the MANIFEST-PF registry.[15]

Winkle et al.[12] and Takigawa et al.[16] reported 1-year RF catheter ablation results for *PAF (PAF)* of 89% and 93%, respectively (Fig. 52.9). The anxiously awaited PULSED-AF trial reported a 1-year success rate with PFA catheter ablation for PAF of 66%.[17] The recent randomized, single-blind, noninferiority ADVENT trial compared 305 patients who had PFA ablation with 302 who had thermal ablation for PAF (Fig. 52.10).[18] The 1-year success rates were 73.1% for PFA ablation and 71.3% for thermal ablation. The authors' conclusions were as follows:

> *"Among patients with paroxysmal atrial fibrillation receiving a catheter-based therapy, pulsed field ablation was noninferior to conventional thermal ablation with respect to freedom from a composite of initial procedural failure, documented atrial tachyarrhythmia after a 3-month blanking period, antiarrhythmic drug use, cardioversion, or repeat ablation and with respect to device- and procedure-related serious adverse events at 1 year."*[18]

Both Winkle[12] and the German Centers Study[19] reported 75% 1-year success rates for RF ablation for *persistent AF,* and the 1-year success rates for PFA ablation were 72% in the MANIFEST-PF registry[15] and 55% in the PULSED-AF trial[17] (Fig. 52.11).

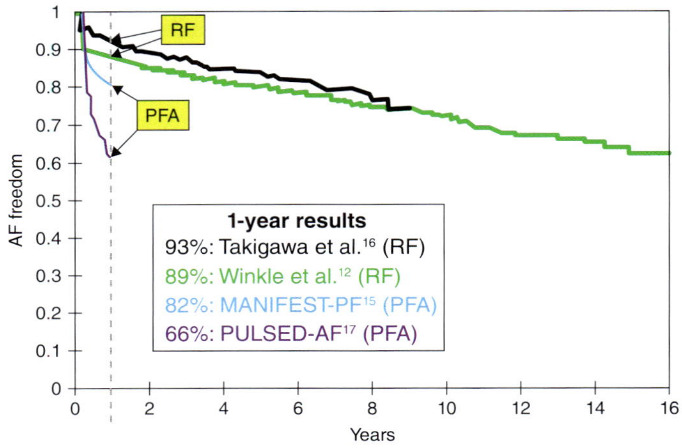

Fig. 52.9 Catheter ablation at 1 year for paroxysmal atrial fibrillation (PAF). In patients with paroxysmal atrial fibrillation (PAF), the 1-year results of PFA catheter ablation are actually *inferior* to those for radiofrequency (RF) catheter ablation. The success rate for RF catheter ablation of PAF was 93% in Takigawa et al.'s series[16] and 89% in Winkle et al.'s report.[12] The 1-year success rates for PFA catheter ablation of PAF were 82% in the MANIFEST-PF registry[15] and 66% in the PULSED-AF trial.[17]

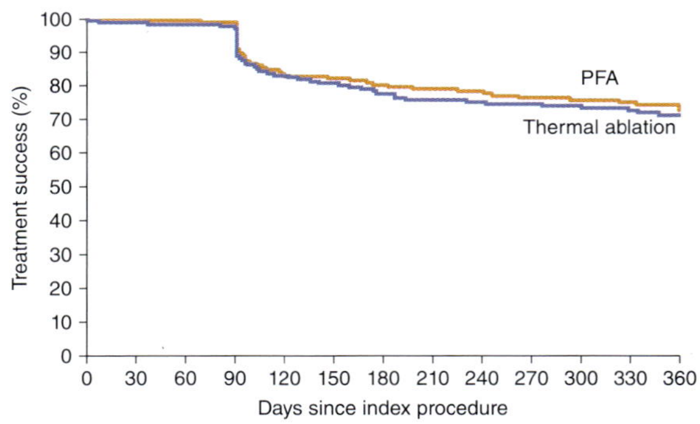

No. at risk					
PFA	301	298	238	228	176
Thermal ablation	296	292	228	219	150
Treatment success (%)					
PFA	993	99.0	79.7	76.4	73.1
Thermal ablation	987	97.3	77.5	74.5	71.3

Fig. 52.10 The ADVENT trial: pulsed-field ablation (PFA) versus thermal energy for paroxysmal atrial fibrillation (PAF). The randomized, single-blind, noninferiority ADVENT trial showed that there was no difference between the efficacy of PFA and radiofrequency ablation for PAF. (Reproduced from Reddy VY, Gerstenfeld EP, Natale A, et al. Pulsed field or conventional thermal ablation for PAF. *N Eng J Med.* 2024;389(18):1660–1671).

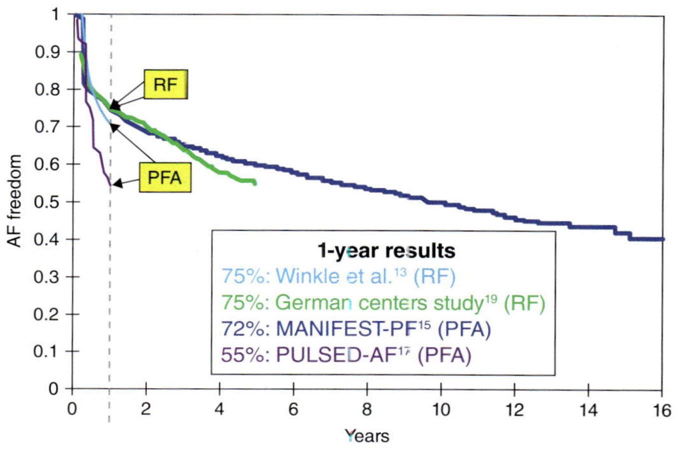

Fig. 52.11 Catheter ablation at 1 year for persistent atrial fibrillation (PAF). In patients with PAF, the 1-year results of pulsed-field ablation (PFA) catheter ablation are also somewhat inferior to those for radiofrequency (RF) catheter ablation. The success rate for RF catheter ablation of persistent AF was 75% in both Winkle et al.'s series[12] and Schreiber et al.'s[19] report from several German centers. The 1-year success rates for PFA catheter ablation of persistent AF were 72% in the MANIFEST-PF registry[15] and 55% in the PULSED-AF trial.[17]

The current enthusiasm for PFA is based on the proposition that it is safer than RF and cryoballoon catheter ablation yet has similar efficacy and ease of use. Indeed, in the introduction to the ADVENT trial, the authors make the statement that "Pulsed field ablation, which delivers microsecond high-voltage electrical fields, may limit damage to tissues outside the myocardium,"[18] confirming that the oft-repeated claim that PFA is "myocardial specific" has yet to be proven, even to their satisfaction. Early studies indicate that not only is PFA *not* more effective than RF or cryothermia for the ablation of AF, but that PFA is associated with adverse side effects that are not associated with either RF or cryoballoon ablation procedures. Although the safety of PFA is still in question, its ease and speed of use are inarguable. However, basing the long-term future of AF catheter ablation on PFA alone is unlikely to be successful if its efficacy is no better than that of RF ablation and some of its adverse side effects are potentially more serious. This appears to be of no concern in the current environment, however, because it is clear that the driving force behind the universal acceptance of PFA as the preferred ablative energy source for the catheter ablation of AF is the speed with which an individual procedure can be completed, leading to the ability to perform two to three times more AF ablation procedures per EP per day than was possible using RF as the ablative energy source. It is obvious that the number of repeat catheter ablation procedures will also increase dramatically in the future.

These limitations of PFA as currently used include (1) a huge loss of administered energy available for tissue ablation into the cavitary blood that is seen on echocardiography as clouds of microbubbles in the left atrial cavity, (2) the subsequent need to administer higher energy levels to drive more ablative energy into the atrial tissue, and (3) coronary artery spasm and skeletal muscle contractions that result from the high energy applied through the ablation catheter. If one is truly wedded to the use of PFA as the primary ablative energy source for AF, it would seem prudent to find a way to prevent the loss of ablative energy into the cavitary blood and thereby increase the depth of penetration of the atrial tissue while simultaneously drastically lowering the required level of energy administration. In fact, this exact scenario has already been accomplished and is described below.

Ultra-Low-Temperature Cryoablation

Cryosurgery for arrhythmias has been used since the mid-1970s. Currently, there are two cryogens available to surgeons: (1) N_2O and (2) argon gas. N_2O cryoprobes, which cool the cryoprobe to −60°C, have been used successfully for the treatment of almost all clinical arrhythmias for over 50 years. N_2O gas cannot be adapted for use in a cryoablation catheter because of the internal pressures required for cooling, but it is used in cryoballoon catheters in which the pressurized gas is contained safely within the cryoballoon itself. Argon gas, which cools the cryoprobes to −160°C, has been in use for some 20 years, but argon gas has not been successfully adapted for use with catheters because of the risk of catheter leak and gas embolism. Both N_2O and argon gases are obviously less dense that liquid cryogens, so their cooling power is less efficient than that of liquid nitrogen. However, in recent years, engineers have learned how to maintain liquid nitrogen near its liquid-vapor critical point ("near-critical nitrogen") at which the nitrogen retains the cooling power of liquid nitrogen (−196°C) but has the low viscosity of a gas, which means it can be delivered through tiny channels smaller than a pencil lead. The pressure required to maintain liquid nitrogen inside a catheter in this gaseous phase (i.e., "near-critical nitrogen") is substantially less than the pressure required for either N_2O or argon gases, making it an ideal cryogen for use in catheters. Furthermore, like liquid nitrogen, near-critical nitrogen cryoprobes are so cold that they are far more efficient than the warmer cryogen cryoprobes. In addition, near-critical nitrogen has now been adapted for use in a cryocatheter.

In full disclosure, the author co-founded Adagio Medical, Inc., in 2011 with the sole intent of *"providing EPs with a tool equivalent to the surgeon's knife"* by developing a cryocatheter that uses near-critical nitrogen as its cryogen and that could be easily formed into any desired shape without changing to a different catheter. The basis of this effort was my belief that the main reason that interventional EPs were unable to treat patients with non-PAF as successfully as they can treat those with all other cardiac arrhythmias is that they do not have the proper tools to do so. Patients with the Wolff-Parkinson-White syndrome, automatic atrial tachycardias, atrioventricular node reentry tachycardia, His bundle ablation, ischemic and nonischemic ventricular tachycardias, and atrial flutter can all be treated successfully by placing *focal* lesions in appropriate sites or in confined regions of the heart. The ability of EPs to treat all of these arrhythmias with the tips of catheters has been spectacularly successful. Although AF is usually induced by a focal trigger, AF is *not* a focal arrhythmia. Rather, it is an arrhythmia whose sustaining mechanisms involve the entirety of both atria and catheters that are capable of creating only focal lesions are simply inadequate to ablate it permanently. We believed that if we could design an appropriate catheter for the EPs, they would have a tool that would allow them to create and position all of the lesions of a full biatrial Maze procedure with a single catheter.

Over the past decade, Dr. Alex Babkin and our colleagues at Adagio Medical, Inc., have been successful in developing just such a catheter that is now in early clinical use (Fig. 52.12).[20,21] The shape of the catheter can be controlled by interchangeable preformed stylets passed through a tiny central channel in the catheter itself so that neither the catheter nor its sheath need be removed to change the shape of the catheter. Thus a focal, circular, or linear cryolesion of any desired size and shape can be created at any desired site anywhere inside either atrium (Fig. 52.13). Although the results of RF, cryoballoon, and PFA ablation for persistent AF are similar,[4,18,21] the 1-year results of this ULTC catheter ablation is superior to all of them (Fig. 52.14).[4,17,21] Indeed, using the ULTC catheter, the success of catheter ablation procedures is no longer limited by the ability to create perfect contiguous, transmural lesions. In addition, because the ULTC

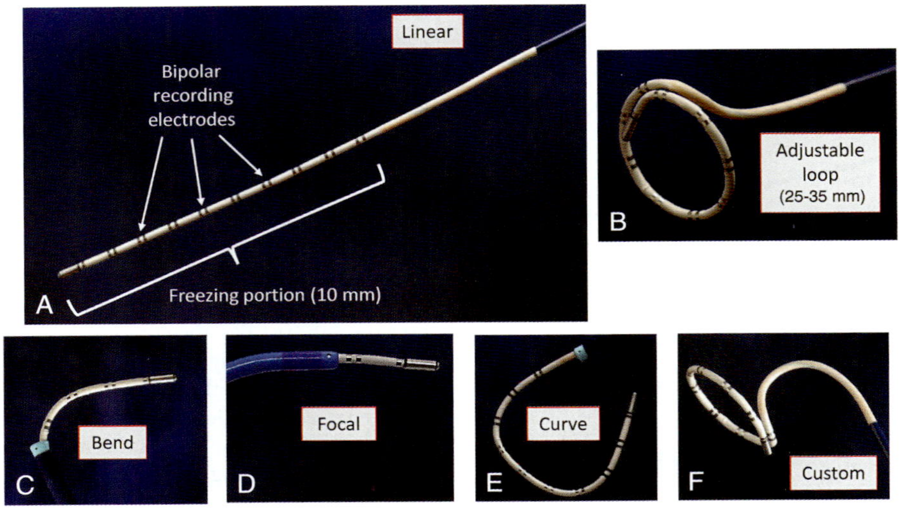

Fig. 52.12 The Adagio linear cryoablation catheter uses near-critical nitrogen as a cryogen that cools the freezing portion of the catheter to −196°C, a technique called "ultra-low-temperature cryoablation" (ULTC). The linear cryoprobe has multiple bipolar electrodes along its 10-cm freezing segment and can create a transmural linear cryolesion in a matter of seconds because of its extremely low temperature. Multiple preshaped stylets can be inserted individually into a tiny central channel of the ULTC catheter so that the catheter can be changed to any desired shape for access to any part of either atrium without removing either the catheter or its sheath. The ULTC catheter can create a 10-cm-long linear lesion, or it can be changed to a loop that is adjustable from 25 to 35 mm in diameter. The "bend" shape is used to create a cavotricuspid isthmus lesion, and the catheter's tip can be used for focal lesions similar to radiofrequency and pulsed-field ablation catheters if so desired.

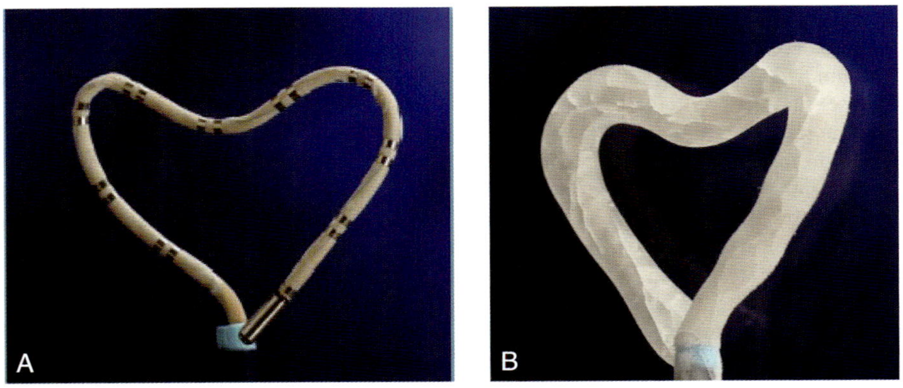

Fig. 52.13 (A) and (B) The range of flexibility of the ultra-low-temperature cryoablation linear cryocatheter in creating cryolesions of any desired shape in the atria.

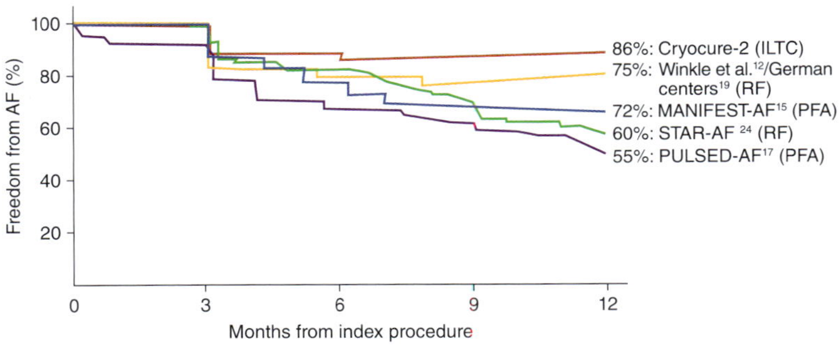

Fig. 52.14 Catheter ablation at 1 year for persistent atrial fibrillation (AF). In patients with persistent AF, the 1-year success rate of 86% using the ultra-low-temperature cryoablation catheter[20,21] is superior to that of either radiofrequency (RF) or pulsed-field ablation (PFA) catheter ablation. The success rates for RF catheter ablation of persistent AF were 75% in both Winkle et al.'s[12] series and in Schreiber et al.'s[19] report from several German centers but only 60% in the STAR-AF II trial.[4] The 1-year success rate of PFA catheter ablation for persistent AF was 72% in the MANIFEST-PF registry[15] but only 55% in the PULSED-AF trial.[17]

linear catheter can be formed into any desired shape and can reach anywhere inside the left and right atria, there is also no longer a need to limit the lesion pattern performed during catheter ablation for AF.

Combined Ultra-Low-Temperature Cryoablation and Pulsed-Field Ablation

There are several advantages of combining cryoablation and PFA ablation, a technique that we refer to as "pulsed-field cryoablation" (PFCA). Most of the side effects of PFA mentioned earlier can be eliminated using PFCA, and it appears to be quicker and more effective than either PFA or cryoablation alone. As mentioned earlier, when PFA alone is administered to the atrial endocardium during catheter ablation, the majority of the PFA energy is lost into the cavitary blood (see Fig. 52.6). This is to be expected because the resistance of the myocardium is less than that of cavitary blood, so most of the electrical current enters the cavitary blood and creates the microbubbles. However, with the PFCA catheter, an iceball is first created around the catheter that *insulates* it from the cavitary blood and prevents *any* PFA energy from leaking into the cavitary blood pool and causing microbubbles. This means that the amount of PFA energy subsequently delivered through the catheter can be decreased 10-fold, thereby eliminating the left atrial bubbles, the coronary artery spasm, and the skeletal muscle contractions associated with current catheter ablation using PFA alone.

Using the same Adagio linear cryocatheter shown in Fig. 52.12 to deliver PFA, the first step is to confirm endocardial surface contact of all electrodes along the linear catheter by continuously recording electrical signals during positioning of the catheter. After contact at all electrode sites is confirmed by the local bipolar electrograms, the linear probe is cooled to a *sublethal* temperature of approximately 0°C. An iceball immediately forms around the linear cryocatheter throughout its length, causing the catheter to adhere to the atrial wall in a fixed position so that the endocardial catheter will not move again until the cryothermia is discontinued. As mentioned, the iceball that forms around the catheter also insulates it from the cavitary blood (Fig. 52.15A). The cryolesion is then cooled enough to create an iceball through the full thickness of the atrial wall (Fig. 52.15B). This is the point at which interventional EPs and surgeons using cryoablation alone must decide how much longer to freeze because of the temperature gradient across the left atrial wall and whether or not to "pulse" the cryothermia to attain greater lesion depth. However, when using PFCA, the PFA is simply turned on at this point, and because of the high resistance of the iceball of frozen myocardium, the PFA will almost instantly travel throughout the frozen tissue to the edge of the cryolesion but no farther (Fig. 52.15C). This characteristic has several immediate salutary effects. First, even if the temperature of the subepicardium encompassed by the cryolesion has not yet reached the critical lethal temperature of –30°C, the PFA will fill the entire iceball and destroy all of the myocardial cells within it (Fig. 52.15D).

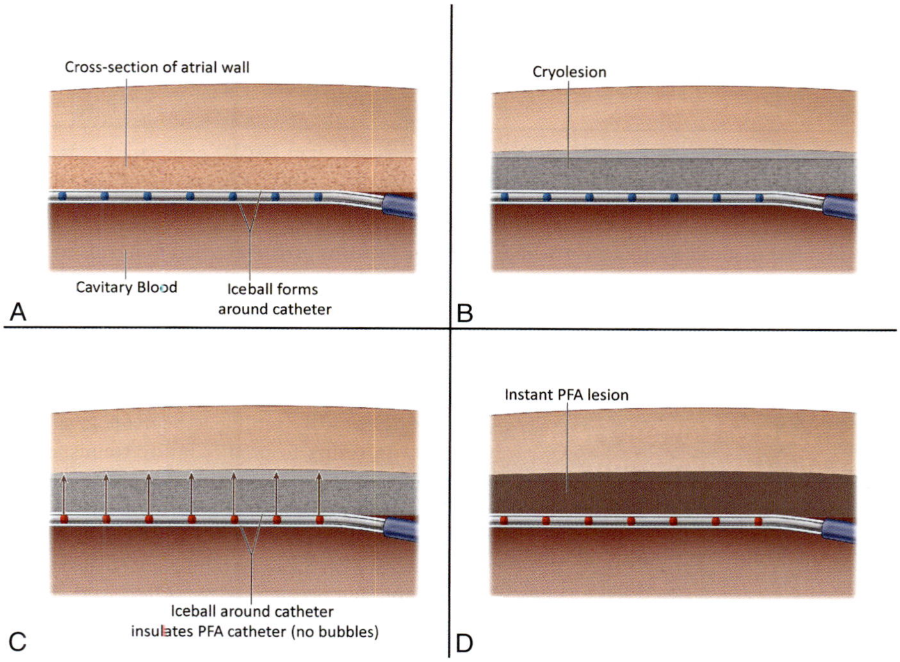

Fig. 52.15 The ultra-low-temperature cryoablation (UTLC) catheter, which uses near-critical nitrogen as its cryogen, can also deliver pulsed-field ablation (PFA) energy, a technique called pulsed-field cryoablation (PFCA). (A) The ultra-low-temperature cryoablation (UTLC) catheter is first positioned against the atrial endocardium with contact all along the catheter confirmed by recording bipolar electrograms from the catheter's multiple electrodes. The cryogen is then initiated which "fixes" the linear cryoprobe to the atrial endocardium and the iceball around the catheter also insulates the catheter from the cavitary blood. (B) The cryolesion *(white area)* is then extended transmurally to the epicardial surface, though the subepicardium does not necessarily reach the critical lethal temperature of –30°C. (C) The catheter input is then switched from cryothermia to PFA energy *(brown arrows)*, which does not leak into the cavitary blood because of the insulation of the iceball around the catheter. Because the frozen myocardium within the iceball has a higher impedance than the nonfrozen myocardium, the PFA instantly conducts throughout the cryolesion but not beyond it. (D) The combination of pre-freezing the myocardium with the ULTC and then delivering PFA into the cryolesion (PFCA) drastically reduces the amount of PFA energy required yet results in the lesions penetrating deeper into the atrial wall than a PFA lesion alone. The catheter insulation and the use of far less PFA energy also prevent the formation of atrial cavitary microbubbles, skeletal muscle contractions, and coronary artery spasm.

Thus the fundamental advantage of PFCA over PFA alone is due to the effect of pre-freezing the target tissue before initiating the PFA. The target tissue of the atrial wall is the conductor for the electrical energy delivered from the endocardium to the epicardium during the creation of a PFA lesion. According to Ohm's law, the electric current through a conductor between two points is directly proportional to the voltage across the two points. When the constant of resistance is added, Ohm's mathematical equation becomes V = IR, in which I is the current through the conductor, V is the voltage measured across the conductor, and R is the resistance of the conductor. The conductor in this case is the atrial wall between the endocardium and epicardium because the energy is applied from the endocardium but must reach the epicardium to create a transmural lesion. The voltage necessary to destroy myocardium using PFA alone is relatively constant, so as the resistance of the target tissue increases, the current needed to reach the voltage to destroy the myocardium decreases. Because pre-freezing the target tissue before administering PFA greatly increases the resistance of the target tissue, far less PFA current is needed to provide the voltage necessary to create the ultimate lesion. During PFA alone, the required current is 10 to 30 amps, but it is less than 1 amp after creation of a cryolesion. This low level of PFA current kills the cells throughout the entire cryolesion because the frozen tissue has far higher resistance than non-frozen tissue. However, this low level of PFA current is incapable of penetrating the myocardium or any other non-frozen tissue because of their lower resistances. Because the depth of the ultimate lesion can be controlled by adjusting the amount of tissue that is pre-frozen, the lesions created by PFCA may be deeper than those with PFA alone despite using only one-tenth the administered electrical current (Fig. 52.16).

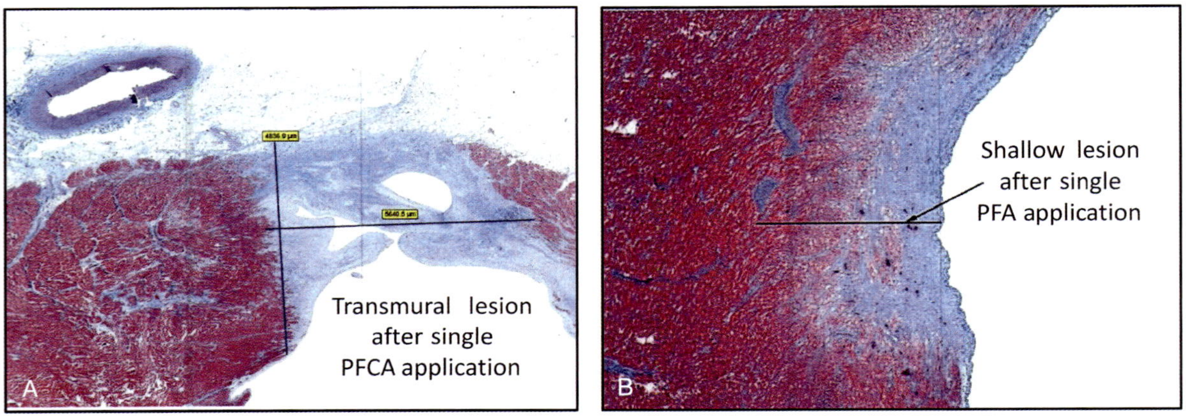

Fig. 52.16 Preclinical studies document that pulsed-field cryoablation (PFCA) consistently creates deeper pulsed-field ablation (PFA) lesions (A) than PFA alone (B).

Another benefit of PFCA is that less that one amp of electrical current applied to the endocardium of the atrium does not cause left atrial microbubbles, skeletal muscle contraction or coronary artery spasm. Thus PFCA holds even greater promise than PFA alone for improving catheter ablation safety and efficacy in the future (Table 52.1).

TABLE 52.1 Comparison of Pulsed-Field Ablation and Pulsed-Field Cryoablation

Parameter	Pulsed-Field Ablation	Pulsed-Field Cryoablation
Procedure time	Short	Shorter
Cost of catheters	Similar	Similar
Multiple catheter changes	Yes	No
Left atrial microbubbles	Yes	No
Skeletal muscle contraction	Yes	No
Coronary artery spasm	Yes	No
Chronic coronary changes	Yes	No
Lesion depth	Shallow	Transmural

CLOSING COMMENTS

Whether these new energy sources and more maneuverable catheters will become the standards of AF catheter therapy in the future remains to be seen, but if they do, it would represent another stepwise improvement, not a paradigm shift. The development of methods to ablate AF by focusing crossed radiation beams to ablate critical areas of the atria from outside the body, the ongoing laboratory efforts to develop gene therapy for the treatment of AF, an increased understanding of the relationship between the heart's neural input and arrhythmias, and even potential progress in pharmacologic therapy all hold the possibility of creating a paradigm shift in AF therapy. Until then, we can except that progress will continue to be made in small steps.

In trying to predict future trends, one is obligated to observe the ancient axiom suggesting that only by learning from the past can a reasonably educated guess be made about the future. Trends in the interventional treatment of patients with AF in the past have consistently focused on the overarching goal of decreasing the invasiveness of interventional procedures regardless of their relative effectiveness in treating the problem. These trends favor catheter ablation over off-pump hybrid procedures, which are favored over minimally invasive surgical procedures, which are favored over open surgical procedures. It is ironic that these clinical preferences are in the exact reverse order of the efficacy of these procedures. Indeed, perhaps more than in any other field, evolution of the interventional treatment of AF has overwhelmingly prioritized lowering the degree of invasiveness over improving the degree of therapeutic success. Although this choice is anathema to most surgeons, we should not expect these trends to change in the foreseeable future.

REFERENCES

1. Cox JL, Schuessler RB, D'Agostino JrHJ, et al. The surgical treatment of atrial fibrillation: III. development of a definitive surgical procedure. *J Thorac Cardiovasc Surg*. 1991;101:569–583.

2. Haïssaguerre M, Jais P, Shah DC, et al. Spontaneous initiation of atrial fibrillation by ectopic beats originating in the pulmonary veins. *N Eng J Med*. 1998;339(10):659–666.
3. Van der Heijden CAJ, Vroomen M, Luemans JG, et al. Hybrid versus catheter ablation in patients with persistent and longstanding persistent atrial fibrillation: a systematic review and meta-analysis. *Eur J Cardio-Thorac Surg*. 2019;56:433–443.
4. Verma A, Jiang C, Betts TR, et al. Approaches to catheter ablation for persistent atrial fibrillation. *N Engl J Med*. 2015;372:1812–1822.
5. McCarthy PM, Cox JL, Kislitsina ON, et al. Surgery and catheter ablation for atrial fibrillation: history, current practice, and future directions. *J Clin Med*. 2021;11(1):210.
6. Daniels CS, Rubinsky B. Cryosurgery with pulsed electric fields. *PLoS One*. 2011;6(11):e26219.
7. Zhang C, Neuzil P, Petru J, et al. Coronary artery spasm during pulsed field vs radiofrequency catheter ablation of the mitral isthmus. *JAMA Cardiol*. 2024;9(1):72-77. https://doi.org/10.1001/jamacardio.2023.4405.
8. Knight BP, Pfenniger A. Invited commentary: pulsed field ablation—will coronary spasm lead to iconoclasm? *JAMA Cardiol*. 2023. https://doi.org/10.1001/jamacardio.2023.4441.
9. Higuchi S, Im SI, Stillson C, et al. Effect of epicardial pulsed field ablation directly on coronary arteries. *JACC Clin Electrophysiol*. 2022;8(12):1486–1496.
10. Cvetkoska A, Macek-Lebar A, Trdina P, Miklavacic D, Rebersek M. Muscle contractions and pain sensation accompanying high-frequency electroporation pulses. *Sci Rep*. 2022;12(1):8019.
11. Neven K, Futing A, Byrd I, et al. Absence of (sub-) acute cerebral events or lesions after electroporation ablation in the left-sided canine heart. *Heart Rhythm*. 2021;18(6):1004–1011.
12. Winkle RA, Mead RH, Engel G, et al. Very long term outcomes of atrial fibrillation ablation. *Heart Rhythm*. 2023;20:680–688.
13. Packer DL, Mark DB, Robb RRA, et al. Effect of catheter ablation vs antiarrhythmic drug therapy on mortality, stroke, bleeding, and cardiac arrest among patients with atrial fibrillation: the CABANA randomized clinical trial. *JAMA*. 2019;321(13):1261–1274.
14. Duytschaevver M, De Potter T, Grimaldi M, et al. Parosysmal atrial fibrillation ablation using a novel variable-loop biphasic pulsed field ablation catheter integrated with a 3-dimensional mapping system: 1-year outcomes of the multicenter inspire study. *Circ Arrhythm Electrophysiol*. 2023;16(3):e011780. https://doi.org/10.1161/CIRCEP 122.011780.
15. Turagam MK, Neuzil P, Schmidt B, et al. Safety and effectiveness of pulsed field ablation to treat atrial fibrillation: one-year outcomes from the MANIFEST-PF registry. *Circulation*. 2023;148:35–46.
16. Takigawa M, Takahashi A, Kuwahara T, et al. Long-term follow-up after catheter ablation of paroxysmal atrial fibrillation. *Circ Arrhythm Electrophysiol*. 2014;7:267–273.
17. Verma A, Haines DE, Boersma LV, et al. Pulsed field ablation for the treatment of atrial fibrillation: PULSED AF pivotal trial. *Circulation*. 2023;147:1422–1432.
18. Reddy VY, Gerstenfeld EP, Natale A, et al. Pulsed field or conventional thermal ablation for paroxysmal atrial fibrillation. *N Eng J Med*. 2024;389(18):1660–1671.
19. Schreiber D, Rostock TR, Frolich M, et al. Five-year follow-up after catheter ablation of persistent atrial fibrillation using the stepwise approach and prognostic factors for success. *Circ Arrhythm Elecctrophysiol*. 2015;8:308–317.
20. Klaver MN, De Potter TJR, Iliodromitis K, et al. Ultralow temperature cryoablation using near-critical nitrogen for cavotricuspid isthmus-ablation, first-in-human results. *J Cardiovasc Electrophysiol*. 2021;32(8):2025–2032.
21. De Potter T, Klaver M, Babkin A, et al. Ultra-low temperature cryoablation for atrial fibrillation: primary outcomes for efficacy and safety: the Cryocure-2 study. *JACC Clin Electrophysiol*. 2022;8(8):1034–1039.

INDEX

Note: Page numbers followed by "*f*" indicate figures, "*t*" indicate tables, and "*b*" indicate boxes.